SMART MEDICINE FOR HEALTHIER LIVING

JANET ZAND, LAc, OMD
ALLAN N. SPREEN, MD, CNC
JAMES B. LaVALLE, RPh, ND

AVERY PUBLISHING GROUP

Garden City Park • New York

The information and advice in this book are based on the training, personal experiences, and research of the authors. Its contents are current and accurate; however, the information presented is not intended to substitute for professional medical advice. The authors and the publisher urge you to consult with your physician or other qualified health-care provider prior to starting any new treatment, or if you have any questions regarding a medical condition. Because there is always some risk involved, the author and publisher cannot be responsible for any adverse effects or consequences resulting from the use of any of the suggestions, preparations, or procedures described in this book.

Cover design: Rudy Shur
Editor: Amy C. Tecklenburg
Original illustrations: Mircea Catusanu
Front Cover Photo Credit: SuperStock, Inc.
Back Cover Photo Credits: SuperStock, Inc. and PhotoDisc, Inc.
Typesetters: Gary Rosenberg and Richard Morrock

Avery Publishing Group, Inc.
120 Old Broadway
Garden City Park, NY 11040
1–800–548–5757
www.averypublishing.com

Library of Congress Cataloging-in-Publication Data

Zand, Janet.
  Smart medicine for healthier living : a practical z-to-z reference
to natural and conventional treatments for adults / Janet Zand,
Allan Spreen, James B. LaValle.
    p. cm.
  Includes bibliographical references and index.
  ISBN 0-89529-867-8 (pbk.)
  1. Medicine—Popular Encyclopedias. 2. Alternative medicine
Encyclopedias. I. Spreen, Allan. II. LaValle, James B.
III. Title.
RC81.A2736 1999
610'.3—dc21   99-24547
                                                         CIP

Copyright © 1999 by Janet Zand

All rights reserved. No part of this publication may be reproduced, stored in a retrieval system, or transmitted, in any form or by any means, electronic, mechanical, photocopying, recording, information storage system, or otherwise, without the prior written permission of the copyright owner, except for the inclusion of brief quotations in a review.

Printed in the United States of America

10 9 8 7 6 5 4 3 2

Contents

Part Three: Therapies and Procedures
Techniques for Using Conventional and Natural Treatment

Introduction, 586

Acknowledgments

To the teachers who inspired me, to the students who challenged me, and to the patients who taught me, I would like to express my endless gratitude.

Thank you to Rudy Shur, my publisher, whose vision and support were instrumental in the creation of this book, and to Amy Tecklenburg, my editor, who relentlessly and brilliantly put this all together. Thank you to Nikki Antol for her dedication, and to my co-authors, Drs. Allan Spreen and Jim LaValle.

And many thanks to my husband, Michael, and my two sons, Christopher and William, for their love, support, and much-needed comic relief.

"The marvelous pharmacy that was designed by nature and placed into our being by the universal Architect produces most of the medicines that we need." (Norman Cousins)

J.Z.

Many factors conspire to make a manuscript of this magnitude a reality. However, deserving of special mention are the efforts of Rudy Shur, publisher extraordinaire, who pushed to bring the whole project together; Amy Tecklenburg, editor extraordinaire, whose knowledge of nutrition assisted in a function far beyond that of normal editing; and Nikki Antol, whose behind-the-scenes input was invaluable.

Finally, I'd like to acknowledge my sister Cathy for the support needed to get this career going in the first place.

A.N.S.

I would like to thank my family for their lifelong, never-ending support and love, even when it was considered "strange" to be in natural medicine.

To my new family, Laura, Libby, Jill Beth, and my soon-to-be-born child, for giving me a deeper understanding of love and commitment, and for the spiritual growth they have stimulated in me.

I want to acknowledge my mentors: Alexander Wood, D.C., N.D., the most talented teacher and practitioner of natural medicine that I have had the pleasure of working under; David Polen, D.C., for sharing his in-depth knowledge and understanding of health and disease; Bob McKinney, N.M.D., President of Central States College of Naturopathic Medicine, whose commitment to natural medicine is a commitment to all; and J. Richard Wuest, R.Ph., Pharm.D., Professor of Pharmacy Practice at the University of Cincinnati College of Pharmacy, who helped me to develop the skills I needed to become an effective communicator.

To the partners and staff of Natural Health Resources—your never-ending support is the backbone of the success of our company. Thank you also to my friends Debbie, Asbjorn, and Kelly.

J.B.L.

Preface

In the history of human thinking, the most fruitful developments frequently take place at those points where two different lines of thought meet.

Werner Heisenberg
1932 Winner, Nobel Prize for Physics

Some of the most important decisions we ever have to make concern health care. Yet often, people are not aware of the full range of choices available to them. The goal of this book is to offer information on a variety of approaches that will help you create and maintain vibrant good health. The authors believe in an integrated approach to health care that considers all treatment possibilities and draws on what works. Sometimes this will be an herb, sometimes an antibiotic, sometimes both. We believe it is just as significant that a particular therapy has been used effectively for hundreds or thousands of years as it is that a scientific paper substantiates a particular approach. Taking advantage of one form of knowledge does not necessarily preclude using another.

This book outlines and describes the application of conventional medicine, dietary modifications, nutritional supplements, herbal medicine, homeopathy, and acupressure. We believe that understanding and integrating the full range of health-care options offers the most complete and responsible way to a healthy life. We hope to foster an awareness that natural healing therapies and conventional medical treatment, two apparently divergent approaches, can—and should—work together.

Natural healing sciences (including herbal medicine, homeopathy, diet, nutritional supplements, and acupressure) are sometimes called "complementary" medicine. As that name implies, natural medicine and conventional medicine can be used to complement and support each other in helping to create health. Complementary medicine is gaining increasing acceptance in the United States, as evidenced by the many multidisciplinary clinics in which medical doctors, naturopathic physicians, acupuncturists, nutritionists, homeopaths, chiropractors, and counselors work together in an integrated manner, treating the patient as a whole person. Even the United States

government has taken notice of these developments. In the fall of 1992, the Office of Alternative Medicine was established at the National Institutes of Health to study the effectiveness of various types of alternative health care. Among the subjects being studied there are homeopathy, acupuncture and acupressure, herbal medicine, reflexology, chiropractic, biofeedback, hypnosis, and relaxation and visualization techniques.

Natural healing systems are much more widely used than many people suppose. The World Health Organization, established in 1948 as a specialized agency of the United Nations, reports that 80 percent of the world's population relies on natural healing as their primary form of health care. And in 1997, according to an article in *The New York Times*, 42 percent of Americans tried some form of alternative treatment. In fact, more visits were made to alternative-care practitioners in that year than to primary-care physicians, even though most of these visits were not covered by health insurance and had to be paid for out of pocket.

More and more medical doctors are recognizing the safety and effectiveness of natural medicines. There are physicians who prescribe herbal medicines and homeopathic remedies; many more recommend dietary changes for their patients. By now, a clear link has been established between diet and health. The American Heart Association, the American Cancer Society, and the United States government have all published dietary guidelines to promote health. Conventional and complementary health-care practitioners alike emphasize the role of nutrition as fundamental to the healing process. Indeed, a 1988 report of the Surgeon General of the United States found that two-thirds of all deaths in this country are nutrition related.

Homeopathy is an accepted form of medical practice in many parts of the world. Generation after generation of

Asian families have turned to acupuncture and acupressure for relief of illness. Even modern pharmacology has deep roots in herbal medicine. The use of the herb ma huang (ephedra), for example, dates back several thousand years; ephedrine, one of its primary ingredients (and pseudoephedrine, a synthetic version of it) is used by pharmaceutical companies today in many over-the-counter cold and allergy medicines.

"The physician treats, but nature heals." This is an often-quoted saying from Hippocrates—known as the "Father of Medicine"—who recognized that the body has a natural tendency toward health and vitality. To nurture this tendency, we need to treat illness in ways that support and strengthen the body's natural processes. Using a complementary approach to health care, we can draw on modern conventional medicine, natural medicine, and ancient healing traditions to find what is most effective and supportive in curing and preventing illness.

Conventional medicine generally works with drugs or surgery to suppress or correct a specific condition. And sometimes, that is exactly what is needed. At other times, however, a natural medical approach makes more sense. Natural medicine works by supporting the body in healing itself. While antibiotics can be used to kill harmful bacteria, for example, the herbs echinacea and goldenseal boost the immune system so that the body is better able to resist or fight infection on its own. These herbs strengthen and support the body in its ability to defend itself against bacterial invasion.

When you are suffering from a cold, you can choose to take over-the-counter or prescription medications, such as decongestants or cough medicines, to suppress the symptoms. However, cold medicines can cause side effects, and they do little to strengthen the immune system or address the underlying reason for the cold. Some commonly used ingredients in cold medications can cause restlessness, insomnia, drowsiness, or headaches. And there is nothing in these products that can actually *cure* the cold. In contrast, when a cold is treated with herbs to soothe the respiratory tract and boost the immune system, homeopathy to ease the discomforts and prevent recurrences, acupressure to open blocked energy channels, and soups and teas to maintain adequate hydration, the body is supported and strengthened as it works to restore health. For many of the illnesses that afflict us, natural medicine is gentle, effective, and safe. It is an important way to work with the body's ability to heal itself.

In his book *Health and Healing* (Houghton Mifflin, 1988), Dr. Andrew Weil wrote, "The only prerequisite for learning to take responsibility for one's own health is to discard concepts that stand in the way and adopt more useful ones. . . . Anyone who comes to see healing as an innate capacity of the body, rather than something to be sought outside, will gain greater power over the fluctuations of health and illness."

Being willing to accept responsibility is central to taking an integrated approach to health care. Develop greater faith in your body's ability to heal itself, when supported and nourished by natural medicines. When faced with illness, use this book to learn and understand the many options for care and healing. Observe how the natural and conventional medical treatments you choose affect your health and well-being. Be both responsible and willing to explore health-care options.

With the information in this book, you can learn to be an active participant in your health care. As you gain confidence and understanding in the use of natural healing systems, in concert with conventional medicine when necessary, you will gain greater confidence in optimizing health and minimizing illness. We invite you to discard the concept that health care is an either-or proposition. It's not. Integrated health care is a remarkably effective and exciting hands-on endeavor.

Using an integrated approach to health care will strengthen your capabilities. Taking care of yourself in this way will promote a healthy and responsible relationship between you and your health-care practitioner. Learn to pay attention to your body, and to appreciate your own uniqueness and vitality.

The human body is wonderfully responsive. When the body is supported with thoughtful integrated care, the best of natural and conventional medicine, it works quickly to attain full health. By giving nature a nudge—by supporting, nurturing, and nourishing the body's capacity to heal itself—you can help yourself achieve vibrant good health.

How to Use This Book

This is an in-home guide that will help you maintain your health through a unique approach that seeks to combine the best of conventional medicine, herbal medicine, homeopathy, acupressure, diet, and nutritional supplementation. Written by a naturopathic physician, a medical doctor, and a registered pharmacist and naturopath, it offers advice and explanations of the full spectrum of options available today.

This book is intended to help you make informed health-care decisions. The information and suggestions presented here are meant to be used in conjunction with the services of a physician or other qualified health-care providers. This book is not meant to replace appropriate consultation with health-care practitioners, medical investigation or treatment, or emergency first-aid training by qualified professionals. In fact, we strongly suggest that everyone who is able to do so complete an emergency first-aid course that includes instruction in artificial respiration and cardiopulmonary resuscitation (CPR). Then, should you ever be called upon to practice these techniques, the emergency instructions we provide will help you through the procedure.

The subjects in this book have been divided into three parts. Part One, The Elements of Health Care, discusses the basic history, theories, and practices of conventional medicine, herbal medicine, homeopathy, Bach flower remedies, acupressure, and aromatherapy. It also covers issues in diet and nutrition, nutritional supplementation, and exercise.

Part Two, Common Health Problems, contains an alphabetic directory of common illnesses, and outlines the different kinds of treatments appropriate for each. Each entry begins with a discussion of the problem, its causes, and how to identify the signs and symptoms. Treatment options follow, including recommendations for emergency treatment, if appropriate, followed by information about conventional medical treatment, dietary guidelines, and information on nutritional supplementation, herbal treatment, homeopathy, Bach flower remedies, acupressure, and aromatherapy. Each entry also includes a section on general recommendations that gives a brief summary of the most commonly helpful natural treatments, plus a section on prevention.

Part Three, Therapies and Procedures, gives specific instructions to help you use the diagnostic and treatment procedures suggested in Part Two. The use of special diets, the preparation of herbal and aromatherapy treatments, the locations of acupressure points, and other techniques are explained and illustrated so that you will be able to take advantage of the various kinds of treatments available to you.

Also included, in an appendix, are a list of references; a glossary of some of the terms used in this book; a list of common medical abbreviations; a list of recommended suppliers of herbal, homeopathic, and nutritional products; a list of helpful resource organizations, with addresses and telephone numbers; and a bibliography for further reading.

Part One

The Elements of Health Care

The Nuts and Bolts of
Conventional and Natural Treatment

Introduction

Each of us plays an invaluable role in his or her wellness care. While you may rely on professionals to help you manage certain aspects of health care, the fact is that you yourself are the best judge of your own health. Building on the understanding you have of your body and how it functions, you can learn to move from general observation toward identifying the signs and symptoms that reveal an illness or other health problem. Even having a vague sense that something is just "not quite right" is valid and important. You know your body. You know when something is wrong.

When we are ill, we want to ease the discomfort quickly and effectively. But conventional and natural therapies alike can seem confusing and overwhelming, just when they are needed most. The approaches to medicine covered in this book include conventional medicine, herbal medicine, homeopathy, acupressure, nutritional supplements, and diet. In Part One you will find historical information, tables, diagrams, and guidelines to help you understand each system of medicine from a conceptual and practical perspective.

Each of the healing systems offers advantages and benefits. Each has drawbacks. This section provides a clear, unbiased look at all protocols. It will help you gain the insight you need to choose an effective course of action and become confident in your ability to provide yourself with effective, comforting, and gentle health care.

Conventional Medicine

When most Americans think of health care, they think of conventional medicine. It is without question the dominant approach to medicine in the United States today, and it permeates (often without our being aware of it) even our basic understanding of sickness and health. For example, many people think of health as being the absence of disease, and when they don't feel well, they are apt to ask, "Is there something I can take for this?" Both of these ideas reflect the assumptions of modern conventional medicine, which tends to be oriented toward identifying diseases and prescribing cures, usually in the form of drugs.

THE HISTORY OF CONVENTIONAL MEDICINE

The story of the development of the conventional medical science we know today weaves through many centuries and many cultures. If we go back to the dawn of history, we find that the earliest doctors were shamans, and the first medicines were plants.

It is generally accepted that the history of today's conventional medical science starts with Hippocrates, the Greek physician revered as the "Father of Medicine." Up to the time of Hippocrates (c. 460–370 B.C.E.), illness was believed to be caused by supernatural forces. Hippocrates taught that all disease was of earthly origin, not visited upon the sufferer by some wrathful god.

It was Hippocrates who set the stage for the scientific procedures of today. He began the practice of bedside observation. He listened to and recorded each patient's story—today, we would call it a case history—and considered the effects of diet, emotion, occupation, even climate, in his diagnosis and treatment. Through careful observation and logical reasoning, Hippocrates showed that it was possible to determine the cause of illness, and thereby discern the cure.

Hippocrates believed that health was the result of good balance between a person's internal nature and external environment. Illness indicated an imbalance. To restore balance in his patients, Hippocrates designed special diets, mandated exercise, and prescribed botanical medicines, including an occasional purgative or emetic. For digestive troubles (possibly stomach ulcers), he ordered bland drinks. Hippocrates also recognized the importance of stress reduction. He was known to have recommended to certain patients that they relocate to calmer surroundings, or that they take a glass of wine with supper.

Galen (c. 130–200), who was known as the "Great Physician," added to the knowledge of medicine and anatomy. He performed experiments and dissections, and wrote prolifically about his discoveries. For example, he is credited with discovering that blood is carried through the body by means of the arteries. Although a Greek by birth, Galen lived and practiced in Rome, where he was personal physician to several Roman emperors.

With the collapse of Rome in the fifth century, Europe descended into a period of turmoil. The anatomical studies and the emphasis on observation and logic of the ancient Greeks and Romans were lost to most of the continent for nearly 500 years. During this time, European medical knowledge for the most part amounted to a mixture of folk art and superstition. The heirs to the knowledge of Hippocrates and Galen were not Europeans, but Arabic and Jewish scholars (although some of the classical practice was preserved in southern Italy). It was through these sources that the medical knowledge of Greece and Rome was eventually reintroduced to Europe. By the year 1000, the medical school at the University of Salerno had an established reputation, and for centuries to come, Italy remained the focal point for medical science in Europe. However, the study of medicine remained primarily an academic discipline, rather than an area of active inquiry, experimentation, or practical application. Not until the Renaissance—when invention, intellectual pursuits, and creativity flourished—did this approach begin to change significantly, ushering in the beginning of what we might recognize as medical science.

Leonardo da Vinci (1452–1519), considered by many to be the first modern anatomist, extensively studied and diagrammed anatomy. Following his initial contributions, other scholars continued to perform dissections and study anatomy, adding to the knowledge of the inner workings of the body. Reason, logic, and observation once again became the foundation of medical learning. The practice of surgery also has its beginnings during this time—despite the lack of anesthesia.

In the century that followed, the mechanisms of blood circulation and respiration came to be understood. Inventions such as the clinical thermometer and the microscope made it possible to observe the workings of the body on an entirely new level, and anatomical details such as lymph nodes and red blood cells were appreciated. Certain illnesses were also distinguished, including diabetes mellitus, diabetes insipidus, rickets, scarlet fever, measles, and gout. In the eighteenth century, medical schools were founded in Vienna, Edinburgh, and Glasgow. Although the course of study at the time still emphasized the assimilation of knowledge rather more than experimentation or invention, progress was made in the practice of surgery, amputation, and the treatment of bone fractures, and new diagnostic methods were developed, such as percussion and pulse-taking. Modern immunology also traces its origins back to this period. In 1796, Edward Jenner, an English physician, began a series of experiments that proved that inoculating a person with cowpox provided immunity against smallpox, a dreaded disease that had erupted in epidemics throughout history.

Further dramatic advances and discoveries followed, including the invention of the stethoscope, which made possible more precise diagnosis of heart and lung problems. Huge strides were made in the understanding of anatomy and physiology. Robert Koch—whose bacteriological culture techniques are still used today—identified the bacteria that cause many serious infectious diseases, including anthrax, tuberculosis, and cholera. His work led to an understanding of the importance of water filtration in the prevention of cholera and typhoid. Louis Pasteur made tremendous contributions to our understanding of the causes of disease and the means by which infectious illnesses spread. His study of the activity of bacteria disproved the theory of spontaneous generation (the belief that living organisms can develop from nonliving material) and led to the acceptance of his germ theory of infection. He also invented anthrax and rabies vaccines, as well as the process that bears his name, pasteurization, by which potentially illness-causing microorganisms in food are killed. Soon, many different types of bacteria were identified, including those that cause tetanus, leprosy, typhoid, diphtheria, and gonorrhea.

The acceptance of the germ theory made it possible for surgery to make great leaps forward, because it led to an appreciation of the necessity for sterile conditions during surgery. This new emphasis on aseptic (sterile) technique, plus the development of anesthesia, helped to establish surgery as a viable treatment option, rather than a desperate last resort. (Prior to this time, many people died during or after surgery from infections that were a direct result of a lack of attention to cleanliness.) The germ theory also had great implications for public health policy, which now involved vaccination programs, quarantine measures, and attention to the cleanliness of the water supply.

As understanding of the workings of the body and its systems grew, the latter half of the nineteenth century saw the birth of the fields of neurology (the study of the brain and nervous system), psychiatry, and endocrinology (the study of glands and hormones). In 1895, x-rays were discovered. Medical science continued to follow a path that emphasized the importance of the scientific method—logical study that produces reliable results that can be duplicated. In the last few decades, medicine has made progress that would have been unthinkable just three or four generations ago. The use of insulin injections has allowed people with diabetes to live long and relatively healthy lives; the discovery of antibiotics like penicillin and streptomycin has improved the treatment and prognosis for people with bacterial infections; the polio vaccine was developed and has largely eliminated this dreaded disease; and organ transplantation has become an accepted, viable treatment for certain conditions. Increasingly sophisticated diagnostic tools and advances in treatment have been developed. In addition, the course of conventional medicine has included the creation of huge drug companies, health insurance programs, and government agencies like the National Institutes of Health. All of these developments have played a role in shaping the health-care system we know today.

Because of the many successes in the treatment of infectious diseases, the emphasis in medical research has now shifted toward the chronic and degenerative diseases, which remain less curable. Heart disease, the various forms of cancer, and acquired immune deficiency syndrome (AIDS) are among the health problems that pose the greatest challenges to medical science today. Since chronic and degenerative diseases are usually the cumulative result of many factors, rather than a reaction to a single agent, practicing preventive medicine—eating a healthful diet, exercising regularly, reducing stress, and making healthy lifestyle choices such as not smoking and limiting alcohol intake—is becoming more and more central to taking care of our health.

CONVENTIONAL MEDICINE TODAY

Most of us grew up with conventional medicine, also called "orthodox," "Western," or "modern" medicine. In the United States, conventional health care usually means a visit to your family or primary-care physician. Depending on the nature of the problem, your doctor may run tests, prescribe a drug, recommend dietary changes and exercise, refer you to a specialist or surgeon, or merely tell you to get extra rest and drinks lots of fluids.

Many sophisticated diagnostic tools are available to medical doctors today. Some are familiar, such as the stethoscope, otoscope, and x-ray. More recent advances also include computerized axial tomography (CAT) scanners, magnetic resonance imaging (MRI), and other laboratory tests. Yet like all healing systems, conventional medical science evolved from a long tradition of careful observation. Even with the tremendous advances of the last 100 years, the most important tool your physician has is still his or her willingness to listen closely and observe carefully.

WORKING WITH YOUR DOCTOR

Physicians are here to help you make appropriate decisions regarding your health care, to work with you. Even if you favor a natural approach to health care, there may come a time when only conventional medicine has the cure you need. A physician who knows you well is a wonderful backup in case of crisis. When choosing a physician, consider the following guidelines:

- Choose a physician who keeps up to date with the latest treatments. A concerned and knowledgeable physician is an absolute must. New drugs come on the market all the time. The side effects of drugs—especially new ones, which do not have long track records—should be understood and carefully considered.

- Find a physician who is open-minded about natural and complementary therapies. Your physician does not necessarily have to prescribe natural medicine, but he or she should at least be willing to listen to your ideas and explore options.

- Find a physician who will work with you as a partner, who believes in making decisions with you, rather than for you.

- Choose a physician who is a good communicator. It is important that a doctor be able not only to explain situations and treatments to you, but also to listen well to your concerns. You want a physician who is competent and supportive, one who will give you enough time so you can ask questions and learn.

- Choose a physician who looks at the big picture. It is essential to work with someone who acknowledges that you are not just a case of high blood pressure, but a person who has interests and responsibilities, who is involved with life, *and* who has high blood pressure.

- Find a physician who is willing to see you and interact with you as the intelligent, worthwhile person that you are.

In this age of specialization and managed care, the old-fashioned family doctor who knows and treats all members of the family from birth through old age has become something of a rarity. It is up to you, therefore, to take an active role in developing the kind of relationship with any doctor or doctors you consult that will serve your health-care needs best. This presents you with certain responsibilities. First, it is up to you to seek medical advice promptly. Don't procrastinate. Many people put off going to a doctor because they are shy of baring their less-than-perfect bodies, or they really don't want to hear what the doctor may say. Even in the face of serious symptoms, some people would rather let nature take its course than see a physician.

If you are concerned about something, make an appointment. The longer you wait, the more you will worry, and the more you worry, the worse you will feel. Your doctor may find that you are basically healthy but would feel better if you made some lifestyle adjustments, such as moderating your diet, learning to manage stress more effectively, and getting regular exercise. If you do have a health problem, an early diagnosis often means an early cure.

Second, when you make your first visit to a particular physician, be prepared to fill out a form that includes details of your medical history and a list of all the medications you are currently taking. Bring all of this information with you. Most doctors will review your history and talk with you before examining you physically. Third, no matter how trivial or even silly you think they are, write down all your questions at home and bring the list with you. Don't hold back. No matter what is troubling you—mentally or physically—share it with your physician. Remember that your mental state affects your physical being. Very likely even those things you consider too embarrassing to reveal to another living soul trouble dozens of your doctor's other patients as well. We humans share many of the same problems, both physically and psychologically. Your doctor has heard it all.

Finally, if you do not understand something your doctor tells you, ask him or her to repeat it, more than once if need be, or to explain it in terms that you can understand. Only if you have full understanding and information about your condition can you participate fully in the program proposed for your recovery. A good doctor will want his or her patients to be fully informed regarding their conditions and treatments. Similarly, if your doctor gives you instructions, make sure you understand exactly what it is that you are to do. If the instructions are not perfectly clear in your mind, ask the doctor or a nurse, assistant, or secretary to write them down for you.

There may be a time when your doctor recommends a comprehensive health-care program for you. A good doctor will work with you in formulating a regimen that is both manageable and effective. Make sure you fully understand all phases of any program your doctor is suggesting. Ask as many questions as necessary. Don't just agree passively to diet, medication, or lifestyle changes that will be immensely difficult or perhaps even impossible to carry out. Airing your fears and concerns is an important part of your responsibility. Without your input, your doctor has no way of knowing that you find a program difficult or impossible to implement. If for any reason you cannot carry out the program, or can handle only a portion of it, tell your physician. There are probably workable alternatives.

A good doctor recognizes that a physician-patient partnership is of immense benefit. The physician you choose should want to know you, welcome your questions, take the time to explain and advise, and be willing to explore natural treatment options. A physician who will work with you in taking an integrated approach to health care is invaluable.

TREATMENT WITH CONVENTIONAL MEDICINES

When you choose conventional medical treatment, an important part of your responsibility as patient is to thoroughly understand the appropriate use of the medications, both prescription and over-the-counter, recommended by your physician.

If you are given a prescription for medication, do not leave your doctor's office until you fully understand its purpose, the benefits it offers, the effect it should achieve, and how long it will take before you can expect an improvement in symptoms. Ask about any possible side effects that should be reported to the doctor. For example, the development of a skin rash might be an early warning sign of sensitivity to a particular drug. Unless you are aware that a rash may signal "danger," you could overlook it. If you are taking other drugs or natural medicines, ask about any possible drug interactions. Certain drugs are not compatible with others. If you have been diligent in providing a list of all the medications you take, both prescription and over-the-counter, your doctor will be able to avoid prescribing a drug that might cause an adverse reaction in combination with something else you are taking. Once you begin taking a prescribed drug, do not take any new over-the-counter medicines without first checking with your physician or pharmacist to make sure it is safe to do so. Even a product that has been manufactured expressly to combat a certain condition may not be suitable for you.

When talking with your doctor or pharmacist about a medication or over-the-counter product, ask about *all* of the ingredients in it. Many medicines contain significant and often unnecessary amounts of preservatives, dyes, and alcohol. Some prescription and nonprescription medicines also contain sugar. Your doctor or pharmacist should be able to tell you what additives are in a prescribed medication. When selecting an over-the-counter product, read the label carefully. The label should tell you exactly what the product contains, including the sugar content and additives (often listed as "inert ingredients"), as well as how to administer it and possible side effects. If you have any doubts about the safety of a particular medication, ask your physician or pharmacist for any further

information you need to feel comfortable. We also recommend that you buy or have access to a good reference book on drugs, such as *The People's Pharmacy* by Joe Graedon (St. Martin's Press, 1996).

Be sure to take all medications as directed. The failure to take drugs as prescribed is a serious problem. The National Council on Patient Information and Education reports that over 50 percent of people with high blood pressure fail to take their medication as prescribed; 42 percent of people with diabetes do not take their medication as scheduled; and 39 percent of adults with asthma do not follow the regimen of drugs set by their doctors. The cost of such failure to comply with doctors' instructions has been estimated at more than $100 billion a year in additional doctor visits, medications, and hospitalization. The costs in terms of people's health are even higher. Statistics show that over 250,000 adults are hospitalized each year because they failed to take medication as directed, and as many as half of these people die as a result.

Unless there have been complicating side effects, always continue to take a prescribed medication—whether a natural or conventional medication—for the full course of treatment ordered by your physician. This is particularly important with antibiotics. If you are on a fourteen-day course of an antibiotic but stop taking it after ten days because your symptoms have lessened, your symptoms may return within a short time. This can happen because the weaker bacteria are quickly destroyed by the medication, but the more hardy ones may not be. Then, when you stop the medication early, these stronger members of the species can—and in many cases do—evolve into a drug-resistant strain that is harder to kill. Once they have time to multiply, the illness returns in a magnified form and a more powerful antibiotic or combination of antibiotics is required to combat it.

If for any reason you miss a scheduled dose of medicine, take the next dose at the scheduled time. Do not double the next dose. It is dangerous to skip a dose, but it can be doubly dangerous to take two doses at once. Many people complain that they simply forget to take their medication as scheduled. If you find it a nuisance to keep an eye on the clock, invest in a watch with a beeper alarm and set it to go off when it's time for your next dose. If you are taking several different drugs, you may understandably find it difficult to keep track of what you've taken in the course of a day. In that case, it may be worthwhile to buy a pill dispenser that has a different compartment for each day of the week. By looking at the current day of the week, you can tell at a glance what you have taken and what you still must take to complete your daily dosages. There are even dispensers with several compartments for each day, so that each scheduled dose gets its own compartment. Most drugstores sell these inexpensive dispensers. Or you can use a medication chart to keep track of what you have taken. (More about this in HOME AND PERSONAL SAFETY, later in Part One.)

Never take a drug that was prescribed for someone else, even if your symptoms are identical to those the drug is designed to combat. Even if you come down with the same condition as a friend or another member of your family, you cannot assume that a drug prescribed for one person will be safe for another. No drug is equally safe or effective for all people.

Another factor to remember when you are taking prescription drugs is that different drugs interact with each other. When you have a new prescription filled, your pharmacist should give you printed information on the prescribed drug, including a list of any other drugs and/or foods that should not be taken with that medication. You may be surprised to learn that some common foods can decrease the effectiveness of certain drugs, and other common foods can give rise to uncomfortable and even downright dangerous side effects if taken with particular drugs. Most pharmacies have computer programs that track all the drugs being taken by each customer, even if the prescriptions were written by more than one physician. This is an immensely important safeguard. When you have a prescription filled, the pharmacist can call up your computerized records and alert you to any possible danger, should you be taking drugs that are incompatible with each other. You may also get a call from your pharmacist if you fail to request a refill when one is due.

Your pharmacist should inform you as to how a drug should be stored. This is especially important for drugs taken on an ongoing basis. Many drugs lose their effectiveness more quickly if kept in a high-humidity environment, such as that of a bathroom. Others lose their effectiveness when exposed to sunlight, and some require refrigeration. If your pharmacist doesn't mention any specific storage instructions when you pick up your prescription, ask if humidity is a factor, and be sure to check the bottle. If special storage conditions are needed for a particular medication, you should find a label on the bottle that advises you of storage requirements.

Don't try to stockpile medications. Drugs undergo chemical changes as they age. Most often this renders them ineffective, but certain drugs can actually become toxic over time. All prescription drugs carry expiration dates for your protection. Always dispose of outdated medications. Similarly, dispose of any medications that undergo a change in appearance or develop an unusual odor. It's safer to replace them with a new prescription.

Get all your prescriptions filled at the same pharmacy. This allows for an accurate record of all the medications you are taking. You should also notify your pharmacist concerning any natural medicines you may be taking so that he or she can keep a complete record for you.

If a drug that once was helpful to you becomes less effective over time, alert your doctor. The body can build up a tolerance to many drugs, especially sleeping pills and pain medications. Increasing the dosage in an attempt to regain the original effect can be extremely dangerous. In all likelihood, you don't need a higher dose of the original drug, you need a different prescription.

If at any time during the course of treatment you develop signs of an allergic reaction, such as a rash or difficulty breathing, stop taking the medication and call your doctor immediately. If you experience any other new symptoms while taking a drug (such as headache or stomach pains), notify your doctor or call your pharmacist promptly and ask for advice. It may be advisable to discontinue the medication, or there may be other measures you can take to minimize side effects.

When prescribing medication, a doctor may be interested primarily in the effectiveness of a drug, not its cost. Your doctor may not even know what a given medication costs, but it is fair and important for you to ask. Drugs can be very expensive. You may wish to ask if a lower priced generic preparation can adequately be substituted for a brand-name product.

Common Conventional Medications

The most commonly prescribed conventional medications include analgesics (painkillers), antibiotics, cold and allergy medicines, and drugs to combat stomach problems, anxiety, depression, diabetes, arthritis, and cardiovascular disorders, especially high blood pressure. When your doctor writes a prescription or recommends an over-the-counter preparation, refer to the table on pages 10–21 for a quick review of some of these medications, their purposes, and possible side effects.

Taking Conventional Medication

Some medications are better taken with food to minimize side effects, and some also work better if taken with a meal. In other cases, however, mixing food with a drug may impede or alter its absorption, making it less effective. Some drugs are fine in combination with certain foods, but not with others (see Food and Drug Interactions, page 8). Always ask your doctor or pharmacist about the best way to take any medication that is prescribed for you.

There are also medications that are designed with a timed-release factor that makes certain ingredients exit the stomach and enter the bloodstream at different times. If you dislike swallowing pills or capsules, and prefer to open or crush them and mix the contents with food or liquid, check with your doctor or pharmacist to make sure that form of administration is both safe and suitable for that particular medication. If you crush or cut a sustained-release pill or capsule, for example, you may receive all at once a medication that is meant to be absorbed slowly. These types of medicines should always be taken whole.

Be especially careful if you are taking more than one preparation at the same time, whether the medications are conventional or natural, prescription or over-the-counter. Always be sure that your doctor knows about *all* the substances you are taking.

Following are general recommendations for taking different types of medicines.

Liquid Medicines

Many medications are available in sweetened and flavored liquid form. These are easy to take. If the taste is too strong, simply dilute the appropriate dosage in a little water, juice, or herbal tea. Many liquid medications, both prescription and over-the-counter, are high in sugar, so if you have diabetes, consult your physician before using them.

Tablets

Medications in tablet form are generally meant to be swallowed whole. Some people, however, find it difficult to swallow tablets. If you have this problem, you may be able to crush the tablet and mix it with a spoonful of fruit-flavored yogurt or applesauce, or dissolve it in tomato or vegetable juice. You should be aware, though, that some tablets are enteric-coated, and should not be crushed. These tablets are meant to pass through the stomach whole and are absorbed in the intestines. Before crushing tablets, check with your doctor or pharmacist to make sure it is safe and appropriate to do so.

Capsules

Capsules slide down much more easily than tablets do. Most people can swallow capsules even if they can't quite manage to swallow dry tablets. Unless your physician has

---

Food and Drug Interactions

If your diet includes everything from bananas and Brussels sprouts to sour cream and pork sausage, indigestion might not be your only worry. All of these foods can cause problems in combination with certain medications. Medicine, like food, must be broken down by the body before its active components can go to work. However, certain foods and drugs compete with one another to be absorbed or metabolized by the body. This can diminish a drug's effectiveness and/or cause an adverse reaction. For example, dairy products and alcohol interfere with the action of some antibiotics, and salt consumption influences how well the antidepressant lithium is absorbed.

Finding out exactly which foods can interfere with which drugs has been the focus of many medical studies. Recent studies have shown that taking medicine with grapefruit juice can cause some drugs to stay in the body longer, and at higher levels, than taking them with plain water. While this property of grapefruit juice appears to be beneficial for people taking the antirejection drug cyclosporine (it can reduce the need for high doses), it can dangerously multiply the effect of some blood-pressure medicines. At the same time, grapefruit juice has been shown to compete with some antibiotics (such as erythromycin [also sold under the brand names ERYC, Ilotycin, and others]), certain sedatives and antianxiety agents (such as the sleeping medication triazolam [Halcion]), as well as the calcium-channel blocker felodipine (Plendil). Anyone taking any of these drugs should avoid grapefruit juice altogether.

A well-known type of food-drug interaction occurs with a class of drugs known as monoamine oxidase (MAO) inhibitors, commonly prescribed for depression.

Examples include isocarboxazid (Marplan), phenelzine (Nardil), and tranylcypromine (Parnate). People who take these drugs can suffer potentially serious consequences—including headaches and sharp, sudden rises in blood pressure—if they consume foods that contain a substance called tyramine. Tyramine is found in aged, fermented, and smoked foods, including beer, wine, cheese, yogurt, sour cream, and soy sauce, as well as avocados, raisins, bananas, and chocolate. Also avoid anything containing caffeine.

Another drug for which it is critical to follow food-interaction guidelines is the anticoagulant warfarin (Coumadin). Vegetables such as asparagus, broccoli, spinach, Brussels sprouts, and all leafy greens contain vitamin K, which, if eaten in significant amounts, may decrease the effectiveness of this drug. This does not mean you must completely banish these nutrient-packed vegetables from the menu, but you should eat only moderate amounts (ask your doctor what specific limit he or she would set, if any).

Finding out which beverages or foods should be avoided or consumed in moderation only with each medication is a matter of asking your doctor and/or pharmacist. Pharmacists are required by law to offer patients medical counseling with each prescription they dispense, and most are happy to do so. Unless your doctor directs otherwise, you should assume that the optimum drink for swallowing medicine is water. It is best to drink at least four to eight ounces with each dose to aid the medication in reaching its destination.

The following table indicates some of the most common food-drug interactions and recommendations on how to avoid them.

FOOD AND DRUG INTERACTIONS

Type of Drug	Example(s)	Food Interaction	Recommendation
Angiotensin-converting enzyme (ACE) inhibitors, used to treat high blood pressure	Benazepril (Lotensin, Lotrel); captopril (Capoten); enalapril (Vasotec); fosinopril (Monopril); lisinopril (Prinivil, Zestril); quinapril (Accupril); ramipril (Altace)	Consuming too much potassium can lead to too-high levels of this mineral in the body, which can result in heart irregularities and other problems.	Limit your consumption of bananas, green leafy vegetables, oranges, orange juice, and licorice.
Some antianxiety medications	Alprazolam (Xanax); chlorazepate (Tranxene); chlordiazepoxide (Librium); diazepam (Valium); lorazepam (Ativan); meprobamate (Miltown); oxazepam (Serax)	Consumption of alcohol can cause flushing, rapid heartbeat, and/or shortness of breath.	Avoid alcoholic beverages while taking this drug.
Anticoagulants (blood-thinners)	Warfarin (Coumadin)	Eating foods high in vitamin K can counteract the effects of this drug, decreasing its effectiveness.	Limit your consumption of green leafy vegetables such as spinach, broccoli, Brussels sprouts, and others.
Some antiprotozoals/ antibiotics, used to treat parasitic and bacterial infection	Metronidazole (Flagyl, Protostat)	Consumption of alcohol can cause flushing, abdominal cramps, nausea, vomiting, and/or headaches.	Avoid alcoholic beverages while taking this drug and for three days thereafter.
Blood sugar lowering drugs, used in the management of diabetes	Glipizide (Glucotrol); glyburide (Diaßeta, Glynase, Micronase)	Consumption of alcohol can cause flushing, headache, rapid heart rate, and low blood sugar, and interfere with control of blood-sugar levels.	Limit consumption of alcoholic beverages while taking this drug.
Bronchodilators, used to treat asthma	Theophylline (Quibron, Slo-Phyllin, and others)	Consuming food or beverages containing caffeine can cause nervousness, shakiness, anxiety, and/or insomnia.	Avoid coffee, tea (except caffeine-free herbal teas), colas, cocoa, chocolate, and anything else containing caffeine.
Insulin, used in the management of diabetes	Various preparations and brand names	Consumption of alcohol can cause a low blood sugar reaction.	Limit alcoholic beverages if you must use insulin.
Monoamine oxidase (MAO) inhibitors, used to treat depression	Isocarboxazid (Marplan); phenelzine (Nardil); tranylcypromine (Parnate)	Eating foods high in the amino acid tyrosine or a related compound, tyramine, can result in severe headache and dangerously high blood pressure.	Avoid avocados, raisins, bananas, liver, meat tenderizers, caffeine, and chocolate, as well as any foods that have undergone aging, pickling, smoking, or fermentation, including cheeses, dry sausage (salami, pepperoni), sour cream, yogurt, yeast extract, beer, and wine.
Tetracycline antibiotics, used to treat bacterial infections	Demeclocycline (Declomycin); doxycycline (Doryx, Monodox, Vibramycin, Vibra-Tabs); minocycline (Dynacin, Minocin); tetracycline (Achromycin)	Foods high in calcium can interfere with the absorption of this drug, decreasing its effectiveness.	Limit your consumption of milk and other dairy products. Consume these foods at least two hours away from taking the antibiotics.

given prior approval, *do not* open a capsule and mix the contents with food. If you have difficulty swallowing capsules, try tilting your head forward as you swallow. Since capsules float, they will move to the back of your mouth with this maneuver.

Suppositories

If you are vomiting and unable to hold anything down, your doctor may prescribe a suppository. To use a sup-pository, gently insert it into your rectum. To give the suppository time to melt, hold your buttocks together for about five minutes.

Because they are designed to melt easily, suppositories should be stored in the refrigerator. To make insertion more comfortable and to shorten melting time after insertion, take a suppository out of the refrigerator about thirty minutes before the scheduled time of administration, so that it can come to room temperature. You can also bring

COMMON CONVENTIONAL MEDICATIONS

Any medication can cause an allergic reaction. An allergic reaction can happen with the first exposure or after you have taken the medication several times. Symptoms of an allergic reaction can include rash, swelling, itching, and/or difficulty breathing. If you think you are having an allergic reaction, call your physician. If you expe-

Medication	Effects	How Taken	How Available
ANALGESICS (PAINKILLERS)			
Acetaminophen (Tylenol, Datril, and others)	Relieves pain; reduces fever.	By mouth in liquid, chewable, or pill form; in suppository form for infants.	Over the counter.
Nonsteroidal anti-inflammatories (aspirin [Bayer, Ecotrin, and others]; ibuprofen [Advil, Motrin, Nuprin, and others]; ketoprofen [Orudis, Oruvail]; diclofenac [Voltaren]; fenoprofen [Nalfon]; tolmetin [Tolectin]; others)	Relieve pain; reduce pain, inflammation.	Tablet, capsule, liquid, suppository, depending on particular drug.	Over the counter and by prescription, depending on potency.
Narcotics (codeine; hydrocodone [in Hydrocet, Lortab, Vicodin, and others, often combined with aspirin or ibuprofen]; hydromorphone [Dilaudid]; oxycodone [in OxyContin, Percocet, Percodan, and others, often combined with aspirin or ibuprofen]; petazocine; propoxyphene [Darvon]; others)	Relieve pain by binding with receptors to block the brain's perception of it.	Tablet, capsule, liquid, injection.	By prescription.
ANTIBIOTICS			
Cephalosporins (cefaclor [Ceclor]; cefixme [Suprax]; ceftriaxone [Rocephin]; cephalexin [Keflex]; others)	Fight bacterial infection.	Tablet, capsule, liquid, injection.	By prescription.
Combination antibiotics (sulfamethoxazole + trimethoprim [Bactrim, Septra]; others)	Fight bacterial infection.	Tablet, liquid, injection.	By prescription.
Macrolide antibiotics (erythromycin [ERYC, Ilotycin, and others]; azithromycin [Zithromax]; others)	Fight bacterial infection.	Tablet, capsule, chewable tablet, liquid, injection. Also gel and liquid for topical use.	By prescription.
Metronidazole (Flagyl, Metric, Protostat)	Fight bacterial and protozoal infection.	Tablet, injection.	By prescription.

a suppository to a suitable temperature more quickly by rolling it between the palms of your hands. Make sure you unwrap the suppository before inserting it.

Injections

Injection of a drug is usually done by a nurse or physician. Should you ever have an ongoing need for an injectable drug, such as insulin for diabetes, your doctor should make sure you have the training you need to handle injections at home.

Conventional medicine is a broad, ever expanding field of health care. It is the dominant form of health care in North America, and can be particularly useful in helping you through health crises and acute problems. Develop a trusting working partnership with your doctor. Ask questions, state your concerns and needs, listen, learn—be active in your health care. Your health can best be supported by integrating conventional medicine with natural medicine.

rience difficulty breathing, go to the emergency room of the nearest hospital. Always follow your doctor's prescription and read package directions carefully to be sure you are taking the medication properly and in the correct dose.

Possible Side Effects	Contraindications	Comments
Reportedly none if taken in recommended doses. Can be fatal if overdosed.	Do not take if you have liver disease, such as hepatitis or mononucleosis.	In excessive amounts, this drug can cause liver damage. Be careful not to exceed the proper dosage.
Stomach upset, heartburn, increased chance of gastric bleeding. Aspirin can cause an allergic reaction in susceptible individuals.	Do not take in late pregnancy. Aspirin should not be taken by children or teenagers unless specifically recommended by a doctor.	Take with a full glass of water. Take with food to prevent or lessen stomach upset.
Drowsiness, lightheadedness, sedation, upset stomach, constipation, skin rash.	Do not take if you have a known allergy to codeine or another medication in this family, such as morphine or meperidine.	Take with food to relieve or prevent stomach upset. Do not exceed the recommended dosage. Can be habit-forming.
Diarrhea, skin rash (hives), yeast infection, allergic reaction, slowed blood clotting. May cause nausea and vomiting after alcohol consumption.	Do not take if you have a known allergy to these drugs. If you are allergic to penicillin, you may also be allergic to cephalosporins.	Take 1 hour before or 2 hours after a full meal. If you develop side effects, call your doctor.
Upset stomach, skin rash, anemia, depressed immune system, severe allergic reaction.	Do not take if you have folate-deficiency anemia or a known allergy to this drug.	Take with food to relieve stomach upset.
Upset stomach, skin rash; allergic reaction. Erythromycin can cause liver dysfunction.	Do not take if you have a known allergy to these drugs. Poorly tolerated if you already have nausea or are vomiting.	Do not cut or crush the coated tablets. Talk to your pharmacist about whether or not the brand you are buying can be taken with food. If you experience intense stomach pain, discoloration of the skin or eyes, dark urine, or fatigue, call your doctor.
Nausea, vomiting, upset stomach, metallic taste in the mouth, headache, dizziness, dark urine, numbness in extremities.	Do not take if you have a known allergy to this drug.	Take with food to lessen stomach upset. Avoid alcohol when taking this drug.

Medication	Effects	How Taken	How Available
ANTIBIOTICS (continued)			
Penicillins (amoxicillin [Amoxil, Augmentin, Polymox, Trimox, Wymox]; ampicillin [Omnipen, Polycillin]; penicillin [Bicillin, Pentids, Pen-Vee, Pfizerpen, Veetids, Wycillin]; others)	Fight bacterial infection.	Tablet, capsule, chewable tablet, liquid, injection.	By prescription.
Antifungals (griseofulvin [Fulvicin, Grifulvin, Grisactin]; nystatin [Mycolog, Mycostatin, Mytrex, Nilstat, Nystex]; others)	Fight fungal infection.	Tablet, liquid, cream, powder, depending on individual product.	By prescription.
Anthelmintics (mebendazole [Vermox]; ivermectin [Stromectol]; niclosamide [Niclocide]; praziquantel [Biltricide]; pyrantel pamoate [Antiminth]; thiabendazole [Mintezol]; others)	Fight worm infection.	Tablet, chewable tablet, liquid, depending on product.	By prescription.
ASTHMA DRUGS			
Bronchodilators (albuterol [Proventil, Ventolin]; metaproterenol [Alupent, Metaprol]; terbutaline [Brethine, Bricanyl]; theophylline [Aerolate, Elixophyllin, Slo-Phyllin, and others]; others)	Open the airway.	Tablet, capsule, liquid, injection, aerosol inhaler, depending on product.	By prescription.
Cromolyn sodium (Intal, Nasalcrom)	Prevents spasm of the airway.	Capsule, aerosol inhaler.	By prescription.
Steroids (beclomethasone [Beclovent, Vanceril]; flunisolide [AeroBid]; prednisone; triamcinolone [Azmacort])	Reduce inflammation of the airway.	Tablet, liquid, aerosol inhaler, depending on product.	By prescription.
CARDIOVASCULAR AGENTS			
Thiazide and related diuretics (chlorothiazide [Diuril]; hydrochlorothiazide [HydroDiuril]; metolazone [Zaroxolyn]; others)	Increase excretion of fluid; reduce blood pressure.	Tablet.	By prescription.
Loop diuretics (furosemide [Lasix]; ethacrynic acid [Edecrin]; bumetanide [Bumex]).	Remove excess fluid from the body by increasing excretion of fluids; reduce blood pressure.	Tablet, injection.	By prescription.
Potassium-sparing diuretics (amiloride [Midamor]; dyrenium [Triamterene]; spironolactone [Aldactone])	Remove excess fluid from the body by increasing excretion of fluids; reduce blood pressure.	Tablet, capsule.	By prescription.

Possible Side Effects	Contraindications	Comments
Diarrhea, skin rash (hives), yeast infection, allergic reaction.	Do not take if you have a known allergy to any drugs in this class. If you are allergic to cephalosporin drugs, you may also be allergic to penicillin.	Best taken 1 hour before or 2 hours after a full meal (food can decrease absorption). If you develop side effects, call your doctor.
Upset stomach, nausea, vomiting. Griseofulvin can cause skin rash and increased sun sensitivity.	Do not take if you have a known allergy to these drugs. If you are allergic to penicillin, you may also be allergic to griseofulvin.	Tablets are best taken with food. For oral thrush, swish the medicine around in your mouth for a couple of minutes. If you are treating a skin infection, cleanse the area before applying the cream.
Diarrhea, nausea, abdominal pain, fever.	Do not take mebendazole during pregnancy.	Tablets can be taken at any time during the day. May be chewed, crushed and mixed with food, or swallowed whole. These drugs should not be taken by a child under 2 years of age.
Nervousness, dizziness, headache, increased heart rate, flushed face, chest pain, nausea, diarrhea.	Do not take if you have heart disease or a known allergy to these drugs. Do not take albuterol or metaproterenol if you are taking monoamine oxidase (MAO) inhibitors, tricyclic antidepressants, or stimulants.	If you use an inhaler, follow instructions for use that come with the product. Do not use if solution turns brown or contains any solid particles. Terbutaline can be taken when needed, but keep doses 2 to 3 hours apart. If asthma is triggered by exercise, a dose can be taken 30 minutes before activity to prevent an attack. Certain drugs may increase or decrease the effectiveness of theophylline; consult your doctor. Take it exactly as prescribed. If using liquid form, shake well before using. If using a sustained-release form, do not crush.
Throat irritation, dry mouth, nose irritation, stomach upset, chest tightness.	Do not take if you have a known allergy to this drug.	Capsule form used only as an inhalant. Do not stop therapy suddenly unless directed to do so by your doctor.
Inhaled types: Oral yeast infection. Oral types: Suppression of the immune system, fluid retention, insomnia, increased appetite.	May be risky in cases of serious infections, such as pneumonia, but may be used for bronchitis-complicating asthma.	Inhaled steroids are currently conventional treatment of choice for asthma. Oral types can cause withdrawal symptoms if stopped abruptly; dosage must be tapered off gradually.
Nausea, vomiting, diarrhea, yellowing of the skin or eyes.	Do not take if you have a known allergy to these drugs, sulfa drugs, or oral diabetes medicines. Avoid if you have kidney or liver disease.	Take early in the day, at the same time each day. Do not stop taking this medicine without talking to your doctor. Avoid sudden changes in posture. Use caution when driving and performing tasks requiring alertness.
Stomach upset, diarrhea, sun sensitivity, dizziness or lightheadedness, restlessness.	Do not take if you have a known allergy to these drugs, sulfa drugs, or oral diabetes medicines.	Used in treatment of edema due to heart failure. Not usually used to treat high blood pressure, but may be for some patients. Take early in the day—this medication increases urination. Take with food or milk if stomach upset occurs. Use a sunscreen or protective clothing if sun sensitivity occurs.
Nausea, vomiting, diarrhea, fatigue, dry mouth, dizziness or lightheadedness.	Do not take if you have a known allergy to these drugs.	Used alone in treatment of edema due to heart failure. Used in combination with thiazide diuretics to treat high blood pressure. Take early in the day, at the same time each day. Do not use salt substitutes without checking with your doctor. Do not stop taking this drug without talking to your doctor. Avoid sudden changes in posture. Use caution when driving and performing tasks requiring alertness.

Medication	Effects	How Taken	How Available
CARDIOVASCULAR AGENTS (continued)			
Beta-blockers (atenolol [Tenormin]; metoprolol [Lopressor]; nadolol [Corgard]; propranolol [Inderal]; others)	Lower heart rate and contraction; lower blood pressure; help to maintain stable heart rhythm; aid in management of angina and prevention of migraines.	Tablet, capsule.	By prescription.
Calcium-channel blockers (amlodipine [Norvasc]; diltiazem [Cardizem]; felodipine [Plendil]; nifedipine [Adalat, Procardia]; verapamil [Calan]; others)	Relax peripheral blood vessels; lower blood pressure; aid in managing angina and maintaining stable heartbeat.	Tablet.	By prescription.
Angiotensin-converting enzyme (ACE) inhibitors (benazepril [Lotensin, Lotrel]; captopril [Capoten]; enalapril [Vasotec]; fosinopril [Monopril]; lisinopril [Prinivil, Zestril]; quinapril [Accupril]; ramipril [Altace]; others)	Dilate (open) veins and arterioles; lower blood pressure.	Tablet.	By prescription.
Angiotensin II receptor antagonists (losartan [Cozaar]; valsartan [Diovan])	Relax blood vessels; lower blood pressure.	Tablet.	By prescription.
Alpha-blockers (doxazosin [Cardura]; prazosin [Minipress]; terazosin [Hytrin]; others)	Dilate (open) blood vessels; lower blood pressure.	Tablet, capsule.	By prescription.
Central alpha agonists (clonidine [Catapres], methyldopa [Aldomet], guanfacine [Tenex])	Reduce constriction of blood vessels; lower blood pressure.	Tablet, patch, injection.	By prescription.
Neuron blockers (guanethidine [Ismelin]; others)	Stop release of nerve stimulators; lower blood pressure.	Tablet.	By prescription.
Direct vasodilators (hydralazine [Apresoline]; minoxidil [Loniten]; nitroglycerin; others)	Dilate blood vessels; lower blood pressure.	Tablet.	By prescription.
Nitrates (nitroglycerin [Deponit, Nitro-Bid, Nitrostat, and others]; isosorbide dinitrate [Dilatrate-SR, Isordil, Sorbitrate]; isosorbide mononitrate [Imdur, Ismo, Monoket]; sodium nitroprusside)	Dilate blood vessels; used to treat angina.	Tablet, capsule, sub-lingual tablet, patch, spray, depending on product.	By prescription.
Bile-acid sequestrants (cholestyramine [LoCholest, Questran]; colestipol [Colestid])	Prevent absorption of fats; lower blood-cholesterol levels.	Powder, tablet.	By prescription.
Fibric-acid derivatives (clofibrate [Atromid-S], gemfibrozil [Lopid])	Reduce blood-cholesterol levels.	Tablet, capsule.	By prescription.
HMG-CoA-reductase inhibitors (fluvastatin [Lescol]; lovastatin [Mevacor]; pravastatin [Pravachol]; simvastatin [Zocor]; others)	Inhibit production of cholesterol; lower blood-cholesterol levels.	Tablet, capsule.	By prescription.

Possible Side Effects	Contraindications	Comments
Dizziness, fatigue, depression, slowed heart rate, bronchospasm, shortness of breath, diarrhea, rash, itching, swelling.	Do not use if you have asthma, lung disease, liver dysfunction, overactive thyroid, or a known allergy to these drugs.	Read drug insert information carefully. Take at the same time each day. Do not interrupt or stop taking without contacting your doctor. Avoid sudden changes in posture, and use caution when driving and performing tasks requiring alertness.
Headache, fatigue, nausea, dizziness, weakness, flushing, shortness of breath, chest pain, heart failure, swelling of the hands, legs, or feet.	Do not use if you have a known allergy to these drugs. Use with caution if you have heart failure or liver or kidney dysfunction.	Read drug insert information carefully. Take at the same time each day. Do not stop taking this medicine abruptly. Avoid sudden changes in posture, and use caution when driving and performing tasks requiring alertness.
Headache, lightheadedness, dizziness, fatigue, cough, rash, itching, kidney or liver damage, nausea, impotence.	Do not use if you have a known allergy to these drugs. Do not use if you are pregnant or nursing. Use with caution if you have kidney or liver disease.	Read drug insert information carefully. Take at the same time every day. Do not use salt substitutes. Do not stop taking this medicine without talking to your doctor. Avoid sudden changes in posture, and use caution when driving and performing tasks requiring alertness.
Cramps, insomnia, nausea, vomiting.	Do not use if you have a known allergy to this drug. Do not use if you are pregnant. Use with caution if you have heart failure or liver or kidney disease.	Read drug insert information carefully.
Fainting, dizziness, fatigue, headache, nasal congestion.	Use with caution if you are an older adult, a pregnant woman, or a nursing mother.	Read drug insert information carefully. Avoid sudden changes in posture.
Sedation, drowsiness, rash, constipation, joint pain.	Use with caution if you are an older adult or have liver disease.	Read drug insert information carefully. Do not stop taking this medicine abruptly. Avoid sudden changes in posture, and use caution when driving and performing tasks requiring alertness.
Swelling, diarrhea, sexual dysfunction, depression.	Do not use if you have ulcers or a history of depression.	Read drug insert information carefully. Avoid sudden changes in posture, and use caution when driving and performing tasks requiring alertness.
Blood changes, rash, fluid retention, increased heart rate. Minoxidil can cause unwanted hair growth.	Do not take if you have a known sensitivity to these drugs.	Not usually used on their own, but may be added if other blood-pressure medications are not effective.
Headache, dizziness, angina, nausea, rash, low lood pressure.	Use with caution if you have suffered a recent heart attack or have heart failure or low blood pressure, or are pregnant or nursing.	These drugs have many interactions with other drugs; make sure your doctor knows about all the medicines you are using, even if they are for unrelated conditions.
Constipation, abdominal pain, gas, nausea.	Do not take if you have a known allergy to these drugs.	Drink lots of fluids. Do not take in the dry powder form—mix it in water or noncarbonated beverage. Take other medicines at least 1 hour before or 4 to 6 hours after this medicine.
Upset stomach, stomach pain, nausea, vomiting, diarrhea, fatigue, rash.	Do not take if you have a known allergy to these drugs, or active liver disease.	Follow your doctor's instructions on diet and exercise.
Stomach pain, muscle pain, constipation, nausea, vomiting, diarrhea, headache. May also cause sensitivity to sunlight and upset coenzyme-Q_{10} levels.	Do not take if you have a known allergy to these drugs, or active liver disease.	Follow your doctor's instructions on diet and exercise.

Medication	Effects	How Taken	How Available
COLD AND ALLERGY MEDICATIONS			
Over-the-counter antihistamines (chlorpheniramine [Chlor-Trimeton, Teldrin, and others]; clemastine [Tavist]; diphenhydramine [Benadryl and others]; others)	Fight allergic reaction and can aid sleep. Diphenhydramine also inhibits coughing.	Tablet, capsule, liquid, cream.	Over the counter.
Prescription antihistamines (astemizole [Hismanal]; azatadine [Optimine, Trinalin]; cetirizine [Zyrtec]; cyproheptadine [Periactin]; fexofenadine [Allegra] hydroxyzine [Atarax, Vistaril]; loratidine [Claritin]; promethazine [Phenergan])	Relieve allergy symptoms of runny nose, itching, red and watery eyes, sneezing, and hives.	Tablet, capsule, syrup, depending on product.	By prescription.
Decongestants (phenylpropanolamine [in Allerhist, Congesprin, Triaminic, and others]; pseudoephedrine [Novahistine, Sudafed, and others])	Ease nasal and sinus congestion.	Tablet, capsule, liquid.	Over the counter.
Nonnarcotic cough suppressants (dextromethorphan [in many Comtrex Cough, Triaminic Multi-Symptom, many others])	Inhibit coughing.	Liquid; lozenge.	Over the counter and by prescription, depending on formula.
Narcotic cough suppressants (codeine [Brontex, Dimetane-DC, and others]; hydrocodone [Codiclear DH, Hycodan, and others])	Inhibit coughing.	Tablet, capsule, liquid.	By prescription.
Expectorants (guaifenesin [Duratuss, Humibid, and others]; others)	Aid in clearing mucus from the respiratory tract.	Tablet, capsule, liquid.	Over the counter and by prescription.
DIGESTIVE MEDICATIONS			
Antacids (various formulas; examples include milk of magnesia, Tums, Riopan, Mylanta, Maalox, many others)	Neutralize stomach acid to relieve heartburn, sour stomach, and acid indigestion.	Tablet, liquid.	Over the counter.
Stomach-acid reducers (cimetidine [Zantac]; famotidine [Mylanta AR, Pepcid]; nizatidine [Axid]; ranitidine [Zantac]; others)	Decrease the amount of acid produced by the stomach, thereby relieving or preventing heartburn, acid indigestion, and sour stomach brought on by consuming foods or beverages.	Tablet, liquid, injection, depending on the product.	Over the counter and by prescription, depending on potency.
Bismuth subsalicylate (Pepto-Bismol)	Binds with toxins and bacteria to relieve diarrhea, heartburn, indigestion, upset stomach, and nausea from overindulgence in food and drink.	Tablet, chewable tablet, liquid.	Over the counter.
Kaolin-pectin (Donnagel, Kaopectate, Parapectolin, others)	Binds with noxious substances and solidifies stool.	Liquid.	Over the counter.

Possible Side Effects	Contraindications	Comments
Dry mouth, drowsiness; cream can cause hives, rash, itching.	Do not use on an allergic skin disorder such as poison ivy. Do not use, except as directed by a doctor, if you have glaucoma, cardiovascular disease, high blood pressure, or asthma.	Can be taken with food. Use caution when driving and performing tasks requiring alertness.
Headache, thirst, dry mouth or nose, blurred vision, dizziness, nervousness, drowsiness.	Do not take if you have a known allergy to these drugs.	Read drug insert information carefully. Chew gum or suck on hard candy if your mouth is dry. Use a sunscreen or protective clothing if sensitivity to sunlight occurs. Use caution when driving and performing tasks that require alertness. Avoid alcohol and sedatives while taking these drugs, and check with your doctor before taking medicines for cold, cough, insomnia, asthma, or weight loss.
Headache, restlessness, insomnia.	Do not take if you have a known allergy to these drugs, and use with caution if you have heart disease or high blood pressure.	Take 30 minutes to 1 hour to work.
None reported.	Do not take if you have a known allergy to these drugs.	Drink plenty of fluids while taking these drugs.
Nausea, sleepiness, lightheadedness, dizziness, headache, heart-rhythm disturbances, constipation, and others. Narcotics can also be highly addictive.	Do not take if you have a known allergy to these drugs. Do not use if you are pregnant or nursing.	Read drug insert information carefully. Avoid alcohol and sedatives. Check with your doctor before taking any other medications. Use caution when driving and performing tasks requiring alertness.
Stomach upset.	Do not take if you have a known allergy to these drugs.	Drink plenty of fluids to increase expectoration.
Diarrhea, constipation.	None known.	If you take prescription drugs, do not take an antacid within 2 hours without first checking with your doctor. Do not take continuously for more than 2 weeks without the advice of a doctor.
At low doses, side effects are rare. At higher doses, can cause constipation, diarrhea, headaches, dizziness, rash.	Do not take if you have a known allergy to these drugs.	At low doses, used to relieve or prevent heartburn, acid indigestion, and sour stomach related to diet. At higher doses, used to treat ulcers and diseases in which the stomach produces too much acid. Do not take for indigestion for longer than 2 weeks at a time unless directed by your doctor. If you have trouble swallowing or persistent abdominal pain, see your doctor promptly. For ulcers, if dose is once daily, take at bedtime. Take antacids at least 1 hour before taking this medicine.
Constipation.	Do not take if you are allergic to aspirin.	Do not use without checking with your doctor if you are taking blood-thinners or drugs for diabetes or gout. If you develop ringing in the ears, stop taking and talk to your doctor. May cause dark stools. Takes 30 minutes to 1 hour to work.
None reported.	Do not take if you have a known allergy to kaolin or pectin.	Takes 1 to 4 hours to work.

Medication	Effect	How Taken	How Available
DIGESTIVE MEDICATIONS (continued)			
Loperamide (Imodium AD, others)	Slows intestinal motility and movement of water into stool to control diarrhea and cramping.	Tablet, liquid.	Over the counter.
Bulk-forming laxatives (psyllium fiber [Metamucil and others]; Citrucel, FiberCon, others)	Increase the amount of bulk in the intestines, soften stool, and initiate contractions of the intestines to relieve constipation (irregularity).	Powder, tablet.	Over the counter.
Saline laxatives (Epsom salts, magnesium hydroxide [milk of magnesia]; magnesium citrate; others)	Draw fluid into the intestines to soften stool and initiate bowel movement.	Powder, liquid.	Over the counter.
Stimulant laxatives (bisacodyl [Dulcolax]; senna extract [Senokot]; others)	Stimulate bowel movement.	Tablet, suppository, liquid.	Over the counter.
Stool softeners (docusate [Colace]; others)	Soften stool to promote bowel movement.	Capsule, liquid.	Over the counter.
Antiemetics (dimenhydrinate [Dramamine]; meclizine [Antivert, Bonine]; promethazine [Phenergan]; prochlorperazine [Compazine]; Trimethobenzamide [Tigan]; others)	Prevent and relieve nausea, vomiting, and dizziness, especially that associated with motion sickness.	Tablet, liquid, suppository, injection.	Over the counter and by prescription, depending on the product.
PSYCHOTHERAPEUTIC DRUGS			
Antianxiety agents (alprazolam [Xanax]; chlordiazepoxide [Librium]; diazepam [Valium]; lorazepam [Ativan]; oxazepam [Serax]; others)	Reduce anxiety.	Tablet, capsule, liquid, injection.	By prescription.
Selective serotonin reuptake inhibitors (SSRIs) (fluoxetine [Prozac]; fluvoxamine [Luvox]; paroxetine [Paxil]; sertraline [Zoloft])	Alleviate depression; may be useful in managing obsessive-compulsive disorder and treating bulimia.	Tablet, capsule, liquid.	By prescription.
Tricyclic and similar antidepressants (amitriptyline [Elavil]; amoxapine [Asendin]; clomipramine [Anafranil]; desipramine [Norpramin]; nortriptyline [Aventyl, Pamelor]; imipramine [Tofranil]; bupropion [Wellbutrin, Zyban]; venlafaxine [Effexor]; nefazodone [Serzone]; others)	Alleviate depression. Clomipramine may be useful in managing obsessive-compulsive disorder.	Tablet, capsule, liquid.	By prescription.
Monoamine oxidase inhibitors (MAOIs) (isocarboxazid [Marplan]; phenelzine [Nardil]; tranylcypromine [Parnate])	Alleviate depression.	Tablet.	By prescription.
Antipsychotics (chlorpromazine [Thorazine]; trifluoperazine [Stelazine]; haloperidol [Haldol]; fluphenazine [Prolixin]; thiordazine [Mellaril]; others)	Reduce anxiety, depression, and agitation; induce/promote sleep. Used to reduce fears in older adults and behavior problems in children.	Tablet, capsule, liquid, suppository, injection.	By prescription.

Possible Side Effects	Contraindications	Comments
Abdominal pain, contipation, dizziness, drowsiness, fatigue, dry mouth, nausea, vomiting, rash.	Do not take if you have a known allergy to this drug. Do not use if you have bloody diarrhea or temperature over 101°F. Use with caution if you have ulcerative colitis.	Drink plenty of clear fluids to prevent dehydration. Use caution when driving and performing tasks requiring alertness. If you develop a distended abdomen, discontinue use.
Diarrhea, bloating, gas, abdominal pain.	Do not take if you have a known allergy to these drugs. Do not take if you have an intestinal blockage.	Use 2 hours before or after taking other medicines. Take with plenty of liquid. Do not use for longer than 1 week unless directed by your doctor.
Abdominal cramps.	Do not take if you have kidney disease, abdominal pain, or nausea, or if you are vomiting.	Do not use for longer than 1 week unless directed by your doctor.
Abdominal cramps.	Do not take if you have abdominal pain or nausea, or are vomiting.	Do not use for longer than 1 week unless directed by your doctor.
None reported.	None known.	Do not use for longer than 1 week unless directed by your doctor.
Drowsiness, dry mouth.	Do not use if you have a known allergy to these drugs. Do not use dimenhydrinate or meclizine if you have a breathing problem, like emphysema or chronic bronchitis, or if you have glaucoma or difficulty urinating due to an enlarged prostate.	Do not exceed the recommended dose. Avoid alcohol and sedatives while taking these drugs. Use caution when driving and performing tasks requiring alertness.
Drowsiness, lightheadedness, dry mouth, depression, headache, constipation, diarrhea, irregular heartbeat.	Do not take if you have a known allergy to these drugs.	Do not stop taking suddenly or change the dose without checking with your doctor. Avoid sudden changes in posture. Use caution when driving or performing tasks requiring alertness.
Anxiety, nervousness, insomnia, headache, loss of appetite, dizziness, nausea, diarrhea, sweating, frequent yawning, sexual dysfunction.	Do not take if you have a known allergy to these drugs.	Avoid alcohol while taking these drugs. Use caution when driving or performing tasks that require alertness.
Drowsiness, fatigue, weight gain, dizziness, dry mouth, blurred vision, constipation, sexual dysfunction, difficulty urinating.	Do not take if you have a known allergy to these drugs. Should be used with caution by people with heart disease. Not generally recommended for people with bipolar (manic) depression.	Avoid alcohol, diet medicines and medicines for cough, colds, and allergy while taking these drugs. Use caution when driving or performing tasks that require alertness.
Anxiety, nervousness, sleep disturbances, drowsiness, fatigue, headache, dizziness, tremors, nausea, vomiting, difficulty urinating, dry mouth.	Do not take if you have a known allergy to these drugs or a history of liver or heart disease. Do not take if you are taking other drugs for depression or using an inhaler for asthma.	These drugs have many potentially serious interactions with other drugs, both prescription and over the counter, as well as with foods. Discuss dietary and drug restrictions thoroughly with your doctor or pharmacist. Use caution when driving or performing tasks that require alertness.
Drowsiness, dry mouth, blurred vision, fever, jerky movements of the head, face, or mouth.	Do not take if you have severe depression, blood problems, liver damage, or known allergy to these drugs.	Chew gum or suck on hard candy if your mouth is dry. Use caution when driving or performing tasks requiring alertness.

Medication	Effects	How Taken	How Available
SKIN PREPARATONS			
Burow's solution	Acts as a drying agent for skin problems; fights infection.	Powder, mixed with water and used as a soak.	Over the counter.
Calamine	Acts as a drying agent; relieves itching.	Cream; lotion.	Over the counter.
Topical hydrocortisone (Alphaderm, Cort-Derm, Cortisporin, Cortril, Hytone, Lacti-Care, Nutracort, Renecort, Synacort, others)	Fights inflammation.	Cream, ointment.	Over the counter and by prescription, depending on potency.
OTHERS			
Anticonvulsants (phenytoin [Dilantin]; carbamazepine [Tegretol]; divalproex sodium [Depakote]; clonazepam [Klonopin]; topiramate [Topamax]; lamotrigine [Lamictal]; others)	Prevent seizures.	Tablet, capsule, liquid.	By prescription.
Antispasmodics (procyclidine [Kemadrin]; trihexyphenidyl [Artane]; benztropine [Cogentin]; others)	Inhibit tremors and relax muscles; aid symptoms of Parkinson's disease.	Tablet, liquid, injection.	By prescription.
Anti-Parkinsonian agents (levodopa [Larodopa]; levodopa/carbidopa [Atamet, Sinemet]; amantadine [Symadine, Symmetrel]; bromocriptine [Parlodel]; selegiline [Eldepryl]; pergolide [Permax]; others)	Counteract Parkinson's disease and its symptoms.	Tablet, capsule, liquid.	By prescription.
Hormone replacement therapy agents (estrogens [Climara, Vivelle, Estraderm, Premarin, Estratab, Ogen, diethylstilbestrol (DES), others]; estrogen/progestin combinations [Premphase, Prempro, others])	Help to ease symptoms of menopause and prevent and treat osteoporosis in menopausal and postmenopausal women.	Tablet, capsule, patch, vaginal cream, injection.	By prescription.
Oral contraceptives (Demulen, Lo/Ovral, Ortho-Novum, Triphasil, others)	Prevent pregnancy. Also used to treat hormonal and menstrual problems.	Tablet.	By prescription.
Insulin (Humulin, Iletin, Novolin, NPH, others)	Controls blood-sugar levels in people with diabetes.	Injection.	Over the counter.

Possible Side Effects	Contraindications	Comments
None reported.	None known.	Good for weeping eczema and other "wet" skin disorders.
Burning skin rash.	Do not use on open or blistered skin.	Put a thin layer of the cream or lotion on clean skin.
Long-term use can make the skin become very thin and fragile, especially with the high-potency prescription forms.	Do not use on large areas or open areas. Do not use for more than a few days unless directed by your doctor.	Put a light layer on the skin. Leave skin open to air after applying. If the area worsens or shows no improvement after several days of use, call your doctor. Avoid long-term use, especially on the face.
Drowsiness, headache, dizziness, blurred vision, decreased muscle coordination, nausea, vomiting. Phenytoin can cause overgrowth of gums.	Do not take if you have a known allergy to these drugs.	Do not stop taking suddenly—if necessary, your doctor will adjust the dose slowly. Use caution when driving and performing tasks requiring alertness. Avoid alcohol and medicines that make you drowsy.
Constipation, dry mouth, nausea, vomiting, difficulty urinating, blurred vision.	Do not take if you have a known allergy to these drugs.	Avoid alcohol. Use caution when driving and performing tasks that require alertness.
Nausea, dizziness, lightheaded-ness, stomach pain, dry mouth, confusion.	Do not take if you have a known allergy to these drugs.	Avoid alcohol. Avoid sudden changes in posture. Use caution when driving and performing tasks that require alertness.
Nausea, stomach cramps, bloating, breast tenderness, changes in vaginal bleeding, headaches, depression.	Do not use if you have breast cancer or estrogen-dependent tumors. Do not take if you are pregnant.	Read drug insert information carefully and follow the instructions there. Take at the same time each day.
Nausea, stomach cramps, spotting or light bleeding, breast tenderness.	Do not use if you have breast cancer, estrogen-dependent tumors, blood clots, or some types of heart disease. Do not take if you are pregnant. Not generally recommended for women who are over thirty-five and/or who smoke.	Read drug insert information carefully and follow the instructions there. Take at the same time each day.
Hypoglycemic (low blood sugar) reaction; symptoms can include sweating, dizziness, irregular heartbeat, tremor, restlessness, headache, anxiety.	Do not take if you have a known allergy to these drugs.	Read drug insert information carefully and follow the instructions there. Measure each dose accurately. Do not change the amount or switch to another insulin without talking to your doctor. Rotate injection sites. Follow storage directions carefully.

Herbal Medicine

Herbalists use the leaves, flowers, stems, berries, and roots of plants to prevent, relieve, and treat illness. From a "scientific" perspective, many herbal treatments are considered experimental. The reality is, however, that herbal medicine has a long and respected history. Many familiar medications of the twentieth century were developed from ancient healing traditions that treated health problems with specific plants. Today, science has isolated the medicinal properties of a large number of botanicals, and their healing components have been extracted and analyzed. Many plant components are now synthesized in large laboratories for use in pharmaceutical preparations.

THE HISTORY OF HERBAL MEDICINE

The history of herbology is inextricably intertwined with that of modern medicine. For example, salicylic acid, a precursor of aspirin, was originally derived from white willow bark and the meadowsweet plant. Vincristine, which is used to treat certain types of cancer, comes from periwinkle. Digitalis, a heart regulator, comes from the foxglove plant. Cinchona bark is the source of malaria-fighting quinine. The opium poppy yields morphine, codeine, and paregoric, a treatment for diarrhea. Laudanum, a tincture of the opium poppy, was the favored tranquilizer in Victorian times. Even today, morphine—the most important alkaloid of the opium poppy—remains the standard against which new synthetic pain-killers are measured.

Prior to the discovery and subsequent synthesis of antibiotics, the herb echinacea (which comes from the plant commonly known as purple coneflower) was one of the most widely prescribed medicines in the United States. For centuries, herbalists prescribed echinacea to fight infection. Today, research confirms that the herb boosts the immune system by stimulating the production of disease-fighting white blood cells.

The use of plants as medicine is older than recorded history. As mute witness to this fact, marshmallow root, hyacinth, and yarrow were found carefully tucked around the bones of a Stone Age man in what is now Iraq. These three medicinal herbs continue to be used today.

In 2735 B.C.E., the Chinese emperor Shen Nung wrote an authoritative treatise on herbs that is still in use today. Shen Nung recommended the use of ma huang (known as ephedra in the Western world), for example, against respiratory distress. Ephedrine, extracted from ephedra leaf, is widely used as a decongestant. You can find its synthetic form, pseudoephedrine, in many allergy, sinus, and cold medications produced by large pharmaceutical companies.

The records of King Hammurabi of Babylon (c. 1800 B.C.E.) include instructions for using medicinal plants. Hammurabi prescribed the use of mint for digestive disorders. Modern research has confirmed that peppermint does indeed relieve nausea and vomiting by mildly anesthetizing the lining of the stomach.

The entire Middle East has a rich history of herbal healing. There are texts surviving from the ancient cultures of Mesopotamia, Egypt, and India that describe and illustrate the use of many medicinal plant products, including castor oil, linseed oil, and white poppies. In the scriptural book of Ezekiel, which dates from the sixth century B.C.E., we find this admonition regarding plant life: " . . . and the fruit thereof shall be for meat, and leaf thereof for medicine." Egyptian hieroglyphs show physicians of the first and second centuries of the Common Era treating constipation with senna pods, and using caraway and peppermint to relieve digestive upsets.

Throughout the Middle Ages, home-grown botanicals were the only medicines readily available, and for centuries, no self-respecting household would be without a carefully tended and extensively used herb garden. For the most part, herbal healing lore was passed from generation to generation by word of mouth. Mother taught daughter; the village herbalist taught a promising apprentice.

By the seventeenth century, the knowledge of herbal medicine was widely disseminated throughout Europe. In 1649, Nicholas Culpeper wrote *A Physical Directory*, and a few years later produced *The English Physician*. This respected herbal pharmacopeia was one of the first manuals that the layperson could use for health care, and it is still widely referred to and quoted today. Culpeper had studied at Cambridge University and was meant to become a great doctor, in the academic sense of the word. Instead, he chose to apprentice to an apothecary and eventually set up his own shop. He served the poor people of London and became known as their neighborhood doctor.

The first *U.S. Pharmacopeia* was published in 1820. This volume included an authoritative listing of herbal drugs, with descriptions of their properties, uses, dosages, and tests of purity. It was periodically revised and became the legal standard for medical compounds in 1906. But as Western medicine evolved from an art to a science in the nineteenth century, information that had at one time been widely available became the domain of comparatively few. Once scientific methods were developed to extract and synthesize the active ingredients in plants, pharmaceutical laboratories took over from providers of medicinal herbs as the suppliers of drugs. The use of herbs, which for most of history had been mainstream medical practice, began to be considered unscientific, or at least unconventional, and to fall into relative obscurity.

HERBAL MEDICINE TODAY

Today, the *U.S. Pharmacopeia*, with its reliance on herbal compounds, has been all but forgotten by most modern physicians. They rely instead on the *Physician's Desk Reference*, an extensive listing of chemically manufactured drugs. In addition to specifying the chemical compounds and actions of particular drugs, the companies that list their products in this book also include contraindications and possible side effects.

Rather than using a whole plant, pharmacologists identify, isolate, extract, and synthesize individual components, thus capturing the active properties. This can create problems, however. In addition to active ingredients, plants contain minerals, vitamins, volatile oils, glycosides, alkaloids, bioflavonoids, and other substances that are important in supporting a particular herb's medicinal properties. These elements also provide an important natural safeguard; isolated or synthesized active compounds may become toxic in relatively small doses, while it usually takes a much greater amount of a whole herb, with all of its components, to reach a toxic level. Herbs can have powerful effects, however, and they should not be taken lightly. The suggestions for herbal treatments in this book are not intended to substitute for consultation with a qualified health-care practitioner, but rather to support and assist you in understanding and working with your physician's advice.

There are over 750,000 plants on earth. Only relatively few of the healing herbs have been studied scientifically. And because modern pharmacologists look for one active ingredient and seek to isolate it to the exclusion of all the others, most of the research that is done on plants continues to focus on identifying and isolating active ingredients, rather than studying the medicinal properties of whole plants. Herbalists, however, consider that the power of a plant lies in the interaction of all its ingredients. Plants used as medicines offer synergistic interactions between ingredients both known and unknown.

The efficacy of many medicinal plants has been validated by scientists abroad, from Europe to eastern Asia. Thanks to modern technology, scientists have identified some of the specific properties and interactions of botanical constituents. With this scientific documentation, we now know why certain herbs are effective against certain conditions. However, almost all of the current research validating herbal medicine has been done in Germany, Japan, China, Taiwan, and Russia. And for the most part, the U.S. Food and Drug Administration (FDA), which is responsible for licensing all new drugs (or any substances for which medicinal properties are claimed) in the United States, does not recognize or accept findings from across the sea. Doctors and government agencies generally want to see American scientific studies before recognizing the effectiveness of a plant as medicine. Yet until recently, drug companies and laboratories in the United States have not chosen to put much money or resources into botanical research. The result is that herbal medicine does not have the same place of importance or level of acceptance in this country as it does in other countries.

WORKING WITH AN HERBALIST

There is no national licensing or certification for herbalists in the United States. If you wish to locate a qualified herbalist, the best place to start is probably in your local herb shop or health-food store. The staff there may be able to refer you to a knowledgeable herbalist who can advise you. If you are unable to locate an herbalist this way, you may wish to contact the Herb Research Foundation, located at 1007 Pearl Street, Boulder, Colorado 80302 (telephone 303–449–2265) for suggestions. Today, many doctors, pharmacists, and nurses are getting training in the use of herbal medicines as well.

After making an evaluation of your needs, an herbalist can be expected to suggest individual herbs or herbal combinations known to be beneficial for your particular condition. An herbalist will often recommend herbs or herbal combinations both to strengthen the underlying system or organ and to relieve symptoms. Ask your herbalist when the preparation can be expected to effect an improvement in your condition. When you start taking an herbal prescription, promptly report improvement, lack of improvement, or any side effects to your herbalist. If the specified amount of time passes without any change in your symptoms, it is important to report this, too. A change in prescription may be indicated.

TREATMENT WITH HERBS

The power and potency of the healing herbs are very real.

Every herbal treatment suggested in this book has specific healing properties, carefully balanced to create a particular action within your body.

When you take an herbal preparation, pay close attention to how it makes you feel. Watch for signs that symptoms are easing. Using herbal treatment requires observation, coupled with good judgment. Natural herbal preparations are generally well tolerated, even by children. Most herbs are nontoxic, with few, if any, harmful side effects. However, it is important to know the actions and possible side effects of an herb before you take it. Although it is very unusual, some people may show signs of sensitivity to a particular herb. Reactions can include a headache, an upset stomach, or a rash. If you have a reaction, discontinue use of the herb.

If you are responding favorably to the herb, but the reaction is too intense, either decrease the dosage or discontinue use of the herb. For example, say you are constipated and you take a laxative herb. If you begin having diarrhea, you have obviously achieved relief of constipation. It's the right idea, but the reaction is too intense. Use your judgment and discontinue the herb. Likewise, if you are taking an herb with expectorant properties and you begin coughing up large quantities of mucus, you should consider decreasing the dose so expectoration is manageable.

Herbal treatment is useful for both acute and chronic conditions. It is also valuable in maintaining health and preventing illness. Many of the herbal preparations recommended in this book will help boost the immune response and help arm the body against recurrent infections.

Common Herbs and Herbal Preparations

Herbs are available in a variety of forms, including fresh, dried, in tablets or capsules, or bottled in liquid form. You can buy them individually or in mixtures formulated for specific conditions. Whatever type of product you choose, the quality of an herbal preparation—be it in capsule, tablet, tea, tincture, bath, compress, poultice, or ointment form—is only as good as the quality of the raw herb from which it was made.

Generally, herbs fall into two categories: wild-grown and farm-grown. A wild-grown herb is one that grows naturally, without human intervention. As a result of natural selection, plants tend to be found in places with conditions that optimize their growth. For example, horsetail grows best in moist, swampy areas, while arnica thrives at high altitudes in alpine meadows. The process of gathering herbs from their natural habitats is called *wildcrafting*.

The disadvantage of wild-grown herbs is that there is no guarantee that the plants haven't been exposed to chemicals and pesticides. Herbs harvested from a meadow, for example, may have been exposed to chemical drift from a crop-dusted farm nearby. Exhaust fumes from passing traffic may have settled invisibly on plants growing near a country road. Water-loving plants, like horsetail, may be rooted in the bank of a polluted stream.

Because of the possibility of contamination, unless you are very sure of the source of wildcrafted herbs, organic herbs grown commercially may be a better choice. Wildcrafted herbs also have greater variability in terms of the active ingredients they contain than cultivated plants do. This variability makes it more difficult to guarantee the consistency of the end product. Organic farm-grown herbs are becoming increasingly available, as more and more herb farms are being established. With careful management, organic herb farms can provide a steady supply of quality herbs to the consumer.

To produce top-quality products, herb farmers require a great deal of specialized knowledge. For maximum potency, it is important that particular herbs be harvested at the optimum moment. For example, echinacea is gathered in the spring, winter, and fall, but not in summer, when the plant's energies are concentrated on growth and flowering.

Responsible farmers use compost and organic matter to fertilize and replenish the health of the soil. For obvious reasons, we favor the use of certified organically grown herbs, produced without the use of synthetic fertilizers or chemical pesticides. Not all states have agencies inspecting and certifying organic growers, so to be sure you are getting pure, pesticide-free herbs grown without chemical contamination, check the label for the words "certified organic" before you make a purchase. The name of the certifying agency should be specified on the label. There are over thirty private and state organizations currently involved in certifying organic produce. Most use standards similar to those of the National Organic Standards Board (NOSB). Federal legislation on requirements for labeling a product "organic" has been passed, but is not yet being fully implemented and the proposed federal guidelines for organic labeling are generating a great deal of controversy. These are considerably less stringent than those of the NOSB, and would also prohibit labeling of organic produce by the specific farming procedures used. It is currently best to look for certification from an organization such as the Organic Growers and Buyers Association, California Certified Organic Farmers, or the Texas or Washingon state Department of Agriculture.

The herbal treatments recommended in Part Two of this book include teas, baths, compresses, poultices, oils, and ointments. In some instances, you may need to start from scratch and preparing herbal treatments yourself (instructions on how to prepare your own herbal treatments are given in Part Three, Therapies and Procedures). Some of the most commonly used herbal treatments and their applications are reviewed in the table beginning on page 27.

Using Herbal Treatments

Herbs and prepared herbal compounds are available in different forms, each of which has its own particular characteristics. Your pharmacy or health-food store will have individual herbs as well as complex herbal formulations, including raw herbs, tinctures, extracts, capsules, tablets, lozenges, and ointments. Here's a look at what's available.

Tinctures

If the label says *tincture,* the preparation contains alcohol. In a tincture, alcohol is employed to extract and concen-trate the active properties of the herb. Alcohol is also a very effective natural preservative. Because tinctures are easily assimilated by the body, this can be a very effective way to administer herbal compounds. Tinctures are concentrated and cost-effective. However, the full taste of the herb comes through very strongly in a tincture. Some people may find the taste of some herbs unpleasant. Goldenseal, for example, is bitter-tasting.

Another concern when using tinctures is the presence of the alcohol. If you wish to lessen the amount of alcohol in a tincture, mix the appropriate dose with one-quarter cup of *very* hot (just short of boiling) water. After about

---

Standardized Extracts:
Modern Science Meets Traditional Wisdom

Herbal products are available almost everywhere you turn. But the quality of these products can vary greatly; with plants, there is a natural amount of variability in the active compounds they contain. As a result, in the past, there was often no way to figure out what exactly you were paying for. Fortunately, this is changing. Today, modern techniques are being used to process herbal products. These manufacturing steps are as elaborate as those used to produce manufactured pharmaceutical products—sometimes, in fact, even more elaborate.

Applying the principles of pharmaceutical manufacturing is done for good reason. Over the past forty years, scientists have worked to identify active ingredients and substances termed *marker compounds* in herbs. A marker compound may not necessarily be an active ingredient itself, but for a substance to serve as a marker compound, it must be known that an herb with a certain percentage of that compound has therapeutic activity. Identifying active ingredients and/or marker compounds permits supplement producers to guarantee that their herbal preparations have a known percentage of active constituents and a known dosage. This process is called *standardization.* Standardized extracts also undergo a concentration process. For example, if 50 pounds of ginkgo leaves will end up making one pound of the final extract, it is termed a 50:1 extract.

In addition to allowing consumers to know what they are getting, standardization permits researchers to conduct valid scientific studies to determine the therapeutic effects of herbal treatment. Most studies of herbs that are quoted in the scientific literature were done with standardized extracts. The most reliable herbal products are those that have been tested and proven to have benefits in human trials, and that can be produced in such a way as to deliver the same strength of active ingredient every time.

When evaluating herbal products, it is important to know what to look for. Some companies quote scientific studies to support the use of certain herbs, but do not actually use the same extracts in their products that were used in the studies. Some other companies do indeed put quality extracts in their products—but not enough to be effective. Still others misuse the word *standardized* to mean that their capsules weigh the same amount every time, not that they contain the same amount of active ingredient. It is therefore necessary to read the label of any herbal product carefully before you buy it. Look for the following information:

- The name of the compound the standardization is based on.
- The percentage of that compound the extract contains.
- The extract ratio (for example, 50:1 or 4:1).
- The weight of each capsule or tablet.
- The number of capsules, tables, or ounces per bottle.
- The recommended daily dosage (in therapeutic levels).
- The expiration date and product code (for tracking purposes).
- The producer's name, address, telephone number, and/or website (so that you can contact the company for further information about the product).

A reputable company should also screen the product for the presence of pesticides, heavy metals, parasites, and fungal contamination, and determine the stability and consistency of the finished product.

Standardized extracts are the most advanced form of herbal therapy available today. By being an informed consumer and knowing what to look for, you can be sure that you're getting what you pay for with herbal remedies.

five minutes, most of the alcohol will have evaporated away, and the mixture should be cool enough to drink. Also, some herbs do not extract well in alcohol, and some compounds may not stay stable in tincture form, so tinctures may not always have the desired potency.

Extracts

Extracts can be made with alcohol, like tinctures, or the essence of the herb can be leached out with water. When purchasing a liquid extract of an herb, the only way to be certain of the extraction process (alcohol or water) is to read the label. Extracts offer essentially the same advantages and disadvantages that tinctures do. They are concentrated and therefore cost-effective, and they are easy to administer, but they have a strong herbal taste.

Standardized extracts are currently the most advanced form of herbal therapy. They allow you to be sure that the product you buy contains consistent doses of active herbal components (*see* Standardized Extracts, page 25).

Capsules and Tablets

Capsules and tablets contain a ground or powdered form of raw herb. They are easy and convenient to use, and most people prefer them. In general, there seems to be little difference between the two in terms of clinical results. Because finely milled herbs degrade quickly, it is important that herbs be freshly ground and then promptly encapsulated or tableted, within twenty-four hours of being powdered. When making your selection, read the label to make sure fresh herbs have been used in the product.

Teas

There are many delicious blends of herbal teas on the shelves of your health-food store; they need no introduction here. You'll find loose herbs ready for steeping, herbal formulations aimed at specific conditions, and convenient pre-bagged teas. Some are just for sipping; some are medicinal. When you are ill, a comforting cup of herbal tea (medicinal or not) is a wonderful way to take additional liquids. However, teas can deliver inconsistent doses, so they are not recommended as the primary form of using herbs for specific health problems.

Lozenges

Herbal-based, nutrient-rich, naturally sweetened lozenges are readily available in most health-food shops. You'll find cold-fighting formulas, natural cough suppressants, some with decongestant properties. Many are boosted with natural vitamin C. Choose lozenges made without refined sugar.

Ointments, Salves, and Rubs

From calendula ointment (for broken skin and wounds) to goldenseal (for infections, rashes, and skin irritations) to aloe vera gel (to cool and speed the healing of minor burns, including sunburn) to heat-producing herbs (for muscle aches and strains), there is a wealth of topical herbal-based products on the market. Your selection will depend on the condition you are treating.

The Treatment and Care entries in Part Two of this book offer recommendations for herbal treatments for common conditions. When using herbal treatments, you can follow the same basic suggestions that you would for conventional medications. If the taste of an herb is too strong, dilute the appropriate dosage in a little juice or water. Tableted herbs or capsules can be swallowed whole, opened or crushed and mixed with a spoonful of fruit-flavored yogurt or applesauce. Herbal teas can be sweetened with honey. For instructions on how to make and use different types of herbal preparations, *see* **PREPARING HERBAL TREATMENTS** in Part Three of this book.

When taking herbal remedies, use your judgment and common sense. The herbal treatments recommended in this book are gentle. It is still possible, however, for any herb to cause adverse reactions. If you develop a rash, a stomachache, a headache, or any other new symptom after treatment with an herbal remedy, discontinue using the herb and consult with your health-care provider.

Adverse reactions are unusual if herbal remedies are used in recommended doses. Problems are more likely to occur if an herb is overused—if the dosage is too high or if the herb is taken continuously for too long. Chamomile, for example, may cause an individual to develop an allergy to ragweed if taken on a daily basis for too long; the prolonged use of licorice can lead to elevated blood pressure. An herb may also interact with another medication you are taking. This is why, even if an herb is beneficial for a chronic condition, it is not usually recommended that an herbal remedy be taken on an ongoing basis, but rather that it be used for set periods of time, or alternated with another remedy or remedies. When using herbal treatment—as with most other aspects of a healthy life—moderation is the key. If you have any question about the use of a particular herb, consult with a qualified herbalist or health-care professional.

Herbal medicine has a long history, and a time-tested, valuable place in the treatment of many common health problems. When using herbs to treat an illness, often you not only help to alleviate symptoms, but also address an underlying problem and strengthen the overall functioning of a particular organ or system. Herbs are readily available—they can even be grown in your own back yard. To be sure you are getting the best and purest product possible, however, we recommend that you use herbal products formulated by reputable manufacturers. The more you use herbs, the more comfortable you will become with this gentle, effective form of health care.

COMMON MEDICINAL HERBS

Any medication, including herbs, can cause an allergic reaction. An allergic reaction can happen with the first exposure or after you have taken the preparation several times. Symptoms of an allergic reaction can include rash, swelling, itching, and/or difficulty breathing. If you think you are having an allergic reaction, call your physician. If you experience difficulty breathing, go to the emergency room of the nearest hospital.

Always read package directions carefully to be sure you are taking the preparation properly and in the correct dose. Note that with herbal medicines, side effects are more likely to occur in the case of overdose. When taken in recommended doses, toxicity is unlikely.

Herb	Medicinal Use	Plant Part Used	How Taken	Possible Side Effects	Comments
Aloe vera	Topically: Pain reliever, excellent for burns, sore nipples, itching. Internally: Relieves stomach inflammation and constipation.	Pulp from inside leaf.	Liquid applied topically to affected area or taken internally.	None known.	Topically: Use pulp from inside plant leaf. Internally: Use prepared food-grade liquid.
American ginseng	Helps strengthen overall constitution; helpful in relieving fatigue or debilitation after an illness.	Root.	Standardized extract, tea, tincture.	Nervousness, insomnia, diarrhea.	Do not take if you have a fever.
Astragalus	Immunotonic; reduces fatigue; used for colds and flu.	Root.	Standardized extract, liquid extract, tea.	None known.	Do not take if you have acute inflammation or fever.
Bilberry	Antioxidant; helps strengthen capillaries and blood vessels, good for eyesight.	Fruit.	Standardized extract.	None known.	Use with caution if you have a bleeding problem or are taking anticoagulants.
Black cohosh	Balances female hormones and strengthens the female reproductive organs, lowers blood sugar. Also used for arthritis, rheumatism, and tinnitus.	Rhizome.	Standardized extract, tea.	In excessive amounts, may cause nausea, vomiting, headache, dizziness, slow pulse.	Do not use if you are allergic to aspirin.
Black currant	Has anti-inflammatory and anti-oxidant actions, and benefits the skin; used for chronic inflammation, diabetes, PMS, and skin diseases.	Seed oil.	Capsules, liquid oil.	None known.	Contains balanced essential fatty acids.
Borage	Has an anti-inflammatory effect and benefits the skin; used for chronic inflammation, diabetes, PMS, and skin diseases.	Seed oil.	Capsules, liquid oil.	None known.	Contains omega-6 essential fatty acids.
Bupleurum	Liver detoxifier; strengthens immune system; helpful in treating chronic conditions such as allergies.	Root.	Tincture, capsule (taken in combination with other herbs).	None known.	Most commonly used in combination with other herbs, not by itself. Do not take if you have a fever or other signs of acute infection. Do not use if you have high blood pressure.
Burdock	Blood purifier and cleanser.	Root.	Tincture, tea, capsule, fresh cooked root.	Dilated pupils, dry mouth.	Do not take for more than 2 consecutive weeks. Alternate 2 weeks on, 2 weeks off.
Calendula	Antiseptic; speeds tissue healing; useful for cuts, blisters, burns, abrasions.	Flower.	Lotion, cream, or tincture, applied topically to the affected area.	None known.	
Chamomile	Soothes upset stomach; calms nerves and relaxes.	Flower.	Standardized extract, tea, tincture.	Allergic reactions in sensitive individuals.	Use with caution if you are allergic to ragweed.

Herb	Medicinal Use	Plant Part Used	How Taken	Possible Side Effects	Comments
Chinese (Korean) ginseng	Helps strengthen overall constitution; helpful in relieving fatigue or debilitation after an illness.	Root.	Standardized extract, liquid extract, tea.	Nervousness, insomnia, diarrhea.	Take in cycles—three weeks on, two weeks off.
Cordyceps	Antioxidant; strengthens the immune system; increases oxygen supply to body systems; protects the lungs.	Mushroom.	Standardized extract.	None known.	Use with caution if you are having a bleeding problem or are taking anticoagulants.
Dandelion	Promotes excretion of fluids; used as a diuretic.	Leaf.	Liquid extract, fresh plant juice, fresh leaf.	May cause fluid loss if used in high doses.	Contains vitamins and minerals, especially vitamin A and potassium.
Dong quai	Blood tonic and hormonal regulator used for problems such as PMS and menopausal symptoms; also has a mild sedative effect.	Root.	Standardized extract, liquid extract, tea.	May cause increased sensitivity to the sun.	Contains phytoestrogens. Do not use if you have a bleeding problem.
Echinacea	Antibiotic; boosts immune system. Useful in treating many infections, insect bites, and stings.	Root.	Standardized extract, tea, tincture, salve.	None known.	Long-term use not advised. Best used for 5 days to 1 week at a time. Alternate 1 week on, 1 week off.
Evening primrose	Has an anti-inflammatory effect and benefits the skin; used for chronic inflammation, diabetes, PMS, and skin diseases.	Seed oil.	Capsule, oil.	May cause minor stomach upset or rash in sensitive individuals.	Contains omega-6 essential fatty acids.
Flax	Soothing to the digestive tract; relieves constipation.	Seed.	Tea, capsule, oil.	Agitation, excitement, rapid breathing.	Contains balanced essential fatty acids. Seeds are safe when cooked; leaves can be toxic and are not normally used.
Garlic	Antibiotic, antiseptic, antiworm; lowers blood pressure and cholesterol.	Clove.	Fresh whole herb, standardized extract, capsule, liquid.	Stomach upset, contact dermatitis, flatulence.	Fresh cloves may be used, but odorless capsule form may be more palatable for some people. Use with caution if you have a bleeding problem or are taking anticoagulants.
Ginger	Aids digestion; relieves congestion; promotes perspiration and relieves fever; soothes achy muscles.	Root.	Standardized extract, tincture, tea, bath or oil for achy muscles.	Diarrhea, nausea.	Use with caution if you have a bleeding problem or are taking anticoagulants.
Ginkgo biloba	Increases blood flow to the brain and extremities; used for Alzheimer's disease and other conditions requiring increased blood flow, as well as for asthma, ringing in the ears, and mild depression.	Leaf.	Standardized extract.	May cause minor stomach upset, rash, or headache in sensitive individuals.	Do not use if you have a bleeding problem. Use with caution if taking nonsteroidal anti-inflammatory drugs (NSAIDs) such as ibuprofen.
Goldenseal	Antibiotic; tonifies mucous membranes of the respiratory and digestive system; used to treat many infections.	Root.	Standardized extract, tea, tincture, capsule.	Irritation of mouth and throat, nausea, vomiting, diarrhea.	Do not take during pregnancy. Do not take for more than 1 week to 10 days at a time. This is now classified as an endangered species. Oregon grape root can be used as a substitute.
Gotu kola	Enhances mental performance and improves learning ability; topically, used for wound healing of skin and connective tissues.	Whole plant.	Standardized extract, liquid extract, capsule, topical aerosol spray.	May cause rash in sensitive individuals.	Works well in combination with ginkgo.

Herb	Medicinal Use	Plant Part Used	How Taken	Possible Side Effects	Comments
Green tea	Antioxidant; protects against effects of radiation exposure; has anticarcinogenic properties; blocks the body's absorption of dietary cholesterol.	Leaf.	Standardized extract, tea.	In tea form, can cause jitteriness and insomnia if taken in excess.	
Hawthorn	Antioxidant; general heart tonic.	Leaf, flower, berry.	Standardized extract.	None known.	If you are currently taking prescription medicine for a heart condition, use only under the supervision of a physician.
Horsetail	Diuretic; good source of silica; used for health of skin, hair, and nails.	Spring shoots.	Standardized extract.	May deplete vitamin B_6.	Take a multiple vitamin when taking this herb.
Kava kava	Eases anxiety, nervousness, and tension; may be helpful for insomnia.	Root.	Standardized extract, capsule, root.	May interact with prescription medicines for anxiety. Prolonged use of high doses can cause skin rash.	Do not use if you have Parkinson's disease. Avoid alcohol while using this herb. Use caution when driving and performing tasks requiring alertness.
Licorice	Tonic; expectorant; soothing to respiratory tract; tonic for the adrenal glands; increases energy; used for symptoms of peptic ulcer.	Root.	Standardized extract, tincture, capsule, chewable tablet, tea, liquid extract.	Can lead to loss of potassium and high blood pressure with long-term use unless DGL form is used.	Do not take if you have high blood pressure or heart disease. Use with caution during pregnancy.
Marshmallow	Demulcent; helpful for sore throat and lung congestion.	Root.	Tea, capsule.	None known.	May decrease absorption of some medications; check with your pharmacist.
Milk thistle	Detoxifies the liver; used for chronic liver problems.	Seed.	Standardized extract.	None known.	If you have chronic liver disease, use only under the supervision of a physician.
Nettle	Leaf used for allergies and hay fever; root used for prostate problems.	Leaf, root.	Standardized extract, tea, capsule.	None known.	Leaf should be freeze-dried.
Oat straw	Calming; may help decrease cravings for nicotine and opiates; used for nervous conditions and addictive disorders.	Whole plant.	Capsule, liquid extract, tea.	None known.	
Parsley	Increases urination; helpful in treating bladder infection.	Leaf.	Tea, capsule.	Dizziness, headache, warmth, nausea, vomiting, itching.	Use with caution during pregnancy. Excessive amounts can stop milk production in nursing mothers.
Passionflower	Calms and relaxes; used for nervous conditions, stress, insomnia.	Vine.	Standardized extract (liquid or capsule).	None known.	May interact with other medications used for anxiety and insomnia. Avoid alcohol while using this herb. Use caution when driving and performing other tasks requiring alertness.
Peppermint	Aids digestion; relieves nausea; reduces fever; relieves diarrhea, gas, heartburn.	Leaf.	Tincture, tea, capsule.	In large doses, can cause stomach irritation and coldness of the body.	Do not use if you are taking homeopathic remedies.

Herb	Medicinal Use	Plant Part Used	How Taken	Possible Side Effects	Comments
Red clover	Blood purifier; helpful in treating skin infections; mild sedative.	Flower.	Tincture, tea, capsule.	None known.	Do not use if you have a bleeding disorder.
Red raspberry	Astringent; used for excessive menstrual bleeding.	Leaf.	Liquid extract, capsule, tea.	None known.	Tea is an excellent uterine tonic for pregnant women.
Rosemary	Antispasmodic, stimulating tonic; helpful in treating colds, sore throats, headaches; increases circulation.	Leaf.	Tea, in soup.	Nausea, diarrhea.	A strong tea can also be used topically to enhance scalp health and hair growth.
Sage	Increases urination; aids digestion; antiseptic; helpful for nasal discharge, sore throat.	Leaf.	Tincture, tea, capsule, topically on cuts or abrasions. Can also be used as a gargle for sore throats.	Dry mouth, local irritation.	Do not use during pregnancy. May decrease milk production in nursing mothers.
Saw palmetto	Beneficial for the male reproductive system; used for benign prostatic hypertrophy (BPH).	Berry.	Standardized extract.	None known.	
Shiitake	Enhances immunity; used for stress and fatigue.	Mushroom.	Standardized extract.	None known.	Do not use if you have a fever or other sign of acute infection.
Siberian ginseng	Helps the body cope with stress; enhances energy, immunity, and mood.	Root.	Standardized extract.	May cause nervousness and restlessness in some individuals. May increase digoxin levels in those taking this drug.	Take in cycles—four weeks on, two weeks off. If you are taking medication for a heart condition, take only under the supervision of a physician.
Skullcap	Sedative, nerve tonic.	Leaf.	Tincture, tea, capsule.	Giddiness, irregular heartbeat.	Best used in combination with other calmatives
Slippery elm	Helpful in treating constipation, diarrhea, irritated/inflamed gastrointestinal tract.	Bark.	Capsule, powder.	None known.	
St. John's wort	Antiviral; used for mild depression; used topically for bruises and sprains.	Flowering buds.	Standardized extract, topical oil.	May cause increased sensitivity to the sun.	If you are currently taking prescription medication for depression, use only under the supervision of a physician. Do not use if you are taking a monoamine oxidase (MAO) inhibitor.
Thyme	Antiseptic; relieves lung congestion, diarrhea, lack of appetite, colic, flatulence; useful for peptic ulcer disease.	Leaf.	Capsule, tea, in soup.	In large doses, can cause diarrhea.	May be used as a mouthwash.
Turmeric	Antioxidant; used for inflammatory conditions such as arthritis; may lower blood cholesterol levels.	Root.	Standardized extract.	May cause minor stomach upset or rash in sensitive individuals.	Do not use if you have a bleeding disorder or peptic ulcer. Do not take nonsteroidal anti-inflammatory drugs (NSAIDs) such as ibuprofen when taking this herb.
Yellow dock	Detoxifier; mild laxative; antiworm; relieves cough and lymphatic congestion.	Root.	Tincture, tea, capsule.	In large doses, can cause nausea, vomiting, diarrhea.	Encourages perspiration.

Homeopathy

Homeopathy is a system of treatment that uses dilutions of plant, mineral, and animal substances, as well as some chemicals, to stimulate the defensive systems of the body in a very subtle way. It is widely used in Europe, but not as well known in the United States. The theoretical and empirical basis of homeopathy is a concept called the Law of Similars, often summarized as "like cures like." Perhaps more than anything else, what distinguishes the practice of homeopathy from other approaches to medicine is that instead of focusing on the specific *causes* of disease (such as viruses and bacteria), it focuses on the specifics of the *symptoms* of disease, *as they are experienced by the individual person.*

THE HISTORY OF HOMEOPATHY

Samuel Hahnemann (1755–1843) of Leipzig, Germany, created the practice of homeopathy. A medical doctor, Hahnemann did in-depth studies and wrote extensively on chemistry, pharmacology, and medicine. His study of arsenic, written in 1796, remains an authoritative text.

In 1790, Dr. Hahnemann began to question the accepted medical theories of the time. *Cinchona officinalis,* or Peruvian bark, had been the treatment of choice for malaria since 1700. Conventional medical thought attributed its beneficial action to its bitter and astringent properties. Hahnemann rejected this explanation. He observed that other plants and botanicals had even greater bitterness and stronger astringency, yet did nothing to relieve malaria. In an attempt to better understand how cinchona worked, he experimented by taking some himself. After taking the cinchona compound, Hahnemann promptly developed the symptoms of malaria.

This inspired him to further experimentation with many different plants, chemicals, and minerals. Hahnemann experimented first on himself, then on his family and friends. As his work continued, he noted the same remarkable effect again and again: Derivatives of certain extracts produced symptoms in the body similar to those produced by certain diseases. Pressing on with his experimentation, Hahnemann found that systematically diluted doses of extract actually produced the opposite effect. Instead of causing the symptoms of a particular disease, the well-diluted extract reversed the course of the disease.

This led Hahnemann to his observation that "like cures like"—that is, a substance that causes a certain set of symptoms in a healthy person will, in minute doses, cure a sick person of those same symptoms. He called this phenomenon the Law of Similars.

Many of Hahnemann's colleagues argued against his practice of using himself as a guinea pig, predicting dire consequences. But the doctor refused to heed their warnings, saying, "He knows with greatest certainty the things he has experienced in his own person." Through his experiments, Hahnemann learned that a minute dose of a substance would cause illness in a healthy person but, paradoxically, effect a cure in a sick individual. For example, a remedy that caused fever, chills, and leg cramps in a healthy person would cure a sick person of similar fever, chills, and leg cramps when given in microdoses.

HOMEOPATHY TODAY

Homeopathy is accepted as an effective form of medicine in many parts of the world today, including Great Britain, France, Germany, Greece, India, and South America. The British royal family has been under the care of homeopathic physicians since the time of Queen Victoria.

This systematic and precise form of natural medicine can address both physical and emotional symptoms. It recognizes that each person is unique and will have an individual disease pattern. The experimentation, documentation, in-depth testing, and recording of the effects of homeopathic remedies did not end with Dr. Hahnemann. Diagnosis of a specific disease is not the primary concern when using homeopathics. Rather, the correct remedy is chosen according to the specific symptoms and emotions you are experiencing.

Homeopathic remedies stimulate the body's vital force, enhancing its ability to heal itself. The "vital force" described by Hahnemann cannot be precisely identified. Even today's most technologically advanced medical detectives do not really understand the ways in which body and mind work together. A complex interrelationship between immune factors and regenerative biological systems, the essential life force locked within body and mind remains a mystery.

Homeopathic remedies work by, in effect, "turning on a switch" that affects particular functions in the mind or body. Homeopathic compounds somehow send a healing and normalizing message throughout the body. They spark unbalanced internal systems so that they are better able to perform their functions.

Increasingly, the effectiveness of homeopathy is being backed up by scientific research. In 1997, the British medical journal *Lancet* published a comprehensive review of such research that looked at 186 separate scientific studies. The majority (119) were double-blind and/or randomized placebo-controlled studies, meaning that they were designed according to the same scientific principles as studies of pharmaceutical drugs. Of these, 89 were considered rigorously controlled enough to include in the review. As a group, these research studies demonstrated that homeopathic remedies had an effect 2.45 times greater than that of placebos. Among the health problems treated in these studies were respiratory and other infections, digestive disorders, allergies, arthritis, and psychological problems.

Other studies have supported the underlying principle of homeopathy—that the same substance will have opposite effects depending on whether it is given in ordinary doses or in homeopathic microdoses. It is well known, for example, that taking common aspirin decreases the blood's tendency to form clots, but a French scientist working at the School of Pharmacy of Bordeaux demonstrated that microdoses of acetylsalicylic acid (aspirin's active ingredient) actually shortens bleeding time. Similarly, in studies on animal subjects, ordinary doses of thyroxine (thyroid hormone) were shown to speed up metabolic processes, while highly dilute doses slowed them down. As yet, there is no satisfactory scientific explanation for this phenomenon; however, the effectiveness of homeopathic treatment is widely accepted around the world.

WORKING WITH A HOMEOPATHIC PHYSICIAN

Remedies that may be appropriate for a variety of common health problems are recommended in Part Two of this book. However, because the deeper concepts of homeopathy and the intricacies of the remedies can be difficult to master, you may find it helpful to consult a homeopathic physician. Often, a homeopathic physician can determine a constitutional remedy that will help to balance your entire system.

Homeopathy is on the upswing in the United States. Many different types of health-care practitioners use homeopathy. You will find medical doctors, naturopathic physicians, acupuncturists, herbalists, chiropractors, nurse practitioners, physician assistants, and laypeople who are knowledgeable in the field. Homeopathic pharmacies, even major health food stores, are other resources to explore. They may be able to tell you how to find a practicing homeopath in your area.

There are national organizations throughout the United States that can provide you with a list of homeopaths as well. If you cannot readily find a homeopathic physician in your area, you may wish to contact the International Foundation for Homeopathy, the National Center for Homeopathy, or Foundation for Homeopathic Education and Research (see the Resources section at the end of the book).

When choosing a homeopath, it is important to select a physician with whom you feel very comfortable. This doctor will question you closely, asking you to reveal very intimate information. Much of homeopathic diagnosis and treatment depends on your ability to observe and relate specific details, some of which may even seem absurd or irrelevant to you at first. For example, if you have a runny nose or are coughing up phlegm, your homeopath will want to know the color, smell, and consistency of the discharge. You will probably be asked if it is heavier in the morning or evening, after eating, or before eating.

Your homeopath will also consider your temperament and the way you respond emotionally to illness. Do you want company when ill, or prefer to be left alone? Do you become irritable and demanding, or quiet and passive? Do you sleep a lot, or become restless and wakeful? Do you want the window open to admit cool, fresh air, or do you feel chilly even snuggled under a cozy comforter?

How the other members of your household respond to your illness is something else your homeopath will ask you to reveal. When a loved one is ill, some family members become irritated and annoyed, some nervous and anxious. The very fortunate have a deep well of calm and certainty on which to draw. Be truthful when your doctor inquires about this. Emotional responses are not something people can necessarily control consciously. Faced with a hectic schedule, many of us have difficulty mustering up as much patience as we would like. All of the physical and emotional factors surrounding you must be taken into account in determining the appropriate remedy. Because the emotional response of those around you will unavoidably have an impact on you, your homeopathic physician may prescribe a helpful remedy for other members of the household as well.

TREATMENT WITH HOMEOPATHIC REMEDIES

Of all the remedies commonly used in the various medical protocols, homeopathic remedies are unique in that they are symptom-specific. That is, the correct remedy is determined not by the disease, but by the specific complex of physical and emotional symptoms you are experiencing. The choice of homeopathic remedies takes into consideration your temperament and emotional responses as well as the most minute details of your physical condition.

For example, the cold that infects you and a neighbor may be caused by the same virus, but each of you will exhibit a unique set of symptoms and emotions. One of you may have a headache and a runny nose, feel completely exhausted, and want to eat when not napping. The other may be clogged and congested, feel restless, be unable to sleep, and refuse food. Consequently, although infected by the same virus, you will require entirely different remedies.

Homeopathy respects the complexity and uniqueness of each individual. To identify the correct homeopathic remedy, you must carefully observe your unique—even quirky—behaviors and responses. Choosing the appropriate remedy requires you and the homeopathic physician to match your symptoms, both obvious and subtle, with the remedy. Today, some practitioners also select homeopathic remedies based on their effectiveness for specific conditions.

Based on your overall physical, emotional, and mental constitution, your homeopathic physician may prescribe a constitutional remedy. An appropriate constitutional remedy can help prevent illness, as well as maintain and support optimal health. For example, if you are subject to recurrent colds, sinusitis, allergies, or digestive disorders, a constitutional homeopathic remedy may be extremely helpful.

The correct constitutional remedy can help strengthen and stimulate the vital life force. The response to the remedy will be at once subtle and profound, on the physical, emotional, and mental levels. Prescribing a constitutional remedy is a complicated art, however. To discover the most helpful constitutional remedy, consult a homeopathic physician or other health-care practioner experienced in homeopathy.

Common Homeopathic Remedies

Homeopathic remedies are prepared according to the standards of the *United States Homeopathic Pharmacopoeia*. All remedies are derived from naturally occurring plant, mineral, or chemical substances. Some of the most useful homeopathic remedies and their common indications are described in the table on page 34.

Homeopathic remedies come in different potencies. Of all of the issues in homeopathy, Dr. Hahnemann's concept of potency is probably the one that has evoked the most questions, because it seems somewhat paradoxical at first. The term *potency* means something different in homeopathy than in conventional medicine. Homeopathic remedies undergo a systematic series of dilutions. After each dilution, the remedy is succussed (shaken with impact or force). Each time a remedy is succussed, it is considered to have been potentiated. Thus, the more times a remedy has been succussed, the greater its potency.

Commonly available homeopathic remedies come in several forms: the mother tincture, x potencies, and c po-tencies. Homeopathic tablets are made by mixing diluted remedies with lactose (milk sugar) to make solid pellets. There are also homeopathic creams, ointments, and salves, made by mixing diluted remedies with a cream or gel base.

Mother Tincture

The mother tincture is an alcohol-based extract of a specific substance, as it comes from the original plant, animal, or mineral. Mother tinctures are generally used topically or in a fashion similar to herbal tinctures.

X Potencies

In homeopathic remedies, the x (derived from the Roman numeral decimal system) represents 10. It indicates that the mother tincture has been diluted to one part in ten. The number preceding the x indicates how many times the remedy has been diluted and succussed. Thus, a 6x potency represents six such dilutions/succussions, beginning with the mother tincture. Remember that the more times a homeopathic remedy has been succussed, the more potent it is. So a 6x potency remedy, which has been diluted and succussed six times, is more potent than a 3x potency compound, which has been diluted and succussed only three times.

C Potencies

The c, also derived from the Roman numeral decimal system, represents 100. A c potency indicates that a mother tincture has undergone dilutions to 1 part in 100; the number preceding the c indicates how many dilutions it has undergone. Thus, a 3c potency indicates that the substance has been diluted to 1 part in 100 and succussed three times. As with x potencies, the higher the number, the stronger the remedy.

In home treatment, it is usually sufficient to use the lower potencies, such as 12x, 30x, 6c, and 9c. Many homeopaths agree that once you have identified the correct remedy, it will work regardless of potency.

If you are lucky, you may live in an area where you have access to a homeopathic pharmacy that specializes in homeopathic remedies. If not, check with your local health-food store. Major health-food stores across the United States usually carry a comprehensive selection of homeopathic remedies. If you cannot find what you are looking for, many health-food shops will special-order for you. A list of recommended suppliers of homeopathic remedies is also provided in the Appendix.

Proper storage and handling of homeopathic remedies is extremely important. They are sensitive, and a certain amount of care must be taken in order not to diminish their potency or interfere with their action. Keep remedies out of sunlight and extreme heat, and away from strong smells. Avoid touching homeopathic remedies with your

COMMON HOMEOPATHIC REMEDIES

Remedy	Indications	Remedy	Indications
Aconite	Very often the first remedy for acute problems, especially if fright or shock is part of the picture.	Hepar sulfuris	Hypersensitivity to pain; yellow mucus; symptoms that feel worse from cold drafts, better with warmth.
Antimonium tartaricum	Rattling cough with breathlessness.	Hypericum	Nerve pain; trauma to nerve endings, especially of the fingers and toes.
Apis mellifica	Insect bites that are red and swollen.	Ignatia	Anxiety; digestive disorders related to or exacerbated by stress or distress.
Argentum nitricum	Stomach upset from eating sweets; nervousness; for a person who craves sweets and fatty foods; for a person who craves stimulation.	Lachesis	Headache that begins or is worse in the left side of the head; symptoms of menopause or PMS; sore throat localized on the left side; symptoms that are worse upon awakening.
Arnica	Bruises; sprains; strains. Can be taken internally or administered topically (but do not use topically if the skin is broken).	Ledum	Black-and-blue bruises; puncture wounds; black eye.
Arsenicum album	First remedy for food poisoning; diarrhea with anxiety; a cold with restlessness.	Lycopodium	Problems affecting the right side of the body; reactions to food.
Aurum muriaticum	Depression, distress , agitation, anxiety, nervousness, uterine discomfort.	Magnesia phosphorica	Menstrual cramps that feel better with heat on the lower abdomen, especially cramps on the right side of the body; diarrhea.
Belladonna	Fever; acute problems with sudden onset, red face, dilated pupils; headache.	Mercurius corrosivus	Diarrhea or vaginal discharge with a very strong odor; illness accompanied by sore throat.
Berberis vulgaris	Low back pain, pain in the gallbladder area that is worse with pressure. Remedy of choice for disorders affecting the kidneys.	Mercurius solubilis	Bad breath, mouth sores, lingering illness that resists treatment, illness accompanied by sore throat and/or offensive-smelling body odor, stool, and/or urine.
Bryonia	Dry cough; constipation; achiness; irritability.		
Calcarea carbonica	Dyspepsia; skin eruptions; for a person who craves milk and eggs.	Natrum muriaticum	Dehydration; emotional upset with strong desire for salty foods; acne; canker sores.
Cantharis	Burns; burning sensation associated with urinary tract infections.	Nux vomica	Hypersensitivity and irritability; indigestion; for a person who likes to go to bed late; for a person who craves rich foods.
Carbo vegetabilis	Digestive problems such as acid indigestion, heartburn, burning pain in the center of the stomach, abdominal gas, nausea.	Phosphorus	Sore throat; tiredness during the day and difficulty sleeping at night; for a sensitive person.
Chelidonium majus	Pain in the upper right quadrant of the abdomen; pain in the arms and shoulders, particularly the right shoulder.	Phytolacca	Sore throat, swollen glands in the neck, pain in the neck, jaw, and/or chest.
China	Anemia due to blood loss, abdominal gas and/or bloating, digestive difficulties accompanied by tiredness or weakness.	Pulsatilla	Nasal congestion with yellow mucus; cold symptoms; earache; for a person who cries easily.
Coffea cruda	Difficulty falling asleep due to racing thoughts, such as might occur the night before a major event.	Rhus toxicodendron	Chickenpox; poison ivy; joint pain associated with arthritis.
Colocynthis	Menstrual cramps that are sharp and stabbing; diarrhea cramps.	Ruta graveolens	Tendinitis; sprains of wrist or ankle.
Euphrasia	Burning, tearing eyes, especially accompanied by nasal discharge; swollen eyelids; eyestrain; allergy or cold that affects the eyes; hayfever; feeling of pressure in or behind the eyes.	Sepia	Menstrual cramps; constipation; for a person who feels better with exercise.
Ferrum phosphoricum	Mild fever; nosebleed.	Silicea	Pain and soreness affecting the legs and feet; for a person who feels cold, tired, and weak.
Gelsemium	Cold symptoms that include heavy, droopy eyes, weakness, achy muscles, chills; nervousness before a performance.	Spongia	Laryngitis; hacking cough.
		Staphysagria	Urinary tract infection; for a person who is irritable and/or angry.
Graphites	Skin disorders with a clear or yellow discharge, a tendency to gain weight easily, thick, brittle, cracked and rough nails, possibly with inflamed nail beds.	Sulfur	Pinworms; skin infections; ringworm.
		Thuja	Warts; athlete's foot; after vaccinations; thrush.

hands, and do not put any pellets that fall out of the bottle back in. Also, never touch the inner rim or the inside of a remedy bottle or lid.

Taking Homeopathic Remedies

Many common health problems can be treated effectively and gently with homeopathy. Home use of homeopathic remedies is ideally suited for acute situations—conditions that attack suddenly—rather than conditions medically termed chronic (illnesses that develop slowly and persist over a long period of time).

When you take the right remedy, it will work quickly. Experienced homeopathic physicians say that using the "wrong" remedy will usually cause no harm. Once the symptoms improve, discontinue the remedy. It is possible to experience an aggravation or increase in the symptoms being treated, an effect sometimes caused by the Law of Similars. Should your symptoms be increased by a remedy, stop taking it.

Homeopathic remedies come in pellet, tablet, and liquid form. You should avoid touching them with your hands, as this can decrease their effectiveness. Shake pellets or tablets into a clean spoon or the top of the bottle, and then place them directly into your mouth and let them dissolve rather than chewing them. Homeopathic pellets and tablets are mostly sweet milk sugar (lactose) that melts in the mouth, so they are generally very easy to take.

The liquid remedies—homeopathic tinctures—are not generally preferred because of their high alcohol content. However, as with herbal tinctures, if you put them in very hot water and let the mixture sit for five minutes, much of the alcohol will evaporate.

Homeopathic remedies work best when taken at least thirty minutes before or after eating. Clinical experience suggests that strong flavors (such as mint products), odors (paints, perfumes), foods and beverages that contain caffeine, and camphor or camphor-containing products (mothballs or deep-heating ointments)—all decrease the effectiveness of the remedies, so all of these substances should be avoided when using homeopathic remedies.

Unless the treatment recommendations in Part Two specify otherwise, use the following guidelines when administering homeopathic remedies.

- **For a severely acute situation.** For a problem such as a headache or fever, take one dose, as directed on the product label, every fifteen minutes for one hour. If you see no change after four doses, you probably have the wrong remedy and should choose another.

- **For a less acute situation.** For a problem such as a runny nose or a sore throat, take one dose, as directed on the product label, every two hours. Once symptoms start to improve, you can continue the remedy at less frequent intervals. During this stage, take one dose, three times daily.

A homeopathic remedy should be taken for as long as it is needed. For example, if a headache is gone fifteen minutes after you take a headache remedy, stop taking the remedy. If the headache returns four hours later, try the same remedy again. Once you feel better, there is no longer any need to take the remedy.

Homeopathy is a form of treatment that offers a first line of defense for common complaints. It is ideal for people who cannot use certain over-the-counter drugs or herbs, whether because of other health problems or because they must take other medications on a regular basis. Because everyone in the household can use the same remedies, homeopathy is cost-effective, and the remedies are clearly labeled to indicate the conditions they are designed to treat, making it easy to select the right ones.

Bach Flower Remedies

The world of natural treatment also includes emotion-balancing flower preparations. This system of healing was developed by Dr. Edward Bach (1897–1936). Dr. Bach believed that physical problems were secondary to emotional problems—that physical illness was a manifestation of emotional imbalance. He taught that physical symptoms could be relieved by altering or alleviating destructive emotions. The various remedies he devised are used to treat illness by easing quite specific types of emotional and mental distress.

The Bach flower remedies are dilute essences of plants. Unlike chemical mood-altering drugs, the flower remedies—while effective—are gentle and easy to use. Although beneficial and benign, these natural flower essences have remarkable emotional and mental balancing effects. Because they act quite gently, they can be used freely whenever you think they may help you feel better.

When choosing a Bach essence, match your overall temperament, personality, and fears, as well as the particular emotional distress you are experiencing. If no single remedy seems to address all of these concerns, you may combine up to three remedies. (Although there is no danger in blending more than three remedies at any one time, their effectiveness can be diminished in a blend that is too complicated.)

CHOOSING A REMEDY

Once you have identified the primary emotional distress you are experiencing, use the table on pages 37–39 to find an appropriate remedy. Match your personality, temperament, fears, and emotional upset with the suitable Bach flower remedy. Bach flower remedies are available at many health-food stores. If you cannot get them at a store near you, you can obtain them through Nelson Bach USA, Inc. (see the Resources section at the end of the book).

USING BACH FLOWER REMEDIES

Bach flower remedies are essences of flowers that come in tincture form (see page 25). The bottled remedy you buy at your health-food store is called the mother tincture, and is the most concentrated form available. There are two different ways you can take a Bach remedy:

- Place a drop of the mother tincture into a small glass of noncarbonated spring water and sip it over a period of a few hours. For added benefit, swish the mixture around in your mouth before swallowing it.

- If you prefer, you can make a diluted mother tincture. Fill a two-ounce glass bottle with spring water. Add three drops of mother tincture and shake gently to blend. When using a diluted mother tincture, take two droppersful, three times daily.

After taking a flower remedy, monitor your response. As your emotional response and behavior change, the need for a particular remedy may cease to exist. Take a remedy until the situation has been resolved. Once your mood and emotions have been gently altered, you may need to select another remedy to complete and sustain the alteration. Once any destructive emotions have eased sufficiently and you feel your emotional and mental state has come into balance, discontinue the remedy.

Of all the Bach flower remedies, the overwhelming favorite of many people is Rescue Remedy. This is a premixed combination remedy made from the essences of cherry plum, clematis, impatiens, rock rose, and star of Bethlehem. It is useful in many crisis situations, such as after hearing bad news, before a major or anxiety-provoking event in your life, or after an injury. It helps to relieve apprehension and restore calm when you are nervous, panicked, or tense. Rescue Remedy is particularly good when the cause of the distress is not clear—when you feel overwhelmed and/or intensely frustrated yet cannot say precisely why. Put two or three drops in half a glass of water and sip it as needed.

Bach flower remedies are dilute essences of plants that treat emotional, mental, and physical distress. As with homeopathic remedies, choosing a flower remedy involves paying close attention to your emotional state, and then selecting the remedy that matches your observations. Although science is still baffled by the Bach flower remedies, anecdotal results over the past fifty years have been impressive. Many people report that these gentle preparations are excellent for alleviating stress and making them feel better when they are sick, uncomfortable, or unhappy.

BACH FLOWER REMEDIES

Flower Remedy	Primary Expression of Emotion	Underlying Emotional Concerns
Rescue Remedy (a combination of cherry plum, clematis, impatiens, rock rose, Star of Bethlehem)	Fear; panic; apprehension; inconsolable crying; anxiety; tension; night terrors.	This premier flower remedy is excellent for alleviating any crisis-caused stress, major or minor. It helps to calm, restore balance, and ease apprehension. Whether the cause is an accident, bad news, anxiety over an upcoming event, or anything else, Rescue Remedy calms and alleviates stress. It is particularly useful in acute situations where you are feeling overwhelmed, desolate, and/or intensely frustrated. Of all the Bach remedies, many people report being most appreciative of Rescue Remedy.
Agrimony	Outwardly, smiling and brave; inwardly, anguished and suffering.	A determination to appear cheerful, despite suffering going on underneath. The anguish may be due to a family trauma, a significant disappointment, or anything else you view as a failure.
Aspen	Fearfulness.	Fears that you can't (or won't) name, often resulting in bad dreams or difficulty falling asleep.
Beech	Impatience; intolerance.	A tendency to be a perfectionist and to keep to yourself. You are drawn to order, precision, and pure reason, have little patience with others, and rail against upsets in schedule.
Centaury	Shyness; feelings of intimidation.	A weak-willed nature. You often find yourself being pushed around by others, have great difficulty standing up for yourself, and don't want to be noticed.
Cerato	Need for constant affirmation.	Lack of self-confidence; low self-esteem. You often feel as if the things you do are not quite right somehow. You don't like trying new things and are reluctant to go anywhere alone.
Cherry plum	Fearfulness.	Fear of situations over which you have no control. You may be afraid of air travel, for example.
Chestnut bud	Incorrigible behavior.	An inability (or unwillingness) to understand cause and effect or learn from past mistakes. For example, you may continue self-defeating actions even though you know the aftereffects will be unwelcome. Chestnut bud is especially helpful in alleviating this type of behavior.
Chicory	Need for constant attention; selfishness; possessiveness; easily hurt feelings.	Insecurity and fear of being rejected. You have difficulty sharing things, especially the people you love. Your feelings are easily hurt and you often feel rejected.
Clematis	Indifference; apathy; short attention span.	A tendency to daydream. You become distracted and preoccupied easily, and often appear indifferent to your surroundings. It can be difficult to capture and hold your attention.
Crabapple	Excessive neatness; compulsive behavior.	An inability to tolerate disorder or untidiness, which may be related to feelings of shame about your physical condition or appearance. Your striving for neatness may border on compulsive behavior.
Elm	Feelings of incompetence.	Fundamental feelings of inadequacy. You may often complain of being incapable of doing things you want (or need) to accomplish.
Gentian	Need for much praise and encouragement.	A tendency to become discouraged by any setback, no matter how minor. You require a great deal of encouragement to accomplish anything. You typically try something once, and if success is not immediate, you are unwilling to try again. Gentian is especially helpful for someone who is discouraged at work or school.
Gorse	Feelings of deep despair, usually after a serious family trauma.	Following a traumatic situation, such as a death or divorce, you worry that nothing will ever be the same again, and fear that you will never be able to be happy and carefree again. Gorse can help to ease such feelings during this period.
Heather	Self-centeredness.	Utter self-absorption. You tend to talk exclusively (and at length) about your problems and concerns. Others may have commented that you seem to believe the world begins and ends with you.

BACH FLOWER REMEDIES

Flower Remedy	Primary Expression of Emotion	Underlying Emotional Concerns
Holly	Anger; fits of temper.	Insecurity and jealousy that come out in displays of anger and bad temper.
Honeysuckle	Obsession with happy times from the past; homesickness.	A feeling that past times were perfect, and you can't stop yourself from comparing them with the imperfect present. You often talk of times when you were particularly happy, when everything was going well. Honeysuckle is also helpful if you are suffering from homesickness.
Hornbeam	Exhaustion.	Fatigue and tiredness that keep you from accomplishing everyday tasks or joining in normal activities.
Impatiens	Impatience; nervousness; hyperactive behavior.	Feelings of impatience and tension. You tend to be nervous and easily irritated. Impatiens is also an excellent remedy for the type-A person who simply cannot sit still.
Larch	Lack of self-confidence.	Low self-esteem. You are self-effacing and fear calling attention to yourself. A job interview, a speech, or an important presentation is an ordeal. Taken before an event, Larch will help bolster self-confidence.
Mimulus	Frequent expression of fears of one thing or another.	Fearfulness, shyness, and timidity. You often feel afraid and express fear of particular things. You blush easily. Unlike the Aspen individual, who has fears he or she cannot name, the Mimulus person has fears that are identifiable and well articulated.
Mustard	Sadness.	Sorrow and depression. The cause may not be readily apparent, but often these feelings are related to a loss of some kind.
Oak	Constant busyness and bustling.	A "type-A" personality; a relentless drive to achieve. You feel you must be a role model for others; you are an overachiever who presses on without letup.
Olive	Exhaustion.	Continual fatigue; a sense of being exhausted to the very core. Gently stimulating olive is the remedy of choice.
Pine	Feelings of guilt.	A deep, internalized sense of shame and remorse. You may feel you have done something so awful it can never be forgiven; you may blame yourself for everything that goes wrong. Even when the fault lies elsewhere, you feel guilty inside.
Red chestnut	Inappropriate worrying.	Excessive concern over the well-being of others. You worry constantly.
Rock rose	Absolute terror; panic.	Irrational fears. You often suffer from terrifying nightmares.
Rock water	Inflexibility; unwillingness to forgive.	A rigid, unforgiving nature, and a need to strive for perfection. You are very hard on yourself, as well as on others.
Scleranthus	Feelings of uncertainty; vacillation.	An inability to make a decision, to choose between different courses of action. You often feel torn between choices and ask, "Should I do this?" "Should I do that?"
Star of Bethlehem	Emotional shock following a life-changing experience.	A traumatic and possibly life-changing event, such as sudden or shocking sad news, a severe scare, an accident, or a significant disappointment, that causes feelings of shock and loss. Star of Bethlehem is excellent for alleviating the physical and emotional shock associated with traumatic experiences.
Sweet chestnut	Anguish and torment.	Feelings of exhaustion and alienation. For whatever reason, you are in torment and feel very much alone.
Vervain	Tension; drivenness.	Perfectionism that causes you to strive so hard that you become nervous and tense. You may have difficulty sleeping normally.
Vine	Selfishness; ruthlessness.	A need to have your own way, no matter what. You will do and say anything to swing others your way, and can be utterly ruthless in pursuit of your desires.
Walnut	Tendency to be very easily influenced.	A nature that is sensitive and easily cowed. Even if a proposed course of action is not to your liking, you tend to "follow the leader" rather than following the dictates of your own head and/or heart.

BACH FLOWER REMEDIES

Flower Remedy	Primary Expression of Emotion	Underlying Emotional Concerns
Water violet	A tendency to be alone, removed from peers.	An asocial nature that feels no need or desire to associate with others. You prefer to be alone, aloof, and removed, "above" the daily hurly-burly.
White chestnut	Obsessive thinking.	A tendency to dwell on ideas or events without letup. Long after others thought the subject had been forgotten, you may still be fixated on the same idea. This remedy is very helpful for someone who obsesses about being accepted socially.
Wild oat	Indecisiveness.	A tendency to be fearful and anxious, especially about the future. This remedy is especially helpful for someone at a crossroads who is fearful and indecisive over future plans.
Wild rose	Apathy; resignation.	Feelings of tiredness, a lack of vitality. You feel resigned to just soldier on, placing one foot in front of the other, buffeted by the winds of fate.
Willow	Refusal to be pleased or satisfied.	Resentfulness, bitterness, feelings of dissatisfaction and jealousy. Nothing is ever quite "good enough." When ill, you can be very difficult to deal with. You may even refuse to admit to being helped or eased.

Acupressure

Acupressure is a gentle, noninvasive form of the ancient Chinese practice of acupuncture. In acu*puncture,* thin needles are inserted into the body at specific points along lines called meridians. In acu*pressure,* thumb or finger pressure is applied at these same points, but the body is not punctured. In both practices, the aim is to effect beneficial changes and achieve harmony within the body's systems and structure.

THE HISTORY OF ACUPRESSURE

Because acupressure evolved from acupuncture, an ancient Chinese healing practice, the history of this form of treatment begins with traditional Chinese philosophy as it applies to the healing arts. The fundamental principle of Chinese philosophy is the concept of *yin* and *yang.* The yin and yang are two opposite, yet complementary, forever-entwined forces that underlie all aspects of life. Yin and yang is depicted as the subtly curved light and dark halves of a circle. Both proceed from the *t'ai chi* (the Supreme Ultimate).

According to this philosophical system, the human body, like all matter, is made up of five elements: wood, fire, earth, metal, and water. Each element corresponds to an aspect of the body, such as the organs, senses, tissues, and emotions, as well as to aspects of nature, such as direction, season, color, and climate (see inset, page 41). The five-element theory, combined with the principle of yin and yang, forms the basis of the Chinese concept of balance. The intention is to balance yin and yang and to balance the energies of the five elements.

Yin is earthy, female, dark, passive, receptive, and absorbing. It is represented by the moon, the tiger, the color orange, a broken line, and the shady side of a hill. Yin is cool, inward, still, and soft.

Yang is represented by the sun, the dragon, the color blue, an unbroken line, and the sunny side of a hill. Yang is hot, outward, moving, aggressive, and bright.

Because yin and yang are intertwined halves of the same whole, all things, and all people, contain elements of both, although at any one time, one or the other will be predominant. Thus, a child is more yin; an adult more

The Yin-Yang Circle

yang. When you assert yourself, it is your yang that is coming to the fore.

The sun is yang, the moon is yin. We awaken in the morning and greet the sun. It is natural to be active and moving throughout the daylight. As twilight descends into night, we become more passive and quiet. Nighttime expresses the qualities of yin.

Chinese medical theory teaches that the two branches of the body's nervous system, the sympathetic and parasympathetic, correspond to the two halves of the yin-yang circle. The sympathetic branch is the part of the nervous system that mobilizes our bodies to respond to stress. It initiates the fight-or-flight response, a more yang part of the cycle. The parasympathetic branch replenishes and supports the body during rest, the yin part of the cycle. These two branches oppose and balance each other to create stability and health. When the yin and yang are balanced within the body, all the body's functions are healthy. Illness is caused by an imbalance between yin and yang.

Conventional Western medicine typically pinpoints and directly treats only the affected part of the body. Chinese medical philosophy encompasses the entire universe. Everything that affects the patient is considered, including emotion, environment, and diet.

Chinese philosophy proposes a way of life based on living in accordance with the laws of nature. This profound connection with nature is reflected in the language used to describe illness. For example, you might be diagnosed with a "wind invasion" or "excess heat." Acupuncture (or acupressure) points may be chosen to "disperse wind," "remove summer damp," or "disperse rising fire."

In traditional Chinese medicine, every aspect of health is described in terms of a balance between yin and yang. For example, yin illnesses are caused by excessive expansion (overweight as a result of eating too much sugar, for example), while yang illnesses are caused by excessive contraction (sunstroke or fever). An imbalance of yin and yang factors can be demonstrated by showing how red blood cells respond to different substances. When red

The Five Elements and Their Correspondences in Nature and the Human Body

In traditional Chinese philosophy, all matter is considered to be composed of five elements (wood, fire, earth, metal, and water). The elements in turn have correspondences in various aspects of the natural world, including the human body. According to this philosophy, health is achieved when yin and yang, and the energies of the five elements, are all in proper balance. The elements and some of their corresponding characteristics and parts of the body are illustrated in the table below.

ELEMENT	THINGS IN NATURE					THE HUMAN BODY				
	Direction	Taste	Color	Growth Cycle	Environmental Factor	Season	Organs	Sense Organ	Tissue	Emotion
Wood	East	Sour	Green	Germination	Wind	Spring	Liver, gallbladder	Eye	Tendon	Anger
Fire	South	Bitter	Red	Growth	Heat	Summer	Heart, small intestine	Tongue	Vessel	Joy
Earth	Middle	Sweet	Yellow	Ripening	Dampness	Late summer	Spleen, stomach	Mouth	Muscle	Meditation
Metal	West	Pungent	White	Harvest	Dryness	Autumn	Lung, large intestine	Nose	Skin and hair	Grief and melancholy
Water	North	Salty	Black	Storing	Cold	Winter	Kidney, bladder	Ear	Bone	Fright and fear

blood cells are placed in water (yin), they absorb the water, expand, and finally burst. When red blood cells are placed in a concentrated saline (salt) solution (yang), they contract, shrink, and shrivel. In a solution of normal saline (0.9 percent salt), the yin and yang are perfectly balanced and the cells remain virtually unchanged. An example of how the ancient yin-yang theory can be used to describe concepts in conventional medicine can be found in the treatment of breast and prostate cancer: Female hormones (yin) help control prostate cancer (yang); male hormones (yang) help control breast cancer (yin). The interplay of the yin and yang—as one increases, the other decreases—describes the process of the universe and everything in it. In more familiar Western terms, as modern physical science teaches, "For every action, there is an equal and opposite reaction."

In Chinese philosophy, the energy that pulses through all things, animate and inanimate, is called *chi*. Health exists when there is a harmonious balance under heaven of both internal and external forces. Each bodily organ must have the right amount of *chi* to function. Too much or too little *chi* causes an imbalance, resulting in illness or disease. *Chi* flows through all things, enters and passes through the body, creating harmony or disharmony.

Chinese medicine works directly with the natural, vital energy—or *chi*—of the body. The goal of acupuncture and acupressure is to normalize the body's energies. *Chi* can be tapped at specific points along channels known as meridians. Activating one key point sets up a predictable reaction in another area. By tonifying (increasing energy

in) a specific area, the yin-yang balance is treated. Moving an excess of *chi* from one area and directing it to another, weaker area, corrects the yin-yang balance.

Acupuncture is an ancient protocol. As a component of Oriental medicine, it has been practiced for centuries. The *Huangdi Neijing* (Canon of Medicine), written about 500–300 B.C.E., is the oldest surviving medical text. Among other medical practices, it describes the use of acupuncture.

ACUPRESSURE TODAY

Acupressure is a form of body work in which pressure is applied to specific acupuncture points to balance internal function. Acupressure is practiced around the world.

The Chinese have a very descriptive term for taking advantage of a combination of two or more healing systems—a practice this book advocates. They say the patient is "walking on two legs." A two-year study conducted jointly by the Northwestern University Medical School and Evanston Hospital in Evanston, Illinois, employed a combination of acupuncture and acupressure. In this study, patients suffering from chronic headaches of all types, including migraine, cluster, whiplash, and tension, were first treated with acupuncture. The patients were then individually instructed in specific acupressure techniques to use when a headache seemed imminent. The researchers reported that the need for prescription painkillers and other drugs was eliminated entirely in most patients—thus verifying the effectiveness of "walking on two legs."

COMMON ACUPRESSURE POINTS

Point	Effect	Indications
Back Shu points	Stimulate all internal organs.	Fatigue; sluggishness; anxiety.
Bladder 23	Increases circulation to the urinary tract and reproductive organs.	Lower back pain; urinary tract infection; vaginitis.
Bladder 28	Master point for the bladder.	Urinary tract infection; edema.
Bladder 60	Increases circulation to the urinary tract and reproductive organs.	Urinary tract infection; vaginitis; protatitis; urethritis.
Conception Vessel	Holds reproductive "energy."	Reproductive system problems.
Four Gates	Calms the nervous system.	Chickenpox; fever; hay fever; herpes; motion sickness; pain; poison ivy; sleeplessness; weight problems.
Kidney 3	Strengthens the bladder and kidneys; increases circulation to the reproductive organs.	Incontinence; urinary tract infection; vaginitis.
Kidney 7	Strengthens the bladder and kidneys.	Incontinence.
Large Intestine 4	Beneficial to the head and face; relieves congestion and headaches; removes energy blocks in the large intestine; clears heat.	Acne; allergies; common cold; fever; headache; menstrual cramps; sore throat; toothache.
Large Intestine 11	Relieves itching; reduces allergic reactions.	Allergies; chickenpox; constipation; hay fever.
Large Intestine 20	Decreases sinus congestion.	Allergies; hay fever; sinusitis.
Liver 3	Quiets the nervous system; relaxes muscle cramps and spasms.	Asthma; eye pain; headache; menstrual cramps.
Lung 7	Clears the lungs; moistens the throat.	Asthma; common cold; sore throat.
Neck and Shoulder Release	Relaxes the muscles of the neck and shoulders; relaxes the body.	Headache; weight problems.
Pericardium 6	Relaxes the chest; relieves nausea; relaxes the mind.	Asthma; motion sickness; sleeplessness; stomachache; vomiting.
Points along either side of the spine	Improve circulation; relax the nervous system; balance the respiratory system; relax the spine.	Anxiety; common cold; insomnia; menstrual cramps; nervousness.
Spleen 6	Reduces uterine cramping.	Menstrual cramps.
Spleen 10	Detoxifies the blood.	Acne; boils; herpes; poison ivy; vaginitis.
Stomach 36	Tones the digestive system; strengthens overall well-being.	Allergies; constipation; diarrhea; indigestion; vomiting.
Ting points	Increase circulation.	Shock; cold hands and feet; circulatory problems.
Triple Warmer 5	Improves hormonal function.	In combination with other points, used for hormonal problems.

WORKING WITH AN ACUPRESSURIST

There are professionally trained and college-educated acupressurists, just as there are acupuncturists. If you wish to consult a trained acupressurist, check the yellow pages of your telephone book. You'll find this category listed in most large cities.

For the most part, though, the gentle form of acupressure recommended in the Treatment and Care entries in Part Two of this book is something you can do yourself, at home.

TREATMENT WITH ACUPRESSURE

In *The Chinese Art of Healing* (Bantam, 1972), author Stephan Palos identifies the hand as "man's original medical tool." We instinctively use our hands to alleviate pain. When we suffer a bump or bruise, have a cramp, or hurt anywhere inside, we rub, knead, or massage the painful spot.

When you are ill, gently working the acupressure points recommended in the appropriate entry in Part Two will probably be beneficial (the illustrations in Part Three provide guidelines for locating all of the acupressure points recommended). Massaging a particular point helps relieve symptoms as well as strengthen and balance the yin-yang in the body. For example, applying acupressure to the point identified as "Large Intestine 11" helps relax the intestine, thus relieving constipation. Another related point is Stomach 36; massaging Stomach 36 helps tone an upset digestive tract. When you are ill, the appropriate acupressure points, as well as other areas of the body, will be tender. Use your intuitive sense. Notice what feels good.

Common Acupressure Points

In acupressure, there are twelve lines called meridians that run along each side of the body. Each pair of meridians corresponds to a specific organ. For example, there is a pair of Lung meridians, Spleen meridians, Stomach meridians, and Liver meridians. Acupressure points are named for the meridian they lie on, and each is given a number according to where along the meridian it falls. Thus, Spleen 6 is the sixth point on the Spleen meridian. The table on page 42 lists some of the acupressure points most often recommended in the entries in Part Two of this book.

Administering Acupressure

When you give an acupressure treatment, your tools are your hands, notably your thumbs and fingers, and occasionally your palms. For the most part, you will be using the balls of your thumbs and fingers, never the nails. Before administering acupressure, make sure your finger-nails are clipped short, so that you do not inadvertently scratch yourself.

Choose a time of day when you are most relaxed, perhaps after a warm bath and just before bedtime. Take a few deep breaths. This aids relaxation and will automatically focus your attention inward on your body. Be calm and unhurried. Make sure to keep warm throughout the treatment. You can apply pressure to the points directly onto the skin, or through a shirt or light sheet.

Work right-side and left-side acupressure points at the same time. Use your fingers or thumbs to apply *threshold pressure* to the point. Threshold pressure is firm pressure, just on the verge of becoming painful. The idea is to stimulate the point without causing the body to tighten up or retract from the pain. The pressure you exert should not hurt. Firm but gentle is the rule.

Apply from one to five minutes of continuous pressure. Or apply pressure for ten seconds, release for ten seconds, reapply pressure for ten seconds, release for ten seconds. Repeat this cycle five times.

Specific acupressure points helpful for different conditions are included in the Treatment and Care entries in Part Two of this book. To learn how to locate specific acupressure points, *see* ADMINISTERING AN ACUPRESSURE TREATMENT in Part Three.

Acupressure is a wonderful hands-on way to stimulate the body to heal. By using the acupressure points described in this book, you will be working to relieve the underlying cause of illness.

Aromatherapy

Aromatherapy is the art of using essential oils to stimulate beneficial changes within the body. Essential oils are liquid essences distilled from the flowers, leaves, and other parts of certain plants, and they are intensely concentrated. For example, it takes 150 pounds of lavender flowers to produce a single pound of essential lavender oil, and 5,000 pounds of rose petals to produce a pound of essential rose oil. There is a significant difference between the essential oils used for aromatherapy and the type of fragrant oils used most often as perfumes. Essential oils are usually extracted by steam distillation from a single plant source, such as a certain type of tree, grass, flower, leaf, gum or resin, root, or seeds. They are typically seventy times more concentrated than the plant or herb from which they are derived.

Aromatic essential oils have been used for centuries as inhalants and in baths, massage oils, and compresses to gently alter mood, restore energy, and enhance pleasure. The ancients even applied essential oils directly to the skin to treat certain disorders, a method of administering medicinal substances that has been validated scientifically. Today, many medications are introduced into the body by means of drug-impregnated skin patches, among them hormone replacement therapy and nicotine for those who want to stop smoking without the usual uncomfortable withdrawal symptoms.

The use of essential oils to promote health has not received extensive scientific study, but there is some research that demonstrates beneficial effects. Tests have shown that active constituents contained in the oils can be detected in the bloodstreams of laboratory animals one hour after exposure. An article in the British medical journal *Lancet* reported that people suffering from insomnia fell asleep more readily when breathing in the fragrance of lavender. Memorial Sloan-Kettering Cancer Center in New York has experimented with aromatherapy on patients undergoing magnetic resonance imaging (MRI) scans who complained of claustrophobia while spending an hour in the magnetic capsule. Patients exposed to the scent of vanilla reportedly felt less anxiety and discomfort during the procedure. Fragrant vanilla, an undeniably pleasant scent, may even qualify as an aphrodisiac. It has been reported to increase blood flow to the penis. (Interestingly, certain essential oils have long been reputed to be aphrodisiacs, but vanilla is not among them.)

While studies substantiating the effectiveness of essential oils are few, advocates say the effects they provide are sufficient to explain their popularity. One of the most promising uses of aromatherapy seems to be in the treatment of emotional and stress-related disorders. Think of the refined ladies of past centuries who pressed lavender-scented handkerchiefs to their noses when they were agitated or felt as if they were about to swoon. The fragrance of lavender is a known calmative. Michel Eyquem de Montaigne, the great French philosopher, wrote in his *Essais* in 1580 that certain essences could make him happy, excited, contemplative, or peaceful. The same is true for us today.

The table on pages 45–46 provides an introduction to some of the most popular essential oils used in aromatherapy. Pure essential oils can be purchased in special aromatherapy stores and some health-food stores. They can also be ordered by mail (see the Resources section at the end of the book for suppliers).

You can use essential oils in a variety of different ways: as inhalants, in massage, in baths, and in compresses (*see* PREPARING AROMATHERAPY TREATMENTS in Part Three for instructions). You should not, however, apply them directly to your skin, as they can be quite irritating if not properly diluted. And *never* take essential oils internally. Always store them in glass bottles, away from heat, light, and moisture—and, of course, out of the reach of children.

COMMON ESSENTIAL OILS

Essential Oil (Plant Source)	Traditional Use	Properties and Effects
Basil (*Ocimum basilicum*)	To calm the nerves and treat respiratory complaints.	Stimulates or restores energy, depending on individual chemistry. Helps open nasal passages.
Bergamot (*Citrus bergamia*)	To strengthen the stomach and calm the nerves.	Restores appetite, relieves flatulence. Eases depression.
Chamomile (*Chamaemelum nobile, Matricaria chamomilla,* or *Anthemis mixta*)	To induce calm, aid digestion, and heal the skin.	Relaxes the nerves; promotes sound sleep; reduces inflammation; soothes irritated skin; helps combat depression, anxiety, irritability, and stress.
Elemi (*Canurium luzonicum*)	To improve overall well-being and to calm the nerves.	Calms nerves and promotes harmony within; an aid to meditation. A rejuvenating stimulant that fortifies against stress.
Frankincense (*Boswellia thurifera* or *B. carteri*)	To calm the nerves.	Eases anxiety, tension, and stress. This stabilizing "centering" fragrance helps bring a feeling of serenity and comfort to those in emotional distress.
Geranium (*Pelargonium graveolens*)	To calm the nerves.	Combats depression, eases mental tension, and simultaneously calms and energizes. Said to balance passive/aggressive characteristics. Some people say this scent eases their fear of speaking in public.
Jasmine (*Jasminium officinalis* or *J. grandiflorum*)	To calm the nerves and enhance sexual desire.	Sensual and inspirational, jasmine encourages optimism, banishes depression, and elevates the spirit.
Lavender (*Lavandula officinalis*)	To calm the nerves and promote sound sleep.	Eases emotional problems, including depression, irritability, mood swings, and nervous tension. This fragrance reportedly can neutralize sensory overload and restore balance by calming a racing mind or stimulating a sluggish one. Lavender is a documented aid to restful sleep.
Myrrh (*Commiphora myrrha* or *Balsamodendron myrrha*)	To calm the nerves and cool the body.	Cools and calms agitated emotions and promotes feelings of empowerment and motivation. The fragrance of myrrh is said to build the resolve needed to overcome emotional upsets of all types.
Neroli (*Citrus aurantium, C bigaradia,* or *C. vulgaris*)	To calm the nerves, soothe anxiety, and promote sound sleep.	Neroli (orange blossom) oil comes from the bitter orange tree, not the supermarket variety. This scent is said to alleviate the false angina caused by anxiety. It is helpful for many mental ills, including depression, desperation, melancholy, anxiety, nervousness, and insomnia.
Orange (*Citrus sinensis*)	To aid respiratory problems and digestive difficulties, normalize body temperature, and benefit the skin.	Calms an upset stomach, promotes the elimination of excess fluid from the body, soothes inflamed and irritated skin, acts to balance the emotions by either relaxing or stimulating, as needed.
Patchouli (*Pogostemon patchouli* or *P. cablin*)	To calm the nerves and enhance sexual desire.	The fragrance of patchouli is said to improve concentration, calm the nerves, and ease depression. It can either be calming (in mild concentrations) or stimulating (in heavier concentrations). The earthy, musky scent of patchouli is reputed to stimulate and enhance sexual desire.
Peppermint (*Mentha piperita*)	To calm the nerves, increase energy, and relieve congestion.	Peppermint cools anger and eases nervousness. It energizes the brain, relieves mental fatigue, and clarifies confused thought. This scent is said to clear the head, cool a fever, and open up clogged sinuses.

COMMON ESSENTIAL OILS

Essential Oil (Plant Source)	Traditional Use	Properties and Effects
Pine (*Pinus sylvestris*)	To relieve congestion, aid in clearing mucus from the respiratory tract, and calm the nerves.	Scotch pine is considered helpful for all respiratory conditions. It is even said to counteract the effects of heavy smoking. It is invigorating, bracing, and strengthening, and it is reputed to stabilize conflicting emotions.
Rose (*Rosa damascena* or *R. gallica*)	To calm the nerves, relieve pain, and enhance sexual desire.	The heady fragrance of rose oil is reported to balance mood swings, ease the pain of grief, and alleviate sadness. The scent helps eliminate jealousy and resentment and is supposedly helpful in removing emotional blocks. Some say the scent increases feelings of both love and desire.
Sandalwood (*Santalum album*)	To calm the nerves and enhance sexual desire.	This once-sacred oil relaxes body, mind, and spirit, and helps clear confused thoughts. The scent of sandalwood is at once earthy, sultry, and erotic. Sandalwood incense has been burned for centuries to heighten desire.
Tea tree (*Melaleuca alternifolia*)	To fight infection and clear congestion.	A relative of eucalyptus, this versatile oil is good for respiratory problems; skin disorders, and in first aid for cuts, bites, blisters, and burns. Its aroma is spicy and pungent.
Thyme (*Thymus vulgaris* or *T. citriodoria*)	To relax and calm the nerves, and to increase energy.	Thyme eases nervousness and can overcome some stress-related emotions. This fragrance is reported to enhance memory and increase concentration. Thyme has a normalizing effect. It is reported that this fresh, clean scent can either foster alertness or bring sleep, depending on your body's needs.
Vetiver (*Vetiveria zizanoides, V. odorata,* or *Andropogon muricatus*)	To calm the nerves.	Vetiver oil has an earthy, woodsy scent that can ease nervousness and restore calm. This fragrance is said to bring clarity and focus to thoughts and actions. It is reputed to be an energizer that can restore purpose to those suffering from emotional exhaustion.
Ylang Ylang (*Cananga odorata*)	To calm the nerves and enhance sexual desire.	This seductive floral scent reportedly calms the nerves, lifts depression, and fosters feelings of love and serenity. Ylang ylang is an ancient aid to sexual release that is said to relieve feelings of inadequacy and increase arousal.

Diet and Nutrition

Food provides the energy the body needs to function. It provides the nutrient base necessary for building, maintaining, and repairing a strong and healthy body. Food also provides immediate information to the body. It can make you feel full and energized, or tired, jumpy, and irritable. The breakfasts you eat, the lunches and snacks you select, the dinners you prepare—all provide the fuel required by every cell in your body.

THE HISTORICAL USES OF DIET

Hippocrates, the "Father of Medicine," wrote, "Let food be your medicine. Let your medicine be your food." This recommendation is as important for us today as it was in ancient Greece. Food was a primary form of medicine in ancient cultures and has continued to be used as such through the ages. Warm teas and soups for colds, prune juice for constipation, toast and crackers for diarrhea—all are well-known and time-tested "medicines."

Food is important not only for curing illness, but for preventing it. Today, the importance of diet in maintaining health—and conversely, in contributing to the development of disease—is increasingly evident. A proper diet is therefore useful in treating acute and chronic illness as well as in promoting and enhancing optimal health.

THE AMERICAN DIET TODAY

A hundred years ago, food was prepared in a very different way than it generally is today. Most important, food was prepared and served more simply. In the last several decades, thanks to food-processing technology, we have seen the development of a vast selection of quick-fix packaged, canned, frozen, boil-in-a-bag, and microwavable foods that get us in and out of the kitchen fast. Few people cook in the traditional sense of the word, at least on a regular basis. It's easier and more convenient to stir water into the contents of a package, open a can, heat up a frozen dinner, or "nuke" a prepackaged meal in the microwave.

Highly processed junk food is a billion-dollar-a-year industry. The shelves of American supermarkets are weighted down with candy, cookies, and all kinds of packaged baked goods; snacks loaded with sugar, fat, and salt; sodas, colas, and "juices" and punches made with more chemicals and additives than fruit; and artificially flavored and colored cereals.

The typical American diet is in need of an overhaul. Most of us eat too much fat, too little fiber, and too many empty calories, and are deficient in vitamins and minerals. The typical American gets about 42 percent of total calories from fat, with 16 percent coming from saturated fats and 26 percent from unsaturated fats. Compare this with the recommended amounts: a maximum of 30 percent of total daily calories from fat, with 10 percent from saturated fats (such as meat and dairy products), 10 percent from monounsaturated fats (such as olive oil), and 10 percent from polyunsaturated fats (such as corn, safflower, and soybean oils).

The typical American gets about 22 percent of total calories from complex carbohydrates (such as those in grains and legumes), 6 percent of calories from naturally occurring sugars (such as those found in fruits and honey), and 18 percent of calories from refined and processed sugars (such as those found in sodas, candy bars, and many processed foods). Yet it is recommended that 40 percent of the calories we consume should come from complex carbohydrates and naturally occurring sugars, and no more than a quarter of that from refined and processed sugars.

One of the most significant steps you can take toward feeling healthier, improving your energy level, and reducing your risk of potential disease is to improve your diet. And this change costs nothing. You can make a good start toward a better diet by focusing on five basic dietary goals:

1. Increase your intake of fresh vegetables.

2. Decrease your intake of refined and processed sugars.

3. Decrease your consumption of cooked fats, and make sure the majority of fats you eat are healthy fats, such as those in olive and flaxseed oil.

4. Limit your salt intake.

5. Eat adequate amounts of quality protein.

In addition, base your diet on nutritious whole foods.

Don't depend on processed, packaged foods for your nutrition—it is a disservice to your health. Save food items containing refined and processed sugars for *occasional* treats only.

FOOD ADDITIVES AND OTHER CHEMICALS

Too much of what passes for food in the United States contains chemicals such as manufactured sweeteners, processed fats and/or fat substitutes, artificial flavorings and colorings, plus vast quantities of preservatives. Preservatives are nothing new. Salting down and pickling meat and vegetables were common practices centuries ago, as was the drying (dehydrating) of various foodstuffs. Foods preserved this way lasted a very long time, which was important in an era before refrigeration and efficient transport of fresh foods. But these natural methods took so much time and care that they were not easily adaptable to mass production. As the prepared-food industry grew by leaps and bounds, other time-saving and more cost-effective—if less healthy—methods of preserving foods were developed by the major food manufacturers.

Food additives and preservatives undergo exhaustive testing, on an individual basis. During the testing phase, laboratory animals are given megadoses of a single additive at a time. It's easy enough for manufacturers to explain away any adverse reactions by pointing out that a human will ingest only a tiny bit of a particular additive per serving. But few studies have been conducted on how different food additives interact with each other or what these interactions do to the human body—even though it is virtually impossible to find a processed food product that contains only one additive.

And what about the effects over the long term? Current scientific research cannot tell us what the cumulative effects of ingesting a single food additive will be—let alone what the ever-present chemical combinations of multiple additives may do over a period of many years. Today's food products often contain more chemical additives than basic food ingredients. Always read the labels! Trying to find additive-free products can be an exercise in frustration. Preparing fresh, whole foods is a good beginning and a way to avoid the frustration.

Another problem with the American food supply today stems from the fact that farmers often use pesticides and chemicals in their fields that contaminate even what look like healthy fresh foods. These toxic chemicals do not disperse and decay harmlessly. They contaminate the food we eat, pollute the air we breathe, and seep into the water we drink. And these chemicals are all pervasive, often mysteriously traveling far from the areas where they were actually used.

DDT (dichlorodiphenyltrichloroethane) is a case in point. It was banned in 1972, yet nearly every American still carries traces of DDT in his or her body. DDT has even been detected in wild animals roaming free in the Antarctic, a place once thought free of man-made chemical contamination.

Each year more than 2.5 billion pounds of chemicals are sprayed or dumped on agricultural crops, spread in forests, and used to treat ponds and lakes or "green" lawns and parks. Farmers, pest-control companies, and homeowners spend billions of dollars annually on such chemicals. A 1987 study released by the National Cancer Institute showed that children living in homes where pesticides are routinely used are seven times more likely to develop childhood leukemia than are children who live in chemical-free households. In 1989, the Natural Resources Defense Council (NRDC) reported on a comprehensive two-year study of the impact on children of pesticide residues in food. It showed that, compared with adults, the average child receives four times more exposure to eight cancer-causing pesticides in food. Apples, apple products, peanut butter, and processed cherries that have been treated with the chemical growth regulator daminozide (better known as Alar) were named as foods posing the greatest potential risk. The average exposure of a child under six to daminozide and to UMDH, the carcinogenic compound it forms in the body, has been found to be 240 times the level that poses what the Environmental Protection Agency (EPA) calls an "acceptable" cancer risk after a *lifetime* of exposure to this toxic chemical.

The NRDC study targeted only eight widely used chemicals. But you should be aware that the EPA has identified *sixty-six* different carcinogenic pesticides that turn up in the average person's diet. To date, the EPA has not acted to restrict the use of these chemicals.

Only about 1 percent of the produce, domestic or imported, in your supermarket has been tested for pesticide residues, and tests currently used can detect only around 40 percent of the possible chemical contaminants. Many dangerous metabolites (chemical compounds that form as the source chemicals break down in the body) cannot be detected at all.

The General Accounting Office (GAO) reports that it takes the FDA close to a month, on average, to complete a laboratory analysis of a food sample. During that time, a suspect food stays on the market. In more than 50 percent of the instances where the FDA has found violations, the GAO says, the contaminated food was not recovered. By the time the FDA had completed lab testing, unsuspecting consumers had eaten the "evidence."

GENETICALLY ENGINEERED FOODS

Genetic engineering is a technique that is applied to food crops for a number of different reasons: to increase yield by speeding up the growing process; to increase resistance to plant pests and viruses; and to slow down the ripening process so that the product stays fresh-looking longer. To

Food Safety and the FDA

In the early 1990s, Dr. Harvey W. Wiley tested some commonly used early chemical preservatives, including deadly formaldehyde, and demonstrated their toxicity. The federal Pure Food and Drug Act, pioneered by Dr. Wiley, became law in 1906, creating the first real protection for the commercial food consumer. In 1928, Congress authorized the creation of the Federal Food, Drug, and Insecticide Administration. Three years later the organization's name was changed to the Food and Drug Administration, as we know it today.

In 1958, the federal Food, Drugs, and Cosmetics Act was passed. The Food Additives Amendment to this law required food and chemical manufacturers to demonstrate the safety of their products by running extensive tests on additives before they were marketed. Test results had to be submitted to the FDA, which made rulings on particular substances based on the data supplied by the manufacturers. This marked a significant change; previously, the agency had not been permitted to ban the use of a food additive on the grounds that it had been inadequately tested, or even because it was suspected of being unsafe for human consumption. In addition, the Delaney clause, written by Representative James Delaney, was part of the 1958 law. This clause specifically prohibits the use of any food additive that has been shown to cause cancer.

These developments would seem to justify consumer confidence in the safety of the foods we buy. However, since it was enacted, the Delaney clause has repeatedly been attacked and circumvented. Consider the case of saccharin, an artificial chemical sweetener in use since 1879. In 1977, researchers demonstrated that saccharin caused cancer in laboratory animals. The FDA responded by announcing a ban on the use of the substance in foods and beverages. In the six months following the FDA announcement, industry lobbyists such as the Calorie Control Council spent over $1 million fighting the ban. As a result of their efforts, people from all over the country bombarded their congressional representatives with requests to keep saccharin on the market.

In response to this overwhelming pressure, and despite the research implicating saccharin as carcinogenic, the FDA has continually postponed imposing its ban on this substance. And even though saccharin has now largely been superseded by the proliferation of aspartame, another questionable artificial sweetener (it is suspected of causing nervous system problems, including headaches and seizures; may break down into toxic compounds when heated; and is potentially disastrous for people with PKU, a relatively common genetic disorder), saccharin is still around today, decades after it was identified as carcinogenic.

---

accomplish these seemingly desirable goals, scientists take genes from other living organisms (including pigs, bacteria, and viruses) and splice them onto the genes of certain food crops.

Although many people think of genetic engineering as the stuff of science fiction, this technology is already in use. Genetically altered corn, potatoes, and tomatoes may already be in your supermarket, on the produce shelves and/or in the canned and frozen foods section. Processed foods, including canola and soy oils and some canned sodas, may also contain genetically altered material. At least 15 percent of the U.S. soybean crop currently consists of genetically altered soybeans, and more than 60 percent of processed food products contain soy derivatives.

There are many reasons to be concerned about these developments. First and foremost, genetically engineered foods have not been subjected to long-term testing. Changing the genetic composition of foods can reduce their nutritional value. For people with food allergies, there is reason to fear that genetic engineering may introduce allergens from allergenic foods into previously "safe" foods. Moreover, a large percentage of field-tested genetically altered plants are food crops that were engineered specifically to withstand heavier doses of toxic herbicides. Scientists say that the existence of these herbicide-tolerant plants could make it possible for U.S. farmers to triple their use of herbicides. Another concern is that cross-pollination is bound to occur as insects, birds, and the wind pollinate natural and genetically engineered crops growing in adjacent fields. Engineered living organisms can reproduce and migrate, creating unwanted mutations, and adding still more uncertainty to the end results.

In addition to the effects we can anticipate, genetically engineered foods may very well have serious but as-yet-unknown side effects. It is impossible to predict what effects genetically engineered foods may have on the human body, on livestock and poultry fed altered foods, and on the environment. Yet the FDA does not require that genetically engineered foods be labeled as such, so there is no way to know whether the produce you pick up in the supermarket is in its natural form or not. Unless you buy organic foodstuffs exclusively, there is no sure way to protect yourself against the potential dangers posed by engineered foods. Unfortunately, most people are unaware that the food chain is being so profoundly changed, perhaps irrevocably.

There are organized groups speaking out against genetically altered foodstuffs in general, and many grass-roots groups are demanding that these foods carry identifying labels. If this issue concerns you, get involved and spread the word. As much as possible, choose organically produced foods, including meat, poultry, eggs, and dairy products. For more information about this issue, you can contact The Pure Food Campaign (see the Resources section at the end of the book).

CHOOSING FOOD AND WATER

Your shopping habits have an important and powerful influence on your diet. After all, you will eat whatever you stock in the refrigerator and cupboards. In this section we will offer guidelines to help you provide yourself with a healthy, balanced, nutrient-rich diet.

Buy Organic Food

Whenever possible, we recommend that you buy organically grown produce and grains, and buy meat and poultry from animals raised without hormones or antibiotics. Buying organically grown foods reduces your risk of exposure to pesticides and chemical fertilizers. Certified organic foods are grown without the use of synthetic chemicals. They are absolutely the healthiest choice both for us and for the earth and air.

Contaminants in the air, food, and drinking water of the nation are a major concern. By testing rainwater samples from twenty-three states, a recent study by the U.S. Geological Survey found that agricultural chemicals end up in the atmosphere. Along with eliminating the pesticide residues that linger on commercially farmed foods, organic farming spares the earth from these unnecessary and destructive toxins.

There are currently no national regulations in force governing the production or sale of organic foodstuffs. However, a fourteen-member panel called the National Organics Standards Board has been created by Congress. Its purpose is to devise national standards for organic foods and then (1) to advise the U.S. Department of Agriculture (USDA) on how to implement the federal rules and regulations that will insure the standards have been met and (2) to govern the production and sale of organic foodstuffs.

The recommendations under consideration include requiring that any food product labeled organic contain at least 95 percent organically produced ingredients. If at least half of the ingredients in a product are produced organically, its label could include the statement "contains organic ingredients." Organically raised livestock, including poultry, would have to be fed organically grown feed, allowed access to the outdoors and direct sunlight, and not kept in overcrowded barns and pens. They might be given antibiotics if they became sick, but not routinely, to promote growth. If implemented, such recommendations would require federal certification of everyone and everything involved in every step in every process involved in bringing an organic product to market, including the farmer, the fields, the handler, the processor, and the marketer. It is universally agreed that the term "organic" could not be applied to genetically altered and engineered foods. The recommended fine for knowingly mislabeling a product as organic would be $10,000.

The National Organics Standards Board's recommendations are just that—recommendations. They are not yet the law of the land, and they may not be for some time. Some states already have certification programs governing organic farmers in place, and more states are following suit. If you don't know how your state stands on this important issue, call your state agriculture department and inquire. Whether your state provides official certification or not, almost every community has a number of markets where guaranteed organic produce, meats, eggs, and milk are sold. If you have difficulty finding a source of organic foods, ask your local grocery to carry certified organic produce and grains. Or look under the word "Organic" in your local Yellow Pages for sources.

If you can afford the additional cost—it's true that organic foods are more expensive—it is very much worth your while to eat clean. If you cannot buy organic fruits, vegetables, and grains, wash everything thoroughly. Use a mixture of warm water and vinegar (one-quarter cup of vinegar for each gallon of water). Vinegar accelerates the breakdown of some pesticides. When serving vegetables like cabbage and lettuce, always remove the outer leaves, which often contain much more chemical residue than the inner leaves do. Root vegetables (carrots, potatoes, turnips, and the like) should be scrubbed and peeled. Any fruit or vegetable that has been waxed (this is often done to apples, cucumbers, eggplants, peppers, tomatoes, and citrus fruits to make them look shinier and more attractive) should be peeled as well.

Eat a Balanced Diet

The best diet is one in which 40 to 65 percent of your daily calories come from complex carbohydrates, 15 to 30 percent from protein, and 20 to 30 percent from fats. Of the complex carbohydrates, 45 to 50 percent should be in the form of vegetables; 15 percent, whole grains (wheat, rye, barley, rice, oats, millet, and others); 15 percent, legumes (dried beans, peas); and 20 to 25 percent, whole fruits. The sugars found in complex carbohydrates are more gradually absorbed into the bloodstream than those from processed refined sugars. A diet rich in complex carbohydrates will help you feel more alert and energetic during the day. Of course, individual nutritional needs vary somewhat, depending on your activity level and other factors.

Complete proteins are found in milk, cheese, eggs,

meat, fish, poultry, nuts, and most legumes. Combining grains and vegetables will also provide complete protein. Proteins are essential for the growth and repair of all body tissues, including organs, muscles, bone, skin, blood, and nerves. Each cell in the body requires protein.

Fats are essential for metabolizing fat-soluble vitamins (A, D, E, and K), for normal growth and development, and for maintaining healthy skin, hair, and nails. Fats regulate digestion, influence blood pressure, and are needed for the production of prostaglandins, chemical "messengers" that are present throughout the body. It is important to remember, however, that all fats are not created equal. We recommend using unrefined, minimally processed, cold-pressed organic oils. Use flaxseed, linseed, pumpkinseed, soybean, and walnut oils in order to get important essential fatty acids. Safflower, sunflower, canola, and olive oils are also acceptable sources of fat. Polyunsaturated oils should be kept refrigerated after opening. Try to avoid products containing hydrogenated and partially hydrogenated oils. Margarine and solid shortenings are usually manufactured with partially hydrogenated oils (*see* The Hydrogenation Process, page 56). Despite what many people have been led to believe, a small amount of butter is probably better for you than any amount of margarine.

Another key to a balanced died is to eat a variety of foods. Along with the fun of trying new and different foods, variety ensures that you will get the full range of nutrients your body needs. Next time you shop, buy something new. Include vegetables and grain with each lunch and dinner. At a minimum, you should eat five servings of fresh vegetables and fruits each day. Seven to nine servings is even better. This may sound like a lot, but a serving is generally defined as only one cup of raw leafy vegetables, one-half cup of other vegetables (cooked or chopped raw), or one medium piece of whole fruit, such as an apple, pear, banana, or orange.

Prepare your food simply. Foods that are steamed, baked, or broiled are easily digested. Use water, lemon juice, broths, flavorful herbs, and juices to steam, bake, or broil. Avoid frying your food. Fried foods are difficult to digest; heated oils and fats turn rancid quickly; and oils and fats add calories.

Make sure you have three meals a day, with healthy snacks as necessary. Healthful snacks might include any of the following:

- Almond butter and celery

- Carrot sticks/carrot chips

- Low-fat cheese (made from skim or almond milk or soy-based) and whole-grain crackers

- Low-fat cream cheese and celery with raisins on top

- Hard-boiled eggs

- Fruit sticks or fruit kabobs, or a piece of fresh fruit

- Hummus and whole-grain crackers

- Jicama and peanut butter or almond butter

- Millet or rice toast and fruit-sweetened jelly

- Fresh nuts and/or seeds

- Rice cakes with peanut, almond, or sesame-seed butter and, if desired, fruit-sweetened jelly

- Smoothies (plain yogurt, fruit, and a dab of honey mixed in a blender) or fruit freezes (fruit, ice, and a dab of honey mixed in a blender)

- Fresh raw vegetables and onion dip (use yogurt in place of sour cream for the dip)

- Plain yogurt with fresh fruit and nuts

To supply the fuel your body needs, make breakfast and lunch the larger meals; eat lighter foods at dinner to support your body as it slows down and prepares to rest for the night. Allow at least two hours between dinner and bedtime. Sleeping on an overly full stomach can cause restless sleep and a groggy feeling in the morning.

Shun Sugar

The third basic recommendation for a healthy diet is to reduce your consumption of refined sugars—or, better yet, eliminate them from your diet completely. Admittedly, this is a great challenge for many people. About half of the carbohydrates eaten by the typical American are sugar. The average adult eats about 150 pounds of sugar each year; the average teenager eats a whopping 300 pounds annually.

The ingestion of sugar has many adverse effects on the body. It increases the excretion of valuable minerals, including calcium, magnesium, chromium, copper, zinc, and sodium. The reduction in the amount of calcium in the blood in turn prompts the secretion of parathyroid hormone, which causes the release of calcium from the bones, accelerating bone loss and, possibly, the development of osteoporosis. Sugar also causes blood-sugar levels to soar. In response, the pancreas steps up its production of insulin to drive the blood-sugar level back down. Many people may react to these changes in blood sugar with jitteriness, agitation, and an inability to concentrate, followed by tiredness and irritability. In addition, if this cycle is repeated over and over, the pancreas becomes overworked and fatigued, and the body's cells can become resistant to insulin—ultimately resulting in diabetes. Sugar impairs immune function by competing with vitamin C for transport into white blood cells. This reduces the ability of the white blood cells to destroy aggressive bacteria, making the body more prone to infection. Sugar promotes the

Phytochemicals

Mother was right: You'd better eat your veggies. Phytochemicals, compounds present in fruits and vegetables, are a relatively recent focus of nutritional research. Scientists are only beginning to identify them and their properties—there are thousands of phytochemicals that have been isolated and, no doubt, many more that will be—but research has already confirmed their positive effects. Many of them are powerful substances that offer proven health benefits. Some are antioxidants that fight free radicals. Others have other beneficial properties. Many of the entries in Part Two single out certain fruits and vegetables as beneficial for specific conditions because of the phytochemicals they contain. Here's a quick summary of some of the phytochemicals that have been scientifically studied:

• Acemannan, extracted from the aloe vera plant, appears to be one of its most active ingredients. It is used both orally and intravenously, and has uses from antiviral, antifungal, and antibacterial to helping with symptoms from AIDS and cancer.

• Acetylated acidic polysaccharide and galatluronic acid, two compounds that combine to form the gooey texture okra is known for, are very soothing to the digestive tract.

• Allicin, found in raw garlic, has antibiotic and antiviral properties, lowers cholesterol, and reduces the risk of blood clots. Ajoeine and adenosine, present in cooked garlic, also reduce the risk of blood clots.

• Anthocyanidins (also called phenols) found in grapes—and therefore in red wine, grape juice and grapeseed extract—are strong antioxidants that fight cancer, reduce levels of low-density lipoproteins (LDL, or "bad cholesterol") in the blood, strengthen blood vessels, thin the blood, aid the immune system, and fight allergies.

• Calcium pectate, a type of soluble fiber present in carrots, may help lower cholesterol levels. In one study, people who ate seven ounces of carrots a day for a three-week period experienced, on average, an 11-percent reduction in serum cholesterol.

• Capsaicin, the compound that makes hot peppers hot, has been shown to be an anticoagulant, and may help to prevent heart attacks and strokes due to abnormal blood clots.

• Curcumin, found in the herb turmeric, has been compared against the nonsteroidal anti-inflammatory drug (NSAID) phenylbutazone, with good results. It seems to have some antioxidant and, possibly, anticancer effects as well.

• Ellagic acid, found in many berries (including blackberries, blueberries, cranberries, raspberries, strawber-

---

overgrowth of yeast in the gastrointestinal tract. And we all know the association of sugar with tooth decay and obesity.

There are alternatives to refined sugar. Honey, rice syrup, molasses, barley malt, and maple syrup are fair substitutes. But these too should be used sparingly, as in excess they add little to the diet except calories.

Food advertising promotes many products that are laden with refined sugars—soda, candy, cookies, and breakfast cereals, among others. Processed foods frequently contain surprisingly large amounts of sugar. Even foods that don't seem like sweets, such as spaghetti sauce or peanut butter, often contain sugar. Thus, by decreasing your use of processed foods, you can significantly decrease your refined-sugar consumption. It is important to read food labels carefully so you know exactly what you are eating.

If you can't eliminate sugar entirely, limit it to early in the day. If you eat sugary sweets before bed, you may have difficulty settling down for sleep and may wake up groggy and tired the next morning.

Drink Plenty of Clean Water

To keep all of your body's systems functioning efficiently, you need to drink at least six to eight 8-ounce glasses of water every day. Water accounts for approximately two-thirds of the average adult's body weight. That means that if you weigh 120 pounds, you're carrying 80 pounds of water; if you weigh 180 pounds, your body contains 120 pounds of water. Water is more important to life's essential processes than any other substance we know of. An adult human can live for up to forty days without food, but for no more than seven days without water.

In the United States, it has long been a point of pride that people can safely drink their tap water. Most community water systems supply water that is—though heavily chlorinated—considered to be both safe and of acceptable quality. Yet between 20,000 and 100,000 people become ill every year from drinking tap water, and some die. The very young, the elderly, and people with compromised immune systems are particularly at risk. Because the symptoms associated with drinking contaminated water often mimic those of the flu, the cause of the ries, huckleberries, and loganberries), is believed to have anticancer properties.

• Genistein, an isoflavone present in soybeans, soy flour, soymilk, tofu, and textured soy protein, helps reduce blood cholesterol and fights cancer. It works in much the same way as the cancer drug tamoxifen. It also eases menopausal problems, including hot flashes, and may help in building bone density.

• Glycyrrhizin, found in licorice, has been used to decrease inflammation in people with arthritis.

• Indoles, which are present in the cruciferous vegetables (broccoli, Brussels sprouts, cabbage, cauliflower, and their relatives) are antioxidants that boost the immune system and aid the body in disarming and excreting toxins. It is believed they also can render inactive a type of estrogen that has the potential to support the growth of breast tumors. Researchers have observed that people who eat cabbage frequently have a lower incidence of colon and breast cancer than those who do not.

• Liminene, a substance found in lemons and limes, is a strong antioxidant.

• Lycopenes, found in tomatoes, have antioxidant properties, protect against cancer (notably prostate and pancreatic cancers), and stimulate the brain.

• Lutein, found in dark leafy greens such as kale, spinach, and collard greens, is an antioxidant carotenoid with more power than its better known cousin, beta-carotene. It fights free-radical damage, and has been shown to reduce the risk of macular degeneration, a common cause of blindness in older people.

• Oleuropein, found in extracts from the olive leaf, has been shown to have antifungal, antiviral, and antibacterial effects.

• Quercetin, found in red and yellow onions, red wine, broccoli, and tea, fights cancer, viruses, bacteria, and fungi. This antioxidant bioflavonoid also lowers cholesterol and reduces the risk of unwanted blood clots.

• Pectin, found in apples and other fruits, is a type of fiber that has been shown to be effective in lowering cholesterol levels.

• Sulforaphane, found in broccoli and broccoli sprouts, has demonstrated cancer-preventing properties.

Since nearly every fruit, vegetable, grain, and legume that has been tested contains phytochemicals, it is unlikely that all of these beneficial compounds will be identified anytime soon. Thus, while some manufacturers are producing concentrates of known phytochemicals, it is impossible to get their full benefits in supplement form. Eating a diet that includes generous amounts of a wide variety of fresh produce is still the best way to ensure that you are getting the fullest possible range of phytochemicals and in the balance that nature intended.

---

problem is seldom identified. Most people will simply ignore an upset stomach, a mild case of diarrhea, or a temporary unidentified digestive disturbance, or treat these symptoms with an over-the-counter remedy of some kind without thinking much about it.

Although the chlorine that is added to most municipal water supplies does destroy waterborne bacteria, including the bacteria that cause typhoid fever, cholera, and dysentery, it can be dangerous to your health. Chlorine injures red blood cells and damages their ability to carry life-giving oxygen where it is needed. Some studies suggest that chlorine may contribute to high blood pressure. Chlorine also destroys vitamin E.

Research has linked chlorine-based chemicals to certain forms of cancer, as well as infertility and other reproductive problems. The chemical structure of some chlorine-based chemicals is very close to that of the human sex hormone estrogen. As a result, research suggests, these chemicals may either block the action of natural estrogen, or, in some cases, actually amplify its effect. In the early 1990s, researchers found that certain cancers, infertility

problems, and reproductive abnormalities had one frightening thing in common: All can be caused by exposure to chlorine-based and other chemicals that mimic the effects of human estrogens. Recent years have seen certain alarming health trends in the general population, including a 50-percent drop in the sperm count of the average man; a 50-percent increase in the rate of testicular cancer; and a doubling of the incidence of breast cancer among American women. All of these conditions can result from excessive estrogen exposure. While there is no consensus among researchers that estrogen exposure is indeed to blame, or that chlorine in drinking water is implicated, Greenpeace and the American Public Health Organization have called for a ban on chlorine, and the Environmental Protection Agency (EPA) has proposed a study of this chemical's possible health hazards.

Fluoride is added to the water supply in more than half the cities in the United States, ostensibly to improve dental health. Yet there is still no conclusive evidence proving that this actually works. On the other hand, there is considerable evidence that fluoride itself creates health

A Word About Fat

Many people have come to think of fat as a dirty word. It isn't. In fact, fats are necessary nutrients, just as proteins and carbohydrates are, and it is impossible to be truly healthy without an adequate supply of them. It is important, however, that the dietary fat you consume be the right kind.

Fats are the most energy-dense of the three major nutrient types. That is, they contain more calories per gram than either proteins or carbohydrates do. Fats are therefore a major source of energy for the body. They have other vital functions as well. They help the body to maintain its temperature in cold weather; they act as a "cushion" for vital organs; and they are necessary for healthy nerve function, healthy skin, and proper wound healing. In infants, a lack of the right types of fats slows growth and development, particularly the development of the brain.

Fat molecules are composed of a fatty acid or acids plus glycerol, the slippery substance that makes soap soapy. The general scientific term for a fat molecule is *glyceride*. Depending on the number of fatty acids they contain, specific fat molecules may be designated monoglycerides (one fatty acid), diglycerides (two fatty acids), or triglycerides (three fatty acids). Most dietary fats are triglycerides. Triglycerides do not dissolve in water.

Fatty acids are basically chains of carbon atoms with hydrogen and oxygen atoms attached. They differ from one another both in the number of carbon atoms in their carbon chains and in the number of hydrogen atoms attached to the carbon chain. A fatty acid that contains the maximum possible amount of hydrogen is called *saturated*. In foods, triglycerides with saturated fatty acids are generally solid at room temperature, like butter. Saturated fats occur mostly in foods from animal sources, as well as in coconut oil, palm kernel oil, and cocoa butter. A fatty acid that contains less than the maximum possible amount of hydrogen is referred to as *unsaturated*. Depending on how many pairs of hydrogen atoms are missing, an unsaturated fatty acid may be either *monounsaturated* (one pair missing) or *polyunsaturated* (more than one pair missing). Unsaturated fats are generally liquid at room temperature, and are usually found in foods of vegetable origin, such as vegetable oils. Many fats and oils, both of animal or vegetable origin, contain mixtures of saturated and unsaturated fatty acids. Still another type of fat found in some foods does not occur in nature, but as a result of food-processing technology (*see* The Hydrogenation Process, page 56). These are known as trans-fatty acids.

Saturated and trans-fats (hydrogenated and partially hydrogenated fats and oils) have been linked to a number of serious health problems, including cardiovascular disease and cancer. These are the so-called "bad fats." A number of the polyunsaturated fatty acids, on the other hand—the "good fats"—have been designated *essential fatty acids*. This means that they are required for health and that the body is unable to synthesize them, so they must be obtained in the diet. Essential fatty acids fall into two groups, depending on molecular structure, the omega-3 and the omega-6 essential fatty acids. The omega-3 essential fatty acids include alpha-linolenic and eicosapentaenoic acid (EPA), and are found in flaxseed oil and fish oils. These fatty acids help to lower blood-fat levels and prevent the development of blood clots, thus decreasing the risk of heart disease. The omega-6 essential fatty acids include linoleic acid and gamma-linolenic acid, and are found in black currant seed oil, borage oil, and evening primrose oil, among other sources. The omega-6 oils play a part in nerve function, growth, skin health, and wound healing.

How much fat should you eat? Most nutritionists agree that, for most people, fat intake should fall in the range of 25 to 30 percent of total dietary calories. Thus, if you normally take in about 2,800 calories a day, between 700 and 900 of those calories should be from fat. Since fat contains 9 calories per gram, 900 calories from fat translates into a total of 100 grams of fat.

To figure out the amount of fat you should consume each day, do the following:

1. Figure out approximately how many calories you eat in a day.

2. Multiply this number by 0.25.

3. Divide the result from Step 2 by 9.

This will give you the number of grams of fat that will give you 25 percent of your daily dietary calories. You may find that, like most people in industrialized Western countries, you are consuming more fat than you should. More serious, however, is the fact that, as a group, we consume too much bad fat and not enough of the good fats. So the solution to the "fat problem" is not simply to cut out fat, but to change your diet so that you eat more good fat and less bad fat. One easy way to do this is to increase the amount of fish in your diet. Besides being an excellent source of good fats, fish also provides good-quality protein. Eating just two fish meals per week will help to keep your heart and circulatory system in good health. Types of fish highest in omega-3 fatty acids (a 3.5-ounce serving contains more than 1 gram of EFAs) include anchovies, carp, herring, lake trout, mackerel, salmon, sardines, scad, sturgeon, tuna, and whitefish. Types of fish that contain somewhat less (a 3.5-ounce serving contains 1/2 to 1 gram of EFAs) include bass, bluefish, eel, hake, halibut, oysters, pompano, rainbow trout, rockfish, shark, and smelts.

problems. There is a higher incidence of Down syndrome, cancer, osteoporosis, osteomalacia, mottled teeth, and deaths from all causes in areas where fluoride intake is high. Fluoride also destroys vitamin C. Moreover, sodium fluoride and fluosalicic acid—the compounds used to fluoridate water—are byproducts of aluminum manufacture. They are not found in nature.

Any health professional will tell you that drinking eight glasses of water every day is a standard prescription for good health. Unfortunately, tap water cannot be considered healthy unless proven to be so by laboratory tests. Boiling tap water for three to five minutes will kill bacteria and parasites, but the boiling process concentrates heavy metals, and it cannot eliminate certain pollutants or destroy the chlorine and fluoride.

For a very long time, we have recommended that people drink only pure spring water from a reputable source, and that is the recommendation you will find in most entries in this book. It is important to use quality water not only for drinking, but also to make ice cubes, to reconstitute juices, and for cooking, particularly for cooking grains, such as rice, that absorb water as they cook. It is even advisable to use the purest water possible to brush your teeth, and to filter the water you bathe or shower in. (There are water filters for shower heads made just for this purpose.) Spring water is preferable to distilled water, which has little to no mineral content. Distilled water is the ultimate in soft water, and for reasons not yet fully determined, drinking softened water over time can lead to a measurable increase in high blood pressure and increased risk of heart attack and stroke. This was reported in the *Journal of the American Medical Association* as far back as 1974, based on data covering millions of people on both sides of the Atlantic over a period of decades, though little was made of the news.

Along with the chlorine and fluoride that are routinely added to tap water, there are many other substances that sneak through the purification processes. Most of the pollutants that contaminate drinking water are tasteless, odorless, colorless, and invisible. These substances can include viruses, bacteria, parasites, inorganic chemicals, asbestos fibers, lead, pesticides, herbicides, radioactive particles, methanes, and other poisonous agents. You can't taste them, smell them, or see them. The only way they can be detected is by laboratory analysis.

You should be aware, however, that while many companies advertise their products as "natural spring water," there is no legal definition of what constitutes a spring, and "natural" means only that the mineral content of the water has not been altered. It can be hard to really tell what you're getting. Indeed, the differences between the different types of water available today are a mystery to many. Here's how to find out how your water sources measure up:

- *Tap water.* Contact your local water department or local health department and ask how the water supply is cleaned and treated. Some state agencies will test your tap water free of charge. However, most test only for bacteria, not toxins, pollutants, or parasites. If you really want to find out what is in your tap water, you might have to pay for an independent analysis conducted by a commercial laboratory.

- *Filtered water.* There are three common types of water filters: absorbent filters, microfilters, and ion-exchange filters. Absorbent filters, usually made of charcoal, are designed to pick up and hold contaminates as water passes over them. Microfilters, which can be fashioned of any of a number of different materials, have tiny holes designed to catch and eliminate contaminants as water passes through them. Deionization or demineralization is accomplished with ion-exchange filters, which are designed to remove heavy metals, including lead. None of these filters can remove all contaminants. To remove parasites such as potentially deadly cryptosporidia, a microfilter must have a guaranteed pore size of one micron or smaller, according to the National Sanitation Foundation. Also available are reverse-osmosis filtration systems. These utilize semipermeable membranes similar to those used in kidney dialysis machines to remove impurities. The pores in the reverse-osmosis membrane are so tiny that most contaminants in water (including chlorine and fluoride) are trapped, but hydrogen and oxygen molecules pass through easily. This is one of the most efficient all-around methods of filtration available.

- *Distilled water.* The steam distillation process starts with boiling water. As the water boils, steam rises and is funneled through tubing into a condensing chamber, where it cools and condenses back into water. The steam is pure water vapor. Most of the contaminants remain behind. If you regularly boil water in a teakettle, you have probably noticed the scale that builds up on the bottom of a well-used kettle. That's what happens in the distillation process. However, a lot of the buildup consists of the healthy minerals that give water its taste. That's why distilled water tastes flat.

- *Bottled water.* Bottled water can be purchased in supermarkets in gallon bottles or delivered to your home in five- or six-gallon jugs. Any bottled water you buy should carry a label showing the original source of the water (spring, well, public water supply, etc.) and the type of treatment (filtration, distillation, deionization, ultraviolet-light treatment, ozonation) it has undergone, as well as listing all the elements present in the water (hydrogen, oxygen, minerals). If it doesn't, choose another brand or contact the bottler directly for

The Hydrogenation Process

Hydrogenated and partially hydrogenated fats are vegetable or seed oils that have been subjected to elaborate processing. Hydrogenating an oil means saturating its carbon molecules with hydrogen. This is accomplished under tremendous pressure at temperatures of up to 410°F in the presence of a metal catalyst (nickel, platinum, copper) for as long as eight hours.

A liquid oil can be transformed into a solid or semi-solid fat by adjusting the length of the hydrogenation process. When the desired degree of hardness is attained, the process is stopped. Margarines, "soft" margarines, and solid shortenings are manufactured with partially hydrogenated oils.

Hydrogenation destroys the nutritional value of the oil. A hydrogenated product doesn't spoil, because it is a completely inert (dead) substance. It can be heated for cooking without decomposing. However, it contains chemically altered metabolites—some of which may be harmful—plus traces of the metal catalyst.

Even though logic might suggest otherwise, partially hydrogenated products are in some ways worse than completely hydrogenated products. The molecules in oil being bombarded with hydrogen become saturated (hydrogenated) erratically, and when the process is stopped, a proliferation of strangely altered molecules called trans fatty acids are left behind. Many of these chemically altered elements are harmful because they interfere with the body's normal metabolism. Others have not been scientifically researched. Studies have shown that trans fatty acids are at least as bad for you as saturated fats. What's worse, when saturated fats raise cholesterol levels, they tend to raise the level of high-density lipoproteins (HDLs, the so-called "good cholesterol"). This is not the case with trans fatty acids. Two major studies, one published in the *Journal of the American Medical Association* and the other in *The New England Journal of Medicine,* showed trans fatty acids to be the worst type of fat in terms of heart-attack risk.

this information. If you are considering having bottled water delivered to your home or business, we suggest you ask for written documentation from several different companies attesting to the cleanliness and purity of the water each offers, and choose the supplier whose water is the cleanest. If you have bottled water delivered, be aware that the cooler or ceramic jug you use to dispense the water should be cleaned regularly. Use a mixture of equal parts hydrogen peroxide and baking soda once a month to clean the jug. Run this mixture through the spigot, too. Or, as an alternative, you can use grapefruit-seed extract (*see* WATER PURIFICATION in Part Three). Before refilling, rinse well with tap water, and dry it with a clean towel.

For more information about drinking water and water treatment systems, you can contact the Water Quality Association (see the Resources section at the end of the book).

BASIC NUTRIENTS YOUR BODY NEEDS

The four basic building blocks of the diet are water, complex carbohydrates, proteins, and fats. A proper balance of these essentials is necessary for optimum health. The table on page 57 provides a brief introduction to fundamental dietary requirements, as well as a guide to the functions and food sources of these four dietary elements. A diet based on a wide variety of simply prepared whole foods is most likely to meet your basic nutritional needs.

Vegetarians must take special care to provide adequate protein for tissue growth, maintenance, and repair by eating a nutrient-rich and protein-adequate diet. Many plant foods do not contain the full spectrum of eight amino acids that make up a complete protein. At one time it was thought that to provide a complete protein, certain foods—such as rice and beans—had to be combined and eaten at the same time. Now we know that a diet based on a variety of vegetables, legumes, and grains will provide adequate protein. However, it is important that vegetarians eat a varied, balanced diet in order to get the full spectrum of amino acids, and therefore complete protein.

Also necessary for good health are nutrients that together are classified as *micronutrients,* which include vitamins and minerals.

Vitamins

Vitamins are essential to normal body function. They are not a form of energy or fuel, as foods are. But they play an indispensable role in the normal metabolism, growth, maintenance and repair of the body.

Vitamins are classified as either water-soluble or fat-soluble, depending upon which type of molecule (fat- or water-based) transports them in the bloodstream. Water-soluble vitamins include all of the B complex and vitamin C. These vitamins are quickly used by the body or excreted in urine, so they must be replenished daily. Water-soluble vitamins may leach out of foods during cooking, be damaged by overprocessing, or be destroyed when foods are overcooked.

The fat-soluble vitamins—A, D, E, and K—are fairly stable during low-temperature cooking. However, antibiotics, mineral oil, and certain drugs (steroids, for example)

BASIC NUTRIENTS

Nutrient	Function	Requirements	Signs of Deficiency	Food Sources
WATER/FLUIDS				
The body is two-thirds water by weight. Water is a primary need and essential nutrient.	Water is involved in every bodily function. It transports nutrients in and out of cells, removes toxins, and is necessary for all digestive, absorption, circulatory, and excretory functions. Water is necessary for the utilization of water-soluble B-complex and C vitamins, and for maintaining proper body temperature.	2 to 2⅔ ounces every hour, or 48 to 64 ounces in 24 hours.	Pale yellow urine shows a healthy state of hydration. Dark or scanty urine, thirst, and dry mouth are early signs of dehydration. Chronic dehydration can result in chronic constipation, weight gain, elevated cholesterol, a decreased threshold of pain, decreased ability to clear toxins from the body. Severe acute dehydration can cause disorientation, kidney failure and shock, and can be life threatening.	Best: Pure and clean spring water. Next best: Purified bottled water. Good: Herbal teas, diluted fruit juices. Limit: Alcoholic beverages, beverages containing caffeine, sodas. Avoid: Prepackaged punches, colored drinks, and packaged gelatin products.
COMPLEX CARBOHYDRATES				
Complex carbohydrates contain many vitamins plus healthy fiber.	Complex carbohydrates provide the body with energy. They are needed for the digestion and assimilation of food.	40 to 65 percent of total calories.	Lack of energy; exhaustion; mineral imbalances; breakdown of proteins in tissues.	Whole grains, vegetables, legumes (dried beans, peas), fruits.
PROTEIN				
Proteins are composed of amino acids, 22 of which are essential for normal growth and repair of tissues. The body can make 14 of them; the other 8 must be obtained in the diet.	Protein is essential for growth and repair of tissues. It provides the body with energy and heat, and is needed for the manufacture of hormones, antibodies, and enzymes. It also maintains the body's acid/alkali balance.	15 to 30 percent of total calories.	Diarrhea; vomiting; lack of appetite; edema (buildup of fluids in tissues); fatty liver; poor wound healing; depressed immunity; skin problems.	Complete protein: Milk, eggs, cheese, fish, meat, poultry. Good protein: Whole grains, nuts, beans, peas.
FATTY ACIDS				
The body does require fat, but it must be the right kind. The typical American diet is top-heavy in fats but deficient in the essential fatty acids required for normal function.	Fatty acids carry fat-soluble A, D, E, and K vitamins. The essential fatty acids (EFAs) are linoleic, linolenic, and arachidonic. They help manage cholesterol, regulate body temperature, and help control blood pressure. EFAs are essential for healthy skin, hair, and nails.	20 to 30 percent of total calories.	Skin, hair, and nail disorders; impaired metabolism of fats and fat-soluble vitamins. Eczema may be associated with EFA deficiency.	Best: Cold-expeller-pressed olive and flaxseed oils. Next best: Canola, safflower, sunflower, pumpkin, and walnut oils. Acceptable: Butter. In moderation only: Saturated fats found in animal products such as meat and dairy products, tropical oils such as palm and coconut oil. Not recommended: Margarine, hydrogenated or partially hydrogenated oils or products containing them.

Know Your Greens

Throughout this book, we talk about the importance of various types of vegetables, particularly green vegetables. Nutritionally speaking, though, some greens are better for you than others. Here we will compare the nutritional value of several different types of green vegetables.

SALAD GREENS

Most salad greens are a good source of vitamin C, beta-carotene (the precursor of vitamin A), iron, calcium, folic acid, and dietary fiber. Generally, darker green means more nutrition. For example, the dark green leaves of romaine lettuce have up to six times the vitamin C and five to ten times the beta-carotene of an equal amount of iceberg lettuce. And arugula, an even greener green, has about four times the vitamin C and three times the beta-carotene of romaine. Compare the nutritional values of ten popular salad greens (figures are for 3.5 ounces, or about two cups):

SELECTED NUTRIENT CONTENT OF TEN SALAD GREENS					
Green	**Calories**	**Beta-Carotene (IU)**	**Vitamin C (mg)**	**Calcium (mg)**	**Iron (mg)**
Arugula	23	4	91	309	1
Belgian endive	15	trace	0	18	1
Bibb lettuce	13	0.6	8	35	2
Boston lettuce	13	0.6	8	35	2
Chicory	23	2	4	19	1
Escarole	17	1	7	52	1
Iceberg lettuce	13	0.2	4	19	1
Mache	21	4	38	38	2
Romaine lettuce	16	2	24	68	1
Watercress	11	3	43	120	<1

OTHER GREENS

Many other types of green plants, especially kale, collards, and dandelion greens, are rich in carotene, vitamin C, flavonoids, and other substances that help protect against degenerative diseases. They are also a good source of fiber and many minerals, particularly iron and calcium. Ounce for ounce, fresh collard greens, kale, and mustard greens have about as much calcium as whole milk, and dandelion and turnip greens actually have more. Such green leafy vegetables as turnip greens, collards, green and red Swiss chard, beet greens, kale, dandelion greens, mustard greens, broccoli raab, and sorrel should all be included in a healthy diet. For example, just 3.5 ounces of beet greens can supply more than the daily requirement of vitamin A, 50 percent of the daily requirement of vitamin C, and 15 percent of the daily requirement of calcium. Consider the following figures:

SELECTED NUTRIENT CONTENT OF SEVEN LEAFY GREENS					
Green	**Calories**	**Beta-Carotene (IU)**	**Vitamin C (mg)**	**Calcium (mg)**	**Iron (mg)**
Beet greens	19	4	30	119	3
Collards	19	2	23	117	0.6
Dandelion greens	45	8	35	187	3
Kale	50	5	120	135	2
Mustard greens	26	3	70	103	1
Swiss chard	19	2	30	51	2
Turnip greens	27	5	60	190	1

Note that leafy greens lose much of their volume when cooked. For example, a pound of raw greens will yield only about $\frac{1}{2}$ cup of cooked leafy greens. Recommended preparation methods include steaming, simmering, blanching, braising, and quick sautéing—in other words, almost anything except frying.

"PRIZE" VEGETABLES

There are a number of "prize" vegetables that really stand out for the impressive nutrition they offer. Kale is one of them. A single 3.5-ounce serving of kale supplies nearly twice the recommended daily allowance of both vitamin A and vitamin C, as well as 50 percent of the RDA of vitamin E, 15 to 20 percent of the RDA of vitamin B_6, folic acid, calcium, and iron, and 10 percent of the RDA of magnesium. Other "prize" vegetables are all the members of the cabbage family, including red and green cabbage, savoy cabbage, bok choy and napa cabbage, broccoli, radishes, cauliflower, and Brussels sprouts.

interfere with their absorption from the digestive tract. Frying foods alters the fat-soluble vitamins in them as well.

For a review of the vitamins you need every day, as well as their respective functions and food sources, see the table on pages 61–62.

Minerals

Minerals are part of all body tissues and fluids. They are essential in nerve responses, muscle contraction, maintenance of the body's fluid balance, and the internal processing of nutrients. Minerals influence the manufacture of hormones and regulate electrolyte balance throughout the body. The term *electrolyte* refers to the form in which various minerals circulate in the body. Calcium, potassium, and sodium are examples of important electrolytes. Calcium, for example, is not only an important constituent of bones and teeth; it is also involved in the transmission of nerve impulses, the transmission of energy from cell to cell, and the contraction and relaxation of muscles, including the heart. Calcium, potassium, and magnesium together control the continuous cycle of contraction and relaxation of the heart muscle and blood vessels. If these electrolytes are out of balance, resulting fluid shifts may cause swelling or dehydration, the neuromuscular system may become irritable, or an irregular heart rhythm may develop.

Minerals are excreted daily and must be replaced either through the diet or in supplement form. For a quick review of the minerals you need every day, as well as their functions and food sources, see the table on pages 63–64.

Diet and nutrition together make up a huge subject that deserves your time and attention. Read more, experiment with new and different foods, use cookbooks devoted to whole-foods cooking, and ask lots of questions. The more you understand about food and nutrition, the more committed you will be to making sure you eat a healthy, wholesome diet.

WORKING WITH A NUTRITIONAL COUNSELOR

There are many different kinds of professionals, with varied educational backgrounds and philosophies, who can recommend dietary programs and nutritional supplements. Registered dietitians, nutritionists, naturopathic physicians, pharmacists, chiropractors, medical doctors, and nurses—to name only a few—may all practice nutritional medicine. When interviewing a nutritional counselor, whatever the individual's professional credentials, find out about his or her educational background, work experience, and nutritional philosophy.

Nutrition is a broad and constantly changing field. Eating a healthy, well-balanced, allergen-free diet, along with nutritional supplements when needed, is one of the most important things you can do to support your health. You may need assistance planning the optimum diet. Choose a counselor you feel you can work with, a person who believes in the fundamental importance of a healthy diet. As with any health-care practitioner, choose a person who knows the current research, who is compassionate, and who will work with you as a partner to create the healthiest, most manageable plan possible.

NUTRITIONAL SUPPLEMENTS

While they should not be used as a substitute for a varied, healthy diet, nutritional supplements can help to ensure that you are getting an adequate supply of all the basic nutrients your body needs. They can also be helpful in supporting the body during illness. For example, in many of the entries in Part Two we suggest boosting the body's infection-fighting capability with three specific vitamins. Vitamin C is a well-documented anti-inflammatory that eases the common cold. Bioflavonoids help fight infection, reduce inflammation, and decrease allergic reactions. Beta-carotene, which the body uses to manufacture vitamin A, helps mucous membranes to heal.

In addition to vitamins and minerals, many of the entries in Part Two contain a recommendation for probiotic supplements. Probiotic (meaning "life-promoting") bacteria are the friendly bacteria that live in healthy intestines. There are different types of bacteria that normally inhabit the digestive system. *Lactobacillus acidophilus* is specific to the small intestine; *Bifidobacterium bifidum* is specific to the large intestine. These friendly bacteria are termed *resident bacteria* because they form colonies and do their work inside the body.

Acidophilus bacteria perform many essential functions. They produce the enzyme lactase, required for the digestion of lactose (milk sugar), and aid in the digestion of other nutrients as well. Some strains fight undesirable microorganisms that invade their territory, aid in the destruction of dangerous disease-causing bacteria by producing natural antibiotics, and help reduce the levels of low-density lipoproteins, the so-called "bad cholesterol." When acidophilus colonies are present in sufficient strength, they inhibit the proliferation of *Candida albicans*, a fungal organism (yeast) that can cause a host of problems.

Bifidobacteria produce lactic and other acids that increase the acidity of the region they inhabit and make the area inhospitable to dangerous bacteria. They prevent harmful bacteria from converting compounds known as nitrates (ingested in food or water) into related compounds called nitrites. Nitrites in turn can be converted into nitrosamines, which are known cancer-causing agents. When present in sufficient numbers, bifidobacteria prevent disease-causing bacteria and fungi from forming colonies in their territory and send them on their way. Bifidobacteria also aid in the production of B vitamins and assist in the dietary management of certain liver conditions.

The body can lose its stores of friendly bacteria in many ways. For example, if you must take antibiotics, these drugs not only destroy harmful bacteria, but kill off the essential bacteria as well. Birth-control pills, certain over-the-counter drugs, the chlorine and fluoride in tap water, environmental pollutants, mental and physical stress, chemotherapy and radiation therapy, tobacco, and alcohol also reduce normal levels of beneficial bacteria. Even just getting older causes a loss of the friendly bacteria you need to stay healthy.

Because friendly bacteria have the astonishing ability to rid the body of disease-causing bacteria before they can create a problem, probiotic supplements have become virtually a necessity today. If you must take a prescribed course of antibiotics, supplementing your diet with yogurt is helpful, and taking lactobacilli for at least ten days after the treatment is very important. The bacteria found in true cultured yogurt—as opposed to the commercially produced variety—do not remain in the body for long, but they too enhance digestion and help inhibit undesirable microorganisms.

When selecting probiotics supplements, choose products cultured from "super strains." Good manufacturers will have independent research available concerning their products' ability to survive in an acid environment, specifics about the strain of bacteria they contain, and other characteristics. Also, make sure the product you select has an expiration date stamped or printed on the label. Many live bacteria die in the container. Without an expiration date, there is no way to tell whether you are purchasing living bacteria that will colonize your intestines and deliver full benefit, or inactive bacteria that will do you no good at all. If you are allergic to milk, choose a dairy-free product.

Another food supplement recommended for various conditions is chlorophyll. Chlorophyll, the green pigment found in plant tissue, is a natural deodorizer and contains many useful trace nutrients, especially magnesium. It is helpful when treating ailments as varied as bad breath, canker sores, chronic constipation, menstrual cramps, vaginitis, and mononucleosis, as well as in rebuilding blood after a major bleed or in rebuilding bone tissue after a break.

CHOOSING DIETARY SUPPLEMENTS

Vitamin and mineral supplements are either isolated from food sources or manufactured synthetically. Synthetic and natural vitamins and minerals have identical chemical structures and supposedly do the same work within the body, although there is some controversy over which are more effectively absorbed and used. It is true that, for example, vitamin B_1 (thiamine) is the same molecule however it is made. However, a natural vitamin-B complex contains all of the B vitamins in addition to other coenzymes and as-yet-unidentified compounds that may support the B vitamins' functioning in the body. Similarly, synthetic vitamin E contains a single compound, whereas natural vitamin E contains a mixture of different but related substances known as tocopherols. Recent studies have reported that taking natural vitamin E results in higher blood levels that last longer.

Whether you select a natural or synthetic formula, be aware that the contents of any supplement have to be altered in some way to put them into pill, powder, or capsule form. Many vitamin and mineral formulas contain refined sugars or artificial sweeteners, such as sucrose, mannose, xylitol, and aspartame (NutraSweet). Some health-care practitioners question whether artificial sweeteners are carcinogenic. To be safe, select a formula that does not include them. To avoid stomach upset, it is best to take vitamins and minerals with food. Minerals are best taken at the beginning of a meal. Vitamins are best taken at the end of the meal, when your stomach is full. If you are using a combination vitamin and mineral supplement, take it after a meal.

The dosages of nutritional supplements recommended in this book are therapeutic dosages. That is, they are meant to be taken for limited periods of time to address specific health concerns. They are generally higher than the recommended daily allowances (RDAs) set by the U.S. Food and Drug Administration. RDAs represent the minimum amount of nutrients needed to prevent nutrient-deficiency disease—the equivalent of the "minimum wage" for health. Many researchers agree that levels above the RDAs allow for greater health benefits.

When taking nutritional supplements, you should be aware that if a formula appears to be helping support your body, it does not follow that "more is better." Toxic overdoses of vitamins or minerals are rare, but they can occur, especially with products containing iron. Reactions to appropriate doses of vitamin and mineral supplements are likewise rare; however, you should be responsible and careful in taking them. If you develop an upset stomach or any adverse reaction, decrease the dosage or stop taking the supplement.

Follow the storage instructions on product labels. In general, you should store vitamin and mineral supplements away from heat, tightly capped, and out of reach of children. Keep vitamins A and E in the refrigerator. These two vitamins are usually oil-based and will keep longer in a cool environment. Check the expiration dates on any

formula you buy. A vitamin or mineral formula that has passed its expiration date will not have full potency.

Paying attention to diet and nutrition is perhaps the single most important supportive measure you can take for your health. A good diet will optimize health, just as a poor diet will chip away at your overall health and well-being. A healthy, nutritious diet based on clean, lean protein foods, fresh vegetables and fruits, whole grains, and legumes will increase energy, strength, and vitality—and will help your body to resist illness. Bring home food from the produce section; limit your use of prepared foods that come in boxes, cans, or frozen packages. Look for organic farmers in your area and support them, or ask your grocer to stock organic produce (or, if you can, grow your own!). Take the time to learn about preparing foods that are life enhancing—abundant in essential vitamins, minerals, and trace elements.

VITAMINS AND MINERALS

Vitamin	Function	Signs of Deficiency	U.S. RDA	Optimum Daily Intake	Food Sources
FAT-SOLUBLE VITAMINS					
Vitamin A/ Beta-carotene	Strengthens mucous membranes, the immune system, adrenal glands, and eyes.	Night blindness; eye problems; increased susceptibility to infection.	Men: 1,000 mg (333 IU) Women: 800 mg (266 IU)	10,000–35,000 IU. Do not exceed 4,000 IU during pregnancy.	Fish liver oil; dark green leafy vegetables; yellow fruits and vegetables; vitamin A-fortified milk; butter; egg yolks.
Vitamin D	Supports bone and tooth formation and muscle function. Necessary for proper absorption of calcium, phosphorus, magnesium, and zinc. Supports the healthy functioning of the thyroid gland.	Bone and tooth problems.	Men 15–24: 10 mg 24 and up: 5 mg Women 15–24: 10 mg 24 and up: 5 mg Pregnant/nursing: 10 mg	200–400 IU.	Fish liver oil; fortified milk; salmon; herring; sardines; butter; eggs. Sunshine is the best source.
Vitamin E	Aids in tissue healing. Essential for normal cell structure. Helps maintain normal enzyme function; involved in the formation of red blood cells. Believed to slow the aging of cells. Helps protect tissues from damage by pollutants.	Dry skin.	Men: 10 IU Women General: 8 IU Pregnant: 10 IU Nursing: 12 IU for the first 6 months, then 11 IU	50–800 IU.	Wheat germ oil; wheat germ; egg yolks; butter; most vegetable oils; liver; nuts; whole wheat flour; green leafy vegetables.
Vitamin K	Essential for blood clotting. Necessary for bone formation.	Blood-clotting difficulty.	Men 15–18: 65 mcg 19–24: 70 mcg 25 and up: 80 mcg Women 15–18: 55 mcg 19–24: 60 mcg 25 and up: 65 mcg Pregnant/nursing: 65 mcg	Same as RDA.	Liver; dark green leafy vegetables; vegetable oils.

VITAMINS AND MINERALS

Vitamin	Function	Signs of Deficiency	U.S. RDA	Optimum Daily Intake	Food Sources
WATER-SOLUBLE VITAMINS					
Vitamin B₁ (Thiamine)	Supports healthy functioning of the heart, muscles, and nerves. Plays a role in the breakdown of carbohydrates. Helps maintain normal enzyme function.	Fatigue; memory loss; irritability; depression.	Men 15–50: 1.5 mg 50 and up: 1.2 mg Women 15–50: 1.1 mg 51 and up: 1.0 mg Pregnant: 1.5 mg Nursing: 1.6 mg	5–10 mg.	Brewer's yeast; kidney; liver; wheat germ; peas; peanuts; whole grains; nuts; rice bran; brown rice.
Vitamin B₂ (Riboflavin)	Plays a role in the breakdown and use of carbohydrates, fats, and proteins; involved in cell energy production; supports the production of adrenal hormones; helps the body utilize other vitamins; supports the eyes.	Light sensitivity; reddening of the eyes; dry skin; depression; cracks at the corners of the mouth.	Men 15–18: 1.8 mg 19–50: 1.7 mg 51 and up: 1.4 mg Women 15–50: 1.3 mg 51 and up: 1.2 mg Pregnant: 1.6 mg Nursing: 1.8 mg for the first 6 months, then 1.7 mg	6–15 mg.	Brewer's yeast; kidney; liver; heart; milk; broccoli; Brussels sprouts; asparagus; green leafy vegetables; wheat germ; almonds; cottage cheese; yogurt; eggs; tuna; salmon.
Vitamin B₃ (Niacin)	Involved in the breakdown of carbohydrates and fats, healthy functioning of the nervous and digestive systems, and the production of sex hormones; helps maintain healthy skin.	Fatigue; irritability; insomnia; emotional instability; blood-sugar fluctuations; arthritis.	Men 15–18: 20 mg 19–50: 19 mg 51 and up: 15 mg Women 15–50: 15 mg 50 and up: 13 mg Pregnant: 17 mg Nursing: 20 mg	25–100 mg.	Brewer's yeast; liver; poultry; fish; peanuts; eggs; milk; whole grains.
Vitamin B₆ (Pyridoxine)	Involved in the breakdown of proteins, carbohydrates, and fats; involved in healthy functioning of the nervous and digestive systems; involved in the production of red blood cells and antibodies; helps maintain healthy skin.	Premenstrual tension; irritability; depression.	Men: 2 mg Women 15–18: 1.5 mg 19 and up: 1.6 mg Pregnant: 2.2 mg Nursing: 2.1 mg	10–20 mg.	Soybeans; liver; kidney; poultry; tuna; fish; bananas; legumes; potatoes; oatmeal; wheat germ.
Vitamin B₁₂ (Cobalamin)	Involved in growth and development; involved in production of red blood cells; helps the body use folic acid; supports healthy functioning of the nervous system.	Megaloblastic anemia; irritability; loss of coordination.	Men: 2 mcg Women General: 2 mcg Pregnant: 2.2 mcg Nursing: 2.6 mcg	10–100 mcg.	Liver; oysters; poultry; fish; clams; eggs; dairy products.
Biotin	Involved in metabolism of fatty acids, carbohydrates, and protein; involved in maintaining health of skin, hair, sweat glands, nerves, and bone marrow.	High cholesterol; skin problems; muscle cramps.	None established.	Not known.	Liver; kidney; egg yolks; milk; yeast; whole grains; cauliflower; nuts; legumes.
Folic Acid	Involved in growth, development, and reproduction; involved in production of red blood cells; supports healthy functioning of the nervous system; supports hair and skin.	Anemia; digestive problems; fatigue.	Men: 200 mcg Women General: 180 mcg Pregnant: 400 mcg Nursing: 280 mcg for the first 6 months, then 260 mcg	400–1,000 mcg.	Liver; salmon; eggs; asparagus; green leafy vegetables; broccoli; sweet potatoes; beans; whole wheat.

VITAMINS AND MINERALS

Vitamin	Function	Signs of Deficiency	U.S. RDA	Optimum Daily Intake	Food Sources
WATER-SOLUBLE VITAMINS (continued)					
Pantothenic acid	Involved in the breakdown and use of carbohydrates and fats; supports normal growth and development; involved in production of adrenal and sex hormones; helps the body use other vitamins; supports sinuses.	None known for pantothenic acid alone, but deficiency of any B vitamin usually means deficiency of others.	None established.	10–100 mg.	Liver; kidney; heart; fish; egg yolks; cheese; bran; whole-grain cereals; cauliflower; sweet potatoes; beans; nuts; brewer's yeast.

Vitamin C	Helps maintain normal enzyme function; important for healthy growth of teeth, bones, gums, ligaments, and blood vessels; involved in production of neurotransmitters and adrenal gland hormones; plays an important role in immune response to infection and in supporting wound healing; helps in absorption of iron from the digestive tract.	Slow wound healing; bleeding gums; recurrent infections; allergies.	Men: 60 mg
			Women
			  General: 60 mg
			  Pregnant: 70 mg
			  Nursing: 95 mg
			    for the first
			    6 months,
			    then 90 mg
				250–3,000 mg.	Rose hips; sweet peppers; broccoli; cauliflower; kale; asparagus; spinach; tomatoes; lemons; strawberries; papayas; cantaloupe; oranges; grapefruit; kiwis; liver.

BULK MINERALS					

Calcium	Plays a role in bone and tooth formation, blood clotting, heart rhythm, nerve transmission, muscle growth and contraction, proper functioning of cell membranes.	Muscle cramps; irritability; insomnia.	Men
			  15–24: 1,200 mg
			  25 and up: 800 mg
			Women
			  15–24: 1,200 mg
			  25 and up: 800 mg
			  Pregnant/nursing: 1,200 mg
				1,000–1,500 mg.	Collards; turnip greens; broccoli; kale; yogurt; milk and dairy products; tempeh; tofu.

Magnesium	Involved in blood sugar metabolism and energy maintenance; plays a role in metabolism of calcium and vitamin C; involved in structuring of basic genetic material (DNA and RNA).	Depression; muscle tension; irritability; nervousness and hyperactivity; constipation; premenstrual tension; fatigue; muscle cramps.	Men
			  15–18: 400 mg
			  19 and up: 350 mg
			Women
			  15–18: 300 mg
			  19 and up: 280 mg
			  Pregnant: 320 mg
			  Nursing: 355 mg for the first 6 months, then 340 mg
				400–600 mg	Soybeans; whole grains; shellfish; salmon; liver; almonds; cashews; molasses; bananas; potatoes; milk; green vegetables; honey.

Phosphorus	Involved in bone and tooth formation, cell growth and repair, energy maintenance, heart contraction, kidney function, healthy activity of nerves and muscles, the body's use of vitamins.	Muscle cramps; dizziness; bone problems.	Men
			  15–24: 1,200 mg
			  25 and up: 800 mg
			Women
			  15–24: 1,200 mg
			  25 and up: 800 mg
			  Pregnant/nursing: 1,200 mg
				800–1,200 mg	Fish; poultry; eggs; whole grains; yellow cheese.

Potassium	Involved in healthy, steady functioning of the nervous system; supports the heart, muscles, kidneys, blood.	Muscle fatigue; general fatigue; swelling in extremities; irregular heartbeat.	None established.	Not known, but the recommended number of servings of fruits and vegetables supplies about 3,500 mg per day.	Dried apricots; cantaloupe; bananas; citrus fruit; lima beans; potatoes; avocados; broccoli; liver; milk; peanut butter.

VITAMINS AND MINERALS

Mineral	Function	Signs of Deficiency	U.S. RDA	Optimum Daily Intake	Food Sources
BULK MINERALS (continued)					
Sodium	Helps maintain normal fluid levels in the body; involved In healthy muscle functioning; supports blood and lymph system.	Fainting; intolerance to heat; muscle cramps; swelling in extremities.	None established.	Not known, but most nutritionists recommend 3,000 mg per day or less.	Most foods and water, especially salt; salted foods; soy sauce; cheese; milk; seafood.
TRACE ELEMENTS					
Boron	May help maintain bone strength.	Unknown.	None established.	Not known.	Present in many foods, but content varies depending on soil content.
Chromium	Involved in maintaining blood-sugar level and in healthy functioning of the circulatory system.	Blood-sugar fluctuations; high cholesterol level.	None established.	200 mcg.	Brewer's yeast; liver; cheese; legumes; peas; whole grains; black pepper; molasses.
Cobalt	Involved in healthy function-ing of red blood cells.	Pernicious anemia; weak-ness; nausea; loss of appetite; bleeding gums.	None established.	Not known.	Organ meats; milk; beet greens; spinach; cabbage.
Copper	Plays a role in bone formation, hair and skin color, healing processes, red blood cell production, and mental and emotional processes.	Anemia; inflammation; arthritis.	None established.	2–3 mg.	Shellfish; liver; poultry; cherries; nuts; cocoa; gelatin; whole grains; eggs; legumes; peas; avocados.
Iodine	Important for thyroid health, support of metabolic rate, and health of skin, hair, and hails.	Goiter (swelling of thyroid); cold extremeties, fatigue; depression.	Men: 150 mcg Women General: 150 mcg Pregnant: 175 mcg Nursing: 200 mcg	250 mcg.	Kelp; sea vegetables; iodized salt.
Iron	Supports growth and develop-ment in children; involved in the production of hemoglobin; helps build resistance to disease.	Fatigue; anemia; intolerance to cold; intellectual impairment.	Men 15–18: 12 mg 19 and up: 10 mg Women 15–50: 15 mg 51 and up: 10 mg Pregnant: 30 mg Nursing: 15 mg	Men: 10 mg Women Pre-menopausal: 20 mg Postmeno-pausal: 10 mg	Blackstrap molasses; liver; eggs; fish; spinach; asparagus; prunes; raisins; sea vegetables.
Manganese	Maintains strong bones, aids metabolism and activation of enzyme systems.	Poor muscular coordination; glandular dysfunctions.	None established.	Not known.	Yeast; beets; bananas; blueberries; whole grains.
Selenium	Involved in healthy functioning of cell membranes; may be in-volved in increasing resistance to cancer; supports pancreatic functioning; helps the body use vitamin E effectively.	Poor tissue repair; dry flaky scalp; skin problems; cancer.	Men 15–18: 50 mcg 19 and up: 70 mcg Women 15–18: 50 mcg 19 and up: 55 mcg Pregnant: 65 mcg Nursing: 75 mcg	200 mcg.	Whole grains; soy-beans; tuna; seafood; Brazil nuts; brown rice; pineapples.

VITAMINS AND MINERALS

Mineral	Function	Signs of Deficiency	U.S. RDA	Optimum Daily Intake	Food Sources
TRACE ELEMENTS (continued)					
Silicon	Involved in bone formation; supports skin, major blood vessels, connective tissue, and thymus gland.	Bone deformities; connective tissue disorders; muscle cramps; irritability; insomnia.	None established.	Not known.	Foods high in fiber (apples, celery, etc.).
Sulfur	Enhances hair, nail, skin, and nerve structure formation.	None known, but may lead to premature aging of skin.	None established.	Not known.	Egg yolks, fish, poultry, milk.

Zinc	Promotes burn and wound healing; supports the immune system; involved in carbohydrate and protein digestion; plays a role in reproductive organ growth and development.	White spots on fingernails; stretch marks on skin; loss of sense of smell or taste; joint pains, poor sex drive; menstrual irregularities; prostate problems; slow wound healing; recurrent infections; acne.	Men: 15 mg
			Women
			  General: 12 mg
			  Pregnant:15 mg
			  Nursing: 19 mg for
			    the first 6 months,
			    then 16 mg.
				15–35 mg.	Brewer's yeast; liver; seafood; wheat germ; bran; oatmeal; nuts; peas; carrots; spinach; sunflower seeds.

Home and Personal Safety

We're all familiar with the saying that most accidents happen in the home. Well, it's true. It makes sense, therefore, to do everything you can to prevent household accidents. Most accidents happen when we are simply too busy, too tired, or too short of time to pay proper attention to what we are doing. When you are simultaneously talking on the telephone and trying to prepare dinner after an exhausting day at work, for example, it's easy to let your attention wander from the sharp paring knife in your hand and accidentally cut yourself. If you're running out the door because you're late for an appointment, you may suddenly find yourself slipping and stumbling on the stairs. Children, older people, and people with physical and mental disabilities are particularly prone to accidental injury.

Not all accidents can be prevented, of course, but many can be. The following are some recommendations that can help you reduce the chance that you will suffer an accidental injury. You may have already taken many of the measures discussed here, but some of them may surprise you.

❏ Make sure every room in your home has a working smoke detector. If detectors are wired in, it is a good idea to have a battery-operated backup in case of a power outage. Check and replace batteries as needed, at least once a year.

❏ Install a carbon-monoxide detector in your home. Carbon monoxide is a potentially deadly gas that can accumulate in the home as a result of a malfunctioning heating system, among other things. You can't see it or smell it, so the best way to be sure your home is safe is to use a detector.

❏ Have your furnace and chimney (as well as fireplaces and/or woodstoves, if you have them) inspected and cleaned annually by a qualified professional.

❏ Keep a fire extinguisher in a handy location near the stove (if you have children, mount it high enough to be out of their reach).

❏ If you have any electrical appliance with a frayed or damaged cord, do not use it. Either replace the appliance or have a qualified person replace the cord.

❏ Apply nonslip surfaces to the bottoms of bathtubs and showers. Installing a handrail in the bath or shower is also a good idea.

❏ Anchor area rugs securely with nonslip padding and/or carpet tape.

❏ Make sure sliding glass doors have opaque etching, or affix colored decals to the glass to make it visible.

❏ If you must take medication on an ongoing basis, take measures to ensure you take the drug on schedule and avoid an accidental overdose. One way to do this is to use a pill dispenser with a different compartment (or multiple compartments) for each day of the week. Another way is to use a medication chart to keep track of what you have taken. You may be able to obtain such a chart from your doctor, or you can create a simple chart yourself. Simply draw a grid listing the days of the week in the first column and the times you are supposed to take the medication across the top. Post the chart in a convenient place, such as on the inside of the door of the cabinet where you store your medications, and after you take each dose, place a check in the appropriate box in the grid. This is particularly valuable if you must take more than one type of medication. Keep a separate chart for each medication you take.

❏ Store all medications in their original bottles, away from heat and moisture. Throw away old prescriptions and any over-the-counter medications that have passed their expiration dates.

❏ If you take several different prescriptions, affix color-coded labels to the bottles to aid you in telling them apart to minimize the risk that you will take the wrong pill by mistake. If you have a problem with color vision, use different-shaped labels instead. Or place a different number of drops of glue on each bottle and allow the drops to dry to give yourself tactile cues.

❏ Eat slowly and chew your food thoroughly. This helps to avoid choking (it's also good for weight control).

❏ Never store nonfood items such as household cleaners in empty food containers. This can lead to dangerous mistakes.

❏ If you have a chronic medical condition such as diabetes, a seizure disorder, or severe allergies to certain drugs or other substances, obtain a Medic Alert bracelet or pendant and wear it at all times. Should you become ill and unable to speak for yourself, this will ensure that you get appropriate care. (*See* Medic Alert below).

❏ Wear appropriate protective gear, particularly a helmet, for such activities as bicycling and roller-blading. Wear goggles when operating power tools, including lawn-mowers.

❏ Learn to swim and practice water safety. Even if you are a good swimmer, wear a personal flotation device (PFD) for boating, canoeing, kayaking, or waterskiing.

❏ Before skating on a frozen pond, check with local authorities to make sure the ice is safe.

❏ Do not play with fireworks. Most states prohibit the sale of fireworks to individuals, but people still manage to obtain them. Every year, a number of people suffer severe burns—and worse—from accidents connected with fireworks.

❏ Never mix alcohol or any other substance that can impair awareness with driving, bicycling, boating, operating machinery, or any other activity that requires motor skill.

❏ It may sound obvious, but try to avoid undue haste. Use handrails when climbing stairs. Focus on whatever task you are performing, make sure you have sufficient light, and use the appropriate tool(s) for the job. Untold numbers of accidents are the result of nothing more than a moment's inattention or poor judgment.

In addition to taking measures to prevent accidents, it is important to be prepared for emergencies. Not all accidents can be prevented, even by the most conscientious person, so this is an important safety precaution. Learn cardiopulmonary resuscitation (CPR) and first aid. The Red Cross offers courses in these subjects, as do many hospitals. The important thing is to learn these procedures *before* you need to use them.

Post emergency telephone numbers near every telephone in your home. This can save precious time in an emergency. We urge you to take this precaution now, while you are thinking about it. Post numbers for your local fire department, Poison Control Center, police, and your doctor and dentist. If your telephone is the type that allows you to program numbers for automatic dialing, enter these emergency numbers into the phone as well, and label the appropriate keys clearly. Some telephone models come with keys already labeled for police, fire, and other emergency numbers, which makes this even easier. However, you should not consider this a substitute for keeping emergency numbers on hand in written form. It is possible for programmed numbers to be erased accidentally, so you should still keep a list of emergency telephone numbers in a convenient location.

Assemble and keep, in a convenient but secure location, a home health kit stocked with the basics for dealing with illness and injury (see page 68). Check expiration dates periodically and replace any outdated products promptly. If you know that what you need is ready and on hand, you can save yourself from frantic searching and scrambling. This translates into faster treatment and a less anxiety-filled experience, both invaluable parts of health and healing.

Medic Alert

More than 220,000 Americans are rushed to emergency rooms every day, and over 13,000 of them face life-threatening delays and potentially serious complications because the attending doctors lack information about their medical histories and/or allergies. This is particularly true in the case of people who are too badly injured or too ill to give the necessary information to the physician.

One way to make sure medical personnel have access to the information they need is to wear a Medic Alert bracelet or pendant. The company says that since it was founded in 1956, its bracelets have saved more than 80,000 lives. The individualized bracelets provide instant identification of existing medical conditions, as well as noting any allergies, and they are also engraved with your name and address, thus providing immediate identification. In addition, Medic Alert maintains a central registry of vital medical and personal facts that can be accessed by medical personnel in seconds. This vital information helps paramedics and doctors to provide safe and appropriate emergency care. Simply because necessary information is immediately available, a person wearing a Medic Alert bracelet is likely to receive faster and more comprehensive medical attention. The bracelet or pendant can, and should, be worn at all times.

More than 2 million Americans and over 1.5 million people abroad are members of the organization. Many of these people have diabetes, while others have asthma, seizure disorders, heart problems, and a variety of other conditions. Still others have blood-clotting disorders or severe allergies that could lead to a life-threatening reaction if they are exposed to a particular allergen, be it a drug or other substance.

Anyone with a serious medical condition and/or known allergies would be well advised to wear a Medic Alert bracelet or pendant at all times. The membership cost is quite reasonable, particularly when you consider the life-saving potential of this service. For more information, contact Medic Alert (see the Resources section at the end of the book).

Assembling a Home Health Kit

Assembling a home health kit will give you a good base for treating common illnesses and injuries. Begin putting it together now, so that if you do get hurt or sick, the right treatments and remedies will be close at hand. Use the checklist below as a guide to some of the most important elements for different treatment approaches.

BARE ESSENTIALS

- Ace bandage.
- Adhesive bandages (Band-Aids).
- Hot water bottle.
- Ice bag.
- Rubbing alcohol, hydrogen peroxide, or witch hazel, for disinfecting wounds and sterilizing needle and tweezers.

- Prescription insect bite kit containing adrenaline (such as Ana-Kit or epiPen) if you have a history of severe allergic reactions.
- Scissors with rounded tips.
- Sling and safety pins.
- Sterile gauze pads and adhesive tape.
- Sterile razor blade.

- Sterilized needle.
- Syrup of ipecac.
  Caution: Syrup of ipecac should not be used except at the direction of a doctor or Poison Control Center.
- Thermometer.
- Tweezers.

CONVENTIONAL MEDICINE

- Aspirin, acetaminophen (Tylenol or the equivalent), or ibuprofen (Advil, Nuprin, or the equivalent).
- An antihistamine (such as Benadryl or Chlor-Trimeton).

- An antiseptic ointment (such as bacitracin or Betadine).
- An antacid (such as Maalox or Mylanta).
- A decongestant (such as Sudafed).
- Emetrol syrup.

- Milk of magnesia.
- Pepto-Bismol.
- An antidiarrheal such as loperamide (in Imodium AD and other products).

HERBAL MEDICINES

- Aloe vera gel.
- Calendula cream or ointment.
- Chamomile tea or extract.
- Collagen gel such as Smart Gel.
- Cranberry capsules.
- Echinacea capsules and liquid extract.

- Elderberry extract.
- Flaxseed tea.
- Garlic, in capsules or fresh.
- Ginger root, in capsules or fresh.
- Goldenseal capsules or liquid extract.
- Grape-seed extract.

- Licorice root extract.
- Olive leaf extract.
- Peppermint tea or extract.
- Slippery elm powder.
- Turmeric or feverfew.
- Umeboshi plum paste.

HOMEOPATHIC REMEDIES

- *Aconite.*
- *Apis mellifica.*
- *Argentum nitricum.*
- *Arnica.*
- *Arnica* ointment.
- *Arsenicum album.*
- *Belladonna.*
- *Bryonia.*
- *Calcarea carbonica.*

- *Cantharis.*
- *Carbo vegetabilis.*
- *Chamomilla.*
- *China.*
- *Colocynthis.*
- *Ferrum phosphoricum.*
- *Gelsemium.*
- *Hepar sulphuris calcareum.*
- *Hypericum.*

- *Hypericum opintment.*
- *Ignatia amara.*
- *Kali bichromicum.*
- *Lachesis.*
- *Ledum.*
- *Lydopodium.*
- *Magnesia phosphorica.*
- *Mercurius solubilis.*
- *Natrum muriaticum.*

- *Nux vomica.*
- *Phosphorus.*
- *Pulsatilla.*
- *Rhus toxicodendron.*
- *Ruta graveolens.*
- *Sulfur.*
- *Thuja.*
- *Urtica urens.*
- *Urtica urens* ointment.

BACH FLOWER REMEDIES

- Rescue Remedy.

NUTRITIONAL SUPPLEMENTS

- Vitamin A.
- Vitamin-B complex.

- Vitamin C with bioflavonoids.
- A probiotics supplement (acidophilus and/or bifidobacteria).

- A calcium and magnesium combination formula.
- Zinc lozenges.

MISCELLANEOUS

- Fruit-flavored yogurt, applesauce, or tomato or vegetable juice to mix with herbs or crushed tablets.

- Grapefruit-seed extract for purifying water in emergencies (*see* WATER PURIFICATION in Part Three).
- Honey, barley malt, or rice bran syrup.

- Save•A•Tooth solution (*see* TOOTH, BROKEN OR KNOCKED OUT, in Part Two).
- Smelling salts.

Pets and Your Health

For many people, one of the most delightful aspects of life is interacting with pets. Having the companionship of a domestic animal usually brings a unique type of unconditional love into a person's life. But in some circumstances, pets can be implicated in human health problems. Allergies are probably the most common type of pet-related condition, but there are also a number of diseases that can be transmitted from pets to humans.

Infectious and parasitic diseases in humans can be caused by viruses, bacteria, fungi, protozoa, worms, insects, or mites living on or in an animal. Pet-borne diseases—especially the more serious ones—are rare, but they do occur. When animals transmit diseases or parasites to humans, it is usually through saliva or by direct contact. Ticks, mites, and fungi living in an animal's fur or feathers can be transferred to a person who hugs or strokes an animal. Fleas will jump from an infested area onto a human if no animal host is available. Worm eggs or parasites infesting contaminated animal feces can be accidentally transmitted to humans by fingers or food.

The transmission of serious diseases from animals to humans can be prevented by practicing common sense and good hygiene. To make sure that you do not accidentally come in contact with animal feces, which may be contaminated, designate a separate, fenced outdoor area as your dog's toilet facility, and "scoop" the area regularly to keep it clean so that he doesn't bring bits of fecal matter into the house on his feet. Keep a cat's litter box scrupulously clean; sift out feces regularly and sweep up and carefully dispose of any litter that spills outside the box. This task should *not* be performed by a woman who is, or plans to become, pregnant (see Toxoplasmosis, below).

Make sure your pets get good routine health care, including regular worming and flea treatment. Avoid unnecessary handling of any animal that is obviously ill, and take a sick pet to the veterinarian promptly for treatment.

Following is a discussion of some of the diseases that humans can contract through contact with animals.

DISEASES TRANSMITTED BY DOGS

Hookworms. Hookworms typically infect the lower intestine, but can also cause pneumonia. People who have walked barefoot in areas where worm-containing dog feces have been dropped are particularly at risk of a hookworm infestation. Symptoms include a red and intensely itchy rash that develops around the site where the larvae penetrate the skin, typically on the feet. Treatment consists of drugs that rid the body of the worms. If you become anemic, a common consequence of more than mild infection (the worms attach themselves to the wall of the small intestine and suck blood there), you may require supplemental iron. In the case of an ex-tremely serious, long-lasting infestation, a blood transfusion may become necessary.

Ticks. A tick is a blood-sucking arachnid. Barbs on its proboscis, or feeding snout, enable a tick to attach itself to the skin of its victim to feed. Ticks are extremely tenacious. Even when fully engorged with blood, they seldom let go spontaneously. Because the barbs are deeply embedded, it is useless to try to pull a tick off with your fingers. Even if you manage to pinch off the body completely, the head and feeding proboscis can remain attached. The most effective way to remove a tick is to use a pair of tweezers. Grasp the tick's head as close to your skin as you can, then pull back slowly and firmly until the tick pulls free. Once the tick is removed, thoroughly wash and rinse the site of the injury. To reduce the risk of infection, apply rubbing alcohol or calendula tincture, followed by an antibiotic ointment, such as bacitracin, Betadine, or goldenseal.

DISEASES TRANSMITTED BY CATS

Cat-scratch disease. Cat-scratch disease (also known as cat-scratch fever) begins with a scratch or a claw puncture that becomes infected and resembles a small boil. The scratch may be deep and obvious, or it may not leave a mark at all. Cat-scratch disease is most commonly reported in children under ten years of age. The probable cause is a microbe called *Bartonella* (formerly *Rochalimaea*) *henselae,* which may be transmitted from cat to cat by fleas. Symptoms include swollen lymph nodes, weakness, nausea, chills, loss of appetite, headache, and low-grade fever. Some people run a fever; others break out in a measles-like rash. The symptoms can last for months and, in rare cases, can progress to encephalitis, an inflammation of the brain.

Conventional antibiotics show varying but limited effectiveness against cat-scratch disease, although trimethoprim-sulfa (Bactrim or Septra) and erythomycin are sometimes tried in complicated cases. Standard treatment includes washing the site of a cat scratch well, applying a disinfectant promptly, and keeping the area clean. Natural treatments (such as those recommended under SURGERY, RECOVERY FROM in Part Two of this book) can help support your body as it fights off the infection.

Toxoplasmosis. A central nervous system disease, toxoplasmosis is caused by a single-celled organism, the protozoan *Toxoplasma gondii,* which is particularly fond of cats. Symptoms can include fever, blurred vision, swollen lymph nodes, muscle aches, and an enlarged spleen. This disease is usually transmitted to humans through infected cat feces, although inadequately cooked meat may also be a source. Toxoplasmosis is especially dangerous to children *before* they are born. If a mother-to-be becomes infected with toxoplasmosis, there is a possibility the parasite may migrate through the placenta to the fetus. A toxoplasmosis infection in early pregnancy can cause a miscarriage or severe malformation of the unborn child; in later pregnancy, it can result in serious damage to the developing child's nervous system. A child infected with toxoplasmosis as a fetus may become blind in early childhood.

In adults, the infection is not usually serious, though it can last for up to two months. Many people experience either no symptoms at all or a mild illness with episodes of achiness and fever resembling mononucleosis. However, for people with compromised immune systems, such as those with cancer or HIV disease, or persons who must take immunosuppressive drugs, this infection can present a recurrent problem and can affect the brain, causing seizures, confusion, headaches, and/or various nerve-deficit problems. In some cases, the heart, lungs, or liver—or even several organs at once—may be affected.

Treatment of toxoplasmosis is complicated and involves multiple medications, and it should be handled by a medical doctor with expertise in this condition. To prevent fetal infection, a pregnant woman should never change a cat's litter box.

DISEASES TRANSMITTED BY BOTH DOGS AND CATS

Fleas. Flea bites are usually more of a nuisance than a serious health problem, although they do itch and may become infected if they are scratched. Fleas prefer animal hosts. But if any fleas get left behind when the household pet is out, they will feed on whatever human is handy. Treatment for flea bites begins with thorough cleansing of the site. To reduce the itching that can prompt you to scratch, you can use calamine or Caladryl lotion, or witch hazel.

Rabies. On the opposite end of the scale, rabies is a deadly disease. Any animal bite can cause bleeding and shock, but a person who is bitten by a rabid animal requires immediate vaccination (*see under* BITES, ANIMAL AND HUMAN in Part Two of this book). The animals most likely to be affected are dogs, cats, skunks, raccoons, and bats. Rats, mice, chipmunks, squirrels, hamsters, guinea pigs, gerbils, and rabbits are rarely implicated. Any animal suspected of carrying rabies should be quarantined for at least ten days.

Ringworm. A surprising number of ringworm infections come from family pets, especially cats. Unlike infected dogs, which are afflicted with hair loss and bare patches, cats rarely show obvious signs when carrying this infection. To check a cat for ringworm, examine its coat closely under ultraviolet (UV) light. UV rays cause the fungus to glow, making it visible on infected skin and hair (*see* RINGWORM in Part Two).

Toxocariasis. This is a serious parasitic disease. You can contract toxocariasis through accidental ingestion of worm eggs, which are present in infested dog or cat feces. Children, especially the few who eat dirt, are particularly at risk. As the worm passes through the body, it can cause asthma-like and other allergic symptoms, respiratory difficulties, an enlarged liver, and skin rashes. Drug therapy is not very useful in fighting this disease, but most people recover on their own. In rare cases, a worm egg can infect an eye, causing deteriorating vision or even blindness. This manifestation of toxocariasis is most likely to occur in children who frequently play in soil or sand that has been contaminated by infected dog or cat feces. It must be treated by an ophthalmologist.

DISEASES TRANSMITTED BY BIRDS

Psittacosis. This is a serious chlamydial disease that can be life-threatening if untreated. The first symptoms—fever, chills, and body aches—are similar to those of many other infectious diseases. Rapid breathing and coughing develop as the condition progresses to pneumonia. Psittacosis is usually treated successfully with antibiotics and cough suppressants, although some people develop difficulty breathing during the course of the disease and may have to be supported with oxygen therapy. The most serious cases can involve endocarditis, or inflammation of the inner lining of the heart. It can take weeks, even months, to achieve full recovery.

Psittacosis can be contracted by inhaling dust that comes from the feathers or droppings of infected birds. Parrots, parakeets, and related species are more likely to be infected than other types of birds. There is a simple blood test that can be performed to determine whether a bird has, or has been exposed to, psittacosis. Therefore, the best way to prevent this disease is to have all birds examined and tested by an avian veterinarian (a veterinarian who specializes in birds). If a bird is found to be infected, it can be treated; if found to be free of infection, it will remain so unless exposed to an infected bird at a later time.

DISEASES TRANSMITTED BY REPTILES

Salmonellosis. Salmonellosis is a bacterial disease that can be picked up from handling certain pets, particularly turtles and lizards, including iguanas. Symptoms most often include abdominal pain and cramping followed by diarrhea. It is treated with antibiotics.

Many reptiles normally carry the *Salmonella* bacteria in their systems without becoming ill, so it is wise to assume that any reptile pet you have probably is carrying the bacteria, and take steps to protect yourself. The single most important thing you can do is to practice meticulous hygiene. Always wash your hands thoroughly, scrubbing well around the fingernails, after handling the animal, and do not permit it on countertops or any areas where foods are prepared. Also, keep the animal's living quarters as clean as possible. Ask your veterinarian for recommendations concerning how, and how often, to clean and/or sterilize items your pet comes into contact with regularly.

Part Two

Common Health Problems

Disorders from A to Z
with Recommendations for
Conventional and Natural Treatment

Introduction

Part One introduced you to the basic practices of conventional and a variety of natural health-care approaches, as well as the importance of diet and nutrition, exercise, and personal safety precautions. In Part Two you will find an alphabetic listing of common health problems and available treatments for them. These entries include conventional medical approaches as well as natural treatments you can use at home to speed healing and keep yourself more comfortable.

Each individual entry contains a description and explanation of the disorder, followed by discussions of possible treatments. Information about emergency treatment, where appropriate, is given first. Recommendations for conventional medical treatment, diet, nutritional supplements, herbal treatment, homeopathy, Bach flower remedies, acupressure, and aromatherapy follow. Also included are general recommendations for measures that fall outside the range of other treatment approaches and advice on prevention. Because not every treatment category is useful for each problem, not all entries include recommendations for all therapies. For example, acupressure is not useful in the treatment of athlete's foot, so no acupressure techniques are recommended in that entry.

The authors believe that you should be responsible, curious, and thoughtful in making your health-care choices. Ask questions, read, learn everything you can. By using the guidelines that follow, you can determine when you require conventional care, when you might try natural medicines, and how to develop an integrated approach combining the best of both.

A Guide to Common Symptoms

The guide below lists some of the more common symptoms people experience, together with possible causes, to help you decide which entries may be most helpful to you in a particular circumstance. Although you may be experiencing one or some of the symptoms listed here, you may or may not have any of the illnesses mentioned. Disorders are listed here because they *can* cause the particular symptom, and they are listed in alphabetical order, not in order of the likelihood of occurrence. This chart is not meant to substitute for the advice of a qualified health-care provider. Always consult with your doctor or other practitioner for a professional diagnosis.

Symptom	Possible Causes
Abdominal pain	Anxiety, appendicitis, candida infection, celiac disease, cirrhosis, constipation, Crohn's disease, diarrhea, diverticular disease, drug reaction or withdrawal, endometriosis, fibroids, food allergies, food poisoning, gallbladder problems, gas, hepatitis, hiatal hernia, indigestion, intestinal obstruction, intestinal parasites, irritable bowel syndrome, kidney disease, kidney stones, menstrual problems, motion sickness, nausea, pelvic inflammatory disease, peptic ulcer, premenstrual syndrome, urinary tract infection.
Anal itching	Candida infection, contact allergy, gonorrhea, hemorrhoids, intestinal parasites, local irritation, rectal fissure, scabies, sexually transmitted disease, trichomoniasis.
Increased appetite	Anxiety, bulimia, depression, diabetes, drug abuse, drug reaction, hyperthyroidism, hypoglycemia, intestinal parasites, nicotine withdrawal, premenstrual syndrome.
Loss of appetite	Anemia, appendicitis, cancer, chronic fatigue syndrome, cirrhosis, constipation, Crohn's disease, depression, hepatitis, HIV disease, hyperthyroidism, kidney disease, secondary syphilis, tuberculosis, virtually any viral or bacterial infection.
Backache	Kidney disease, kidney stones, low back pain, menstrual problems, muscle strain, premenstrual syndrome, prostatitis, stress, urinary tract infection.
Bad breath	Diabetes, poor digestion, oral herpes, poor oral hygiene, postnasal drip, tonsillitis, sinusitis, strep throat, tooth decay.
Painful bowel movement	Constipation, Crohn's disease, hemorrhoids, irritable bowel syndrome, rectal fissure/tear.
Breast pain/tenderness	Cancer, fibrocystic breast disease, hormonal fluctuations, premenstrual syndrome.
Difficulty breathing/ shortness of breath	Anaphylactic shock, anemia, acute anxiety, asthma, cardiovascular disease, inhaled foreign object (choking), emphysema, hyperthyroidism, pneumonia, shock.
Chest pain/discomfort	Acid reflux, acute anxiety, candida infection, cardiovascular disease, hiatal hernia, pneumonia.
Difficulty concentrating	Anxiety, chronic fatigue syndrome, concussion, drug abuse/withdrawal, drug reaction, nutritional deficiencies.
Loss of consciousness	Anaphylactic shock, concussion, drug abuse, drug reaction/withdrawal, meningitis, seizure, shock, stroke.
Cough	Acid reflux, allergies, bronchitis, candida infection, common cold, flu, food allergy, hay fever, inhaled irritant, pneumonia, sore throat, stress, tuberculosis, viral or bacterial infection.
Diarrhea	Anatomical deformity, candida infection, celiac disease, colitis, Crohn's disease, diverticular disease, drug reaction/withdrawal, fatigue, food allergy/sensitivity, food poisoning, hepatitis, HIV disease, intestinal parasites, irritable bowel syndrome, pancreatitis, any viral, bacterial, fungal, or parasitic infection.

Symptom	Possible Causes
Dizziness	Anemia, anxiety, cardiovascular disease, concussion, diabetic insulin reaction, drug abuse/withdrawal, drug reaction, eating disorders, fever, fibromyalgia, high blood pressure, hormonal fluctuations, hypoglycemia, Meniere's disease, motion sickness, multiple sclerosis, shock, stroke, temporomandibular joint syndrome.
Earache	Common cold, ear infection, Meniere's disease, mumps, sinusitis, temporomandibular joint syndrome.
Difficulty eating	Cancer, canker sores, dry mouth, HIV disease, thrush.
Eye inflammation/watering/itching	Allergies, blepharitis, chalazion, common cold, conjunctivitis, contact-lens problems, corneal abrasion, food allergies, hay fever, onset of measles, stye.
Eye pain	Contact-lens problems, dry eyes, eyestrain, acute glaucoma, uveitis.
Fatigue/weakness	Anemia, anxiety, cancer, candida infection, cardiovascular disease, chronic fatigue syndrome, cirrhosis, Crohn's disease, depression, diabetes, drug reaction, eating disorder, flu, HIV disease, hyperthyroidism, hypoglycemia, hypothyroidism, insufficient sleep, intestinal parasites, lupus, Lyme or other tickborne disease, menopause, menstrual problems, mononucleosis, multiple sclerosis, poor nutrition, premenstrual syndrome, seizure, shock, sleep apnea, stress, stroke, any viral or bacterial infection.
Fever	Certain types of cancer, Crohn's disease, dehydration, diverticulitis, drug reaction/withdrawal, flu, inflamed gallbladder, heatstroke, hepatitis, HIV disease, kidney disease, lupus, meningitis, pelvic inflammatory disease, pneumonia, prostatitis, sinusitis, secondary syphilis, tuberculosis, any viral or bacterial infection.
Fluid retention/bloating/swelling	Allergies, candida infection, cardiovascular disease, celiac disease, cirrhosis, food allergies, hormonal fluctuations, kidney disease, lymphedema, premenstrual syndrome.
Hair loss	Drug reaction, heredity, hormonal fluctuations, lupus, nutritional deficiencies, physical trauma, ringworm, shingles, stress, secondary syphilis, thyroid disorders, tuberculosis.
Headache	Anemia, cancer (brain tumor), chronic fatigue syndrome, concussion, diabetic insulin reaction, drug reaction/withdrawal, eyestrain, fibromyalgia, food allergies, acute glaucoma, high blood pressure, hormonal imbalance, hypoglycemia, Lyme disease, meningitis, menopause, migraine, mononucleosis, mumps, premenstrual syndrome, sinusitis, stress, stroke, temporomandibular joint syndrome, uveitis.
Hearing loss/disturbance	Ear infection, Meniere's disease, stroke, temporomandibular joint syndrome, tinnitus.
Irregular heartbeat/heart palpitations	Anaphylactic shock, anemia, anorexia nervosa, anxiety, bulimia, cardiovascular disease, drug abuse/withdrawal, drug reaction, fibromyalgia, hyperthyroidism, Lyme disease, menopause, shock, stress.
Irritability/agitation/restlessness	Alcoholism, Alzheimer's disease, onset of anaphylactic shock, anxiety, diabetes, drug abuse/withdrawal, drug reaction, hyperthyroidism, hypoglycemia, meningitis, menopause, premenstrual syndrome, stress, shock.
Jaw pain	Injury, mumps, sinusitis, temporomandibular joint syndrome, tetanus, tooth decay.
Joint pain	Arthritis, bunion, bursitis, candida infection, chronic fatigue syndrome, fibromyalgia, gout, intestinal parasites, lupus, Lyme or other tickborne disease, rheumatic fever, sprain, secondary syphilis.
Light sensitivity	Blepharitis, concussion, corneal abrasion, drug abuse/withdrawal, drug reaction, glaucoma, hyperthyroidism, onset of measles, onset of migraine, photophobia, uveitis.
Enlarged lymph nodes	Chronic fatigue syndrome, genital herpes, HIV disease, Lyme or other tickborne disease, mononucleosis, any viral or bacterial infection.

Symptom	Possible Causes
Malaise (general body-wide discomfort)	Anxiety, chronic fatigue syndrome, depression, fever, fibromyalgia, food poisoning, hepatitis, intestinal parasites, lupus, mononucleosis, any viral or bacterial infection.
Memory lapses	Alcoholism, allergies, Alzheimer's disease, anxiety, systemic candidiasis, chronic fatigue syndrome, concussion, drug abuse, drug reaction, fibromyalgia, inattention, stress.
Abnormal/heavy menstrual bleeding	Cancer, endometriosis, fibroids, hypothyroidism, pelvic inflammatory disease.
Absence of menstrual bleeding	Cancer, eating disorders, hyperthyroidism, menopause, severe weight loss, stress.
Mood/personality changes	Alcoholism, Alzheimer's disease, anxiety, chronic fatigue syndrome, chronic pain, depression, drug abuse/withdrawal, drug reaction, fibromyalgia, hormonal fluctuations, hypoglycemia, manic-depressive disorder, menopause, multiple sclerosis, premenstrual syndrome, stress.
Mouth sores	Canker sores, oral herpes, HIV disease, onset of measles, nutritional deficiencies, thrush.
Muscle aches and pains	Candida infection, chronic fatigue syndrome, fibromyalgia, hypothyroidism, Lyme or other tickborne disease, menopause, multiple sclerosis, muscle strain, overexertion, restless legs syndrome, sprain, tendinitis, any viral or bacterial infection.
Muscle rigidity	Multiple sclerosis, Parkinson's disease, seizure, tetanus.
Runny/stuffy nose	Allergies, bronchitis, candida infection, common cold, drug abuse, drug reaction/withdrawal, food allergies, hay fever, sinusitis.
Numbness/tingling sensations	Anxiety, candida infection, carpal tunnel syndrome, concussion, drug reaction, hypothyroidism, multiple sclerosis, Raynaud's phenomenon, restless legs syndrome, seizure, stroke.
Altered sex drive	Alcoholism, anxiety, depression, drug abuse, drug reaction, menopause, chronic pain, premenstrual syndrome, stress.
Painful sexual intercourse	Chlamydia, endometriosis, fibroids, pelvic inflammatory disease, trichomoniasis, vaginitis.
Skin rash, lesions, or bumps	Acne, allergies, athlete's foot, boils, bruises, candida infection, chickenpox, dandruff, dermatitis, eczema, heat rash, herpes, insect bites, intestinal parasites, lupus, Lyme or other tickborne disease, measles, poison ivy, psoriasis, ringworm, rosacea, scabies, seborrhea, shingles, skin cancer, sunburn, syphilis, varicose veins, warts.
Difficulty sleeping	Anemia, anxiety, chronic fatigue syndrome, chronic pain, depression, drug abuse/withdrawal, drug reaction, fibromyalgia, hyperthyroidism, irregular schedule, jet lag, menopause, restless legs syndrome, sleep apnea, snoring, stress.
Bloody stools/rectal bleeding	Cancer, colitis, Crohn's disease, diverticular disease, hemorrhoids, rectal tear/fissure.
Sweating	Onset of anaphylactic shock, acute anxiety, cardiovascular disease, drug abuse/withdrawal, drug reaction, diabetic insulin reaction, heat exhaustion, high blood pressure, HIV disease, hyperthyroidism, hypoglycemia, overexertion, shock.
Testicular pain	Cancer, epididymitis, mumps.
Excessive thirst	Dehydration, diabetes, drug reaction/withdrawal.
Tremors	Anxiety, drug abuse/withdrawal, drug reaction, hyperthyroidism, hypoglycemia, Parkinson's disease, seizure, stress, stroke.
Difficult/painful urination	Chlamydia, fibroids, gonorrhea, genital herpes, prostate disorders, trichomoniasis, urinary tract infection, vaginitis.

Symptom	Possible Causes
Frequent urination	Diabetes, excessive fluid intake, kidney stones, enlarged prostate, urinary tract infection.
Bloody/dark urine	Dehydration, hepatitis, kidney disease, kidney stones, prostate disorders, urinary tract infection.
Vaginal/vulvar itching	Candida infection, chlamydia, local irritation, trichomoniasis, vaginitis.
Vaginal discharge	Candida infection, chlamydia, fibroids, gonorrhea, pelvic inflammatory disease, trichomoniasis, vaginitis.
Vision loss/disturbance	Cataracts, floaters, glaucoma, hypoglycemia, macular degeneration, onset of migraine or seizure, multiple sclerosis, photophobia, presbyopia, retinal disorders, stroke, uveitis.
Vomiting	Anxiety, celiac disease, drug abuse/withdrawal, drug reaction, cirrhosis, food allergies, food poisoning, fatigue, hepatitis, HIV disease, kidney disease, Meniere's disease, migraine, motion sickness, overeating, poisoning, shock, stress, virtually any systemic viral or bacterial infection.
Weight gain	Poor eating habits, hypothyroidism, slowed metabolism, premenstrual syndrome.
Weight loss	Anorexia nervosa, anxiety, cancer, celiac disease, cirrhosis, Crohn's disease, depression, diabetes, drug abuse, poor eating habits, HIV disease, lupus, tuberculosis.
Wheezing	Anaphylactic shock, allergies, asthma, bronchitis, hay fever.

A Word About Dosages
of Nutritional Supplements

For many of the treatments that are recommended in this section, dosage instructions may be found on the products themselves, whether as part of the product label or your doctor's prescription. This is particularly true of conventional medicines and homeopathic remedies. There is one category of treatment where label information may not be sufficient, however: nutritional supplements. Many supplements come in a variety of dosages. Moreover, we believe that the usual recommended daily allowances (RDAs) given for vitamins and minerals are too low in many circumstances.

The dosage levels specified in the individual entries in Part Two are *therapeutic doses*. That is, they do not necessarily represent the amounts of these nutrients you require on an ongoing daily basis, but rather higher than normal amounts that may be helpful for certain conditions when taken for limited periods of time. Note that some dosages are given in international units (IU); others in milligrams (mg); and still others in micrograms (mcg, the equivalent of $1/1000$ milligram). Because there are different forms of many supplements available—for example, a supplement labeled "vitamin E" may contain d-alpha-tocopherol, dl-tocopheryl acetate, and/or mixed tocopherols, among others—the table below lists the preferred forms of various supplements and a safe daily intake for each. These safe levels assume that you are a basically healthy average adult, and not pregnant or nursing.

While nutritional supplements are, for the most part, readily available over the counter, the authors believe they should be used judiciously. The same is true of herbal products and homeopathic remedies. When taking them, particularly in the case of chronic conditions, it is a good idea to choose one that seems to be right for your condition and/or symptoms. Try it for a period of time—say, a week—and see how you feel. Then, if you like, add something else. By proceeding in this fashion, you accomplish two things. First, you will be aware of how each supplement or remedy makes you feel. Second, your body will have time to adjust to each addition.

Unless otherwise indicated, the recommendations in this book are for adults. For information about treating children's health-care problems with a combination of natural and conventional approaches, we recommend consulting *Smart Medicine for a Healthier Child* (Avery, 1994).

PREFERRED FORMS AND SAFE DAILY DOSES OF NUTRITIONAL SUPPLEMENTS

Supplement	Preferred Form	Safe Daily Intake
VITAMINS		
Beta-carotene	Both natural and synthetic forms have been said to have protective properties. Natural preparations may be more bioavailable and often offer additional carotenoids for more protection.	500–200,000 IU.
Vitamin A	Vitamin A palmitate is effective, but mycellized preparations are more bioavailable.	5,000–25,000 IU. Under medical supervision, up to 100,000 IU daily. If you are pregnant, or if you have liver disease, consult your physician for advice. Pregnant women should not ingest a total of more than 25,000 IU per week from all supplements.
Vitamin B₁ (thiamine)	Thiamine HCl is effective, but for obvious deficiency, choose thiamine pyrophosphate.	10–300 mg.

Supplement	Preferred Form	Safe Daily Intake
VITAMINS (continued)		
Vitamin B$_2$ (riboflavin)	Riboflavin.	10–100 mg.
Vitamin B$_3$ (niacin)	Niacin. To avoid the "niacin flush," use inositol hexanicotinate or niacinamide.	Niacin: 10–200 mg. Inositol hexanicotinate: 100–3,000 mg (under a doctor's supervision). Niacinamide: 10–300 mg.
Vitamin B$_6$ (pyridoxine)	Pyridoxine HCl.	10–200 mg. Long-term use of over 200 mg daily requires a doctor's supervision.
Vitamin B$_{12}$	Hydroxycobalamin.	50–3,000 mcg. Take with folic acid.
Folic acid	Folic acid.	400–3,000 mcg. Take with vitamin B$_{12}$.
Pantothenic acid	Pantothenic acid. To detoxify the liver, use pantethine.	10–1,000 mg.
Vitamin C	Ascorbic acid or a buffered form such as calcium ascorbate.	250–10,000 mg, depending on individual tolerance.
Vitamin D	Cholecalciferol.	400 IU, but not normally necessary if you get 20 minutes or more of sun exposure daily.
Vitamin E	D-alpha-tocopherol or mixed tocopherols. Avoid dl- forms.	100–1,200 IU. If you have high blood pressure, 400 IU except under a doctor's supervision.
Vitamin K	Leafy green vegetables, green-foods supplements such as chlorella and spirulina.	50–150 mcg.
MINERALS		
Calcium	Calcium carbonate, calcium citrate, calcium chelate, or calcium aspartate.	1,000–1,500 mg.
Chromium	Chromium nicotinate, chromium picolinate, or chromium chelate.	100–400 mcg.
Copper	Copper citrate or copper chelate.	1 mg for every 15 mg of zinc ingested.
Iron	Iron glycinate.	10–30 mg. You should not take supplemental iron unless blood tests reveal deficiency, however.
Magnesium	Magnesium citrate, magnesium chloride, magnesium oxide, magnesium aspartate, or magnesium glycinate.	400–800 mg.
Manganese	Manganese chelate, manganese aspartate, or manganese picolinate.	2–5 mg.
Potassium	Potassium aspartate or potassium citrate. Also foods such as bananas, orange juice, and vegetables.	99–300 mg.
Selenium	Sodium selenite.	100–400 mcg.
Zinc	Zinc picolinate, zinc chelate, zinc aspartate, zinc sulfate, zinc oxide, or zinc gluconate.	15–100 mg. If you take more than 50 mg daily, you should take 1 mg of copper for every 15 mg.
OTHER		
Coenzyme Q$_{10}$	Coenzyme Q$_{10}$.	25–100 mg.
Cysteine	N-acetylcysteine.	500–1,500 mg.
Glutamine	L-glutamine.	500–2,000 mg.
Lysine	L-lysine.	500–2,000 mg.
Taurine	Taurine.	500–2,000 mg.
Tyrosine	L-tyrosine.	500–1,500 mg.

Abscess

An abscess is a collection of pus contained in a small area walled off from the rest of the body by inflammatory cells and decaying tissue. Pus is a thick white to yellowish fluid, composed primarily of dead white blood cells, that forms as a result of infection. Abscesses actually represent an attempt on the part of tissues at a local site to insulate the body from invading organisms. They can occur just about anywhere in the body, from the brain to the abdomen to the area around the toenails, but they are most common in the skin.

The infecting organisms responsible for the formation of abscesses vary. *Staphylococcus* (staph) bacteria are prevalent in skin abscesses, but a multitude of other organisms, including viruses, bacteria, fungi, amoebas, and worms, can be involved as well, depending on the site of the abscess. In some cases, the cause is unknown.

Most abscesses cause local pain and tenderness. If they are close enough to the surface of the skin, there is likely to be redness and swelling. Deeper abscesses can cause fever, fatigue, and loss of appetite. If an internal organ is involved, there can be symptoms resulting from disruptions in the functioning of that organ.

Even a small, localized skin abscess should be treated rather than being left to resolve itself on its own. Otherwise, it may tax the body's immune mechanisms, and infection may spread. Also, leaving an abscess to resolve itself can occasionally result in the formation of a fibrous lump, or possibly a calcified mass, in the area.

CONVENTIONAL TREATMENT

■ Effective treatment requires physical removal of the pus and elimination of the pocket it accumulated in. At the skin surface, this can be accomplished fairly simply, using applications of heat and pressure or anesthetizing the site and cutting into the abscess with a scalpel. The common medical term for this procedure is *incision and drainage* (or I and D). For a deeper abscess, a doctor may need to use ultrasound or a CT scan to locate it and to guide him or her in placing a drain into the site to remove the pus. Abscesses deep within internal organs such as the liver may even necessitate full surgery.

■ Though antibiotics alone are not usually a satisfactory treatment, they are often used in conjunction with incision and drainage. For this reason, the pus may be cultured so that the infectious organism can be identified. Unfortunately, recent years have seen an increase in the number of antibiotic-resistant organisms, which makes this type of treatment more difficult and also potentially more toxic, since higher doses and more potent types of drugs must be used to overcome these "superbugs."

■ An abscess that breaks loose into the system from a deep location can be life threatening, requiring prolonged hospitalization.

DIETARY GUIDELINES

■ Drink at least ten 8-ounce glasses of pure water daily until the abscess heals.

■ Eat plenty of steamed leafy green vegetables and sea vegetables to ensure a good supply of vitamins and minerals needed for healing.

■ Eat fresh pineapple. Fresh pineapple contains bromelain, which is very effective at reducing inflammation.

■ Eliminate from your diet all fried foods and anything containing refined sugar, which slow healing.

NUTRITIONAL SUPPLEMENTS

■ Blue-green algae contains many trace minerals that are needed for healing and that are missing in the average diet. Take 300 milligrams two or three times daily.

■ Colloidal silver is a liquid mineral supplement that fights infection. Take 10 drops three to four times daily.

■ If you must take antibiotics, restore the body's "friendly" bacteria by taking a probiotic supplement, such as acidophilus and/or bifidobacteria, as recommended on the product label. If you are allergic to milk, select a dairy-free formula. Colostrum is another effective probiotic that can be taken on a rotating basis with acidophilus and bifidobacteria. Take 300 milligrams three times daily, between meals.

■ Vitamin C and bioflavonoids improve the immune response and help to reduce inflammation. Take 1,000 milligrams of vitamin C three to five times daily and 500 milligrams of mixed bioflavonoids three to four times daily.

HERBAL TREATMENT

■ Cat's claw enhances the immune response and has antibacterial properties. Take 500 milligrams of standardized extract three times a day until the abscess clears.

Note: Do not use cat's claw if you are pregnant or nursing, or if you are an organ-transplant recipient. Use it with caution if you are taking an anticoagulant (blood thinner).

■ Echinacea and goldenseal have antibacterial properties and also boost the body's natural immune response. They are helpful for fighting virtually any type of infection. Take one dose of an echinacea and goldenseal combination formula supplying 250 to 500 milligrams of echinacea and 150 to 300 milligrams of goldenseal three to four times daily for up to one week.

Oregano has antibacterial properties and helps to fight infection. Take 75 milligrams of standardized extract three times a day.

Pine-bark and grape-seed extracts have antioxidant and anti-inflammatory properties. Take 50 milligrams of either four times daily for ten days.

HOMEOPATHY

Hepar sulphuris calcareum is for an abscess that is painful and sensitive to the slightest touch. You are likely also feeling chilly and irritable. Take one dose of *Hepar sulphuris calcareum* 12x or 6c three times daily for three days.

Choose *Mercurius hydrargyrum* if you have an abscess and are unable to tolerate heat or cold, and your breath and perspiration have a very strong smell. Take one dose of *Mercurius hydrargyrum* 12x or 6c three times daily for three days.

BACH FLOWER REMEDIES

Crabapple is useful if you find yourself feeling something like shame about your physical condition—as if you are "unclean" somehow. Take it as directed on the product label. If the abscess is on the skin, you can also apply the remedy directly to the affected area twice daily.

ACUPRESSURE

For the locations of acupressure points on the body, *see* ADMINISTERING AN ACUPRESSURE TREATMENT in Part Three.

Liver 3 and Large Intestine 4 relax the body.

Spleen 10 detoxifies the blood.

Acidosis

Acidosis is a condition that falls into a category of problems known as *acid-base disorders*. It is characterized by an increase in the acidity of the blood. Normally, if this happens, the body is able to solve the problem on its own and bring itself back into balance. If it is unable to do so, however, various problems can result.

There are two primary types of acidosis: respiratory (due to breathing difficulties) and metabolic (due to chemical changes within the body). Sometimes both factors exist simultaneously. Respiratory acidosis occurs when, for whatever reason, the body cannot adequately expel carbon dioxide (CO_2) through the breath. Anything that adversely affects the ability to breathe—lung disease, an overdose of sedatives, extreme obesity, muscular prob-

lems, or anything else—can cause chronic respiratory acidosis. Acute respiratory acidosis can be a result of a foreign body stuck in the airway, an overdose of medication, trauma, or heart attack, among other things. Symptoms can include headache, drowsiness, muscle twitching or tremors, and/or changes in consciousness that can progress to coma if the situation is not corrected.

Metabolic acidosis occurs when there are chemical changes to the body's normal state that occur too fast for the body to cope with them. Possible causes include fluid loss due to vomiting, insulin-dependent diabetes, severe blood loss or shock, overdoses of certain drugs, chemical toxicities, true starvation, severe alcoholism, serious kidney disease, and prolonged diarrhea. Symptoms can include nausea, vomiting, feelings of weakness, frequent yawning, and breathing that is deeper and/or more rapid than normal, though some people with mild acidosis have no symptoms at all. If the condition is severe, it can lead to shock.

CONVENTIONAL TREATMENT

■ Treatment for acidosis depends on the underlying cause. Acute acidosis usually requires hospitalization, with sophisticated laboratory testing and measures to correct the body's imbalance. Chronic acidosis that is not too severe may be handled on an outpatient basis. In either case, maintaining proper levels of fluids and electrolytes such as sodium and potassium is also an important part of treatment.

DIETARY GUIDELINES

■ The most important dietary measure to take is to avoid refined sugar of any kind. This means not only table sugar, but all processed and refined food products that contain sugar. Be aware that, on food labels, sugar may show up under other names, including brown sugar, corn syrup, dextrose, fructose, glucose, high-fructose corn syrup, invert sugar, lactose, maltose, mannitol, sorbitol, sucrose, and xylitol.

■ Sharply reduce your consumption of acid-forming foods, or eliminate them from your diet entirely until your body regains its natural balance. The following are common acid-forming foods: alcohol, beans, carbonated beverages, catsup, chocolate, coffee, cranberries, eggs, fish, meat, milk, mustard, olives, pepper, prunes, sugar, tea, tomatoes, and vinegar. Emphasize instead foods that are alkalinizing to the body, including corn, dates, most fresh fruits, most fresh vegetables, honey, maple syrup, molasses, raisins, and soy products.

NUTRITIONAL SUPPLEMENTS

■ Green-foods supplements such as spirulina, barley

greens, chlorella, and blue-green algae are very alkaline. Often, this type of supplement will alkalanize the body fairly quickly. Take a green-foods supplement as directed on the product label.

Probiotic bacteria help to neutralize toxic metabolites and indirectly help to adjust the body's acid/alkaline balance. Take a probiotic supplement as recommended on the product label. If you are allergic to milk, select a dairy-free formula.

The B vitamins help with the transformation and transportation of nutrients. Take a B-complex supplement supplying 25 milligrams of each of the major B vitamins three times daily.

HERBAL TREATMENT

Hyssop tea is a mild blood cleanser and also helps to reduce acidity. Take a cup of hyssop tea two or three times daily until your condition improves.

Peppermint tea improves digestion and reduces acidity. Take a cup of peppermint tea with meals.

HOMEOPATHY

Carbo vegetabilis is good for acidosis accompanied by digestive problems such as acid indigestion, gas, and bloating. Take one dose of *Carbo vegetabilis* 12x, 30x, 6c, or 15c three times daily for two to three days, until your body's pH returns to normal.

Sulfur can be helpful for acidosis that causes a burning sensation with urination and/or bowel movements. The stool is very odorous, and you may tend to feel warm and flush easily. Take one dose of *Sulfur* 30c three times daily for up to two days.

BACH FLOWER REMEDIES

Select the remedy that most closely fits your emotional tendencies and concerns, and take it as needed, following the directions on the product label.

Choose Agrimony if you tend to maintain a smiling appearance despite inner feelings of anguish.

Beech helps to relax a tendency to be perfectionistic and impatient.

Holly tames anger that tends to burst out in fits of temper.

ACUPRESSURE

For the locations of acupressure points on the body, *see* ADMINISTERING AN ACUPRESSURE TREATMENT in Part Three.

■ Stomach 36 improves digestion and overall well-being.

AROMATHERAPY

For specific instructions on how to use aromatherapy, *see* PREPARING AROMATHERAPY TREATMENTS in Part Three.

■ Essential oils of chamomile, lavender, rosemary, and peppermint are soothing and balancing. Use any or all of them as inhalants or in baths, diffuse them into the air, or add a few drops to massage oil.

GENERAL RECOMMENDATONS

■ Consider learning and practicing yoga. Yoga helps to improve circulation and digestion, relieves stress, and requires deep breathing, which is alkalinizing.

Acid Reflux

See under HERNIA, HIATAL; INDIGESTION.

Acne

Acne is an inflammatory condition of the skin marked by pimples, whiteheads, and blackheads. It is caused by a problem with the sebaceous glands, the oil-secreting glands that lubricate and moisturize the skin. These are found in large numbers on the face, chest, and back. Acne is particularly common among teenagers. As a result of hormonal shifts associated with adolescence, there is an increase in the number of sebaceous glands, with a consequent increase in the production of oil, or sebum. Normally, sebum passes through glandular canals to the surface of the skin. But when the glands suffer hormonal overload, the oils can harden and obstruct a glandular canal, preventing sebum from reaching the surface of the skin as it should. Hormone production also causes an abnormal increase in the population of *Propionibacterium acnes*, normally benign bacteria that live in the glandular canals. The combination of the increased bacteria count stimulated by hormonal shifts and the obstruction of sebum causes inflammation to occur, leading to the characteristic tender red, swollen bump we call a pimple.

The skin is quickly affected by any hormonal imbalance. Hormone production increases during puberty, which explains why so many teenagers suffer from acne. Hormonal shifts also occur before, during, and after pregnancy; before, during, and after menstruation; and before, during, and after menopause. It is not unusual for women to experience acne outbreaks during these times, but they are usually short-lived. Emotional stress is another contributor to acne.

Acne can also be caused by external irritation, or it may occur following the ingestion of an irritating substance. There is one form of acne that appears as hard, cone-shaped plugs at the corners of the mouth and affects the surrounding skin. There is also a more severe form of acne, often called cystic acne, that produces abscesses, cysts, and thick, raised scars. Rosacea, a chronic skin condition sometimes seen in adults, resembles acne, but is a separate disorder (*see* ROSACEA).

Even newborn babies can get acne. Sometimes, in response to withdrawal from the mother's hormones, an infant's oil glands become enlarged and small pimples develop on his or her nose, cheeks, forehead, back, and/or chest. The pimples look just like a miniature version of teenage acne, which is exactly what they are; the same oil glands are involved.

Both teenage and adult acne may require intervention. Chronic acne, as opposed to the occasional pimple, is a trying experience. If you suffer from long-term acne, prompt attention may be needed in order to avoid the pockmarks and scars that may ensue if the condition remains untreated. Understanding why acne develops and what to do about it is the first step toward eliminating it.

It is important to realize that most often acne is *not* a result of poor hygiene. All the washing and scrubbing in the world will not alter the underlying condition. Acne can, however, be aggravated by many commonly used cosmetic products, especially moisturizers, which often contain oils, such as mineral oil or petrolatum, that block the oil glands. Other potential culprits are ammonia, artificial colors, ethanol, EDTA, formaldehyde, nitrates, polyvinylpyrolidone (also known as PVP and Povidone), and artificial fragrances.

CONVENTIONAL TREATMENT

■ For ordinary, superficial acne, a number of conventional medical products, some available by prescription and others over the counter, may be effective:

- Benzoyl peroxide is a topical nonprescription antibacterial used in many over-the-counter acne preparations. It helps to decrease the growth of bacteria and works to open and clean out clogged pores. Benzoyl peroxide is available in lotion, cream, and gel forms. The gel is considered the most effective, but it can also be the most irritating. Benzoyl peroxide has a drying action and can cause redness and scaling. If it causes irritation, try applying it only every other day.
- Tretinoin (Retin-A, or topical retinoic acid) is a naturally occurring derivative of vitamin A that acts by thinning the outer layer of the skin and opening up clogged pores. It is available by prescription in gel, cream, and liquid forms. Six to twelve weeks of therapy may be necessary before any improvement is noticed. Like

benzoyl peroxide, tretinoin can be very drying to the skin. Also, it is important to avoid the sun when using this medication, as it makes it much easier to get sunburned.

- Topical preparations of the antibiotics erythromycin (Benzamycin, Erygel, and others), clindamycin (Cleocin, Clinda-Derm), and tetracycline are available by prescription and may be useful against acne, especially if benzoyl peroxide and tretinoin prove ineffective by themselves. As with all antibiotics, an allergic reaction is possible and may be difficult to distinguish from simple contact irritation. Even when applied to the skin, these drugs are absorbed into the bloodstream. In rare cases, these antibiotics can cause a dangerous form of diarrhea or colitis.

■ If you develop cysts or pustules in addition to ordinary pimples, it may be time to consult a doctor. Depending on the severity of the condition, and on your physician's expertise with skin problems, it may be necessary to seek advice from a specialist in dermatology for chronic acne. Dermatologists often prescribe oral antibiotics such as tetracycline (also sold under the brand name Achromycin), minocycline (Dynacin, Minocin), doxycycline (Doryx, Monodox), and erythromycin (ERYC, Ilotycin) for significant inflammatory acne. Antibiotics work to decrease the amount of bacteria on the skin and have an anti-inflammatory action. Usually improvement can be noted in one to three months, but oral antibiotics are often recommended for a six- to twelve-month period to ensure success. Tetracycline can cause discoloration in developing teeth. It should therefore not be taken by children who do not have all of their permanent teeth, or by pregnant women. Also, be alert for developing signs of abdominal distress. These antibiotics can cause a rare but very dangerous form of diarrhea or colitis.

■ Isotretinoin (better known by its brand name, Accutane) is a synthetic compound that resembles vitamin A. It can be extremely effective against acne, but it can also have such severe side effects as arthritis, elevation of blood fats, liver toxicity, nosebleeds, cracking at the corners of the mouth, and extreme dryness of the eyes. Most significantly, it is known to cause birth defects in a very high percentage of fetuses exposed to it. So serious is this danger that doctors often recommend that any woman of childbearing age who takes this drug use multiple forms of birth control and take pregnancy tests monthly. If, despite these measures, pregnancy does occur, therapeutic abortion may be recommended. We believe that if pregnancy is even a remote possibility, this drug should be not be used. In general, isotretinoin is a treatment of last resort for disfiguring cystic acne that does not respond to other treatments.

■ Steroid injections introduced directly into a cystic acne

lesion help decrease the size and inflammation of the lesion. They also help reduce the unsightly scarring and pitting that occurs in severe cases of this type of acne. Steroid injections are painful, however, and have potentially serious side effects, so they are generally recommended only for very severe cases of cystic acne that do not respond to other treatment.

■ For severe cases of acne that result in deep scarring, dermabrasion may help to improve the appearance of the skin. This technique can cause a significant amount of discomfort, however. Longer-lasting problems with dermabrasion can include pigmentation problems, with patches of skin ending up either darker or lighter than surrounding areas, and scarring. Darker skinned people seem to encounter these problems more frequently than those with lighter complexions.

DIETARY GUIDELINES

■ Eat a nutritious, well-balanced diet. This is very important for the health of the skin. The Chinese believe that acne is tied to inefficient and incomplete digestion, which results in toxic metabolites that show up on the skin. A skin-healthy diet emphasizes raw and lightly cooked vegetables, especially green leafy vegetables that contain valuable trace minerals and are rich in fiber. Fresh green vegetables are essential. Also include in your diet lean protein sources and complex carbohydrates, such as rice, whole-grain bread, potatoes, and legumes (legumes may be omitted if they cause a digestive problem). These fiber-rich foods help ensure a clean gastrointestinal tract, which is especially important in the management of acne. Eat three healthy meals daily to provide important nutrients and to decrease your appetite for sugary or greasy fried foods.

■ Drink plenty of spring water every day to help flush toxins from your body.

■ Limit your intake of animal fats and hydrogenated oils for at least one or two months. This means cutting back on (or eliminating) dairy products, margarine, fatty red meats, unskinned poultry, and all fried foods. This step alone can sometimes result in a dramatic improvement.

■ Avoid foods that contain additives and preservatives. These chemicals contribute to the amount of toxins in the body.

■ Avoid alcohol, sodas, chocolate, fried foods, and refined sugar. Each of these contributes to an acidic internal environment, which may foster the development of acne.

■ Excessive amounts of iodine in the diet can be a problem for some people with acne. Many dermatologists believe that consuming over 1,000 micrograms (1 milligram) of iodine daily will eventually cause a problem. Significant quantities of iodine are commonly found in fast foods (the iodine content of a fast-food meal is often

twenty to thirty times the recommended daily allowance of 150 micrograms). Shrimp and shellfish are also high in iodine, as are sea vegetables such as nori, hijiki, arame, and kombu. Keep your consumption of these foods to a low level (or avoid them entirely). Also avoid using iodized salt at the table and in cooking. Eating foods high in zinc, such as whole grains, may be helpful as well.

■ There is some debate as to whether specific foods are involved in causing acne. If you think a certain food is making trouble, try giving it up for a month or so, then see what happens when you reintroduce it.

NUTRITIONAL SUPPLEMENTS

■ Acidophilus and bifidobacteria are important supplements that restore friendly bacteria in the intestines and normalize bowel action. Constipation fosters the development of acne and can worsen an already existing condition. In combination with a fiber-rich diet, acidophilus and bifidobacteria help to keep the bowels regular. Friendly flora in the bowel cleanse and strengthen the intestinal function. Probiotics are particularly important if you are taking antibiotics, as these drugs destroy both good and bad bacteria. Take a probiotic supplement as recommended on the product label until your skin improves. If you are taking antibiotics, take these supplements at least one hour before or after taking the medication.

■ Beta-carotene, which the body uses to manufacture vitamin A, helps to heal the skin. While vitamin A can be toxic in large doses, beta-carotene appears to be extremely safe (the only side effect of taking too much is that your skin may temporarily turn a slightly orange color). Take 25,000 international units of beta-carotene and 5,000 international units of vitamin A, twice daily, five days a week, for one month. If you are pregnant, or intend to get pregnant, or if you have liver disease, consult your doctor before taking supplemental vitamin A. Pregnant women should not ingest a total of more than 25,000 international units of supplemental vitamin A *per week* from all sources.

■ Calcium and magnesium are very helpful for acne-prone individuals who are nervous and crave sugar. These minerals relax a stressed nervous system and often decrease the desire for sweets. Take 500 milligrams of calcium and 250 milligrams of magnesium twice daily, either between meals or at the beginning of a meal.

■ Chromium helps balance blood sugar and decreases sugar cravings, especially those that strike between meals. Take 200 micrograms of chromium twice daily for one month. Then reduce the dosage to 100 micrograms twice daily for one month.

■ Vitamin C and bioflavonoids help to clear acne. Vitamin C helps strengthen connective tissue; bioflavonoids act as a natural anti-inflammatory. Take 500 milligrams of each three times a day, between meals, for one month. After that, take 500 milligrams of each twice daily for one month. Then reduce the dosage to 500 milligrams of each once a day.

■ Zinc has a healing effect on disturbed skin cells and mucous membranes. Take 25 milligrams of zinc chelate or zinc picolinate twice daily for two weeks, and then once daily for two months.

Note: Take zinc with food to prevent stomach upset. If you take over 30 milligrams of zinc daily for more than one or two months, you should also take 1 to 2 milligrams of copper each day to maintain a proper mineral balance.

HERBAL TREATMENT

■ Cucumber refreshes oily skin. Slice a fresh cucumber and put the slices on your skin for five to ten minutes daily.

■ Pine-bark and grape-seed extracts are high in bioflavonoids, which enhance the healing action of vitamin C and are natural anti-inflammatory agents that are very helpful in clearing acne. Take 25 milligrams of either three times daily for one month.

NUTRITIONAL/HERBAL/HOMEOPATHIC COMBINATION TREATMENT

■ A combination of herbal, homeopathic, and nutritional treatments often yields very good results against acne. Over a twelve-week period, take the following remedies in the sequence given. Take acidophilus and bifidobacteria supplements during the entire period. The program may be repeated as needed.

Week 1: Take one dose of an echinacea and goldenseal combination formula supplying 250 to 500 milligrams of echinacea and 150 to 300 milligrams of goldenseal two to three times daily, plus 200 micrograms of chromium picolinate twice a day.

Week 2: Take 500 milligrams of burdock root three times a day, plus 25,000 international units of beta-carotene and 10,000 international units of vitamin A twice daily.

Week 3: Take one dose of an echinacea and goldenseal combination formula supplying 250 to 500 milligrams of echinacea and 150 to 300 milligrams of goldenseal three times daily, plus 200 micrograms of chromium picolinate twice a day.

Week 4: Take 500 milligrams of burdock root three times a day, plus 250 micrograms of pine-bark or grape-seed extract three times daily.

Week 5: Take one dose of homeopathic *Sulfur* 12x or 6c two to three times a day, plus 500 milligrams of calcium, 250 milligrams of magnesium, and 25 milligrams of zinc chelate or zinc picolinate twice daily.

Week 6: Twice a day, take one dose of homeopathic *Natrum muriaticum* 6x plus 500 milligrams of evening primrose oil, 25,000 international units of beta-carotene, and 10,000 international units of vitamin A.

Week 7: Take one dose of homeopathic *Berberis aquifolium* 6x twice a day, plus 500 milligrams of evening primrose oil, 500 milligrams of calcium, 250 milligrams of magnesium, and 25 milligrams of zinc chelate or zinc picolinate twice daily, between meals or at the beginning of a meal.

Week 8: Take one dose of *Kali bromatum* 12x or 6c twice a day, plus 25 to 50 milligrams of pine-bark or grape-seed extract three times daily.

Week 9: Take one dose of an echinacea and goldenseal combination formula supplying 250 to 500 milligrams of echinacea and 150 to 300 milligrams of goldenseal twice daily, plus 25,000 international units of beta-carotene and 10,000 international units of vitamin A twice a day.

Week 10: Take 500 milligrams of burdock root twice a day, plus 500 milligrams of calcium and 250 milligrams of magnesium twice daily (between meals or at the beginning of a meal).

Week 11: Take one dose of an echinacea and goldenseal combination formula supplying 250 to 500 milligrams of echinacea and 150 to 300 milligrams of goldenseal twice a day, plus 250 milligrams of vitamin C and 250 milligrams of bioflavonoids twice daily. Also take 500 milligrams of calcium, 250 milligrams of magnesium, and 25 milligrams of zinc chelate or zinc picolinate twice a day, between meals or at the beginning of a meal.

Week 12: Take 500 milligrams of burdock root twice a day, plus 50 milligrams of pine-bark or grape-seed extract three times daily.

Note: If you experience any digestive disturbances, such as gas, bloating, or an upset stomach when following this regimen, take a full-spectrum digestive-enzyme supplement with each meal. If you are pregnant, or intend to get pregnant, or if you have liver disease, consult your doctor before taking supplemental vitamin A.

■ Try the following vitamin/mineral/herbal formula to fight acne. This is a clear solution that is not noticeable on the skin.

Add the following to 1 pint of water: $\frac{1}{2}$ cup plus 2 tablespoons of aloe vera gel; $2\frac{1}{2}$ teaspoons of herbal calendula extract; 2,000 milligrams of powdered vitamin C; 50 milligrams of zinc (open a capsule, crush a tablet, or use 2 tablespoons of liquid); and 2,400 micrograms of folic acid powder (open three 800-microgram capsules). Blend all the ingredients together well. Using a clean cotton ball, apply this mixture to the skin morning and night. Folic acid, one of the B-complex vitamins, helps renew and restore tissue. Zinc aids in healing skin tissue and helps prevent scarring. Calendula is a soothing, healing, and antibacterial herb, and vitamin C protects the skin and is mildly anti-inflammatory. Aloe vera is soothing and restorative.

BACH FLOWER REMEDIES

■ Crabapple can be taken internally and/or applied directly to the skin twice daily to clear acne. Flower remedies work on the emotional as well as on the physical level. An individual who feels "dirty" or feels a desire to "get rid of something bad" in his or her body will often improve with this Bach remedy. (*See* BACH FLOWER REMEDIES in Part One.)

ACUPRESSURE

For the locations of acupressure points on the body, *see* ADMINISTERING AN ACUPRESSURE TREATMENT in Part Three.

■ Large Intestine 4 has a beneficial effect on the head and face.

■ Spleen 10 works to detoxify, or take the "heat" out of, the blood.

AROMATHERAPY

For specific instructions on how to use aromatherapy, *see* PREPARING AROMATHERAPY TREATMENTS in Part Three.

■ An aromatherapy facial steam treatment made with essential oil of frankincense, lavender, myrrh, and/or tea tree is helpful for opening blocked pores and reducing inflammation. Use this treatment once or twice a week until you see results.

■ Five-percent solution of tea tree oil, applied topically to the skin twice daily, has been shown to have effects similar to those of benzoyl peroxide.

GENERAL RECOMMENDATIONS

■ Never pick at, pinch, or squeeze a pimple. Not only does this make the area redder and more sensitive, but irritating the skin increases the chance of infection and scarring. If necessary, apply hot compresses or use steam treatments to help open and drain larger pustules.

■ Keeping your skin clean is important, but too-vigorous scrubbing will further irritate the area and can actually contribute to the spread of acne. Using mild soap and water, wash gently no more than three times daily. Castile and hypoallergenic soaps, or ones made with calendula or chamomile, are best for acne.

■ Exercise vigorously enough to break into a sweat. Many toxins are excreted through the skin. Exercise also speeds up blood circulation and increases the rate at which toxins are excreted.

■ Green clay, taken internally, helps to balance an acidic body. If you eat too much sugar and fat, your internal environment is likely to be highly acidic, a condition that fosters the development of acne. Drink 1 teaspoon of green clay in a glass of water, twice daily, for one week.

■ A clay masque is especially beneficial for anyone with excessively oily skin. Mix 1 teaspoon of kaolin, bentonite, or green clay in a little water, until a pastelike consistency is achieved. Apply this mixture to the skin, and allow it to remain in place for fifteen minutes. Wash it off with warm water.

■ If you wear makeup, use only water-based preparations. Avoid greasy and oil-based cosmetics and skin- or hair-care products, which can further clog the skin and worsen the problem. If a moisturizer is called for, be sure to choose a water-based product. It is particularly important not to wear oil-based makeup or other cosmetic products during exercise. The oils will clog the pores and may worsen the skin condition.

■ Avoid using skin- or hair-care products containing mineral oil or petrolatum, as well as ammonia, artificial colors, ethanol, EDTA, formaldehyde, nitrates, PVP, or artificial fragrances. All of these substances can aggravate acne. Always read the labels of skin- and hair-care products before you buy them.

PREVENTION

■ The causes of acne are so many and so varied that preventing an outbreak may not be possible. Conscientious skin care is one important way to guard against the development of acne, but even people who diligently maintain scrupulously clean skin may suffer from acne.

■ A clean, simple diet is important to healthy skin (*see* Dietary Guidelines in this entry). Constipation contributes to acne because it slows the elimination of toxins through the intestinal tract, which in turn can cause skin eruptions. A fiber-rich diet augmented with acidophilus and bifidobacteria supplements helps to ensure proper elimination and bowel regularity.

■ Regular exercise helps skin cells stay healthy. An exercise program promotes the release of toxins through the sweat glands and improves blood circulation.

Addiction

See ALCOHOLISM; DRUG ABUSE; NICOTINE ADDICTION.

Addison's Disease

See under ADRENAL INSUFFICIENCY.

Adrenal Insufficiency

The adrenal glands sit atop the kidneys. They are very small, but their functions are immense. The inner portion of each gland, or adrenal medulla, produces and stores adrenaline (also known as epinephrine), the "fight-or-flight" hormone. The outer portion, or adrenal cortex, has three separate areas. One area secretes aldosterone, which helps to control the balance of the body's electrolytes (circulating minerals such as potassium and sodium) by helping the kidneys retain sodium and excrete potassium. If aldosterone levels fall, the kidneys may become unable to regulate the body's salt and water balance, resulting in a drop in blood volume and blood pressure. Another area of the adrenal glands manufactures sex hormones, or androgens. Possibly most important is the area that manufactures cortisol, the body's natural cortisone. This hormone, which belongs to a class of hormones called glucocorticoids, has a multitude of purposes. Its most important job is to assist the body in dealing with stress. It also regulates the metabolism of carbohydrates, maintains adequate blood pressure, and controls the body's response to injury and the process of tissue repair. Obviously, if the adrenal glands become weakened or injured and cannot function properly, a multitude of problems may result.

Weakness of the adrenal cortex that comes on suddenly and rapidly can be life-threatening. This situation is called, appropriately, *adrenal crisis.* It can occur as a result of serious stress or trauma, whether from direct injury, surgery, a tumor, or abrupt cessation of high-dose cortisone therapy, and is most likely to occur in individuals whose adrenal glands are already somewhat weak. It can also occur if a person with weak adrenals takes thyroid medication. Symptoms of adrenal crisis include low (and falling) blood pressure with high fever, extreme weakness, confusion, sluggishness, nausea, vomiting, diarrhea, headache, and severe abdominal and/or lower back pain. This situation requires emergency treatment.

Less severe but chronic weakness of the adrenal glands is called Addison's disease. This is a rare disorder that affects about 1 in 100,000 people. It occurs in all age groups and afflicts men and women in equal numbers. Symptoms may include low blood pressure, weakness (worse after exercise or use of thyroid hormone), weight loss, loss of appetite, nausea, vomiting, nervousness, and

irritability. Joint and muscle pains are common, and the skin in many areas of the body may develop hyperpigmentation (darkening). Also, since cortisol regulates carbohydrate metabolism by counteracting the effects of insulin, low cortisol levels can result in bouts of low blood sugar. Some people with Addison's disease have symptoms all the time; others seem to be fine most of the time, but develop symptoms when they are under stress.

Adrenal insufficiency is diagnosed on the basis of symptoms and blood tests to measure the levels of adrenal hormones. Since the symptoms of Addison's disease are similar to ones caused by other disorders, including anorexia nervosa, gastrointestinal disease, and even hidden cancers, those possibilities must be ruled out before a firm diagnosis can be made. There is some question in conventional medicine as to whether it is possible to have chronic subclinically weak adrenal function—that is, adrenal insufficiency that is not severe enough to be detected by conventional testing, but that can nevertheless cause symptoms.

EMERGENCY TREATMENT

■ If you develop signs of adrenal crisis, call for emergency help or have someone take you at once to the emergency room of the nearest hospital. This condition requires immediate, rapid treatment that includes hospitalization and the administration of hydrocortisone, salt, and sugar, and, possibly, other intravenous medication.

CONVENTIONAL TREATMENT

■ The primary treatment for adrenal insufficiency is oral hydrocortisone, taken once or twice daily, to support the underfunctioning glands. Other hormones may be needed as well to help control sodium and potassium levels. If aldosterone is deficient, it is replaced with oral doses of fludrocortisone acetate (Florinef), which is taken once a day. Supplemental sodium may also be necessary.

■ If an infection triggered the problem, it is necessary to track down the nature of the infection and treat it aggressively with appropriate antibiotics.

■ If you suffer from chronic adrenal insufficiency, you should seek out and work closely with an endocrinologist or other physician who specializes, or at the very least has considerable experience, in the treatment of this condition.

DIETARY GUIDELINES

■ To keep your blood-sugar level on an even keel, eat a balanced diet. Eating five or so small meals at regular, more frequent intervals is better than eating two or three large meals daily.

■ A low-carbohydrate diet, sometimes useful for helping to control low blood sugar, is *not* recommended. If you have low adrenal function, it may actually make your blood-sugar problems worse.

■ Do not limit your salt intake. Doing so can increase the stress on the adrenals by making them produce more aldosterone in an effort to maintain sodium levels (aldosterone is a hormone that causes the body to retain sodium).

■ Avoid caffeine and alcohol, which place unnecessary stress on the body.

NUTRITIONAL SUPPLEMENTS

■ It is a good idea to consult with a nutritionally oriented physician who can develop a program of nutritional supplementation specifically for your condition.

■ To be sure you are providing your body with all the basic nutrients it needs, take a high-potency multivitamin and mineral supplement twice daily. Choose a formula that contains at least 25 milligrams of each of the major B vitamins per dose. The B vitamins are essential for adrenal function.

■ Raw adrenal and raw adrenal cortex glandular extract may be helpful. This supplement supplies many components used by the adrenal glands. Take 50 to 150 milligrams twice daily, or follow the directions on the product label.

■ Chromium picolinate can help to regulate blood sugar and prevent fluctuations in blood-sugar levels, which can make symptoms of Addison's disease worse. Take 100 micrograms twice a day for two months. This works best in conjunction with a balanced diet of frequent small meals (*See under* Dietary Guidelines, above).

■ Pantothenic acid supports the adrenal glands, and both pantothenic acid and vitamin B_{12} are important for relieving feelings of fatigue. Take 250 to 500 milligrams of pantothenic acid and 500 micrograms of vitamin B_{12} twice daily.

■ The adrenal glands have the highest level of vitamin C of any organ in the body. Vitamin C is also a natural anti-inflammatory. Take at least 500 milligrams (and up to 2,000 milligrams) of vitamin C with bioflavonoids three times daily.

■ Dehydroepiandrosterone (DHEA), a hormone produced by the adrenal glands, is available in supplement form. However, if you are interested in using DHEA, we recommend that you consult a health-care professional experienced in its use who can determine the proper dosage and monitor its effects.

HERBAL TREATMENT

■ Licorice contains compounds that slow the breakdown of steroid hormones by the liver, easing the adrenal glands' task of making more. While in general it is neces-sary to be cautious about using this herb because it can raise blood pressure, if you have adrenal insufficiency, it can help your pressure approach a normal level. Take 250 to 500 milligrams three times daily.

■ Pine-bark and grape-seed extracts are natural anti-inflammatories. Take 25 milligrams of either three times daily.

■ Siberian ginseng helps to strengthen and regulate adrenal function. Choose an extract standardized to contain 0.5 percent eleutheroside E and take 100 milligrams twice daily, in morning and afternoon.

HOMEOPATHY

■ Chronic adrenal insufficiency is a complicated problem that can cause a variety of symptoms. The best approach to treating it homeopathically is to consult a homeopath who can prescribe a constitutional remedy. There are homeopaths who not only treat this problem constitutionally, but who also report success using homeopathic pituitary, hypothalamus, and adrenal extracts.

BACH FLOWER REMEDIES

Select the remedy that fits your emotional tendencies and concerns, and take it as needed, following the directions on the product label.

■ Hornbeam is helpful for feelings of being exhausted and overextended.

■ Olive helps to counteract feelings of continual fatigue and being fatigued to the very core.

GENERAL RECOMMENDATIONS

■ One of the most important things you can do if you have adrenal insufficiency (whether suspected or diagnosed) is to lower the amount of stress in your life. This takes a load off the adrenals by reducing the amount of cortisol required for daily functioning. *See* STRESS for a discussion of ways to eliminate and manage stress.

■ Don't smoke, and avoid secondhand smoke. Exposure to tobacco smoke adds to the amount of stress your body must bear. If you have adrenal insufficiency, your body's mechanisms for coping with stress are impaired.

■ Get regular exercise, but take care not to overstress yourself, especially at first. For example, two twenty-minute walks a day are initially better than thirty minutes of intense aerobics. Eventually, more strenuous exercise will be easier. Most people can attempt more intense exercise after a month or so of mild exercise.

■ An excellent book on the adrenal glands and treating them with natural substances is *Safe Uses of Cortisol*, second edition, by Dr. William Jeffries (Charles C. Thomas Publisher Ltd., 1996).

Aging

Aging is not a disease, but a normal part of life. However, it brings with it certain changes in the body that most of us would like to keep at bay for as long as possible, including a decline in the acuity of the senses and visible changes in appearance, such as wrinkling of the skin and thinning of the hair. The likelihood of developing certain disorders, including arthritis, macular degeneration, memory problems, Parkinson's disease, Alzheimer's disease, cardiovascular disease, and many types of cancer, also increases with age. Humans have been searching for the mythical "fountain of youth" for millennia. Yet aging remains a process that, sooner or later, will affect all of us. It proceeds slowly, and begins at the cellular level.

The human body is composed of literally trillions of cells. In a constant dynamic process, individual cells die and are replaced with new ones. For the most part, cells are replaced through *mitosis*, in which a single healthy cell divides in half and "gives birth" to an identical brand-new cell. Cells use the raw materials drawn from the nutrients you provide to repair, rebuild, and renew themselves.

Why do cells die? There is a limit to the number of times a cell can undergo mitosis—most cells can undergo only some twenty to thirty divisions, after which they die, to be replaced by new cells. Cells can also die as a result of injury, whether that injury takes place on a level you can see (a burn or a cut, for instance), or on a microscopic level. Thanks to their ability to divide and multiply, the dead and dying cells are normally replaced, and the total number of cells in your body remains pretty much the same throughout your adult life. As we age, however, the process of cell division slows down, and the rate of cell death may outstrip the body's ability to produce replacement cells. Eventually, the body's tissues—which are composed of cells—begin to suffer, and start to malfunction in various ways.

Our bodies seem to be programmed to age. Yet much of what we think of as normal aging may in fact be *premature* aging. In recent years, much attention has been focused on the role of free radicals in aging. Free radicals are atoms or molecules that are highly chemically reactive. This is because they contain within their structures one or more unpaired electrons. Since electrons normally occur in pairs, an unpaired one will always be "looking" for another electron to join with, even if it must steal one from another molecule.

Even though most free radicals exist for only a fraction of a second, they can have dramatic effects. In the body, free radicals can attack cell membranes and can even change the genetic material of cells, resulting in mutations

and a higher than normal rate of cell death. Obviously, anything that accelerates cell death would be implicated in the aging process. Free radicals also can interact with other substances in the body, such as cholesterol, which then becomes more likely to adhere to the walls of blood vessels. Thus, hardening of the arteries, commonly associated with aging, may be more a result of free-radical damage than the simple passage of time.

It is important to note that not all free radicals harm the body. For example, the immune system produces free radicals that destroy certain bacteria and viruses. It is a free-radical reaction that enables hemoglobin, the red pigment in the blood, to bind to oxygen and carry it throughout the body. Other free radicals are involved in the production of energy, and some help produce hormones and special enzymes important to the processes of life. The body also produces free radicals in the normal course of breaking down food.

Since the body produces free radicals, you would expect that it would have a way of coping with them. And it does. Indeed, under normal circumstances, the body produces other substances that neutralize free radicals and prevent them from doing any harm. But if there are too many of them roaming around, the body becomes unable to deal with them all, and the free radicals become more likely to start causing damage. This is an increasing problem today, because in addition to those produced by the body, we are subjected to free radicals from a variety of other sources, including high levels of fat in the diet; exposure to pollutants such as automobile exhaust, tobacco smoke, and a large variety of other chemicals, including chlorine in drinking water; and exposure to radiation, including that from the sun—something to think about as we hear of the thinning of the earth's protective ozone layer.

Finally, many common conditions often attributed to age can sometimes be traced to nutritional problems. For example, a lack of the B vitamins, especially vitamin B_{12}, can give rise to a number of neurological symptoms, including memory loss, dizziness, weakness, uncertain balance, and disorientation, that are easily mistaken for signs of senility. This type of problem may be due to insufficient intake or to poor absorption; many older adults no longer secrete sufficient digestive juices to digest and assimilate nutrients well, so that even with a good diet, they may develop deficiencies.

In 1900, the average life expectancy for an American man was forty-seven, while the average American woman could expect to reach age fifty. Thanks to greatly improved sanitation, inoculation against childhood diseases, and the development of antibiotics, a child born today can reasonably expect to reach his or her seventies. That's the good news. The bad news is that while we are living *longer*, we are not necessarily living *better*. Simply by making changes in lifestyle, you can reduce your risk of developing many of the health problems commonly associated with old age. The younger you are when you start applying these strategies, the better.

The focus of this entry is on preventing age-related problems from arising. If you take adequate precautions—that includes eating right, taking protective supplements, and exercising—you actually can keep your body younger longer. However, if you have already developed some age-related problems, this entry (and the entries that target your specific ailments) can help you overcome them.

CONVENTIONAL TREATMENT

■ Conventional medicine tends to focus not on ways to slow the aging process, but on treating "diseases of aging" or other signs of the aging process as they arise. For the most part, the only preventive measure recommended is the annual physical examination to look for developing problems so that they may be treated early.

DIETARY GUIDELINES

■ Eat a diet that is high in fiber and includes plenty of lean, clean protein foods such as chicken, fish, and soy products. A high-fiber diet, including plenty of vegetables, fruits, and whole grains, prevents constipation, keeps the gastrointestinal tract healthy, and has been shown to help prevent heart disease, cancer, and all gastrointestinal tract disorders. We recommend that you get 30 to 35 grams of fiber daily. Soy-based foods such as tofu, tempeh, miso, and sprouts help reduce cholesterol, thus reducing the risk of heart disease. They also contain genistein, a phytochemical believed to be a potent cancer preventive.

■ Enjoy the cruciferous vegetables (broccoli, cabbage, kale, cauliflower, and Brussels sprouts) often. These vegetables have powerful antioxidant agents, including the enzyme superoxide dismutase (SOD), that work to prevent premature aging by protecting against the ongoing cellular damage caused by free radicals. They also contain phytochemicals that have been shown to be active against the development of cancerous cells.

■ Eat plenty of leafy greens and yellow-orange vegetables, including carrots, peaches, cantaloupe, pumpkin, sweet potatoes, and apricots. These foods contain phytochemicals called carotenes. Beta-carotene, the best known of this group, has been found to provide protection against the sun's ultraviolet (UV) rays, which initiate free-radical formation that leads to both premature aging of the skin and skin cancer. Carotenes also help the body fight other types of cancer and reduce the formation of the atherosclerotic plaque that clogs arteries. And in one study, people who ate foods rich in beta-carotene were found to have 39 percent fewer cataracts than those on an average diet.

■ If you like garlic and onions, enjoy them to your heart's content. These foods contain alliin, a phytochemical known to help regulate blood pressure and aid in the production of red blood cells. Dialylsulfide, another phytochemical found in these vegetables, has been shown to deactivate some cancer-causing agents in animals. These vegetables also stimulate the production of glutathione, a potent antioxidant agent that fights premature aging.

■ Include in your diet sardines, salmon, wheat germ, asparagus, spinach, and white mushrooms. These foods are rich in the nucleic acids DNA and RNA, which improve skin color and texture, help fade age spots, and increase energy levels.

Note: If you eat these foods regularly, be sure to drink at least eight glasses of pure spring water daily. Foods rich in DNA and RNA can increase uric acid levels, which increases the risk of some forms of arthritis, notably gout.

■ Grape juice and red wine contain compounds that act as antioxidants and protect the blood vessels. Enjoy a glass of either daily.

■ Drink green tea often. Green tea contains potent antioxidant agents that protect against premature aging. It is rich in polyphenols that are destroyed in the fermenting processes used to produce ordinary black tea. Studies show that green tea helps to ward off heart disease, reduce the risk of stroke and cancer, bring down high blood pressure, combat cold and flu symptoms, and even fight dental decay and bad breath. One double-blind European study showed that drinking two cups of green tea every day can help decrease excess body fat as well.

■ Reishi mushrooms, long considered a delicacy in East Asia, fight the effects of aging on normal immune function. They also fight viruses and bacteria, inhibit tumor growth, lower cholesterol, and reduce blood pressure. You can buy them dried and add them to many of your favorite recipes (soak the dried mushrooms for half an hour before using them). Reishi is also available in supplement form.

■ Eat live-culture yogurt to protect against gastrointestinal problems, including constipation and diarrhea. People who eat live-culture yogurt regularly have substantially fewer colds than those who do not. One or two servings per day has been shown to be an effective amount.

■ Avoid foods and beverages containing caffeine and/or refined sugars. These substances stress the body and can deplete valuable nutrients. If you consume alcohol, do so in moderation only.

NUTRITIONAL SUPPLEMENTS

■ Acidophilus is a probiotic supplement that boosts the immune system. Probiotic supplements provide essential friendly bacteria that benefit the entire gastrointestinal tract, helping to prevent constipation, control diarrhea, and protect against digestive upsets, food poisoning, viral and bacterial invasions, and some parasites. Take a probiotic supplement as recommended on the product label. Colostrum, a very effective probiotic, may be rotated with acidophilus as well.

■ Bioflavonoids are phytochemicals found in many fruits and vegetables. Rutin, a bioflavonoid found in the white connective membranes of citrus fruits and bell peppers, helps to prevent the oxidation of low-density lipoproteins ("bad" cholesterol), which accelerates the deposition of cholesterol in the blood vessels. It also slows down the action of some cancer-causing substances. Quercetin, present in red and yellow onions, helps reduce the inflammation associated with allergies, and also inhibits the action of several known carcinogens. Lycopene, found in red fruits and vegetables such as tomatoes, red grapefruit, and red peppers, is another excellent antioxidant with anticarcinogenic properties. The bioflavonoids work with vitamin C and enhance its antioxidant action as well. Unless you eat all of the foods mentioned here regularly, take 500 to 1,000 milligrams of mixed bioflavonoids three times daily.

■ Boron helps create stronger bones. Taking supplemental boron has been shown to reduce losses of calcium and magnesium from the body in postmenopausal women. It may also have a positive effect on estrogen levels. A deficiency of boron may result in depressed mental alertness. Take a supplement providing 1.5 to 3 milligrams of boron daily.

■ Carnitine is very helpful for cardiovascular function, and improves physical stamina and endurance during exercise. Brain tissue is rich in carnitine, which may explain why some studies suggest that it may slow the progress of Alzheimer's disease. Carnitine is found primarily in red meat, lamb, and dairy products. Since we do not recommend including large amounts of these foods in your diet, you may want to include carnitine in your supplement program. Take 500 milligrams of L-carnitine twice daily.

■ Choline increases the speed with which nerve impulses are transmitted and is a noted memory-booster. Good food sources include soybeans, cauliflower, and cabbage. If these foods are not regularly featured on your menu, take 250 to 1,000 milligrams of supplemental choline daily.

■ Chromium improves glucose tolerance and regulates blood-sugar levels. It has been shown to lower the level of various fats circulating in the blood. If you are exercising regularly—and you should be—chromium can help you build muscle. Take 200 to 400 micrograms of chromium picolinate daily.

■ Coenzyme Q_{10} is a substance found in every cell in the body. It is essential for the processes that provide cells with energy and oxygen. It is also a strong antioxidant that inhibits the peroxidation of lipids, a process that contributes to heart disease, cancer, and premature aging. Take at least 30 milligrams three times daily.

■ The amino acid cysteine is a powerful antioxidant that neutralizes free radicals. Take 250 milligrams of N-acetylcysteine (NAC) daily.

■ Dehydroepiandrosterone (DHEA) is a hormone produced by the adrenal glands. The production of DHEA falls as the body ages, which some scientists theorize may be related to the increasing risk of cancer, heart disease, high blood pressure, Parkinson's disease, osteoporosis, diabetes, nerve degeneration, and other disorders that occur with aging. In studies on laboratory animals, DHEA therapy has been found to increase lifespan by as much as 50 percent. However, some researchers caution that taking DHEA in supplement form can damage the body's ability to manufacture this hormone. In addition, taking too much DHEA can cause serious damage to the liver. Therefore, we advise that DHEA be taken only under the supervision of a physician experienced in its use. If you do decide to experiment with this hormone on your own, start with a small amount, such as 5 milligrams daily, and monitor your reaction. If you experience adverse symptoms such as headaches or irritability, discontinue the supplement.

■ The nucleic acids DNA and RNA are required by every cell in the body for cellular metabolism, respiration, and repair. Several studies have found that laboratory animals injected with the nucleic acids lived measurably longer than those not given the injections. Take 100 milligrams of a DNA/RNA supplement daily.

Note: If you take DNA/RNA supplements, be sure to drink at least eight glasses of pure water daily.

■ Flaxseed and fish oils contain omega-3 essential fatty acids, which may reduce the risk of heart disease by up to 40 percent. These essential fatty acids work against heart disease, stroke, arthritis, and cancer, and also can yield noticeable improvements in skin clarity and tone. Take 500 to 1,000 milligrams twice daily.

Note: If you are taking blood-thinning medication or taking aspirin daily, do not use an omega-3 supplement without first discussing it with your physician. In conjunction with blood-thinners, excessive amounts of omega-3 essential fatty acids can lead to problems with bleeding.

■ Gamma-linolenic acid, an essential fatty acid found in black currant seed oil, borage oil, and evening primrose oil, helps to prevent cardiovascular disease and often relieves the inflamed and painful joints common in arthritis. Choose one of these oils and take 500 to 1,000 milligrams twice a day.

■ Glutathione is an antioxidant that has anticancer properties, boosts the immune system, and is a natural anti-inflammatory agent. Low levels of glutathione are associated with premature aging and depressed immunity. Take 500 milligrams twice a day.

■ Lipoic acid works against the normal aging process by enhancing the antioxidant action of vitamin C, vitamin E, and glutathione. It also assists in the digestive process by aiding the action of enzymes crucial to the conversion of nutrients into energy. Take 50 milligrams twice a day.

■ Melatonin is a hormone produced by the pineal gland in the brain. It is vital to the maintenance of normal body rhythms, especially the sleep-wake cycle. It also has antioxidant properties and is believed to reduce stress and improve immune function. If you wish to improve your sleep pattern, take 3 milligrams each evening, between one-half hour and two hours before retiring for the night. For the antioxidant and anti-aging properties of this hormone, take 500 micrograms daily, at bedtime. Do not take melatonin during the day, as it may interfere with your body's normal rhythms and cause drowsiness.

■ Pancreatin enhances digestion and utilization of nutrients. Take 350 milligrams three times daily, with meals.

Note: Long-term supplementation with pancreatin is not advised, as it can cause your pancreas to reduce its own production of this important enzyme. Overuse also has the potential to cause nausea or diarrhea. After two months on pancreatin, discontinue use and monitor your reaction. If you find that digestive problems recur, discuss pancreatin supplementation with your health-care provider.

■ Phosphatidylserine, a type of lipid, is an important nutrient for the brain. It can help restore and preserve brain function, including memory. Take 50 to 100 milligrams twice a day.

■ Pregnenolone is a hormone the body uses to create numerous other hormones, including DHEA, estrogen, and testosterone. Taken in supplement form, it can elevate mood, improve memory, and increase energy. Start by taking 10 milligrams daily, then gradually increase the dosage to 30 milligrams daily. Take it for three weeks at a time, then stop for one week.

■ Royal jelly is a milky, nutritionally rich substance fed to bee larvae to make them mature into queen bees. (Ordinary bee larvae, denied royal jelly, mature into the sexless workers of the hive.) Royal jelly is high in hormones and contains vitamins A, C, D, and E; all of the B-complex vitamins; and numerous minerals, enzymes, and amino acids. It is also a natural source of pure acetylcholine, an important neurotransmitter. Take 20 milligrams daily.

■ Superoxide dismutase (SOD) is an antioxidant enzyme that neutralizes superoxide, one of the most dangerous of all free radicals. As a result, it inhibits the cellular destruction common to the aging process. Because SOD must be protected against digestive acids and enter the small intestines intact in order to be effective, select a supplement that is enteric coated. Take it as directed on the product label.

■ Vitamin C is a potent antioxidant. It is essential for the formation of collagen, an important protein that is a constituent of bone, skin, and connective tissue. Used topically, vitamin C may help fight wrinkles by stimulating the production of collagen. Taken internally, it helps to protect against heart disease. This primary antioxidant also helps raise glutathione levels, thereby providing double protection against free-radical damage and premature aging. Take 1,000 milligrams three times daily.

■ Vitamin E is an antioxidant that prevents the oxidation of lipids, thus helping to protect the membrane of every cell in the body. It boosts the immune system, helps prevent cardiovascular disease, and improves the utilization of oxygen. Choose a product containing mixed tocopherols, and start by taking 200 international units in the morning, then gradually increase the dosage until you are taking 200 to 400 international units in the morning and again in the evening.

Note: If you have high blood pressure, limit your intake of supplemental vitamin E to a total of 400 international units daily. If you are taking an anticoagulant (blood thinner), consult your physician before taking supplemental vitamin E.

■ Selenium works synergistically with vitamin E and is needed by the body to convert harmful substances called peroxides into water. It helps maintain healthy blood cells, and protects the heart, liver, and lungs from free-radical damage. Take 50 to 100 micrograms twice a day.

■ Zinc supports the immune system, speeds the healing process, promotes the absorption of vitamins A and E, and is important for glandular health in both men and women. Zinc is also a component of superoxide dismutase (SOD). Take 15 to 50 milligrams daily, with food.

Note: Both selenium and zinc enhance the action of vitamin E. These three nutrients should be taken together. Take zinc with food to prevent stomach upset. If you take over 30 milligrams of zinc on a daily basis for more than one or two months, you should also take 1 to 2 milligrams of copper each day to maintain a proper mineral balance.

HERBAL TREATMENT

■ Aloe vera has anticarcinogenic properties and helps prevent or correct constipation, which in turn reduces the body's exposure to toxins. Be sure to use a food-grade product. Take ¼ cup of aloe vera juice two or three times daily.

Astragalus stimulates the production of T-lymphocytes (T-cells), key components of the immune system, thereby enhancing immune response. It also helps to protect the body from cardiovascular disease by improving the flow of blood to the heart. Take 500 milligrams (or 2 droppersful of liquid extract) of astragalus daily for two weeks out of every month.

■ Bilberry contains bioflavonoids called anthocyanidins that help strengthen the smallest blood vessels and protect against capillary fragility. Bilberry is especially good for the eyes. Choose a product containing 25 percent anthocyanidins (also called PCOs) and take 20 to 40 milligrams three times daily.

Burdock has anticancer, antibacterial, and antifungal properties. It assists in the production of bile, which is required for the breakdown of fats. Burdock is a common condiment in Japan, where it is taken as a digestive aid. Anecdotal evidence suggests that it is effective against rheumatism, arthritis, and gout. Take 500 milligrams twice a day for one or two weeks out of each month.

If you are a woman over forty-five and are *not* on hormone replacement therapy, consider taking dong quai, a noted hormonal regulator with mild sedative action that is effective against stress. Take 500 milligrams twice daily.

Fo-ti (also known as *ho shou wu, shou wu shih,* and *Polygonum multiflorum*) helps prevent cardiovascular disease. It has anti-inflammatory action and can relieve the inflamed and painful joints typical of arthritis. Take 500 milligrams or one cup of tea once or twice daily.

Ginger has been used for 3,000 years for a wide variety of ailments associated with aging. It helps prevent inappropriate blood clotting, thus protecting against heart disease and stroke; it has anti-inflammatory activity, which eases inflamed joints; and it aids digestion, improving the absorption of nutrients. Choose a standardized extract containing 5 percent gingeoles and take 200 milligrams three times daily. Or take one cup of ginger tea three times daily.

Ginkgo biloba has antioxidant properties, guards against blood clots, improves circulation, and is known as an aid to improved memory and mental clarity. Choose a product containing at least 24 percent ginkgo heterosides (sometimes called flavoglycosides) and take 40 milligrams three times daily.

All types of ginseng are whole-body energizers. These tonic herbs have antioxidant properties, may help protect against heart disease and cancer, and fight stress. Take a ginseng formula as recommended on the product label.

Note: Do not use ginseng if you have high blood pressure, heart disease, or hypoglycemia.

Gotu kola is excellent for all circulatory disorders. It improves circulation, eases depression, fights fatigue, helps improve appetite, and also speeds the healing of all wounds. Choose a standardized extract containing 16 percent triterpenes and take 200 milligrams two to three times daily.

■ Hawthorn benefits the cardiovascular system, strengthens the heart muscle, helps regulate heartbeat, and acts to reduce high blood pressure. German studies have shown that hawthorn is very effective in the treatment of angina. Choose a standardized extract containing 1.8 percent vitexin-2 rhamnosides and take 100 to 200 milligrams two or three times a day.

■ Milk thistle contains silymarin, a potent flavonoid that protects cells against free-radical damage. It is particularly valuable for reducing inflammation in the liver and protecting against liver damage inflicted by toxins, including alcohol. Choose an extract standardized to contain 80 percent flavonoids (silymarin) and take 200 to 300 milligrams three times daily for one or two months out of the year.

■ Pine-bark and grape-seed extracts contain flavonoids called proanthocyanidins that work synergistically with vitamin C. Research suggests that these compounds help vitamin C to enter the cells and protect against oxidative damage. They can also help to protect against heart disease and cancer, strengthen the capillaries, and maintain collagen. Take 50 to 100 milligrams of pine-bark or grape-seed extract twice daily.

■ Schizandra is a Chinese herb with a reputation for promoting longevity. This tonic herb helps increase stamina, reduces fatigue, and has been used to treat stress and depression for centuries. It also is considered to be an aphrodisiac. Take 150 to 250 milligrams upon arising and again at bedtime.

■ The following is a four-week herbal program formulated especially for men in their forties and fifties. It has been designed to support the changes men experience during midlife, particularly with regard to the prostate. It can be used three to four times a year.

Week 1: Twice a day, take 160 milligrams of saw palmetto extract standardized to 80 to 90 percent essential fatty acids and sterols, plus an antioxidant formula supplying 10,000 international units of vitamin A, 15,000 international units of beta-carotene, 3,000 milligrams of vitamin C, 1,500 milligrams of bioflavonoids, 200 micrograms of selenium, and 25 milligrams of zinc daily.

Week 2: Three times daily, take one dose of a ginseng and fo-ti combination formula as recommended on the product label. Or take 100 milligrams of Siberian ginseng twice daily.

Week 3: Twice a day, take one dose of saw palmetto plus an antioxidant combination formula (*see under* Week 1, above).

Week 4: Three times daily, take one dose of a ginseng and fo-ti combination formula. Or take 100 milligrams of Siberian ginseng twice daily.

Note: If necessary for relief of chronic symptoms related to enlarged prostate, you can take the saw palmetto three times daily both during the entire four-week program and at other times. If you suffer from persistent or recurrent infections in conjunction with prostate problems, take one dose of an echinacea and goldenseal combination formula supplying 250 to 500 milligrams of echinacea and 150 to 300 milligrams of goldenseal daily for one week per month to support your immune system. Omit the ginseng if you have high blood pressure, heart disease, or hypoglycemia.

■ The following is a four-week herbal program formulated especially for women in their forties and fifties. It is designed to support women during the changes they experience in midlife, particularly with regard to the decline in hormonal production that occurs during menopause. You can use this program three or four times a year.

Week 1: Twice a day, take one dose of a dong quai and chaste tree (*Vitex agnus-castus*) combination formula supplying 500 milligrams of each herb, plus an antioxidant combination supplying 10,000 international units of vitamin A, 15,000 international units of beta-carotene, 3,000 milligrams of vitamin C, 1,500 milligrams of bioflavonoids, and 200 micrograms of selenium daily.

Week 2: Three times daily, take 200 milligrams of dong quai or 20 milligrams of black cohosh and 500 milligrams of red raspberry leaf.

Week 3: Twice a day, take one dose of a dong quai or black cohosh and chaste tree combination formula, plus an antioxidant combination (*see under* Week 1, above).

Week 4: Three times daily, take one dose of dong quai or black cohosh and red raspberry leaf (see under Week 2, above).

Note: You should also use a calcium and magnesium combination formula providing at least 1,000 milligrams of calcium and 500 milligrams of magnesium daily throughout the month. If you suffer from persistent or recurrent infections, take one dose of an echinacea and goldenseal combination formula supplying 250 to 500 milligrams of echinacea and 150 to 300 milligrams of goldenseal daily for one week per month to support your immune system.

■ The following is a four-week herbal and nutritional support program for people of either sex in their forties and fifties who are on health and fitness programs that include a low-fat, high-fiber diet and aerobic exercise. You can use this program three or four times a year. You can also supplement this program with garlic (the equivalent of 500 milligrams of fresh garlic three times daily) for one

to two weeks per month. Garlic helps detoxify the body and boost the immune system.

Week 1: Twice a day, take an antioxidant combination supplying 5,000 international units of vitamin A, 7,500 international units of beta-carotene, 1,500 milligrams of vitamin C, 750 milligrams of bioflavonoids, 100 micrograms of selenium, and 25 milligrams of zinc.

Week 2: Twice a day, take 100 milligrams of standardized Siberian ginseng extract and 500 milligrams of L-carnitine.

Week 3: Take an antioxidant combination (*see under* Week 1, above) plus 500 milligrams of hawthorn extract three times daily.

Week 4: Three times a day, take 100 milligrams of Siberian ginseng extract plus 500 milligrams of hawthorn extract.

HOMEOPATHY

■ See a homeopathic practitioner for a constitutional remedy. A constitutional remedy designed for your personal needs will help to maintain and enhance your vitality and health as you grow older.

BACH FLOWER REMEDIES

■ Select remedies that most closely fit your emotional tendencies and concerns, and take the remedies as needed, following the directions on the product label. These remedies can be immensely helpful. Start by using one remedy alone. If this does not bring about the changes you want, you can add or substitute another. (*See* BACH FLOWER REMEDIES in Part One for more information about using these remedies.)

ACUPRESSURE

For the locations of acupressure points on the body, *see* ADMINISTERING AN ACUPRESSURE TREATMENT in Part Three.

■ Acupressure (and massage) enhance circulation and increase vitality. Scheduling regular (daily, if possible) acupressure or massage treatments provides the most benefit. All acupressure points are pertinent during midlife, but Stomach 36 is the most important. It strengthens digestion and absorption or nutrients.

AROMATHERAPY

For specific instructions on how to use aromatherapy, *see* PREPARING AROMATHERAPY TREATMENTS in Part Three.

■ Essential oils of peppermint, rosemary, and vetiver help to energize and sharpen thinking and concentration. You can use either or both as an inhalant or diffuse them into the air in your home. Or you can add a few drops of peppermint oil to massage oil and use it in conjunction with massage.

Gender Differences in Aging

The average woman today can expect to outlive her mate by seven years. Science has long been puzzled by the longevity gap that exists between men and women. The latest theory that attempts to explain this gender gap has been put forth by gerontologist Royda Crose in her book *Why Women Live Longer Than Men* (Jossey-Bass, 1997). Crose speculates that some of the blame for men's shorter life span may be attributed to the sex hormone testosterone. Men have higher levels of testosterone in their bodies than women do, and this hormone fosters aggressive tendencies that can lead men to engage in risky adventures that may lead to injury or premature death. Crose also hypothesizes that this "macho" hormone may explain why men are more likely to feign invincibility and spurn help when they need it. This generates a great deal of stress, which many men attempt to ignore or hide—thereby only increasing the stress they are under. Stress contributes to many diverse health problems. Women, Crose says, are more likely to be able to release stress by talking about what is bothering them.

Further, women often live more diversified lives than men do. They tend to develop close relationships with many different people, whereas men are often shy about expressing deep feelings with anyone, with the possible exception of their spouses. In addition, many men focus most of their energies on their careers, while women are more likely to put equal emphasis on many different parts of their lives—family relationships, friendships, career, and community. As a result, when women retire or are widowed, they usually have good support networks to supply meaningful pursuits and human companionship, whereas men are more likely to feel disoriented and isolated in retirement and/or widowhood. Obviously, the more meaningful a person's life is—at whatever age or stage—the more zest for life he or she is apt to have. Research has shown that psychological factors such as life satisfaction have very real effects on physical health.

Another factor that may help women in the longevity game is that they tend to pay greater attention to their bodies. When a woman has a health problem, she is usually quick to consult a health-care professional. Many men feel threatened by signs of illness or interpret them as a kind of weakness, so they either ignore them or try to tough them out. Yet most people acknowledge that successful treatment is more likely if health problems are found in their early stages. The sex hormone estrogen may also play a role. At least until menopause, women have relatively high levels of estrogen in their bodies, and this appears to offer protection against a number of health problems, most notably cardiovascular disease. Finally, men are more likely to smoke and to drink too much than women are, and both smoking and excessive alcohol consumption are dangerous to health.

Closing the gender gap would please women all over the world. Most women want to keep their men with them for as long as possible. Unfortunately, nine out of ten women today survive their mates. Fortunately, we know of many ways men can change their lifestyles to increase their chances of living longer. Simply by eliminating known health risks—paying more attention to a healthy diet, regular exercise, cholesterol levels, and blood pressure; learning ways to reduce and deal with stress effectively; and avoiding harmful habits such as smoking and alcohol abuse—men can go a long way toward increasing their average life span.

■ Geranium, jasmine, myrrh, neroli, and vetiver oils are good for counteracting the visible signs of aging. Make a skin oil using one or several of these oils, or add a few drops of them to your favorite skin-care products (no more than 10 drops per ounce of product).

GENERAL RECOMMENDATIONS

■ Eliminate the known risk factors that contribute to serious health problems associated with aging. Keep your weight within a healthy range, and pay attention to your diet. Avoid exposure to toxins such as tobacco smoke and dangerous chemicals, and to excessive amounts of sun-light. A fourteen-year study of 10,000 Mormon men and women revealed that those who follow church teachings—which include avoiding all alcohol, caffeine, tobacco, and recreational drugs, and practicing premarital chastity and postmarital monogamy—are among the healthiest and longest-lived people in the United States.

■ Have regular physical checkups. This is the only way to keep track of your cholesterol count and blood pressure. If any danger signs are detected during your checkup, take immediate steps to remedy them.

■ Exercise regularly. Regular exercise maintains strength

and flexibility, boosts circulation, and improves a person's overall quality of life. Schedule at least twenty to thirty minutes of exercise at least three times a week.

■ Don't vegetate. Participate. For a very long time, scientists believed that it was impossible for the brain to generate new nerve cells or repair itself in any way. Ongoing research at the Salk Institute in La Jolla, California, however, suggests that new nerve cells can be generated in the hippocampus—an area of the brain involved in memory, learning, reasoning, and emotion—throughout life, as long as the brain is stimulated and challenged.

■ Pay attention to your spiritual side. Studies have shown that a strong faith in a higher power and, especially, regular participation in worship are associated with a longer life.

■ Hypothyroidism is a fairly common problem in people over the age of fifty. Common symptoms include fatigue, feeling cold, and unexplained weight gain. (*See* HYPO-THYROIDISM.)

AIDS

See HIV DISEASE.

Alcoholism

Alcoholism is a condition characterized by dependence, physical and/or psychological, on alcohol. Chronic alcoholism most often results from the regular consumption of ever-increasing amounts of alcohol over a long period of time. Some alcoholics engage in drinking binges that alternate with periods of sobriety; some are never completely sober.

This condition affects more than twice as many men as women. Experts say that at least 9 percent of adult men and 4 percent of adult women in the United States are alcohol-dependent—an estimated one out of every thirteen people. Alcohol dependence can occur at any age. Most active alcoholics are between the ages of thirty-five and fifty-five, but many teenagers and young adults are either alcohol-dependent or on their way to becoming so. Statistics show that three times as many college students today drink purposely to become intoxicated as did so just twenty years ago.

No one knows why some people are able to consume moderate amounts of alcohol for years without developing problems, while others become alcoholics. It is known,

however, that the children of alcoholic parents are more apt to use alcohol (and other recreational drugs) than people whose parents are teetotalers or controlled social drinkers. Studies have shown that even if children of alcohol-dependent parents are adopted by nondrinkers, they are still significantly more likely to grow up to abuse alcohol than biological children of nondrinkers. This suggests a genetic component in the tendency toward substance abuse and dependence.

Although alcoholism usually starts slowly and progresses gradually from social drinking to heavy drinking to dependence, it can progress with lightning speed, depending on an individual's tolerance for alcohol. Alcoholism typically develops in four main stages. In stage I, a social drinker develops an ability to drink a greater quantity of alcohol before experiencing any ill effects or becoming obviously intoxicated. This person is sometimes described as having a "hollow leg" because of a capacity to "hold his (or her) liquor," and may even be admired for it in some settings.

In stage II, the drinker begins to experience blackouts and has trouble remembering what occurred during a drinking binge. These memory lapses can be frightening, and they cause some drinkers to cut back on their consumption. An alcoholic in the making, however, usually either laughs off or ignores such episodes.

In stage III of the disease, the drinker no longer has the ability to stop drinking, even if he or she wants to. If confronted, he or she will either vehemently deny the existence of a problem, or promise to stop. Holding down a job is a challenge most stage-III alcoholics cannot meet. In many instances, a deep feeling of shame sets in, and the drinker will go to great lengths to hide the addiction—employing such tactics as stashing bottles in handy places and adding alcohol secretly to harmless beverages (such as coffee, tea, juice, and soda). Drinking in the morning and throughout the day becomes a necessity. A person in stage III undergoes sometimes frightening personality changes, with such traits as moodiness, irritability, jealousy, selfishness, and uncontrolled anger coming to the fore.

In stage IV, the final stage of alcoholism, the drinker suffers from mental and physical complications. Because of the calories coming from alcohol, he or she is likely to have no appetite for food. Personal appearance often suffers, and a formerly fastidious person may become a complete slob. The liver, which is responsible for metabolizing alcohol, suffers damage, which may include fatty degeneration, hepatitis, cirrhosis, and/or cancer. The heart muscle may suffer damage as well. In addition, prolonged heavy drinking increases the risk of high blood pressure, breast cancer, cancer of the mouth and/or esophagus, stroke, and impotence. The digestive system suffers from consumption of large amounts of alcohol (and insufficient

Alcohol and Pregnancy

A pregnant woman who drinks as little as two drinks per day (the equivalent of two ounces of liquor, eight ounces of wine, or sixteen ounces of beer) risks bearing a child with fetal alcohol syndrome. Children with this disorder are usually shorter than average, have smaller than normal eyes and small jaws, often are of lower than average intelligence, and may suffer birth defects such as a cleft palate or heart problems. Occasional "binge" drinking can also cause problems, even if a woman drinks very little during most of the nine months she is pregnant. Even if a woman drinks only small quantities, and only occasionally, there are still risks. Because a proportion of any alcohol a pregnant woman consumes will reach the developing fetus, even small amounts can affect normal development and also increase the risk of miscarriage. Fortunately, alcohol-related birth defects and other problems are completely preventable: If you are pregnant, or planning on becoming pregnant, do not take alcohol in any form.

intake and depletion of nutrients) and responds with gastritis, pancreatitis, and ulcers. Because alcohol acts as a diuretic and increases urine output, long-term heavy drinking can lead to kidney failure. Facial flushing, including that characteristic red nose, can become a permanent condition in heavy drinkers.

Alcohol also impairs the central nervous system. Symptoms such as confusion, disturbances of speech, an unsteady gait, pain, cramps, numbness, tingling, and weakness in the hands and legs are common. Alcoholism contributes to anxiety and psychiatric disorders, including severe depression. The incidence of both attempted and successful suicides is higher among alcoholics than any other group. Prolonged alcohol abuse can permanently injure the brain and central nervous system. This disease has social effects as well as physical ones. Alcoholism is a major factor in crime, marital breakdown, domestic violence, absenteeism, and accidents, both on the road and in the home.

When a serious alcoholic quits drinking, he or she may experience a type of withdrawal known as *delirium tremens,* or, colloquially, "DTs." This is a state characterized by confusion, tremors, heavy sweating, heart problems, hallucinations, and other uncomfortable symptoms. Seizures may also occur, and low magnesium and potassium levels are common. Delerium tremens usually begins within two days after the person starts abstaining from drink, and can last from two to ten days. As long as the person continues to avoid alcohol, chances are good that he or she will then recover.

Another potential alcohol-related problem is the state known as *alcoholic hallucinosis,* in which the person experiences hallucinations, usually auditory and laced with paranoia, and sometimes leading to aggressive outbursts. Alcoholic hallucinosis can accompany or follow heavy drinking. Recovery can take as long as several weeks, and the affected individual may or may not have to abstain from all alcohol in order to remain healthy afterwards.

Successful treatment depends entirely on the desire of the alcoholic to overcome the addiction. The earlier he or she acknowledges the condition, the earlier treatment can begin, and the greater the chance for a successful recovery. This entry focuses on what you can do to help yourself regain your health and control of your life.

CONVENTIONAL MEDICINE

■ In severe cases, detoxification may require medical supervision in a hospital setting in order to alleviate the worst reactions to withdrawal. This can include the use of tranquilizers such as diazepam (Valium) or alprazolam (Xanax) to control seizures, certain vitamins (particularly vitamin B_1, vitamin C, and folic acid) to address deficiencies and prevent complications, and rehydration therapy. Monitoring to prevent accidental injury may be necessary, and counseling is a standard part of treatment as well.

■ Disulfiram (Antabuse) is sometimes prescribed for persons who are motivated to quit drinking. If a person taking this drug drinks even a small quantity of alcohol, he or she will experience a toxic reaction whose symptoms include intense nausea, vomiting, severe headaches, blurred vision, and a feeling of impending death. Needless to say, as long as a person continues to take this drug, he or she will have great motivation to avoid alcohol in any form.

■ Naltrexone (Trexan) is a drug that blocks the pleasurable effects of alcohol. Some studies have shown that people who took this drug were three times as likely to stay with their recovery programs as those who did not. This drug is not suitable for people with liver disease, however.

■ Counseling and support are considered very helpful, if not vital, to the recovery process. Participation in Alcoholics Anonymous (AA, for the patient), Al-Anon (for the spouse), and Alateen (for adolescent children) has helped many people to deal with alcoholism in themselves and in their families. There are also other group approaches, such as Women for Sobriety, that can help. Private psychological and/or religious counseling can be beneficial as well.

DIETARY GUIDELINES

■ A healthy, well-balanced diet is very important. Alcoholics often get more of their daily calories from alcohol than from nutrient-dense food. Moreover, alcohol itself depletes the body of certain nutrients, particularly the water-soluble vitamins (the B-complex vitamins and vitamin C) and minerals such as calcium and magnesium. As a result, alcoholics are likely to suffer from multiple nutritional deficiencies. *See* DIET AND NUTRITION in Part One for information about healthy eating.

■ Particularly during the withdrawal period (about two to four weeks for most people, though it can continue for up to a year in some cases), eat five small, nutrient-dense meals daily, plus a nutritious snack or two as needed, to keep your blood-sugar level on an even keel. Alcohol raises blood sugar levels quickly, so when a person who is used to consuming large quantities of alcohol stops drinking, his or her blood-sugar level is likely to become unbalanced. Detoxification involves bringing the blood-sugar regulating mechanism back into balance. For the same reason, avoid foods containing sugars and other refined carbohydrates.

NUTRITIONAL SUPPLEMENTS

■ Alcohol is a source of free radicals and is damaging to many cells in the body. Antioxidants, including vitamins A, C, and E; the mineral selenium; and the amino acid cysteine, are nutrients that fight free-radical damage. Take 5,000 international units of vitamin A, 200 to 400 micrograms of selenium, and 500 milligrams of N-acetylcysteine (NAC) daily. Also take 1,000 milligrams of vitamin C with bioflavonoids three times daily and 400 international units of vitamin E (in mixed-tocopherol form) twice daily.

Note: If you are pregnant or have liver disease, consult your doctor before taking supplemental vitamin A. If you have high blood pressure, limit your intake of supplemental vitamin E to a total of 400 international units daily. If you are taking an anticoagulant (blood thinner), consult your physician before taking vitamin E.

■ Most alcoholics are deficient in the B vitamins, which are required to strengthen and restore the nervous system. Serious deficiency of the B vitamins is also a factor in delirium tremens. Take a B-complex supplement that supplies 25 milligrams of each of the primary B vitamins two to three times daily.

■ Carnitine, a substance related to the B vitamins but often grouped with the amino acids, has been shown to restore normal transport of fatty acids from the liver. It helps to reduce free fatty acid levels and reduces elevated triglycerides and liver enzymes. Start by taking a dose of 250 to 500 milligrams of L-carnitine with breakfast. After one week, add a second dose, with lunch. After another week, add a third dose, so that you are taking 250 to 500 milligrams with each meal. Continue taking L-carnitine for three to four months.

■ Chromium helps to even out blood-sugar levels and prevent hypoglycemia, which can be a problem for recovering alcoholics. Take 200 micrograms of chromium once or twice a day.

■ Choline helps restore normal liver function. Take 500 milligrams of choline twice daily.

■ Glutathione is an amino-acid compound that aids in detoxification of the liver. It is required by many of the body's systems for healthy functioning. Take 500 milligrams of glutathione twice a day.

■ Alcohol depletes the body of magnesium, which is required by the central nervous system. Take 250 milligrams of magnesium twice daily to correct deficiency and ease nervousness.

■ If you have an underactive thyroid (whether markedly so or whether tests show your thyroid functioning in the low-normal range), you are likely to feel very sluggish and very tired when you stop drinking. To counteract those symptoms, take 500 milligrams of the amino acid L-tyrosine twice daily, one dose before breakfast and the other before lunch, for up to three weeks.

Caution: If you are taking a monoamine oxidase (MAO) inhibitor, a type of drug often prescribed for depression, do not take supplemental tyrosine, as this may lead to a sudden and dangerous rise in blood pressure.

■ Vitamin A and beta-carotene help to repair the liver and strengthen liver function. Take 5,000 international units of vitamin A and 25,000 international units of beta-carotene twice a day.

Note: If you are pregnant, or intend to get pregnant, or if you have liver disease, consult your doctor before taking supplemental vitamin A. Pregnant women should not ingest a total of more than 25,000 international units of supplemental vitamin A *per week* from all sources.

■ Most alcoholics suffer from a deficiency of zinc. The body requires zinc to manufacture the enzymes essential for the detoxification of alcohol. Low levels of this mineral therefore make it difficult for the liver to metabolize alcohol, leading to more toxicity and a greater risk of cirrhosis. Take 25 milligrams of zinc twice a day.

Note: Take zinc with food to prevent stomach upset. If you take over 30 milligrams of zinc daily for more than one or two months, you should also take 1 to 2 milligrams of copper each day to maintain a proper mineral balance.

HERBAL TREATMENT

A two-week herbal detoxification program is helpful for cleansing the body at the beginning of the recovery process. The program may be repeated as needed.

Week 1: Take one dose of an echinacea and goldenseal combination formula supplying 250 to 500 milligrams of echinacea and 150 to 300 milligrams of goldenseal three to four times daily for three days. This combination helps detoxify the blood and the lymphatic system quickly.

Week 2: Two or three times daily, take 100 milligrams of standardized Siberian ginseng extract containing 0.5 percent eleutheroside E. Siberian ginseng restores energy and helps regulate blood sugar and the hormonal system.

Milk thistle is the primary herb for all diseases that involve the liver. It contains silymarin and other substances that restore and protect liver function. Choose an extract standardized to contain 80 percent flavonoids (silymarin) and take 200 to 300 milligrams three times daily for three months.

Bupleurum and dragon bone is an old Chinese herbal remedy that is helpful for anxiety caused by withdrawal from alcohol. Take a bupleurum and dragon bone combination formula as directed on the product label.

Dandelion is a mild liver-protective remedy. It enhances the flow of bile, thereby relieving liver congestion. Take 500 milligrams or one cup of dandelion-root tea three times a day for six weeks. Stop for one month, then repeat.

HOMEOPATHY

Lachesis helps to relax the female social alcoholic who often awakens with a headache. This individual can talk endlessly, and doesn't like tight clothing around her waist. Take one dose of *Lachesis* 30x or 15c three times daily for five days.

Nux vomica helps to detoxify the body. Take one dose of *Nux vomica* 30x or 15c, as directed on the product label, three times daily for three days. Stop for one week, then repeat.

Quercus is a homeopathic remedy that reduces the craving for alcohol. Take one dose of *Quercus* 12x or 6c three times a day for five days. Thereafter, take one dose as needed to counteract cravings.

Zincum metallicum is for the person who is hypersensitive to light and noise, and who has a low sex drive. Take one dose of *Zincum metallicum* 30x or 15c three times a day for three days. Stop for three days, then take one dose three times a day for another three days.

BACH FLOWER REMEDIES

Select the remedy that most closely fits your emotional tendencies and concerns, and take it as needed, following the directions on the product label.

■ Holly is the remedy for feelings of frustration that are displayed with anger and fits of temper.

■ Impatiens is for nervous tension, impatience, and irritability.

ACUPRESSURE

For the locations of acupressure points on the body, *see* ADMINISTERING AN ACUPRESSURE TREATMENT in Part Three.

■ Gallbladder 34 relaxes the muscles.

■ Large Intestine 4, 10, 11 detoxify the body.

■ Liver 3 relaxes the nervous system and restores the liver.

■ Spleen 10 helps to detoxify the blood.

AROMATHERAPY

For specific instructions on how to use aromatherapy, *see* PREPARING AROMATHERAPY TREATMENTS in Part Three.

■ Many essential oils can be used to reduce stress and help restore balance. The oils best known for these effects include bergamot, elemi, frankincense, lavender, neroli, thyme, and ylang ylang. You can use one or more of these as an inhalant or diffuse them into the air in your home.

GENERAL RECOMMENDATIONS

■ Avoid alcohol in any form. Be aware of "hidden" sources of alcohol. For instance, it is an ingredient in many different food products, mouthwashes, and over-the-counter cold medicines. Ironically, beverages marketed as "nonalcoholic" wines and beers very often do contain some alcohol, so it is best simply to avoid these. The only way to know is to read labels or, in the case of foods served in restaurants or in the homes of other people, to ask your chef, waiter, or host.

■ If you are not already a member of Alcoholics Anonymous (AA), join. There is no greater support for alcoholics who want to stop drinking than AA, as millions of recovering alcoholics will attest.

■ Many alcoholics suffer from reactive hypoglycemia and/or thyroid malfunction. Discuss these possibilities with your doctor. *See* HYPOGLYCEMIA and/or HYPOTHYROIDISM for additional information and recommendations.

■ When cravings start, don't give them time to build. Take a dose of homeopathic *Quercus* 12x or 6c and immediately begin engaging in the form of exercise of your choice. Anything from jumping jacks in the living room (or your workplace) to a jog around the block or a walk around the mall will help blunt the craving for alcohol.

■ For additional help and information, contact Alcoholics Anonymous (call the number listed in the White Pages of your local telephone directory or write or call their headquarters in New York) or call the Alcohol and Drug Helpline (see the Resources section at the end of the book).

Allergic Rhinitis

See ALLERGIES; HAY FEVER.

Allergies

An allergy is a hypersensitive reaction to a normally harmless substance. There are a variety of substances, termed allergens, that may trouble a sensitive individual. Common allergens include pollen, animal dander, house dust, feathers, mites, chemicals, and a variety of foods. Some allergies primarily cause respiratory symptoms; others can cause such diverse symptoms as headache, fatigue, fever, diarrhea, stomachache, and vomiting. This entry addresses respiratory allergies, both chronic and seasonal (for a discussion of allergic reactions caused by foods, *see* FOOD ALLERGIES).

If you have allergies, you may suffer from a stuffy and/or runny nose, sneezing, itchy skin and eyes, and/or red, watery eyes. Needless to say, it can be very uncomfortable. These symptoms occur because, in the presence of an allergen, the immune system releases chemicals called histamines to fight what it perceives as an invader. Histamines cause a string of reactions, including the swelling and congestion of nasal passages and increased mucus production. This is essentially a hypersensitive, or overactive, response by the body to an external stimulus.

Whether allergies are seasonal or chronic depends on the particular allergen or allergens involved. Seasonal allergies tend to be caused by pollen (*See* HAY FEVER). Ongoing or chronic allergies are usually caused by factors that are present in the environment year-round, such as animal dander, dust, or feathers. Chronic allergic rhinitis is a persistent inflammation of the mucous membrane lining the nasal passages that is caused by an allergic reaction. It is characterized by a stuffy, runny nose, frequent sneezing, and a tendency to breathe through the mouth. The eyes may be red and watery. Headache, itchiness, nosebleeds, and fatigue may be secondary complications. Dark circles under the eyes (called "allergic shiners"), along with a puffy look to the face, are frequently seen. Whether symptoms occur seasonally or chronically, there is often a family history of allergies; many times a parent or grandparent of an allergy sufferer also had allergies.

Allergies can contribute to other chronic health problems, such as acne, asthma, eczema, incontinence, irritability, and even difficulty maintaining concentration. Allergic reactions can occur immediately after exposure to the offending substance, or take days to surface. A delay in the onset of an allergic reaction can make it more difficult to pinpoint the allergen.

EMERGENCY TREATMENT

■ Occasionally, an allergic reaction is so severe it can be life threatening. If you develop rapidly spreading hives or have difficulty breathing, especially if you have a history of severe reactions, have someone take you immediately to the emergency room of the nearest hospital, or call for emergency help and stress the urgency of the situation. Seconds count. If you have an emergency adrenaline-injection kit, such as Ana-Kit or EpiPen, administer it immediately, either as you are on your way to the hospital or while you wait for help to arrive.

CONVENTIONAL TREATMENT

■ Conventional medical treatment of allergies often begins with tracking down the offending substance. There are several tests your physician may recommend to identify the particular allergens that are making your life miserable:

• Scratch testing consists of placing a small amount of diluted allergen on a lightly scratched area of skin. If a bump develops there within fifteen minutes, you are probably allergic to that substance.

• Intradermal testing is done by injecting the skin with suspected allergens at timed intervals. A control injection (one containing no allergen) is also given. If an allergen produces a wheal (a red, itchy bump), you are allergic to that substance. An intradermal test is more accurate than a scratch test, but there is a greater risk that you might suffer a severe reaction.

• Blood testing (a radioallergosorbent test, or RAST) measures total and specific levels of IgE and IgG, which are antibodies produced by the body's immune system. An elevated level of either of these may indicate an allergic reaction to the substance being tested.

■ Once testing has been completed, treatment may be recommended. Antihistamines are the medications most commonly used for respiratory allergies. They work by blocking the action of the histamines that cause swelling and congestion of nasal passages and increased mucus production. Brompheniramine (in Allerhist and Dimetane, among others), diphenhydramine (Benadryl), and chlorpheniramine (Chlor-Trimeton) are common over-the-counter antihistamines suggested for respiratory allergies. Possible side effects include drowsiness and dry mouth.

■ Prescription antihistamines include azatadine (Optimine, Trinalin), clemastine (Tavist), astemizole (Hismanal), and promethazine (Phenergan). Astemizole does not cause the drowsiness that other antihistamines do, but has been implicated in causing serious heart-rhythm problems that, in some cases, led to death. Do not take these medications at the same time as the antibiotic erythromycin (ERYC, Ilotycin) or the antifungal ketoconazole (Nizoral), as this seems to magnify the problem. Loratidine (Claritin) is a newer antihistamine that seems to avoid the heart-rhythm problem, but you still may have to deal with fatigue, headache, dry mouth, abdominal pain, anxiety, and other side effects that are common to antihistamines.

■ Cromolyn sodium (Intal or Nasalcrom) is a medication that can be taken as a nasal spray to prevent the symptoms of respiratory allergies. It works by coating the membranes of the nose and stabilizing the white blood cells so that they do not react to foreign substances. In some cases this drug can cause gastrointestinal upset or throat and nose irritation, but it usually produces very few side effects and is generally considered one of the safer medications. Its major drawback is that it must be used consistently, as many as six times a day for at least two weeks, before it begins to take effect.

■ Decongestants decrease nasal congestion and swelling by constricting the blood vessels in the nasal membranes, thus allowing the mucus to drain more effectively. Decongestants are available as pills, nasal drops, and nasal sprays. These include oxymetazoline (in Afrin, Dristan, Sinex, and others), phenylephrine (in Alconefrin, Allerest, and others), phenylpropanolamine (found in many common over-the-counter formulas, including Contac, Coricidin D, Sine-Off, and Sinutab), and pseudoephedrine (Neo-Fed, Sudafed, and others). These medications have a number of common side effects, including restlessness and insomnia. Also, if a spray or drop form is used for more than three or four days in a row, it creates a dependency that results in a rebound—or worsening of symptoms—when the medicine is stopped.

■ If allergy symptoms include shortness of breath, theophylline may be helpful in opening these passageways (See ASTHMA). Side effects can include heart rhythm problems, headache, nausea, irritability, convulsions, rashes.

■ An increasing trend has been to use steroid inhalant sprays such as triamcinolone (Azmacort, Nasacort) and beclomethasone (Beclovent, Beconase, Vanceril, Vancenase). They are especially useful for people who suffer from chronic allergic rhinitis. These are powerful anti-inflammatories, and decrease swelling and mucus pro-

duction as well as the oral antihistamines do, without causing sedation.

■ If antihistamines offer no relief, desensitization is sometimes recommended for the relief of allergies. This involves the injection of gradually increasing amounts of allergen into the body over a period of time. However, the procedure is complicated and costly, requires careful supervision by a physician, and is not always effective. It should be tried only if no other form of treatment affords any relief.

■ In some cases, a chronic runny nose may not be the result of an allergic reaction, and should be distinguished from a more serious underlying illness, such as chronic sinusitis. This is a task best performed by a health-care professional.

DIETARY GUIDELINES

■ Drink lots of water to thin secretions and ease expectoration.

■ If you have respiratory allergies, you may be allergic to certain foods. In addition to dairy products and wheat, common culprits include eggs, chocolate, nuts, seafood, and citrus fruits and juices. Try eliminating one of these foods for two weeks and watch for an improvement. Use an elimination or rotation diet to discover and work with food allergies (See ELIMINATION DIET or ROTATION DIET in Part Three). Or keep a diary recording your symptoms and the foods eaten.

■ Try eliminating dairy foods from your diet. Dairy foods can thicken mucus and stimulate an increase in mucus production. If your allergies are seasonal, it may also be helpful to avoid whole wheat during the allergy season; many allergy sufferers are sensitive to wheat.

■ Cut out cooked fats and oils. When your body is under any type of stress, including the stress of an allergic reaction, the digestive system is not as strong as usual, and fats—which are difficult to digest at the best of times—can put a strain on the digestive system. Also, undigested fats contribute to mucus production and foster a toxic internal environment.

■ Monitor the ratio of different types of foods you eat to one another. Eating either too much fat or too much carbohydrate (or both) can cause allergic symptoms.

NUTRITIONAL SUPPLEMENTS

■ Calcium and magnesium are important nutrients for the allergy sufferer. They help to relax an overreactive nervous system. While symptoms are acute, take a supplement containing 750 to 1,000 milligrams of calcium and 500 milligrams of magnesium twice a day. Then take the same dosage once a day for two months.

■ Allergies are often related to the transformation and

transportation of foods in the digestive system. Taking a digestive-enzyme supplement will enhance the assimilation and utilization of nutrients. Take a full-spectrum digestive-enzyme supplement providing 5,000 international units of lipase, 2,500 international units of amylase, and 300 international units of protease, plus 500 to 1,000 milligrams of pancreatin immediately after each meal.

Note: Long-term supplementation with pancreatin is not advised, as it can cause your pancreas to reduce its own production of this important enzyme. Overuse also has the potential to cause nausea or diarrhea. After two months on pancreatin, discontinue use and monitor your reaction. If you find that your problems recur, discuss pancreatin supplementation with your health-care provider.

■ Essential fatty acids such as those found in black currant seed, borage, evening primrose, and flaxseed oils help to regulate the inflammatory response. Take 500 to 1,000 milligrams of any of these oils twice each day for one month.

■ Methylsulfonylmethane (MSM) is a good source of sulfur, a trace mineral that may help to reduce the severity of the allergic response. Take 500 milligrams three or four times daily, with meals.

■ Selenium is an antioxidant and works synergistically with vitamin E. Take 50 to 100 micrograms twice a day during the allergy season.

■ Thymus glandular extract helps to strengthen immune function and diminish the allergic response. Take a product supplying 30 milligrams of pure thymus polypeptides twice a day, with breakfast and lunch, for six weeks.

■ The B-complex vitamins help to support adrenal function and strengthen the immune system. For seasonal allergy symptoms, take a B-vitamin complex supplying at least 25 milligrams of each of the major B vitamins each day (between or before meals) for two to three months.

■ Pantothenic acid, one of the B vitamins, is exceptional for resolving the acute symptoms of a respiratory allergic reaction. Take 250 to 500 milligrams three to four times daily for one week, then reduce the dosage to 250 milligrams three to four times daily, as needed, for an additional week. You can also take pantothenic acid in anticipation of the hay fever season to prevent symptoms before they start. When taking individual B vitamins, it is a good idea to take a balanced B-complex supplement separately, at a different time of day.

■ If you suffer from allergic rhinitis coupled with fatigue and constipation, vitamin B_{12} may be helpful. Take 500 micrograms once a day for one week.

■ Vitamin C has anti-inflammatory properties. During acute flare-ups, take 1,000 milligrams five times a day for four to five days. Follow this with 1,000 milligrams three times a day for three weeks; then take 1,000 milligrams a day for two months. Some people with allergies find mineral ascorbate vitamin C or esterified vitamin C (Ester-C) easier to tolerate than simple ascorbic acid.

■ Bioflavonoids are potent anti-inflammatories with specific antiallergenic effects and are best taken with vitamin C. Bioflavonoids are chemically related to cromolyn sodium (*see under* Conventional Treatment in this entry). Take 1,000 milligrams three times a day for two weeks.

HERBAL TREATMENT

■ Astragalus is a Chinese herb that helps to strengthen the overall constitution. Take 500 milligrams daily for one month before the hay fever season begins.

Note: Do not take astragalus if you have a fever or any other signs of acute infection.

■ If your nasal mucus is green or yellow, you may have an infection on top of allergies. Take one dose of an echinacea and goldenseal combination formula supplying 250 to 500 milligrams of echinacea and 150 to 300 milligrams of goldenseal two to three times daily for five to seven days to help resolve the infection.

■ If you enjoy herbal teas, prepare a blended tea of fenugreek, thyme, and licorice (*see* PREPARING HERBAL TREATMENTS in Part Three). These herbs act as mild decongestants and work to relieve nasal and sinus congestion. Take one cup of tea twice daily, as needed.

Note: Do not take licorice on a daily basis for more than five days in a row, as it can elevate blood pressure. If you have high blood pressure, omit the licorice entirely.

■ Nettle can be very helpful for drying out the sinuses. It can be highly effective for chronic allergies. Take 150 to 500 milligrams two or three times daily, as needed, for two weeks.

Note: Some people experience stomach upset as a result of taking nettle. If this happens, stop taking the herb.

■ Turmeric is an East Indian herb with natural anti-inflammatory properties. It is an excellent remedy for those who suffer from fatigue coupled with allergies. Take 500 milligrams three times daily.

HOMEOPATHY

Homeopathy can work simply and effectively in resolving allergy symptoms. Select a symptom-specific remedy and, unless otherwise noted, take one dose (as directed on the product label) three times daily for three days. If there is no improvement after thirty-six hours, try another remedy. When you do notice an improvement, discontinue the remedy. If your symptoms return, resume taking one dose, three times daily, for another two days. If the problem is not resolved, it may be helpful to consult a homeopathic practitioner who can prescribe a constitutional remedy.

■ *Allium cepa* 30x or 9c is good if you experience bouts of sneezing with a burning sensation in the nose that affects the upper lip, and if your symptoms improve in the outdoors or when you splash your face with cold water. *Allium cepa* is homeopathic onion. It is for an allergic reaction similar to the one many people have when cutting or peeling an onion—red, teary eyes, for example.

■ *Ammonium muriaticum* 30x or 9c is good if you have a watery discharge that burns your upper lip and the inside of your nose. You may have the feeling that your nose is stopped up even though your nose is running. You may also lose your sense of smell and/or experience a tickling feeling in your throat.

■ *Arsenicum album* 30x or 9c can be helpful if you are sneezing, with nasal burning, and if you feel better with hot compresses on the sides of your nose and when breathing into a warm humidifier. Restlessness, fatigue, cold hands and feet, and waking in the night with great distress are symptoms of the *Arsenicum* individual. Chances are you are not only allergic to dust and mold, but highly sensitive to cats as well. You may also have food allergies to milk, wheat, or sugar, and tend to be high-strung.

■ *Calcarea carbonica* 30x or 9c should be beneficial if you are pale and sweat a lot, especially around the head, and are sensitive to drafts. Swollen glands may accompany your runny nose. You may have digestive problems as well.

■ *Euphrasia* 30x or 9c, which is homeopathic eyebright, is good if you have burning tears and a nonacrid nasal discharge. There is a good chance you often develop conjunctivitis along with your allergies. You are very sensitive to light and prefer to stay indoors in a dimly lit room.

■ Take *Hydrastis* 12x or 6c if you have a thick yellow or yellow-green discharge from the nose. Very often mucus will form crusts around the nose. *Hydrastis* is homeopathic goldenseal.

■ *Natrum muriaticum* 12x or 6c is recommended if you feel that the inside of your runny nose hurts or burns. You will likely have thick mucus; you may have a sore or pustule between your nose and upper lip; and your lips are dry and cracked. You probably like—perhaps even crave—salty foods.

■ *Pulsatilla* 30x or 9c will help if you feel much worse in a stuffy room and better in the cool, open air. As a result, you prefer to sleep with the window open. Your nasal passages are congested and dry at night, with a nonirritating yellow discharge during the day. *Pulsatilla* is homeopathic windflower (anemone). For the person whose moods and symptoms change like the wind, homeopathic windflower works wonders.

■ Try *Sabadilla* 30x or 9c if you experience spasmodic sneezing with a lot of nasal discharge and a peculiar itching of the nose and soft palate that makes you want to scratch your upper palate. Exposure to flowers often increases the itching and sneezing.

■ If you often have a runny nose, take *Thuja* 30x or 9c twice a day for two days. This remedy is helpful for people who are sensitive to cold and humidity, and have a tendency to develop warts.

■ If none of the above remedies seems to match your situation, there are homeopathic combination formulas available that may be useful.

ACUPRESSURE

For the locations of acupressure points on the body, *see* ADMINISTERING AN ACUPRESSURE TREATMENT in Part Three.

■ Four Gates helps to calm the nervous system.

■ Gallbladder 20 helps to relieve head congestion.

■ Large Intestine 4 helps to relieve head congestion.

■ Large Intestine 11 reduces the severity of allergic reactions.

■ Large Intestine 20 clears the nose and decreases sinus congestion.

■ Stomach 36 strengthens overall well-being.

AROMATHERAPY

For specific instructions on how to use aromatherapy, *see* PREPARING AROMATHERAPY TREATMENTS in Part Three. Note that it is possible for some essential oils to cause allergic reactions in susceptible individuals. You may wish to start with only 1 drop of each. If your symptoms seem to worsen, discontinue use of the suspect oil.

■ Essential oils of basil, eucalyptus, peppermint, and pine help to ease congestion. You can use them as inhalants, diffuse them into the air, or make a steam inhalation treatment with them.

■ Relaxing the nervous system is very important in controlling allergies. To help yourself relax, try a bath prepared with 3 drops of lavender oil plus 3 drops of either chamomile or clary sage oil.

■ If your allergies cause cold- or flulike symptoms, try a bath with 2 drops of rosemary oil, 2 drops of grapefruit oil, and 2 drops of juniper or tea tree oil.

GENERAL RECOMMENDATIONS

■ Avoid contact with plants that cause an allergic reaction, especially during their pollination seasons.

■ Investigate and eliminate possible environmental factors that may be contributing to the problem. Environmental triggers include dust, molds, and cigarette smoke. Wood- and/or coal-burning stoves and fireplaces can also be a source of respiratory irritation. In extreme cases, it may be necessary to eliminate feather pillows and household items that collect and hold dust, such as knickknacks, rugs, draperies, and even upholstered furniture.

■ If animal dander causes a reaction, keep pets outside. Above all, do not permit pets in your bedroom.

■ Saline nasal irrigation is valuable for a chronic runny nose. Use the procedure described under NASAL SALINE FLUSH in Part Three, then suck out the mucus with a bulb syringe.

■ Allergies usually cause a clear, thin nasal discharge. If you develop a discharge that is thick and yellowish or greenish in color and that does not seem to go away, you may have a different problem, such as a sinus infection. Consult your physician.

PREVENTION

■ There is no known way to prevent allergies from developing. However, if you suffer from allergies, you can prevent acute flare-ups of allergic symptoms by identifying those things you are allergic to and then avoiding them. If this fails (or is not possible), use the suggestions in this entry to help you alleviate symptoms.

Alopecia

See HAIR LOSS.

Alzheimer's Disease

Alzheimer's disease is a progressive brain disorder in which the nerve cells degenerate and the size of the brain shrinks, resulting in dementia—a deterioration in mental functioning. Alzheimer's disease is the cause of more than 75 percent of documented cases of dementia in North Americans over sixty-five years of age. At the current time, some 5 million Americans suffer from Alzheimer's disease, but as the population ages in the coming years, this figure is expected to rise—to 15 million by the year 2020, according to some experts.

Alzheimer's disease strikes some people in their forties and fifties, but this is rare. Most people who develop the condition are over sixty. Although it is not a result of the normal aging process, the incidence increases steadily with age.

There are three broad stages that characterize the progression of Alzheimer's disease. In stage I, the individual becomes increasingly forgetful, and may even joke about it. The progressive loss of short-term memory often triggers compulsive list-writing, as the affected person seeks to overcome this frightening problem. He or she feels understandably anxious, and may become depressed.

In stage II, memory loss continues. Although memories of the past may remain sharp during this period, the person experiences increasing difficulty remembering events that occurred the previous day, or even what happened on a favorite television show the minute it goes off the air. In this stage of the disease, the first signs of disorientation appear. The individual may become confused just visiting a neighbor he or she has known for years. The ability to master numbers declines, concentration slips, and finding the right word to complete a sentence becomes a challenge. This is a particularly difficult time. The affected person is very much aware of his or her decline, very anxious over what will come next, and frustrated by the knowledge that there is no way to prevent the degeneration taking place. Mood changes are sudden and unpredictable. Personality changes are inevitable.

In stage III, the disease takes over. Unmistakable signs of nerve damage begin to appear. Hallucinations and delusions are common. Incontinence becomes an issue. Some people in this stage of the disease become passive and compliant, while others become violent and strike out. During a violent episode, the person may be a danger to him- or herself and to others. People with this insidious disease sooner or later lose all their treasured memories, can no longer recognize loved ones, and forget everything, from their own names to how to tell time or tie a shoelace. Although many people with Alzheimer's disease continue to live on in this state for a number of years, some fall into a coma and slip away.

No one knows what causes Alzheimer's disease to develop. Some scientists theorize, however, that it may be linked to damage caused by free radicals. Free radicals are unstable molecules or parts of molecules that form as a result of cellular metabolism as well as exposure to certain substances, such as tobacco smoke. These unstable compounds can interact with cells, including brain cells, and damage them. The body has certain natural defenses against free radicals, namely substances known as antioxidants, which deactivate the free radicals and prevent them from doing any harm. Unfortunately, however, there are often more free radicals present than the body can deactivate, resulting in cellular damage. Science has identified a number of different vitamins, minerals, enzymes, and other substances that act as antioxidants. As people grow older, however, deficiencies of important nutrients become quite common, and more serious. It has been demonstrated that people with Alzheimer's disease are usually deficient in antioxidants.

In addition to revealing signs of shrinkage, microscopic examination of the brains of people affected by Alzheimer's disease shows a loss of nerve cells, the development of neurofibrillary tangles (tangles of nerve fibers) wrapped around the brain's memory center, and accumulations of bits of debris. Buildups of beta-amyloid, a type of protein, have been found clogging brain tissue. These protein clogs were once thought to be a result of the disease, but more recently, scientists have begun to believe that they may actually be involved in causing it. Studies show that a lack of acetylcholine, a chemical that facilitates the transmission of messages between nerve cells, fosters the formation of the deposits that clog brain tissue. Certain natural hormones that may inhibit this buildup are currently under investigation.

There is some controversy over whether exposure to aluminum may play a role in the development of Alzheimer's. However, it is true that autopsies of people who have died of Alzheimer's disease show abnormally high levels of aluminum in the brain. In this connection, it is interesting to note that patients undergoing kidney dialysis sometimes develop a syndrome called dialysis dementia, which is believed to be a result of high concentrations of aluminum in the brain coming from aluminum in the water used for dialysis.

Obtaining a reliable diagnosis of Alzheimer's disease is difficult. There are certain tests that can suggest the presence of the disease—an electroencephalogram (EEG) may show increasingly slow brain waves, or a computerized tomography (CT) or magnetic resonance imaging (MRI) scan may show evidence of shrinkage of the brain, for example—but there is no single definitive test that can be performed on a living person. Diagnosis is generally made based on symptoms and by a process of elimination. A physician must first rule out such problems as hypothyroidism, pernicious anemia, vitamin deficiencies, brain tumor, and subdural hematoma (an accumulation of blood in the brain), any of which can cause similar symptoms. Lyme disease also can cause Alzheimer's-like symptoms, as can a "silent" (undiagnosed) stroke. Further, the effects of drugs and drug interactions must be considered. Many older people regularly take multiple prescription and nonprescription drugs that can affect mental function. Some people who exhibit signs of dementia are actually suffering from what doctors call *pseudodementia*, which is a form of depression and is treatable. If all these conditions have been investigated and ruled out, the diagnosis of Alzheimer's may be made, based on physical and symptomatic evidence.

CONVENTIONAL TREATMENT

■ If you or a loved one suffers from Alzheimer's disease, you should seek out and work closely with a neurologist or other physician who specializes, or at the very least has considerable experience, in the treatment of this illness.

■ All medications that are not absolutely necessary should be discontinued, as many drugs have detrimental effects on mental processes.

■ Tacrine (Cognex) is a prescription drug that short-term studies have found to be "reasonably efficacious" in treating Alzheimer's disease. However, only about a third of patients seem to respond to it, and even then appreciable improvement is less than outstanding. The results of long-term treatment with tacrine are as yet undetermined, and careful weekly liver function studies are mandatory, as liver damage is a not-uncommon side effect.

■ Ergot mesylate (Hydergine) has been tried as a treatment for Alzheimer's, with mixed results. Some patients appear to experience improved mood, and may be able to care for themselves somewhat better while taking this drug, but there is no proof that it brings about any demonstrable mental improvement.

■ The hormone estrogen may help relieve symptoms of Alzheimer's disease in postmenopausal women. In research released by the Society for Neuroscience, estrogen administered in skin-patch form increased memory ability and concentration and dramatically enhanced mental activity in elderly women suffering from Alzheimer's disease. Estrogen appears to promote the growth of brain cells and enhance the connections between them, thereby improving memory and lengthening the attention span. However, these effects are specific to women.

■ Treatment with hyperbaric oxygen (putting the person in a closed chamber with a high-pressure oxygen atmosphere) has been tried for Alzheimer's disease. Unfortunately, it does not seem to provide significant improvement in most cases.

■ No matter how beloved the person with Alzheimer's disease is, in the end stage of the disease, home care almost always is an impossibility. If the individual is bedridden, as is often the case, additional complications such as bedsores, feeding difficulties, and the possibility of pneumonia arise. The time will come when full-time hospital and/or nursing-home care is required, for the welfare of both the patient and his or her family.

DIETARY GUIDELINES

■ A person with Alzheimer's disease should eat healthy, well-balanced meals and increase his or her consumption of vegetables and fruits. Smaller, more frequent meals are recommended to keep blood sugar levels on an even keel.

Four to six small meals per day are better than three large meals.

■ Anyone who has Alzheimer's disease should *avoid* alcohol, nicotine, and excessive amounts of caffeine.

NUTRITIONAL SUPPLEMENTS

■ All the antioxidants help fight free radicals, which have been implicated in the development of this disorder. A person with Alzheimer's disease should take 5,000 international units of beta-carotene and 100 micrograms of selenium twice a day, plus supplements of pine-bark or grape-seed extract as directed below.

■ The B vitamins are necessary for the proper functioning of neurotransmitters. Many people with Alzheimer's disease have low levels of the B vitamins, especially vitamin B_{12}. A person with Alzheimer's disease should take a B-complex supplement that supplies at least 25 milligrams of each of the primary B vitamins twice a day, plus an additional 500 micrograms of vitamin B_{12} three to four times daily. Although the oral form of B_{12} is acceptable, injections are more easily assimilated. Ask your doctor about weekly injections of vitamin B_{12}.

■ Carnitine assists in the utilization of fats. When fats are digested more efficiently, nerve tissue stays healthier. Carnitine has been shown to have an impact on the attention span and may aid concentration. A person with Alzheimer's disease should take 500 milligrams of L-carnitine twice daily. Research has shown that L-acetylcarnitine (a form of carnitine chemically bound to acetic acid) can significantly enhance brain function and energy in people with Alzheimer's disease. This form of carnitine is more expensive than regular L-carnitine, but it seems to have benefits specific to this disorder. When taking any form of carnitine, it is best to start by taking a dose of 250 to 500 milligrams of L-carnitine with breakfast. After one week, add a second dose, with lunch. After another week, add a third dose, so that you are taking 250 to 500 milligrams with each meal.

■ Choline stimulates the production of acetylcholine, which helps boost short-term memory. The recommended dose is 500 milligrams three times daily.

■ Coenzyme Q_{10} helps to increase the supply of oxygen to the brain. A person with Alzheimer's disease should take 50 milligrams of coenzyme Q_{10} twice daily.

■ A good digestive-enzyme supplement helps to ensure complete utilization of all nutrients. A person with Alzheimer's disease should take a full-spectrum digestive-enzyme supplement containing lipase, amylase, protease, and betaine hydrochloride (HCl) immediately before each meal, following the dosage directions on the product label.

■ Lecithin contains choline, and is a fat emulsifier. Take 1,200 milligrams twice daily, with meals.

■ Lipoic acid helps defuse toxic metabolites created during imperfect liver metabolism. A person with Alzheimer's disease should take 100 milligrams three times daily.

■ A deficiency of magnesium, in conjunction with high concentrations of aluminum in the brain, can result in progressive dementia. In addition, many people with Alzheimer's disease suffer from constipation. Magnesium can either alleviate or prevent constipation, as needed. A person with Alzheimer's disease should take 250 milligrams of magnesium twice daily. If loose stools result, reduce the dosage.

■ Low levels of phosphatidylserine, an important brain nutrient, are associated with impaired mental function and depression. The recommended dosage is 100 milligrams taken three times daily.

■ The person with Alzheimer's should take 500 milligrams of vitamin C with bioflavonoids three times daily. This combination acts against inflammation and fights free-radical activity.

■ A two-year study of Alzheimer's patients given megadoses of vitamin E (2,000 international units daily) showed that this vitamin slowed the loss of function by about 25 percent, and delayed the necessity of committing the patients to nursing-home care by an average of about seven months. In contrast, the usual therapeutic dose of vitamin E is 400 international units administered twice daily. The best way to start taking vitamin E is to begin with 100 or 200 milligrams and gradually increase to the recommended amount.

Note: Persons with high blood pressure should limit their intake of supplemental vitamin E to a total of 400 international units daily. Anyone who takes an anticoagulant (blood thinner) should consult his or her physician before taking supplemental vitamin E.

■ Zinc and evening primrose oil have been shown to help some Alzheimer's patients. Evening primrose oil and flaxseed oil are good anti-inflammatories and sources of essential fatty acids. Zinc helps prevent degeneration of nerve tissue and has been shown to prevent the deposition of lead in the tissues, which can lead to the characteristic neurofibrillary tangles found in the brains of Alzheimer's patients. Zinc deficiency also causes abnormal functioning of certain enzymes, resulting in abnormal DNA production, which may promote the formation of the tangles. A person with Alzheimer's should take 25 milligrams of zinc and 500 to 1,000 milligrams of evening primrose or flaxseed oil twice daily.

Note: Zinc should be taken with food to prevent stomach upset. Anyone who takes over 30 milligrams of zinc daily for more than one or two months should also take 1 to 2 milligrams of copper each day to maintain a proper mineral balance in the body.

HERBAL TREATMENT

■ Chinese (or Korean) ginseng protects the cells of the brain, increases mental alertness, and boosts serotonin levels. Begin by taking half the manufacturer's recommended dose, then gradually work up to the dose as directed on the product label.

Note: Chinese ginseng should not be taken by anyone with high blood pressure, heart disease, or hypoglycemia. If you are sensitive to the effects of caffeine and other stimulants, you may want to consult with a qualified herbalist before using ginseng.

■ Ginkgo biloba helps increase the blood supply to the brain. Choose a standardized extract containing at least 24 percent ginkgo heterosides (sometimes called flavoglycosides). The recommended dosage is 50 to 80 milligrams three times a day.

■ Gotu kola has been used for centuries in India to increase the efficiency of the brain. Choose a standardized extract containing 16 percent triterpenes and take 200 milligrams three times a day.

■ Pine-bark and grape-seed extracts contain antioxidant and help support liver function. A person with Alzheimer's disease can take 25 milligrams of either two or three times daily.

■ Siberian ginseng increases cerebral circulation. Choose a standardized extract containing 0.5 percent eleutheroside E and take 100 milligrams in the morning and again in the afternoon.

■ A person who is undergoing chelation therapy, either oral or intravenous, should be aware that this treatment can put an extra burden on the kidneys. Herbs that support kidney function include parsley root, parsley leaf, and marshmallow root.

HOMEOPATHY

■ If exaggerated constipation is a problem, use one dose of *Alumina* 200x or 30c daily for three to four days.

■ A person with Alzheimer's disease would be wise to see a homeopathic physician. Although the symptoms of this condition cannot be reversed, they can sometimes be alleviated if a proper homeopathic remedy tailored to the individual's specific difficulties is prescribed and administered in the early stages of the disease.

BACH FLOWER REMEDIES

Select the remedy that most closely fits your emotional tendencies and concerns, and use it as needed, following the directions on the product label.

■ Chestnut bud is for childlike, incorrigible behavior, and a seeming inability (or unwillingness) to understand cause and effect.

■ Chicory is helpful for feelings of insecurity, a constant craving for attention, and feelings that are easily hurt.

■ Heather is good for counteracting self-centeredness and a tendency to talk exclusively about one's own concerns, as if nothing else is important.

■ Holly helps to ease anger and fits of temper.

■ White Chestnut is especially helpful for obsessive thoughts, for example, for a person who is obsessed with the disease and cannot stop thinking about what is coming.

ACUPRESSURE

For the locations of acupressure points on the body, *see* ADMINISTERING AN ACUPRESSURE TREATMENT in Part Three.

■ All inner and outer Bladder points improve circulation and relax the nervous system.

■ Gallbladder 20 improves circulation to the head.

■ Stomach 36 supports and improves circulation and digestion.

AROMATHERAPY

For specific instructions on how to use aromatherapy, *see* PREPARING AROMATHERAPY TREATMENTS in Part Three.

■ Rosemary oil stimulates mental function; elemi, lavender, and neroli can calm and ease agitation. You can use one or more of these oils as inhalants or diffuse them into the air in your home.

■ If fatigue is a problem, try an aromatherapy bath prepared with 3 drops of rosemary oil, 2 drops of thyme or grapefruit oil, and 1 drop of pine oil.

GENERAL RECOMMENDATIONS

■ Whatever remedies you use, whether conventional or natural, they will be of greatest benefit if begun early, at the earliest sign of symptoms.

■ Avoid exposure to aluminum. Acid rain has contributed a lot of aluminum to tap water. Other everyday sources of aluminum include aluminum cookware, canned drinks, some antacids, and antiperspirants.

■ A new kind of therapy called audio presence intervention has proved helpful for end-stage Alzheimer's patients who become so severely agitated that they require tranquilizers or restraints to prevent them from hurting themselves. It has been found that hearing the recorded voice of a loved one can calm a frustrated and/or violent individual more effectively than medication. In this type of treatment, family members provide at least four tapes on which they reminisce about happy times, talk about the person's favorite holidays, sing a familiar song, give news of the family's doings, and so on. These one-sided conversations are then played for the patient through headphones hooked up to a personal tape player. According to early reports, the tapes work so well that it has been possible to reduce the medication given some patients.

■ Chelation therapy has proven helpful in enhancing cognitive function in many Alzheimer's patients. In chelation therapy, certain agents are administered to bind with toxins such as heavy metals and cause the body to excrete them. There are oral chelation formulas available over the counter. Intravenous chelation employs ethylenediaminetetraacetic acid (EDTA).

Note: Intravenous chelation therapy must be administered and monitored by a qualified doctor. Laboratory tests are required before commencing treatment. Because chelation affects the kidneys, kidney function must be monitored during the course of the treatment.

PREVENTION

■ Unfortunately, there is no known way of preventing Alzheimer's disease. Taking therapeutic doses of certain nutrients may help, however. Vitamins A, C, and E; the minerals zinc and selenium; the enzyme superoxide dismutase (SOD); plus pine-bark or grape-seed extract and bioflavonoids protect against the type of free-radical damage that is associated with this disease. Magnesium protects against abnormal DNA production, which may be involved in the formation of the characteristic neurofibrillary tangles in the brain.

Anaphylactic Shock

Anaphylactic shock is a severe and violent allergic response that may occur as a result of contact with an allergen. Possible allergens include chemicals, medicines, vaccines, particular foods or food additives—such as sulfites—and insect venom. Anaphylactic shock may cause severe breathing distress and can be life-threatening.

In anaphylactic shock, the body's reaction to an allergen can cause a swelling of the air passages, with a consequent narrowing of the airway, resulting in extreme difficulty in breathing. In rare instances, the tongue and air passages may swell to the point where the airway closes and breathing becomes almost impossible.

Symptoms usually come on rapidly, most often within one to fifteen minutes of contact with an allergen. The more quickly a reaction begins, the more severe it is likely to be. The first signs of a reaction can include a sense of uneasiness, agitation, weakness, sweating, flushing, and shortness of breath, accompanied by intense fear and anxiety. Another early sign may be the presence of itchy hives that begin to spread rapidly all over the body. Other symptoms may include restlessness, falling blood pressure, shock, uneven heartbeat, wheezing, trouble swallowing, nausea, and diarrhea.

This kind of an allergic reaction is frightening. But don't panic. As you seek help, try to remain as calm as possible. An agitated state makes breathing even more difficult. It is important to reassure yourself that the situation will be resolved.

EMERGENCY TREATMENT

■ At the slightest sign that you may be having difficulty breathing due to a severe allergic reaction—especially if you have a history of such reactions—have someone take you immediately to the emergency room of the nearest hospital. If there is no one available to transport you, call for emergency help and stress the gravity of the situation. Seconds count. If an emergency adrenaline-injection kit such as Ana-Kit or Epi-Pen is available, administer it immediately, either as you are on your way to the hospital or while you are waiting for assistance. *Do not* take anything to eat or drink while you are experiencing breathing distress.

■ Rely on emergency personnel to take appropriate measures. They will probably administer an injection of epinephrine (Adrenalin or Sus-Phrine, a long-acting form) at once. Bronchodilators (such as Alupent or Bronkosol) are sometimes used as well to counteract the allergen, decrease inflammation, and open the airway to restore free breathing, and intravenous fluids are often given to maintain adequate blood pressure, which can lower considerably. Antihistamines (such as Benadryl), oxygen, and even corticosteroids (hydrocortisone or prednisone) may be required later in treatment, depending upon the extent of the attack.

HERBAL TREATMENT

■ Following the trauma of anaphylactic shock, you will probably feel chilly or cold for a day or two. If you do, take a cup of hot ginger tea one to three times a day, with meals, for two days. Ginger is a warming and stimulating herb.

HOMEOPATHY

■ Once the crisis is over and it is safe to take something by mouth, take one dose of Aconite 200x, 30c, or 200c to help allay the emotional distress that inevitably follows such an episode.

107

BACH FLOWER REMEDIES

■ After emergency medical personnel have administered treatment, take one dose of Rescue Remedy. This remedy helps to ease anxiety and fright.

■ Once you are home from the hospital, take one dose of Mimulus each day for one week after the incident.

GENERAL RECOMMENDATIONS

■ If you have reason to suspect that you may be susceptible to anaphylaxis—based on previous reactions or family history, for example—ask your doctor to prescribe a home emergency kit containing epinephrine, such as the Ana-Kit or EpiPen, and be sure you learn how to administer it correctly. Having a supply of epinephrine on hand may someday save your life.

■ There are natural remedies that can help support your full recovery from an episode of this nature once the immediate crisis has passed and the source of the reaction has been diagnosed. See ALLERGIES; ASTHMA; BITES AND STINGS; and/or FOOD ALLERGIES for appropriate suggestions.

PREVENTION

■ Unfortunately, there is often no way to know ahead of time that you may be allergic to a particular substance. Should you ever suffer a dangerous allergic reaction, however, it goes without saying that you should guard against any future contact with the allergen.

Anemia

Anemia is a general term for conditions characterized by an inadequate oxygen-carrying capacity of the blood, and therefore an insufficient supply of oxygen to the tissues. The classic symptoms include fatigue, paleness, general breathlessness, difficulty breathing during activity, and heart palpitations. Dizziness, headache, an unsettled stomach, poor appetite, insomnia, irregular heartbeat, and heart murmur may also occur.

Anemia can come about from a variety of causes. Oxygen is transported in the blood by means of molecules of hemoglobin, a red pigment found in red blood cells. Each healthy red blood cell circulating in the body carries between 200 and 300 molecules of hemoglobin. Therefore, anything that causes a lack of hemoglobin or of red blood cells can lead to anemia. The most commonly diagnosed cause is iron deficiency. Iron is essential for the formation of hemoglobin. *Iron-deficiency anemia* can result from inadequate consumption or absorption of iron or from blood loss such as may occur during surgery or following a

heavy menstrual period. Pregnancy also draws hemoglobin from the body. For obvious reasons, women are more susceptible to this form of anemia than men are.

Other nutrient deficiencies can lead to anemia as well. Like iron, vitamin B_{12} and folic acid are essential for the formation of hemoglobin, so a deficiency of either of these vitamins can cause anemia. In the case of vitamin B_{12}, very little is required for hemoglobin production, so *B_{12}-deficiency anemia* takes much longer to develop than iron-deficiency anemia, up to two years in some cases. Because vitamin B_{12} is found almost exclusively in foods of animal origin, vegetarians have a higher risk of developing this form of anemia. People with Crohn's disease and celiac disease, conditions that interfere with the absorption of vitamins from the intestinal tract, are at increased risk as well. In addition to the classic symptoms of anemia outlined above, symptoms of B_{12}-deficiency anemia can include yellowish skin and, in some cases, abdominal pain, weight loss, tingling in the arms and legs, and neurological impairment resulting in disorientation and depression. *Pernicious anemia* is a related condition that mainly affects older adults. It results from a deficiency of the substance that activates cyanocobalamin, which is part of vitamin B_{12}. As a result, B_{12} cannot be utilized and the production of red blood cells in bone marrow ceases.

Folate-deficiency anemia most often affects older adults and pregnant women; the need for folic acid is higher during pregnancy, in infancy, and in elderly people. Folate-deficiency anemia can develop very quickly, in a matter of weeks. A poor diet or absorption problems, such as occur in celiac disease, are likely causes of folic-acid deficiency. Stress also depletes folic acid.

By far the most common form of anemia is *nutritional anemia*, although it is often not diagnosed as such. Like all types of anemia, it is characterized by the inadequate production of red blood cells, and it causes all the classic symptoms. Nutritional anemia is directly caused by a lack of sufficient quantities of all the nutrients mentioned here—iron, folic acid, and vitamin B_{12}. This condition is common in older people, who often eat poorly and who may have absorption problems, and in people whose diet consists primarily of fast food and junk food.

Some types of anemia develop not because of a lack of nutrients but because of a defect in the body's ability to produce hemoglobin, even if all the required raw materials are available. *Sickle cell anemia* is a serious, incurable condition characterized by the abnormal formation of hemoglobin, which in turn results in the red blood cells being abnormally shaped. Normal red blood cells are tiny round, flat disks with an indentation in the center. Sickle cells are crescent-shaped. These distorted cells can get stuck in small blood vessels, causing a serious deficiency of oxygen in the area. Sickle cell disease can cause joint pain, blood clots, fever, long-term anemia, enlargement of the spleen, lack of energy, and weakness. In people with sickle cell disease, certain conditions, such as infection or surgery, can lead to acute flare-ups termed crises, during which the pain may be severe and there is a high risk of infection.

Sickle cell disease is an inherited condition that primarily affects people of African or West Indian descent. If an individual inherits a defective copy of the gene that governs hemoglobin production from both parents, he or she will have sickle cell disease and, consequently, sickle cell anemia. If a person inherits a defective gene from one parent and a normal one from the other parent, he or she is said to have sickle cell trait. Such an individual will not suffer from anemia, but may pass the defective gene on to his or her children. If a couple both have the trait, their children have, statistically, a 25-percent risk of being born with sickle cell disease.

Thalassemia is an inherited form of anemia that mostly affects people of Middle Eastern, East Asian, and Mediterranean ancestry. People with thalassemia produce fewer red blood cells than normal and hemoglobin whose content is not fully matured. Further, this defective hemoglobin is destroyed more quickly than ordinary hemoglobin. Children born with thalassemia may grow poorly, and puberty may be reached much later than normal. This condition can also have indirect effects on the bones, heart, spleen, and liver. The most severe form of thalassemia, known as *Cooley's anemia,* is associated with a significantly shortened life span.

In *aplastic anemia,* the bone marrow produces insufficient quantities of both red and white blood cells, as well as platelets. This problem can have a variety of causes, including cancer of the bone marrow, exposure to radiation, and the use of certain drugs, including cancer chemotherapy agents. This condition results in easy bruising and extreme vulnerability to infection.

Another type of anemia is *hemolytic anemia.* This term encompasses a group of disorders that cause the premature destruction of red blood cells. Normally, red blood cells have a life span of 120 days; after that, they are broken down by the body, primarily in the spleen. However, if the body starts destroying some red blood cells before the normal 120 days, anemia can result. If the bone marrow is able to step up production, the anemia may be slight. However, in most cases, red blood cells are destroyed more rapidly than they are created, resulting in all the classic symptoms of anemia, plus jaundice and dark urine. Hemolytic anemia can occur with some infectious diseases or in response to certain drugs or toxins. In rare cases, it results from an autoimmune disorder—an inappropriate response of the immune system that causes the body to create antibodies that attack red blood cells.

If you suspect you may be anemic, you should consult a physician for a proper diagnosis and appropriate treatment.

CONVENTIONAL TREATMENT

■ Conventional treatment of anemia depends on the underlying cause. A number of different blood tests may be done to determine the exact type of anemia and the cause.

■ Anemia resulting from nutritional deficiencies is usually treated with supplemental forms of the missing nutrients. Iron may be taken in either tablet or injection form. If the iron depletion is very severe, a blood transfusion may be necessary. Vitamin B_{12} is usually taken by mouth, but if the deficiency is serious, injections are preferred. For folate-deficiency anemia, high doses of supplemental folic acid are prescribed. When nutritional anemia is addressed with dietary corrections and proper supplementation, there is almost always fast improvement.

■ Pernicious anemia is treated with injections of vitamin B_{12}. This successfully counteracts the effects of the disorder, but it does not actually cure it, so treatment must be continued for life.

■ There is no treatment that can cure sickle cell anemia. Treatment focuses on managing the acute crises. During an episode, antibiotics and painkillers, possibly narcotics, may be prescribed. Occasionally, transfusions may be necessary to manage complications.

■ Mild cases of thalassemia generally require no treatment. Severe cases are treated with periodic blood transfusions. In some cases, surgery to remove the spleen may be recommended.

■ Treatment for aplastic anemia generally begins with the administration of antibiotics to treat any existing infection and drugs to stimulate the marrow's production of red blood cells. Transfusions may be necessary and, in extreme cases, bone-marrow transplantation may be advised.

■ With hemolytic anemia, the first step in treatment is identifying the cause of red blood cell destruction. If it is found to be a response to a drug, the drug is discontinued; if it is determined to be an autoimmune problem, steroids may be prescribed to suppress immune function. Another option is surgical removal of the spleen.

DIETARY GUIDELINES

■ Include in your diet plenty of foods that are rich in iron. These include green leafy vegetables, blackstrap molasses, dried fruits, cherries or cherry juice, eggs, fish, and poultry. Eat generous servings of green vegetables daily. The best source of dietary iron is organic calf liver. If you are watching your cholesterol, choose the clean, lean protein of chicken, fish, and lean red meat.

■ Folic acid is found in dark-green leafy vegetables, root vegetables, whole grains, brewer's yeast, milk, salmon, and organ meats. Increase your consumption of this nutrient by basing your diet on vegetables and whole grains.

■ Dietary sources of vitamin B_{12} include whole grains, legumes, blackstrap molasses, egg yolks, nuts, brewer's yeast, and meat, especially organ meats.

NUTRITIONAL SUPPLEMENTS

■ To remedy an iron deficiency, take a liquid iron supplement as recommended by your physician. If you find you are unable to tolerate a liquid supplement, try taking 15 to 20 milligrams of iron succinate twice daily in pill form.

Note: Excessive amounts of iron are associated with a variety of health problems, including an increased risk of cardiovascular disease. Do not take supplemental iron unless a deficiency has been diagnosed by your healthcare provider, and do not take the supplement in higher amounts or for a longer period of time than he or she prescribes.

■ To remedy a vitamin-B_{12} deficiency, take 1,000 to 2,500 micrograms (1 to 2.5 milligrams) twice daily.

■ To remedy a folic-acid deficiency, take 400 micrograms two or three times a day.

■ Vitamin C is an antioxidant that fights free-radical damage, aids in the absorption of iron, and helps strengthen the blood vessels. Take 500 milligrams twice daily.

HERBAL TREATMENT

■ Chinese ginseng is a revitalizing tonic herb that has long been used for anemia. It also helps reduce the body's sensitivity to stress. Select a standardized extract containing 7 percent ginsenosides and take 100 milligrams twice daily for two to three weeks.

Note: Do not use Chinese ginseng if you have high blood pressure, heart disease, or hypoglycemia. If you are sensitive to the effects of caffeine and other stimulants, you may want to consult with a qualified herbalist before using ginseng.

■ Dandelion, nettle, and yellow dock are botanical sources of bioavailable iron. Dandelion also helps regulate liver function. Take 500 milligrams of dandelion extract or one cup of dandelion-root tea three times a day for six weeks; 500 milligrams of nettle twice daily; and/or 250 to 500 milligrams of yellow dock twice daily for six weeks.

■ Dong quai is a Chinese herb traditionally used against anemia. It is a premier blood tonic. Take 500 milligrams twice a day for three weeks.

HOMEOPATHY

■ *China* will help if you are suffering from anemia due to blood loss, either as a result of surgery or because of heavy menstrual periods, possibly from oncoming menopause. You may have digestive difficulties and lower abdominal discomfort, feel very cold and tired, and be hypersensitive and prone to having your feelings hurt. Take one dose of *China* 30x or 15c, as directed on the product label, twice daily for five days. Stop for five days, then repeat for five days.

■ *Ferrum phosphoricum* is for the very sensitive individual who has a pale face but flushes easily. Take one dose of *Ferrum phosphoricum* 30x or 15c twice daily for five days. Stop for five days, then repeat for five days.

■ Choose *Natrum muriaticum* if you are constipated and suffer from headaches and dry lips and mouth, and have a tendency to cold sores. You may also crave salt. Take one dose of *Natrum muriaticum* 30x or 15c twice daily for five days. Stop for five days, then repeat for five days.

■ *Picricum acidum* is for the person who is pale and physically and mentally fatigued, and who has difficulty carrying plans through to completion. Take one dose of *Picricum acidum* 30x or 15c twice daily for five days. Stop for five days, then repeat for five days.

BACH FLOWER REMEDIES

Select the remedy that most closely fits your emotional tendencies and concerns, and take it as needed, following the directions on the product label.

■ Centaury helps ease feelings of intimidation.

■ Hornbeam will prove helpful if you have withdrawn from all activity due to supreme exhaustion.

■ Mimulus is for shyness and timidity, and a feeling of being intimidated by and fearful of everything.

■ Use Olive if you are fatigued and feel exhausted to the very core.

ACUPRESSURE

For the locations of acupressure points on the body, *see* ADMINISTERING AN ACUPRESSURE TREATMENT in Part Three.

■ Spleen 6 helps to strengthen the blood.

■ Stomach 36 supports and improves circulation and digestion, and gradually improves the absorption of nutrients.

GENERAL RECOMMENDATIONS

■ As soon as you are able, begin a regular program of gentle exercise. Yoga and yoga breathing exercises can be especially helpful.

PREVENTION

■ Not all forms of anemia are preventable, but those

caused by nutritional deficiencies can be avoided by maximizing your intake of foods containing iron, vitamin B_{12}, and folic acid, or by taking supplements of these nutrients.

Angina

See under CARDIOVASCULAR DISEASE.

Ankle, Sprained

See under MUSCLE SPRAIN, STRAIN, AND PAIN.

Ankylosing Spondylitis

See under ARTHRITIS.

Anorexia Nervosa

Anorexia nervosa is a disorder characterized by an abnormal fear of being fat and a consequent refusal to eat. It is seen mainly in teenage girls and young women. Experts believe that between 1 and 2 percent of the female population in these age groups is affected.

The onset of anorexia often occurs during puberty. Although the trigger that causes a seemingly normal person to become anorexic is far from clear, a phobic fear of becoming fat may be related to a distorted self-image, a wish to remain childlike in form, or a desire to maintain control over some part of life at least. It has been noted that many people with anorexia come from close families that put many demands on them, and that as a result they may feel ineffective and be abnormally anxious to please.

Many physicians see anorexia as a symptom of a mental or emotional problem, such as anger, fear, stress, and/or depression, rather than as a separate disorder. Some scientists believe that the condition may arise as a result of a problem with the hypothalamus, the portion of the brain that controls hunger, thirst, and body temperature, among other things. More recently, it has been suggested that a serious deficiency of zinc may be involved.

A person with anorexia sees him- or herself as "fat" even though he or she is painfully thin—even emaciated—to objective eyes. Most anorexics deliberately starve themselves, but some overuse laxatives and/or induce vomiting after eating to keep from gaining weight. Some do all three of these things. The most obvious physical sign of anorexia is an increasingly serious loss of weight. A person with this disorder may lose more than one third of his or her normal body weight. With the weight loss come other problems, including weakness, dizziness, low blood pressure and a faltering or irregular heartbeat. In girls and women, menstruation ceases as the extreme lack of nutrients disrupts normal hormone production. In anorexics who also induce vomiting, other symptoms may include a swollen neck, broken blood vessels on the face, and damage to the enamel of the back teeth.

Anorexia nervosa is an extremely serious, potentially life-threatening condition. While almost half of those who develop it ultimately outgrow the disorder, more than 30 percent battle the condition all their lives. Relapses are common. Those who refuse treatment or give up the battle very often die prematurely.

CONVENTIONAL TREATMENT

■ Initial treatment is aimed at correcting metabolic imbalances caused by insufficient nutrition. Hospitalization and intravenous feeding may be necessary.

■ Once your nutritional status has been stabilized, psychotherapy or family counseling will be recommended to help you work to restructure your behavior. Your therapist and medical doctor should work together to help you reestablish healthy eating habits. This may take some time.

■ If depression or an anxiety disorder is part of the picture, medication to combat those conditions may be prescribed.

DIETARY GUIDELINES

■ Controlling your blood-sugar level is very important. To keep blood-sugar levels in balance, eat five small well-balanced meals daily. If you can, eat several small high-protein snacks as well.

■ An impaired digestive system is associated with anorexia. To help improve your digestion, eat slowly and chew each bite thoroughly.

■ To be certain you are receiving a good balance of all the nutrients you need, consult a nutritionist. The advice of a professional can be very valuable.

■ Avoid all alcohol, caffeine, and sugar.

NUTRITIONAL SUPPLEMENTS

■ To help keep your blood-sugar level in balance, take 200 micrograms of chromium twice daily for six weeks, then reduce to a maintenance dosage of 200 micrograms once a day.

■ Magnesium ensures bowel regularity and also eases a stressed nervous system. Take 500 to 1,000 milligrams of magnesium daily, preferably in the form of magnesium glycinate.

■ To aid digestion, take a good-quality probiotic supplement daily, as recommended on the product label. If you are troubled by constipation, take acidophilus. If chronic indigestion is troublesome, take bifidus.

■ The B vitamins are required for the healthy functioning of the hormonal and nervous systems. Take a good-quality B-complex supplement supplying 25 milligrams of each of the major B vitamins every day.

■ Vitamin E assists in balancing hormonal function, which is adversely affected by anorexia. Choose a product containing mixed tocopherols and start by taking 200 international units daily, then gradually increase the dosage until you are taking 400 international units twice daily.

Note: If you have high blood pressure, limit your intake of supplemental vitamin E to a total of 400 international units daily. If you are taking an anticoagulant (blood thinner), consult your physician before taking supplemental vitamin E.

■ Most people with anorexia have serious zinc deficiencies. Take 25 milligrams of zinc twice a day.

Note: Take zinc with food to prevent stomach upset. If you take over 30 milligrams of zinc daily for more than one or two months, you should also take 1 to 2 milligrams of copper each day to maintain a proper mineral balance.

HERBAL TREATMENT

■ Astragalus helps improve digestion, enhances energy production, and eases feelings of fatigue. Astragalus may be combined with a variety of herbs, including Siberian ginseng, cordyceps, and codonopsis. If fatigue is a problem, take an astragalus combination formula as recommended on the product label.

■ Bupleurum and dong quai is a 2,000-year-old Chinese formula that improves the utilization of nutrients and helps relax the nervous system. Take 1,000 milligrams of a bupleurum and dong quai combination formula two or three times daily for two weeks out of every month (if you are a woman, take it for the two weeks prior to the anticipated onset of your menstrual period).

■ Kava kava helps relax the nervous system. It is most helpful during the first six to eight weeks of recovery, especially if anxiety is an issue. Choose a product containing 30 percent kavalactones and take 200 milligrams twice a day.

Note: In excess amounts, this herb can cause drowsiness. Do not exceed the recommended dose. Do not use kava kava if you are pregnant or nursing, if you have

Parkinson's disease, or if you are taking a prescription medication for depression or anxiety.

■ To combat blood-sugar swings, take a cup of licorice tea once or twice a day for the first week of therapy.

Note: Do not take licorice on a daily basis for more than five days in a row, as it can elevate blood pressure. Do not take it at all if you have high blood pressure.

■ Although some forms of ginseng are too strong for people with anorexia, Siberian ginseng is a tonic herb that will increase energy levels gently. Choose a standardized extract containing 0.5 percent eleutheroside E and take 100 milligrams in the morning and again in the afternoon.

HOMEOPATHY

■ If you have anorexia, you will likely benefit most from an individualized constitutional remedy. Consult a homeopathic physician.

■ *Lycopodium* is the remedy of choice for dyspepsia and bloating. Take one dose of *Lycopodium* 30x or 15c three times daily for a total of up to ten doses.

■ *Natrum muriaticum* is especially helpful if you are feeling a vague sense of loss and melancholy. You may also crave salt. Take one dose of *Natrum muriaticum* 30x or 15c three times daily for a total of up to ten doses.

■ *Nux vomica* is helpful for nausea and/or indigestion. Take one dose of *Nux vomica* 30x or 15c three times daily for a total of up to ten doses.

■ *Pulsatilla* is for the person who cries easily, and who frequently lapses into helpless sobs. Take one dose of *Pulsatilla* 30x or 15c three times daily for a total of up to ten doses.

BACH FLOWER REMEDIES

Select the remedy that most closely fits your emotional tendencies and concerns, and take it as needed, following the directions on the product label.

■ Aspen is a valuable remedy for vague feelings of fear, especially fear of the unknown.

■ Larch is good if you are feeling helpless and ineffectual. This remedy helps restore self confidence and self esteem.

■ Mimulus is helpful for battling concrete fears of known origin.

■ White Chestnut helps ease obsessive thoughts and compulsions.

ACUPRESSURE

For the locations of acupressure points on the body, *see* ADMINISTERING AN ACUPRESSURE TREATMENT in Part Three.

■ All back Bladder points relax and tone the nervous system.

■ Liver 3 relaxes the nervous system.

■ Pericardium 6 relaxes the chest and upper digestive tract.

■ Stomach 36 improves digestion.

AROMATHERAPY

For specific instructions on how to use aromatherapy, *see* PREPARING AROMATHERAPY TREATMENTS in Part Three.

■ Essential oils of bergamot and peppermint help to stimulate the appetite. Bergamot oil also helps combat depression. You can use either or both as an inhalant or in an aromatherapy bath, or diffuse them into the air.

■ Elemi oil promotes inner harmony and eases feelings of stress. Jasmine oil helps to combat depression and elevate mood. Use them in inhalants or baths, or diffuse them into the air.

GENERAL RECOMMENDATIONS

■ Thyroid problems and food allergies can contribute to anorexia. If these conditions have not already been ruled out, discuss these possibilities with a health-care professional.

■ Relaxation techniques, such as biofeedback, yoga, and meditation, can be extremely helpful. *See* RELAXATION TECHNIQUES in Part Three.

■ Begin a program of regular exercise to improve circulation and enhance mood. Ten to fifteen minutes of mild exercise a day should make a noticeable difference.

Anxiety Disorders

Anxiety disorders are conditions that manifest themselves in feelings of anxiousness, fear, excessive worry, and dread, without any apparent external cause. The symptoms can range from a mild disquiet to intense, even incapacitating, anxiety and panic. These problems affect over 10 million people in the United States alone.

When you are faced with threatening situations, you experience stress. The body's response is to send out a flood of hormones in what is called the *fight-or-flight response.* Your muscles tense, your heart beats faster, and you breathe more rapidly as your body prepares to deal with the threat. However, if neither "fight" nor "flight" is possible, a feeling of anxiety is generated.

Everyone experiences a certain amount of anxiety at times. Anxiety, tension, and stress are all part of daily life.

Feeling worried and anxious over an impending deadline, for example, is normal and can even be of benefit. As the deadline looms, you are motivated to buckle down and focus your attention on the project, bringing about a satisfactory conclusion. As the work goes forward, your anxiety level goes down proportionately and appropriately.

In contrast, an anxiety disorder involves unfounded worry that can last for six months or more. People suffering from anxiety disorders tend to feel threatened all the time, even though most often they cannot identify or name what it is that is threatening them. This disorder may begin with initial vague feelings of unease that come and go, and then may escalate to the point where severe anxiety or even panic takes over. The distress may become so intense that you can no longer carry on with your normal daily activities.

In addition to being tense, nervous, and severely stressed, people with anxiety disorders often experience mood swings and can be restless, easily irritated, and impossible to please. They may also be forgetful and have difficulty concentrating, and often become exhausted out of proportion to the amount of energy they expend. Sleep disturbances are common. Some people want to sleep all the time, while others have trouble falling asleep and sleeping through the night. Instead, they toss and turn throughout the night and awaken unrefreshed.

Panic attacks are an extreme manifestation of an anxiety disorder. A person having a panic attack experiences a sudden and intense feeling of dread and terror, accompanied by a pounding heart, shortness of breath, dizziness, nausea, cold sweats, trembling and weakness, and/or a tingling sensation in the extremities. It is not uncommon for a person in the midst of such an attack to believe that he or she is having a heart attack or stroke and is about to die, or that he or she is going crazy. Needless to say, panic attacks can be quite incapacitating.

Anxiety can also be a symptom of other physical and psychological disorders. Depression, for instance, can be experienced as (or accompanied by) a feeling of anxiety, but is more often characterized by despair. Mitral valve prolapse is sometimes associated with symptoms similar to those of a panic attack. A person who is beginning to have an anaphylactic reaction to an allergen may experience a sudden wave of anxiety as well. Posttraumatic stress disorder is a condition that can cause extreme anxiety. This syndrome, a reaction to a specific overwhelmingly disturbing and disorienting event—rape, natural disasters, traumatic accidents, and experiences in war, among others—causes a person to relive the event over and over again in the form of waking or sleeping nightmares, and leaves him or her in a state of chronic anxiety. Anxiety can also be a result of medication reactions, substance abuse, glandular disorders, hypoglycemia, drug withdrawal, heart disease and other illnesses. Such problems should be ruled out before a diagnosis of anxiety disorder is arrived at. Phobias also may be at the root of anxiety. Phobias are characterized by a persistent, often irrational fear of a person, object, place, or situation. Agoraphobia, a fear of open or public spaces, is quite common in the United States, and 75 percent of those who suffer from it are women. People with agoraphobia may experience intense anxiety or even full-blown panic attacks when placed in such common situations as visiting a shopping mall or boarding a bus, train, or airplane.

CONVENTIONAL TREATMENT

■ For many years, the drugs of choice for anxiety disorders have been members of the benzodiazepine class of tranquilizers. This group includes clonazepam (Klonopin), diazepam (Valium), lorazepam (Ativan), and oxazepam (Serax), among others. They can be effective in reducing feelings of anxiety, but these drugs also have considerable potential for creating dependency, especially if used over a long period. They can also cause a range of more immediate side effects, including drowsiness, dizziness, weakness, and memory impairment. In some people, they can cause liver damage. If you must take one of these drugs, you should avoid all alcohol.

■ Buspirone (BuSpar) is an antianxiety drug that belongs to a different class than the benzodiazepines. It does not appear to have the dependency potential of the benzodiazepines, but it can take longer for its effects to be felt—up to three weeks, in some cases. Possible side effects include dizziness, headache, nausea, ringing in the ears, and—paradoxically—anxiety.

■ There are a variety of psychotherapeutic and stress-reduction approaches that may be helpful, including traditional "talk" therapy or counseling, group therapy, relaxation techniques, and hypnotherapy. Your physician should be able to refer you to a qualified mental-health professional who can help.

DIETARY GUIDELINES

■ Maintaining a steady blood-sugar level is extremely important. A drop in blood sugar can cause or exacerbate nonspecific feelings of anxiety. To keep your blood sugar in balance, eat five small meals a day rather than the usual three large ones, and avoid all refined sugars. If snacks are a passion, try a handful of fresh nuts or seeds or a piece of fruit.

■ Make sure each meal includes a preponderance of fresh fruits and vegetables and sufficient clean, lean protein. Try not to eat all-carbohydrate meals, so that your blood-sugar level remains within narrower limits.

■ Beverages containing caffeine can increase nervousness and anxiety. Avoid coffee, tea (except for herbal varieties), and caffeinated soft drinks.

NUTRITIONAL SUPPLEMENTS

■ The B vitamins are important nutrients needed by the nervous system. Take a good B-complex formula that supplies at least 25 milligrams of each of the major B vitamins daily.

■ Calcium and magnesium are vital to a stable nervous system. Take a calcium and magnesium combination formula that supplies 400 milligrams of calcium and 200 milligrams of magnesium three times daily.

■ Chromium helps to even out blood-sugar levels and keep them in balance. Take 100 milligrams of chromium twice daily.

■ People who suffer from anxiety are often deficient in folic acid. Take 800 micrograms twice daily for one month, then once daily for one month. Thereafter, take a maintenance dose of 400 to 800 milligrams daily.

■ (GABA) Gamma-aminobutyric acid (GABA) is a neurotransmitter (a substance that transmits information from one nerve cell to another in the brain) that has calming effects. It is often very helpful for anxiety. GABA has been shown to be effective for mild panic disorder as well as for anxiety associated with perimenopausal symptoms. Take 500 milligrams two or three times daily.

HERBAL TREATMENT

■ Bupleurum and dragon bone combination formula is an old Chinese remedy with strong calmative powers. This formula is especially useful for people suffering from anxiety caused by withdrawal from caffeine, nicotine, or alcohol. Take one dose twice a day, as directed on the product label.

Note: If you have a troublesome and/or weak digestive system, select another remedy. This formula is very strong.

■ Kava kava is the herb of choice if your anxiety is not due to overproduction of adrenaline for physical reasons but is primarily emotionally induced. Chose a product containing 30 percent kavalactones and take 200 milligrams twice a day.

Note: In excess amounts, this herb can cause drowsiness. Do not exceed the recommended dose. Do not use kava kava if you are pregnant or nursing, if you have Parkinson's disease, or if you are taking a prescription medication for depression or anxiety.

■ Passionflower is an excellent relaxant. Choose an extract standardized to contain 0.7 percent flavonoids and take 250 milligrams in capsule form two or three times daily.

■ Many studies have shown that St. John's wort has note-worthy calming and antidepressant effects. It can be very helpful for anxiety accompanied by depression. Choose a product containing 0.3 percent hypericin and take 100 milligrams two to three times daily. Take the second dose at least six or seven hours before bedtime. Taking a dose of kava kava in the evening is good for easing anxiety and aiding sleep.

Valerian is a strong calmative that is useful for the physical manifestations of anxiety. Studies show it is also helpful for insomnia. Select a product containing 0.5 percent isovalerenic acids and take 200 to 300 milligrams one-half hour before bedtime.

HOMEOPATHY

Coffea cruda helps relieve anxiety associated with obsessive thoughts. Take one dose of *Coffea cruda* 12x or 6c twice during the day and once before bedtime for up to ten days.

Ignatia is good if you have suffered a panic attack. It is also useful if you are restless and have difficulty sleeping. Take one dose of *Ignatia* 30x or 15c twice during the day and once before bedtime for up to ten days.

Passiflora is helpful for nervousness and difficulty falling asleep. Take one dose of *Passiflora* 12x or 6c twice during the day and once before bedtime for up to ten days.

BACH FLOWER REMEDIES

Select the remedy that most closely fits your emotional tendencies and concerns, and take it as needed, following the directions on the product label.

Rescue Remedy is the first choice to alleviate any crisis-caused stress that results in fear, panic, anxiety, tension, and/or apprehension.

Aspen is good for anxiety and vague, nameless fear.

Cherry Plum will help if you become fearful and excessively anxious when placed in situations where you have no control.

Mimulus helps to ease shyness and timidity, as well as apprehension or dread of upcoming events.

Rock Rose is good if you experience irrational terror, panic, and/or horrendous nightmares.

Sweet Chestnut should relieve feelings of anguish, torment, alienation, and isolation.

Choose Wild Oat if you are fearful and anxious over what the future may bring. You may be at a crossroads in your life and dread making the wrong decision.

ACUPRESSURE

For the locations of acupressure points on the body, *see* ADMINISTERING AN ACUPRESSURE TREATMENT in Part Three.

■ All Bladder points relax the nerves.

■ Liver 3 brings energy down from the head.

■ Pericardium 6 relaxes the chest and upper digestive tract.

■ Massaging the points along either side of the spine relaxes the nervous system.

AROMATHERAPY

For specific instructions on how to use aromatherapy, *see* PREPARING AROMATHERAPY TREATMENTS in Part Three.

■ There are many essential oils that have a calming and anxiety-reducing effect. Among the best known are bergamot, frankincense, geranium, lavender, myrrh, neroli, vetiver, and ylang ylang. Any of these oils can be used in a wide variety of ways to help combat anxiety; they can be inhaled directly from the bottle, added to relaxing baths, diffused into the air, or added to massage oil. You can also put a drop or two on a clean tissue or handkerchief and inhale it that way as needed.

GENERAL RECOMMENDATIONS

■ Exercise. A program of regular exercise is best, but even an occasional brisk walk around the block can ease the physical manifestations of anxiety.

■ When anxious feelings strike, try to pin down exactly what it is that is causing you to feel edgy. This may be difficult at times, but keep in mind that it is much easier to deal with concrete fears than with vague, undefined feelings of unease. Sometimes, simply identifying the trigger can ease anxiety.

■ Anxiety can be a symptom of underlying depression. *See* DEPRESSION to help you assess whether this is the case for you.

■ If you need professional help, seek it. Talking with a therapist has worked wonders for many people, even people once incapacitated by anxiety disorders.

Aphthous Ulcer

See CANKER SORES.

Apnea

See under SNORING.

Appendicitis

Appendicitis is an acute inflammation of the appendix, a thin, tube-shaped structure that protrudes from the first section of the large intestine. The appendix can become inflamed due either to an anatomical obstruction or a blockage of hardened feces. This inflammation can rapidly develop into an infection.

Symptoms of appendicitis usually begin with pain around the navel that intensifies over several hours and moves to the lower right quadrant of the abdomen. This area will be very tender to even light pressure, and you may find yourself instinctively holding or protecting it. Many people also experience decreased appetite, vomiting, and fever. You may have diarrhea as well, and extending your right leg may make the pain worse.

An inflamed appendix can burst, causing a life-threatening infection of the abdominal wall. If this happens, you will rapidly become very ill, with a fever, pale color, and severe abdominal pain. Although continuous abdominal pain is a key indicator of appendicitis, some people experience a milder onset of pain that comes and goes over several days before settling in as constant and severe. If you suspect appendicitis, seek immediate medical care.

In order to diagnose appendicitis, a doctor will want to know details of when the pain began and the location and quality of the pain. Your doctor will do an abdominal and rectal exam, take a sample of blood to look for signs of an infection, and might order an x-ray or ultrasound scan to look for signs of blockage or inflammation.

CONVENTIONAL TREATMENT

■ If your doctor confirms a diagnosis of appendicitis, surgery to remove the inflamed appendix is the recommended course of treatment. Because of the danger that the appendix may rupture, surgery is usually done soon after the diagnosis is made.

■ To lower the risk of infection, you may be given antibiotics both before and immediately after surgery. If your appendix has ruptured, intravenous antibiotics will be administered. You may need to be hospitalized for one to two weeks after surgery.

■ Because of the surgery and the manipulation of your digestive tract, your intestines will slow down and may even stop moving for a day or two. You may have a nasogastric tube, a tube placed in the nose and down into the stomach, that uses suction to pull the contents of the stomach out of the body. This prevents nausea and vomiting. Except for an occasional ice chip, you will not be able to eat or drink anything until your intestines begin working

again. Intravenous fluids to prevent dehydration and pain medication to help relieve discomfort will be administered.

■ You will have to get up out of bed and walk the day after surgery. Even though this may seem like a daunting task, the importance of movement cannot be overemphasized. Among other things, walking helps the intestines to begin working again, and helps to prevent pneumonia from developing.

DIETARY GUIDELINES

■ Even after your doctor gives you full permission to eat, you may have little or no appetite. Begin slowly, with clear liquids such as broth, juices, and herbal teas.

■ To allow your gastrointestinal tract to readjust to food, gradually work up to a full diet. Eat whole, well-cooked foods that are full of the many vitamins and minerals the body needs to heal and regain energy. Homemade applesauce and soups are excellent "starter" foods for anyone who has undergone surgery. Foods high in beta-carotene, such as squash and cooked greens, are also important.

■ Avoid eating any gas-producing foods, such as nuts and legumes, for the first two weeks after surgery.

NUTRITIONAL SUPPLEMENTS

■ Acidophilus and bifidus are both very good for restoring bowel health after the trauma of surgery and potent antibiotics. Follow the dosage directions on the product label and take one dose three times a day for ten days. Then take one dose twice a day for two weeks. After that, take one dose once a day for one month.

■ If postoperative complications result in constipation, take 250 milligrams of magnesium at breakfast and another 250 milligrams at bedtime for one month.

■ Surgery for appendicitis disturbs the normal intestinal flora, resulting in lower than normal absorption of vitamin B_{12}. This vitamin is an especially important part of the B complex that restores strength. Take 500 micrograms of vitamin B_{12} sublingually (place the tablet under your tongue and allow it to dissolve and be absorbed that way) twice daily for one month. If you find you have trouble digesting it, ask your doctor for a vitamin-B_{12} injection once weekly for one month. In addition to the B_{12}, take a B-complex supplement once a day for one month as directed on the product label.

■ Vitamin C and bioflavonoids aid in tissue repair and in decreasing inflammation. Take 1,000 milligrams of vitamin C and 500 milligrams of bioflavonoids three times a day for two weeks, then reduce to the same dosage twice daily.

■ Vitamin E is an antioxidant nutrient and a mild but effective natural anti-inflammatory. Choose a product containing mixed tocopherols and start by taking 200 international units daily, then gradually increase the dosage until you are taking 400 international units twice a day. Maintain that dosage for one month.

Note: If you have high blood pressure, limit your intake of supplemental vitamin E to a total of 400 international units daily. If you are taking an anticoagulant (blood thinner), consult your physician before taking supplemental vitamin E.

■ Zinc hastens wound and tissue healing and supports the immune system. Take 25 milligrams of zinc twice a day for two weeks. Then take 25 milligrams once a day for two weeks.

Note: Take zinc with food to prevent stomach upset, and do not exceed 100 milligrams daily from all supplements.

HERBAL TREATMENT

Herbal treatment for appendicitis is intended to support recovery from surgery. It is not meant to be a substitute for surgical treatment. If you suspect appendicitis, seek medical treatment immediately.

■ Once the crisis is over, follow this regimen below to help your body recover.

Days 1–4: Take one dose of an echinacea and goldenseal supplying 250 to 500 milligrams of echinacea and 150 to 300 milligrams of goldenseal three times daily. Echinacea and goldenseal help to detoxify the blood after anesthesia. They also support the immune system and can help prevent a possible infection in a surgical wound.

Days 5–8: Take 500 milligrams of astragalus three times daily. With its rich concentration of trace minerals and micronutrients, this herb helps to strengthen the immune system. Do not take astragalus if you have a fever, however. If you have a fever, continue taking echinacea and goldenseal until the fever is gone.

Days 4–14: Take 50 to 75 milligrams of pine-bark or grape-seed extract three times a day. These herbal extracts are high in bioflavonoids and act as natural anti-inflammatories.

Days 8–12: Take 100 milligrams of standardized Siberian ginseng extract containing 0.5 percent eleutheroside E thirty minutes before breakfast and another thirty minutes before lunch. This is another excellent source of trace minerals and micronutrients, and will help strengthen your internal defenses.

Note: Do not take this herb if fever or any other signs of acute infection are present.

Days 13–16: Take one dose of a gentian and dandelion root combination formula supplying 250 to 300 milligrams of each herb three times daily. If your digestion is impaired, continue taking them for one month.

■ Once the incision has closed and healing has begun,

and your surgeon gives you the okay, gently rub vitamin-E oil, castor oil, or evening primrose oil into the wound to minimize scarring.

HOMEOPATHY

Homeopathic treatment for appendicitis is intended to support recovery from surgery. It is not meant to be a substitute for surgical treatment. If you suspect appendicitis, seek professional medical treatment immediately.

■ If you seem to have had an adverse reaction to anesthesia, take one dose of *Nux vomica* 30x or 200x, as directed on the product label, as soon as possible after surgery, to help lessen the side effects. Then follow this regimen to aid recovery from surgery:

Days 1–2: Take one dose of *Arnica* 30x or 9c three or four times daily. Arnica helps to decrease inflammation following surgery and speeds the healing process.

Days 3–4: Take one dose of *Staphysagria* 30x or 15c three times a day to help the incision heal.

Day 4: To further hasten healing, take one dose of *Ledum* 12x or 6c three times during the day.

Days 5–6: For nerve pain following surgery, take one dose of *Hypericum* 6x or 5c three times a day.

Days 7–9: To help digestion and to relieve lower bowel gas, take one dose of *Lycopodium* 3x or 15c twice daily.

ACUPRESSURE

For the locations of acupressure points on the body, *see* ADMINISTERING AN ACUPRESSURE TREATMENT in Part Three.

■ Massaging the Stomach meridian, particularly Stomach 36 and 37, as well as Liver 3, will help tone the digestive tract and speed recovery.

GENERAL RECOMMENDATIONS

■ To ensure a full and strong recovery after surgery, adequate rest is essential. Limit visitors and create a calm and familiar environment.

■ Once you are discharged from the hospital, expect periods of fatigue. As soon as your doctor permits, resuming your daily routine is fine, although you may need more rest than usual until you fully recover your strength. To help increase your energy level, you can take a B-complex supplement for two weeks. Taking 500 milligrams of American ginseng at approximately 11:00 AM each day can also be helpful.

Note: Do not use American ginseng if you have high blood pressure, heart disease, or hypoglycemia. If you are sensitive to the effects of caffeine and other stimulants, you may want to consult with a qualified herbalist before using ginseng.

■ Contact sports, heavy lifting, and abdominal exercises

must be avoided for as long as your doctor recommends, probably for six to eight weeks after surgery.

Arrhythmia

See under CARDIOVASCULAR DISEASE.

Arteriosclerosis

See under CARDIOVASCULAR DISEASE.

Arthritis

Arthritis is the name given to inflammatory diseases that affect the joints. It is not a single disease, but many. No matter what form arthritis takes, the overall symptoms include inflammation, pain, and stiffness in the joints. The pain can be a mild, manageable achiness or truly torturous—or anything in between. Any joint in the body can be affected. In its most severe forms, arthritis can cause a joint or joints to become misshapen and deformed.

Osteoarthritis, which typically begins in middle age, is the most common form of this disease. Almost 80 percent of all people over the age of fifty have some degree of osteoarthritis. Osteoarthritis is considered a degenerative disease brought about by wear and tear on the joints, and it becomes progressively worse with age. It primarily affects the weight-bearing joints—the hips, knees, and spine—and, because the hands are in constant use, it may also strike the finger joints. In this type of arthritis, the pain typically improves with rest.

Osteoarthritis develops in several stages. Where bones come together to form a working joint, they are shielded from one another by a layer of the dense connective tissue known as cartilage, and the entire joint is surrounded by the synovial membrane, a thin membrane that encloses a layer of lubricating fluid. As the joint is subjected to wear or injury, that cartilage shield wears down. When the aging body fails to replace it, the bones that interact at the joint start to grind together whenever the joint is used. The greater the loss of cartilage, the greater the degree of inflammation and pain. The friction caused by the scraping of bone against bone irritates the periosteum, the thin protective membrane that sheathes the bones. The periosteum fights back by causing the growth of bony knobs, leaving the working joint to scrape against the knobs with every movement. As the disease progresses, movement is impaired and the joint may become deformed. A diagnosis of osteoarthritis is made based on symptoms plus x-rays that show characteristic changes in the joint, including narrowing of the joint space and increasing bony growth.

Rheumatoid arthritis is a type of arthritis classified as an autoimmune disorder, which means that it is a result of the immune system mistakenly attacking the body's own tissues. The joints most often affected include the hands, feet, wrists, ankles, and knees. Rheumatoid arthritis begins with irritation and inflammation of the synovial membrane, causing pain, stiffness, and swelling. The inflamed membrane responds by sending out enzymes that cause the cartilage of the joint to break down. The cartilage is then replaced with fibrous tissue that can calcify and form bony knobs that may fuse the joint and restrict movement.

The onset of rheumatoid arthritis commonly occurs between the ages of twenty and forty, but it can affect people of any age. The course of the disease is impossible to predict. In up to 20 percent of those affected, it simply disappears on its own and never returns. In others, it remains for life and causes varying degrees of disability. Multiple joints are usually involved, with warmth, redness, pain, and stiffness, often improving during the day. Besides localized joint pain, diagnosis hinges on the presence in the blood of a specific protein called *rheumatoid factor*; the development of rheumatoid nodules, characteristic roundish lumps that occur under the skin, often near joints; and, possibly, signs of inflammation in other parts of the body, including the heart, lymph glands, and other sites.

Ankylosing spondylitis is a form of arthritis that affects the spine. In this autoimmune disease, the vertebral (spine) joints become inflamed. At its most severe, this condition can cause the joints to fuse together. Ankylosing spondylitis can spread to other joints and, once contracted, may affect the hips, though in 50 percent of cases it resolves on its own. Diagnosis involves an evaluation of symptoms, including low back pain and a limited range of motion; x-rays to detect changes in the sacroiliac joint, in the extreme lower back; and blood tests.

Other types of arthritis include gout, psoriatic (psoriasis-related) arthritis, and septic arthritis, which is a result of infection of a joint. Disorders such as lupus and Lyme disease can cause arthritis-like symptoms as well. Localized inflammatory syndromes, including inflammatory bowel disease and Reiter's syndrome, which affects the eyes, urinary tract, and skin, can also affect the joints to differing degrees.

CONVENTIONAL MEDICINE

■ The mainstay of conventional treatment for arthritis, in

general, is the use of painkillers and anti-inflammatory drugs. Some are available over the counter, including acetaminophen (Tylenol, Datril, and others), aspirin (Bayer, Ecotrin, and others), and the nonsteroidal anti-inflammatories (NSAIDs) ibuprofen (Advil, Motrin IB, Nuprin, and others), ketoprofen (Orudis), and naproxen (Aleve). Other members of the NSAID class of drugs are available by prescription. These include diclofenac (Voltaren), diflunisal (Dolobid), fenoprofen (Nalfon), indomethacin (Indocin), piroxicam (Feldene), and tolmetin (Tolectin), as well as higher strength versions of ibuprofen (Motrin, Ibu-Tabs), ketoprofen (Oruvail), and naproxen (Anaprox, Naprelan, Naprosyn). These medications, though commonly used in therapy, should be respected, as they can (and sometimes do) cause ulceration, bleeding, and perforation of the gastrointestinal tract—sometimes without any warning. They can also lead to kidney damage and liver dysfunction. Other adverse reactions include (but unfortunately are not limited to) abdominal pain, indigestion, constipation, diarrhea, nausea, mouth sores, headache, dizziness, itching, rashes, ringing in the ears, bloating, shortness of breath, and palpitations.

■ For mild to moderate arthritis, a supervised exercise program may be prescribed to improve joint function without aggravating the situation.

■ Some people find relief with the injection of synthetic corticosteroids into the most affected joint spaces. This helps to minimize the use of oral forms of these drugs, which have a greater risk of causing such systemic effects as fluid retention and suppression of adrenal and immune function.

■ If destruction progresses to the point that pain or lack of mobility becomes unbearable, joint-replacement surgery may be recommended.

■ For rheumatoid arthritis, alternating applications of heat and cold, alternating rest and exercise therapies, and splints and other assistive devices may be prescribed.

■ Methotrexate (Rheumatrex) is a cancer chemotherapy drug that inhibits the synthesis of DNA, thus interfering with cell replication, particularly in fast-growing cells. Why it helps people with rheumatoid arthritis is not known, but it can be effective within about a month of treatment, sometimes highly so. However, it is also highly toxic, causing bone-marrow suppression, liver damage, and severe lung damage, among other serious side effects. Its use must be very closely monitored by a physician experienced with this kind of therapy.

■ Gold salts, most often administered by injection, are sometimes used to treat rheumatoid arthritis if other drugs have failed. Examples of these drugs include aurothioglucose (Solganal), gold sodium thiomalate (Myochrysine), and auranofin (Ridaura). As with methotrexate, its mode of action is unknown. About half the people who receive this treatment experience improvement, but they rarely improve completely, and side effects are not uncommon. These include suppression of the bone marrow and resulting blood abnormalities, kidney damage, liver damage, lung damage, colitis, rashes, skin pigment changes, itching, nausea, and nerve damage.

■ The antimalarial drug hydroxychloroquine (Plaquenil) also is used in some cases of rheumatoid arthritis. The reason for this drug's effect on rheumatoid arthritis is not understood. It results in improvement in fewer than half the cases treated and can take up to 6 months for effect; however, it is considered less toxic than some other drugs used for this condition. Nevertheless, it can cause side effects, including skin rash, itching, hair loss, skin pigment changes, nausea, weight loss, blood abnormalities, and irreversible vision damage.

■ Penicillamine (Cuprimine, Depen) is a chelating agent that may be prescribed for some people with severe rheumatoid arthritis. Here again the mechanism of action is not understood. Potential side effects are considerable and common—up to half of those who take it experience adverse effects, including blood abnormalities, kidney damage, autoimmune disorders, rashes, mouth ulcers, and loss of the sense of taste.

■ Sulfasalazine (Azulfidine) is a common second-line drug tried for rheumatoid arthritis. That is, it is generally reserved for cases in which other therapies fail, due to its potential toxicity. Blood counts should be taken frequently, as blood abnormalities are frequent.

■ If none of the standard treatments works, your doctor may recommend more exotic, experimental treatments deliberately aimed at suppressing the immune system. These involve the use of such agents as cyclophosphamide (Cytoxan) or chlorambucil (Leukeran). These are cancer chemotherapy drugs with extremely powerful and serious effects. Side effects can be severe, including blood abnormalities, bone-marrow suppression, serious lung disease, and—paradoxically—cancer, among others.

■ Even many conventional physicians today consider it acceptable to experiment with treatments such as fish-oil and oral cartilage supplements. (*See* Nutritional Supplements, below, for further information.)

■ Some women experience arthritic symptoms around the time of menopause. If this happens to you, consult with your gynecologist or other health-care practitioner. Often, balancing a woman's hormones can quickly reduce these aches and pains.

DIETARY GUIDELINES

■ Eat a diet that is high in fiber and that is not tainted with chemicals, which stress the body. Maximize your intake of fresh vegetables, fruits, fish, nuts, seeds, and whole grains.

Make sure your menu includes cold-water fish such as salmon and halibut. The oils in these fish are beneficial to the joints and act as natural anti-inflammatories.

■ Avoid saturated fats, hydrogenated and partially hydrogenated oils, rich fatty foods, fried foods, and refined sugar. These substances make the internal environment more acidic. Acid in the joints promotes inflammation, which worsens symptoms and increases pain.

■ Avoid alcohol and caffeine, which also create acid.

To flush toxins from your body, be sure to drink at least six to eight glasses of pure water daily.

NUTRITIONAL SUPPLEMENTS

To correct possible nutritional deficiencies, take a good multivitamin and mineral complex daily.

Bromelain, an enzyme derived from pineapple, has a notable anti-inflammatory action. It is as useful in sports injuries as in arthritis. Take 200 to 400 milligrams three times daily, between meals.

■ Black currant seed oil, borage oil, evening primrose oil, fish oil, and flaxseed oil contain essential fatty acids that increase the production of anti-inflammatory prostaglandins. Take 500 to 1,000 milligrams of any of these oils twice daily. Be aware that it may take several weeks to notice an improvement in symptoms.

Glucosamine, a compound of the simple sugar glucose and the amino acid glutamine, has been shown to be an effective natural means of slowing cartilage breakdown and encouraging cartilage repair. With continued use, it helps to relieve joint pain and stiffness. Several studies have shown that glucosamine sulfate can be a more effective pain reliever than ibuprofen for arthritis. Take 500 milligrams of glucosamine sulfate three times daily. Be aware that it may take as long as six to eight weeks to attain maximum relief.

Lactobacillus acidophilus and *Bifidobacterium bifidum* are friendly bacteria that are essential to the efficient functioning of the entire gastrointestinal tract. Take them as recommended on the product labels.

■ Magnesium is essential to the central nervous system and protects against muscular excitability and tremors. Take 250 milligrams twice daily.

■ Many people with arthritis are deficient in manganese, a trace element that activates important enzymes and is necessary for normal skeletal development. Take 5 milligrams twice daily for one month.

Methylsulfonylmethane (MSM), a natural source of sulfur, can help relieve arthritis pain and maintain joint health. Sulfur is an essential component of proteins that make up connective tissue. Take 500 milligrams three or four times daily, with meals.

■ Pancreatic enzymes are important for digestion. Choose 10X strength non-enteric-coated enzyme tablets or capsules, and take 500 milligrams immediately before each meal. Make sure the label states that the tablet or capsule contains amylase (an enzyme that breaks down starch molecules into smaller, more easily digested sugars), lipase (an enzyme that assists in the digestion of fats), and proteases (enzymes that break down proteins).

■ S-adenosylmethionine (SAM or SAM-e) is an amino-acid derivative that has been shown in clinical trials to be comparable in effect to the combination of glucosamine and chondroitin. Like glucosamine, SAM plays a role in the formation of cartilage. It also exerts a mild analgesic effect. Try taking it as follows:

Week 1: Take 400 milligrams three times a day.

Week 2: Take 400 milligrams twice a day.

Week 3: Reduce to a maintenance dosage or 200 milligrams twice a day.

■ Selenium is a powerful antioxidant that fights free-radical damage. Take 200 micrograms of selenium daily.

■ Shark cartilage may be useful in treatment of this disease, but it takes time. This is not inexpensive, unfortunately. Each day, take one 750-milligram capsule per 11 pounds of body weight (or 1 gram of powder per 15 pounds of body weight), divided into three equal doses. Once you have achieved relief of pain, reduce the dose to one 750-milligram capsule per 30 pounds of body weight (or 1 gram of powder per 40 pounds of body weight).

■ People with arthritis, particularly rheumatoid arthritis, are often deficient in pantothenic acid. Further, studies have shown that supplementation with this B vitamin can improve symptoms of pain, stiffness, and limitation of motion. Take 100 to 250 milligrams of pantothenic acid twice daily for three weeks.

■ Vitamin E protects against muscle-wasting and is essential in cellular respiration, thus helping remove toxins. Choose a product containing mixed tocopherols and start by taking 200 international units daily, then gradually increase the dosage until you are taking 400 international units twice daily, once in the morning and again at bedtime.

Note: If you have high blood pressure, limit your intake of supplemental vitamin E to a total of 400 international units daily. If you are taking an anticoagulant (blood thinner), consult your physician before taking supplemental vitamin E.

HERBAL TREATMENT

■ Aloe vera encourages healthy bowel function and

helps detoxify the bloodstream and the lymphatic system. Select a food-grade product and take $1/4$ cup three times daily for two weeks, then reduce the dosage to $1/4$ cup twice daily.

■ If you have swelling and are retaining water, try the following: 250 to 500 milligrams of bladderwrack two or three times daily, 250 to 500 milligrams of horsetail twice daily, and 250 to 500 milligrams of juniper berry twice a day. You can take them singly or in any combination.

Capsaicin, an extract of the cayenne pepper (capsicum), is available over the counter in cream form as Dolorac and Zostrix. Applied twice daily to affected areas, it increases local blood flow, warms the skin, and numbs the area. The same kind of therapy is available (at less cost) with over-the-counter products like Heet.

Devil's claw is a good anti-inflammatory agent. Take 1,000 milligrams (1 gram) twice daily.

Feverfew has been used for centuries for arthritis. Some studies have found that the anti-inflammatory effects of this herb are greater than those achieved by NSAIDs. Take 250 milligrams once or twice daily.

Siberian ginseng helps to strengthen the immune system and improve adrenal function. Choose a standardized extract containing 0.5 percent eleutheroside E and take 100 milligrams in the morning and again in the afternoon.

Yucca also has anti-inflammatory action. Take 1,000 milligrams (1 gram) twice daily.

Note: The remarkable effects of the anti-inflammatory herbs are cumulative. Expect results to build over a period of two months.

HOMEOPATHY

Choose *Bryonia* if you feel worse after activity, such as taking a short walk. You may also be irritable and have a tendency to constipation. Take one dose of *Bryonia* 30x or 9c as needed.

Rhus toxicodendron will help if you feel better with movement, such as after a short walk. Take one dose of *Rhus toxicodendron* 30x or 9c as needed.

See a homeopathic practitioner for a constitutional remedy tailored to your specific symptoms.

ACUPRESSURE

For the locations of acupressure points on the body, *see* ADMINISTERING AN ACUPRESSURE TREATMENT in Part Three.

All back Bladder points help improve circulation and stimulate the internal organs.

■ Gallbladder 34 helps to relax muscles and tendons.

■ Large Intestine 4 and Liver 3 are relaxing to the body.

Spleen 6 helps strengthen the blood.

■ Stomach 36 helps improve absorption of nutrients and benefits overall well-being.

AROMATHERAPY

For specific instructions on how to use aromatherapy, *see* PREPARING AROMATHERAPY TREATMENTS in Part Three.

■ Soothing aromatherapy baths and massages can help to ease the pain and inflammation of arthritis. Choose one or more of the following essential oils to add to bath water or massage oil: basil, black pepper, elemi, eucalyptus, myrrh, and pine.

GENERAL RECOMMENDATIONS

■ Studies have shown that exercise can both increase ease of movement and reduce pain and stiffness. Gentle stretching exercises, mild yoga, and tai chi can all be helpful. *See* STARTING AN EXERCISE PROGRAM in Part Three.

■ Although there are no studies to support their use, many people with arthritis claim they get a measure of relief from wearing a copper bracelet. You may wish to try this simple prescription yourself and see if it works for you.

PREVENTION

■ There is no sure way to prevent arthritis, but there are a number of measures that may help. Seek treatment promptly for any suspected injury involving a joint, and follow your doctor's recommendations concerning any limits on activity while the joint is healing. Ignoring injuries and/or overstressing the joints contributes to the later development of arthritis.

Asthma

Asthma is an inflammatory respiratory illness characterized by mild to severe difficulty in breathing. This is caused by constriction and swelling of the airways, along with an increase in secretions of mucus, which plugs up the smaller passages. As a result, air cannot get into or out of the lungs as easily as it usually does. Wheezing results as air squeaks through the narrowed and inflamed air passages. An asthma attack can cause such shortness of breath and poor oxygen intake that a person may need to be hospitalized.

Asthma can be triggered by a variety of things, including exposure to pollen, dust, feathers, molds, animal dander, pollution, cigarette smoke, or cold dry air, as well as upper respiratory infection, exercise, excitement, and stress. Sometimes a susceptible individual will develop an asthma attack for no apparent reason.

An asthma attack causes coughing, wheezing, an increased respiratory rate, a feeling of tightness in the chest, and difficulty breathing. Early signs of an asthma attack can include an itchy throat, a change in breathing pattern, fatigue, paleness, nervousness, a runny nose, or moodiness. It is important to seek early treatment if you feel an asthma attack coming on. If you have any doubts as to your breathing, don't hesitate to call your doctor.

If you suffer from asthma, one simple way to monitor your breathing is with an instrument called a peak flow meter, available at many large drugstores and through medical-supply catalogs. These are relatively inexpensive, simple-to-use devices that measure how much air pressure you can exert with a full exhalation. The meter's indicator can be used to compare how your air flow changes from day to day. By monitoring yourself in this way, you will have a more reliable means of determining whether your condition is getting better or worse. Your physician will help you determine what to watch for.

EMERGENCY TREATMENT

■ In the event of a severe asthma attack, you need to seek immediate medical care. If your asthma is not resolving with the treatments you know, have someone call your doctor and take you to the emergency room of the nearest hospital or call for emergency medical assistance.

■ At the hospital, you will probably be given an inhaled medication that sprays a bronchodilator (a substance that opens air passages to restore normal breathing) directly into the airways. If this does not help, you may receive other drugs, such as intravenous steroids or theophylline, and you may need to be hospitalized. Some people need to receive oxygen to ease the work of breathing.

CONVENTIONAL TREATMENT

■ The mainstay of conventional treatment is medication, primarily with oral or inhaled bronchodilators like albuterol (Proventil, Ventolin), isoetharine (Bronkometer, Bronkosol), isoproterenol (Isuprel), metaproterenol (Alupent), and terbutaline (Brethaire, Brethine, Bricanyl). These medications work to open up the airways, easing breathing. They can cause a variety of side effects, including nervousness, increased heart rate, tremors, increased blood pressure, and dizziness.

■ In more advanced or chronic cases of asthma, corticosteroids may be prescribed, in either oral or inhaled form. Inhaler forms include beclomethasone (Beclovent, Vanceril, Vancenase, Beconase), fluticasone (Flovent), and triamcinolone (Azmacort, Nasacort). Prednisone is the most commonly prescribed oral form. These medicines work by decreasing the swelling and inflammation of the airways, but they do have several disadvantages. First, they have an adverse affect on the functioning of the immune system

and the adrenal glands. Oral yeast infections can be a problem with inhaler forms. All steroids have the potential to cause significant side effects, especially when taken over the long term, that need to be understood. Talk this over with your doctor or pharmacist.

■ A relatively new class of drugs known as *antimediators* are now often used to prevent acute attacks. They work by stabilizing mast cells in the body. In response to certain stimuli, mast cells release chemicals that set in motion a chain of biochemical reactions that can lead to constriction of the airways; by stabilizing the mast cells, you may be able to stop this entire process before it begins. These drugs are comparatively nontoxic. In fact, they are slightly altered, patented forms of bioflavonoids, which are used in conjunction with vitamin C in nutritional therapy for allergy, colds, and asthma. Drugs of this type include cromolyn sodium (Intal, Nasalcrom) and nedocromil sodium (Tilade). Another type of antimediator is called the *leukotriene receptor antagonist* (LTRA). These drugs also inhibit the action of chemicals that can initiate an asthma attack. Examples include montelukast (Singular) and zafirlukast (Accolate). Possible side effects include headache, liver stress, fatigue, fever, and gastrointestinal distress.

■ Theophylline and related drugs, once commonly prescribed for asthma, are less often used today because they are more likely to cause side effects such as restlessness, insomnia, headache, loss of appetite, increased heart rate, dizziness, nausea, and vomiting. Long-term use of theophylline may also be associated with behavioral problems and learning disabilities, although the evidence for this is not conclusive.

DIETARY GUIDELINES

■ Eat a healthy whole-foods diet based on lean protein foods, such as fish; fresh vegetables and fruits; and whole grains. Fatty fish such as salmon, sardines, and tuna, which are high in omega-3 essential fatty acids, have natural anti-inflammatory properties. Eating fish three or four times a week can be very beneficial.

■ Include onions in your diet. Onions contain diphenylthiosulfinate, an anti-inflammatory compound with anti-asthmatic effects. Moreover, some researchers believe that asthma has its roots in infection by an organism known as *Chlamydia pneumoniae,* and onions have natural infection-fighting properties as well.

■ Avoid saturated fats, hydrogenated and partially hydrogenated oils, and simple carbohydrates, such as refined sugar.

■ If you have a sensitivity to dairy foods, avoid them. Remember that dairy foods tend to increase the production of mucus.

■ Beware of foods such as nuts, citrus fruits, whole-wheat products (especially yeasted breads), seafood, and foods containing additives like preservatives or food dyes, as well as contact with animals. Any of these things can cause or exacerbate an allergy-induced asthma attack.

■ Certain food additives, especially metabisulfite, can be dangerous for individuals with asthma. Sulfites are commonly found in commercially prepared foods such as dried fruits. They are also used by many restaurants to keep fruits and vegetables at salad bars looking fresh and attractive. If you have asthma, it's best to avoid salad bars and to buy only unsulfured dried fruits. Monosodium glutamate (MSG) can also cause problems for some people with asthma, so avoid food products prepared with this additive. You should also be aware of "hidden" sources of MSG. These often show up on food labels as "hydrolyzed protein," "autolyzed yeast," "sodium caseinate," and "calcium caseinate."

■ Following an asthma attack, drink plenty of fluids once your condition is stable enough for you to do so. It is important to thin secretions so that they are easily coughed out.

■ If you suffer from fatigue, hair loss, dry skin, constipation, and have difficulty losing weight, ask your physician to check your thyroid function. Asthma is often exacerbated by low thyroid function.

NUTRITIONAL SUPPLEMENTS

Nutritional supplements for asthma are intended to prevent or support recovery from an asthma attack, rather than to treat an acute episode. In the event of an acute asthma attack, seek immediate medical treatment.

■ Allergy-induced asthma is often related to imperfect digestion. Supplementing your diet with digestive enzymes will improve your absorption and utilization of nutrients. Take a full-spectrum digestive-enzyme supplement providing 5,000 international units of lipase, 2,500 international units of amylase, and 300 international units of protease, plus 500 to 1,000 milligrams of pancreatin, with each meal.

Note: Long-term supplementation with pancreatin is not advised, as it can cause your pancreas to reduce its own production of this important enzyme. Overuse also has the potential to cause nausea or diarrhea. After two months on pancreatin, discontinue use and monitor your reaction. If you find that your problems recur, discuss pancreatin supplementation with your health-care provider.

■ Omega-3 and omega-6 essential fatty acids (EFAs) help to regulate the inflammatory response. Flaxseed and fish oils are good sources of omega-3 EFAs; good sources of omega-6 EFAs include black currant seed oil, borage oil, and evening primrose oil. Take 500 to 1,000 milligrams of any of these oils twice daily for two to three months. A combination of omega-3 and omega-6 may be more effective for some people.

■ Magnesium has a bronchodilating effect if taken in the proper dosage. Some doctors give magnesium sulfate by injection to treat acute asthma attacks. Try taking 500 milligrams of magnesium twice a day. If you develop loose stools, reduce the dosage.

■ Pantothenic acid, one of the B vitamins, supports adrenal function and the nervous system. Take 250 to 500 milligrams three times a day for one month. If you take any of the B vitamins individually, you should also take a B-complex supplement at a different time of day.

■ Quercetin is an antioxidant flavonoid that has properties similar to those of cromolyn sodium (see under Conventional Treatment in this entry). Take 30 to 100 milligrams twice a day.

■ A deficiency of vitamin B_{12} has been linked to some types of asthmatic conditions. Taken in either oral or injectable form, this vitamin can help to prevent asthma attacks. Discuss this with a nutritionally oriented physician.

■ Many adults with asthma suffer from compromised adrenal function but are unaware of it. You may find it helpful to take adrenal glandular extract for short periods of time. Take 150 milligrams three times daily, with meals, for three weeks.

■ If you suffer from frequent colds and flu in addition to asthma, consider taking immune-enhancing thymus glandular extract. Take 300 milligrams with breakfast and lunch for three weeks.

HERBAL TREATMENT

Herbal treatments for asthma are intended to prevent or support recovery from an asthma attack, rather than to treat an acute episode. In the event of an acute asthma attack, seek immediate medical care.

■ Astragalus is a Chinese herb that helps to increase what the Chinese call *wei chi,* or a person's own protective energy. It also helps strengthen the lungs. Take 500 milligrams twice a day for two weeks out of every month for three months following an asthma attack.

Note: Do not take this herb if you have a fever or any other signs of infection.

■ Ginkgo biloba has been shown to have anti-allergy and anti-asthmatic properties. It appears to relieve constriction of the bronchi, the main air passages. Choose a product containing at least 24 percent ginkgo heterosides (sometimes called flavoglycosides) and take 80 milligrams two or three times daily.

■ Licorice, horehound, thyme, hyssop, mullein, and lungwort are helpful in strengthening the respiratory system. Although these herbs may be taken individually, they work best in combination. Look for a combination herbal remedy and take it as directed on the product label.

■ Turmeric helps strengthen immune function, acts as a natural anti-inflammatory, and enhances energy. Take 500 milligrams twice a day for one month.

HOMEOPATHY

Homeopathic treatments for asthma are intended to prevent or support recovery from an asthma attack, rather than to treat an acute episode. In the event of an acute asthma attack, seek immediate medical care.

■ If you suffer from chronic asthma, consult a homeopathic physician to determine an appropriate constitutional remedy.

■ *Antimonium tartaricum* is a homeopathic remedy for the individual who is wheezing, with a tight feeling in the chest. There may be mucus, but it is difficult to cough up. If your symptoms match this description, take one dose of *Antimonium tartaricum* 12x, 30x, 6c, or 9c every hour until symptoms lessen. Then take one dose three times a day for several days or until symptoms subside.

  Note: Do not use this remedy if you have a fever.

■ *Arsenicum album* 30x, 200x, 9c, or 30c is recommended if you are tired, anxious, and cold-sensitive, and your symptoms are often worse in the middle of the night or when lying down. Take one dose three times a day for several days or until symptoms subside.

■ *Chamomilla* 30x or 9c is helpful for asthma that is triggered or accompanied by anger and irritability. Take one dose three times a day for several days or until symptoms subside.

■ *Pulsatilla* 30x or 9c is for asthma that is often triggered by an upper respiratory tract infection. There is little or no mucus. You probably have more difficulty breathing in a closed, stuffy room, and feel more comfortable outside. Take one dose three times a day for several days or until symptoms subside.

ACUPRESSURE

The points listed below can be massaged on a daily basis to help balance your entire system. In the event of an acute asthma attack, seek immediate medical care (you can work these points as you are on your way to the hospital). For the locations of acupressure points on the body, *see* ADMINISTERING AN ACUPRESSURE TREATMENT in Part Three.

■ Conception Vessel 17 relaxes the chest.

■ Liver 3 helps to quiet the nervous system.

■ Lung 7 clears the lungs.

■ Pericardium 6 relaxes the chest.

AROMATHERAPY

For specific instructions on how to use aromatherapy, *see* PREPARING AROMATHERAPY TREATMENTS in Part Three.

■ Essential oils that can help ease breathing include basil, frankincense, lavender, myrrh, peppermint, pine, rose, and tea tree. Choose one or more of these oils and use them as inhalants or in steam inhalation treatments. Start by using one at a time, however, as it is possible that you may be sensitive to one or more essential oils.

GENERAL RECOMMENDATIONS

■ Avoid contact with any foods or environmental allergens that you suspect, based on past experience, may trigger an episode.

■ Follow the regimen prescribed by your physician. Be sure you understand exactly when and how to take the medicines prescribed. Going off medication without careful supervision can result in a severe asthma attack and hospitalization, and should not be attempted.

■ Yoga, relaxation, and deep-breathing techniques are invaluable for people with asthma. In addition to building physical strength and flexibility, yoga teaches slow, steady, controlled deep breathing, which helps to strengthen the respiratory system. Using relaxation and visualization exercises at the beginning of an asthma attack can help calm you and ease breathing (*See* RELAXATION TECHNIQUES in Part Three).

■ Get regular exercise to improve lung function. Swimming is particularly good, and the humidity helps to keep the mouth and air passages from drying out. (Make sure, however, that you do not swim in an excessively chlorinated pool, since high levels of chlorine can produce allergic reactions in some people.) Depending on the severity and type of your asthma, you may need to take medication before activity to prevent respiratory distress. Discuss this with your physician.

■ Be aware that using steroid-containing asthma inhalants can increase the risk of glaucoma (or the conditions that usually precede glaucoma) by as much as 44 percent. This is a particular concern for older adults. Discuss your use of inhalants with your doctor.

Athlete's Foot

Athlete's foot (or *tinea pedis*) is a fungal infection caused by any of several related organisms. It is similar to the condition known as ringworm. People often develop athlete's foot after prolonged exposure to warm and moist environments, such as shower floors, locker rooms, and sweaty socks. Although it is contagious, athlete's foot seems most likely to occur in predisposed individuals.

Symptoms of athlete's foot include burning, itching, scaling, cracking, sores, and tiny blisters between the toes and on the soles of the feet. Athlete's foot can usually be treated successfully at home. However, it is possible for a bacterial infection to develop alongside a fungal infection. If the condition persists or gets worse after treatment, see your doctor for further help.

CONVENTIONAL TREATMENT

■ A number of over-the-counter antifungal creams are available that may help with athlete's foot, among them miconazole (in Micatin-Derm and Monistat-Derm), tolnaftate (Tinactin, Dr. Scholl's), undecylenic acid (Desitin), and clotrimazole (Lotrimin, Mycelex). There are also prescription varieties of these medications, including ketoconazole (Nizoral), econazole (Spectazole), sulconazole (Exelderm), oxiconazole (Oxistat), naftifine (Naftin), terbinafine (Lamisil), and ciclopirox (Loprox). Normally these creams are applied twice daily. They can produce results in as little as three to four days, but it may be necessary to use them for up to a month in persistent cases.

■ If the skin is cracked, open, or oozing, aluminum-solution soaks (aluminum chloride, aluminum acetate, Burow's solution) can be helpful as an antiseptic and astringent. These are over-the-counter products usually sold as powder and diluted for use on the skin.

■ If the infection involves a lot of redness and swelling, your doctor may prescribe a combination antifungal/steroid preparation, such as Lotrisone. While there is little difference in potency between the over-the-counter products and most of the prescription medications used for this condition, there are individual differences in susceptibility, so if all else fails it may be worth trying a prescription cream. Bear in mind that topical steroids can cause thinning and wasting of the skin at the site; can be absorbed into the bloodstream, causing stress on the adrenal glands; and rarely make any difference as to whether the condition becomes chronic.

■ There are a number of oral antifungal drugs that may be effective for acute outbreaks. However, they are usually no more effective at preventing recurrences than the over-the-counter preparations, and they are more expensive. Available by prescription only, these include fluconazole (Diflucan), griseofulvin (Fulvicin, Grifulvin), itraconazole (Sporanox), ketoconazole (Nizoral), and terbinafine (Lamisil).

DIETARY GUIDELINES

■ Avoid sugary foods, including soft drinks and commercially processed foods. Sugar encourages the growth of fungus.

■ Make sure your menu includes plenty of vegetables.

■ Because fruits are full of natural sugars, it is best to limit your intake of fruits until the condition is resolved.

NUTRITIONAL SUPPLEMENTS

■ Acidophilus and bifidobacteria are probiotic supplements that restore the friendly bacteria necessary to fight a fungal infection. If you have been taking antibiotics, a probiotic supplement is especially valuable. Antibiotics strip the body of beneficial bacteria that help keep fungal infections under control. Take a probiotic supplement as recommended on the product label. If you are allergic to milk, select a dairy-free product.

■ Methylsulfonylmethane (MSM) is a good source of sulfur, a trace mineral that helps to fight parasites and fungi. It can be applied directly to the affected area in cream or spray form. Follow the directions on the product label.

■ Vitamin A and beta-carotene protect mucous membranes and fight infection. Take 5,000 international units of vitamin A and 15,000 international units of beta-carotene twice daily for two weeks.

Note: If you are pregnant, or intend to get pregnant, or if you have liver disease, consult your doctor before taking supplemental vitamin A. Pregnant women should not ingest a total of more than 25,000 international units of supplemental vitamin A *per week* from all sources.

■ Zinc helps to heal skin tissue. Take 15 milligrams twice a day for two weeks to one month. Take zinc with food to prevent stomach upset.

HERBAL TREATMENT

■ If your feet are itchy and red, try using alternate applications of aloe vera gel and calendula (in ointment form if the athlete's foot is dry, in lotion form if the skin is damp). Both of these herbs are very soothing and healing for the skin.

■ If you are prone to infection, make a blend of equal parts of aloe vera liquid and calendula, echinacea, and goldenseal extracts. Rub the mixture well into the affected area. This liquid mixture is a good antifungal, relieves itching, and is very soothing.

■ Rub a washcloth dipped in apple-cider vinegar briskly between your toes to remove the soggy skin and scales. It feels like scratching and relieves the itch. A soak in warm water with a liberal amount of apple cider vinegar added also helps.

■ Cat's claw enhances the immune response and has antifungal properties. Take 500 milligrams of standardized extract three times a day until the condition resolves.

Note: Do not use cat's claw if you are pregnant or nursing, or if you are an organ-transplant recipient. Use it with caution if you are taking an anticoagulant (blood thinner).

■ Echinacea, goldenseal, oat straw, and yellow dock are antifungal, antibacterial, and have a soothing effect on the skin. Take one cup of tea brewed with the blended herbs, or 1,000 milligrams of the combined extracts three times a day for two weeks.

■ Garlic is a powerful fungicide. Cut a few slivers of raw garlic and put them in your socks, or dust your shoes with garlic-based foot powder. The medicinal properties are absorbed through the skin.

■ Dust between your toes with an absorbent powder, such as green clay, to help keep these problem areas dry.

HOMEOPATHY

■ *Thuja* is an effective treatment for athlete's foot. Morning and evening, rub a few drops of undiluted liquid homeopathic *Thuja* directly on the affected areas of your feet. If you see improvement after one month, continue the treatment, as it is likely the infection will continue to clear. If you see no change after thirty days, it is best to try another approach.

AROMATHERAPY

For specific instructions on how to use aromatherapy, *see* PREPARING AROMATHERAPY TREATMENTS in Part Three.

■ Tea tree oil is an effective treatment for athlete's foot. It speeds healing and quickly relieves the intolerable itching. Tea tree oil is considered one of the most powerful botanical antifungal remedies. Twice a day, add 10 drops of tea tree oil to 1 quart of warm water and soak your feet in the treated water for ten minutes. After each soak, dry your feet thoroughly, especially between the toes. After drying, use a cotton swab to paint the affected area with undiluted tea tree oil. Continue these soaks for ten days. You should notice considerable improvement, marked by decreased tenderness, scaling, and blistering. Continue applying undiluted tea tree oil to the affected area for another ninety days. Although most cases of athlete's foot will improve in three weeks, some cases of fungal infection are more stubborn. If you don't have time to sit and soak, applying the undiluted oil twice daily can be effective.

GENERAL RECOMMENDATIONS

■ Expose your feet to the air as much as possible. If weather permits, this is the time for open sandals. Non-porous leather shoes and rubber-soled shoes hold in heat and moisture, creating the perfect environment for athlete's foot. When your feet get hot and sweaty, the healing process is inhibited. Fungi thrive in a warm, moist environment.

■ Practice good hygiene. Dry your feet thoroughly, taking extra care between the toes.

■ White cotton socks allow the feet to breathe and do not contain any irritating dyes. To kill the fungus and prevent reinfection, wash your socks in chlorine bleach after each wearing. If you are extremely active and sweat a lot, change your socks two or three times a day.

■ It can be difficult to do, but try not to scratch. Scratching athlete's foot breaks the blisters and spreads the fungus, making the infection worse. Applying a topical calendula gel will help reduce the itching.

PREVENTION

■ Keep your feet clean and dry, especially between the toes.

■ When you will be in the type of environment where athlete's foot flourishes, such as a public locker room, wear shoes or slippers. Socks alone do not provide sufficient protection.

■ Make sure your socks are dry before putting on your shoes. Many people run around the wet floor of a locker room in stocking feet, resulting in damp—and possibly fungus-contaminated—socks. Putting shoes on over damp socks creates the perfect environment for the athlete's foot fungus to grow and thrive.

■ If you discover that you have athlete's foot, alert the authorities responsible for any communal area where the fungus might be lurking.

Babesiosis

See under LYME AND OTHER TICKBORNE DISEASES.

Back Pain and Strain

Over 80 percent of Americans suffer from back pain at some point in their lives. This entry addresses lower back pain, the most common of all back problems.

Lower back pain, sometimes called *lumbago,* is typically concentrated below the waist, in the small of the back, and there the pain remains. It does not spread. Most people speak of pain that comes on after exercising or lifting something, but it also can occur after such simple activities as vacuuming, picking something up from the floor, twisting awkwardly, or coughing—or even for no apparent reason at all. It can be experienced as a nagging ache that develops gradually and never quite disappears, or as an instantaneous eruption of agonizing pain. Once the pain begins, you may freeze in position and be reluctant to move for fear of making it worse. The pain is likely to be more bearable when you are standing or lying down and worse when you are sitting, because sitting increases the pressure on the back muscles.

Many people assume an aching back is an inevitable part of growing older, but that isn't necessarily so. It is true that advancing age and certain conditions account for some backaches, but most are caused by stress, muscle spasms, and/or muscular weakness.

This condition most often strikes people in their thirties and may then recur, off and on, for the rest of their lives. "Weekend athletes"—people who get significant exercise only occasionally—are particularly at risk. People who live sedentary lives, whether by choice or because their occupations keep them chained to a desk during the week, are usually out of shape. An occasional game of basketball with friends, a run around the park, or a friendly set of tennis can trigger painful muscle spasms as lax muscles are pushed to perform athletic feats and cannot respond adequately.

Others at risk for back pain include those whose jobs alternate between sedentary and strenuous. Many truck drivers, for instance, must endure long periods of sitting interspersed with heavy lifting. Nurses are constantly required to alternate between doing paperwork and chores like lifting and turning patients. Sometimes, all it takes is one wrong move for one or more of the power muscles of the back to protest, with pain, spasm, and weakness. Lifting things improperly is a major cause of lower back problems.

Lower back pain can also be linked to sleeping in a bed that is too soft, sitting for too long in a poorly designed chair, or spending long hours behind the wheel—driving a bus, for example. This type of back pain is sometimes called *posture pain*. Other common factors in back pain include pregnancy and obesity. People carrying extra weight tend to have weaker abdominal muscles, which puts added strain on the back muscles. Stress has been identified as a major factor in back pain as well.

While most back pain is muscular in nature, there are a number of other conditions that can cause this kind of pain. These include disorders of the kidneys and problems with the bones, disks, muscles, ligaments, tendons, nerves, and joints of the spine. If back pain does not begin to improve within a few days, see your doctor.

CONVENTIONAL MEDICINE

■ A doctor is likely to recommend painkillers to make you more comfortable. There are different classes of pain medication that may be used. If the pain is not too severe, acetaminophen (Tylenol, Datril, and others) may be sufficient. If not, do not take more than the recommended dosage in an attempt to get relief, but try a different medication. While acetaminophen is generally considered

quite safe in recommended doses, taking too much can cause liver damage.

■ When the body is injured, its natural response is to send more blood and fluids to the area, and to sensitize the nerves there. The result is pain and inflammation. Nonsteroidal anti-inflammatory drugs (NSAIDs) decrease this response. This class of drug includes aspirin (Bayer, Ecotrin, and others), ibuprofen (Advil, Motrin, Nuprin, and others), indomethacin (Indocin), naproxen (Aleve, Anaprox, Naprelan, Naprosyn), and sulindac (Clinoril). Some of these drugs are available over the counter, others by prescription. All of them have the potential to cause side effects, including nausea, vomiting, diarrhea, constipation, liver or kidney damage, and gastrointestinal irritation, particularly with long-term use.

■ For severe, incapacitating pain, a narcotic such as codeine, hydrocodone, or oxycodone (all sold under many brand names, often combined with acetaminophen, aspirin, or ibuprofen) or meperidine (Demerol) may be prescribed. These are powerful drugs that block the body's perception of pain. Possible side effects include drowsiness, nausea, constipation, dizziness, itching, and low blood pressure. In addition, with all of these drugs, there is a tendency to develop tolerance—a situation in which stronger and stronger doses are required to achieve the same effect—as well as physical dependence.

■ Muscle relaxants, like carisoprodol (Soma), chlorzoxazone (Parafon), cyclobenzaprine (Flexeril), and methocarbamol (Robaxin), are sometimes prescribed to interrupt the painful spasms that occur with strained muscles. Potential side effects of these drugs include drowsiness, dizziness, weakness, and blurred vision. There is also a fairly high potential for abuse with these medications.

■ Physical therapy may be worth trying, if your health-insurance policy provides coverage for it.

■ Surgery is not appropriate for muscular or other soft-tissue injuries, but is reserved for cases of true damage to the disks or vertebrae.

DIETARY GUIDELINES

■ Avoid eating large meals. Consuming a lot of food at one time causes the digestive system to go into overdrive, which makes your back more vulnerable.

■ Eat a diet that is high in fiber. A good, well-balanced diet keeps the bowels regular. Constipation aggravates lower back pain.

NUTRITIONAL SUPPLEMENTS

■ Calcium is required by the nerves and muscles; magnesium plays an important role in neuromuscular contractions and helps ensure regular bowel movements.

Take 1,000 milligrams of calcium and 500 milligrams of magnesium daily. If your back pain is accompanied by constipation, increase the amount of magnesium to 1,000 milligrams daily.

■ Glucosamine sulfate helps to relieve inflammation, strengthen the integrity of the joints, and enhance circulation in the muscles. Take 500 milligrams three times a day.

■ Lower back pain sometimes benefits from high doses of vitamin C. Take 1,000 milligrams of vitamin C and an equal amount of bioflavonoids three times daily.

HERBAL TREATMENT

Pine-bark and grape-seed extracts are high in natural bioflavonoids that fight inflammation. Take 50 to 75 milligrams of either three times daily.

Valerian is a calmative herb that can help if you have difficulty relaxing. It is especially useful if you have a problem falling asleep. Choose a standardized extract containing 0.5 percent isovalerenic acids and take 200 to 300 milligrams one-half hour before bedtime.

HOMEOPATHY

Select an appropriate symptom-specific remedy and, while the pain is acute, take one dose, as directed on the product label, every fifteen minutes for one hour. Once your symptoms start to improve, cut back to one dose three times daily. If your symptoms do not start to improve after twenty-four hours, discontinue the remedy and try another.

Arnica 30x or 15c is the remedy of choice for acute pain.

Berberis vulgaris 6x or 3c is particularly helpful for lower back pain, especially if the urine is concentrated and has a strong odor.

Bryonia 12x or 6c relieves pain that is worsened by movement, and that is usually concentrated on the right side. The pain may be accompanied by constipation.

Rhus toxicodendron 12x or 6c is helpful for pain that is relieved by moving around, and is usually concentrated on the left side.

BACH FLOWER REMEDIES

Select the remedy that most closely fits your emotional tendencies and concerns, and take it as needed, following the directions on the product label.

■ Rescue Remedy quickly helps to ease acute pain.

Beech helps to tame perfectionism and a tendency to be impatient with circumstances and other people.

Oak helps to ease a tense, restless type-A personality with a relentless drive to succeed.

Vervain is the remedy for the tense and nervous perfectionist.

ACUPRESSURE

For the locations of acupressure points on the body, *see* ADMINISTERING AN ACUPRESSURE TREATMENT in Part Three.

■ Bladder 23 increases circulation to the lower back.

■ Bladder 60 brings circulation down from the lower back and helps resolve stagnation.

■ The inner and outer Bladder points on the lower back improve local circulation.

AROMATHERAPY

For specific instructions on how to use aromatherapy, *see* PREPARING AROMATHERAPY TREATMENTS in Part Three.

■ Peppermint oil, added to a hot bath and/or mixed with base oil and used in massage, is soothing to painful muscles.

■ Many essential oils help to reduce stress, a major contributor to back pain. Some of the best known for this purpose are elemi, frankincense, geranium, jasmine, lavender, myrrh, and neroli. Choose the one (or the combination) you like best and use it as an inhalant or diffuse it into the air in your home.

GENERAL RECOMMENDATIONS

■ When pain strikes, a measure of relief can often be attained by lying down on one side or the other.

■ It can be difficult to do, but try to relax and have patience. Most cases of lower back pain resolve themselves with rest and time. If you respond to the pain by becoming tense and anxious, you will only make it worse.

■ Consult a chiropractor. Many people find relief from lower back pain with chiropractic treatment. Chiropractors are particularly helpful in alleviating posture pain and sudden pain of unknown origin.

■ If you typically awaken with an aching back that eases during the day, it may be time to shop for a new mattress.

PREVENTION

■ Exercises that strengthen the stomach muscles, such as sit-ups and crunches, are important. If your stomach muscles are strong, it is not necessary for your back muscles to carry the whole load.

■ To reduce the strain on your back muscles, be careful when lifting anything heavy. Bend your knees, go into a squatting position, and keep your back relaxed. Grasp the object, straighten your legs, and stand up. This transfers the strain to your leg muscles and relieves your back.

■ Be equally careful when moving something heavy. Instead of bending your back, leaning forward, and pushing with your arms, push backwards. With the object behind you, reach back with your arms to guide it, bend your knees slightly, and push with your legs.

■ If you must sit for long periods, watch your posture. Don't slump. Slouching pushes your lower back forward and puts an added strain on the muscles. Sit up straight, with your spine resting on the chair back and your feet flat on the floor in front of you.

■ Don't be a couch potato, but don't be a weekend warrior, either. You cannot make up for a sedentary lifestyle with on-again, off-again bursts of physical activity. One of the best things you can do for your all-around good health is to fit a regular (daily if possible) exercise period into your schedule, and then stick to it. (*See* STARTING AN EXERCISE PROGRAM in Part Three.)

Bad Breath

Bad breath is an embarrassing problem. A person with bad breath may be offensive without realizing it, as all the advertisements for breath mints, mouthwashes, and toothpastes are so quick to point out. In some cases, an unusual breath odor may be a sign of illness, such as a herpes infection of the mouth, diabetes, postnasal drip, tonsillitis, sinusitis, dental infection, strep throat, liver or kidney failure, or a lung abscess. Most of the time, however, bad breath—medically termed *halitosis*—is not the result of any major health problem. It is usually related to poor oral hygiene or poor digestion, sometimes both.

If a friend or family member (or you yourself) notice a bad smell on your breath, especially if the breath has a persistent or unusual odor, consult your physician. He or she will be able to determine whether or not your bad breath is related to an underlying infection or other illness. One particularly helpful—though, unfortunately, not often recommended—diagnostic test is a comprehensive stool analysis, which can be used to determine problems with digestion and assimilation, the presence of parasites, or the overgrowth of abnormal bacteria in the digestive tract.

CONVENTIONAL TREATMENT

■ If your doctor rules out other causes, the problem is most likely related to an oral health problem, whether gum disease, extensive cavities, or inadequate hygiene. In this case, it is best to see your dentist without delay.

■ Believe it or not, if you persistently complain of having bad breath and do not accept your doctor's assurances that there are no grounds for the complaint, you may be referred for psychiatric evaluation.

DIETARY GUIDELINES

■ Limit the amount of sugar in your diet. Base your diet on healthy whole foods.

■ If you have a "sour stomach," bad breath may be related to digestive difficulties. Limit your intake of fried foods and refined sugar. Better yet, eliminate these items from the menu entirely.

NUTRITIONAL SUPPLEMENTS

■ Take an acidophilus and bifidobacteria supplement daily to establish and maintain favorable intestinal flora and healthy digestion. If you are allergic to milk, select a dairy-free product.

■ Chlorophyll tablets help freshen the breath because they have a cleansing effect in the intestines. Take a chlorophyll supplement, as directed on the product label, after each meal and again at bedtime.

■ If you suspect bad breath related to poor digestion, try supplementing your diet with digestive enzymes. There are a number of over-the-counter products available that use natural enzymes—bromelain (from pineapple) or papain (from papaya)—which may be helpful. Follow the dosage directions on the product label.

■ Sometimes bad breath is a result of poor stomach function. To strengthen the gastrointestinal tract, you may want to try taking duodenal extract with vitamin A as directed on the product label.

HERBAL TREATMENT

■ Choose an herbal-based toothpaste or tooth powder formulated without sugar. If this type of product is not available in your local drugstore, check a health-food store. Merfluan is a baking-soda-based tooth powder that is very popular in Europe. It comes in several different flavors.

■ The Chinese patent medicine Fare You is a cabbage extract that helps to heal and strengthen the stomach lining. If bad breath originates from compromised stomach function, consider trying Fare You. Follow the dosage directions on the product label.

■ Chew on a small sprig of parsley to freshen your breath. Parsley is rich in the natural deodorizer chlorophyll, and also sweetens the digestive tract.

■ If bad breath is an occasional problem related to poor digestion, typically accompanied by upset stomach, diarrhea, constipation, or a lot of burping, sipping a cup of peppermint tea after meals should help to ease digestion. Or try taking a cup of ginger tea twice a day, with meals, to enhance digestion.

HOMEOPATHY

■ For bad breath related to oral herpes (cold sores), take

one dose of *Natrum muriaticum* 30x or 9c three times daily for three days. Follow up with one dose of *Mercurius solubilis* 12x or 6c twice daily for three to five days. If there is no improvement in this time, stop taking the remedy.

■ For sour breath caused by acid indigestion, *Carbo vegetabilis* is the answer. Take one dose of *Carbo vegetabilis* 30x or 15c as needed.

■ For bad breath caused by overeating, take one dose of *Nux vomica* 30x or 15c each day for two days.

GENERAL RECOMMENDATIONS

■ See a dentist and dental hygienist regularly, and make sure you practice good oral hygiene, including effective brushing and flossing. Teaching oral hygiene is an important part of a dental hygienist's responsibilities. Use a sugar- and saccharin-free toothpaste and an herbal mouthwash. The mouthwash should be used at least once a day.

■ A simple mouthwash of 1 teaspoon each of hydrogen peroxide and baking soda diluted in 2 ounces of spring water will cleanse and deodorize the mouth. The combination of peroxide and baking soda is an effective antibacterial combination. Undiluted, the combination makes an excellent toothpaste.

■ A mouthwash made with folic acid, herbal extracts, and essential oils can be helpful. Dissolve 1,200 micrograms of folic acid, 1 tablespoon of hawthorn berry extract, 1 tablespoon of echinacea extract, 40 drops of peppermint oil, and 10 drops of thyme oil in 24 ounces of spring water. Swish this mixture around in your mouth after thoroughly brushing your teeth (and tongue). Folic acid heals gum tissue and helps reduce plaque; hawthorn berry is astringent and helps tighten gum tissues; echinacea cleanses the mouth and kills bacteria; peppermint oil tastes great and leaves the breath smelling fresh and clean.

■ If simple, natural treatments do not freshen your breath promptly and keep it fresh, see your physician to rule out the possibility of an underlying condition.

Bedsores

Known to doctors as *decubitus ulcers*, bedsores (or pressure sores) are the result of skin being suffocated beneath the weight of the body. These lesions are caused by continuous extended pressure on the skin, usually in an area over a prominent bone or cartilage structure such as the hips or tailbone. This pressure restricts the flow of blood, and therefore the supply of oxygen and nutrients, to that part of the skin. Ultimately, the smaller blood vessels clot and a sore red patch of skin appears. If not attended to, it can crack open and develop into a painful wound.

The first sign of a developing pressure sore is reddening of the skin. There may be local swelling or hardening of the tissue as well. Eventually, if the pressure is not relieved, the skin breaks down and ulcerates, and infection may take hold. Obviously, people who are confined to bed for long periods are most at risk for this problem. Wheelchair users also have an increased risk of developing pressure sores. An individual who suffers from impaired wound healing, common in older adults and people with diabetes, can develop bedsores rather quickly.

When it comes to bedsores, prevention is better than treatment. It is also necessary to rule out the possibility that another disorder might be mimicking a bedsore, especially if the sore appears to be spreading at an unusually fast rate. Herpes lesions, bacterially induced ulcers, and even skin cancers can look like bedsores, but require different treatment.

CONVENTIONAL TREATMENT

■ As soon as you suspect a pressure sore may be developing, take steps at once to relieve the pressure on that part of the body, and keep it clean and dry. Clean foam underlays may help lower pressure at the site. If the problem is not too advanced, this may be all that is needed, and the developing sore may heal on its own.

■ If more aggressive treatment is called for, absorbent foamlike bandages may be applied and changed frequently. There are also special dressings with a water-based suspension that may be used as a covering to protect the site. Topical antibiotic ointment may be applied to prevent infection.

■ If the area is moist, topical zinc oxide ointment can help to dry the sore out.

■ For more advanced sores, debridement (surgical trimming away of dead tissue) may be required. Your doctor may also prescribe systemic antibiotic treatment to fight infection.

DIETARY GUIDELINES

■ Keep your diet simple. Eat plenty of fresh fruit and green and yellow vegetables to ensure a good supply of vitamin C, vitamin A, minerals, and phytonutrients.

■ Drink plenty of pure water to ensure that you stay well hydrated.

NUTRITIONAL SUPPLEMENTS

Although bedsores can improve dramatically with the help of supplementation, it is imperative to consult a health-care practitioner if bedsores develop. This is especially important if you have diabetes or another condition that makes bedsores able to intensify rapidly.

■ People with bedsores are often deficient in one or more

basic nutrients. Take a good multivitamin and mineral supplement daily.

■ Vitamin C is an anti-inflammatory and is vital for the health of the skin and blood vessels. A study reported in the *British Medical Journal* found that bedridden patients with bedsores had significantly lower levels of vitamin C in their blood than did similar patients who were free of bedsores. Take 500 milligrams of vitamin C and an equal amount of bioflavonoids three times daily.

■ Zinc supports the immune system and promotes wound healing. Take 15 milligrams three times daily. Take zinc with food to prevent stomach upset. If you take over 30 milligrams of zinc on a daily basis for more than one or two months, you should also take 1 to 2 milligrams of copper each day to maintain a proper mineral balance.

HERBAL TREATMENT

The following suggestions should be used only if the wound is closed. Open wounds should be attended to by a health-care practitioner.

■ Aloe vera, applied topically in ointment, gel, or cream form, is effective in healing sores.

■ Topical calendula cream is very soothing and healing to wounds. Use it as directed on the product label.

■ Goldenseal is a natural antiseptic; vitamin E is healing and soothing to the skin. Make a paste by combining the contents of three 500-milligram capsules of goldenseal (or 1 teaspoon of goldenseal powder) and 800 international units of vitamin E (pierce capsules and squeeze out the oil). If the resulting mixture is too dry, add a few drops of olive oil. Apply this to the affected area three times daily.

HOMEOPATHY

■ *Petroleum* is good for sores that itch and burn, with skin that is dry, sensitive, rough, and cracked, almost leathery. Take one dose of *Petroleum* 12x or 6c three times daily for up to three days.

■ *Graphites* is helpful for sores that ooze. The skin appears cracked, and there is burning and stinging pain. Take one dose of *Graphites* 12x or 6c three times daily for up to three days.

ACUPRESSURE

For the locations of acupressure points on the body, *see* ADMINISTERING AN ACUPRESSURE TREATMENT in Part Three.

■ The back Bladder points, Gallbladder 34, Large Intestine 4, Liver 3, and Stomach 36 all enhance circulation. Gently work any of these points that can be reached easily.

GENERAL RECOMMENDATIONS

■ If you are in a situation in which pressure sores are a possibility, be vigilant in monitoring your skin for any signs of reddening, and treat any possible sores aggressively.

■ Exposure to fresh air and natural light is important.

PREVENTION

■ Prevention of pressure sores is based on limiting the amount of time any area of skin is subjected to pressure. Most doctors recommend moving every fifteen minutes. If this is impossible, as in the case of a bedridden person, he or she should be turned at least every hour, and both bed linens and skin should be kept clean and dry. Keeping the bedclothes as unwrinkled as possible is important. The softest bed surface possible is also desirable. If you use a wheelchair, a pressure-reducing pillow can help minimize pressure on susceptible areas. Even so, you should shift your position in the chair frequently (four or more times each hour). Wear loose, clean cotton clothing.

Bee Sting

See under BITES AND STINGS, INSECT AND SPIDER.

Bites, Animal and Human

If you suffer a bite that breaks the skin, prompt medical care is essential. This applies whether the bite is from a wild or stray animal, the family pet, or even an angry toddler. Animals' mouths are heavily populated with bacteria and other microorganisms that thrive on food residue and debris. These organisms can be transmitted by bites and produce infection, especially if there is extensive tissue damage.

For reasons that are not clear, cat bites are more likely to cause infection than dog bites. Estimates vary, but up to 50 percent of cat bites may become infected, whereas dog bites cause infection only 5 percent of the time. The potential for infection from a human-inflicted bite falls somewhere between the two. Bites from children tend to cause infection less often than those from adults, principally because adults can cause deeper injuries that allow more serious infections to establish themselves.

Most bite-related infections are treatable. However, certain dangerous viruses, including hepatitis and herpes viruses as well as human immunodeficiency virus (HIV) are present in the saliva of infected individuals, and could conceivably be transmitted by a bite that breaks the skin. It is worth noting, however, that there have been no documented cases of HIV being transmitted this way.

EMERGENCY TREATMENT

■ If you suffer a bite that breaks the skin, immediately and thoroughly disinfect the area with lots of water, soap, and hydrogen peroxide. Bite wounds that break the skin can easily become infected. This is true of human as well as animal bites. Human saliva is often alive with infectious bacteria.

■ If you have been bitten by an animal, try to confine the animal so it can be tested for rabies. If the animal belongs to someone, be sure you can identify the owner. If you can determine that the animal is not rabid, you can be spared the very uncomfortable (but otherwise necessary) treatment with rabies vaccine. If the animal is wild and you cannot capture it, you will have to be treated for rabies.

■ Call your physician, go to the emergency room of the nearest hospital, or call for emergency help. Anyone who suffers a bite wound that breaks the skin should be examined and treated by a doctor.

CONVENTIONAL TREATMENT

■ The bite wound will be cleansed, treated with a topical antibiotic such as Betadine, bacitracin, or Neosporin, and bandaged. You will probably be instructed to change the dressing daily, with a new application of antibiotic at each change. Depending on the nature and location of the bite, the wound may be stitched closed. If the wound is very deep, involves the hands or knuckles, or involves damage to tendons that must be repaired, surgery may be recommended to thoroughly clean the affected tissues and close the wound before bandaging. Even wounds that look small and/or clean must be meticulously cleansed using high-pressure washing. If you are bitten by an animal with long incisor teeth, the site of the injury will have to be carefully explored in case there is deep injury that is not readily visible. A wound culture may be ordered to check for infectious organisms.

■ After emergency first aid has been administered, you may be given an injection to update your immunity to tetanus. Tetanus is a deep infection, as the organism that causes it proliferates where there is little access to air or oxygen. It is rarely a problem with superficial wounds, but in accordance with the "better-safe-than-sorry" rule, your doctor will probably recommend a tetanus shot if it has been more than five years since you last had one.

■ If you are bitten by an animal, the issue of rabies will have to be considered. A bite from a rabid animal is life-threatening unless you receive immediate medical treatment. The types of animals that are most likely to carry this disease vary somewhat from one area of the country

to another, but, in general, the possibility of rabies is of particular concern in bites from raccoons, skunks, foxes, coyotes, and bats. Rabbits and rodents, including squirrels, as well as dogs, cats, and ferrets, are somewhat less likely to be infected. Regardless of the type of animal involved, however, unless its owner has proof that it has been vaccinated against rabies, it will have to be quarantined for observation (for household pets) or euthanized and autopsied (for wild animals). If neither of these measures is possible, you will have to receive a series of rabies injections over a period of twenty-eight days and possibly again at ninety days. There are different types of injections available for this purpose, rabies immune globulin for "passive" immunization, and a vaccine, either human- or horse-derived, for "active" immunization. Sometimes these two approaches are used in conjunction with one another. If the equine (horse-derived) version is the only type of vaccine available, you should first be tested for sensitivity to it.

■ Once the wound is thoroughly cleansed and bandaged, and any necessary immunizations have been given, an oral antibiotic such as ampicillin (also sold under the brand name Omnipen), cephalexin (Keflex), clindamycin, or dicloxacillin may be prescribed to prevent infection. Many doctors prescribe two-drug therapy to be on the safe side. If any signs of infection are already present, plan on extended use of these drugs, as such infections can be resistant to treatment. Once the results of the wound culture come back, your doctor may switch you to a more appropriate antibiotic.

■ Until it heals, the wound will need to be checked every few days for signs of infection, and treated accordingly.

DIETARY GUIDELINES

■ Limit your consumption of sugar and fried foods while the tissue is healing.

■ Make sure to eat plenty of dark-green and yellow vegetables to increase your intake of beta-carotene.

NUTRITIONAL SUPPLEMENTS

■ Bioflavonoids fight infection and inflammation. Take 500 milligrams three times daily for two weeks.

■ Bromelain, an enzyme derived from pineapple, helps to reduce inflammation. If there is swelling in the area of the bite, take 400 milligrams of bromelain three times daily, between meals.

■ Pantothenic acid is helpful in strengthening adrenal function, thus aiding the body in handling stress. Taking 250 milligrams three or four times daily for the first two or three days after an injury is often helpful in recovery.

■ Vitamin A and beta-carotene help the skin to heal.

Take 5,000 international units of vitamin A and 15,000 international units of beta-carotene twice daily for two weeks.

Note: If you are pregnant, or intend to get pregnant, or if you have liver disease, consult your doctor before taking supplemental vitamin A. Pregnant women should not ingest a total of more than 25,000 international units of supplemental vitamin A *per week* from all sources.

■ Vitamin C is a mild anti-inflammatory and helps detoxify the blood. Take 1,000 milligrams three times daily for two weeks.

Zinc aids in wound healing. Take 15 milligrams twice a day for two weeks. Take zinc with food to prevent stomach upset.

HERBAL TREATMENT

Echinacea and goldenseal help to detoxify the blood and prevent infection. Take one dose of an echinacea and goldenseal combination formula supplying 250 to 500 milligrams of echinacea and 150 to 300 milligrams of goldenseal three times daily for three to five days.

Garlic has antibiotic properties, and helps to detoxify the blood. Take 500 milligrams at least three times a day for one week. If you like garlic, you can use fresh garlic instead of the capsule form.

HOMEOPATHY

Arnica 30x or 9c is useful if there is tissue damage or bruising. Take one dose every hour for the first three hours. Then take one dose three times a day for two days.

Hypericum 12x or 6c is recommended if there is nerve pain following the trauma. Take one dose four times daily for the first day or two after the injury.

Ledum 12x or 6c is good if there is bruising surrounding the bite. Take one dose three times daily for two days. *Ledum* is useful for all puncture-type wounds.

PREVENTION

It can be dangerous to tease or roughhouse with animals. Even a beloved family companion or usually-friendly neighborhood pets can become provoked.

If possible, get to know neighborhood pets. Identify any animals, such as guard dogs, that may jump a fence and become aggressive or dangerous.

■ Before embarking on a camping trip, check with local authorities regarding animal life in the area where you plan to set up camp. Use common sense in wilderness areas; don't attempt to approach wild animals, and don't store food in your tent.

Bites, Snake

Being bitten by a snake raises greater concern than being bitten by most other animals because of the possibility that the bite may be poisonous. While most of the snakes in the world are *not* venomous, there are many varieties of poisonous snakes. Consequently, prompt medical care for snakebite is essential.

Symptoms caused by a poisonous snakebite range from mild to severe, and can include a racing pulse, with swelling and discoloration around the area of the bite. You may feel weak and be short of breath, will probably feel nauseated, and may vomit. If the venom is very strong, you can experience severe pain and much swelling. Your pupils dilate, and shock and convulsion may occur. You may twitch uncontrollably, and your speech may become slurred. After a severe snakebite, a person can become paralyzed and lose consciousness. If you are bitten by a snake, act fast.

EMERGENCY TREATMENT

■ Have someone take you immediately to the emergency room of the nearest hospital, or call for emergency medical personnel. Medical intervention is essential.

■ If medical care is not immediately available, stay calm, and do the following:

1. Lie down and remain as still as possible. Activity can spread the venom throughout the body. Try to keep the affected limb at the same level as your heart.
2. If a venom extractor is available, have someone begin applying suction immediately. It takes at least three minutes to begin adequate poison extraction. Continue suctioning out the venom for at least fifteen minutes and as long as an hour, or until you can secure medical care.
3. *Do not* let anyone make an incision into the bite, suck the poison out with his or her mouth, or apply a tourniquet, and do not take any medications of any kind. These actions create more problems than they solve.
4. *Do not* use an ice pack on the wound. Cold therapy is not recommended for snake bites, as it can damage tissues.
5. Have someone call your local Poison Control Center for instructions on how best to treat you.
6. Seek medical care as soon as possible.

CONVENTIONAL TREATMENT

■ Seek emergency treatment (see above). Rely on medical personnel to take the appropriate measures. The primary treatment for poisonous snakebite is the use of intravenous antivenin for the correct class of snake, given as soon as possible after the injury.

Many people have reactions to the antivenin. If this occurs, you may need treatment with epinephrine and/or prednisone during or after treatment for the poison.

■ Once the wound has been treated and you have recovered sufficiently from the effects of the injury to leave the hospital, medical personnel will advise you on the proper way to care for yourself as you recover.

If you are bitten by a snake known *not* to be poisonous (a household pet, for example), the bite will be treated much like any animal bite (*see* BITES, ANIMAL AND HUMAN).

DIETARY GUIDELINES

Once emergency medical care has been administered and you are well enough to leave the hospital, support recovery by avoiding sugar, saturated fats, hydrogenated and partially hydrogenated oils, and all fried foods to promote a healing internal environment.

Increase the amount of green and yellow vegetables in your diet so that you get plenty of important vitamins and minerals.

NUTRITIONAL SUPPLEMENTS

The nutritional supplements below are intended to support recovery from the bite once appropriate emergency medical care has been administered and you are well enough to leave the hospital. In the case of snakebite, seek emergency medical care immediately.

Bioflavonoids fight infection and inflammation. Take 500 milligrams three or four times daily for one week.

Vitamin A and beta-carotene help heal mucous membranes and fight infection. Take 5,000 international units of vitamin A and 15,000 international units of beta-carotene twice a day for two weeks.

Note: If you are pregnant, or intend to get pregnant, or if you have liver disease, consult your doctor before taking supplemental vitamin A. Pregnant women should not ingest a total of more than 25,000 international units of supplemental vitamin A *per week* from all sources.

Vitamin C helps detoxify the body. Take 1,000 milligrams three times a day for one week.

■ Vitamin E is an excellent antioxidant that improves the utilization of vitamin A. Choose a product containing mixed tocopherols and take 200 international units three times daily for two weeks following the bite.

Note: If you have high blood pressure, limit your intake of supplemental vitamin E to a total of 400 international units daily. If you are taking an anticoagulant (blood thinner), consult your physician before taking vitamin E.

■ Zinc helps a wound to heal. Take 15 milligrams twice a day for two weeks. Take zinc with food to prevent stomach upset.

HERBAL TREATMENT

Herbal treatments for snakebite are intended to support recovery from the bite once appropriate emergency medical care has been administered and you are well enough to leave the hospital. In the case of snakebite, seek emergency medical care immediately.

■ Echinacea and goldenseal help to prevent and/or treat infection. Both herbs have antibiotic properties and help to boost the immune system. Take one dose of a combination formula supplying 250 to 500 milligrams of echinacea and 150 to 300 milligrams of goldenseal three times a day for five days. Then take one dose twice daily for five days.

■ Garlic has antibacterial properties, and helps detoxify the blood. Take 500 milligrams (or eat one clove) three times a day for two weeks.

HOMEOPATHY

Homeopathic treatments for snakebite are intended to support recovery from the bite once appropriate emergency care has been administered and medical personnel advise you that you are well enough to take something by mouth. In the case of snakebite, seek emergency medical care immediately.

■ Follow these three steps, in sequence:

1. Take one dose of *Aconite* 30x, 200x, or 30c, as directed on the product label, to ease the shock and fright.
2. Take one dose of *Arnica* 12x, 30x, 200x, 7c, or 30c every hour, for a total of three doses, to help the injured tissue begin to heal.
3. Take one dose of *Lachesis* 30x or 9c, three times a day, for two to three days. *Lachesis* will help alleviate the symptoms of the bite.

ACUPRESSURE

Acupressure treatments for snakebite are intended to support recovery from the bite once appropriate emergency medical care has been administered and you are well enough to leave the hospital. In case of snakebite, seek emergency medical care immediately. For the locations of acupressure points on the body, *see* ADMINISTERING AN ACUPRESSURE TREATMENT in Part Three.

■ Four Gates will help to relax you. This can be helpful immediately following emergency treatment for the bite.

■ Spleen 10 helps to detoxify the body.

GENERAL RECOMMENDATIONS

■ Make sure you know how to identify any types of venomous snakes that are indigenous to your area. Should a medical emergency arise, knowing the species of the snake that attacked you will save precious time.

■ Along with your usual first aid supplies, keep a snakebite kit readily available, especially when camping out. We recommend The Extractor from Sawyer Products, which is available in many camping and outdoor equipment stores or directly from the company (see the Resources section at the end of the book).

PREVENTION

■ Most snake bites occur on unprotected ankles and legs. Shorts and sneakers do not provide adequate protection. Wear tough hiking boots and suitable pants, such as heavy jeans, for tramping through the woods or going on a hiking trip.

■ Do not poke sticks into holes or stick your hands blindly into underbrush.

Bites and Stings, Insect and Spider

Bites and stings from most common insects, such as mosquitoes, gnats, fleas, flies, and ants, as well as from common spiders, can cause itchy welts on arms and legs. A bee, wasp, or hornet sting can cause swelling and stinging at the site. Usually, bites and stings are no more than an annoyance and cause only slight local swelling and irritation.

There are exceptions, however, such as a bite from a venomous spider like the brown recluse or black widow spider, or a severe allergic reaction to a bee sting. A bite from a tiny deer tick may cause a large circular lesion that progresses into a rash of small round lesions. The deer tick is the insect responsible for transmitting Lyme disease, and the characteristic rash is often the first sign of that illness (see LYME DISEASE).

If you are stung by a bee, wasp, or hornet, or bitten by an insect you suspect may be poisonous (such as the black widow or brown recluse spider), emergency medical treatment may be necessary (see page 137). If you know you are allergic to bee venom, seek immediate medical care in the event of a sting. At any time, if you develop respiratory symptoms, such as wheezing or difficulty breathing, have someone take you immediately to the emergency room of the nearest hospital. People rarely have a problem with a first bee sting. However, if you have a family history of allergies, or if you exhibit a strong reaction to a first bee sting, you may be more likely to develop a serious allergic response after a later incident.

EMERGENCY TREATMENT

See the inset on page 137.

CONVENTIONAL TREATMENT

For most insect bites and stings, home treatment is usually all that's needed. Begin with the following suggestions.

■ If you are stung by a bee, wasp, or hornet, examine the area for a visible stinger. Remove the stinger by gently scraping it out with your fingernail or the back of a knife blade, rather than by pulling on it. The stingers of these insects are barbed. Pulling the stinger out directly can squeeze more venom into the wound.

■ If you find a tick on any part of your body, do not try to pull it off with your fingers. The barbs on a tick's proboscis (feeding snout) become deeply embedded in its victim, so that even if you pull off the body, the head remains. To remove a tick, use a pair of tweezers to grasp the head, as close as possible to the spot where it is attached to the skin. Pull back slowly and firmly until the tick pulls free. Once the tick is removed, wash, rinse, and disinfect the site of the bite thoroughly with rubbing alcohol. Then apply an antibiotic ointment, such as bacitracin or Betadine.

■ For minor insect bites, apply ice or a cold compress to the area to reduce the spread of histamines and other body chemicals that cause itching and swelling. For spider bites and stings of most bees, wasps, and fire ants, apply ice to the bite to help numb the area and relieve pain, then follow up with applications of an ointment containing a steroid, an analgesic, and/or an antihistamine.

■ Take an oral antihistamine such as diphenhydramine (Allerdryl, Benadryl, and others) or chlorpheniramine (Chlor-Trimeton) to help counteract itching and swelling. Follow the directions on the product label.

■ Witch hazel, calamine lotion, or a low-dose cortisone cream such as Lanacort or Cort-Aid may be applied to the area as needed for one or two days to relieve itching. Creams or lotions that contain an antihistamine such as diphenhydramine can also help relieve the itching of minor insect bites. Apply a thin layer of any of these medications to the area around the bite, but do not put them on open wounds.

■ Scorpion stings usually are only locally bothersome. Applying ice can help to relieve pain.

■ If you have ever had a serious allergic reaction to a bite or sting, you should carry a prescription epinephrine kit and an antihistamine with you at all times. Epinephrine, which can open the airways and restore free breathing in a crisis, is available for home use as the Ana-Kit or EpiPen. These kits contain a syringe with a premeasured dose of medication. Your doctor may also recommend a desensitization program.

DIETARY GUIDELINES

■ Make sure to get plenty of fluids, including pure spring water, light soups, and diluted natural juices, to help your body flush out residual toxins.

NUTRITIONAL SUPPLEMENTS

To help relieve the pain of a bad bite or sting, take calcium and magnesium combination formula to calm and soothe your nervous system. Take 250 milligrams of calcium and 125 milligrams of magnesium two to three times daily for four days.

Vitamin C and bioflavonoids are helpful in relieving the toxicity of all bites and stings, and also have anti-inflammatory properties. Take 1,000 milligrams of vitamin C three times a day and 500 milligrams of bioflavonoids twice daily for two days. If you develop loose stools, cut the dosage in half. Vitamin C can also be used topically to reduce inflammation. Mix a bit of powdered vitamin C with just enough water to make a paste, and apply it to the bite as needed.

HERBAL TREATMENT

Aloe vera gel is very soothing for minor insect bites that are stinging and burning. Apply the gel to the area as needed.

Taken internally, aloe vera extract is a mild anti-inflammatory that soothes from the inside out. Be sure to choose a food-grade product and take 2 tablespoons three times daily for one week.

Calendula gel or cream helps to soothe and relieve the irritation of insect bites. Apply it directly to the bite as needed.

Echinacea is highly effective for wounds and stings. Take 250 to 500 milligrams every two to three hours for the first day after a bad bite or sting. Then take the same dose three or four times daily until the swelling subsides, up to five days.

Plantain leaves and comfrey can help draw out the poison and relieve the itching of an insect bite. Prepare and apply a poultice of plantain leaves and comfrey (see PREPARING HERBAL TREATMENTS in Part Three). Tobacco leaves also make a time-honored poultice for bites and stings. If these herbs are not readily available, try applying an echinacea and goldenseal combination formula directly to the site.

HOMEOPATHY

■ Apply *Natrum muriaticum* 6x (preferably in liquid form) immediately to the bite. This homeopathic remedy lessens itching and relieves the burning sensation. If the liquid form is unavailable, dissolve a few pellets in a small amount of distilled water and apply the resulting solution.

■ *Apis mellifica* 12x, 30x, 6c, or 9c helps decrease the swelling and stinging sensation associated with a bee sting. Take one dose, as directed on the product label, every hour until the swelling diminishes, up to a total of four doses.

■ *Ledum* 12x, 30x, 6c, or 9c reduces the bruising, swelling, and general discomfort of an insect bite. Take one dose three times daily. Or apply homeopathic Ledum ointment directly to the bite.

AROMATHERAPY

For specific instructions on how to use aromatherapy, *see* PREPARING AROMATHERAPY TREATMENTS in Part Three.

■ Tea tree oil is a strong antiseptic and aids healing. It also has insect-repellent properties. Add 8 to 10 drops of tea tree oil to 1 quart of cold water and soak a clean cotton cloth or cotton ball in the mixture. Apply the compress to the bite for ten to fifteen minutes four times daily. If you prefer, you can substitute bergamot, lavender, or pine oil for tea tree oil.

GENERAL RECOMMENDATIONS

■ An old standby for treating minor bites and stings that cause swelling is to mix 2 teaspoons of baking soda and 2 teaspoons of Epsom salts with just enough water to make a paste, and apply this mixture directly to the affected area. Allow the paste to remain in place for twenty to thirty minutes. Often, a single application results in noticeable improvement.

■ If you have a severe allergy to bites or stings, wear a Medic Alert bracelet (see the Resources section at the end of the book). Should you suffer a severe reaction, the information the bracelet carries will help ensure you get prompt, appropriate treatment. Also, ask your doctor for a prescription for emergency medication for quick administration.

■ If you are prone to stings, it may be worthwhile to invest in The Extractor, a device that can be used to extract venom from a bite or sting. It is available in many camping and outdoor equipment stores or directly through the manufacturer, Sawyer Products (see the Resources section at the end of the book).

■ Sweating increases the discomfort of most skin irritations. Try to keep your skin cool and dry.

PREVENTION

■ There are many commercial insect repellents sold over the counter. Deet (diethyl toluamide) is generally considered the most effective, although it is potentially quite toxic. Read and follow package directions carefully.

Emergency Treatment for Insect and Spider Bites and Stings

■ **For venomous spider bites, get immediate help.** If you suspect that you have been bitten by a venomous spider, such as the black widow or brown recluse spider, have someone take you immediately to the emergency room of the nearest hospital. If no one is available to take you, call for emergency help and explain the situation. In the beginning stages, the only way you will know that you have been bitten by a poisonous spider is if you see the spider in the vicinity. If possible, capture the spider and have it ready to show the doctor for quick identification. If you are bitten by an insect or spider you cannot identify, call your local Poison Control Center for instructions on how best to proceed.

■ **For black widow spider bites.** The poisonous venom of the black widow spider causes sweating, stomach cramps, nausea, headaches, and dizziness. There is an antivenin available for treatment of black widow bites. The antivenin itself, however, can cause an allergic reaction in some people. Otherwise healthy adults are usually monitored and given painkillers, muscle relaxants, antianxiety agents such as diazepam (Valium), and/or intravenous calcium to relieve muscle pain and spasms.

■ **For brown recluse spider bites.** A bite from the poisonous brown recluse spider will cause a characteristic bull's-eye marking—a blister surrounded by white and red circles. Pain, nausea, fever, and chills are common. Medical care is essential. If the bite is untreated, a large amount of the surrounding tissue can die, requiring surgical excision. An antivenin for brown recluse spider bites has been developed, but is not yet commercially available. The bite may be treated with injections of steroids, although their effectiveness is controversial. A drug called dapsone may be used in some cases.

■ **For bee, wasp, or hornet stings.** Should you be stung by a bee, wasp, or hornet, remove the stinger by gently scraping it out, then wash and rinse the area thoroughly. Be alert for signs of an allergic reaction, such as hives, difficulty breathing, or redness that begins spreading rapidly outward from the area of penetration. Reactions can occur within minutes or after several hours, so be vigilant.

At the first sign of a severe allergic reaction, especially if you are having difficulty breathing, have someone take you to the emergency room of the nearest hospital, or call for emergency help and stress the gravity of the situation. Seconds count. If you have an emergency adrenaline kit such as the Ana-Kit or EpiPen, administer it immediately. These kits, which are available by prescription only, contain a syringe filled with a premeasured dose of epinephrine, a hormone that opens the airways and restores free breathing to combat a life-threatening allergic reaction.

■ **For common insect bites.** Monitor your reactions. If you should suffer a serious allergic or toxic reaction after a bite or sting from a common insect, have someone take you at once to the emergency room of the nearest hospital. If you feel listless or unlike your normal self following a bite or sting, call your physician.

■ **For scorpion bites.** Most scorpion stings are merely painful, not dangerous. However, if you have been stung by an Arizona centruroides (bark) scorpion, you should seek treatment. There is no antivenin as yet approved by the U.S. Food and Drug Administration (FDA), but if the reaction is serious enough, some doctors may use an unapproved version from Arizona Poison Control.

Be aware that these formulas may not be safe for children.

■ Citronella and pennyroyal are safe, natural repellents that may be applied to the skin. Oils of citronella and pennyroyal are usually available in health-food stores.

Caution: Do not use pennyroyal during pregnancy.

■ Garlic helps to repel insects. Take the equivalent of 500 milligrams of fresh garlic twice a day for three days before a wilderness outing and throughout the trip.

■ Spray permethrin (available as Nix, Permanone, or Duranon) on clothing. This is a medication normally used to get rid of head lice. It is very effective and virtually non-toxic when used this way as an insect repellent. One spraying can last for up to two weeks.

■ Liquid vitamin-B complex, taken orally, is effective in preventing some insect bites. The B vitamins are excreted through the skin and are believed to leave a bad taste in the mouths of mosquitoes and fleas. Three days before an outdoor trip or outing, start taking a good B-complex supplement supplying 50 milligrams of each of the major B vitamins twice daily, and continue taking it throughout the trip.

■ Do not chase bees, wasps, or hornets. If you spot a nest built by one of these stinging insects, stay away from it.

■ Don't swat at or squash a yellow jacket. Studies have shown that the body of a crushed yellow jacket exudes a chemical that attracts and stimulates other yellow jackets in the area to attack. If you are being bothered by a yellow jacket, it's better to leave the area.

■ Cologne, shiny jewelry, and even perfumed suntan lotions all attract insects, so it's best not to use or wear them when spending time outdoors.

Black Eye

See under BRUISE.

Bladder Infection

See under URINARY TRACT INFECTION.

Bleeding, Minor

See CUTS AND SCRAPES.

Bleeding, Nose

See NOSEBLEED.

Bleeding, Severe

We all suffer cuts and scrapes from time to time. For the most part, these minor injuries can be treated at home (see CUTS AND SCRAPES). But if you receive a severe external wound that spurts or causes a great deal of steady bleeding, it is possible that an artery or vein has been cut. Arteries carry oxygen-rich blood from the lungs and heart to the rest of the body; veins carry oxygen-poor blood back to the heart and lungs. If an artery is cut, it will bleed oxygenated blood that is bright red in color. Oxygen-poor blood coming from a cut vein is a dark, bluish red.

Hundreds of miles of blood vessels run to every living organ and tissue (except for the cornea of the eye). If blood flow to any part of the body is cut off, that part will die. Brain cells die after three to four minutes without a fresh supply of blood.

If you are bleeding heavily, emergency treatment is necessary.

EMERGENCY TREATMENT

See the inset on page 139.

CONVENTIONAL TREATMENT

■ Seek emergency medical treatment (see page 000). Rely on medical personnel to take over and do what is necessary and appropriate to stop the bleeding and stabilize your body. You may require a blood transfusion or the administration of intravenous saline solution to maintain fluid levels.

■ On reaching the hospital, you may require sutures (stitches) or surgery to repair the damage that caused the bleeding.

■ Once the wound has been treated and you are well enough to leave the hospital, medical personnel will advise you on the proper way to care for yourself as you recover from your injury. Ask your doctor for recommendations regarding diet, activity level, special exercises, and any measures necessary to guard against complications.

■ A substance known as type II collagen (sold under the brand name Hycure) can be applied as a gel or powder to protect the injury, speed healing, and reduce scarring.

DIETARY GUIDELINES

■ While you are recovering from a blood loss, make sure your diet includes lots of green leafy vegetables, squashes, and fresh fruits, as well as liquids, to provide necessary vitamins and minerals and restore fluid balance.

■ If you are taking supplementary iron (see under Nutritional Supplements, below), your diet should also include extra fiber and liquids to prevent constipation, which is an occasional side effect of iron supplementation.

NUTRITIONAL SUPPLEMENTS

The nutritional supplements recommended here are intended to support recovery once appropriate emergency medical care has been administered and you are well enough to leave the hospital. If you are bleeding profusely, seek emergency medical care immediately.

■ Chlorophyll has trace minerals that assist the body in rebuilding blood. Take a chlorophyll or sea-greens supplement, such as spirulina and blue-green algae, for two to three months. Follow the dosage directions on the product label.

■ If your physician determines that the blood loss has resulted in anemia, he or she may prescribe an iron sup-

Emergency Treatment for Severe Bleeding

In the case of a severe external wound, have someone call immediately for emergency help.

■ Cover the bleeding wound with a clean cloth or gauze, and quickly apply very firm, steady pressure. If there is no clean cloth or gauze readily available, use your bare hand to apply pressure. Even if the pressure hurts, continue applying very firm, steady pressure. It is necessary to stop the bleeding.

■ If there is no suspicion of a spinal injury, raise the wound above the level of your heart to help minimize the amount of blood that spurts from the wound with every beat of your heart. Signs of a spinal injury include pain at the site of the injury, weakness or numbness in an extremity, inability to move an extremity, or lack of feeling in an extremity. If any of these signs are present, do not allow anyone to move you. Any movement may worsen the injury.

■ If the blood soaks through the cloth pad or gauze, put more cloth or gauze over the old pad and continue applying pressure. It is best not to remove the original blood-soaked pad. Any early clotting may become dislodged if you attempt to change the bandage.

■ If emergency medical personnel are not already on their way to you, have someone take you to the emergency room of the nearest hospital. If you are alone, call for emergency assistance.

■ Despite what you may have seen in the movies, tourniquets are to be *avoided*. Because it cuts off the blood supply, a tourniquet deprives the tissues below the wound of oxygen, creating the risk of losing a limb. Continue to apply enough pressure to stem the bleeding while you wait or go for emergency help.

---

plement to help build up your blood. If possible, select a chelated form (ferrous chelate). Ferrous gluconate and ferrous fumarate are also acceptable. Avoid ferrous sulfate, which can cause stomach irritation and constipation. Take this supplement as prescribed by your physician.

Note: Excessive amounts of iron are associated with a variety of health problems, including an increased risk of cardiovascular disease. Do not take supplemental iron unless a deficiency has been diagnosed by your health-care provider, and do not take the supplement in higher amounts or for a longer period of time than he or she prescribes.

■ The B vitamins, especially vitamin B_{12} and folic acid, are very important for restoring healthy blood. Take a B-complex supplement containing 50 milligrams of each of the major B vitamins three times a day for two weeks, plus 500 micrograms of vitamin B_{12} twice a day for two to three months.

■ Vitamin C and bioflavonoids are helpful for wound healing. Vitamin C also helps the body to absorb iron. Take 500 milligrams of vitamin C and an equal amount of mixed bioflavonoids twice a day for two to three months.

HERBAL TREATMENT

The herbal treatments that follow are intended to support recovery once appropriate emergency medical care has been administered and you are well enough to leave the hospital. If you are bleeding profusely, seek emergency medical care immediately.

■ A person who has suffered a blood loss may become anemic. Floradix formula is an herbal iron supplement that can be used to slowly help replace some of the iron lost through bleeding. Follow the dosage directions on the product label and take it for two to three months. Floradix is best for mild anemia. If a blood test has determined that you have an anemic condition, a more concentrated nutritional iron supplement may be a better way to rebuild your blood.

■ Nettle and yellow dock help build healthy blood cells. After the crisis is over, take 300 to 500 milligrams of nettle and/or 250 to 500 milligrams of yellow dock twice daily for one to two weeks.

Note: Some people experience stomach upset as a result of taking nettle. If this happens, stop taking it.

HOMEOPATHY

Homeopathic treatment is intended to support recovery once appropriate emergency medical care has been administered and you are well enough to leave the hospital. If you are bleeding profusely, seek emergency medical care immediately.

■ *Arnica* is helpful for trauma and inflammation. Take one dose of *Arnica* 12x or 6c three times daily for up to three days.

■ *Ferrum phosphoricum* helps the body recover from a major blood loss. Take one dose of *Ferrum phosphoricum* 12x or 6c, as directed on the product label, three times daily for five days.

■ *Hypericum* and *Ledum* promote wound healing. Take one dose of *Hypericum* 12x or 6c or *Ledum* 12x or 6c three times daily for five days.

GENERAL RECOMMENDATIONS

■ Once the crisis is over and you are well enough to leave the hospital, ask your doctor for recommendations regarding diet, activity restrictions, and other measures to support recovery.

■ For additional suggestions regarding natural therapies that aid in recovery from a major blood loss and speed healing, *see* SURGERY, RECOVERING FROM.

PREVENTION

■ The best way to prevent an injury that causes severe bleeding is to take sensible precautions to avoid accidents. For example, drive defensively, and always wear your seat belt. Don't drink and drive. If you own a gun, keep it unloaded and locked up. Wear proper protective gear when operating power tools, including lawnmowers. For additional suggestions, *see* HOME AND PERSONAL SAFETY in Part One.

Blepharitis

Blepharitis is an inflammation of the eyelids that affects the oil glands of the lids and the eyelashes. There are two forms of this condition, ulcerative and nonulcerative. In its nonulcerative form, it causes symptoms including swelling, itching, burning, watering, and redness, accompanied by the formation of crusts of dried mucus on the lids. In fact, this condition was once referred to as "granulated eyelids." Nonulcerative blepharitis is a cousin of dandruff and eczema, and may be a complication of psoriasis. It is often linked to seborrhea of the scalp, the eyebrows, and the skin around the eyes.

In ulcerative blepharitis, a *Staphylococcus* infection at the roots of the eyelashes causes sticky crusts to form on the lid margins, followed by small sores, or ulcers. The eyes become reddened and abnormally sensitive to light.

Both forms of blepharitis can be contagious. Severe blepharitis can lead to corneal problems. This condition should not be neglected.

CONVENTIONAL TREATMENT

■ Sores on the eyelids call for an evaluation by an ophthalmologist. Topical antibiotic ointment applications may be adequate treatment, but let an expert decide.

■ Infection of structures adjacent to the eyelids may require oral, instead of topical, antibiotics, and/or drainage of inflamed glands.

■ Occasionally, topical steroid ointments are used to reduce inflammation, but these drugs must be used with great care. If there is even a suspicion of a viral infection, such as a herpes infection, steroids should *not* be used. Steroids suppress the local immune response, allowing a herpes infection to become more aggressive. Use of these drugs also creates a risk of increased pressure within the eyeball, which can lead to glaucoma as well as to cataracts, perforation of the cornea, and damage to the optic nerve.

DIETARY GUIDELINES

■ Be sure to eat plenty of fresh fruits and vegetables. These healthy foods contain antioxidant phytochemicals that can protect all the cells of the body, including those of the eyes, from free-radical damage.

■ Eat clean, lean protein foods, such as chicken and fish. Protein is needed for healing and to maintain healthy eyes.

■ Limit your intake of sugar and caffeine. These substances contribute to eye irritation and worsen the symptoms caused by many eye problems.

NUTRITIONAL SUPPLEMENTS

■ Alpha-lipoic acid is an antioxidant and detoxifier. Take 100 milligrams three times daily.

■ Beta-carotene is a strong antioxidant that prevents free-radical damage. It is related to vitamin A and has many of the same properties, but it does not become toxic in large doses. Take 10,000 to 25,000 international units of beta-carotene daily.

■ The essential fatty acids (EFAs), found in black currant seed oil, borage oil, evening primrose oil, and flaxseed oil, are required by every cell in the body. They have been shown to reduce pain, inflammation, and swelling. EFAs also help counteract the hardening effects of cholesterol on cell membranes. Take 500 to 1,000 milligrams of any of these oils twice daily.

■ Selenium is an excellent antioxidant that helps prevent free-radical damage throughout the body, including the eyes. While symptoms are acute, take 100 micrograms twice daily. When symptoms improve, reduce the dosage to 100 micrograms once daily.

■ Vitamin A protects against free-radical damage and is especially important to the eyes. Without sufficient vitamin A, the eyes are more susceptible to infection and ulceration. Take 5,000 international units of vitamin A three times a day for two months. Then reduce to a maintenance dosage of 5,000 international units twice daily.

Note: If you are pregnant, or intend to get pregnant, or if you have liver disease, consult your doctor before taking supplemental vitamin A. Pregnant women should not ingest a total of more than 25,000 international units of supplemental vitamin A *per week* from all sources.

■ Inadequate intake of the B-complex vitamins can result in itching, burning, bloodshot eyes that water excessively. Combined with vitamins C and E, the B-complex vitamins are especially beneficial to the eyes. While symptoms are acute, take a B-complex supplement that supplies 50 milligrams of each of the primary B vitamins twice daily. When symptoms improve, reduce the dosage to 25 milligrams twice daily.

■ Vitamin C helps to prevent and clear up infections. It also helps strengthen capillaries, maintains collagen, and prevents tissue hemorrhaging, and is notable for speeding healing. Select a vitamin-C formula that includes bioflavonoids, especially rutin; these nutrients work best together. While symptoms are acute, take 1,000 to 3,000 milligrams of a vitamin-C complex three times daily. When symptoms improve, reduce the dosage to 500 to 1,000 milligrams three times daily.

■ Vitamin E is an antioxidant and is essential in cellular respiration. Choose a product containing mixed tocopherols and start by taking 200 international units daily, then gradually increase the dosage until you are taking 400 international units twice a day. Maintain that dose as long as symptoms are acute, then cut back to 200 international units twice daily.

Note: If you have high blood pressure, limit your intake of supplemental vitamin E to 400 international units daily. If you are taking an anticoagulant (blood thinner), consult your physician before taking supplemental vitamin E.

■ Zinc supports the immune system and aids in the healing process. While symptoms are acute, take 25 to 50 milligrams of zinc daily. When symptoms improve, reduce the dosage to 15 to 20 milligrams daily.

Note: Take zinc with food to prevent stomach upset, and do not exceed 100 milligrams daily from all supplements. If you take over 30 milligrams of zinc on a daily basis for more than one or two months, you should also take 1 to 2 milligrams of copper each day to maintain a proper mineral balance.

HERBAL TREATMENTS

■ Bilberry is an anti-inflammatory and antioxidant that promotes circulation to the eyes. Choose a standardized extract containing 25 percent anthocyanidins (also called PCOs) and take 80 milligrams two or three times daily.

■ Cat's claw has anti-inflammatory properties and helps to regulate the immune response. Take 500 milligrams of standardized extract three times daily.

Note: Do not take cat's claw if you are pregnant or nursing, or if you are an organ transplant recipient. Use it with caution if you are taking an anticoagulant (blood-thinner).

■ An eyebright eyewash helps prevent excessive tearing and eases discomfort. Bring 3 ounces of sterile saline solution to a boil, and pour it over 1 tablespoon of dried cut herb (or one eyebright teabag). Allow it to steep for fifteen minutes, then strain out the herb. When the liquid has cooled to a comfortable temperature, use it as an eyewash. Bathe your eyes with the eyewash and/or prepare a compress by moistening a sterile cloth in the warm infusion. Place the compress over the closed eye, pressing down gently to achieve contact with the affected area. Relax for at least ten minutes. Then moisten a fresh sterile cloth in the eyewash tea and wipe away the crusts and scales. Throw away (or sterilize) each cloth after one use. Never reuse the cloth after contact with the eye without first washing it in hot water, preferably with chlorine bleach added. To do so is to invite reinfection.

■ Grapefruit-seed extract is a natural antibiotic. Take 100 milligrams three times a day.

■ Turmeric is a potent anti-inflammatory. Take 500 milligrams of standardized extract three times daily.

HOMEOPATHY

■ *Euphrasia* is good for eyes that are burning and tearing, with inflamed eyelids and, possibly, a feeling of pressure. Take one dose of *Euphrasia* 12x or 6c three times a day for up to three days.

■ *Hydrastis* is good for eyelids that appear infected. Take one dose of *Hydrastis* 12x or 6c three times a day for up to three days.

■ Choose *Phytolacca* if the eyelids are swollen and feel hard. Take one dose of *Phytolacca* 12x or 6c three times a day for up to three days.

GENERAL RECOMMENDATIONS

■ Keep the area scrupulously clean. Soap your hands for at least ten seconds and rinse well before treating your eyes.

■ Avoid touching or rubbing your eyes. That can spread the infection.

■ If you wear makeup, give it up for the duration. Contaminated eye makeup can be a contributing factor to both forms of blepharitis. Once you decide to start using makeup again, replace old cosmetics—especially eye makeup—with fresh products.

■ If you have a related skin condition, such as dandruff, eczema, or psoriasis, see the appropriate entries for additional recommendations.

Blisters

We all get blisters at one time or another, whether from local irritation, burns, insect bites, allergic or drug reactions, infection, trauma, or illness. These little balloons are nature's way of insulating damaged skin under a coating of clear fluid. Medically speaking, if the size is less than $1/5$ inch in size it is called a vesicle; otherwise it qualifies as a blister. Blisters are most common among people who have difficulty finding shoes that fit properly and athletes who may be running or walking long distances.

The fluid inside a blister is serous fluid, which means that its composition is the same as that of the clear portion of the blood (minus the red and white blood cells and clot-forming proteins). As long as a blister is intact, its contents are sterile, and the underlying tissue is protected against infection. Therefore, the longer you can keep the blister intact, the better off the tissue beneath.

CONVENTIONAL TREATMENT

■ Bursting a blister to get the fluid out is not recommended as long as the fluid within remains clear, possibly with a slight yellowish tint. Instead, protect the area for as long as possible using "doughnut"-type pads that surround the blister but are open in the center so the blister itself remains uncovered. Eventually (usually in a week to ten days), the fluid will be reabsorbed by the body and the blister will be healed.

■ If a blister bursts, your doctor may recommend that you apply silver sulfadiazine (Silvadene) and keep the injury covered with a bandage. Silver sulfadiazine is effective against *Pseudomonas* bacteria, the most common type of bacteria found in weeping-type wounds. It is also painless to sensitive raw skin. Other anti-infective agents, such as povidone-iodine (Betadine) and mafenide (Sulfamylon), are generally reserved for more serious and deeply infected wounds, as they can both be painful and tend to slow the growth of new skin.

■ If a burst blister gets badly infected, systemic oral antibiotics may be in order.

DIETARY GUIDELINES

■ Drink at least six 8-ounce glasses of water daily. Dehydration exacerbates blisters and makes the skin more vulnerable. Staying well hydrated can help prevent blisters as well.

NUTRITIONAL SUPPLEMENTS

■ Take a good multivitamin and mineral supplement daily to ensure a supply of all the nutrients necessary for healing.

■ Vitamin C and bioflavonoids speed healing. Take 500 milligrams of each two or three times daily.

HOMEOPATHY

■ *Arnica* can help to resolve initial inflammation. Take one dose of *Arnica* 30x or 15c three times daily for the first twenty-four hours after a blister develops.

■ *Cantharis* is good for blisters that burn and smart, with a feeling of rawness. Take one dose of *Cantharis* 12x or 6c three times daily for the following forty-eight hours.

GENERAL RECOMMENDATIONS

■ Applying tincture of benzoin and covering the area with topical patches, such as Compeed patches, helps to protect active feet that have blisters. This combination is also used by athletes who are trying to prevent blisters from forming. Tincture of benzoin helps to tighten and toughen the skin.

■ Second Skin is a moist bandage that can be used to protect a blister. Johnson & Johnson's Elastikon tape is also very popular among athletes. If you are covering a blister that has burst, be careful to cover the edges so that dirt cannot enter the area.

PREVENTION

■ Many marathon runners use a layering technique to prevent blisters on their feet. Begin with a pair of shoes that are slightly big for your feet. Apply petroleum jelly (Vaseline) to your feet, then put on a pair of thin socks. Then put on a pair of thicker athletic socks before putting on your shoes.

■ Many runners and hikers apply New Skin spray before activity they think might lead to blisters.

Boils

A boil is a bacterial infection that begins deep in a hair follicle or a sebaceous gland, one of the skin's oil-producing glands, and gradually works its way up to the surface of the skin. *Staphylococcus aureus* is the bacteria most frequently responsible for boils.

Boils most often appear on the neck, face, underarms, or buttocks. If you notice a red, elevated, and painful bump, watch the area closely. Should a boil be developing, a pustule will form in the center of the affected area within two to four days.

It is possible, although unusual, for a boil to spread beyond the affected area and cause a more serious systemic infection. For example, nearby lymph glands may become swollen. A boil may also be a sign of an underlying infection in the body that is manifesting itself through the skin. In either case, you need medical attention.

To determine when to call the doctor, pay attention to your body. Do you feel fine otherwise, or do you have other symptoms of illness? If you are overtired, running a fever, not eating well, or just not "up to par," you should see a physician.

CONVENTIONAL TREATMENT

■ Once the boil has localized close to the skin surface, your doctor will probably recommend that it be opened and the contents expressed—a procedure known as incision and drainage, or I and D. This is a procedure that should be done by a medical professional. If the doctor incises the boil, or if it ruptures by itself, it will drain thick pus. A topical antibiotic, such as Betadine or bacitracin, may be prescribed to help clear the infection.

■ Your doctor will probably prescribe an oral antibiotic and do a culture of the contents of the boil. When the results of the culture reveal the particular organism responsible for the infection, your antibiotic prescription may be changed accordingly.

■ If the situation recurs, and the culture determines it to be a staphylococcal infection, close contacts of yours may also need to be treated so that you do not pass the infection back and forth.

DIETARY GUIDELINES

■ Avoid sweets and greasy, fried foods. Keep your diet simple and clean.

■ Make sure your diet includes plenty of dark-green vegetables.

NUTRITIONAL SUPPLEMENTS

■ Bromelain, an enzyme extracted from pineapple, is a good anti-inflammatory. Take 300 milligrams three times a day until healed.

■ Vitamin A and beta-carotene help to heal skin tissue. Take 5,000 international units of vitamin A and 15,000 international units of beta-carotene twice a day for one week or until the boil is healed.

Note: If you are pregnant, or intend to get pregnant, or if you have liver disease, consult your doctor before taking supplemental vitamin A. Pregnant women should not ingest a total of more than 25,000 international units of supplemental vitamin A *per week* from all sources.

■ Vitamin C and bioflavonoids have mild anti-inflammatory properties and help to boost the immune system. Take 1,000 milligrams of vitamin C three times a day and 500 milligrams of bioflavonoids twice a day for one week or until the boil heals.

■ Zinc helps support the immune system and heal skin tissue. Take 15 milligrams twice a day for one week or until healed. Take zinc with food to prevent stomach upset.

HERBAL TREATMENT

■ Cat's claw enhances the immune response and has antibacterial properties. Take 500 milligrams of standardized extract three times a day until the boil clears.

Note: Do not use cat's claw if you are pregnant or nursing, or if you are an organ-transplant recipient. Use it with caution if you are taking an anticoagulant (blood thinner).

■ Echinacea and goldenseal stimulate the immune system and help to clear infection. Echinacea has antiviral properties; goldenseal is an antibacterial herb that also soothes the skin and mucous membranes. Take one dose of an echinacea and goldenseal combination formula supplying 250 to 500 milligrams of echinacea and 150 to 300 milligrams of goldenseal three times daily until the boil improves, up to one week. Goldenseal can also be applied topically to a boil for its antiseptic properties.

■ Ginger-tea compresses help to draw out infection and bring a boil to a head. Prepare a strong ginger tea and soak a clean white cloth in it. Apply this warm, wet compress to the boil for ten to fifteen minutes at least four times daily.

■ Green clay paste helps draw out and dry up infection. Mix 1 teaspoon of green clay with a small amount of water, just enough to make a pastelike consistency. After using a ginger tea compress, apply this paste to the boil.

■ Oregano has antibacterial properties and helps to fight infection. Take 75 to 150 milligrams of standardized extract three times a day.

■ Pine-bark and grape-seed extracts are high in bioflavonoids and natural anti-inflammatory agents. Take 25 milligrams of either three times a day for one week to ten days.

■ Turmeric strengthens immune function and has both anti-inflammatory and antibacterial properties. Take 500 milligrams of standardized extract twice a day for one month.

■ Usnea moss is effective against *Staphylococcus* bacteria. Make a strong usnea tea by boiling 3 tablespoons of the whole herb (or 2 tea bags) in 1 cup of water for three minutes. Remove the mixture from the heat and allow it to steep for another ten minutes. Then soak a clean white cloth in the tea and apply it to the boil for ten to fifteen minutes. Repeat this procedure three or four times daily until the boil heals. Usnea is also available in ointment form.

■ Make an herbal poultice by adding 1 tablespoon each of

plantain, marshmallow root, goldenseal, and/or Oregon grape root to 1 cup of water. Bring to a boil and simmer for twenty minutes. Soak a cloth in the mixture, and apply the poultice to the affected area for twenty to thirty minutes. Do this three times a day for two to three days.

HOMEOPATHY

The following homeopathic remedies will help relieve your discomfort quickly. Please note that they are to be used in stages.

Belladonna helps bring down a boil that is large, red, and hot. When a boil first appears and is red and throbbing, take one dose of *Belladonna* 30x or 9c, as directed on the product label, every three to four hours for one day.

When the pustular head on the boil appears, *Hepar sulfuris calcareum* will help promote discharge. Take one dose of *Hepar sulfuris calcareum* 12x or 6c three times daily after the boil comes to a head.

To speed draining after pus appears, take one dose of *Silicea* 12x or 6c three times daily for two days. *Silicea* can also help to bring a boil to a head.

Myristica encourages boils to open and drain. If you have a stubborn boil that refuses to open, take one dose of *Myristica* 12x or 6c four times daily for one day.

Calcarea sulfurica is used for a boil that is not healing readily. Once the boil does begin to drain, take one dose of *Calcarea sulfurica* 12x three times daily until the boil has emptied.

ACUPRESSURE

For the locations of acupressure points on the body, *see* ADMINISTERING AN ACUPRESSURE TREATMENT in Part Three.

Spleen 10 detoxifies the blood.

AROMATHERAPY

For specific instructions on how to use aromatherapy, *see* PREPARING AROMATHERAPY TREATMENTS in Part Three.

Use tea tree oil compresses. Tea tree oil is a strong antiseptic and helps to resolve infection. Add 8 to 10 drops of tea tree oil to 1 quart of warm water and soak a clean cotton cloth or cotton ball in the mixture. Apply the warm compress to the boil for ten to fifteen minutes four times daily.

GENERAL RECOMMENDATIONS

Do not squeeze or puncture a boil. Opening it prematurely can worsen and spread the infection.

■ Avoid using tape or an adhesive bandage to cover a boil. Covering a boil may increase irritation and can lead to scarring.

PREVENTION

■ Keep your skin clean and dry. Good hygiene is helpful. However, even someone who practices meticulous skin care can still develop a boil, especially in hot and humid environments.

■ Propolis is a natural antibiotic made by bees. Three days each week, take 500 milligrams three times daily to prevent the recurrence of boils.

■ If you are prone to recurrent boils, try the following three-week cycle:

Week 1: Take one dose of an echinacea and goldenseal combination formula supplying 250 to 500 milligrams of echinacea and 150 to 300 milligrams of goldenseal two to three times a day.

Week 2: Take 50 milligrams of pine-bark or grape-seed extract two to three times a day.

Week 3: Take 250 to 500 milligrams of burdock root, red clover, and/or nettle two to three times a day.

Repeat this cycle three times, for a total of nine weeks.

Note: Some people experience stomach upset as a result of taking nettle. If this happens, stop taking it.

Bone, Broken

When people think of bones, they often visualize them as "dead," rather like the dry skeletons that sometimes hang in science classrooms. But bones are really living tissue, with a rich supply of blood vessels and nerves. As a result, a bone fracture is not only painful, it causes shock and trauma to the whole body.

If you have suffered an accident, a bad fall, or a hard blow, you may have broken a bone. Depending on the cause of the break, there may be an open wound near the fracture. You may find yourself lying very still to protect yourself against the pain of movement. An affected limb may appear crooked or bent. The area near a fracture will be painful or tender when moved or touched, and may appear swollen, red, and bruised.

Depending on which bone is broken, there is a possibility of additional damage, including internal bleeding. A broken rib may puncture a lung; a broken vertebra can damage the spinal cord; a skull fracture can cause bleeding into the brain. Broken bones should be taken seriously and treated immediately.

EMERGENCY TREATMENT

■ If you think you may have suffered a serious bone fracture—a broken long bone, rib, or vertebra, or a skull fracture—do not move and do not allow anyone other than trained medical personnel to move you. Movement can cause additional injury. Even if an obvious fracture is visible, it is better not to try to move it back into place. Other structures may be involved in the injury, and manipulating the area may make it worse. Have someone call for emergency help.

■ If possible, without moving the affected area, immobilize it as well as you can, whether it be an extremity or spinal cord. Rolled-up magazines, towels, and blankets can all be adequate temporary splinting materials.

Keep calm and warm. Panic can cause you to hyperventilate or go into shock, altering your mental state and making the situation worse.

If you have broken a smaller bone, apply ice. Have someone take you to the hospital emergency room or your physician promptly.

If you fracture a finger or toe, apply ice or a cool compress to the injury and elevate it above the level of your heart. This will minimize swelling and help relieve pain. Have someone take you to the emergency room or to your physician.

Noses are seldom actually broken. A blow to the nose can be very painful, however. A blood-filled bruise may develop inside the nose, causing a black eye on one or both sides. Apply an ice pack immediately. With the ice pack in place, have someone take you to the emergency room or to your physician for prompt attention.

CONVENTIONAL TREATMENT

If you have any suspicion that you may have broken a bone, you should seek professional medical care immediately. Failure to do so, even for an injury that looks relatively insignificant, may result in permanent disability. A broken bone must be assessed, x-rayed, set, and possibly placed in traction by a physician.

The proper setting and casting of the long bones of the arms and legs are critical. Broken fingers and toes may be splinted, or the doctor may securely tape the injured digit to adjacent fingers or toes. Either method will keep the bone immobilized while it heals.

The possibility of internal damage will be considered. Should any further injury come to light, medical personnel will take the appropriate measures.

If you are in pain, pain medication may be prescribed.

■ If the fracture appears to be too serious a consequence for the circumstances of the accident, bring this to your physician's attention. It may be a *pathologic fracture*—that is, a fracture that is a sign of underlying disease, such as osteoporosis.

DIETARY GUIDELINES

■ Once appropriate medical care has been administered, support the healing process by eating a diet containing plenty of lean protein, plus bone-building foods containing calcium, phosphorus, and vitamin D. Calcium-rich foods include all the familiar dairy products. Green leafy vegetables also provide calcium and valuable trace minerals. Phosphorus is found in bananas, whole-grain breads and cereals, nuts, eggs, fish, and poultry. Vitamin D is present in fortified dairy products, eggs, and saltwater fish, and is synthesized by the body when the skin is exposed to sunshine.

■ If you are recovering from a broken bone, you should not consume any sodas or other foods containing phosphoric acid. This substance actually depletes calcium from the bones. Also avoid alcohol, which is toxic to bone-building tissues.

NUTRITIONAL SUPPLEMENTS

■ Calcium and magnesium help to rebuild bone tissue. Take 250 milligrams of calcium and 125 milligrams of magnesium four to five times daily for a minimum of two months. Calcium microcrystalline hydroxyapatite is a mineral supplement derived from bone that is a good source of absorbable calcium. Products from New Zealand sources are purest. Other good forms of calcium include calcium amino acid chelate (but make sure it is a true chelate form, not merely a tablet coated with soy protein) and calcium citrate. For magnesium, choose magnesium citrate or magnesium aspartate.

■ Vitamin C and bioflavonoids help in the process of bone healing. Take 500 milligrams of each one to three times daily for two to three months.

■ Chlorophyll provides trace minerals that help rebuild bone tissue. Take a chlorophyll or sea-greens supplement, such as spirulina and blue-green algae, following the dosage directions on the product label, for two to three months after a bone break or until the break is healed.

■ Vitamin D improves the absorption of calcium. Take 400 international units of vitamin D every day for two to three months.

HERBAL TREATMENT

Herbal treatment for a broken bone is intended to support recovery once appropriate emergency medical care has been administered and you are well enough to leave the hospital.

■ Horsetail is high in silica, which helps the body absorb the calcium needed for bone tissue healing. Take 500 milligrams three times daily for two weeks.

■ Nettle is high in silica and other trace minerals. It also enhances calcium absorption. Take a cup of nettle tea daily for two to three weeks.

Note: Some people experience stomach upset as a result of taking this herb. If this happens, stop taking it. This herb should not be given to a child under four.

■ Oat straw is high in silica and is a mild relaxant. Take 250 to 500 milligrams twice daily for two weeks.

HOMEOPATHY

Homeopathic treatment for a broken bone is intended to support recovery once appropriate emergency medical care has been administered and you are well enough to leave the hospital.

■ If you suspect that you have broken a bone, take one dose of homeopathic *Aconite* 30x, 200x, 9c, or 30c, as directed on the product label, on the way to the hospital. *Aconite* is excellent for relieving the shock and fright associated with an injury. The cold sweat, fear, dizziness, and nausea you may be experiencing will quickly be alleviated with this remedy.

■ Five minutes after the initial dose of *Aconite*, take one dose of *Arnica* 30x, 200x, 9c, or 30c. Take another dose of *Arnica* every thirty minutes thereafter for a total of three doses. *Arnica* helps lessen the bruising and aching pain associated with a bone fracture. It also aids in healing the injury to the soft tissue and muscle surrounding a break.

■ After the immediate crisis has been handled and you are home from the hospital, take the following remedies in the sequence indicated to help the break knit quickly and to speed healing:

Days 1–2: Three times a day, take one dose of *Arnica* 30x or 9c.

Days 3–5: Three times a day, take one dose of *Ruta graveolens* 12x or 6c to help relieve bone pain.

Days 6–8: Three times a day, take one dose of *Symphytum* 6x to help the bone heal quickly.

Days 9–19: Three times a day, take one dose of *Calcarea phosphorica* 6x or *Calcarea carbonica* 6x to support the healing process.

Days 20–27: Stop all administration of homeopathic remedies for one week.

Days 28–38: Three times a day, take one dose of *Calcarea phosphorica* 6x or *Calcarea carbonica* 6x.

Botulism

See under FOOD POISONING.

Breast Cancer

Breast cancer is the most common type of cancer in women. As with all types of cancer, it is characterized by uncontrolled cell reproduction that leads to the formation of a mass, or tumor. While a thorough discussion of all the facets of and variables involved in this disease is beyond the scope of this book, it is important to be aware of certain common characteristics, signs and symptoms, and risk factors associated with breast cancer so that you can minimize your chances of developing it or, if you do develop it, you can maximize your chances of early detection and cure. It should be noted that, when detected early, breast cancer is considered 70 to 90 percent curable.

Early in the disease, there may be a single small, firm nodular mass in the breast, usually in one breast only. Most tumors are found by women themselves rather than by doctors during a medical exam. A mammogram (breast x-ray) can also detect possible cancerous growths, sometimes before there is any mass that can be felt from the outside. If you divide the breast into four equal parts (as you would divide a pie into quarters), the upper outer quadrant, or section, of the breast is by far where the most cancers occur, although no area of the breast is immune.

There are different subtypes of breast cancer, classified by the type of tissue they arise in and their tendency to spread. By far the most common form of breast cancer, accounting for 70 to 80 percent of all cases, is the infiltrating, or invasive, ductal type, which originates in the milk ducts and spreads to other breast tissue. The invasive lobular type, which originates in the lobules (where milk is produced) and spreads to other tissue, accounts for 6 to 8 percent of cases. Between 4 and 6 percent of breast cancers are noninvasive (less aggressive) lobular and intraductal cancers. There is also a very small percentage of uncommon types.

In addition to being classified according to type, cancers are *staged*, or ranked, according to a physician's estimate of how advanced they are. The common classification system is called the TNM system. It uses a combination of the size of the *t*umor, whether lymph *n*odes in the local area are involved, and whether the tumor has *m*etastasized (spread) to more distant lymph nodes. This system is meant to give an idea of how the disease should be treated and a prognosis as to the likelihood of cure. Staging is hardly an exact science, however, and much controversy exists about it. The rankings range from stage 0, which is the least severe, through stages I, IIA, IIB, IIIA, and IIIB, to stage IV, which has the poorest prognosis. Cancers through stage II are normally considered curable, while those in higher stages are considered more serious, and treatment tends to focus on slowing the progression of the disease rather than curing it.

While the precise cause or causes of breast cancer are not well understood, there are a number of factors that are known to increase the risk. If a woman had her first child after the age of thirty (or never had children), if there is a family history of the disease, or if she began menstruating early, her risk of developing breast cancer increases. Late menopause, fibrocystic breast disease, and a history of uterine cancer are also associated with an increased risk. Other known risk factors include excessive consumption of alcohol, a high-fat diet, obesity, and a history of radiation treatment of the chest with high-dose x-rays. One thing most of these risk factors have in common is that they are associated with an increased lifetime exposure to estrogen. There is evidence that exposure to certain pollutants can increase the risk of breast cancer as well, apparently because these compounds mimic the effect of estrogen in the body. One particularly interesting bit of research, an Israeli study published in 1990, found that in the 1970s, Israeli women had one of the highest mortality rates from breast cancer in the world. In 1976, Israel banned the use of certain pesticides, most notably DDT, and in the ten years that followed, Israeli breast-cancer rates decreased by 20 percent—while they continued to increase in other industrialized nations. Prior to the ban, many dairy products produced in Israel had pesticide-residue levels that were as much as 300 to 500 percent above those in the United States, and pesticide-residue levels in the milk of nursing Israeli mothers were sometimes 500 to 800 percent above those of their American counterparts.

About 5 percent of breast cancer cases are thought to be related to an abnormality in a single gene, dubbed BRCA1. None of these factors is necessary for the disease to occur, however. In fact, more than 70 percent of women who develop breast cancer have no known risk factors. Eighty percent of all breast cancers are found in women over the age of fifty. The average age at the time of diagnosis is around sixty, but breast cancer can occur at almost any age after puberty. And while it is not a common problem, men can get breast cancer, too.

It is worth stressing that not every lump or tender area in a breast is a sign of cancer. In fact, most are not. Benign fatty tumors, cysts, fibroids, inflamed glands, and other conditions can cause you to feel lumps as well. However, any lump should be evaluated by a professional. A physician will likely employ physical examination, ultrasound, and biopsy techniques in making a diagnosis of breast cancer.

CONVENTIONAL TREATMENT

■ If you are diagnosed with breast cancer, you should seek out and work closely with an oncologist (cancer specialist) or other physician who specializes, or at the very least has considerable experience, in the treatment of this disease.

■ Surgery is the primary treatment for breast cancer. The type of surgery likely to be recommended depends on the size, location, and aggressiveness of the tumor. The least drastic technique is lumpectomy (sometimes called breast-conserving surgery). This involves removal only of the tumor itself, plus a margin of healthy tissue. However, in most cases some lymph nodes are surgically removed as well and examined to determine whether the disease has spread. A doctor may also recommend radiation therapy of the breast following lumpectomy to kill any cancer cells that may still be present. The other most common surgical approach is mastectomy, in which the entire breast and lymph nodes are removed. There are numerous studies that indicate long-term survival after mastectomy is no better than after lumpectomy and radiation, but this is not yet completely accepted, and many doctors (and patients) still opt for mastectomy because they feel it offers a better chance of a cure.

■ For cancers through stage II, which are considered curable, chemotherapy is often advised after surgery. Chemotherapy involves the administration of highly toxic drugs to kill any cancer cells that may have metastasized while they are tiny growths, and theoretically most susceptible to these agents. The most common chemotherapy drugs used are cyclophosphamide (Cytoxan), methotrexate (Rheumatrex), and fluorouracil, though there are others, such as melphalan (Alkeran) and doxorubicin (Adriamycin). Sometimes combinations of drugs are used. Chemotherapy regimens vary, but treatment is generally given every three to four weeks for up to six months. By definition, chemotherapy agents are highly toxic. Potential side effects include bone marrow suppression, severe anemia, hair loss, nausea and vomiting, liver damage, kidney damage, heart problems, and, paradoxically, cancer.

■ Hormone therapy may be recommended, especially for premenopausal women and women with tumors found to be sensitive to stimulation by the sex hormone estrogen. The commonly used drug for this purpose is tamoxifen (Nolvadex), which blocks the effects of naturally produced estrogens. Possible side effects include digestive upsets, hot flashes, increased tumor pain, liver damage, blood clots, blood changes, and rash.

■ It is possible to reconstruct a breast after mastectomy using a saline-filled implant. This may be done without fear that you may mask a recurrence of the cancer later on. There are also reconstruction procedures available in which flaps of a woman's own muscle and skin are used.

DIETARY GUIDELINES

■ If you are undergoing radiation and/or chemotherapy

treatment, it is important to consume sufficient protein, at least 1 gram for every 2 pounds of body weight. Thus, if you weigh 120 pounds, you would need to take in at least 60 grams of protein every day. If necessary, there are many excellent whey protein supplements that can be added to your diet in the form of a shake. These are also good if you are having trouble maintaining your weight as a result of either the disease or its treatments.

Keep your intake of fat to no more than 20 percent of your daily calories. Use monounsaturated fats such as olive oil rather than polyunsaturated oils. Avoid saturated, hydrogenated, and partially hydrogenated fats and oils.

A diet rich in green vegetables, which are full of trace minerals and chlorophyll, is very helpful in maintaining vitality in the face of cancer and its treatments.

Onions, garlic, and ginger are important (and tasty) adjuncts to an anticancer diet. Onions and garlic are high in allicin, which has been shown to have immune-stimulating properties. Ginger is very useful for relieving nausea, a common side effect of cancer treatments. It is also helpful for enhancing digestion.

Drink plenty of liquids, including at least six to eight 8-ounce glasses of pure water each day, to flush toxins from your body and maintain adequate hydration. It is especially important not to become dehydrated during cancer treatment.

Avoid caffeine, alcohol, and refined sugar, all of which place added stress on the body.

NUTRITIONAL SUPPLEMENTS

Take a high-potency multivitamin and mineral supplement daily. Choose a formula *without* iron. In some cases, tumors may use synthetic iron to enhance their growth.

The antioxidant nutrients are very important. They combat dangerous free radicals and help to maintain strong immune function. Take 25,000 international units of vitamin A twice daily for two months, then cut back to 25,000 international units daily. In addition, take 25,000 units of a multiple carotene complex twice daily; 500 milligrams of vitamin C with bioflavonoids four times daily; 400 international units of vitamin E twice daily, in morning and evening; and 200 micrograms of selenium daily. Also take 50 milligrams of alpha-lipoic acid three times daily.

Note: If you are pregnant, or intend to get pregnant, or if you have liver disease, consult your doctor before taking supplemental vitamin A. If you have high blood pressure, limit your intake of supplemental vitamin E to a total of 400 international units daily, and if you are taking an anticoagulant (blood thinner), consult your physician before taking vitamin E.

■ Borage and flaxseed oils contain gamma-linolenic acid (GLA), an excellent natural anti-inflammatory. Take 500 to 1,000 milligrams of either or both three or four times daily.

■ Coenzyme Q_{10} is a strong antioxidant that assists in minimizing side effects from chemotherapy. Take 75 to 100 milligrams three times daily while you are receiving chemotherapy and for three months afterward.

■ Proteolytic enzymes are strong free radical scavengers. Take a proteolytic-enzyme supplement as directed on the product label, with and between meals.

■ Soy isoflavones, particularly genistein and daidzein, help to metabolize estrogen and have anticancer properties. Take 500 milligrams twice daily.

■ Superoxide dismutase (SOD) is a strong antioxidant often used as part of a nutritional therapy program for both the prevention and treatment of cancer. Take an SOD supplement as directed on the product label. Since adequate amounts of zinc, copper, and manganese are required for the proper utilization of SOD, it is a good idea also to take a multimineral supplement that includes the trace minerals.

■ Thymus extract helps to stimulate immune function. Take 500 milligrams twice daily.

HERBAL TREATMENT

The herbal treatments listed here cannot cure breast cancer, but they can help to reduce symptoms associated with the disease and its treatment.

■ Astragalus is very helpful before and during chemotherapy. It is known to help stabilize the white blood cell count and improve energy. Take 250 to 500 milligrams twice a day, in morning and afternoon

■ Ginger root tea is excellent for helping to minimize nausea associated with chemotherapy. Take a cup of ginger tea two to three times daily, as needed.

■ Green tea has antioxidant properties and protects cells. Choose a standardized extract containing 50 percent catechins and 90 percent total phenols and take 300 to 400 milligrams daily.

■ Milk thistle protects the liver, which is placed under considerable stress by cancer treatments. Many people have found that milk thistle helps to minimize some of the side effects of chemotherapy. Choose an extract standardized to contain 80 percent flavonoids (silymarin) and take 200 milligrams twice daily while undergoing chemotherapy and for two to three months afterward.

■ Siberian ginseng is worth considering if you are experiencing fatigue. Choose an extract standardized to contain 0.5 percent eleutheroside E and take 100 milligrams three times daily. Take the first dose before breakfast, the second in midmorning, and the third just before lunch.

This should help to combat fatigue and strengthen immune function.

HOMEOPATHY

The homeopathic treatments listed here cannot cure breast cancer, but homeopathy can help to reduce symptoms associated with the disease and its treatments.

■ *Asterias rubens* is helpful for dull aching pain in the breast that may extend down the left arm to the fingers. The pain is worse on the left side. Take one dose of *Asterias rubens* 6x or 3c three times daily for up to three days.

■ *Carbo vegetabilis* is good for symptoms of stomach pain, a sensation of heaviness or fullness, sleepiness, nausea, burping, and a faint feeling in the stomach not relieved by eating. You may suffer digestive distress half an hour after eating. Take one dose of *Carbo vegetabilis* 30x or 15c three times daily, as needed.

■ *Conium maculatum* is for breasts that are painful and hard, and feel better with local pressure. You may feel quite debilitated, and your glands may be enlarged. Take one dose of *Conium maculatum* 200x weekly for four weeks.

■ *Lycopodium* is for weak digestion with bloating and abdominal gas, as well as a desire for sweet things. After you eat, you feel pressure in your stomach and have a bitter taste in your mouth. Eating even the smallest amount creates a sense of fullness. Take one dose of *Lycopodium* 30x or 15c three times daily for up to three days.

■ *Nux vomica* is very effective in reducing nausea associated with chemotherapy. Take one dose of *Nux vomica* 30x or 15c three times daily, as needed.

BACH FLOWER REMEDIES

Everyone responds to the news of breast cancer in her own way. The Bach flower remedies can be very useful during the different phases associated with the discovery, treatment, and recovery from this disease. Select the remedy that most closely fits your emotional tendencies and concerns, and take it as needed, following the directions on the product label.

■ Choose Agrimony if you are smiling and brave outwardly, but inwardly anguished and suffering.

■ Cerato helps to counteract a lack of self-confidence and low self-esteem.

■ Gorse eases feelings of deep despair.

■ Holly helps to tame anger that bursts out in fits of temper.

■ Hornbeam is useful for extreme exhaustion.

■ Mustard helps to lift sadness and depression.

■ Sweet Chestnut is good for feelings of exhaustion and alienation.

GENERAL RECOMMENDATIONS

■ Become familiar with the way your breasts normally feel, and examine them regularly (*see* BREAST SELF-EXAMINATION in Part Three). If you detect anything out of the ordinary, see your doctor. Ideally, you should consult a doctor you have seen regularly. Such a physician will be familiar with your breasts and better able to monitor any changes than would someone who sees you for the first time.

■ Some physicians recommend that all women have a mammogram at around age forty that can be used as a baseline; should any problems be suspected at a later date, this will enable your doctor to compare an early mammogram with a later one and make a more informed diagnosis. There is controversy, however, about whether there is really any benefit for most women in starting mammographic screening before age fifty. On the other hand, women who have a family history of breast cancer should probably begin having annual mammograms earlier than other women, possibly as early as between the ages of twenty-five and thirty-five. You may want to discuss with your physician the approach that seems best for you.

■ Do not smoke, and avoid secondhand smoke. Tobacco smoke contains dangerous toxins and carcinogens.

■ As much as possible, exercise. Regular exercise improves tissue oxygenation and aids recovery.

PREVENTION

■ Keep your weight down. An extensive study reported in the *Journal of the American Medical Association* in 1997 found that a woman's risk of breast cancer increases with every pound she gains after the age of eighteen. Scientists theorize that this is because the more body fat a woman has, the higher her estrogen level is likely to be, and exposure to high levels of estrogen is a known risk factor for breast cancer.

■ Get regular exercise. Exercise not only helps in weight control and promotes overall good health, but may act as a cancer preventive.

■ Vitamin D plays an important role in the prevention of cancer. If you do not get twenty minutes of exposure to sunlight daily, consider taking 200 to 400 international units in supplemental form each day.

■ One theory on the origins of breast cancer focuses on the role of lymphatic drainage in breast health. The lymphatic system is an important part of the body's infection-fighting and cleansing systems, and is the means by which many waste products and toxins are removed from the tissues. Approximately 85 percent of lymphatic fluid flowing from the breasts drains through lymph nodes in the armpits; the remaining 15 percent drains through nodes along the breastbone. According to this theory, wearing clothing, such as a tight bra, that restricts the proper flow of lymphatic fluid can interfere with this process, trapping toxins in breast tissue, which may in turn increase the risk of breast cancer. It is probably a good idea to make sure your underwear and other clothing fit loosely enough to be comfortable, and avoid wearing any garment that constricts the areas of lymphatic drainage on a regular basis or for a long period of time.

Breathing Distress

See ANAPHYLACTIC SHOCK; ASTHMA.

Bronchitis

Bronchitis is an inflammation of the trachea (windpipe) and the large bronchi (air passages) of the respiratory tract. Bronchitis can be caused by a bacterial or viral infection, or it can be triggered by an allergic reaction to molds, pollens, dander, or dust.

Bronchitis begins with a runny nose, fever, a dry cough, and, possibly, wheezing. The cough eventually becomes productive, with clear sputum at first and, later, thick, yellow sputum. Symptoms of allergic bronchitis include a cough that is often worse at night, malaise, loss of appetite, and wheezing. Chronic bronchitis is characterized by a persistent dry cough without other symptoms. A lingering or chronic cough can be debilitating.

CONVENTIONAL TREATMENT

■ In general, a dry cough need not be encouraged and can be treated with a cough suppressant. Dextromethorphan is an ingredient found in many over-the-counter cough preparations. It can usually be identified by the initials DM on the label. Codeine is a narcotic that is included in many prescription cough suppressants. Nearly all cough suppressants are mood-altering and may cause drowsiness.

■ A wet cough indicates that the body is attempting to eliminate excess mucus. In this case, an expectorant, such as guaifenesin (found in Donatussin, Meditussin, and Robitussin, among others) may be helpful. Expectorants help to thin secretions so that they are easier to cough out.

■ A bronchodilator, such as metaproterenol (Alupent) or albuterol (Proventil, Ventolin), may be prescribed to relax the airways, stop wheezing, and ease breathing. These medicines also have a tendency to speed up the heart rate and may make you feel anxious.

■ Unlike pneumonia, bronchitis does not usually require the use of antibiotics. However, if your doctor determines that the bronchitis is caused by a bacterial infection, he or she will prescribe an antibiotic. Since bacterial bronchitis is relatively rare, if your doctor prescribes an antibiotic, be sure to ask why he or she believes that this is an important part of your treatment.

DIETARY GUIDELINES

■ Eliminate potentially mucus-forming foods (such as dairy products, sweets, and fried foods) from your diet until you recover.

■ Take plenty of fluids to thin secretions so that they are easier to cough out.

■ Chicken or vegetable soup made with lots of vegetables (especially carrots, parsley, string beans, and zucchini), and the herbs ginger and garlic, is healing. Chicken soup has been shown to contain an ingredient that helps to thin mucus so that it is easier to eliminate. If you dislike certain vegetables, include them in the cooking process anyway, and strain them out before eating the soup.

NUTRITIONAL SUPPLEMENTS

■ If you must take antibiotics, be sure to take supplemental acidophilus and/or bifidobacteria to restore healthy intestinal flora. Take them as recommended on the product labels, at least one hour away from the antibiotics. If you are allergic to milk, select dairy-free products.

■ Beta-carotene helps to heal mucus membranes. Take 5,000 international units three times a day until you recover.

■ Vitamin C and bioflavonoids have anti-inflammatory properties. Take 500 milligrams of each three times a day until you are better.

■ Zinc helps to boost the immune system and speed recovery. Take 15 milligrams twice a day for as long as symptoms last. Take zinc with food to prevent stomach upset.

HERBAL TREATMENT

■ Astragalus acts to simulate the immune system and also stimulates the regeneration of bronchial cells. Take 500 milligrams three times a day.

■ Yellow and/or greenish mucus is often a sign of infection. Echinacea, goldenseal, and garlic form an antibiotic mixture that is very effective in resolving an infection. Take 250 to 500 milligrams of echinacea, 150 to 300 milligrams of goldenseal, and the equivalent of 500 milligrams of fresh garlic four times a day while the infection is acute. If the infection has not resolved after one week of taking echinacea and goldenseal, consult your health-care provider.

■ A tea of ginger, lemon, licorice, and/or slippery elm can help thin mucus and soothe irritated mucous membranes. Add 1 tablespoon (or 1 tea bag) of each herb to 16 ounces of water. Bring the mixture to a boil, then reduce the heat and simmer for two minutes. Strain and cool to sipping temperature. Take a cup of the tea three or four times a day, as needed.

  Note: Do not take licorice on a daily basis for more than five days in a row, as it can elevate blood pressure. If you have high blood pressure, omit the licorice entirely.

■ Grapefruit-seed extract acts as a natural antibiotic, and may help prevent infection. Take 100 milligrams three times a day.

■ Hsiao Keh Chuan is a Chinese herbal cough medicine. It has a strong taste, but it is very effective in resolving a cough. Follow the dosage directions on the product label.

■ Osha root has traditionally been used by Native Americans in the western part of the United States to treat colds, flu, and other upper respiratory infections. Take 500 milligrams three times daily, as needed.

■ Slippery elm tea can ease a dry cough. Take one cup as needed.

■ Thyme has a mild antimicrobial action and helps to reduce the spasmodic nature of a cough. Try taking 300 milligrams three times a day. This herb has a strong taste. If you find it impossible to swallow, try taking a relaxing bath made with thyme, chamomile, or rosemary.

HOMEOPATHY

Choose the most appropriate symptom-specific homeopathic remedy from the list below and take one dose, as directed on the product label, three times a day until your symptoms improve. If there is no improvement in forty-eight hours, it is unlikely that the remedy will do anything more; discontinue it and try another.

■ If you have a moist, rattling cough and are breathless and pale, take *Antimonium tartaricum* 12x or 6c.

  Note: Do not take this remedy if you are running a fever.

■ *Bryonia* 12x or 6c is recommended if your cough is worse at night and you have pain in your chest or throat. You probably want cold drinks, and may be constipated.

■ *Drosera* 12x or 6c is for a whooping-type cough that is dry and accompanied by wheezing.

■ *Eucalyptus* 12x or 6c promotes loosening of mucus.

■ *Kali bichromicum* 12x or 6c is for a cough accompanied by thick, stringy mucus.

■ Consider *Phosphorus* 30x or 9c if you have a harsh cough that is lingering. The *Phosphorus* person tends to be quite sensitive.

■ Choose *Pulsatilla* 30x or 9c if you have a cough, a runny nose, and thin yellow phlegm. You may feel emotionally vulnerable and cry easily.

■ Take *Rumex crispus* 12x or 6c if you have a cough and a lot of mucus, feel worse at night, and find yourself waking at around 11:00 PM. Your lymph glands may be swollen.

■ *Spongia tosta* 12x or 6c is good if you have a barking cough that increases with excitement, and feels better with hot drinks.

ACUPRESSURE

For the locations of acupressure points on the body, *see* ADMINISTERING AN ACUPRESSURE TREATMENT in Part Three.

■ Liver 3 relaxes the nervous system.

■ Lung 1 and 7 clear the chest.

■ Pericardium 6 relaxes the chest.

■ Massaging along the spine is soothing and relaxing, especially for the chest and nervous system.

AROMATHERAPY

For specific instructions on how to use aromatherapy, *see* PREPARING AROMATHERAPY TREATMENTS in Part Three.

■ A steam inhalation treatment made with basil, eucalyptus, pine, and/or tea tree oil can help to clear mucus and ease breathing. Rubbing a massage oil prepared with any or all of these oils over your chest may also be helpful.

GENERAL RECOMMENDATIONS

■ Rest interspersed with periods of moderate activity is important in treating bronchitis. The moderate activity is helpful in keeping secretions from settling and leading to the development of pneumonia.

■ In addition to taking plenty of fluids, use a humidifier to help thin secretions and soothe the respiratory tract.

■ If you have a "wet" cough with clear sputum that is accompanied by a sore throat, dilute 1 teaspoon of salt in a cup of water and gargle with this mixture every two hours.

■ Place a hot-water bottle on your chest or back for twenty minutes every day. This helps to ease breathing, especially when used in combination with a humidifier.

PREVENTION

■ If you suffer from respiratory allergies, try to prevent

exposure to those things that provoke a reaction, and try to keep any allergic reactions that do occur from escalating into bronchitis (*see* ALLERGIES).

■ Smoke of any kind, whether tobacco smoke or sweet-smelling wood smoke from a fireplace, irritates the respiratory tract and causes the passages to constrict. Nothing is more important than a smoke-free environment.

■ Astragalus strengthens respiratory function and enhances the immune system. Take 250 milligrams three times a day for one month before the cold and flu season begins.

■ To improve respiratory function over the long term, get regular exercise. (*See* BEGINNING AN EXERCISE PROGRAM in Part Three.) Walking is generally recognized as a safe activity for anyone of any age, but don't overdo it at first. If you are a non-exerciser over the age of fifty, see your doctor before embarking on any exercise program.

■ When you catch a cold, begin appropriate treatment promptly (*see* COMMON COLD). This may help decrease the possibility of developing bronchitis.

■ If you are susceptible to respiratory distress, avoid contact with sick individuals as much as possible.

Bruise

When you develop a bruise, it is because an injury to a blood vessel has caused blood to leak into the surrounding tissue. Bruises are usually related to an injury to the small capillaries located near the surface of the skin. These tiny blood vessels heal fairly quickly. As the body reabsorbs the blood, the characteristic mark disappears.

There are many blood vessels in the head. If you suffer a blow to the head, there can be a lot of bleeding into surrounding tissue, causing the classic "goose egg." A blow to the forehead or nose can cause blood to accumulate in the surrounding loose tissues, resulting in the condition commonly known as a black eye. If a mass of blood accumulates in the tissues, it is called a *hematoma*.

A new bruise is tender to the touch and may be swollen. A bruise generally starts out as a red mark, then turns the classic black-and-blue or purple color. As the bruise fades, it becomes lighter and sometimes a bit yellow or brown from residual iron left over after the blood fluids are reabsorbed.

Most bruises are merely a result of everyday bumps and injuries. Nutritional deficiencies such as a lack of vitamin C or vitamin K can lead to easier than normal bruising, however, and in rare cases an underlying illness such as hemophilia, leukemia, or purpura may be behind a ten-

dency to bruise easily and often. In both hemophilia and leukemia, the blood does not clot as it should, so it is more likely to leak out of an injured vessel to form a bruise. *Purpura* is a condition in which bruising can occur even without any particular injury. It is believed to occur because the small blood vessels, for some unknown reason, are more fragile than normal. While the bruises may be unsightly, purpura is not usually considered a serious disorder.

CONVENTIONAL TREATMENT

■ Simple bruising is considered a normal fact of life, and little can be done about it. You may be able to minimize the extent of bruising, however, by doing the following: Immediately after an injury, elevate the affected area. Put ice on the bruise for five to ten minutes. Then take the ice off for fifteen to twenty minutes. Repeat this cycle at least three to five times immediately following the injury, and as much as possible for the first day or two afterward. To avoid causing frostbite damage to the tissues, place a towel or washcloth between the ice and the skin, and be careful not to leave the ice in place too long.

■ People who bruise easily are often deficient in vitamin K, which is necessary for normal blood clotting. There are a number of possible reasons for vitamin-K deficiency. If you have gallbladder disease or difficulty in digesting fats, you may have trouble absorbing this fat-soluble vitamin. In addition, vitamin K is synthesized by "friendly" bacteria in the intestines. If you take a course of antibiotics, these drugs will destroy the friendly bacteria along with the bad, and vitamin-K production may suffer as a result. Other drugs, including aspirin, steroids, anticoagulants, and asthma medication, can also thin the blood and make you more prone to bruising. If you develop a bruise at the slightest injury, or often discover a black-and-blue mark and have no idea how you got it, discuss this with your doctor. He or she may recommend blood testing to check for a possible bleeding disorder. Phytonadione (Mephyton) is a prescription drug that is often recommended to correct low levels of vitamin K.

■ A hematoma may have to be removed or drained surgically, depending on its severity and location.

NUTRITIONAL SUPPLEMENTS

■ To help restore the integrity of blood-vessel walls, take a vitamin-C formula that contains bioflavonoids. Take 500 milligrams of each twice a day for two to three weeks. Then take 500 milligrams daily for one month. If the bruising seems excessive, continue taking vitamin C for an additional two to three more months.

HERBAL TREATMENT

■ Bilberry and grape-seed extracts are rich sources of

bioflavonoids that decrease the fragility of the capillaries. Choose standardized bilberry extract containing 25 percent anthocyanidins (also called PCOs) and take 80 milligrams three times a day. Or take 50 to 100 milligrams of standardized grape-seed extract containing 90 percent PCOs three times a day.

HOMEOPATHY

■ *Arnica* is the classic homeopathic remedy for bruises. To ease the pain and prevent a bruise from becoming larger, take one dose of *Arnica* 30x or 6c, as directed on the product label, immediately after an injury. Then take one dose three to four times daily for the first twenty-four hours. After two or three doses, you should feel less pain.

■ If the skin is not broken, apply a topical *Arnica* oil or gel directly to the bruise. If the skin is broken, a topical homeopathic *Calendula* oil or gel will soothe the hurt and help speed healing.

■ If the bruise is still apparent after forty-eight hours, *Ledum* 12x, 30x, 6c, or 9c, taken orally, will help resolve the discoloration. Take three to four doses daily for two to three days.

AROMATHERAPY

For specific instructions on how to use aromatherapy, *see* PREPARING AROMATHERAPY TREATMENTS in Part Three.

■ Immediately after an injury, prepare a cold compress using geranium, lavender, and/or thyme oil. Apply the compress to the injured area for at least ten minutes, substituting a new cold compress if the original one becomes warm. Repeat as often as possible for the day or two after the injury.

GENERAL RECOMMENDATIONS

■ If you suffer a blow that results in a black eye, be alert for any signs that your vision has been affected. If you suspect any vision impairment, consult an ophthalmologist.

■ If you are prone to bruising at the slightest bump, or if you seem to be bruising more easily than you used to, see your doctor to find out if there is some underlying cause that can be treated.

Bruxism

See under TEMPOROMANDIBULAR JOINT SYNDROME.

Bulimia

Bulimia is an eating disorder characterized by overeating followed by self-induced vomiting, known as the "binge-and-purge" syndrome. The reason for this behavior is an abnormal fear of becoming fat, an obsession with remaining (or becoming) thin, plus a fierce hunger for food. A person with bulimia may binge on food, then purge to expel the food as quickly as possible, once or several times a day. He or she may use high doses of laxatives as well. It is not unusual for someone with this disorder to gorge, leave the dining table, purge, and return to the table for dessert or more food. In an effort to burn off calories, many people with bulimia are also devoted to exercise. They typically carry that behavior to extremes as well.

Bulimia is sometimes, though not always, a variant of anorexia nervosa, in which dieting is carried out to the point of emaciation (*see* ANOREXIA NERVOSA). Although most people with bulimia are extremely thin, some are of normal weight and some are even slightly overweight. Most people with bulimia are females between the ages of fifteen and thirty.

Continual vomiting can lead to dehydration, electrolyte imbalances, and serious malnutrition. Early symptoms include weakness, dizziness, and cramping. Low blood pressure, an irregular heartbeat, and a cessation of menstrual periods occur as the condition continues. A swollen neck, broken blood vessels on the face, and damage to the enamel of the back teeth—all results of excessive vomiting—are characteristic of this disorder as well.

People with bulimia tend to be highly secretive about their behavior. Intellectually aware that he or she is risking serious health damage, but helpless to stop, a person with this disorder may become depressed, even suicidal.

CONVENTIONAL TREATMENT

■ The primary conventional treatment is counseling, particularly cognitive-behavioral therapy, to modify behavior patterns and deal with mental or emotional problems, such as depression and low self-esteem, that are contributing to this behavior.

■ Antidepressants, predominantly fluoxetine (Prozac), are often prescribed, and seem to be helpful not only for relieving depression but combating bulimia. Fluoxetine is a type of drug called a selective serotonin reuptake inhibitor (SSRI). It works by increasing the level of the neurotransmitter serotonin, which is closely tied to mood, in the brain. Besides improving mood, SSRIs tend to depress the appetite. Potential side effects include anxiety, insomnia, tremor, fatigue, nausea, diarrhea, rash, and changes in blood-sugar levels.

The consequences of repeated vomiting may need to be treated. Problems with the teeth should be addressed by a dentist. Chronic inflammation of the throat and esophagus may be treated with liquid antacids or bismuth preparations. Electrolyte imbalances may require treatment with intravenous fluids. Bronchitis, hemorrhoids, and constipation are treated symptomatically.

If you suffer from bulimia, you should have your gastrointestinal tract and thyroid, adrenal, and hormonal functions tested. A dysfunction in any of these important systems can cause a predisposition to bulimia.

Most people with bulimia are deficient in important nutrients. See a physician who can administer the necessary tests to detect nutritional deficiencies.

DIETARY GUIDELINES

If you are working to overcome bulimia, you require substantial support, including a nutritional counselor who can devise a proper diet. You need to eat many *small* meals daily, with appropriate snacks in between.

A food coach who schedules mealtimes, monitors what you eat, and provides encouragement is tremendously helpful. A food coach functions much as an AA sponsor does, keeping in close touch to make sure his or her charge is eating on schedule and taking in enough nourishment. If you should feel the urge to binge and purge, a call to the coach may be enough to overcome the impulse. A doctor experienced in treating bulimia should be able to offer a referral to help you find a qualified coach.

Hidden or low-level food allergies may contribute to bulimia. Discuss the possibility of allergies with your doctor.

NUTRITIONAL SUPPLEMENTS

Calcium and magnesium are essential to the central nervous system. They work best when taken together. Take 400 to 600 milligrams of calcium citrate, amino acid chelate, or microcrystalline hydroxyapatite and 250 to 400 milligrams of magnesium citrate or aspartate twice daily.

To help regulate blood-sugar levels, take 200 micrograms of chromium once or twice daily.

Take a good digestive-enzyme supplement with each meal to ensure good digestion and full assimilation of all important nutrients.

■ The amino acid tyrosine helps strengthen thyroid function and can improve mood. It is better absorbed if not taken with other proteins. Take 500 to 1,000 milligrams of L-tyrosine on arising each morning for up to three weeks.

Note: If you are taking a monoamine oxidase (MAO) inhibitor drug, do not take supplemental tyrosine, as a sudden and dangerous rise in blood pressure may result.

The B vitamins are essential for nutrient metabolism

and help normalize nervous-system function. Take a B-complex supplement that supplies 25 milligrams of each of the primary B vitamins two to three times a day.

■ Pantothenic acid supports adrenal function, which is usually compromised in persons recovering from bulimia. In addition to the B-complex supplement, take 100 milligrams of pantothenic acid three times a day for one month.

■ Most people with bulimia are deficient in zinc. Zinc is essential for reestablishing normal enzyme activity and hormonal function. Take 25 milligrams of zinc twice daily, immediately before meals.

Note: Take zinc with food to prevent stomach upset. If you take over 30 milligrams of zinc on a daily basis for more than one or two months, you should also take 1 milligram of copper each day to maintain a proper mineral balance.

■ Supplements of the amino acid tryptophan are no longer available over the counter because a number of people became ill as a result of taking a contaminated product. Tryptophan is available by prescription, however. This natural substance encourages the production of serotonin, which in turn helps to stabilize mood, combat depression, and ease insomnia. Studies have shown that, in many cases, tryptophan supplementation can significantly lessen the bulimic impulse. The effective dosage is 500 milligrams of L-tryptophan taken three times daily for six weeks. You may want to discuss this finding with your doctor. As an alternative, 5-hydroxytryptophan is available over the counter. The recommended dose is in the range of 250 to 500 milligrams two or three times daily.

HERBAL TREATMENT

■ Astragalus helps strengthen immune function, thereby decreasing vulnerability to the low-grade infections that plague so many people with bulimia in the early stages of recovery. Take 500 milligrams twice a day for two weeks out of every month for three months.

Note: Do not take this herb if you have a fever or any other signs of infection.

■ Kava kava is a calming herb that helps relax the mind and relieve tension. Choose a product containing 30 percent kavalactones and take 350 milligrams as needed, up to three times daily.

Note: In excess amounts, this herb can cause drowsiness. Do not exceed the recommended dose. Do not use kava kava if you are pregnant or nursing, if you have Parkinson's disease, or if you are taking a prescription medication for depression or anxiety.

■ Oat straw restores and strengthens the nervous system. It also helps reduce hypersensitivity to allergens, which may be an important factor if you suffer from allergies. Take 500 milligrams two to three times daily.

■ St. John's wort is an effective antidepressant that also helps ease anxiety. Choose a product containing 0.3 percent hypericin and take 300 milligrams two or three times daily.

■ Siberian ginseng helps strengthen hormonal function, improve energy levels, and even out blood-sugar levels. Choose a standardized extract containing 0.5 percent eleutheroside E and take 100 to 200 milligrams in the morning and again in the afternoon.

HOMEOPATHY

See a homeopathic physician for a constitutional remedy formulated especially for you.

Calcarea carbonica 200x or 30c is good if you are a timid overweight woman who craves eggs and creamy foods; have a sluggish constitution; and find it difficult to concentrate for an extended period of time. Take one dose three times a day for two to three months.

Choose *Natrum muriaticum* 200x or 30c if you dislike being the center of attention, crave salty snacks, and tend to be melancholy. You probably have a thin neck, and if you put on weight, it tends to be concentrated in the thighs and buttocks. Take one dose three times a day for two to three months.

■ *Nux vomica* 200x or 30c is for the person recovering from bulimia who craves rich, spicy foods; has a tendency to constipation; has a type-A personality; and is often irritable and agitated. Take one dose three times a day for two to three months.

Pulsatilla 200x or 30c is good if you cry easily, are extremely sensitive to what other people think, crave sweets, and tend to be uncomfortable unless the windows are open. Take one dose three times a day for two to three months.

BACH FLOWER REMEDIES

Select the remedy that most closely fits your emotional tendencies and concerns, and take it as needed, following the directions on the product label.

Choose Gorse if you are sad and depressed and having difficulty looking forward to a time when all your bulimic impulses will be a thing of the past.

Holly is good if you are furious at yourself over your behavior.

Impatiens should help if you are impatient and in a tremendous hurry to get well.

■ White Chestnut is the remedy for obsessive thinking. In spite of much effort, you find yourself obsessing about gorging and purging.

ACUPRESSURE

For the locations of acupressure points on the body, *see* ADMINISTERING AN ACUPRESSURE TREATMENT in Part Three.

■ The back Bladder points relax and tone the nervous system.

■ Gallbladder 20 relaxes the head and neck muscles.

■ Large Intestine 4 relaxes the nervous system.

■ Liver 3 also relaxes the nervous system.

■ Spleen 6 strengthens the blood.

AROMATHERAPY

For specific instructions on how to use aromatherapy, *see* PREPARING AROMATHERAPY TREATMENTS in Part Three.

■ Acupressure of the back Bladder points is even more effective when used in conjunction with an aromatherapy massage oil containing essential oil of lavender, lemon balm, or orange.

■ Breathing in thyme oil helps regulate liver function.

GENERAL RECOMMENDATIONS

■ See a physician to investigate the possibility of underlying conditions that contribute to bulimia.

■ Join a support group of persons recovering from bulimia and/or talk to a therapist or psychological counselor who can help you uncover the reasons why bulimia became a part of your life.

■ Be aware that withdrawal symptoms, such as anxiety, depression, fatigue, and insomnia, are common. Persevere. These uncomfortable symptoms should fade away in a few weeks.

PREVENTION

■ It has been shown that episodes of bulimia often coincide with uncontrollable stress and low self-esteem. If you are feeling stressed out or worthless, have heavy emotional problems, or fear that your life is out of control, see a therapist. Talking things out with an objective, nonjudgmental professional is the nicest thing you can do for yourself.

Bunion

If the bony structure of the big toe is forced out of normal alignment, the result is a hard bump, or bunion. Described medically as *hallux valgus* (displacement of the great toe toward the other toes), bunions are characterized by enlargement of the joint at the base of the big toe, resulting in that joint protruding abnormally from the foot. In some people, the top of the big toe overlaps one or more of the smaller ones.

A bunion results from continuing inflammation, and subsequent thickening, of the bursa of the joint at the base of the great toe. A bursa is a small fluid-filled sac that acts as a kind of cushion for a joint or other structure. Women in particular are subject to bunions. That's because many fashionable ladies forgo comfort and choose instead stylish shoes that pinch and squeeze. Too-tight, too-small shoes with pointed toes and too-high heels force the toes out of alignment. Although bunions do tend to run in families and it is possible to inherit a weakness of the joint, the primary cause of bunions is wearing shoes that do not conform to the normal contour of the toes. It is no wonder, then, that women are three times more likely to suffer from bunions than men are.

Bunions can be so painful that it becomes difficult to walk normally. Without proper treatment, a bunion that is continually irritated will only get worse.

CONVENTIONAL MEDICINE

■ Many people resort to over-the-counter painkillers such as ibuprofen (Advil, Motrin, Nuprin, and others) or naproxen (Aleve) to help them deal with the pain of bunions. However, because the pain is a result of an anatomic abnormality, this is obviously a temporary solution. For proper treatment, you should see a podiatrist.

■ A small bunion may be corrected by wearing a special device that straightens the big toe and forces it back into alignment.

■ For mild to moderate discomfort, aspirin can be used topically to relieve pain and inflammation. Use a product such as Aspercreme, or crush an aspirin with the back of a spoon. Drizzle in a drop or two of olive oil, and mix it into a paste. Apply the mixture directly to the affected joint. This simple remedy is reported to be amazingly effective.

■ For severe pain and swelling, injections of a steroid or long-lasting anesthetic may be necessary.

■ Surgery to remove the swollen tissue and remodel the bones of the great toe may be the only answer to a painful bunion of long standing. If an operation is required, your foot will be in a cast (or special shoe) for six to twelve weeks afterwards, depending on the extent of the surgery.

DIETARY GUIDELINES

■ Eat a diet that emphasizes steamed and raw green vegetables. Incomplete digestion fosters an acidic environment in the body, which can worsen pain and inflammation. This type of diet won't repair a bunion, but it can help relieve symptoms.

■ Avoid fried foods, and all greasy and fatty foods, especially those containing saturated fat or hydrogenated oils. Foods of this type will worsen symptoms.

NUTRITIONAL SUPPLEMENTS

■ Bromelain, an enzyme extracted from pineapple, has strong anti-inflammatory properties. Take 250 to 500 milligrams two or three times daily, between meals, to help bring down inflammation.

■ Flaxseed oil contains essential fatty acids that reduce the body's inflammatory response. Take 1 tablespoonful daily.

■ Pine-bark and grape-seed extracts also are excellent anti-inflammatory agents. Take 25 to 50 milligrams of either two to three times daily, between meals.

■ Applying a film of vitamin-E oil to the joint at night, then applying a 70 percent solution of DMSO, can be effective for relieving pain and decreasing swelling.

HERBAL TREATMENT

■ Castor oil can be used topically. This soothing treatment often brings relief. Warm a little castor oil and soak a piece of cheesecloth (or a clean white cloth) in the warm oil. Apply this compress to the affected joint. Overwrap it with a towel to hold in the heat.

■ Turmeric is an anti-inflammatory and helps to relieve pain. Take 300 milligrams of standardized extract three times daily.

HOMEOPATHY

■ *Benzoicum acidum* is good for pain that is centered on the joint at the great toe. Take one dose of *Benzoicum acidum* 6x or 3c, as directed on the product label, three to four times daily until the pain is lessened.

■ *Ruta graveolens* is for pain that radiates throughout the foot and ankle. Take one dose of *Ruta graveolens* 12x or 6c three to four times daily until the pain is relieved.

■ *Silicea* is the remedy for pain and soreness in the foot from the instep clear through to the sole. Take one dose of *Silicea* 30x or 15c three to four times daily until the pain is relieved.

BACH FLOWER REMEDIES

Select the remedy that most closely fits your emotional tendencies and concerns, and take it as needed, following the directions on the product label.

■ Holly helps relieve anger. It's easy to be mad at the world when your feet hurt!

■ White Chestnut relieves obsessive thinking. This remedy is for the individual who cannot think about anything but his or her sore bunion.

GENERAL RECOMMENDATIONS

■ Take your oldest, softest, and most comfortable shoes. Cut out an opening over the affected joint so that nothing is pressing on the bunion. Wear these shoes until the pain and inflammation have lessened.

■ If you are shy about leaving the house in cut-out shoes, be sure to wear shoes that provide sufficient space for your toes to lie normally. Depending on the placement of the straps (and the weather), sandals may be the answer.

PREVENTION

■ Wear shoes that conform to the normal contour of your foot.

■ Exercise your feet by picking up a soft ball with your toes. A Nerf ball is a good choice. Many people who are subject to bunions have flat feet. Picking up a ball repeatedly with your toes will strengthen your arches, and that will help keep the bones in alignment.

Burns

You can suffer a burn from dry heat (fire or sun); moist heat (steam or hot liquids); corrosive chemicals; or electricity. An encounter with electricity can be particularly dangerous. A severe electrical shock can knock you unconscious and cause you to stop breathing. There may be deep burns at the point where the current entered your body, as well as internal damage.

Depending on the location, extent, and cause of the burn, you may need immediate medical care. A burn can cause scarring, which may limit functioning of the burned area. Regardless of their size and severity, burns on the face, the palms of the hands or the soles of the feet, or on or near a joint, can have serious implications. Burns in these areas should always be checked by a doctor and watched with special care. Any burn should be watched for signs of a possible infection.

When evaluating a burn, here's what to look for.

- A *first-degree burn* involves only the epidermis, the upper layer of the skin. The area is hot, red, and painful, but without swelling or blistering. Sunburn is usually a first-degree burn. (*See* SUNBURN.)
- A *second-degree burn* involves the epidermis and part of the underlying skin layers. The pain is severe. The area is pink or red and mottled, and is usually moist and seeping, moderately swollen, and blistered.
- Because it involves injury to all layers of the skin, a *third-degree burn* is also called a *full-thickness burn*. This severe burn destroys the nerves and blood vessels in the skin. Because the nerves are damaged, there is little or no pain

at first. The affected area may be white, yellow, black, or cherry red. The skin may appear dry and leathery.
- A *fourth-degree burn* extends through the skin and penetrates into underlying structures, such as muscle and bone. It looks and feels like a third-degree burn, but it does greater damage to the body.

EMERGENCY TREATMENT

See the inset on page 159.

CONVENTIONAL TREATMENT

■ Begin taking emergency measures to cool the burn at once (see the inset on page 159).

■ Silver sulfadiazine (Silvadene) is the treatment of choice for topical therapy of burned skin. This is an antibiotic used to treat an existing infection or to prevent one from developing. Your doctor will instruct you in the correct way to apply it and to dress the wound. Some burn dressings have been treated with a film of silver sulfadiazine as well. Or apply type II collagen (Hycure) as a gel or powder to protect the injury, speed healing, and reduce scarring.

■ More extensive burns, either in depth or surface area, may necessitate treatment to compensate for fluid loss and other supportive care. A deep or extensive burn may need to be debrided, a process that cleanses the area and removes dead skin. This is a procedure that must be done by a medical professional.

■ Depending on the depth and extent of the burn, your doctor may recommend a tetanus shot and/or an oral antibiotic, such as penicillin, to guard against infection.

■ Any burn that affects the mouth should be treated promptly by a doctor or dentist to ensure that it heals properly, without inflicting permanent damage. In some cases, a special appliance may be necessary to prevent the wound from contracting as it heals, leaving the individual with a condition known as *microstomia* (literally, "small mouth").

DIETARY GUIDELINES

■ If you sustain a deep, extensive burn, drink lots of liquids to replace fluids that may have been lost through the burn.

■ After any trauma to the body, a diet high in protein helps promote healing. If eating is difficult, substitute a protein drink.

■ Eat a diet high in green and yellow vegetables to provide ample carotenes, vitamin C, and flavonoids.

NUTRITIONAL SUPPLEMENTS

■ Alpha-lipoic acid is an excellent free-radical scavenger. Take 150 milligrams three times daily.

Beta-carotene and vitamin A help burned skin to heal. Take 5,000 international units of vitamin A and 15,000 international units of beta-carotene twice a day until healing is complete.

Note: If you are pregnant, or intend to get pregnant, or if you have liver disease, consult your doctor before taking supplemental vitamin A. Pregnant women should not ingest a total of more than 25,000 international units of supplemental vitamin A *per week* from all sources.

Coenzyme Q_{10} increases the oxygenation of tissues. Take 30 milligrams four times daily.

The amino acid glutamine promotes wound healing. Take 1,000 milligrams of L-glutamine three times daily for three weeks.

Body fluids are lost after a serious burn, which often results in electrolyte imbalances. Potassium in particular must be replaced. Take 99 milligrams of potassium twice a day for ten days. Weeping of the skin in the affected area is a common symptom of potassium deficiency. Also take a multimineral complex with additional magnesium and potassium citrate.

To support the body during the healing process, take 1,000 milligrams of vitamin C three times daily and 500 milligrams of bioflavonoids twice a day for one to two weeks.

Vitamin C can also be applied topically in a liquid spray. To make a vitamin-C spray, combine 2 tablespoons of powdered vitamin C and $1/2$ cup of aloe vera gel in a 16-ounce spray bottle. Apply this mixture twice a day until the burn heals.

Zinc aids in wound healing. Take 15 milligrams twice a day for one to two weeks. Take zinc with food to prevent stomach upset.

HERBAL TREATMENT

Apply aloe vera pulp, gel, or liquid to the burned area to remove the heat and sting from the burn. The pulp of the aloe vera plant has a long history of use as a soothing, cooling, and healing treatment for burns. It works quickly, minimizes scarring, and is remarkably effective. It is even used in the burn units of some hospitals.

Once the stinging sensation associated with a burn has subsided, apply a calendula preparation topically to help prevent infection. Select either an herbal or homeopathic formula.

■ Apply a comfrey root and goldenseal salve or cream to the affected area. Comfrey root contains allantoin, which promotes tissue growth and is very healing to the skin. Goldenseal is a noteworthy antibacterial herb that can help prevent infection.

■ Echinacea and goldenseal stimulate the immune system, which is important in preventing and fighting infection. Echinacea is antiviral; goldenseal is antibacterial. Take one dose of an echinacea and goldenseal combination formula supplying 250 to 500 milligrams of echinacea and 150 to 300 milligrams of goldenseal three times daily for one week to ten days following a burn.

■ Gotu kola helps to speed healing of skin tissue. Choose a standardized extract containing 16 percent triterpenes and take 200 milligrams three times a day for one to two weeks following a burn.

HOMEOPATHY

■ The following thirty-minute regimen is of tremendous help following a minor burn. After completing this procedure, you should feel considerably better:

1. Begin the process while still running cool water over the burn. Take one dose of *Urtica urens* 12x or 6c, as directed on the product label.

2. Five minutes after taking the *Urtica urens,* take one dose of Bach Flower Rescue Remedy to help ease fear and anxiety.

3. After you have run cool water over the burn for ten minutes, turn off the water and apply aloe vera gel to the wound, as directed under Herbal Treatment, above.

4. Five minutes after applying the aloe vera, apply a second soothing coat of aloe vera to the area and take a second dose of *Urtica urens* 12x or 6c.

5. After ten more minutes have passed, apply a third coat of aloe vera to the burn and take a third dose of *Urtica urens* 12x or 6c. If the burn is simple, you will begin to feel better after the first application of aloe vera and the first dose of *Urtica urens.* If you do not feel considerably better after the third application of aloe vera and the third dose of *Urtica urens,* consult your physician.

■ To help reduce blistering, crush a *Kali muriaticum* 6x pellet in a little distilled water. Apply the mixture topically to the wound one hour after completing the procedure outlined above. Apply the mixture again at bedtime.

■ Take one dose of *Kali muriaticum* 6x by mouth three times a day for the first two days after a burn.

■ To help lessen stinging and promote fast healing, apply homeopathic *Urtica urens* ointment or gel to the burn.

■ If the burn isn't healing as quickly as it should, evaluate the condition of the injury. Choose and administer the appropriate symptom-specific homeopathic remedy:

• *Apis mellifica* 12x or 6c helps to heal a burn that bubbles and resembles a bee sting. Take one dose every thirty minutes, for a total of three doses.

• If the burn remains red and throbbing and isn't calmed by the aloe vera and *Urtica urens* regimen, take one dose of *Belladonna* 30x or 9c every thirty minutes, for a total

Emergency Treatment for Burns

■ **Remove the cause.** All burns should be treated first by removing the cause—putting out flames, washing off chemicals, or breaking electrical contact. If your clothing is on fire, douse yourself with water or wrap yourself in a blanket and roll on the floor to put out the flames.

■ **For electrical burns.** In the case of electrical shock, switch off the current (or have someone do this for you). If that is not possible—as in the case of a live wire—use a nonconductive item, such as a wooden broom handle, to lift or push the source of the current away. Always go to the emergency room for medical evaluation after an electrical burn, even if you seem to have suffered only a minor burn. Electrical burns may be far more extensive than they look.

■ **For chemical burns.** If you suffer a chemical burn from a corrosive liquid, immediately flood the area with cool running water to dilute and wash away the chemical. Then go to the emergency room of the nearest hospital. A chemical burn requires professional medical evaluation. Many chemical burns may continue to damage skin for hours after what may appear to be adequate rinsing.

■ **For third- or fourth-degree burns.** If the burn is deep and severe, you will need immediate medical attention. Do not remove any clothing that is stuck to the burn, but lightly cover the area with a clean white cloth. Call for emergency medical assistance or have someone take you immediately to the emergency room of the nearest hospital. Do not attempt to treat a severe third- or fourth-degree burn at home.

■ **For first- or second-degree burns.** To minimize damage from a first- or second-degree burn, cool the burn as rapidly as possible. Immerse the affected area in cool running water until the stinging and burning sensations lessen. This may take ten minutes or longer. Do not stop prematurely. *Do not* use ice water directly on a burn. Doing so can deepen and worsen the burn.

If the burn occurs through clothing (as in a spill of hot liquid), don't wait to remove the clothing. Immediately immerse the area in cool running water. Remove the wet clothes while cooling the burn.

While cooling the burn, remove any watches, bracelets, rings, belts, or other constricting items from the area before the burn swells.

■ **For burns in sensitive areas.** Go to the emergency room if a burn appears severe or extensive, or if the burned area is on the face, the palms of the hands, the soles of the feet, or on or near a joint.

■ **Avoid worsening the injury.** *Do not* apply butter, oil, grease, lotions, or creams to burns. *Do not* cover burns with adhesive dressings or fluffy materials. *Do not* bandage or cover the affected area tightly. *Do not* use iodine to cleanse raw burn tissue. It can irritate the skin, dry it out, and allow iodine to be absorbed into the body.

of three doses, to help reduce the redness and throbbing pain.

• If the burn appears as if it is becoming infected, call your physician and report a possible infection. Begin taking *Mercurius solubilis* 12x or 6c to help ward off infection. Take one dose three times daily for two days.

AROMATHERAPY

For specific instructions on how to use aromatherapy, *see* PREPARING AROMATHERAPY TREATMENTS in Part Three.

■ For minor burns, lavender oil has healing properties. Once you have cooled the burn, blend 10 drops of lavender oil into an ounce of jojoba oil, and apply the mixture to the affected area several times a day.

GENERAL RECOMMENDATIONS

■ Take appropriate first-aid measures (see the inset above).

■ If a blister forms, *do not puncture it*. Nature knows best. This natural bandage provides the best protection there is.

PREVENTION

■ Keep all flammable substances—including lighter fluid, gasoline, kerosene, and especially matches and lighters—out of the reach of children, preferably in a locked storage area.

■ Make sure that all heat-producing appliances are kept well away from potentially flammable items such as curtains or upholstery. This includes devices such as irons, toasters, and space heaters, as well as coffeemakers, curling irons, and halogen lamps—anything that generates heat when turned on. Always exercise special care when using such appliances. These devices should also be unplugged and their cords tucked away when not in use.

■ Avoid using extension cords, and keep all electrical cords out of the reach of pets and small children.

■ Keep the temperature of your hot-water heater set at no higher 120°F. It takes three minutes for 120°F water to cause a third-degree burn, long enough for you to turn it off or get out of the way. At 140°F, water can cause a third-degree burn in *five seconds*.

Bursitis

Bursitis is an inflammation of a bursa. The bursae are small sacs found in connective tissue, usually in the vicinity of joints. These sacs, or "cushions," are lined with membranes containing *synovia,* a fluid that acts to reduce friction between tendons and bones, between tendons and ligaments, and between other structures where friction is likely to occur. Bursitis occurs as a result of prolonged stress, pressure, friction, or injury to the membrane surrounding a joint, causing the fluid-filled bursa to become inflamed and swollen. When the enlarged sac presses against its neighboring joint, the pressure creates pain, which can be mild or excruciating, or anywhere in between.

Bursitis most often affects the shoulder, the hip, the elbow, and the knee. There are many popular terms for different kinds of bursitis. Computer operators, for example, who sit in one position for long hours at a time, can develop "weaver's bottom," a swelling of the bursae in the hips, which can cause pain when crossing the legs. They may also develop bursitis in the shoulders. If left untreated, this form of bursitis may result in "frozen shoulder." "Student's elbow" results from prolonged pressure of the elbow against a desk or table. Landscapers and gardeners, who kneel to weed flowerbeds and care for plants, are particularly subject to bursitis in their knees. This form of bursitis used to be called "housemaid's knee" because it afflicted those "Mrs. Clean"s who frequently got down on their hands and knees to scrub floors. People with this form of bursitis have a great deal of pain when climbing stairs. You may be surprised to learn that bunions also are the result of long-suffering bursae (*see* BUNION).

Anyone of any age can have bursitis. However, aging is a factor; bursitis is most often caused by overuse, and a bursa that is continually insulted over a long period of time is more likely to develop problems. Injury, arthritis, calcium deposits, and tight muscles can be contributing factors.

CONVENTIONAL MEDICINE

■ The primary treatment for an inflamed bursa is rest. Bursitis will often subside on its own after a few days rest. Resting the area where the bursa is located gives the fluid time to be reabsorbed into the bloodstream, allowing the swelling to subside.

■ Nonsteroidal anti-inflammatory drugs (NSAIDs) may be used to combat pain and inflammation. Examples of this class of drug include aspirin (Bayer, Ecotrin, and others), diclofenac (Voltaren), diflunisal (Dolobid), fenoprofen (Nalfon), ibuprofen (Advil, Motrin, Nuprin, and others), indomethacin (Indocin), ketoprofen (Orudis, Oruvail), naproxen (Aleve, Anaprox, Naprelan, Naprosyn), and piroxicam (Feldene). Some of these drugs are available over the counter, others by prescription only. Potential side effects include abdominal pain, indigestion, constipation, diarrhea, nausea, mouth sores, headache, dizziness, itching, rashes, ringing in the ears, bloating, shortness of breath, and palpitations, as well as ulceration and bleeding of the gastrointestinal tract and kidney damage. In addition, long-term use of these drugs may contribute to joint destruction.

■ If the pain is severe and fails to respond to ordinary measures, your physician may give you a local injection of an anesthetic for pain and/or a corticosteroid to bring down inflammation.

■ If infection occurs, your doctor may prescribe an antibiotic and drain the fluid from the bursa.

■ To stop the swelling from recurring, your physician may apply a pressure bandage.

■ If all else fails and the condition continues to recur, your doctor may recommend a bursectomy. This is a surgical procedure in which the lining of the bursal sac is removed to prevent the condition from coming back.

DIETARY GUIDELINES

■ Eat a healthy high-fiber diet, with an emphasis on whole foods.

■ Eat only a small amount of food at any one time, especially in the late afternoon and evening hours. In Chinese medicine, bursitis is believed to be related to digestive problems. When you eat a large quantity of food, the body's supply of enzymes must concentrate on digesting it. Eating lightly allows the body to use some of its enzymes to control inflammation.

■ Enjoy small amounts of clean, lean protein, such as that found in chicken and fish. Eat plenty of fruits and vegetables, especially steamed greens.

■ To rest the liver and improve digestion, avoid fried foods, red meat, and greasy, fatty foods of all kinds.

■ To flush toxins from your body, drink eight glasses of pure water every day.

NUTRITIONAL SUPPLEMENTS

■ Bromelain, an enzyme derived from pineapple, is a

very effective anti-inflammatory. Take 250 to 400 milligrams four times daily, before or between meals.

■ Calcium and magnesium are essential to the central nervous system and help relax the muscles. Three times a day, take 400 milligrams of calcium and 200 milligrams of magnesium.

■ Borage oil and flaxseed oil have notable anti-inflammatory action. These oils help maintain the integrity of cell membranes, and assist the cells in holding water and vital nutrients. Take 1,000 milligrams of either once or twice daily, or 1 teaspoon twice daily.

■ Glucosamine is a natural alternative to prescription anti-inflammatories. In addition, if taken over a period of months, glucosamine can stimulate the rehabilitation of collagen. Take 500 milligrams of glucosamine sulfate or hydrochloride three times daily (four times daily if you weigh over 200 pounds) for three to four months.

■ Chondroitin sulfate enhances the activity of glucosamine. Take 500 milligrams twice daily.

■ Inositol is required for proper muscle function. This is an important supplement to include if the bursitis is accompanied by neuritis. Take 500 milligrams three times daily for one to two weeks. Inositol works quickly. Relief should be apparent after one week.

■ Proteolytic enzymes work to decrease inflammation and help relieve pain. Take one dose of proteolytic enzymes, as directed on the product label, three times a day, between meals.

HERBAL TREATMENT

■ Burdock root, devil's claw, and yucca all have anti-inflammatory action. Take 500 milligrams of each three times daily. Or brew a tea using equal parts of all three herbs (see PREPARING HERBAL REMEDIES in Part Three) and drink one cup of this decoction three times daily for one month.

■ A topical compress of castor oil provides exceptional relief. Warm a small amount of castor oil to a comfortably hot temperature and saturate a clean white cloth with the oil. Fold the cloth into a pad and apply it to the affected area. If you have a great deal of pain, you can use this compress twice a day for twenty minutes at a time.

■ Cayenne (capsicum) has been used topically since ancient times to relieve pain. Select an ointment containing 0.075 percent capsaicin (the "heat" in this "hot" herb) in a cream base. Four or five times a day, apply a thin layer to the affected area and rub it completely into the skin. Be sure to wash your hands well after using the cream.

■ Horsetail supplies natural silica, which is required for tissue repair and healing. Take 500 milligrams three times daily.

■ Pine-bark and grape-seed extracts are natural anti-inflammatories with antioxidant properties. Take 50 milligrams of either three times daily.

■ Turmeric is a strong natural anti-inflammatory. Take 500 milligrams three times daily.

HOMEOPATHY

■ *Benzoicum acidum* is often recommend for gout, but it is equally effective against bursitis. This remedy is very effective for painful joints that creak with motion, especially painfully swollen knees and wrists. Take one dose of *Benzoicum acidum* 12x or 6c, as directed on the product label, three to four times daily, as needed.

■ *Bryonia* is the remedy for joints that are red and swollen and very painful with pressure, and for the person who feels worse with the smallest movement. Take one dose of *Bryonia* 12x or 6c three to four times daily, as needed.

■ *Chelidonium majur* is recommended for pain in the arms and shoulders, particularly if you suffer more on the right side, and feel worse with a change in the weather. Take one dose of *Chelidonium majur* 13x or 6c three to four times daily, as needed.

■ *Rhus toxicodendron* is for hot, swollen joints accompanied by pain in the tendons, ligaments, and muscles. Take one dose of *Rhus toxicodendron* 12x or 6c three to four times daily, as needed.

■ *Ruta graveolens* is good for pain and stiffness that occur in any joints, but especially the knee. The pain may travel from your knee to your thigh when your leg is straightened. Take one dose of *Ruta graveolens* 12x or 6c three to four times daily, as needed.

■ *Sticta pulmonaria* is good for shooting pains. Take one dose of *Sticta pulmonaria* 12x or 6c three to four times daily, as long as you have symptoms.

BACH FLOWER REMEDIES

Select the remedy that most closely fits your emotional tendencies and concerns, and take it as needed, following the directions on the product label.

■ Holly is helpful if you are angry and given to fits of temper.

■ Impatiens is the remedy to choose if you are impatient, easily irritated, and filled with nervous tension.

ACUPRESSURE

For the locations of acupressure points on the body, see ADMINISTERING AN ACUPRESSURE TREATMENT in Part Three.

■ Gallbladder 21, 34, and 41 help move blood and relax muscles.

■ Liver 3 relaxes the nervous system.

■ Stomach 38 helps to alleviate pain in the shoulder.

GENERAL RECOMMENDATIONS

■ Rest. Allow sufficient time for the swelling to subside.

■ Use alternating applications of hot and cold packs to help relieve the pain.

PREVENTION

■ Avoid subjecting a suffering bursa to continual stress. When you are engaging in any kind of physical activity, whether work-related or recreational, do not continue past the point of comfort. If it hurts, stop!

Cancer

Cancer is not a single disease, but rather a broad category of illnesses characterized by an uncontrolled growth of certain cells in the body. A thorough discussion of the causes, physiology, and treatments of different types of cancer is far beyond the scope of this book. It is important, however, to be aware of certain symptoms, especially lingering symptoms that do not seem to get better with treatment, so that if a malignancy develops, it can be diagnosed promptly.

A cancerous tumor begins in what is called a *primary site*. Cancerous cells can invade and damage surrounding tissue, and then break off from the primary tumor to spread, through the circulatory and lymphatic systems, to other parts of the body. These secondary tumors also can be harmful.

A cancerous tumor can develop in any part of the body. Among men, the most common type of cancer is prostate cancer, followed by lung cancer—which, although it occurs less frequently, nevertheless causes more deaths than prostate cancer. Among women, breast cancer and lung cancer are the two most common cancers. For both sexes, colorectal cancers follow lung cancer in terms of frequency. Other prominent types of the disease include cancers of the urinary tract, the female reproductive organs, and the pancreas, as well as leukemia (cancer of the blood-forming tissues), lymphoma (cancer of the lymphatic system), and skin cancer.

Depending on the location, type, and severity of the illness, each cancer has its own set of symptoms. Possible signs of cancer include a change in the appearance of a wart or mole, a sore that doesn't heal, a cough that persists, obvious changes in bowel or bladder habits, a thickening or lump anywhere on the body, blood in the urine (with no pain on urination), blood in the stool, unusual or exaggerated fatigue, persistent low-grade fever, persistent abdominal pain, loss of appetite, weight loss, recurring nosebleeds, and excessive bruising. However, just because you may have lost your appetite or had a bloody nose two days in a row, that does not necessarily mean you have cancer. Virtually all of these symptoms can have other causes as well. Nonetheless, if you do develop one or more of these symptoms, you should see your doctor without delay.

Tremendous amounts of time, energy, and money have been focused on researching the causes and treatment of cancers. Although the exact causes of most cancers are not well understood, several factors have been identified as probable contributors. Exposure to electromagnetic radiation (especially through nearby power lines and transformers), radiation, certain medications (particularly diethystilbestrol, or DES), pesticides, food additives, and cigarette smoke have all been linked with cancer. Dietary choices, such as the consumption of saturated fats, are another important focus of research, though it may be that the diet-cancer puzzle has more to do with individual responses to dietary factors, which in turn may be linked to a complex mixture of genetics, physiology, and lifestyle. An inherited predisposition or genetic condition may also increase the possibility of developing cancer. For example, people with Down syndrome have a greater risk of developing leukemia than other people do. Some types of cancer appear to have an infectious origin; the sexually-transmitted papillomavirus causes cervical cancer in an estimated one percent of those infected with it.

A diagnosis of cancer is made based on the history of the illness, symptoms, a physical examination, blood tests, x-rays, magnetic resonance imaging (MRI) scans, and other specialized tests, such as tissue biopsy, that look more closely at the bone marrow, spinal fluid, or other body tissues. A physician will look for primary and secondary tumors, as well as for the specific type of cancer that has developed.

The prognosis for an individual diagnosed with cancer depends on the type and location of the cancer, the person's overall health at the time of diagnosis, and his or her response to treatment. In the event that you are diagnosed as having cancer, we urge you to consult an oncologist—a medical doctor who specializes in cancers—as well as a natural health-care provider, to help maximize your healing potential. Herbs, homeopathy, acupressure, diet, and nutritional supplements can all be used to help boost your immune system and ease the discomforts of cancer therapies. Because everyone is unique, and because everyone's response to cancer and its treatments is unique, it is best to work closely with qualified health-care practitioners. We advise you to choose a medical doctor who is willing to work with a natural health-care practitioner (and vice versa). Each of these professionals needs to know what the other is doing, as the interventions of one can affect the treatments prescribed by the other.

Types of Cancer

Different medical terms are used to describe different types of cancers. Most of these terms end in the syllable *oma*, which means "mass" or "tumor." The basic categories of cancer include:

- **Carcinoma.** Cancers of the skin, mucous membranes, glands, and internal organs are often classified as carcinomas.

- **Leukemia.** Leukemias are cancers of the tissues that produce blood cells. Because leukemia results in abnormal blood cell formation, it is often referred to as blood cancer.

- **Lymphoma.** Lymphomas are cancers of the lymph nodes and other lymphatic tissue.

- **Sarcoma.** Sarcomas are primarily cancers of the bones, muscles, and connective tissues.

CONVENTIONAL TREATMENT

Once an accurate diagnosis is made, a treatment plan will be recommended. Depending on the type and location of the cancer, and whether it is in an earlier or later stage of development, treatment options may include chemotherapy, surgery, and/or radiation.

■ If a tumor is localized and can be removed without seriously damaging the body, surgery will probably be recommended.

■ Radiation treatment involves aiming concentrated x-rays directly at a tumor to kill the cancerous cells. Side effects of radiotherapy include fever, headache, nausea, vomiting, irritability, and loss of appetite. Also, the area of the skin that is exposed to radiation may become red, sore, and easily irritated.

■ Chemotherapy is medication given by mouth or by injection into the veins or muscles. It works by either killing the cancer cells or preventing them from reproducing. There are many types of chemotherapy agents. All of them are powerful medicines that cause significant side effects, including nausea, vomiting, hair loss, mouth sores, bleeding, an inability to fight infection, and significant bone marrow loss.

■ Cancer chemotherapy drugs often cause significant anemia, which causes debilitating fatigue and other symptoms. (*See* ANEMIA.) The U.S. Food and Drug Administration (FDA) recently approved the use of a drug called epoetin alfa (Epogen, Procrit), which increases the production of oxygen-carrying hemoglobin. This in turn increases energy levels and improves overall quality of life for people who must undergo chemotherapy, and reduces the risk that a blood transfusion may become necessary.

■ Cancer and its treatments are the subject of much research, and certain avenues of inquiry appear to hold promise. For instance, studies are currently underway using an altered version of the common cold virus that researchers believe has become a "cancer-hunter," with the ability to enter a cancer cell and kill it. Other scientists are working on the development of a new type of cancer test to tell in a matter of hours whether a particular individual's cancer is susceptible to chemotherapy and, if so, to what type. A genetically engineered hormone called megakaryocyte growth and development factor is being investigated for its ability to counteract the harmful effects of cancer chemotherapy on bone marrow. On the treatment front, work has been done on treating liver tumors with cryosurgery. In this technique, liquid nitrogen, at a temperature less than –300°F, is injected directly into the tumor, killing the cancer cells. Preliminary studies suggest this treatment can both lengthen life and decrease discomfort in people with liver tumors. These are just a few examples of the work being done to unravel the mystery of cancer and improve available treatments.

■ The treatment of cancer is a complicated and long-term process. Once treatment is completed and tests show that no evidence of cancer remains in your body, it is said that the disease is in remission. It is vital that you keep follow-up appointments as frequently and for as long as your doctor suggests. Cancer can reappear and treatment may need to be reinitiated.

DIETARY GUIDELINES

■ Eat a high-fiber diet consisting mainly of fresh vegetables, fruits, whole grains, and simple clean, lean protein foods.

■ Include soy foods such as tofu in your diet. Soybeans contain a variety of compounds that act to fight cancer, including natural protease inhibitors, which have been shown to block or reduce the development of colon, oral, lung, liver, pancreatic, and esophageal cancers in laboratory animals; phytosterols, which fight colon cancer by inhibiting cellular proliferation and division; and saponins, which can slow the growth of cancerous cervical and skin cells.

■ Drink tea, especially green tea, regularly. Green tea is high in substances known as catechins, which have anticancer properties. Regular tea drinking has been shown to diminish the likelihood of developing skin, lung, and stomach cancer.

■ Avoid saturated fats, hydrogenated and partially hydrogenated oils, sugar, coffee, caffeine, and alcohol. Minimize your consumption of salt and animal protein. Studies have shown that a "Japanese" diet—a diet low in calories and fat, and containing substantial amounts of fish, soy products, grains, and vegetables—is associated with lower rates of cancer, especially breast cancer.

■ Enjoy grapes regularly. Research shows that a substance called resveratrol, found in grapes, can help keep cells from turning cancerous and inhibit the spread of cells that are already malignant. Experts say that grapes contain the most active anti-carcinogenic compounds yet identified in nature.

■ Enjoy garlic and onions to your heart's content. An article in the *Journal of the National Cancer Institute* reported that a survey of 1,600 Chinese people, one-third of whom had stomach cancer, revealed that those who ate the most garlic and onions were 60-percent less likely to have stomach cancer than those who consumed these vegetables only rarely. You can also take ¹/₂ teaspoon of fresh garlic juice three times daily.

■ Add broccoli sprouts to salads. The young sprouts of the broccoli plant have been found to contain more sulforaphane, the cancer-fighting compound in broccoli, than the mature vegetable. If you cannot find them in your local market or health-food store, you can grow them at home, just as you would alfalfa or bean sprouts.

■ Eat tomatoes often. In a study in Italy, researchers found that people who ate raw tomatoes at least seven times per week cut their risk of developing stomach, bladder, and colon cancers by 50 percent.

■ Consider putting beets on the menu. In a laboratory study of more than sixty fruits and vegetables, the University of Mainz in Germany named beets as the richest source of a pigment called beta-cyanin that was found to be a powerful cancer-fighting agent.

■ Drink only pure water. Most municipal water supplies add chlorine to the water. Chlorine-based compounds can mimic the action of the sex hormone estrogen in the body, and high estrogen levels are a risk factor for breast cancer and other diseases. In men, excess estrogen can cause the sex organs to shrink and the breasts to enlarge, and may be related to the increasing incidence of testicular cancer in recent years.

■ If you consume alcohol, do so in moderation only. Excessive alcohol consumption increases the risk of cancer of the upper and lower digestive tract (including oral cancer), liver, prostate, breast, and colon. Rectal cancer in particular has been linked to heavy beer drinking. Men who drink five or more 12-ounce servings of beer a day have twice the normal risk of developing rectal cancer.

NUTRITIONAL SUPPLEMENTS

■ Take a good multivitamin and mineral supplement daily. Choose a powdered or capsule form for best absorption.

■ The antioxidant nutrients are very important. Take 5,000 international units of vitamin A twice a day; 15,000 international units of a carotenoid complex three times a day; 400 international units of vitamin E once or twice a day; and 200 micrograms of selenium daily. All of these nutrients support the immune system and can help to ease the debilitating side effects of radiation and chemotherapy.

Note: If you are pregnant or have liver disease, consult your doctor before taking supplemental vitamin A. If you have high blood pressure, limit your intake of supplemental vitamin E to a total of 400 international units daily. If you are taking an anticoagulant (blood thinner), consult your physician before taking supplemental vitamin E.

■ Beta 1,3 glucan is a compound derived from the cell walls of yeast. It enhances the immune response, acts as an antioxidant, and helps to protect the body against the adverse effects of radiation. Take 10 to 40 milligrams of beta 1,3 glucan daily.

■ An Oregon State University study in which laboratory animals were exposed to a potent cancer-causing substance found that animals given a chlorophyll supplement prior to exposure developed far fewer tumors than animals who were not given the supplement. The researchers believe that chlorophyll may reduce the risk of developing skin, stomach, colon, and liver cancers. Take a chlorophyll or sea-greens supplement, such as spirulina and blue-green algae, as directed on the product label.

■ Citrus pectin, a substance derived from the peels of citrus fruits, boosts the immune system and decreases the ability of cancerous cells to spread to other parts of the body. Take 5 to 6 grams daily.

■ Colostrum helps to improve the absorption of nutrients from food. Take it twice daily as directed on the product label.

■ Low levels of germanium may be associated with a susceptibility to certain forms of cancer. Add germanium to your list of supportive nutrients. Take 10 milligrams daily.

Note: Do not take germanium if you have, or have a history of, a kidney disorder.

■ Inositol hexaphosphate (IP-6), also known as phytic acid or phytate, is a nutrient derived from fiber that is related to inositol, one of the B vitamins. It has been shown to improve the immune response in laboratory animals.

Take 400 milligrams twice a day, on an empty stomach, together with 500 milligrams of inositol.

Take a multimineral supplement that supplies a total of 1,000 milligram of calcium, 500 milligrams of magnesium, 30 milligrams of zinc, 2 to 5 milligrams of manganese, and silica. Cancer depletes the body of these necessary minerals.

■ Studies have shown that omega-3 essential fatty acids, found in flaxseeds and certain deep-water fish, may help prevent and combat breast cancer. Take 500 to 1,000 milligrams of either twice daily.

Thymus glandular extract helps to enhance immune function. Take 250 to 500 milligrams of thymus extract twice a day.

The B-complex vitamins and the bioflavonoids help to support adrenal function and strengthen the immune system. Twice a day, take a B-complex supplement supplying 25 milligrams of each of the major B vitamins, plus 500 milligrams of mixed bioflavonoids.

Vitamin C boosts the immune system and aids healing. Take 500 to 1,000 milligrams of vitamin C, preferably in mineral ascorbate form, three to four times a day for one week following chemotherapy or radiation treatment and at least once a day at all other times.

Zinc helps to stimulate the immune system. Take 15 to 25 milligrams twice a day, at the beginning of a meal.

Note: Take zinc with food to prevent stomach upset. If you take over 30 milligrams of zinc on a daily basis for more than one or two months, you should also take 1 to 2 milligrams of copper each day to maintain a proper mineral balance.

HERBAL TREATMENT

If you are undergoing chemotherapy, astragalus can be used to support the immune system. It has been shown to diminish some of the side effects of chemotherapy, including poor appetite, hair loss, and depression. Take 500 milligrams two to four times a day, as needed.

Note: Do not take this herb if you have a fever or any other signs of acute infection.

Garlic enhances immune function and has antibacterial and antiviral properties. Take 500 milligrams of fresh garlic twice daily.

A tea of ginger or peppermint, or a combination of the two, helps to lessen the nausea that may be caused by chemotherapy or radiation treatment for cancer. Take one cup of tea as needed.

Note: If you are taking a tea containing peppermint as well as a homeopathic preparation, allow one hour between the two. Otherwise, the strong smell of the mint may interfere with the action of the homeopathic remedy.

■ Green tea contains potent antioxidants. It is particular-

ly useful if you are undergoing chemotherapy. Take 500 milligrams of standardized extract daily.

■ A blend of herbs consisting of red clover, burdock, and chaparral, known as the Hoxsey Combination, has been used since the 1930s as an anticancer formula. Follow the dosage directions on the product label.

■ Milk thistle and dandelion are very effective liver detoxifiers and help to ease the side effects of strong treatments. Take 200 to 300 milligrams of milk thistle extract standardized to contain 80 percent flavonoids (silymarin) and/or 500 milligrams of dandelion-root extract three times daily for six weeks. Stop for one month, then repeat.

■ Some studies have found that shiitake mushrooms have antitumor properties. The whole mushrooms can be added to foods, such as soups. Shiitake is also available in capsule form. Take 250 to 500 milligrams three times a day.

■ If your main difficulty is fatigue, Siberian ginseng is useful. It improves energy and also acts to protect the liver from being damaged by chemotherapy and/or radiation treatment. Choose a standardized extract containing 0.5 percent eleutheroside E and take 100 milligrams once or twice daily, as needed.

HOMEOPATHY

■ The first chemotherapy treatment is always a shock, both physically and mentally. Both you yourself and your family members, especially your primary caregiver, will benefit from taking one dose of *Aconite* 200x or 30c, as directed on the product label, after the first treatment.

■ *Arnica* can help to lessen the achiness associated with chemotherapy treatments. Take one dose of *Arnica* 200x or 30c after each treatment.

■ *Nux vomica* is helpful in lessening the nausea associated with chemotherapy. Take one dose of *Nux vomica* 30x or 6c as needed.

AROMATHERAPY

For specific instructions on how to use aromatherapy, *see* PREPARING AROMATHERAPY TREATMENTS in Part Three.

■ Basil, elemi, geranium, patchouli, peppermint, and vetiver oils have energizing properties, and are useful in combating fatigue. Use them as inhalants or diffuse them into the air.

■ Essential oils of bergamot and peppermint help to stimulate a sluggish appetite, which can result either from cancer itself or from cancer treatment (or both). Bergamot oil also helps combat depression. You can use either or both as inhalants or diffuse them into the air.

GENERAL RECOMMENDATIONS

■ To the greatest extent possible, remove from your life

and your home any known and suspected carcinogens (*see* Prevention, below), and do everything you can to reduce the stress in your life while you must deal with the rigors of cancer and its treatments. For example, if doing math makes you anxious, ask someone else to take over balancing the checkbook for the time being. If you have a neighbor or coworker you find difficult to deal with, avoid that person. Try to minimize your exposure to anything and anyone that causes you unnecessary stress and anxiety.

■ Educate yourself about your particular type of cancer and the treatments that have been found to be the most successful for it. This will help you work with your health-care providers to achieve the best possible outcome.

■ Seek out appropriate support, both emotional and practical. You need friends and family to listen and also, possibly, to help with daily tasks. It is also highly beneficial to find professional support, whether through a social worker, a counselor, a member of the clergy, and/or a support group. Regardless of how strong and stable you feel at the time of diagnosis, you should expect to have feelings of deep grief, confusion, anger, exhaustion, and isolation at times. This is natural. Build up a support network early so that you have a place to express and work with these feelings. Suggest to family members that they do the same. Cancer can put a great deal of stress on a family. Family members, including children, of a person with cancer should do whatever they need to do to stay as physically and emotionally healthy as possible.

PREVENTION

The processes that lead to the development of many types of cancer are not well understood, and for that reason cancer cannot be considered wholly preventable. However, there are measures you can take to help safeguard yourself from known risks that might lead to the development of cancer in the future.

■ Do not smoke, and avoid secondhand smoke. Evidence suggests that secondhand smoke may be even more dangerous than the smoke the smoker breathes. And switching to a low-tar brand may actually increase your risk of lung cancer. People who smoke low-tar cigarettes end up inhaling the smoke more deeply in order to get the desired dose of nicotine, with the result that carcinogens penetrate more deeply into lung tissue.

■ Do not drink tap water. Chlorine-based chemicals used to purify tap water are implicated in the development of several different types of cancer.

■ If possible, buy organically grown foods (or grow your own). The herbicides and pesticides used on commercially grown produce may be carcinogenic. Always wash produce thoroughly before eating it.

■ Keep the amount of fat in your diet to no more than 30 percent of total calories consumed, and eat a diet that is high in fiber. A lifetime of eating too much fat and too little fiber may contribute to the development of colorectal and other cancers. Healthy eating habits and a healthy lifestyle are excellent preventive medicine.

■ Vitamin D, the "sunshine vitamin," may help to inhibit the growth of cancer cells. This vitamin is present in foods such as salmon, sardines, egg yolks, and milk. It is also produced in the skin in response to sun exposure. Unfortunately, the ability to produce vitamin D declines with age. If you are over sixty and do not get at least fifteen minutes of sun exposure on your arms and face three times a week, you may wish to take 400 international units of supplemental vitamin D daily.

■ Women who have a daily intake of at least 400 micrograms of folic acid have been found to have a lower risk of developing colorectal cancer than women who consume less than that amount. Folic acid is present in foods such as green vegetables, beans, and whole wheat. If you do not eat generous amounts of these foods regularly, you may wish to take folic acid supplements.

■ Enjoy green tea frequently. Studies from Japan have shown that in areas where green tea is drunk with regularity, the incidence of cancer in general—and of stomach, esophageal, and liver cancer in particular—is considerably lower than in areas where people drink no green tea.

■ Eating grilled, charcoal-broiled, and fried foods may contribute to colon cancer. Either eliminate these foods from your diet or reduce the amount of them you eat. When you do eat such foods, pick lower fat meats and trim any excess fat from the meat before cooking. Never eat meat that is charred.

■ Aspirin may help stop the production of enzymes required for tumor growth. This does not mean you should start taking aspirin on a regular basis, but if your doctor has prescribed a daily aspirin for cardiovascular reasons, you may be reaping additional benefits.

■ Follow your doctor's recommendations regarding measures for early cancer detection. Some of the most common screening measures include, for women, breast self-examination, mammograms, pelvic exams, and Pap tests; for men, prostate exams and PSA tests; and for people of both sexes, sigmoidoscopy, rectal exams, and stool tests for occult blood.

■ Have your house and water tested for the presence of radon. Radon is a naturally occurring radioactive gas that can seep into your home from the surrounding soil. It is believed to be a common cause of lung cancer as well as of stomach cancer. You can't see or smell it, so the only way to know whether it is present is to use a radon test kit. These are available at many hardware stores. If you find that there is radon in your home, you can usually correct the problem by sealing cracks and improving ventilation in the basement.

■ Guard against sunburn. It has been established that even one case of severe sunburn increases a person's risk of developing malignant melanoma, a dangerous form of skin cancer. (*See* SUNBURN.)

■ Avoid breathing in fumes from paints, solvents, gasoline, pesticides, herbicides, nail polish remover, oven cleaner, glues, and other household chemicals. Many of these substances are known to cause, or are suspected of causing, cancer.

■ A vaccine against human papillomavirus, a sexually transmitted infection associated with cervical cancer, is currently undergoing testing. If it proves to be safe and effective, it should offer a measure of protection against this disease.

Calluses

See CORNS AND CALLUSES.

Candida Infection

Candida albicans is a common yeast that lives in the mouth, the digestive system, the genital tract, and the skin. It is usually a rather lazy, noninvasive sugar-loving organism—just one of the many tiny creatures that normally live within the human body without causing too many problems. This is because a healthy body has the means to keep candida under tight control. As long as the human body has sufficient numbers of "friendly," or probiotic, bacteria—*Lactobacillus acidophilus* and *Bifidobacterium bifidum*—candida remains a benign yeast that neither helps nor harms. The lactobacilli and bifidobacteria limit the growth of yeast colonies and stop them from invading new territories.

Probiotic bacteria also prevent candida from developing into a more aggressive, invasive form. If it does, candida produces rhizoids, long rootlike structures that permit more movement and can penetrate mucous membranes. If the friendly bacteria are weak and low in numbers, candida can escape its usual boundaries and establish new colonies throughout the body.

Candidiasis—the medical term for candida infection—can cause a variety of problems, depending on whether the infection is localized in one particular area or systemic, affecting the entire body. A candida infection in the mouth is called *thrush*, and appears as soft, creamy white patches on the tongue and/or insides of the cheeks. Thrush is not uncommon in babies and young children. When it occurs in adults, it is usually considered a sign of a poorly functioning immune system, although recent years have shown thrush to be more and more common among older people, probably the result of natural aging plus years of treatment with antibiotics and other medications. Candida can also infect the skin, causing inflammation and redness and, often, itching. This type of candidiasis most often occurs in areas where skin rubs against skin—the underarms, groin, and, in women, beneath the breasts. Candida infection of the female genital tract, known as vulvovaginitis (or, more commonly, a yeast infection) causes a sticky white or yellow discharge and, especially, itching and burning.

Symptoms of systemic candidiasis can include allergic reactions; persistent heartburn, constipation, diarrhea, colitis, rectal itching, bloating, abdominal pain and cramps, and/or gas; kidney and bladder infections; muscle and joint pain and/or swelling; sore throat; nasal congestion; cough; numbness and/or tingling in the extremities; skin lesions; and fungal infections of the nails. Persistent fatigue, unexplained weakness, hyperactivity, problems with blood-sugar regulation, headaches, difficulty concentrating, trouble remembering, and depression have also been attributed to candidiasis. A woman with systemic candidiasis may suffer from premenstrual syndrome (PMS), menstrual irregularities, and hormonal imbalances, as well as vaginitis. Although candida infection is not usually sexually transmitted, it can be. The sexual partner of a woman with vaginal candidiasis may develop an infection of the penis. The prostate gland may also be affected. If candida infection spreads through the blood to vital organs, it can become extremely serious.

There are three main factors that predispose a person to an overgrowth of candida. The first is impaired immune function. This problem can be transitory—the result of cancer chemotherapy or immunosuppressive drugs (including steroids), for example—or long-term, as in the case of certain cancers and HIV disease. Second, anything that destroys the friendly bacteria that normally keep candida in check increases the likelihood of an overgrowth of the fungus. Antibiotic therapy is a primary culprit here, but stress and even the natural aging process contribute to a decline in friendly bacteria as well. Third, the presence of an abundance of sugar for the yeast to feed on encourages them to grow. This is why people with diabetes are more prone to these infections than most. People whose diets include large quantities of sugar and yeast-based foods also have an increased susceptibility.

Most of the symptoms of candidiasis, whether localized or systemic, can be caused by other conditions. Also, these organisms normally inhabit the human body, so their presence alone is not sufficient to make a diagnosis of candida infection. For these reasons, candidiasis can be very difficult to diagnose. If you have been treated for one or more of the symptoms described above, with only limited success, you may actually be suffering from candidiasis.

CONVENTIONAL TREATMENT

■ Systemic candidiasis is a condition rarely recognized by conventional medical doctors, except in certain circumstances, such as in people with cancer (or who are undergoing cancer chemotherapy) or HIV disease. However, a systemic antifungal drug can actually be a useful diagnostic tool. If you have symptoms that may be related to candida infection and an antifungal drug makes these symptoms improve quickly, this is a good indication that an overgrowth of candida is behind the problem. Ask your doctor if he or she will consider a trial of fluconazole (Diflucan, at a dosage of 150 milligrams a day for two weeks), or a similar drug, such as itraconazole (Sporanox), ketoconazole (Nizoral), or terbinafine (Lamisil). If you take one of these drugs, your liver function may need to be checked at intervals. Though it is uncommon, these drugs, particularly ketoconozale, can cause liver dysfunction, with nausea, vomiting, and other side effects. If you must take one of these drugs, you should not take the antihistamine astemizole (Hismanal), the digestive stimulant cisapride (Propulsid), or the sedative triazolam (Halcion). Interactions between these antifungals and astemizole or cisapride can result in serious cardiac effects; interactions with triazolam can result in an intensification of that drug's sedative effects.

■ Nystatin (available under the brand names Mycolog, Mycostatin, Nilstat, and others) is an antifungal drug that is very useful for thrush.

■ Vaginal candida infection is usually treated with local applications of butoconazole (Femstat 3), clotrimazole (Gyne-Lotrimin), terconazole (Terazol), or miconazole (Monistat). A single oral dose of fluconazole (Diflucan) may be successful as well.

■ Fungal infections of the skin are treated with topical forms of these drugs. If that is unsuccessful, oral doses of griseofulvin (Gris-PEG, Grifulvin), ketoconazole (Nizoral), or itraconazole (Sporanox) may be necessary.

■ Fungal infections of the nails tend to be resistant to topical treatment. Systemic antifungal treatment with itraconazole or fluconazole, taken orally, has become a more popular conventional approach.

DIETARY GUIDELINES

■ Eat adequate clean, lean protein foods such as chicken and fish.

■ Include olive oil in your diet. Yeasts do not feed well on fats. Olive oil is a healthy monounsaturated dietary fat.

■ Drink at least eight glasses of pure water daily to help flush toxins from your body.

■ Eliminate yeast-based foods and foods containing sugar (including fruits) from your diet for at least thirty days, or until the condition is resolved. Both sugar and yeast feed and strengthen candida.

■ When you are in the midst of an acute candida infection, do not eat foods with a high content of mold, such as cheeses, dried fruit, peanuts, and melons.

■ Avoid alcoholic beverages, which are fermented and contain yeasts. Also, the body breaks alcohol down into sugar, which yeast thrive on. If you feel deprived without an occasional cocktail, choose vodka (but avoid mixing it with fruit juice). Vodka seems to have less impact on candidiasis than other alcoholic beverages.

■ Avoid refined and processed foods. These foods tend to be low in necessary nutrients and most contain food additives that may worsen symptoms.

■ Avoid foods that trigger sensitivities or allergies. Many people have allergies to certain foods, often without realizing it. To find out if you have hidden allergies or sensitivities to particular foods, *see* ROTATION DIET in Part Three and follow the program.

NUTRITIONAL SUPPLEMENTS

■ Calcium and magnesium soothe stressed nerves. Twice a day, take a calcium and magnesium combination supplement that supplies 500 to 600 milligrams of calcium and 250 to 300 milligrams of magnesium.

■ Carnitine is a substance related to the B vitamins, though it is often grouped with the amino acids. It is responsible for the conversion of long-chain fatty acids into energy, and increases tissue oxygenation, thereby increasing energy and physical stamina. It is particularly beneficial for the cardiovascular system. If you have candidiasis accompanied by elevated cholesterol and/or triglyceride levels, take 500 milligrams of L-carnitine two or three times daily.

■ Coenzyme Q_{10} assists in supplying the cells with needed oxygen. Take 30 milligrams three to four times daily.

■ Evening primrose oil and flaxseed oil are rich sources of the fatty acids that help regulate hormone production. Take 500 to 1,000 milligrams of either two or three times daily for three to six months.

■ Fructooligosaccharides (FOS) supply a special form of carbohydrate that can be digested by friendly bacteria but not by yeast. This allows the "good guys" to grow like mad, while the "bad guys" tend to get starved out. FOS and probiotics make a powerful anti-candida combination. Start by taking $1/4$ teaspoon of FOS twice a day and work up to 1 teaspoon twice a day over a period of one to two weeks. (If you start taking too much too quickly, you may develop bowel gas.) Continue taking FOS for three months.

■ Lipoic acid aids the action of enzymes crucial to the conversion of nutrients into energy. If you are fatigued, and particularly if you have a history of compromised liver function, take 50 to 100 milligrams of lipoic acid twice a day.

■ Magnesium and malic acid form a combination that helps initiate the Krebs cycle, which converts nutrients into energy at the cellular level. It is especially helpful if you are suffering from fatigue, a common complication of candidiasis. Magnesium and malic acid help reenergize the system. For as long as the fatigue remains, take a combination formula supplying 100 milligrams of magnesium and 300 milligrams of malic acid twice a day, one-half hour or more before meals.

■ To provide your body with the friendly bacteria that control candida, take high-quality probiotic supplements (acidophilus and bifidus). Take them as recommended on the product labels. If you are allergic to milk, select dairy-free products.

■ Thymus glandular extract strengthens the immune system in a very immediate way. For three to six weeks, take 750 milligrams of thymus extract at breakfast and another 750 milligrams at lunch.

■ People with candidiasis—especially those who can't (or won't) stay away from sugary foods—are usually low in the B vitamins, which are required for the metabolism of sugar. For two weeks, take a B-complex supplement that supplies 25 milligrams of each of the primary B vitamins, plus 400 additional micrograms of vitamin B_{12}, twice daily.

■ Vitamin E defuses free radicals and is a good anti-inflammatory. Choose a product containing mixed tocopherols and start by taking 100 or 200 milligrams at bedtime, then gradually increase the dosage until you are taking 400 international units daily.

Note: If you are taking an anticoagulant (blood thinner), consult your physician before taking supplemental vitamin E.

HERBAL TREATMENT

■ Cat's claw enhances the immune response and has antifungal properties. Take 500 milligrams of standardized extract three times a day until your condition improves.

Note: Do not use cat's claw if you are pregnant or nursing, or if you are an organ-transplant recipient. Use it with caution if you are taking an anticoagulant (blood thinner).

■ Garlic has noteworthy antifungal properties. Take 500 milligrams three or four times daily for four to six weeks.

■ Grapefruit-seed extract contains phytochemicals with antifungal action. Take 100 milligrams two or three times daily for four to six weeks. If you have a sensitive digestive system, start with a smaller amount and gradually work up to the recommended dosage.

■ Pau d'arco helps enhance the oxygenation of red blood cells. Take 500 milligrams twice daily for four to six weeks.

Note: The three herbs outlined above can be taken on a rotating basis. For example, for the first four to six weeks, take one. Then take another for the next four to six weeks, then the third for the following four to six weeks.

■ Echinacea and goldenseal together have antifungal, antibacterial, and antiviral properties. Take one dose of an echinacea and goldenseal combination formula supplying 250 to 500 milligrams of echinacea and 150 to 300 milligrams of goldenseal twice daily for ten days.

■ Oat straw is a calmative herb that helps strengthen the nervous system. Take 500 milligrams twice daily.

HOMEOPATHY

■ Candidiasis is a complex problem that contributes to many different health problems. See a homeopathic practitioner for a constitutional remedy designed for your specific symptoms. Also see the individual entries that address particular problems, such as CONSTIPATION, DIARRHEA, HEADACHES, INDIGESTION, HIV DISEASE, and VAGINITIS, for symptom-specific homeopathic remedies for those conditions.

BACH FLOWER REMEDIES

Select the remedy that most closely fits your emotional tendencies and concerns, and take it as needed, following the directions on the product label.

■ Holly helps to tone down feelings of anger and insecurity as well as fits of temper.

■ Impatiens eases nervousness, impatience, tension, and irritability.

■ Mimulus is good if you are shy and timid, and fearful of many things.

■ Choose Scleranthus if you are feeling uncertain and have trouble making decisions and sticking with them.

■ White Chestnut helps to counteract a tendency to obsess about things long after they should have been forgotten.

ACUPRESSURE

For the locations of acupressure points on the body, see ADMINISTERING AN ACUPRESSURE TREATMENT in Part Three.

■ Gallbladder 41 helps to strengthen the endocrine system.

■ Large Intestine 4 and Liver 3 relax the nervous system.

- Spleen 6 and Stomach 36 strengthen the digestive system and enhance the blood.

- Spleen 10 detoxifies the blood. It is useful if you have skin problems associated with candidiasis.

AROMATHERAPY

For specific instructions on how to use aromatherapy, *see* PREPARING AROMATHERAPY TREATMENTS in Part Three.

- Tea tree oil is an effective antifungal. If candidiasis erupts on the skin, apply a 5-percent solution of tea tree oil directly to the affected area twice a day.

GENERAL RECOMMENDATIONS

- If at all possible, avoid antibiotics and corticosteroid drugs while you are trying to rid your body of candida. If you must take antibiotics for a serious condition, be sure to take acidophilus and bifidus supplements to replace friendly bacteria lost during a course of antibiotics.

- Be aware that birth control pills and hormone replacement drugs foster the growth of candida. If possible, adopt another method of birth control while you are battling candidiasis.

- Avoid damp and moldy environments, such as basements.

- Avoid exposure to toxins, including strong toxic cleansers.

- Don't expect an immediate cure. Conquering a long-standing persistent candida infection takes time.

PREVENTION

- Many studies have demonstrated that taking probiotic bacteria (acidophilus and bifidus) can prevent the overgrowth of candida. These friendly bacteria belong in your supplement program. Take a good-quality probiotic supplement as outlined under Nutritional Supplements, above.

Canker Sores

Canker sores are small, swollen, painful ulcers that occur on the lips or in the mouth. Canker sores hurt. When you develop a canker sore, you may not even want to eat. Acidic foods sting. Even the act of chewing can cause irritation in the area.

A canker sore begins as a small red dot on the lip or the inside of the mouth, which then develops into a vesicle with a white head. Eventually the head will rupture, leaving an open ulcer that can become secondarily infected by yeast or bacteria.

The cause of the original ulcer may be difficult to pinpoint, although food allergies, vitamin deficiencies (especially low levels of vitamin B_{12}), acidic conditions, and small cuts are probable causes. There is also some research that indicates an autoimmune phenomenon may be at work.

Canker sores and cold sores look very much alike. Cold sores, however, are caused by the herpes virus, which is highly contagious. Typically, herpes sores appear on the hard part of the gums or the "dry" part of the lips, while canker sores occur on the "loose" part of the gums, the insides of the cheeks, or the inner lip. Also, cold sores tend to recur at exactly the same place every time, while canker sores can occur anywhere in the mouth.

CONVENTIONAL TREATMENT

- There is no drug that will cure a canker sore, although there are over-the-counter medicines that can be dabbed on the sore to numb the pain. These include Campho-Phenique, Carmex, Anbesol, Herpecin, Zilactin, and Gly-Oxide. Follow the directions on the product label.

- A mouthwash made from equal parts of hydrogen peroxide and water can decrease the superinfection of the ulcer.

- Over-the-counter painkillers such as acetaminophen (Tylenol, Datril, and others), aspirin (Bayer, Ecotrin, and others), or ibuprofen (Advil, Motrin, Nuprin, and others) can help to lessen the pain of canker sores.

- If you are in great distress from canker sores, see your physician. A mouthwash or paste made from triamcinolone (a prescription steroid sold as Kenalog in Orabase) has been shown to be effective in relieving the pain of canker sores, although whether it speeds the healing process is the subject of some debate.

- For severe pain, an anesthetic called lidocaine is sometimes prescribed.

DIETARY GUIDELINES

- Avoid acidic foods, such as sugar, citrus fruits and juices, chocolate, and foods containing caffeine. Acidic foods are very irritating to canker sores.

- Soft foods, such as steamed vegetables or warm soups, will be easier to eat.

- If your tongue or lips are very sensitive, use a straw for drinking.

- Suck on ice chips. The coldness of the ice will block the pain for a time.

NUTRITIONAL SUPPLEMENTS

- Acidophilus and bifidus are friendly bacteria that cleanse your internal environment and help prevent future outbreaks. Take them as recommended on the product labels. If you are allergic to milk, select dairy-free products.

■ Chlorophyll is a blood detoxifier and is high in micronutrients. Take a chlorophyll supplement as directed on the product label.

■ When symptoms are acute, chew a 400- or 800-microgram tablet of folic acid three times daily.

■ A deficiency of the amino acid lysine fosters the development of canker sores. During an outbreak, take 250 milligrams of L-lysine three to four times daily. Take it with water or juice, away from protein foods.

■ Vitamin A and the carotenoids help to heal mucous membranes. Take 5,000 international units of vitamin A and 25,000 international units of a carotenoid complex twice a day for one week.

Note: If you are pregnant, or intend to get pregnant, or if you have liver disease, consult your doctor before taking supplemental vitamin A. Pregnant women should not ingest a total of more than 25,000 international units of supplemental vitamin A *per week* from all sources.

■ Take a B-complex supplement supplying 25 milligrams of each of the major B vitamins, plus an additional 100 micrograms of vitamin B_{12}, twice a day for three weeks.

■ Take 1,000 milligrams of buffered vitamin C with bioflavonoids twice a day (between meals) for five days. Choose a formula made without sugar.

■ Zinc lozenges are very soothing and will help heal the lesion. To help boost your immune system, three days out of the week for two months, take 15 to 20 milligrams of zinc twice a day.

Note: Take zinc with food to prevent stomach upset. If you take over 30 milligrams of zinc on a daily basis for more than one or two months, you should also take 1 to 2 milligrams of copper each day to maintain a proper mineral balance.

HERBAL TREATMENT

■ Swish a bit of aloe vera juice around in your mouth several times daily to soothe the inflamed area. Be sure to use a food-grade product for this purpose.

■ To help clear infection and stimulate your immune system, take one dose of echinacea and goldenseal herbal combination formula supplying 250 to 500 milligrams of echinacea and 150 to 300 milligrams of goldenseal three times a day until the canker sore improves, up to one week.

■ Goldenseal powder can be applied directly to the sore. It can also be diluted and used as a mouthwash.

■ Make licorice-root tea and swish it around in your mouth twice a day. Licorice root has antiviral and antibacterial properties, and is very soothing to canker sores.

The tea can be used either cool or warm. You can also cover the ulcer with a paste or a small "plug" made from licorice-root powder. Even chewing on a piece of a licorice root is helpful.

Note: Do not take licorice on a daily basis for more than five days in a row, as it can elevate blood pressure. Do not take it at all if you have high blood pressure.

■ Propolis lozenges can be used to help fight infection and promote healing.

■ A wet tea bag placed against the sore can be soothing. Use ordinary black tea, which contains tannic acid, an effective astringent.

HOMEOPATHY

■ Take one dose of *Natrum muriaticum* 12x three times daily for up to forty-eight hours. If there is no improvement in that time, discontinue the remedy.

GENERAL RECOMMENDATIONS

■ If you discover a tiny red sore in your mouth, suspect a canker sore and begin treating it.

■ Mix 1 teaspoon of baking soda in 8 ounces of pure spring water and swish the mixture around in your mouth. Baking soda reduces the acidity of the mouth and also promotes healing of irritated tissues.

PREVENTION

■ Keep a diet diary that records what you eat and track your responses. This will help identify foods that may aggravate canker sores. Eliminate those foods from your diet.

■ Take acidophilus and bifidus supplements regularly.

■ If you are prone to canker sores, take 20 milligrams of chewable zinc, in lozenge or tablet form, once daily for two months.

■ Avoid sugary sweets.

■ Including yogurt in your diet may help to prevent canker sores.

Cardiovascular Disease

Cardiovascular disease is a general term that denotes disorders of the heart and blood vessels. There are numerous distinct disorders that fall into this category. This section addresses arteriosclerosis and atherosclerosis, angina, heart attack, and heart failure, as well as arrhythmias, myocarditis, cardiomyopathy, heart murmurs, rheumatic heart disease, valvular disease, and mitral valve prolapse. High blood pressure, which also is a form of cardiovascular disease, is treated separately (*see* HIGH BLOOD PRESSURE).

Arteriosclerosis, sometimes called hardening of the arteries, is a condition in which the walls of the arteries thicken and lose their normal elasticity, interfering with normal circulation. The most common type of arteriosclerosis is *atherosclerosis.* In atherosclerosis, the thickening of arterial walls is due to an accumulation of fatty deposits. While ordinary arteriosclerosis affects both major and minor arteries, and is primarily related to aging, atherosclerosis affects the large and medium-sized arteries, and is strongly related to diet. An additional factor that has only recently been identified as a contributor to the formation of plaque is low-level inflammation of the arterial walls. Although the cause of this inflammation has not yet been identified, researchers believe that a long-term infection, so mild that it produces no symptoms on its own, may be a factor. Atherosclerosis of the coronary arteries (the arteries that serve the heart) is known as *coronary artery disease* (CAD).

Arteriosclerosis progresses slowly and silently. By the time any symptoms appear, the condition is likely to be quite advanced. Arteriosclerosis results in increased blood pressure as the heart works harder to pump enough blood through the narrowed, inflexible vessels. This sets up a vicious cycle in which high blood pressure increases the hardening of the arteries, and the increased hardening of the arteries prompts the body to respond by increasing blood pressure. Eventually, blood flow may be so reduced that not enough oxygenated blood reaches the heart, triggering chest pain that may be mild or severe. This pain is known as *angina.* It is usually (though not always) triggered by exertion and relieved by rest. In some cases, angina is caused not by actual blockage, but by spasms of the coronary arteries. This condition can be difficult to diagnose.

Narrowing of the coronary arteries raises the possibility of blockage—either by the fatty deposits themselves or by a clot that may lodge there—that may precipitate a heart attack. In a heart attack, the amount of oxygenated blood that reaches the heart is so sharply reduced that areas of heart tissue die. The medical term for this process is *myocardial infarction* (MI). The well-known symptoms of a heart attack in progress include crushing or squeezing pain in the chest or upper abdomen that may spread to the neck and shoulders, down the arms, and to the back. Sometimes the pain is excruciating, sometimes dull, and sometimes nonexistent. It is not uncommon for a person having a heart attack to mistake it for the discomfort of indigestion. Other possible symptoms include profuse perspiration, a visible paling or graying of the skin, difficulty swallowing, a drop in blood pressure, shortness of breath, dizziness, faintness, a weak and rapid pulse, and, sometimes, nausea and vomiting.

The consequences of myocardial infarction can be very serious, depending on the extent and location of the damage to the heart. Any suspicion that you may be having a heart attack means that you should call for emergency help *immediately.* Even if the pain eases and the symptoms fade, you need medical evaluation and attention.

Another type of cardiovascular disease is *heart failure* (HF), also known as *congestive heart failure* (CHF). In this disorder, the heart is unable to pump sufficient oxygenated blood to fully supply the body. This leads to increased pressure in the circulatory system, which forces fluid from the blood into the surrounding tissues. This fluid retention is what gives the condition its name. Other symptoms include weakness, fatigue, and shortness of breath with even the slightest exertion. Kidney and liver function may be affected as well. Heart failure can result from anything that causes damage to the heart, including coronary artery disease, a heart attack, alcohol abuse, or an illness such as rheumatic fever or infection of the heart tissue. In some cases, the underlying cause is unknown.

Arrhythmias, or abnormal heartbeats, are another relatively common problem. There are different types of abnormal rhythms, and different causes. They range in severity from almost totally insignificant to very serious. The seriousness of rhythm and/or rate variations depends on how much they affect cardiac output, or the amount of blood the heart can pump. Abnormal heart rhythms can affect different areas of the heart, but in general, the most serious are those connected with the left ventricle, which is the main pumping station for all of the body except for the lungs.

Symptoms of arrhythmia can range from none at all to palpitations to dizziness and fainting, even to sudden death. They are usually diagnosed by means of an electrocardiogram (ECG), which provides a picture of the electrical activity in the heart. Since ECG gives only a "one-shot" look at the heart, longer-term monitoring with a Holter monitor may be necessary to detect intermittent rhythm trouble.

Myocarditis is inflammation of the heart muscle. It can be due to infection (viral, bacterial, fungal, or parasitic), but certain drugs, exposure to radiation, and toxins may also be involved. Medications that can cause this problem include cancer chemotherapy drugs; a class of drugs known as phenothiazines, which are used for psychological conditions and to control vomiting; lithium; and antibiotics to which an individual is hypersensitive. Symptoms usually include chest pain and trouble breathing. In some cases, heart failure can develop, leading to increased difficulty breathing and/or weakness and swelling in the legs and ankles. Myocarditis is usually diagnosed by ECG.

Cardiomyopathy is a serious chronic heart disease that causes heart failure, in which the heart's ability to provide sufficient blood flow to the body is reduced. This can be manifested in shortness of breath, fainting, chest pain, weakness, and/or edema. There are three classes of this condition: *dilated cardiomyopathy*, in which the heart enlarges (though its output does not); *hypertrophic cardiomyopathy*, in which the heart muscle thickens (though heart muscle power does not usually increase), which encroaches on the pumping chambers and also enlarges the heart; and *restrictive cardiomyopathy*, in which the heart is not able to expand normally. Dilated cardiomyopathy may be due to alcohol abuse, inflammation of the heart muscle, the use of certain drugs, or genetic disease. In some cases, the cause is unknown. Hypertrophic cardiomyopathy can be a result of heredity or long-term high blood pressure. Radiation therapy to the chest, open-heart surgery, a history of heart-muscle inflammation, and amyloidosis (an accumulation of an abnormal protein called amyloid in the tissue) are among the factors that can lead to restrictive cardiomyopathy.

Many people have been told they have *heart murmurs*. A murmur itself is not a disorder; rather, it is a sound the heart makes. Identifying a murmur can help a physician to diagnose certain heart conditions. For example, there are characteristic murmurs associated with valvular disease, septal defects (abnormal holes in the heart-chamber walls), and restrictions to blood flow in blood-vessel walls. Not all murmurs are signs of serious trouble, however. Many are quite trivial. In fact, some high-level distance athletes develop murmurs because of their extremely high cardiac output.

Rheumatic heart disease is a possible long-term complication of rheumatic fever in which the valves of the heart become scarred, stiff, deformed, or pulled out of normal position. This decreases the heart's pumping efficiency and disrupts blood flow, which in turn can allow bacteria to establish themselves on heart valves and cause more damage. Rheumatic heart disease can cause heart failure, heart-rhythm disturbances, and other problems, though symptoms may not surface until many years after the rheumatic fever that caused them. This condition is usually diagnosed based on a person's medical history plus a physical exam.

Valvular disease is often a result of rheumatic fever, but there are other possible causes as well, including other types of infection; the formation of calcifications on congenitally abnormal valves (or just from some unknown effect of long life in developed countries); certain genetic syndromes, such as Marfan's syndrome; trauma; tumors; or other deformities within the heart's chambers. The severity of valvular disease depends on the valve involved. The valves must open and shut with every beat of the heart, and their efficiency is extremely significant. The valves most often involved are the mitral valve, the aortic valve, and the tricuspid valve.

The main problem in valvular disease is that of *stenosis,* which is a stiffening and partial closing that reduces a valve's ability to function. This can lead to an inadequate flow of blood into one of the heart's chambers. It can also cause *regurgitation,* in which the valve does not close completely when it should, allowing blood to slip backwards through the defective valve. Diagnosis usually follows the discovery of a murmur and, possibly, echocardiography.

One commonly diagnosed valvular condition, especially among women, is *mitral valve prolapse.* The mitral valve is the one that must close every time the left ventricle (the heart's biggest chamber, and its main pumping station) pumps blood to the body, and must resist considerable pressure changes. In prolapse, the valve protrudes too far into the chamber during pumping. However, this particular situation occurs in an estimated 10 percent of healthy people, and it is not considered a particularly serious condition. Symptoms, when they occur, can include fatigue, nondescript chest pain, shortness of breath, and/or chest palpitations. This condition also causes a characteristic murmur.

More than 75 million Americans have some form of cardiovascular disease. Many of them are unaware of it. While some may not recognize the symptoms, many simply have no symptoms. Unfortunately, it is possible for the first symptom to be a disastrous episode such as a heart attack. An estimated 25 percent of people who have had heart attacks experienced no warning signs. Fortunately, however, we do know of numerous risk factors that can be identified and, in most cases, minimized if not eliminated entirely. Risk factors that contribute to cardiovascular disease include smoking (smoking constricts the blood vessels and exposes the body to toxins), high blood pressure, high blood-cholesterol levels, obesity, lack of exercise, diabetes, stress, age (people over sixty-five are at higher risk), and family history. With the exception of your age and your family history, all of these factors can be addressed and the risk reduced.

One curious fact about cardiovascular disease is that, except in people of Asian or Native American ancestry, the presence of a diagonal crease in the earlobe has been shown to be a more accurate predictor of incipient heart disease than other well-known risk factors, including elevated cholesterol, smoking, and age. While the presence of a crease does not necessarily mean you have heart disease, if you have one, you should be examined and promptly address any underlying problems that may put you at risk.

EMERGENCY TREATMENT FOR HEART ATTACK

■ The symptoms of heart attack may come on instantaneously or develop over a period of hours, and usually involve some combination of the following:

- A feeling of pressure, fullness, squeezing, or pain in the chest.
- Pain that originates in the chest and spreads to the shoulder(s), neck, upper back, and/or arm(s).
- Chest discomfort accompanied by a feeling of faintness or dizziness, a change in skin tone (paling or graying), profuse sweating, nausea, or shortness of breath.

If you experience any of these symptoms, call at once for emergency medical assistance. It is best to have a paramedic or other trained professional attend you as quickly as possible, rather than waiting for medical help until you arrive at the hospital.

■ Expect emergency medical personnel to immediately place you on monitoring equipment consisting of electrodes placed over the chest area and attached to a device that depicts electrical activity within heart muscle. They will likely also establish intravenous access so that medications may be administered directly into the bloodstream, and give you oxygen so as to maximize the delivery of oxygen to tissues that are starving for it. Unless the emergency team deems it necessary to begin other measures, such as cardioversion (administering electrical shock to the heart to restore rhythm), you will then be transported to the hospital, where your heart rhythm will be monitored constantly and other treatments administered as your condition requires.

CONVENTIONAL TREATMENT

■ A heart attack requires emergency medical intervention (*see* Emergency Treatment, above).

■ Ultrasound treatment to stop a heart attack in progress is a new technique being developed in Israel. In this procedure, doctors insert a catheter fitted with an ultrasound probe into an artery, position it at the blockage, and liquefy the clot with bursts of ultrasound. The procedure has worked successfully on thirteen out of fifteen patients in clinical trials. Trials of the procedure in the United States are in the planning stages.

■ Even once the crisis has passed, a heart attack can leave a person with any of an array of arrhythmias. Some are not very significant, while others can be quite serious and necessitate the use of any of several different kinds of drugs. Using drugs to treat abnormal heart rhythm is a bit like walking a tightrope, trying to balance between maintaining adequate output from the heart and holding down stress on the heart muscle, plus handling side effects. In general, doctors are likely to recommend drug treatment only for the most serious arrhythmias or those that cause major symptoms.

■ One treatment for coronary artery disease is coronary angioplasty. In this procedure, a balloon-tipped catheter (a thin, hollow, flexible tube) is threaded into an artery that is damaged by plaque. The balloon is then inflated, pushing the plaque back and increasing the open space within the vessel. Unfortunately, in an estimated 30 to 50 percent of cases, the artery becomes blocked again within six months and the process must be repeated.

■ Coronary artery bypass surgery is a procedure that brings blood to the heart by taking sections of blood vessels from elsewhere in the body and grafting them onto the coronary arteries to create detours around areas of blockage. This often improves quality of life, especially for people with angina, but it does not address the underlying process that led to the blocked arteries in the first place. As a result, nearly 40 percent of bypassed vessels are diseased again within five years.

■ For angina, relaxation and rest may be helpful. A doctor is also likely to prescribe nitrate drugs such as nitroglycerin (Nitro-Bid, Nitro-Dur, Nitrostat), to be used as needed. Beta-blocking drugs, which lower the heart rate and heart-muscle load, may also be prescribed. Examples include propranolol (Inderal), metoprolol (Lopressor), and atenolol (Tenormin).

■ Congestive heart failure is treated first with thiazide diuretics or a related drug, metolazone (Zaroxolyn). These drugs increase the elimination of fluids from the body and ease the heart's workload. In mild cases of heart failure, diuretics may be the only treatment. These drugs have side effects that can include excessive fluid loss, electrolyte imbalances (particularly potassium deficiency), dizziness, increased thirst, skin rashes, kidney problems, liver problems, low white-blood-cell counts, elevated blood sugar, excessive uric acid levels in the blood, and more.

■ For more serious heart failure, with poorer kidney function, a stronger class of drugs known as "loop" diuretics may be prescribed, either alone or in conjunction with the initial diuretic. Examples of loop diuretics include furosemide (Lasix), bumetanide (Bumex), and ethacrynic acid (Edecrin). If you must take one of these drugs, it is vital that you also take additional potassium, as this important mineral is excreted in the urine along with the drug. You will also have to be monitored for increased levels of nitrogen wastes in the blood, volume depletion (an insufficient amount of blood in the circulatory system), and resulting low—sometimes very low—blood pressure. Other possible side effects of these drugs include damage to the auditory nerve, skin rashes, and gastrointestinal complaints such as nausea, vomiting, diarrhea, and abdominal pains.

■ Another type of diuretic, known as "potassium-sparing" diuretics, may be used as well. These are not as strong as other types, but they can further reduce fluid retention without causing additional losses of potassium, which can have serious consequences for the heart. This class of drugs includes spironolactone (Aldactone), triamterene

(Dyrenium), and amiloride (Midamor). These drugs too can have side effects, including kidney damage, excessively high levels of potassium, and gastrointestinal upset. In men, spironolactone can cause breast enlargement, though this does not seem to occur in women.

■ Angiotensin-converting enzyme (ACE) inhibitors are rapidly becoming standard treatment for heart failure. They work by altering hormone levels in the blood to cause the blood vessels to relax and dilate. This lowers blood pressure. Although other drugs can do this as well, ACE inhibitors tend to do it without causing the body to develop a tolerance for the drug—a situation in which progressively higher and higher doses are required over time to achieve the same effect. Agents in this class include captopril (Capoten) and enalapril (Vasotec). Potential side effects include very low blood pressure, kidney problems resulting from an insufficient flow of blood to the kidneys, cough, skin rash, and a low white-blood-cell count. ACE inhibitors can also interact with other drugs in unwanted ways, and should *not* be used by pregnant women.

■ Nitroglycerin, or nitrate therapy, is another popular treatment that causes vasodilation (relaxation of the blood vessels). It is used primarily on a short-term basis, as tolerance is known to develop, making this drug less effective over time. Other undesirable effects include headaches and low blood pressure.

■ Often, combination therapy is used for heart failure—for example, putting diuretics together with ACE inhibitors. This increases the positive effects of the therapy, of course, but unfortunately allows for the possibility of drug interactions and more side effects.

■ Once the major drug used to treat heart failure, digitalis compounds (digitoxin, digoxin) are no longer as widely used. Recent studies have shown that these drugs ultimately had no effect on survival rates for people with heart failure. While the number of deaths from heart failure itself decreased with the use of digitalis, the death rate from arrhythmias (abnormal heart rhythms) increased, negating the positive effect. Moreover, these drugs must be taken at near-toxic levels to be effective.

■ Many doctors recommend a daily aspirin as a preventive measure, particularly in people who have already had one heart attack. Aspirin thins the blood, making it less prone to clotting. Some are now saying, however, that relying on aspirin may not be sufficient. A new blood-thinning drug named clopidogren was shown in a study of 19,000 people to reduce the risk of new heart attacks and strokes by one third. The study also found that those who use aspirin are more likely to suffer digestive bleeding as a side effect than those who take clopidogren. It should be noted, however, that certain individuals may benefit greatly from aspirin's anti-inflammatory effects. This is because

low-level inflammation of the arterial walls has been found to contribute to coronary artery disease. The presence of a type of protein called C-reactive protein is considered to be a sign of inflammation. People with high levels of C-reactive protein in their blood may be able to reduce their risk of a heart attack by taking aspirin.

■ Treatment of infectious heart disorders is based on very aggressive antibacterial therapy. However, surgical replacement of an affected valve may be necessary.

■ Arrhythmias are treated with any of five different types of drugs, depending upon where the electrical activity is abnormal and the specific trait of the rhythm—whether it is too slow, too fast, or irregular. There are also pacemakers, electrical devices that can be implanted or worn externally to override the abnormal impulses within the heart. A technique called *cardioversion* may be used in some cases. This involves applying a controlled electrical shock to the chest region that may jolt the heart back into a more normal rhythm.

■ High doses of magnesium may be effective in calming some arrhythmias, though mainstream medicine is just beginning to explore this kind of treatment. This natural mineral has little to no toxicity, even when taken in huge doses. Unfortunately, such doses must be given intravenously; if taken by mouth, large amounts of magnesium cause diarrhea.

■ Cardiomyopathy is difficult to treat. Beta-blockers such as metoprolol (Lopressor) or propranolol (Inderal) may help in some cases by slowing the heart rhythm and allowing better filling of the heart chambers between beats. Fluid retention may be treated with diuretics. Ultimately, transplantation may be the only option. However, the cost, limited availability, trauma of such massive surgery, and the suppression of the immune system caused by the anti-rejection drugs needed after surgery obviously make this a last resort.

■ People with rheumatic heart disease are usually advised to take preventive antibiotics before elective surgery, dental work, and other invasive procedures to prevent infection from establishing itself on heart valves and worsening the damage. If the damage is severe enough, surgical valve replacement may be necessary.

■ Many valvular problems remain minor, even for years, and require only observation. Mitral valve prolapse generally falls into this category. For some cases of other valvular disorders, a doctor may prescribe anticoagulants (blood thinners) to prevent the formation of clots due to abnormalities in blood flow. Other medical treatments may be necessary for symptoms such as shortness of breath, edema (swelling due to an accumulation of fluid in the tissues), arrhythmias, or other problems. Moderate to severe damage to any one of the valves may require surgical treatment or replacement of the valve to assure adequate blood flow and avoid heart failure. If you must take blood-thinning medication, it is vital that you avoid aspirin, or excessive bleeding may result.

■ If you are diagnosed with any type of cardiovascular disease, it is wise to seek out and work closely with a cardiologist or other physician who specializes, or at the very least has considerable experience, in the treatment of your condition.

DIETARY GUIDELINES

■ If you are overweight, adopt a healthy weight-reduction diet plan and stick to it. Obesity places a strain on the cardiovascular system.

■ Eat a low-fat, high-fiber diet. This will reduce your blood-cholesterol levels, and your arteries may even begin to clear. Take in no more than 25 to 30 percent of daily calories from fat per day—and make sure any fat you consume is "good" fat. Monounsaturated fats, found in olive and canola oil, cause levels of low-density lipoproteins (LDL, the so-called "bad cholesterol") to decline without affecting levels of high-density lipoproteins (HDL, or "good cholesterol"). Saturated fats, found primarily in animal products such as meat and dairy foods, and trans-fatty acids, a group of unnatural fats found in margarine, shortening, and hydrogenated and partially hydrogenated oils, have the opposite effect. These should be avoided. Meat and dairy products are also loaded with cholesterol.

■ Eat a diet rich in fruits and vegetables. Emphasize foods that are rich in the antioxidant substances (beta-carotene, vitamins C and E, and selenium) that fight free radicals. Enjoy fruits, tomatoes, carrots, sweet potatoes, dark leafy greens, alfalfa sprouts, and whole-grain products.

■ Put Concord grapes, eggplant, and red cabbage on the menu. If you drink wine, enjoy a glass of red wine with your dinner. Experts believe that pigments called anthocyanidins in red wine grapes may explain why moderate consumption of red wine can help lower the risk of heart attack and stroke. This substance is known to dilate blood vessels, which helps keep blood flowing freely. Anthocyanidins are found in blue and purple fruits and vegetables.

■ Avoid grilled and barbecued foods. Research shows that people who favor meat cooked over smouldering charcoal are increasing their risk of cardiomyopathy. Carcinogens that form during the browning process are believed to contribute to inflammation of the arteries and the deterioration of the heart muscle.

■ Limit your intake of salt. Salt contains sodium, which increases fluid retention and makes the heart work harder. The average American ingests an average of 8 to 10 grams (8,000 to 10,000 milligrams) of sodium daily. The American Heart Association advises heart patients to limit their sodium intake from all sources to the equivalent of no more than 1 teaspoon of salt daily.

■ If you take aspirin regularly for a heart condition, avoid alcohol and antacids, especially within an hour or so of taking the aspirin. The combination of aspirin and alcohol can easily aggravate the stomach, and it is possible for blood-alcohol levels to become higher than they normally would if aspirin is taken even an hour before. Using antacids can reduce the amount of aspirin circulating in the body.

NUTRITIONAL SUPPLEMENTS

■ Take a good multivitamin and mineral supplement daily. Choose a powdered or capsule form for best absorption.

■ The antioxidant nutrients are very important, and it is difficult to get enough of them from food. Take 5,000 international units of vitamin A and 15,000 international units of beta-carotene daily; 1,000 milligrams of vitamin C three times a day; 400 to 800 international units of vitamin E twice a day; and 200 micrograms of selenium daily.

Note: If you are pregnant, or intend to get pregnant, or if you have liver disease, consult your doctor before taking supplemental vitamin A. If you have high blood pressure, limit your intake of supplemental vitamin E to a total of 400 international units daily, and if you are taking an anticoagulant (blood thinner), consult your physician before taking supplemental vitamin E.

■ Carnitine, a substance related to the B vitamins but often grouped with the amino acids, is responsible for the conversion of long-chain fatty acids into energy. It is very useful for its ability to improve cellular oxygenation, and can be helpful for angina, arrhythmias, and recovery from a cardiac episode such as a heart attack. Carnitine has also been shown to lower triglyceride and total cholesterol levels, while at the same time improving HDL levels. Start by taking a dose of 250 to 500 milligrams of L-carnitine with breakfast. After one week, add a second dose, with lunch. After another week, add a third dose, so that you are taking 250 to 500 milligrams with each meal, and after still another week, add a fourth dose at bedtime.

■ Coenzyme Q_{10} improves oxygenation of tissues. It is involved in the body's energy-producing pathways, and seems particularly to affect heart-muscle function. It is especially helpful for symptoms of mitral valve prolapse. Take a minimum of 100 milligrams of coenzyme Q_{10} daily.

■ Essential fatty acids such as those found in black currant seed oil, borage oil, evening primrose oil, fish oil, and flaxseed oil help to prevent unnecessary blood clotting, reduce inflammation, and regulate blood pressure. Take 500 to 1,000 milligrams of any of these oils twice daily.

■ Magnesium can stabilize an irregular heartbeat. In addition, magnesium deficiencies have been identified in more than 20 percent of people with cardiovascular disease. Take up to 500 milligrams of magnesium daily.

Note: An excess of this mineral can cause diarrhea. If you develop loose stools, reduce the dosage slightly until you arrive at the best dosage for your body.

■ Zinc is an antioxidant that helps maintain proper immune function. Take 15 to 20 milligrams of zinc picolinate, aspartate, or gluconate twice daily.

Note: Take zinc with food to prevent stomach upset. If you take over 30 milligrams of zinc on a daily basis for more than one or two months, you should also take 1 to 2 milligrams of copper each day to maintain a proper mineral balance.

HERBAL TREATMENT

Herbal treatments for cardiovascular disease are not meant to be a substitute for appropriate treatment for heart attack. If you suspect a heart attack, seek emergency medical treatment immediately.

■ Artichoke leaf extract reduces blood cholesterol and protects the liver. This herb has antioxidant activity and may inhibit the oxidation of cholesterol, a factor in atherosclerosis. Take 250 to 300 milligrams two or three times daily.

■ Cat's claw contains a variety of valuable phytochemicals. One of these compounds has shown an ability to inhibit processes involved in the formation of blood clots. By increasing circulation and inhibiting inappropriate clotting, it may help to prevent stroke and reduce the risk of heart attack. Take 500 milligrams three times daily.

■ Fo-ti (also known by its Chinese name, *ho shou wu*, and its botanical name, *Polygonum multiflorum*), has shown effectiveness in combating the symptoms of heart disease, helping to reduce blood pressure and blood-cholesterol levels. Take 500 to 1,000 milligrams once or twice daily.

■ Ginkgo biloba enhances circulation. Choose a product containing at least 24 percent ginkgo heterosides (sometimes called flavoglycosides) and take 40 to 60 milligrams three times daily.

■ Guggul, an Indian herb derived from a type of myrrh tree, lowers blood-fat levels while raising levels of HDLs, the so called "good cholesterol." Take 500 milligrams of standardized extract three times a day.

Note: Do not use this herb if you have a thyroid disorder.

■ Hawthorn (sometimes called by its Latin genus name, *Crataegus*) contains a combination of flavonoids that can protect the heart against oxygen deprivation and the development of abnormal rhythms. It also reduces blood levels of cholesterol and triglycerides, and brings down high blood pressure. Choose a standardized extract containing 1.8 percent vitexin-2 rhamnosides and take 100 to 200 milligrams three times a day.

■ Oat straw and kava kava are tonics for the nervous system. Take 500 milligrams of oat straw twice a day or 150 milligrams of kava kava three times a day.

■ White willow bark contains salicin, an aspirinlike compound, and has been used for centuries much as aspirin is today. If your doctor has recommended that you take aspirin for a cardiovascular condition, but you have found that the drug upsets your stomach and are looking for an alternative, you may want to discuss this herb with your physician.

Note: You should not use this herb if you are allergic to aspirin.

HOMEOPATHY

Homeopathic treatment for cardiovascular disease is not meant to be a substitute for appropriate treatment for heart attack. If you suspect a heart attack, seek emergency medical treatment immediately.

■ *Carduus marianus* is for the heart patient with a history of alcoholism and a propensity for drinking beer. This remedy helps regulate the heart and can slowly reverse symptoms. Take one dose of *Carduus marianus* 3x or 6c three times daily for one week of each month for three months.

■ *Crataegus* is a general remedy that helps regulate the heart. Take one dose of *Crataegus* 3x or 3c twice daily for one week of each month for three months.

BACH FLOWER REMEDIES

Select the remedy that most closely fits your emotional tendencies and concerns, and take it as needed, following the directions on the product label. Bach remedies are not meant to be used as a treatment for heart attack. If you suspect a heart attack, seek emergency medical treatment immediately.

■ Beech is the remedy of choice if you are a perfectionist with a type-A personality and tend to be impatient and intolerant.

■ Holly is helpful if you are often angry and have fits of temper.

■ Impatiens is good if you are nervous and tend to be impatient with others.

■ Mustard will help if you are depressed and full of sadness and sorrow.

■ Choose Willow if you are unsatisfied and feel as if nothing is ever quite good enough.

ACUPRESSURE

Acupressure is not meant to be used as a treatment for heart attack. If you suspect a heart attack, seek emergency medical treatment immediately. For the locations of acupressure points on the body, *see* ADMINISTERING AN ACUPRESSURE TREATMENT in Part Three.

■ Heart 3 and 7 help to stimulate circulation in the chest.

■ The inner and outer back Bladder points improve circulation and relax the nervous system.

■ Liver 3 also helps to quiet the nervous system.

■ Pericardium 6 relaxes the chest and eases agitation.

AROMATHERAPY

Aromatherapy is not meant to be used as a treatment for heart attack. If you suspect a heart attack, seek emergency medical treatment immediately. For specific instructions on how to use aromatherapy, *see* PREPARING AROMATHERAPY TREATMENTS in Part Three.

■ Essential oils of basil, geranium, lavender, neroli, pine, thyme, and vetiver all aid circulation. Use one or more of them as inhalants or diffuse them into the air, or add a few drops to massage oil and use it in conjunction with massage.

■ Elemi and frankincense are good for neutralizing stress, an important factor in cardiovascular disease. Use either or both as inhalants, diffuse them into the air, use them to prepare a relaxing bath, or add a few drops to massage oil.

GENERAL RECOMMENDATIONS

■ Whether you have been treated for cardiovascular problems or wish to prevent them, address and eliminate all possible risk factors: Pay attention to your diet, and keep your weight down. Don't smoke, and avoid second-hand smoke. Get regular exercise (if you have cardiovascular disease, consult your physician before beginning any new exercise program).

■ Look into chelation therapy, a treatment method that is gaining more acceptance as its benefits become better known. This is a type of treatment in which a chemical agent (usually ethylenediaminetetraacetic acid, or EDTA) is administered intravenously and binds to minerals and metals, allowing the body to excrete them in the urine. Tests have shown that many people experience distinct improvement in both exercise tolerance and blood-vessel blockage after this treatment. It usually consists of a series of twenty to thirty three-hour sessions. More information can be obtained from the American College of Advancement in Medicine (see the Resources section at the end of the book).

PREVENTION

■ Eat a low-fat, high-fiber diet. Dr. Dean Ornish, author and advocate of healthy lifestyle changes, reports that clogged coronary arteries continue to widen as people improve their diets.

■ Maintain a lean and fit body. Persons who are 30 percent or more overweight have an increased risk of many diseases, including heart disease.

■ Exercise regularly. Exercise has been shown to increase HDL levels and lower LDLs. Further, studies show that people who get regular aerobic exercise have as much as a 50 percent lower risk of dying from cardiovascular disease than those who do not.

■ Eat plenty of garlic, or take garlic supplements. In a German study, researchers found that taking supplemental garlic regularly has a protective effect on the elasticity of the aorta, the main artery that carries blood away from the heart. It also promotes more efficient heart function. The minimum effective dose in the study was 300 milligrams of standardized garlic powder daily.

■ As much as possible, avoid stress, and learn techniques to manage stress you cannot avoid. Stress is a risk factor for heart disease.

■ If you are a smoker, quit now. Smoking accelerates the development of atherosclerotic plaque, especially in the larger blood vessels. The American Heart Association says smoking is one of the major risk factors for heart disease. A study reported in *The New England Journal of Medicine* found that men who quit smoking in midlife lowered their risk of death from all causes by as much as 41 percent.

■ Taking supplemental vitamin E can reduce the risk of heart disease. A study from Cambridge University found that men at high risk of heart disease were 75 percent less likely to have a heart attack if they were taking vitamin E. A unisex study done at Harvard University found that taking vitamin E reduced the risk of heart disease by 40 percent. Start by taking 200 international units daily, then gradually increase the dosage until you are taking up to 800 international units daily, preferably with 200 micrograms of selenium. Choose the mixed-tocopherol form of vitamin E; this is a natural form of the vitamin and easily absorbed by the body.

Note: If you have high blood pressure, limit your intake of supplemental vitamin E to a total of 400 international units daily. If you are taking an anticoagulant (blood thinner), consult your physician before taking supplemental vitamin E.

■ Studies have shown that drinking *moderate* amounts of alcohol (one or two drinks a day) can cut the risk of heart attack in healthy people. In one study, moderate alcohol consumption after a heart attack reduced cell death by 50 percent, and almost doubled the recovery of muscle function in the heart.

■ Oral contraceptives appear to be safe for young women who do not smoke and who do not have high blood pressure. However, the risk of heart attack increases dramatically in women over thirty-five and in those who smoke, according to a study by the World Health Organization that involved women from seventeen different countries.

■ Heart attacks are a common complication following surgery in those who have underlying coronary artery disease, even if the operation is completely unrelated to the cardiovascular system. After the trauma of surgery, the heart can race at 100 to 110 beats per minute for several days, which can have serious consequences for those with atherosclerosis. Beta-blockers, which are drugs that reduce the speed and force of the heartbeat, may be prescribed after surgery to prevent this.

■ People who have undergone heart surgery face a higher than normal risk of developing heart failure because of damage to the heart tissue. In such cases, a type of drug called an angiotensin-converting enzyme (ACE) inhibitor may be useful in correcting or preventing hormonal imbalances that may precede heart failure.

■ Monitor your blood pressure and make sure it stays within the acceptable range (*see* HIGH BLOOD PRESSURE).

Carsickness

See MOTION SICKNESS.

Carpal Tunnel Syndrome

Carpal tunnel syndrome (CTS) is a condition that results from excessive and continuing pressure on the median nerve. The median nerve carries sensory messages from the thumb and some fingers to the brain, and also instructions from the brain to the muscles in the hand. On its way, it passes into the hand through a narrow gap situated under a ligament at the front of the wrist. This gap is the carpal (wrist) tunnel.

Most cases of CTS can be attributed to repetitive stress injury. Repeatedly making certain motions involving the wrist creates inflammation, which causes the tissue of the tunnel to press on the median nerve. Carpal tunnel syndrome is the result. Symptoms include numbness, tingling, and pain in the thumb, index, and middle fingers. The pain is often worse at night. The condition can affect one or both hands, and is often accompanied by muscle weakness, particularly in the thumbs.

According to the National Institute for Occupational Safety and Health, repetitive stress injuries account for 62 percent of the occupational illness reported in America, and the National Bureau of Labor Statistics says the number of workers affected by repetitive stress injuries increases by 10 percent every year. Carpal tunnel syndrome is the leading contender in repetitive stress injuries.

There are many different types of repetitive motion that can cause injuries. Computer data-entry and cashiering in a supermarket are in the forefront, simply because these occupations require long hours punching keys. Lesser known causes include writing, small-parts assembly, guitar-playing, knitting, crocheting—even playing tennis. Chefs who spend hours each day cutting and chopping sometimes suffer from carpal tunnel syndrome as well.

For reasons unknown, this condition occurs most often among middle-aged women. It occurs more often than usual in women who have just started taking birth control pills, pregnant women, and women who suffer from premenstrual syndrome. Arthritis sufferers of both sexes also seem more likely to be afflicted than other people.

Diagnosis of CTS may involve a type of testing called electromyography (EMG). This procedure involves sending electrical impulses through the arm and measuring the speed at which they travel. Normally, nerve impulses travel at a speed of approximately 136 meters per second. However, if the nerves are damaged or compressed, the speed of transmission is much slower. If the impulse registers in the range of 90 to 95 meters per second, carpal tunnel syndrome is likely.

CONVENTIONAL MEDICINE

■ With rest and elevation, the condition may resolve itself without treatment. In the meantime, applying ice packs can reduce swelling, and splinting the affected hand at night can alleviate symptoms. The splint holds the hand in the correct position and ensures that you don't exacerbate the condition.

■ Anti-inflammatory drugs such as ibuprofen (Advil, Motrin, Nuprin, and others), naproxen (Aleve, Anaprox, Naprelan, Naprosyn), and many others can help relieve pain and bring down swelling. As with all drugs, side effects, including gastrointestinal distress and, possibly, ulceration, are a possibility.

■ If symptoms persist, your doctor may suggest injecting a small dose of a corticosteroid drug directly into the wrist area.

■ Surgery is the treatment of last resort for carpal tunnel syndrome. In this procedure, the physician cuts the ligament that forms part of the carpal tunnel to reduce the pressure on the nerve and, therefore, the pain. Long-term results with this technique are mixed.

DIETARY GUIDELINES

■ Anything that disturbs circulation will worsen the problem. Avoid concentrated saturated fats, which are difficult to digest at the best of times. Also avoid stimulants such as coffee, tea, and alcohol.

■ Limit your intake of salt. Salt contains sodium, which increases the body's tendency to retain fluids, which can be a factor in carpal tunnel syndrome.

NUTRITIONAL SUPPLEMENTS

■ The antioxidants, especially vitamins C, D, and E, and selenium, are essential for the repair and healing of inflamed tissue. Vitamin C in particular is useful for restoring connective tissue. Take 1,000 milligrams of vitamin C and 400 international units of vitamin E twice a day, plus 400 international units of vitamin D and 200 micrograms of selenium daily.

Note: When you start taking vitamin E, begin with 100 or 200 milligrams and gradually increase to the recommended amount. If you have high blood pressure, limit your intake of supplemental vitamin E to a total of 400 international units daily. If you are taking an anticoagulant (blood thinner), consult your physician before taking supplemental vitamin E.

■ To strengthen your nervous system, take 300 to 500 milligrams of calcium and 200 to 250 milligrams of magnesium twice a day until your symptoms improve.

■ Hormonal changes involved in pregnancy, the menstrual cycle, and menopause can cause excess fluid retention. If your symptoms seem worse during these times, take 99 milligrams of potassium chelate, aspartate, or citrate twice daily as long as you have symptoms. This natural diuretic can gently reduce bloating and water retention.

■ Vitamin B$_6$ (pyridoxine) is effective in relieving nerve disorders and fluid retention. Take 50 to 75 milligrams twice daily until symptoms improve. This can take from thirty to ninety days. Then gradually lower the dose, by approximately 25 milligrams a week, to the lowest amount that maintains control. It has been suggested that a deficiency of vitamin B$_6$ may increase the likelihood of developing carpal tunnel syndrome.

Note: If you take any of the B vitamins individually, you should also take a B-complex supplement at a different time of day.

HERBAL TREATMENT

■ Bromelain and papain are digestive enzymes that help

reduce swelling and inflammation. Take 300 to 500 milligrams of each three times daily, between meals.

■ Ginkgo biloba acts to improve circulation, especially to the hands, feet, and brain. Choose a product containing 24 percent ginkgo heterosides (sometimes called flavoglycosides) and take 40 to 60 milligrams three times daily.

■ Pine-bark and grape-seed extracts have excellent anti-inflammatory properties. Take 25 to 50 milligrams of either three times a day.

■ Turmeric contains curcumin, another useful anti-inflammatory. Take 500 milligrams three times daily.

HOMEOPATHY

■ For the first forty-eight hours, when your symptoms are acute, take one dose of *Arnica* 30x or 15c three times a day. Homeopathic *Arnica* may also be used topically to alleviate pain.

■ Take one dose of *Ruta graveolens* 12x or 6c three times a day for three days following the administration of *Arnica*.

ACUPRESSURE AND MASSAGE

For the locations of acupressure points on the body, *see* ADMINISTERING AN ACUPRESSURE TREATMENT in Part Three.

■ Massage warm castor oil along Pericardium 6. If your arm is too sensitive on the side where you have carpal tunnel syndrome, massage the oil along the opposite side only.

■ Gallbladder 34 and Liver 3 relax muscles and tendons.

■ Large Intestine 4 relaxes the nervous system.

■ General massage of the shoulders, arm, and upper back can help by relaxing the area and improving circulation.

GENERAL RECOMMENDATIONS

■ Take care to use your whole hand, not just your wrist, during repetitive motion activities. Change your position frequently.

■ If you work at a keyboard, use a foam wrist rest and a rigid splint to keep your hand supported and in the proper position.

■ Don't smoke, and avoid secondhand smoke. Smoking impairs circulation and makes you more susceptible to a host of disorders.

■ Consider consulting an acupuncturist. Acupuncture has been shown to very effective for carpal tunnel syndrome.

■ If you can find a chiropractor skilled in sports chiropractic techniques, wrist manipulation may be beneficial. It is vital to consult a practitioner who is specifically trained and experienced in this type of work, however.

PREVENTION

■ If your job requires making repetitive motions of the hands or fingers, take scheduled breaks.

■ Talk with your doctor or a physical or occupational therapist about different methods of performing the necessary repetitive motions connected with your occupation. He or she may be able to demonstrate another way of working that can ease the continuing stress connected with carpal tunnel syndrome.

Cataracts

A cataract is a spot on the lens of the eye that has lost its transparency. The lens is the structure within the eye that is responsible for focusing incoming light so that it forms clear images on the retina. When you shift your attention from the fine print in the newspaper to something going on outside your window, it is your lens that makes the adjustment to allow you to see properly. Located just behind the pupil, the lens is a tiny structure, convex on both sides, composed of many tightly packed transparent cells. If something happens to harm the lens, some of these transparent cells may turn an opaque white—much as the white of an egg goes from being a clear liquid to solid white when poached.

Cataracts develop gradually, usually over a period of many years. Almost everyone over the age of sixty-five has some degree of lens opacity, but it is usually minor and does not interfere with vision. However, as more and more transparency is lost over time, vision suffers. The first sign is usually a loss of clarity and detail and, possibly, some blurring. Even at a very early stage, night driving can become a challenge. Many people chalk these symptoms up to the fact that they are getting older. They realize they have cataracts only when vision loss becomes impossible to ignore.

Interestingly, in the early stages of cataract development, the progressive hardening of the center of the lens can cause a person to become nearsighted. A person who was previously farsighted (very common in the age group most likely to develop cataracts) may be delighted to discover he or she is able to read without reading glasses for the first time in many years. This effect is only temporary, however. In the later stages, the perception of color may change. For example, blues may look dull and gray, and reds, yellows, and oranges may appear brighter. Many people find themselves having increasing difficulty telling certain colors apart.

Cataracts usually occur in both eyes. However, in most cases, one eye is more severely affected than the other. Until the condition is well advanced, there is no external sign of any damage. It is only when the lens becomes opaque that the whiteness is visible through the pupil. Cataracts are painless and never cause total blindness. Even a severely affected lens will admit some light.

In people aged seventy-five and over, cataracts are common. In fact, cataracts are so prevalent in older people that the condition is considered a normal part of the degenerative aging process. This may be because people are now living longer, resulting in long-term exposure to free radicals, which increases the likelihood of cellular damage throughout the body, including the eyes. Free-radical damage is believed to be a contributing factor in the development of cataracts.

Other known causes of cataracts include trauma, either by a direct injury to the lens or even a hard blow to the head, and excessive exposure to certain chemicals, such as can occur with prolonged use of steroid drugs or poisoning by substances such as naphthalene (found in mothballs) or ergot (a fungus that can occur on stored grain). High blood-sugar levels, such as occur in severe untreated diabetes, are associated with cataracts. Unless sufficient precautions are taken, exposure to infrared rays or x-rays can lead to cataracts as well.

CONVENTIONAL TREATMENT

■ In the early stages of cataract development, a stronger prescription for corrective lenses may be sufficient. If vision loss starts to interfere with your everyday activities, however, your doctor is likely to recommend surgery. Cataract surgery is one of the most common and most successful operations performed today; as long as the eye is otherwise healthy, cataract removal is successful in 90 to 95 percent of all cases. Cataract surgery involves first removing the affected lens, and then implanting a tiny plastic intraocular lens. The lens can be removed surgically, all in one piece, or, with phacoemulsification, an advanced ultrasound technique, it can be fragmented and removed through a minuscule incision that requires no stitching afterward. The operation may be performed using either general or local anesthesia, but there is no pain in either case. You may or may not require glasses after the operation. The incision takes about a month to heal. Recuperation is faster with the laser technique. Glasses are not fitted until about ten weeks after surgery.

■ If you have a history of other eye diseases in addition to your cataracts, lens implants may be considered unsuitable. If that is the case, contact lenses will be prescribed for you after surgery.

■ It is possible for a cataract to swell and cause acute glaucoma. If you have a developing cataract and experience sudden pain in or behind your eyes, you should consult an ophthalmologist immediately. (*See* GLAUCOMA.)

DIETARY GUIDELINES

■ Follow a healthy high-fiber diet plan with an emphasis on whole foods.

■ Maximize your intake of vegetables and fruits rich in carotenes. Yellow and orange vegetables and fruits, plus green leafy vegetables (including beet greens, spinach, and broccoli), are all rich sources of these phytochemicals.

■ To insure sufficient hydration, drink eight glasses of pure water every day. The membranes of the eye are particularly susceptible to dehydration.

NUTRITIONAL SUPPLEMENTS

The nutritional supplements recommended here are directed at speeding healing after cataract surgery.

Alpha-lipoic acid is a powerful antioxidant. Take 150 milligrams three times daily for one month, then cut back to 150 milligrams twice daily for three more months. Other antioxidants that may help include N-acetylcysteine and coenzyme Q_{10}. Take 250 milligrams of N-acetylcysteine three times daily and 30 milligrams of lipid-soluble coenzyme Q_{10} four times a day.

Lutein is a carotenoid that is concentrated in the pupil. Take 500 to 1,000 micrograms of lutein twice a day.

Many people, especially older people, do not eat as many servings of vegetables as they should, resulting in deficiencies of important minerals. Take a good multimineral formula that supplies a total of 500 milligrams of magnesium, 99 milligrams of potassium, and 200 micrograms of selenium daily. Take these minerals with food.

Take 5,000 international units of vitamin A three times daily, plus 25,000 international units of beta-carotene twice daily, for one month.

Note: If you are pregnant, or intend to get pregnant, or if you have liver disease, consult your doctor before taking supplemental vitamin A. Pregnant women should not ingest a total of more than 25,000 international units of supplemental vitamin A *per week* from all sources.

Vitamin B_2 (riboflavin) can be therapeutic in some cases. Take 50 milligrams of vitamin B_2 daily for six weeks. Then take a high-potency B-complex supplement daily. If you take any of the B vitamins individually, you should also take a B-complex supplement at a different time of day.

Pantothenic acid supports adrenal function and helps ensure a speedy recovery after surgery. Take 200 milligrams of pantothenic acid twice a day for one month.

Vitamin C and bioflavonoids have antioxidant and anti-inflammatory properties, and are important to the healing process. Three times a day, take 500 milligrams of a buffered vitamin-C formula that includes bioflavonoids.

■ Vitamin E fights free-radical damage and is also a good anti-inflammatory. Choose a product containing mixed tocopherols and begin by taking 100 or 200 milligrams at bedtime, then gradually increase until you are taking 400 international units daily.

Note: If you are taking an anticoagulant (blood thinner), consult your physician before taking supplemental vitamin E.

HERBAL TREATMENT

■ Bilberry has been used for over 200 years for eye problems. Experiments have shown that this herb can inhibit retinal degeneration and slow the development of cataracts. The effectiveness of bilberry is tied to certain phytochemicals, called anthocyanidins, that it contains. Select a product containing 25 percent anthocyanidins (also called PCOs) and take 80 milligrams two or three times daily.

■ Pine-bark and grape-seed extracts are valuable against inflammation and also have notable antioxidant effects. Take 25 to 50 milligrams of either three times daily.

HOMEOPATHY

The homeopathic remedies recommended here are directed at speeding healing after cataract surgery.

■ *Causticum* is good if you have inflamed eyelids and feel as if there is a film before your eyes. You may be seeing dark spots and experiencing some motor disturbances. On the emotional level, you are intensely sympathetic, and may be grappling with a sudden emotion or suffering from long-lasting grief. Take one dose of *Causticum* 30x or 12c, as directed on the product label, two to three times daily for one week before and one week after surgery.

■ Choose *Euphrasia* if you blink frequently and your eyes water all the time. The tears may burn, your eyelids may be swollen, and there may be a feeling of pressure behind your eyes. Take one dose of *Euphrasia* 30x or 12c two to three times daily for one week before and one week after surgery.

■ *Phosphorus* is beneficial if your eyes tire easily and you have the sensation that there is a veil over your eyes. Your spirits may be low, and you may feel hungry again soon after eating. Take one dose of *Phosphorus* 30x or 12c, as directed on the product label, two to three times daily for one week before and one week after surgery.

BACH FLOWER REMEDIES

■ Rescue Remedy will help to ease any feelings of anxiety you may have before and after surgery. This is the premier Bach flower remedy against fear and anxiety. Take it as needed.

ACUPRESSURE

For the locations of acupressure points on the body, *see* ADMINISTERING AN ACUPRESSURE TREATMENT in Part Three.

■ Gallbladder 20 and 21 improve circulation to the head and promote healing.

■ Large Intestine 4 has a beneficial effect on the head and face, including the eyes.

■ Liver 3 quiets the nervous system and helps relieve eye pain.

■ Stomach 36 helps tone the digestive tract and speed recovery from surgery.

GENERAL RECOMMENDATIONS

■ Your doctor will give you instructions on how to care for yourself after surgery. To prevent complications, follow these instructions exactly.

■ If you don't already have a good pair of sunglasses to protect your eyes against the ultraviolet rays in sunlight, invest in a pair with polarized lenses that is guaranteed to filter out the sun's ultraviolet (UV) rays, and wear them whenever you are outdoors.

PREVENTION

■ There is a growing body of evidence showing that free-radical damage is a major contributor to degenerative problems such as cataracts. Eating a healthy diet including a wide variety of whole foods is the best way to get the antioxidant nutrients that fight free-radical damage. If you're not going to eat your veggies, take a good antioxidant supplement regularly.

Cavities

See TOOTH DECAY.

Cat-Scratch Disease

See under PETS AND YOUR HEALTH *under* HOME AND PERSONAL SAFETY in Part One.

Celiac Disease

Celiac disease is an illness caused by an intolerance to gluten, a substance found in wheat, rye, barley, and oats. When a person with this intolerance eats these foods, a protein in gluten called gliadin causes a reaction that results in damage to the intestinal wall. This in turn leads to an inability to absorb most nutrients and eventually to malnutrition.

This condition can first appear either in childhood or adulthood, and symptoms can be mild or severe. It is believed to be inherited, although some people begin to show signs of it only after surgery on the stomach. In severe cases, there are symptoms such as weight loss, bloating, diarrhea, abdominal pain, and vomiting in addition to anemia, muscle-wasting, and other problems resulting from nutritional deficiencies. Fluid may accumulate in the tissues of the legs and feet. In children, growth may be severely retarded. Softening of the bones can develop in the later stages of this illness.

Some people experience no abdominal symptoms but do develop signs of nutritional deficiencies. Such cases are more difficult to diagnose, but once a correct diagnosis is made, the condition can usually be managed successfully.

CONVENTIONAL TREATMENT

■ A diet free of gluten is the primary treatment. Foods containing gluten—anything made from wheat, rye, barley, or oats—must be eliminated or severely restricted. Brown rice and other grains are usually acceptable. Celiac disease is a chronic problem and must handled throughout your lifetime. Deviating from the restricted diet at any time can cause a relapse. Following a gluten-free diet usually relieves symptoms quickly. Generally, this diet must be maintained for life, as eating gluten can trigger symptoms and, eventually, malnutrition again. It is possible that once you are symptom-free and tests show that your intestines have healed, you may be able to eat small amounts of gluten on occasion. This should be done only with medical supervision, however.

■ If you have become severely malnourished as a result of celiac disease, you may need to receive intravenous nutrition to help rebuild your body. Vitamin and mineral supplements may also be prescribed if you are unable to absorb nutrients from foods.

■ If dietary restriction proves ineffective, prednisone (Deltasone) may be prescribed. This is a steroid that suppresses the body's inflammatory response. However, it also has adverse effects on immune function and the adrenal gland, so it is best to take the lowest dose that helps, and for the shortest possible amount of time. If abstaining from all gluten-containing foods fails to solve the problem, it may also be worth considering the possibility of another diagnosis (*see* CROHN'S DISEASE and/or IRRITABLE BOWEL SYNDROME).

DIETARY GUIDELINES

■ As discussed under Conventional Treatment, a restricted diet is the primary form of treatment for celiac disease.

Nutritionists and dietitians are good sources of information about which foods have gluten in them, as well as ideas for gluten-free cooking. Gluten is often a hidden ingredient in food products. For example, products that list "cereal fillers" or "hydrolyzed protein" on the labels contain gluten, and so must be avoided. It is best to work with a professional in developing the correct diet for your individual needs.

NUTRITIONAL SUPPLEMENTS

Acidophilus and bifidus supplements contribute to a healthy intestinal tract, reduce the formation of gas, and can help improve digestion and assimilation of nutrients. Take them as recommended on the product labels. If you are allergic to milk, select dairy-free products.

Digestive enzymes can be helpful for breaking down complex carbohydrates before they reach the intestines. These are generally made from cow pancreas and need to be concentrated to be effective. Take one to three capsules with each meal, as directed on the product label.

HERBAL TREATMENT

Aloe vera, taken in small amounts, can help decrease inflammation in the intestines. Be sure to buy the edible (food-grade) form of this plant. Take 1 tablespoon twice a day, as needed.

Slippery elm is soothing to the digestive tract. It can be taken in capsule or tea form, or made into a paste with water and added to food. Slippery elm has a mild taste. Take 500 milligrams twice a day, as needed.

HOMEOPATHY

Consult a homeopathic physician who can prescribe a constitutional remedy. Often a constitutional remedy can enhance digestion and ease the course of this illness.

For relief of acute, diffuse abdominal gas and difficulty digesting food, take one dose of *China* 12x or 5c, as directed on the product label, three times a day for three days.

For short-term relief of low-bowel gas, take one dose of *Lycopodium* 12x or 5c three times a day for three days.

GENERAL RECOMMENDATIONS

Be aware of your reactions to the different foods in your diet. If you seem to be reacting to foods that contain gluten, consult your physician.

If you are diagnosed with celiac disease, stick to your dietary restrictions. Experiment with gluten-free recipes and learn how to prepare gluten-free foods you like.

■ Seek counseling or a support group to help you deal with the emotional stresses of chronic illness.

Cellulitis

Cellulitis is an inflammation of the skin and the tissues just beneath the skin that results from bacterial infection. Any of a number of different bacteria, including staphylococci and streptococci, may be responsible. The infection manifests itself as a painful, hot, red area with an indistinct border, and can spread both sideways and into deeper tissues. Symptoms generally come on suddenly and increase in severity over a twenty-four-hour period. Cellulitis can occur anywhere on the body, though it is most often found in areas where breaks in the skin provide a pathway for bacteria to enter and in places affected by edema (swelling due to fluid retention). The face and lower legs are the most common sites. People with edema (whether lymphedema or ordinary edema) are particularly at risk. Other risk factors include animal or human bites; diabetes; the use of steroid medications; a history of peripheral blood-vessel disease; and recent cardiovascular or pulmonary surgery or invasive dental work. The skin symptoms may or may not be accompanied by fever, chills, heart palpitations, headache, and/or mental confusion.

Deeper, more serious cases of cellulitis can progress to a state called *necrotizing cellulitis-fasciitis*. In this form of the disorder, the infection can destroy tissue at a very rapid rate, and tissue destruction can extend to the fascia, fibrous tissue below the skin. The skin may take on a bluish color, blisters may develop, and systemic symptoms of fever, a rapid heartbeat, and changes in consciousness are likely.

There is also a more superficial version of cellulitis called *erysipelas*. This problem is caused by an aggressive type of streptococcal bacteria called beta-hemolytic streptococci. Erysipelas often affects the face, with a bright-red, sharply bordered painful area of skin, but can progress quickly to cause fever, chills, and an overall ill feeling.

CONVENTIONAL TREATMENT

■ Cellulitis is treated with antibiotics. A seven- to ten-day course of oral cephalexin (Keflex) or dicloxacillin may be adequate, but in some cases, intravenous antibiotics may be needed for the first day or so.

■ Necrotizing cellulitis-fasciitis requires surgical exploration to debride the area (trim away dead tissue) and release pressure on underlying tissues, followed by aggressive antibiotic therapy.

■ Erysipelas is treated with bed rest, hot packs, and

aspirin to relieve symptoms, plus aggressive use of intravenous antibiotics for two days followed by a one- to two-week course of oral penicillin (Bicillin, Wycillin, and others) or erythromycin (ERYC, Ilotycin, and others).

DIETARY GUIDELINES

■ Drink at least eight 8-ounce glasses of pure water every day.

■ Eat plenty of green vegetables, which contain vitamins, minerals, and phytochemicals that benefit the immune response and promote healing.

■ If you like garlic, enjoy it to your heart's content. Garlic has antibacterial properties.

■ Avoid anything containing sugar or caffeine. Bacteria thrive on sugar, and both sugar and caffeine foster an acidic internal environment, which slows healing.

NUTRITIONAL SUPPLEMENTS

■ Bromelain, an enzyme derived from pineapple, has an anti-inflammatory effect and can help reduce swelling. Take 500 milligrams four times daily, between meals.

■ The carotenoids, including beta-carotene, are used by the body to produce vitamin A, which has a healing effect on the skin. Take 25,000 international units of a carotenoid complex twice daily for two weeks.

■ Pine-bark and grape-seed extracts are excellent natural anti-inflammatories. Take 50 milligrams of either three times a day for ten days.

■ Vitamin C and the bioflavonoids boost the immune system and have anti-inflammatory properties. Vitamin C is also important for the production of collagen, a major skin protein. Take 500 milligrams of vitamin C and an equal amount of mixed bioflavonoids four times daily for two weeks.

■ Zinc also boosts the immune system and helps the body fight infection. Take 15 milligrams three times daily for two weeks. Take zinc with food to prevent stomach upset.

HERBAL TREATMENT

■ Cat's claw enhances the immune response and has antibacterial properties. Take 500 milligrams of standardized extract three times a day until the infection clears.

Note: Do not use cat's claw if you are pregnant or nursing, or if you are an organ-transplant recipient. Use it with caution if you are taking an anticoagulant (blood thinner).

■ Echinacea and goldenseal boost the immune response and fight infection. It is currently believed that echinacea increases the level of a blood protein called properdin that activates the complementary pathway, the part of the immune system reponsible for sending disease-fighting white blood cells into infected areas to battle bacteria and

viruses. Take one dose of an echinacea and goldenseal combination formula supplying 250 to 500 milligrams of echinacea and 150 to 300 milligrams of goldenseal four times a day for one week.

■ Garlic helps to fight bacterial infection. Take 500 milligrams of fresh garlic four times daily for ten days.

■ Oregano has antibacterial properties and helps to fight infection. Take 75 milligrams of standardized extract three times a day.

HOMEOPATHY

■ *Apis mellifica* is helpful for swelling with redness, soreness, and sensitivity. Take one dose of *Apis mellifica* 30x or 15c three times daily for up to three days.

■ *Vespa crabro* helps to relieve intense itching and burning, soreness, and a burning and stinging sensation. Take one dose of *Vespa crabro* 12x or 6c three times daily for up to three days.

ACUPRESSURE

■ Spleen 10 takes the "heat" out of the blood.

AROMATHERAPY

■ Add 4 drops of orange oil, 3 drops of tea tree oil, 2 drops of chamomile oil, and 2 drops of thyme oil to a warm bath. Soak in the bath for ten to twenty minutes. Tea tree and thyme oils are antiseptic, and chamomile and orange oils relax the nervous system.

PREVENTION

■ Wear protective clothing when participating in activities, whether for work or for pleasure, that expose you to a risk of cuts, scrapes, and other injuries. Use particular caution if you have diabetes, lymphedema, or any other condition that predisposes you to developing cellulitis.

■ Clean any breaks in the skin carefully, and treat them properly to prevent infection. (*See* CUTS AND SCRAPES.) Be alert for signs of redness, fluid drainage, or other signs of infection. If you develop any of these symptoms, consult your health-care provider.

Cervical Dysplasia

Cervical dysplasia is a condition in which abnormal cells grow in the tissues of the cervix, the narrow lower part of the uterus that joins with the vagina (*dysplasia* means abnormal cell growth). It causes no symptoms in the woman who has it, but can be detected by a doctor's examination. This is important because certain types of abnormal cervical cells can turn cancerous if not treated early and effectively. Without an examination that includes a Pap smear (see page 187), there is no way to tell that cellular changes are occurring.

It is important to realize that while cervical dysplasia may, if untreated, progress to cervical cancer, this is by no means certain. In fact, only one in ten "precancerous" cells of the type detected in a Pap test is likely to develop into cervical cancer. Many cases of cervical dysplasia ultimately return to normal on their own. This does not mean you should not take an abnormal Pap finding seriously, however. If the results of a first Pap smear are inconclusive—the most common "abnormal" result—your doctor will schedule a follow-up test to verify the findings. Between any abnormal reading and a follow-up test, you have time to make improvements in the next reading. You might be surprised to learn that you can do a great deal to help yourself achieve a normal reading in your follow-up Pap smear. The focus of this entry is on using primarily natural means to give your body what it needs to correct abnormal cells and reverse a diagnosis of cervical dysplasia. Any self-treatment for cervical dysplasia should be discussed with a physician.

CONVENTIONAL TREATMENT

■ If your Pap smear shows evidence of cervical dysplasia, your doctor may decide to take a look inside your cervix with an instrument called a colposcope. This instrument has a magnifying lens and is used to identify any abnormal cells that might need to be examined in a biopsy.

■ If colposcopy or biopsy shows precancerous changes, the next step is to destroy the abnormal cells. In many instances, this can be accomplished with heat, by laser or cauterization, or with cold, by cryosurgery. These methods destroy abnormal cells and are performed on an outpatient basis. There are few side effects and healing is usually rapid.

■ A cone biopsy is required to deal with abnormal tissue that extends further up the cervical canal. In this procedure, a cone-shaped section of the cervix is removed. It is both a biopsy in the usual sense and a procedure to remove precancerous cells in the upper reaches of the cervix. Although cone biopsy does require a local anesthetic, it is performed during an outpatient visit. However, you may need to rest for a day afterward to fully recuperate. In certain cases, having had a cone biopsy can predispose a woman to miscarriage in subsequent pregnancies. If you become pregnant after a cone biopsy, be sure to tell your obstetrician that you have had this procedure. Your pregnancy should be closely monitored.

■ A relatively new technique called the loop electrosurgical excision procedure, or LEEP, developed in Britain, offers advantages over a cone biopsy. It can be used only

if the diseased area is completely visible. A small loop of wire, attached to a doctor-controlled electric current, is used to burn around the affected area, both excising the tissue and cauterizing the wound at the same time. Only local anesthesia is required, and there is usually no lingering pain afterward. If your doctor recommends a cone biopsy, you might wish to raise the possibility of LEEP with him or her.

■ Many physicians recommend that women with cervical dysplasia undergo hysterectomy to avoid the risk of cervical cancer. If you are a woman of childbearing age, this is a serious and emotional decision that requires much soul-searching. If you are undecided, seek a second opinion. Many women may undergo hysterectomy too soon, and many of these surgeries may be performed unnecessarily.

DIETARY GUIDELINES

■ Maximize your intake of foods that are rich in folic acid. Cervical dysplasia is more common in women who are deficient in folic acid. Eat a lot of dark-green vegetables, such as beet greens, kale, broccoli, asparagus, and endive. Wheat germ is a good source of folic acid as well.

■ Include in your diet plenty of foods that are rich in beta-carotene and vitamin A. These include carrots, winter squash, sweet potatoes, dark leafy vegetables, and broccoli. These nutrients help healing and act to strengthen mucous membranes.

NUTRITIONAL SUPPLEMENTS

■ If your menu lacks sufficient food sources of folic acid (*see under* Dietary Guidelines, above), take 800 micrograms of folic acid in supplement form three times daily for two months. You should see an improvement in your next Pap smear.

■ Selenium is an excellent antioxidant that is often deficient in women with cervical dysplasia. Take 200 micrograms daily.

■ Soy isoflavones, phytochemicals derived from soy, may aid in maintaining hormonal balance. Take 250 milligrams three times a day.

■ Women with cervical dysplasia are often seriously deficient in vitamin A. Take 20,000 international units of vitamin A daily for six weeks; then 10,000 international units of vitamin A daily until your follow-up Pap smear. Also take 50,000 international units of beta-carotene twice a day for one month.

Note: If you are pregnant, or intend to get pregnant, or if you have liver disease, consult your doctor before taking supplemental vitamin A. Pregnant women should not ingest a total of more than 25,000 international units of supplemental vitamin A *per week* from all sources. Do not

The Pap Smear

The test we know as the Pap smear is named for George Papanicolaou, the physician who developed it. It is a routine part of a pelvic examination. To perform the test, the doctor inserts an instrument called a speculum that holds the vagina open while he or she uses a light to look for abnormal cells of the cervix and vaginal walls. With the speculum in place, a few cells are scraped from the cervix, smeared on a glass slide, and sent to a laboratory for analysis.

A woman should have her first Pap smear at age eighteen or within six months of first having sexual intercourse, whichever comes first, and another within the following six to twelve months. Thereafter, ideally, a Pap smear should be a regular part of a yearly checkup, although some doctors recommend they be performed at one-, two-, or even three-year intervals. More frequent tests are recommended for women who have multiple sex partners, or whose partners have multiple sex partners.

There are two different ways of reporting results. Laboratories generally use a system employing five basic classifications. Class 1 indicates that only normal cells have been found; class 5 indicates that cancerous cells have been found. The problem with interpreting the results arises when there is a reading of class 2, 3, or 4, which represent varying degrees of abnormality. There have been many reported instances in which laboratory analyses of cervical smears have been inaccurate. If the lab is inefficient, or if the doctor interpreting the results is inexperienced, the reading itself is suspect. This is one of the main reasons why doctors often require several tests before arriving at a firm diagnosis.

Increasing numbers of laboratories are now using the Bethesda system to interpret the results of a cervical smear. This system uses standard terminology (for the medical profession) and gives clear diagnostic results. In the Bethesda system, grades 1 and 2 are both considered normal, with grade 1 meaning that no problems were detected and grade 2 indicating the presence of some inflammation. Grades 3 and 4 mean low-grade and high-grade squamous intraepithelial lesion (SIL), respectively. This means that there are abnormal cells in the outer layer of cervical tissue. Grade 5 means cancer. Because of its accuracy, the Bethesda system is preferable to the more common 1 to 5 classification system. It is up to each laboratory to decide what type of analysis to use. You might ask your doctor to send your Pap smear to a laboratory that uses the Bethesda system.

The Pap smear offers a 95-percent chance of detecting cervical dysplasia, which is the best means of preventing cervical cancer. In addition to detecting cervical dysplasia, Pap smears are also useful for identifying viral infections of the cervix, such as herpes simplex and papillomavirus infection, and for assessing the level of hormones in the body, particularly estrogen and progesterone.

---

take over 10,000 international units of vitamin A daily on an ongoing basis unless you are being closely monitored by a knowledgeable nutritionally oriented physician.

■ While you are using vitamin-A therapy, take 30 to 50 milligrams of zinc daily.

Note: Take zinc with food to prevent stomach upset. If you take over 30 milligrams of zinc on a daily basis for more than one or two months, you should also take 1 to 2 milligrams of copper each day to maintain a proper mineral balance.

■ Vitamin C supports the immune system, helps the healing process, and is beneficial for any type of infection. In addition, low blood levels of vitamin C have been shown to increase the risk of cervical cancer. Three or four times a day, take 1,000 milligrams of a vitamin-C formula that includes the bioflavonoids, especially rutin.

■ Vitamin E is an important antioxidant nutrient. Choose a product containing mixed tocopherols and start by taking 200 international units daily, then gradually increase the dosage until you are taking 400 international units in the morning and another 400 international units in the evening.

Note: If you have high blood pressure, limit your intake of supplemental vitamin E to a total of 400 international units daily. If you are taking an anticoagulant (blood thinner), consult your physician before taking vitamin E.

■ Naturopathic physicians often use a course of vaginal suppositories with various nutrients to treat cervical dysplasia. Consider a four-week program: The first week, use vitamin-A suppositories (insert one each night before going to bed); the second week, use suppositories containing vitamin C and herbs. Then repeat the sequence.

■ If you have digestive problems in addition to an irregular Pap result, consider taking a probiotic supplement such as bifidobacteria, acidophilus, or colostrum. Take it as recommended on the product label.

HERBAL TREATMENT

■ Chaste tree berry (also known by its Latin name, *Vitex agnus-castus*) helps to regulate hormonal balance and cycles. Take 200 milligrams of standardized extract two or three times daily.

■ Echinacea and goldenseal have antibacterial, antifungal, and antiviral properties. Select a vaginal pack that includes these two herbs and apply it as directed on the product label.

■ Purchase liquid herbal extracts, and make a mixture containing 3 parts echinacea, 2 parts each goldenseal and ligusticum, 1 part licorice root, and $1/2$ part lomatia. Take 30 to 40 drops (about $1/2$ teaspoon) of the mixture twice a day for three weeks.

HOMEOPATHY

■ The best way to treat cervical dysplasia homeopathically is to see a homeopathic physician for a constitutional remedy.

ACUPRESSURE

For the locations of acupressure points on the body, *see* ADMINISTERING AN ACUPRESSURE TREATMENT in Part Three.

■ Bladder 23 increases circulation to the reproductive organs.

■ Liver 3 quiets the nervous system and relieves muscle cramps and spasms.

■ Stomach 36 tones the digestive system and strengthens overall well-being.

GENERAL RECOMMENDATIONS

■ If you are a smoker, quit now. Research shows that smoking is a factor in the development of abnormal cells in the cervix.

■ Follow your doctor's recommendations regarding follow-up examinations. Cervical dysplasia is considered a precancerous condition. Fortunately, cervical cancer is curable if detected and treated early. Be especially vigilant if you are a woman whose mother took the drug diethylstilbestrol (DES) during pregnancy, as this creates an increased risk of cervical dysplasia. You should also be aware that there is a correlation between cervical cancer and having multiple sex partners.

PREVENTION

■ Cervical dysplasia is associated with low levels of folic acid and poor dietary habits. Follow the dietary guidelines in this entry.

Chalazion

See under STYE.

Chickenpox

Chickenpox is a highly contagious disease caused by the varicella-zoster virus, a member of the herpes family. Very few people escape chickenpox. It spreads quickly. Coughing and sneezing—even laughing and talking—spread the illness.

A person who is coming down with chickenpox is contagious for one or two days before any symptoms show. Anyone who has not had the disease before and who comes in contact with an infected individual during this period will almost certainly catch it. A person is contagious from a few days before symptoms develop until all of the blisters are dry and have formed scabs.

The more intimate and more frequent the exposure to chickenpox, the more severe the case will be. This fact has very important implications, especially within families. People in different stages of the disease should minimize their exposure to each other. With minimal exposure, the next person to become ill is likely to have a less severe case of chickenpox, with less discomfort.

Chickenpox typically begins with a headache, fatigue, achiness, loss of appetite, and fever, much like any other viral illness. A day or two after these early symptoms, a rash of flat, red, splotchy dots erupts, usually beginning on the chest, stomach, and back, and spreading a day or so later to the extremities, neck, face, and scalp.

The red dots of the rash soon come together to form clusters of tiny pimples, which then progress to small, delicate, clear blisters. Some people develop 3 lesions; some develop 300. Once the rash erupts, expect new crops of blisters over the next three to five days. Scabs, which are the last phase of the pox, form five to six days after the blisters develop. These scabs last for one to two weeks before falling off, exposing tender, freshly healed skin.

Over the course of the disease, the rash shows signs of all the different phases of chickenpox, with some areas that are splotchy and red, some areas of new blisters, areas where sores are crusting over and scabbing, and areas of healing. From eruption through healing, each and every pock is very, very itchy. It is the extreme itchiness of chickenpox that causes the greatest torment.

Although most common in childhood, chickenpox can be contracted at any age. Because infected adults tend to feel much sicker and more miserable with this disease than youngsters do, it's probably best to have it as a child. Once you have had chickenpox, it is highly unlikely that you will ever suffer through it again.

Note that the recommended doses of different treatments given in this section are intended for adults. To determine correct treatment regimens for children, consult your physician or *Smart Medicine for a Healthier Child* (Avery, 1994).

CONVENTIONAL TREATMENT

An over-the-counter painkiller such as acetaminophen (in Tylenol, Tempra, and other medications), aspirin (Bayer, Ecotrin, and others), or ibuprofen (Advil, Motrin, Nuprin, and others) is helpful in relieving pain and bringing down fever.

The antihistamine diphenhydramine (found in Benadryl) or chlorpheniramine (Chlor-Trimeton) can help relieve the awful itching of chickenpox. Benadryl is available in pill form as well as in a spray. The pill form is generally more effective at relieving the itching of chickenpox. An antihistamine can also help you to fall asleep, which can be helpful if the itching is keeping you awake at night.

■ Viscous lidocaine (Xylocaine) is a local anesthetic that can be used as a mouth rinse to decrease pain and itching in the mouth. This rinse numbs mucous membranes, making it more comfortable for you to eat, drink, or brush your teeth if you have mouth sores. This is a prescription drug, and it must be used in small quantities because of its potential toxicity.

Burow's solution is a powder available over the counter at most drugstores. Mixed with water and applied as a soak, it is very effective at drying up weeping sores.

■ Calamine lotion can help to relieve itching and dry weeping sores.

For certain cases of chickenpox, the drug of choice is acyclovir (Zovirax), which appears to lessen the severity and length of the illness. However, it is very expensive and shortens the course of the disease by only a few days. It is therefore used primarily for severe cases that occur in individuals with disorders that impair immune-system function. Possible side effects include nausea, vomiting, diarrhea, dizziness, headache, rash, fatigue, and joint pain.

■ If during the course of the disease you develop vaginal or rectal lesions, bad sores in your mouth, a fever consistently over 102°F, an earache, a very painful sore throat, a persistent cough, and/or increased difficulty breathing, call your doctor. You may be developing a complication such as an ear infection, strep throat, or pneumonia.

DIETARY GUIDELINES

■ Drink plenty of fluids so that you stay well hydrated.

■ Eat a simple, clean, whole-foods diet. Include easily digested foods high in vitamins and minerals, such as soups, well-cooked whole grains, and vegetables.

■ If you have lost your appetite and are not eating well, try diluted fruit juices, herbal teas, and soups. Frozen fruit-juice popsicles are also very good.

NUTRITIONAL SUPPLEMENTS

■ Vitamin A aids in healing skin tissue. Take 10,000 international units of vitamin A and 25,000 international units of its precursor, beta-carotene, once a day for ten days to one month.

Note: If you are pregnant, or intend to get pregnant, or if you have liver disease, consult your doctor before taking supplemental vitamin A. Pregnant women should not ingest a total of more than 25,000 international units of supplemental vitamin A *per week* from all sources.

■ Vitamin C and bioflavonoids help to stimulate the immune system and resolve a fever in the initial stages of the illness. The first week, take 500 to 1,000 milligrams of vitamin C in mineral ascorbate form, plus an equal amount of bioflavonoids, three to four times a day. The following week, take the same combination twice a day. Then continue to take the same combination once a day for three to four weeks.

■ Zinc promotes healing and stimulates the immune system. Take 25 to 50 milligrams of zinc twice a day for two weeks.

Note: Take zinc with food to prevent stomach upset. If you take over 30 milligrams of zinc on a daily basis for more than one or two months, you should also take 1 to 2 milligrams of copper each day to maintain a proper mineral balance.

■ If you are restless and having difficulty sleeping, a calcium and magnesium combination supplement may help. Take a dose containing 400 milligrams of calcium and 250 milligrams of magnesium twice during the day and once again at bedtime for one week.

Note: In excessive amounts, magnesium acts as a laxative. If you develop diarrhea, decrease the dosage.

HERBAL TREATMENT

■ Burdock root and red clover are high in many valuable trace minerals. These herbs help to detoxify the body and heal skin lesions. Take 500 milligrams of each three to four times daily for ten days.

■ Echinacea and goldenseal help to clear infection, support the immune system, and soothe the skin and mucous membranes. Echinacea is a powerful antiviral. Take one dose of an echinacea and goldenseal combination formula supplying 500 milligrams of echinacea and 250 milligrams of goldenseal three to four times a day for up to ten days.

If you are feeling very restless, take a cup of chamomile and oat straw tea three times a day, as needed.

Note: Use chamomile with caution if you are allergic to ragweed.

HOMEOPATHY

Homeopathic *Calendula*, in oil or gel form, helps to relieve itching and promote healing. Apply the preparation topically in the morning, in the afternoon, and before going to bed.

Grindelia, applied topically to the pocks in liquid form, helps to relieve itching. Apply the undiluted liquid in the morning, in the afternoon, and again before bedtime.

If the lesions are oozing or weeping, take one dose of *Mezereum* 12x or 6c three times a day for up to three days.

To fight the intense itching of chickenpox, take one dose of *Rhus toxicodendron* 30x or 9c three times daily for forty-eight hours or until symptoms improve. If there is no improvement in forty-eight hours, try a different remedy.

Sulfur 30x or 9c is often useful for very red and very itchy pocks. Take one dose three to four times a day for up to three days.

ACUPRESSURE

For the locations of acupressure points on the body, *see* ADMINISTERING AN ACUPRESSURE TREATMENT in Part Three.

Four Gates is relaxing.

Large Intestine 11 helps relieve itching of the skin.

Spleen 10 is a specific for taking "heat" out of the blood.

Stomach 36 is useful for improving appetite.

GENERAL RECOMMENDATIONS

Avoid scratching the pocks. Since they are extremely itchy, this can be difficult, but scratching or picking at scabs can cause an infection; rubbing open a blister or pulling off a scab before the new skin has formed underneath will leave a scar, a pockmark. If you find yourself scratching in your sleep, wear gloves to bed to prevent this.

Take any and all measures to relieve the itching. The more it itches, the more you will be tempted to scratch, increasing the risk of infection and scarring. Keep yourself clean, quiet, and cool. A soak in bath water treated with chamomile, calendula, or grindelia will soothe and relax. These herbs help relieve itching, too. Oatmeal baths are very soothing to dry and itching skin. Tie a handful of raw oatmeal in a washcloth and swish it around in the bath water. You can also *gently* rub the washcloth full of oatmeal over the itchy places, but be careful not to break the blisters. Adding apple cider vinegar to bath water helps dry lesions and also reduces itching.

■ If the sores are not open, dilute 1 tablespoon of apple cider vinegar in 1 cup of water and dab it on. This acidic solution will help ease the itching and also speeds up the necessary drying process.

■ Occasionally, a few extra-thick scabs refuse to drop off, and skin begins to form around them. Don't try to lift these stubborn scabs off, or you will be left with pockmarks. If you notice some tenacious scabs that seem to be clinging on too long, encourage them to separate from the skin with a soak in one of the hot treated baths suggested above.

■ If a few tiny scars remain after chickenpox is fully healed, apply vitamin E oil to them. Break open a vitamin-E capsule and rub the oil into the pockmark in the morning and at night until it clears. Rubbing castor oil into the scar will also help.

■ Once the chickenpox has cleared, protect your skin from the sun. The areas where pocks have healed are now tender, new skin that will burn and scar easily. Apply a good sun block or high-SPF sunscreen when you go outside.

■ A person infected with chickenpox is no longer considered contagious once all the scabs have been sloughed off. Until then, you should stay away from anyone who has not yet had the disease.

PREVENTION

■ If you know you have been exposed to chickenpox, you may receive preventive treatment with varicella-zoster immune globulin (VZIG). This is normally used in people with impaired immune function, such as people with HIV and individuals undergoing cancer chemotherapy, after a known exposure to the virus. It is not mixed with other therapeutic measures, and is not used prior to exposure.

■ A vaccine that protects against chickenpox is available. As with any vaccine, some people experience negative reactions to it. The most common include fever (over 102°F), rash, irritation at the site of the injection, upper respiratory illnesses, cough, aches, and fatigue.

Chlamydia

Chlamydia is an infection caused by a parasitic microorganism, *Chlamydia trachomatis.* It the most common sexually transmitted disease in the United States. About 4 million new cases are diagnosed every year, and close to 20 percent of American adolescents have had chlamydia.

About 10 percent of men and 70 percent of women have no symptoms at all in the early stages of the infection. As it progresses, both men and women suffer symptoms that include inflammation, itching, difficulty urinating, and pain during sexual intercourse. A vaginal or urethral discharge is common. In men, chlamydia can cause prostatitis (inflammation of the prostate gland) and epididymitis (inflammation of the seminal vesicles). Symptoms of chlamydial prostatitis include painful urination and a discharge of watery mucus from the urethra.

It is not uncommon for chlamydia to occur as part of a combined infection with gonorrhea or another venereal disease. Once the other infection is treated, a previously hidden chlamydial problem may show up.

The danger of this disease lies in the fact that its long-term consequences can be serious and that it often produces no symptoms until it is in the later stages. It is the leading cause of pelvic inflammatory disease in women, which can lead to tubal scarring and resulting infertility. As many as 50,000 American women have become infertile as a result of this disease. If a woman with a chlamydial infection does become pregnant, the disease can cause problems for her baby, including eye and respiratory infections, even pneumonia.

If you have any signs, symptoms, or suspicions of a sexually transmitted disease, especially if you have a discharge from the vagina or urethra, see your doctor promptly. A diagnosis of chlamydia is made by testing a sample of the urine and/or discharge, either vaginal or urethral, to determine the presence of the microorganism. However, since the organism is sometimes hard to confirm in the laboratory, it may be assumed to be there if the symptoms of burning, redness, and/or discharge are present.

CONVENTIONAL TREATMENT

■ Because it is a leading cause of infertility in women, chlamydia is treated aggressively with antibiotics. In general, drugs of the tetracycline class—tetracycline (also sold under the brand name Achromycin), doxycycline (Doryx, Monodox, Vibramycin, Vibra-Tabs), and others—are preferred. If you are pregnant or cannot tolerate tetracycline, erythromycin is used. Some doctors prescribe a more expensive antibiotic called azithromycin (Zithromax). The advantage of this drug is that it can be given in a single dose. If need be, other antibiotics may be used, but tend to be slightly less effective. Treatment is usually prescribed for a period of three weeks. Often, sexual partners are treated as well, even if they have no symptoms whatsoever, as they may still be infected.

DIETARY GUIDELINES

■ Eat a healthy diet that is high in fiber and low in sugar, with an emphasis on whole foods.

■ Avoid refined and processed foods, especially those that are high in sugar and processed fats.

■ To flush toxins from your system and help promote free urination, drink eight glasses of pure water daily.

NUTRITIONAL SUPPLEMENTS

■ Antibiotics wreak havoc on the body's population of beneficial bacteria, leading to an overgrowth of yeast that can manifest itself as a vaginal yeast infection (characterized by a whiter and "cheesier" discharge), oral thrush (yeast in the mouth and on the tongue), or a myriad of gastrointestinal disturbances. Whenever you must take antibiotics, it is important to take a probiotic supplement to avoid having to be treated later for a yeast infection. Also, acidophilus and bifidus have documented antimicrobial action. Take a probiotic supplement as recommended on the product label. Be sure to take probiotics one hour before or two hours after a dose of antibiotics. If you are allergic to milk, be sure to select a dairy-free product.

■ Vitamin A and beta-carotene are needed for healthy mucous membranes and also build resistance to infection. Take 5,000 international units of vitamin A, and 15,000 international units of beta-carotene two to three times daily for one month.

Note: If you are pregnant, or intend to get pregnant, or if you have liver disease, consult your doctor before taking supplemental vitamin A. Pregnant women should not ingest a total of more than 25,000 international units of supplemental vitamin A *per week* from all sources.

■ Vitamin C and bioflavonoids have notable anti-inflammatory action and also enhance the immune system. Most people who contract sexually transmitted diseases (STDs) like chlamydia have compromised immune function. Take 500 milligrams of vitamin C with bioflavonoids three to four times daily.

■ Vitamin E combats inflammation and infection. People with STDs are often low in vitamin E. Choose a product containing mixed tocopherols and begin by taking 100 or 200 milligrams at bedtime, then gradually increase until you are taking 400 international units daily.

Note: If you are taking an anticoagulant (blood thinner), consult your physician before taking supplemental vitamin E.

■ Zinc supports the immune system and speeds healing. Take 20 milligrams of zinc twice a day.

Note: Take zinc with food to prevent stomach upset. If you take over 30 milligrams of zinc on a daily basis for more than one or two months, you should also take 1 to 2 milligrams of copper each day to maintain a proper mineral balance.

HERBAL TREATMENT

■ Cat's claw enhances the immune response and has antibacterial and antifungal properties. Take 500 milligrams of standardized extract three times a day until the infection resolves.

Note: Do not use cat's claw if you are pregnant or nursing, or if you are an organ-transplant recipient. Use it with caution if you are taking an anticoagulant (blood thinner).

Echinacea and goldenseal support the immune system and have effective antimicrobial properties. Take one dose of an echinacea and goldenseal combination formula supplying 200 to 500 milligrams of echinacea and 125 to 250 milligrams of goldenseal three to four times daily for ten days. Stop for ten days, then repeat.

Garlic, nature's antibiotic, has been shown to possess powerful antibacterial, antimicrobial, and even antiviral activity. Take 500 milligrams at least three times daily.

Oregano has antibacterial properties and helps to fight infection. Take 75 milligrams of standardized extract three times a day.

Turmeric is a time-honored anti-inflammatory herb with antibacterial properties. It also acts as an antioxidant that scavenges free radicals. Take 500 milligrams of turmeric three times daily.

HOMEOPATHY

Cannabis sativa relieves a painful urge to urinate with burning on urination. In men, the urine may flow in a split stream, and the urethra is very sensitive. In some acute cases, there can be a buildup of mucus and pus that causes a stoppage of the urethra. Take one dose of *Cannabis sativa* 12x or 6c three to four times daily, as needed, to relieve symptoms.

Cantharis is for the person who has an intolerable urge to urinate constantly, and who experiences burning on urination. This remedy is also valuable for men infected with chlamydia who suffer from painful erections. Take one dose of *Cantharis* 12x or 6c three to four times daily, as needed to relieve symptoms.

Solidago virga is helpful if the urine is scanty and difficult to pass, with an offensive odor. You may also have lower back pain, as well as discomfort in the lower abdomen and bladder. There is probably a bitter taste in your mouth, especially at night, and your tongue may be coated. Take one dose of *Solidago virga* 12x or 6c three to four times daily, as needed to relieve symptoms.

BACH FLOWER REMEDIES

Select the remedy that most closely fits your emotional tendencies and concerns, and take it as needed, following the directions on the product label.

■ Mimulus eases fear and timidity.

■ Vervain relieves nervousness and tension.

■ Olive is the remedy to choose if the condition is accompanied by exhaustion.

ACUPRESSURE

For the locations of acupressure points on the body, *see* ADMINISTERING AN ACUPRESSURE TREATMENT in Part Three.

■ Bladder 23 increases circulation to the urinary tract.

■ Conception Vessel 3 and 4 stimulate circulation to the genitourinary tract.

■ Gallbladder 21, 30, and 41 increase circulation.

■ Liver 3 takes the "heat" out of the liver.

■ Spleen 10 helps to detoxify the body.

AROMATHERAPY

For specific instructions on how to use aromatherapy, *see* PREPARING AROMATHERAPY TREATMENTS in Part Three.

■ Aromatherapy sitz baths prepared with essential oil of lavender, myrrh, and/or tea tree can be soothing and healing to inflamed tissues.

GENERAL RECOMMENDATIONS

■ If you are being treated for any sexually transmitted disease, your partner also should be under treatment. If only one of you is being treated and the other suffers from recurrent infections, it is likely that you are passing the infection back and forth.

■ To give the tissues time to heal, refrain from sexual activity until the infection is cleared.

■ Because a warm, moist environment fosters infections of all kinds, wear loose cotton underwear that permits air circulation. As much as possible, avoid wearing pantyhose or tight, form-fitting jeans or pants.

PREVENTION

■ Practice monogamy. Multiple sexual partners are a danger to both sexes. For the most part, there is no way to tell what you may be exposed to during a casual encounter.

■ If you do have sex with more than one partner, or change partners often, always use a latex condom. Ask your physician how often you should be examined to insure your health. Should you contract an STD, the earlier treatment begins, the more successful it will be.

Choking

If you should accidentally inhale something that gets lodged in your trachea (windpipe), you may become unable to breathe or speak. Needless to say, this is a dangerous situation requiring emergency intervention.

Children, especially those under four years of age, are at the greatest risk of choking because young children tend to put everything in their mouths. In adults, choking most often results from accidental inhalation of a piece of food while eating.

Ideally, everyone should take a course in basic first aid that includes specific instruction in coming to the aid of someone who is choking. The information in this entry cannot—and is not meant to—substitute for a class in which you can learn and practice such critical details of technique as where to place your hands and how much force to use. Rather, it is intended to serve as a refresher in case of emergency.

It is frightening to realize that you are choking. First, make a quick assessment of the situation. If you are able to talk or are coughing forcefully, no intervention is necessary. This indicates that air is getting through the windpipe. Try not to panic. As long as you can breathe, you may be able to expel the material on your own. Often, coughing and sputtering is enough to expel the object.

However, if you become unable to speak, or begin gasping for air or turning blue, act fast.

EMERGENCY TREATMENT

See the inset below.

GENERAL RECOMMENDATIONS

■ Have someone call for emergency help and begin the Heimlich maneuver immediately (see below).

■ Once the crisis is over, take a dose of Bach Flower Rescue Remedy. This will help calm you and stabilize the anxiety, shock, and fright you may be experiencing (*see* BACH FLOWER REMEDIES in Part One.)

PREVENTION

■ Eat slowly and chew thoroughly before swallowing. If you are in a rush to finish a meal, you can choke on a poorly chewed or extra-large bite.

Emergency Treatment for Choking

If you or someone near you begins choking, have someone call for emergency help and go to the choking person's aid quickly. The age of the individual, and whether or not other people are available to help, will determine the measures you must take to relieve choking. Perform the appropriate procedure as outlined below. Do not stop until the foreign material is expelled, *or* the person begins coughing, breathing, and making normal sounds on his or her own, *or* another person can take over for you, *or* medical help arrives.

Standard Heimlich Maneuver:

1. Stand or kneel behind the individual, wrapping your arms around his or her waist.

2. Make a fist with one hand and clasp your other hand over your fist. Position the thumb side of your fist against the person's abdomen, just above the navel and below the rib cage.

3. Use a quick, forceful *upward* push of your fist into the person's abdomen to force air up through the windpipe.

4. Continue doing these thrusts until the person expels the foreign material.

One-Person Variant

If you are alone and find that you have ingested material that you can neither swallow nor cough up, and speaking/breathing are impossible, you can perform a modified version of the standard Heimlich maneuver on yourself as follows:

1. Find a stable, blunt object somewhat below chest height—for example, a chair back, countertop edge, or fence post.

2. Place the soft part of your upper abdomen, just below the breastbone, against the object, and relax the area as much as possible.

3. Without trying to breathe, thrust your abdomen against the object to rapidly increase pressure under the diaphragm, much as in the standard Heimlich maneuver.

4. Continue doing these thrusts until you expel the foreign material.

■ If you have an infant or very young child, keep a close watch. Always supervise a young child when he or she is eating, and cut all foods, including fruits, into very small pieces. Select toys that are well made and appropriate for your child's age, and examine them regularly to make sure that all small parts are secure.

Cholesterol, High

The presence of a high level of cholesterol in the blood is considered a primary risk factor for cardiovascular disease and stroke. High cholesterol is also a factor in impotence, mental sluggishness, and gallstones.

Cholesterol is not technically a fat, but a building block for steroids that plays an important part in the functions of many systems of the body. Because it is soluble in fat and not in water, it is also classified as a lipid. It is a normal and necessary component of most body tissues, including cell membranes, the brain, the nervous system, the liver, and blood. It is required to produce vitamin D, sex and adrenal hormones, and bile, which is necessary for the digestion of fats and the metabolism of fat-soluble vitamins, including vitamins A, D, E, and K. The liver produces up to one and a half grams of cholesterol daily to meet the body's needs.

Because cholesterol does not dissolve in water, it must be transported in the bloodstream by means of carrier molecules called lipoproteins. Lipoproteins consist of an outer coat of protein wrapped around a core composed of cholesterol and triglycerides, a type of fat. An excess of triglycerides in the blood is also recognized as a risk factor for heart disease and stroke.

There are two major types of lipoproteins that carry cholesterol in the blood: high-density lipoproteins (HDLs) and low-density lipoproteins (LDLs). LDLs transport cholesterol from the liver, where it is produced, to other parts of the body. HDLs bind with excess cholesterol in the blood and bring it back to the liver, where it is eliminated or reprocessed. Ideally, the body manufactures all the cholesterol it needs, any excess is returned to the liver, and the system stays in balance. However, if there is more cholesterol present than the body's natural mechanisms can cope with, cholesterol may be deposited on the interior walls of blood vessels, narrowing them. This is atherosclerosis. This process occurs even more readily when cholesterol is oxidized (reacts chemically with oxygen). Because HDL works to rid the body of excess cholesterol, thereby reducing the amount of cholesterol that is deposited on blood-vessel walls, it is sometimes referred to as "good cholesterol." It is also thought that HDL may help protect against oxidation. LDL, which carries a heavy load of cholesterol to body tissues, is known as "bad cholesterol."

An excess of cholesterol can result from a variety of causes. Primary among these is diet. Eating foods high in cholesterol and/or saturated fat results in increased amounts of cholesterol in the blood. Foods that contain cholesterol include meat, shellfish, and dairy products. All foods that are derived from plants are cholesterol-free, although some, like coconut and palm oil, are nevertheless high in saturated fats. Some people suffer from elevated cholesterol levels because of an inherited defect in fat metabolism. Such individuals may have extremely high cholesterol levels.

The total cholesterol level (HDL and LDL combined) that is generally considered safe is 200 milligrams per deciliter of blood (200 mg/dL). A reading between 200 and 240 shows a rising potential for cardiovascular disease, and a reading over 240 is cause for alarm. However, it has been determined that the ratio of HDL to LDL is even more important than the total number. Thus, even if your total cholesterol level is in the low to normal range, if your HDL level is low and your LDL level is high, you face an increased risk of cardiovasular disease and stroke. For adult men, an HDL level of 45 to 50 mg/dL is considered normal; for adult women, an HDL reading of 50 to 60 is considered normal. For persons of either sex, an HDL reading over 70 is considered excellent and one under 35 a danger signal. If you have other risk factors in addition to a low HDL level, the situation becomes even more critical. A combination of low HDL and high LDL coupled with, for example, obesity or high blood pressure, means a sixfold increase in the risk of heart disease. Smoking increases the risk by twenty times.

CONVENTIONAL TREATMENT

■ The first measure to bring down high cholesterol your doctor is likely to suggest is losing weight, by restricting the total number of calories you consume, if necessary, and by keeping your fat intake to no more than 30 percent of total daily calories, keeping your consumption of animal fats to no more than 10 percent of total daily calories, and/or limiting your cholesterol intake to 300 milligrams a day.

■ Since these initial measures are often unsuccessful, the next step is to make the diet even more restricted by attempting to cut out all sources of dietary cholesterol. This is not likely to work, however, because there is an apparent lack of connection between oral intake of cholesterol and subsequent blood levels. This means that whatever amount of cholesterol you eat (or don't eat), it has little to do with altering the level of cholesterol in your bloodstream—for whatever reason, your body is producing high levels of cholesterol on its own.

■ If all dietary measures fail, drug therapy may be recommended. The use of drugs for cholesterol control is common. One type of drug used to bring down cholesterol is the HMB-CoA reductase inhibitor. Examples include fluvastatin (Lescol), lovastatin (Mevacor), pravastatin (Pravachol), and simvastatin (Zocor). HMB-CoA is an enzyme necessary in the early stages of cholesterol synthesis; by blocking its action, these drugs reduce the production of cholesterol in the liver. Because these drugs affect the liver, regular blood tests are necessary to monitor liver function. Potential side effects include muscle pain, tenderness, and weakness; constipation; diarrhea; stomach pain; nausea; flatulence; and bloating. Bring any side effects to your doctor's attention promptly.

■ Another type of agent used to reduce cholesterol is the bile-acid resin. These drugs, which include colestipol (Colestid) and cholestyramine (Questran), absorb cholesterol and prevent it from being passed through the liver. Instead, it is excreted. Possible side effects of these medications include gastrointestinal irritation and bleeding, abdominal pain, belching, flatulence, nausea, vomiting, diarrhea, and hemorrhoidal problems.

■ Fibric-acid derivatives like gemfibrozil (Lopid) lower triglyceride levels and raise HDL levels. Potential side effects include abdominal pain, diarrhea, vomiting, heartburn, fatigue, and skin rash. These drugs may also foster or worsen psoriasis.

■ The very worst cases of high cholesterol have been treated with a drug called probucol (Lorelco). This agent can cause major side effects, including serious heart-rhythm disturbances, nausea, vomiting, diarrhea, abdominal pain, internal bleeding, headache, dizziness, blood abnormalities, rashes, bruising, impotence, blurred vision, and sudden death.

■ Another agent that can be used to lower cholesterol is the B-vitamin niacin (vitamin B3 or nicotinic acid). This is proven to be effective at lowering LDL, raising HDL, and even simultaneously lowering serum triglycerides. Though relatively low in toxicity, it is not used often. The problems with this remarkable nutrient stem from its primary side effect, the "niacin flush" (see under Nutritional Supplements in this entry). It can also irritate the liver if taken in high doses over a long period of time.

Note: Do not take supplemental niacin if you have gout or liver dysfunction.

DIETARY GUIDELINES

■ Reduce your consumption of fats, if necessary, so that you get no more than 20 to 30 percent of your daily calories from fat. In addition to reducing the amount of fat in your diet, make sure that the fat you consume is the right kind. Emphasize monounsaturated fats, found in olive and canola oil. These can reduce LDL without decreasing HDL. Avoid saturated fats, found in meat, shellfish, and dairy foods, and hydrogenated and partially hydrogenated fats, found in margarine, shortening, and hydrogenated and partially-hydrogenated oils. These increase total cholesterol and also increase the proportion of LDL relative to HDL. To avoid dietary cholesterol entirely, take all animal products off the menu.

■ Eat a diet that is high in fiber. Water-soluble dietary fiber helps reduce cholesterol. Oat bran is probably the best source. Several studies have found that LDL levels dropped by 3 to 10 percent in just two to three weeks when people began eating one and a half cups of cooked oatmeal daily. Other good sources of fiber include brown rice bran, barley, beans, and some fruits.

■ Emphasize foods that are rich in antioxidant substances (beta-carotene, vitamins C and E, and selenium) that destroy free radicals. Eat plenty of fruits, tomatoes, sweet potatoes, dark-green vegetables, and whole-grain products.

■ Add garlic and onions to your diet on a regular basis. Consuming 4 grams of garlic daily (the equivalent of one to two cloves, depending on size) has been shown to reduce cholesterol and triglyceride levels.

■ Put carrots on the menu. Studies conducted by the U.S. Department of Agriculture found that volunteers who ate two or three carrots per day saw their cholesterol levels fall an average of 11 percent. This suggests that higher levels of beta-carotene in the blood can help reduce serum cholesterol.

■ Drink green tea with meals. Catechin, a compound found in green tea, has been shown to lower LDL levels. It also seems to keep cholesterol from being metabolized in such a way that it ends up being deposited on artery walls.

■ Here's some good news for chocoholics. Chocolate, like red wine, has been found to contain flavonoids that protect against the oxidation of cholesterol. The bad news? Chocolate is a high-sugar, high-fat, high-calorie food. Enjoy chocolate occasionally. Choose the dark or bitter-sweet varieties, which contain less sugar than milk chocolate.

■ Exercise moderation in your consumption of alcohol.

■ Avoid coffee and other beverages that contain caffeine. Drinking large amounts of coffee increases the amount of cholesterol circulating in the bloodstream.

NUTRITIONAL SUPPLEMENTS

■ Antioxidants defuse free radicals. Take a good antioxidant formula providing 5,000 international units of vitamin A, 15,000 international units of beta-carotene, 3,000 milligrams of vitamin C, 1,500 milligrams of bioflavonoids,

400 international units of vitamin E, and 200 micrograms of selenium daily.

Note: If you are pregnant, or intend to get pregnant, or if you have liver disease, consult your doctor before taking supplemental vitamin A. If you are taking an anticoagulant (blood thinner), consult your physician before taking supplemental vitamin E.

Carnitine improves the metabolism of fatty acids and helps lower total cholesterol and triglyceride levels. Carnitine levels decline with age. Take 250 to 500 milligrams of L-carnitine three times daily.

■ Nutriceuticals are patented versions of nutrients designed to help with a specific medical concern. One nutriceutical, a purified red yeast rice product sold under the brand name Cholestin, has been found, in both animal and clinical (human) studies, to have beneficial effects in lowering both triglycerides and LDL levels, while raising the level of beneficial HDL. As long as you are not sensitive to yeast, it should have minimal side effects and is essentially nontoxic. Recommended doses range from one to four 600-milligram capsules daily.

Coenzyme Q_{10} enhances cellular oxygenation throughout the body. Take 25 milligrams three times daily.

If you have digestive difficulties, take a full-spectrum digestive-enzyme supplement containing lipase, amylase, protease, and pancreatin with each meal.

The essential fatty acids (EFAs) present in flaxseed oil help keep fats fluid and mobile in the bloodstream, an important attribute that aids in preventing the buildup of plaque on artery walls. EFAs are also needed for the transport of oxygen. Take 1 tablespoon (or 500 to 750 milligrams) once or twice daily. Essential fatty acids found in black currant seed oil, borage oil, and evening primrose oil act directly to reduce LDL. Choose one of these oils and take 500 milligrams twice daily.

Kelp is rich in iodine, essential for normal thyroid function. A sluggish thyroid has been linked to high cholesterol levels, especially in women. Take 150 milligrams of kelp with breakfast, and another 150 milligrams with lunch.

Lecithin is a fat emulsifier that helps lower cholesterol. Take 1,200 milligrams (or 1 tablespoon) three times daily, before meals.

Lipoic acid is an antioxidant that works synergistically with vitamin B_1 (thiamine) and vitamin B_3 (niacin), and enhances the properties of selenium and vitamin E. Because it is effective in helping control blood-sugar levels, it is especially helpful if you have elevated cholesterol and are always tired. Take 50 milligrams twice daily.

Take a total of 100 micrograms of selenium twice daily. If your antioxidant formula doesn't provide this amount,

make up the difference with a separate supplement. Statistics show that the incidence of heart disease and stroke is higher among people with low selenium intake.

■ The B vitamins are necessary for complete fat metabolism. Take a B-complex supplement that supplies 50 to 100 milligrams of each of the primary B vitamins three times daily.

■ Niacin-based supplements are often prescribed to lower cholesterol levels. They are effective, but should be taken only under the supervision of a health-care practitioner because they can irritate the liver. The usual recommendation is to take 500 milligrams of vitamin B_3 (niacin) twice daily. To avoid the "niacin flush"—a reddening of the skin accompanied by a tingling sensation—and other side effects, you should start with a small amount such as 50 milligrams and gradually increase to the recommended dosage.

Note: Do not take supplemental niacin if you have gout or liver dysfunction. Niacinamide is a compound related to niacin, but it does not have the same effect on the circulatory system and does not cause flushing. Niacinamide does work on the nervous system and helps to relax the body. Inositol hexaniacinate, a newer compound, does not cause flushing and may be effective at lower doses.

■ Vitamin E has anticoagulant properties similar to those of aspirin, but is not irritating to the stomach lining. It also scavenges free radicals, is an anti-inflammatory, and is required for proper hormonal function. Low levels of vitamin E are associated with a high risk of cardiovascular disease. Choose a product containing mixed tocopherols and start by taking 200 international units, then gradually increase the dosage until you are taking 400 international units in the morning, and another 400 international units in the evening.

Note: If you have high blood pressure, limit your intake of supplemental vitamin E to a total of 400 international units daily. If you are taking an anticoagulant (blood thinner), consult your physician before taking supplemental vitamin E.

HERBAL TREATMENT

■ Artichoke leaf extract reduces blood-cholesterol levels. Take 250 to 300 milligrams two or three times daily.

■ Dandelion thins bile and has been shown to lower cholesterol. Take 250 milligrams two to three times daily for six weeks.

■ Fo-ti (also known as *ho shou wu* and *Polygonum multiflorum*) can help to reduce blood-cholesterol levels. Take 500 to 1,000 milligrams once or twice daily.

■ Garlic reduces cholesterol levels and high blood pressure. Take 500 milligrams three times daily, with meals.

Hawthorn has been shown to both reduce cholesterol levels and decrease the size of existing plaques in the arteries. This herb is high in flavonoids that may reverse the damaging effects of high cholesterol. Hawthorn has been used for extended periods of time with no adverse side effects. Choose a standardized extract containing 1.8 percent vitexin-2 rhamnosides and take 100 to 200 milligrams three times a day.

Siberian ginseng helps the body adapt to stress and has a wide variety of uses. Among other things, it brings down cholesterol levels and is considered preventive medicine for heart disease. Choose a standardized extract containing 0.5 percent eleutheroside E and take 100 to 200 milligrams twice daily, the first dose before breakfast and the second before lunch, for four to six weeks.

HOMEOPATHY

Elevated cholesterol levels seldom produce symptoms, but if this condition is accompanied by symptoms such as indigestion, constipation, diarrhea, or anything else, please see the appropriate entry and select one or more of the symptom-specific remedies listed there.

ACUPRESSURE

For the locations of acupressure points on the body, *see* ADMINISTERING AN ACUPRESSURE TREATMENT in Part Three.

Gallbladder 20, 21, and 34 helps to regulate the functioning of the gallbladder.

Liver 3 and Stomach 36 enhance digestion.

GENERAL RECOMMENDATIONS

Be aware of your cholesterol and triglyceride levels. You cannot manage your cholesterol level efficiently if you don't know what it is. Consult your physician to schedule a cholesterol test.

Adopt an exercise program and stick to it. Regular exercise increases HDL and reduces LDL. The Stanford University Center for Research in Disease studied close to 500 men and women with high LDL profiles and found that those who exercised not only brought their HDL levels up, but reduced their LDL levels by twice as much as those who merely changed their diets. *See* STARTING AN EXERCISE PROGRAM in Part Three for suggestions to help you get started.

PREVENTION

Eat a low-fat, high-fiber diet. A diet rich in fruits, vegetables, and grains results in less circulating cholesterol and lowers your risk of developing arterial plaque.

Exercise. Physical activity boosts HDL. Regular exercise

can cut your risk of atherosclerosis by as much as 50 percent. As little as thirty minutes of aerobic exercise, such as brisk walking, three to five times a week is enough to make a real difference.

■ Research shows that obesity is associated with low levels of HDL, the protective form of cholesterol, and high levels of LDL, the plaque-forming cholesterol. If you need to lose weight, do it now. Simply losing pounds can shift the ratio of HDL to LDL in your favor.

■ Don't smoke. Smoking increases the development of deposits of cholesterol in the large arteries.

Chronic Obstructive Pulmonary Disease (COPD)

See EMPHYSEMA.

Chronic Fatigue Syndrome

Chronic fatigue syndrome (CFS) is a mysterious condition that can cause a wide range of baffling symptoms. The primary and definitive one is extreme and debilitating exhaustion for which no other cause can be found. Accompanying symptoms can include all-over weakness, aching muscles and joints, loss of appetite, headaches, mild fever, sore throat, swollen lymph nodes in the neck and underarms, intestinal problems, jaundice, muscle spasms, and recurrent upper respiratory tract infections. Mental and emotional symptoms produced by CFS can include mood swings, anxiety, depression, difficulty concentrating, forgetfulness, and sleep disturbances. Some people also suffer some degree of memory loss, which is usually temporary, and mental confusion.

Depending on the severity of the symptoms, CFS can make it very difficult to carry on a normal life. As routine tasks become more and more of a challenge, both physically and mentally, your ability to function can be severely curtailed. Weakness and lack of energy can make just getting out of bed to face the day a major accomplishment.

No one knows what causes CFS, but there are numerous theories. It has been noted that many CFS patients carry high levels of Epstein-Barr virus (EBV) antibodies in their blood, showing that they were infected with this virus at some time or another. EBV is a member of the herpes family, and it causes mononucleosis, another debilitating condition. Further, many people with CFS tie the beginning of their symptoms to a lingering infection of one kind of another. However, no definite link between CFS and EBV has ever been established. Fibromyalgia and intestinal parasites also are common among those afflicted with CFS, but neither of these problems has been identified as a cause of the syndrome, either.

Some experts believe chronic fatigue syndrome is related to a problem with the immune system. Others say it may be caused by a dysfunction of the mechanisms that regulate blood pressure. A Johns Hopkins University study found that 22 out of 23 subjects with CFS suffered a drop in blood pressure and a marked slowing of the heart rate after standing for a prolonged period of time. The result was a feeling of dizziness and exhaustion that lasted for days after the study was concluded. Many patients in this study found their symptoms improved after their blood pressure was stabilized. Other research is centered on the possibility that chemical or food sensitivities may trigger CFS.

Whatever the cause or causes, CFS is widespread in the United States. Although it can occur at any age, it primarily affects people between the ages of twenty and forty. It is more common in women than men. The course of the illness varies widely. Some people have symptoms that persist for months, even years. Others enjoy periods of remission, but recurrences are common and can strike without warning. In some people, the disorder never completely goes away. Most people with CFS do eventually recover, however. As symptoms lessen and disappear, most are able to return, gradually, to a normal level of activity.

If you experience fatigue that lasts for longer than two weeks, see a health-care professional. You may have another health problem that requires attention. Conditions that can produce similar symptoms include anemia, cancer, systemic candida infection, chemical dependencies, depression, food allergies or sensitivities, heart problems, hepatitis, HIV disease, hypoglycemia, hypothyroidism, chronic infection, Lyme disease, multiple sclerosis, rheumatoid arthritis, thyroid problems, tuberculosis, and reactions to medications.

Diagnosis of chronic fatigue syndrome is based on the presence of unexplained exhaustion that is not improved by sleep or rest, persists for three to six months, and causes an all-over weakness and lack of energy so severe that it interferes with normal living. The first step in diagnosing chronic fatigue syndrome is to rule out any underlying conditions, including psychological disorders, that may be contributing to the problem.

There is no cure for chronic fatigue syndrome, and it is not considered a dangerous illness. That is small comfort, though, to those who suffer from the debilitating effects of this disorder. CFS has a tremendous impact both on the person who has it and on his or her family. This entry focuses on what you can do to ease the symptoms and regain some control over your life.

CONVENTIONAL MEDICINE

■ If all underlying conditions are ruled out and chronic fatigue syndrome is diagnosed, the conventional approach to treating it centers on providing symptomatic relief. Painkillers such as acetaminophen (Tylenol, Datril, and others), aspirin (Bayer, Ecotrin, and others), and ibuprofen (Advil, Motrin, Nuprin, and others) may be recommended to control inflammation and pain in the muscles and joints, and to treat headaches. Beyond that, your doctor may encourage you to rest as needed and participate in as much activity as you can.

■ Some doctors refer patients with symptoms of chronic fatigue for psychiatric evaluation, implying that the problem is "all in your head." Some may even prescribe antidepressants. While it is true that depression can cause symptoms similar to those of chronic fatigue, true CFS is not a psychiatric condition and should not be treated as such.

DIETARY GUIDELINES

■ Symptoms associated with chronic fatigue, including muscle and joint pain, can be caused by unsuspected food allergies or sensitivities. To make sure you are not eating foods that are causing troublesome symptoms, *see* ROTATION DIET in Part Three and follow the program.

■ Eliminate from your diet excess sugar, processed foods, and all caffeine and alcohol. All these substances worsen symptoms.

■ Drink at least six 8-ounce glasses of pure water daily to flush the body and get rid of toxins. Many people with CFS suffer from impaired digestion, which causes a buildup of toxic metabolites.

NUTRITIONAL SUPPLEMENTS

■ Bromelain, an enzyme derived from pineapple, and proteolytic enzymes help reduce inflammation. Take 500 milligrams of either twice a day, between meals.

■ The digestion and assimilation of nutrients are often compromised in people with chronic fatigue syndrome. Take a full-spectrum digestive-enzyme supplement containing 5,000 international units of lipase, 2,500 international units of amylase, 300 international units of protease, plus 500 to 1,000 milligrams of pancreatin, with each meal.

Note: Long-term supplementation with pancreatin is not advised, as it can cause your pancreas to reduce its own production of this important enzyme. Overuse also has the potential to cause nausea or diarrhea. After two months on pancreatin, discontinue use and monitor your reaction. If you find that your problems recur, discuss pancreatin supplementation with your health-care provider.

■ Flaxseed oil contains valuable essential fatty acids that people with CFS need but sometimes have difficulty digesting. Start with a small amount and gradually increase the dosage until you are taking 1 tablespoon, or 500 to 750 milligrams in capsule form, twice daily.

■ Gamma-aminobutyric acid (GABA) is very useful if the fatigue is associated with anxiety. Take 500 milligrams in the morning and again at bedtime.

   Note: If you are taking melatonin in the evening, eliminate the evening dose of GABA.

■ Glucosamine sulfate relieves joint pain by assisting in the production of cartilage. Take 500 milligrams of glucosamine sulfate three times daily (if you weigh over 200 pounds, take the same dose four times daily). It may take up to eight to twelve weeks to see results, so don't give up too soon.

■ Lipotropics are emulsifiers that help in the digestion of fats. They also assist in the transmission of signals from one nerve cell to another, which is an important consideration if you are experiencing bodywide weakness. Take 1,200 milligrams (or 1 tablespoon) of lecithin twice daily, with meals. Or take 300 to 500 milligrams of a lipotropic complex three times daily, with meals.

■ Magnesium and malic acid assist in initiating the Krebs cycle, a series of biochemical reactions that transform nutrients into energy. Take a combination formula that supplies 100 milligrams of magnesium and 300 milligrams of malic acid three times daily, twenty minutes before each meal, for six to eight weeks.

■ In spite of extreme fatigue, many people with CFS do not sleep well. Melatonin, a natural hormone that regulates sleep, can be helpful. Take 0.5 to 3 milligrams daily, one to two hours before bedtime.

   Note: Melatonin can cause drowsiness. Do not take it during the day.

■ Take a probiotic supplement. The friendly bacteria normalize the intestinal tract, which is often compromised in CFS. They also fight candida infection, another common complication of CFS. Take a probiotic supplement as recommended on the product label. You can also take colostrum on a rotating basis with other probiotics.

■ Fructooligosaccharides (FOS) are a form of carbohydrate that can be utilized by the friendly bacteria but not by yeast, such as candida. They thus enhance the action of probiotic supplements. Start by taking $1/4$ teaspoon of FOS twice a day and gradually work up to 1 teaspoon twice a day over the course of two to three weeks.

■ Sea greens, such as spirulina and blue-green algae, contain many trace minerals that are missing in the normal diet. Take a sea-greens supplement as directed on the product label.

■ Thymus glandular extract enhances immune function, which is often impaired in people with chronic fatigue syndrome. Take 750 milligrams of thymus extract at breakfast and again at lunch.

■ If you have an understanding physician, ask for an injection of vitamin B_{12}. Though your blood level of this nutrients may be normal, there is no danger whatsoever in this treatment—the shot is both tiny and inexpensive—and many people find it helpful. If you feel better, ask to have the shot repeated weekly until it no longer brings about any additional improvement.

■ Vitamin C has strong antibacterial and antiviral properties. Take at least 1,000 milligrams of buffered vitamin C with bioflavonoids three times daily, up to the highest level you can tolerate without developing loose stools.

■ Vitamin E is an anti-inflammatory agent and free-radical scavenger. Choose a product containing mixed tocopherols and start by taking 100 to 200 milligrams at bedtime, then gradually increase until you are taking 400 international units daily. If pain and discomfort are severe, experiment by slowly continuing to increase your intake of vitamin E until you are taking 400 international units three to four times daily. As your symptoms lessen, slowly reduce your intake back to 400 international units a day, taken at bedtime.

   Note: If you have high blood pressure, limit your intake of supplemental vitamin E to a total of 400 international units daily. If you are taking an anticoagulant (blood thinner), consult your physician before taking supplemental vitamin E.

■ Some naturopathic physicians treat CFS with an intravenous solution containing pantothenic acid, vitamin C, and hydrochloric acid (HCl). Many people report remarkable improvement with this treatment.

HERBAL TREATMENT

■ Astragalus helps strengthen the production of white blood cells, required for fighting infection and inflammation. Take 250 milligrams three or four times daily.

■ Cat's claw has anti-inflammatory and immune-promoting properties. Start by taking 250 milligrams of standardized extract three times a day, and gradually increase the dosage over a period of four weeks until you are taking 1,000 milligrams three times daily.

   Note: Do not use cat's claw if you are pregnant or nursing, or if you are an organ-transplant recipient. Use it with caution if you are taking an anticoagulant (blood thinner).

■ Chinese (or Korean) ginseng helps the body fight stress and enhances energy. It also fights viral infection and helps support the immune system. This herb is very powerful. Approach it with respect. Select a standardized extract containing 7 percent ginsenosides and begin by taking half the manufacturer's recommended dose, then gradually increase the dosage until you are taking it as directed on the product label.

Note: Do not use Chinese ginseng if you have high blood pressure, heart disease, or hypoglycemia. If you are sensitive to the effects of caffeine and other stimulants, you may want to consult with a qualified herbalist before using ginseng.

■ Take one dose of an echinacea and goldenseal combination formula supplying 250 to 500 milligrams of echinacea and 150 to 300 milligrams of goldenseal three times daily for five to ten days. This formula is especially valuable if you are battling an acute infection, such as a sore throat.

■ Kava kava is a calmative herb that helps ease the anxiety associated with CFS. Choose a product containing 30 percent kavalactones and take 250 milligrams twice daily, the first dose in the middle of the day and the second before bedtime.

Note: In excess amounts, this herb can cause drowsiness. Do not exceed the recommended dose. Do not use kava kava if you are pregnant or nursing, if you have Parkinson's disease, or if you are taking a prescription medication for depression or anxiety.

■ Olive leaf has antifungal and antiviral effects. Take 250 milligrams of standardized extract two or three times daily.

■ St. John's wort is helpful for chronic fatigue accompanied by depression. Select a product containing 0.3 percent hypericin and take 300 milligrams three times daily.

■ Siberian ginseng increases the body's resistance to stress, fatigue, and disease. It also has been shown to increase mental alertness, and possesses strong antioxidant properties. Choose a standardized extract containing 0.5 percent eleutheroside E and take 100 to 200 milligrams twice daily, in the morning and again in the afternoon.

■ Valerian is a good relaxant that improves the quality of sleep. If insomnia is a problem, valerian can help. Studies show that people taking this herb fall asleep faster, wake up fewer times during the night, and feel refreshed upon awakening in the morning. Select a standardized extract containing 0.5 percent isovalerenic acids and take 200 to 400 milligrams half an hour before bedtime.

HOMEOPATHY

When dealing with chronic fatigue, it is best to consult a homeopathic practitioner for a constitutional remedy. If that is not possible, select among the symptom-specific remedies listed below.

■ Choose *Argentum nitricum* if you are fearful, anxiety-ridden, and secretive, with irrational motives for your acts, which are often kept hidden. You probably have headaches with coldness and trembling, sleep poorly, and often have bad dreams, and you may have lost your sense of smell. Take one dose *Argentum nitricum* 30x or 12c, as directed on the product label, three times daily, as needed, for up to three days.

■ *Phosphoricum acidum* is good if you are feeling emotionally and physically drained and apathetic, perhaps due to grief. Take one dose of *Phosphoricum acidum* 30x or 15c three times daily, as needed, for up to three days.

■ *Picricum acidum* will help if you feel terrible after the least exertion, especially after mental exertion, and have an aversion to food. You may feel so tired that you lack willpower and determination, and you frequently have headaches that are relieved by strong pressure. Take one dose of *Picricum acidum* 3c or 6x three times daily, as needed, for up to three days.

■ *Silicea* is good for headaches and exhaustion caused by overwork. You tend to be chilly and sensitive to cold air, and often have cramps in the calves and soles of your feet. If you are a woman, you may have a vaginal discharge. Take one dose of *Silicea* 30x or 15c three times daily, as needed, for up to three days.

■ Choose *Zincum metallicum* if you are forgetful and tend to repeat things. You are mentally exhausted and very sensitive to noise, grind your teeth while sleeping, and may suffer from chronic constipation. Take one dose of *Zincum metallicum* 30x or 15c three times daily, as needed, for up to three days.

BACH FLOWER REMEDIES

Select the remedy that most closely fits your emotional tendencies and concerns, and take it as needed, following the directions on the product label.

■ Aspen is good if you are fearful but cannot (or cannot bring yourself to) explain your feeling of fright. You may have trouble sleeping because of bad dreams.

■ Holly eases feelings of anger and fits of temper due to insecurity and jealousy.

■ Hornbeam helps alleviate fatigue and utter exhaustion.

■ Impatiens calms impatience, tension, nervousness, and irritability.

■ Mimulus is good if you are shy and timid, and frequently and clearly express your fears.

ACUPRESSURE

For the locations of acupressure points on the body, *see*

ADMINISTERING AN ACUPRESSURE TREATMENT in Part Three.

■ All back Bladder points relax and tone the nervous system.

■ Gallbladder 20 and 21 help to bring down energy from the head and keep it circulating throughout the body to promote healing.

■ Gallbladder 41 helps to regulate hormonal function.

■ Kidney 3 regulates kidney function. In Chinese medicine, a general lack of energy is associated with an imbalance in kidney function.

■ Large Intestine 4, 10, and 11 activate the large intestine, promoting proper elimination of toxins.

■ Liver 3 relaxes the nervous system.

■ Pericardium 6 relaxes the chest and the mind.

■ Spleen 6 strengthens the blood.

■ Stomach 36 improves digestion and absorption of nutrients.

AROMATHERAPY

For specific instructions on how to use aromatherapy, *see* PREPARING AROMATHERAPY TREATMENTS in Part Three.

■ Essential oils of basil, bergamot, geranium, lavender, peppermint, and thyme have stimulating and energizing properties. Bergamot oil also helps combat depression. You can use any or all of these oils as inhalants, in aromatherapy baths, or in massage oil, or you can diffuse them into the air.

GENERAL RECOMMENDATIONS

■ See your doctor to rule out any underlying conditions. There are many other health problems that can cause symptoms similar to those of CFS.

■ Investigate the possibility that you have undetected food allergies or sensitivities.

■ If you are diagnosed with chronic fatigue syndrome, support both your mind and body with all the resources at your command. Above all, be patient. CFS is a complicated condition that cannot be resolved overnight.

■ Giving in and giving up is the worst thing you can do. However, you must give yourself permission to rest. Rest is important.

■ Involve your loved ones in your recovery. They must understand that the condition is real, not imagined.

PREVENTION

■ No one can say with certainty what causes chronic fatigue syndrome. However, it has been observed that a viral infection often precedes the onset of CFS. Including garlic, which has documented antiviral properties, in your regular supplement program may provide a measure of protection.

Cirrhosis

Cirrhosis is a long-term disease of the liver. During the course of this disease, the liver becomes scarred and covered with fibrous tissue, which prevents it from functioning normally.

The liver is the body's largest internal organ. It is responsible for producing bile, which is necessary for the digestion of fats. The liver also processes glucose, proteins, vitamins, fats, and most of the other compounds used by the body. In addition, this complex organ detoxifies and renders harmless substances such as nicotine, alcohol, drug residues, environmental contaminants, and various other poisons, as well as certain harmful substances produced in the intestines.

As cirrhosis progresses, liver function gradually decreases. This affects the manufacture of glucose and some hormones, as well as stomach and bowel function. The free flow of blood through the liver may become blocked. In the early stages, there may be no symptoms at all. The disease is often discovered during a routine physical examination or blood test given for some other reason. Or there may be symptoms including nausea, weakness, stomach pain, bloody vomit, ascites (abdominal swelling caused by an accumulation of fluid in the tissues), and varicose veins. Loss of appetite and resulting weight loss are common. The veins on the face may become noticeably distended as well. Unless the cause of the disease is addressed and treated, bleeding in the bowels and stomach may occur, and kidney failure may result. Mental confusion is common. In addition, toxins that would be detoxified by a healthy liver may accumulate in the brain, causing hepatic encephalopathy, a decline in brain function manifested as speech difficulties, altered sleep, tremors, and other symptoms. Ultimately, cirrhosis can lead to hepatic coma and death.

The most common cause of cirrhosis is long-term alcohol abuse. Alcohol is a toxin that inflicts direct damage on the liver. The risk of damage relates to the amount of alcohol ingested, not the form in which it is consumed. Wine and beer contribute to the problem just as much as hard liquor. Women are more susceptible to alcoholic cirrhosis than men, probably due to their usually smaller body size and lower weight than to any genetic difference. Cirrhosis can also result from exposure to other toxins, as well as chronic hepatitis, malnutrition, or other infections.

Cirrhosis is diagnosed by a combination of physical

examination and x-ray, and confirmed by liver biopsy. Blood tests of liver function are done to monitor the progress of the disease and evaluate the success of treatment.

The liver is a remarkably resilient organ. If exposure to all toxins, particularly alcohol, is removed, the liver can often repair much of the damage if given the proper help and support, unless too much tissue has been destroyed. Recovery of liver function is a very slow process, however.

CONVENTIONAL TREATMENT

In general, treatment is supportive, aimed at removing as much stress on the liver as possible while waiting to see if the liver retains enough regenerative capacity to improve. Alcohol is absolutely prohibited. So is acetaminophen (sold as Tylenol, Datril, and other over-the-counter pain remedies) and any products that contain it. Acetaminophen is irritating to the liver.

Even conventional medicine recommends nutritional supplementation for this illness, particularly supplementation with folic acid and/or iron for certain anemias and vitamin K for bleeding problems.

A balanced diet is recommended, although protein may be restricted if the disease is severe enough that hepatic encephalopathy or coma has occurred.

Ascites is handled first by restricting salt intake. If this proves insufficient, diuretics are prescribed. More severe cases are handled by drawing off the fluid with large needles and administering intravenous doses of serum protein to prevent blood volume from declining too far. Serious cases of ascites that will not improve with other therapies are handled with shunts, which are pipelines implanted surgically to move the fluids back into the circulatory system. This treatment is not without problems of its own. Complications can arise if there is too much fluid in the circulatory system or too many toxins floating around in that fluid, or if the pipeline becomes plugged up.

If hepatic encephalopathy develops, all unnecessary drugs are withheld, though antibiotics are used to kill bacteria that might produce ammonia. Lactulose, a synthetic sugar, may be administered to encourage the bacteria to make a nonabsorbable form of ammonia.

If systemic infection develops, a not-uncommon problem in cirrhosis, antibiotics are prescribed.

In the end stage of this disease, a liver transplant offers the only chance of survival. This is extremely serious surgery, complicated by the fact that there is a tremendous scarcity of available organs. In addition, transplant patients must take antirejection drugs, which wreak havoc on the immune system.

DIETARY GUIDELINES

■ Abstain *completely* from alcohol, including any over-the-counter remedies that contain alcohol, such as certain cough medicines and tinctures.

■ If the cirrhosis is severe, eat only steamed fresh vegetables and fruits until your liver begins to recover.

■ Proper nutrition is essential. To support the liver while it works to heal itself, eat five or six small, nutrient-dense meals that contain clean, lean protein daily. Vegetable protein, such as that found in tofu, legumes, and whole grains, is preferred.

■ Fruits are easy to digest. Grapes, applesauce, watermelon, cantaloupe, and diluted juices are usually welcome and are well tolerated.

■ Lightly steamed greens, including artichokes, collards, and endive, support the healing process. Unless you are anemic, avoid spinach. Spinach contains high levels of iron, which can irritate the liver.

■ To help flush toxins from your body, drink eight glasses of pure water every day.

■ Avoid animal fats completely. Animal fats take longer to break down for absorption than any other nutrients. Most of that work is done by the liver. A compromised liver requires rest.

NUTRITIONAL SUPPLEMENTS

■ Acidophilus and bifidus supplements restore friendly flora in the gastrointestinal tract. Take them as recommended on the product labels. If you are allergic to milk, select dairy-free formulas.

■ The antioxidants—especially beta-carotene, lipoic acid, selenium, and vitamins A and E—fight free-radical damage. Select a good antioxidant formula that provides 2,500 international units of vitamin A, 15,000 international units of beta-carotene, 3,000 milligrams of vitamin C, 1,500 milligrams of bioflavonoids, 400 milligrams of vitamin E, and 200 micrograms of selenium daily. In addition, take 25 milligrams of lipoic acid three times daily. Lipoic acid has a specific oxygenating effect on the liver and helps improve energy.

Note: If you are pregnant, or intend to get pregnant, or if you have liver disease, consult your doctor before taking supplemental vitamin A. If you are taking an anticoagulant (blood thinner), consult your physician before taking supplemental vitamin E.

■ A warm castor-oil pack can reduce acute inflammation and help restore proper liver function. Prepare a warm castor oil pack by saturating several layers of clean white cloth with the oil. Either warm the oil before preparing the pack, or prepare the pack, place it on a clean plate, and warm it in a microwave oven for twenty to thirty seconds. The pack should be warm but not hot. Place the warm pack over the upper right quadrant of your abdomen and leave it in place for fifteen to twenty minutes. Do this once a day for five to seven days.

■ Carnitine, a substance related to the B vitamins but often grouped with the amino acids, helps to reduce free fatty acid levels in people with cirrhosis. It also reduces elevated triglycerides and liver enzymes. Start by taking a dose of 250 to 500 milligrams of L-carnitine with breakfast. After one week, add a second dose, with lunch. After another week, add a third dose, so that you are taking 250 to 500 milligrams with each meal. Continue taking L-carnitine for three to four months.

■ Choline is very beneficial to the liver. Take 500 milligrams a day until recovery is complete.

■ To insure more efficient digestion, take a good full-spectrum digestive-enzyme supplement containing 5,000 international units of lipase, 2,500 international units of amylase, 300 international units of protease, plus 500 to 1,000 milligrams of pancreatin, with each meal.

Note: Long-term supplementation with pancreatin is not advised, as it can cause your pancreas to reduce its own production of this important enzyme. Overuse also has the potential to cause nausea or diarrhea. After two months on pancreatin, discontinue use and monitor your reaction. If you find that your digestive problems recur, discuss pancreatin supplementation with your health-care provider.

■ Green-foods supplements that contain chlorophyll supply trace minerals usually lacking in the diet. They also supply chlorophyll, which helps detoxify the blood and increases energy. Take a green-foods supplement as recommended on the product label.

■ Lecithin helps fat digestion. Take 1,200 milligrams (or 1 tablespoon) of lecithin twice a day, with meals.

■ Studies have shown that N-acetylcysteine has beneficial effects on liver inflammation. Take 250 to 500 milligrams three times a day.

■ The B vitamins help to restore energy. Take a good B-complex supplement supplying at least 25 milligrams of each of the major B vitamins daily.

■ Vitamin C and the bioflavonoids have anti-inflammatory action and help hasten healing. Take 500 to 1,000 milligrams of vitamin C and 500 milligrams of mixed bioflavonoids three times a day.

■ Unless your doctor prescribes one, *avoid* any nutritional supplements containing iron. A stressed liver cannot process iron effectively.

HERBAL TREATMENT

When choosing herbal products, do not select tincture forms. Tinctures contain alcohol, which is strictly off-limits for those with cirrhosis.

■ Bupleurum and dong quai, a Chinese herbal combination formula, improves digestion and relaxes the nervous system. In Chinese medicine, this formula is used to harmonize the liver and pancreas. Take 1,000 milligrams of a bupleurum and dong quai combination formula two or three times daily for two weeks out of every month (if you are a woman, take it for the two weeks prior to the anticipated onset of your menstrual period).

■ Dan shen (red root sage) is a Chinese herb that dilates blood vessels, thereby increasing the flow of oxygen and nutrients to the liver (and the heart). It also helps relieve feelings of nausea and fatigue. Dan shen is also used in China for chronic hepatitis. Take 300 milligrams three times daily.

■ Dandelion enhances the flow of bile, which reduces liver congestion and relieves jaundice. It is also a mild diuretic. Take 250 milligrams or one cup of dandelion-root tea three times daily for six weeks. Stop for one month, then repeat.

■ Jigucao is a Chinese patent medicine that can be effective in bringing down elevated liver enzymes. Take one capsule twice a day, or follow the dosage directions on the product label.

■ Licorice contains glycyrrhizin, which inhibits liver damage produced by a buildup of toxic chemicals. It is also effective against hepatitis. Take 300 milligrams twice a day.

Note: Do not take licorice on a daily basis for more than five days in a row, as it can elevate blood pressure. Do not take it at all if you have high blood pressure.

■ Milk thistle, which contains silymarin, has the remarkable ability to stimulate the growth of new liver cells. Its antioxidant properties help inhibit the free radicals that add to liver damage. Choose an extract standardized to contain 80 percent flavonoids (silymarin) and take 200 to 300 milligrams three times daily.

■ Pine-bark or grape-seed extract and lipoic acid support the liver. Take 50 milligrams of pine-bark or grape-seed extract three times daily and 50 milligrams of lipoic acid two or three times daily.

■ Turmeric contains substances that help prevent the liver from being damaged by toxic chemicals. It also enhances the flow of bile. Take 300 to 500 milligrams of standardized extract two or three times daily.

HOMEOPATHY

■ Cirrhosis is a serious condition. The best approach to treating it homeopathically is to consult a homeopathic physician for a constitutional remedy formulated especially for you.

■ *Chelidonium* is the remedy for pain and discomfort in the liver and gallbladder that radiates to the right shoulder. Take one dose of *Chelidonium* 6x or 3c, as directed on the product label, three times daily, as needed.

■ *Cholesterinum* helps improve fat digestion, which is always a concern when the liver is involved. Take one dose of *Cholesterinum* 12x or 6c three times daily, as needed.

BACH FLOWER REMEDIES

Select the remedy that most closely fits your emotional tendencies and concerns, and take it as needed, following the directions on the product label.

■ Gorse is the remedy to choose if you are in despair and fear nothing will ever be the same again.

■ Holly is good for anger over the the limitations imposed by this condition.

■ Impatiens is helpful if you are impatient to be well and filled with nervous tension.

ACUPRESSURE

For the locations of acupressure points on the body, *see* ADMINISTERING AN ACUPRESSURE TREATMENT in Part Three.

■ Bladder 17, 18, 19, 20, 21, and 23 help to relax and improve the functioning of the digestive system.

■ Gallbladder 34 and 41 regulate gallbladder function.

■ Liver 3 improves liver function.

■ Stomach 36 improves digestion and absorption of nutrients.

GENERAL RECOMMENDATIONS

■ Avoid becoming constipated. Constipation worsens symptoms. (*See* CONSTIPATION.)

■ Be patient. A compromised liver is slow to recover.

PREVENTION

■ Alcohol abuse is the primary cause of cirrhosis. If you drink, do so in moderation only. If you think you may have a problem with alcohol, *see* ALCOHOLISM.

CMV

See CYTOMEGALOVIRUS.

Cold

See COMMON COLD.

Cold Sores

See HERPES.

Colitis, Ulcerative

Ulcerative colitis is one of two common inflammatory bowel diseases (Crohn's disease is the other). In this condition, the lining of the colon (the large intestine) becomes inflamed and areas of ulceration develop. This disorder most often affects the sigmoid colon and rectum (the lower end of the colon), but can also affect the entire colon. The primary symptom is bloody diarrhea, usually without much pain. While symptoms are acute, the diarrhea and blood loss can be extreme and quite serious if not treated quickly. However, most people's symptoms are not so severe, but follow a course of periodic flare-ups followed by remission. Stress seems to play a major role in the onset of acute symptoms.

The underlying cause of ulcerative colitis remains elusive. Many cases seem to be related to an acute infection with bacteria or parasites, particularly amoebic disease. Also, an overgrowth of yeast can directly irritate the intestinal lining or produce substances that do. This condition seems to run in families, although the genetic link is not really understood. Food allergies and hypersensitivities may also play a role. An advanced case of Lyme disease may result in a type of colitis as well.

The possibility of developing nutritional deficiencies is a major concern with ulcerative colitis. When the lining of the colon is inflamed, nutrients cannot be absorbed properly. Absorption is further hindered by diarrhea, which results in a more rapid passage of food through the colon. Deficiencies of amino acids, essential fatty acids, the many B vitamins, the fat-soluble vitamins (A, D, E, and K), and most minerals can be a problem for people suffering from ulcerative colitis.

Ulcerative colitis is diagnosed by barium enema, x-ray, and direct examination of the colon by means of a fiber-optic scope (either the sigmoidoscope or the more complete colonoscope) inserted into the colon through the rectum. If your doctor observes generalized inflammation and blood, especially with localized ulcers in the colon, he or she will diagnose ulcerative colitis.

CONVENTIONAL MEDICINE

■ If you are diagnosed with ulcerative colitis, it is wise to seek out and work closely with a gastroenterologist, internist, or other physician who specializes, or at the very least has considerable experience, in the treatment of this condition.

■ Reducing inflammation, controlling diarrhea, and providing nutritional support are the major elements in the management of ulcerative colitis. The drug sulfasalazine (sold under the brand name Azulfadine) has been used for decades to reduce inflammation in the colon. A newer (and more expensive) derivative of sulfasalazine called mesalamine (Asacol, Pentasa, Rowasa) provides increased delivery of active anti-inflammatory to the colon. It is available in rectal suppositories and enema solution as well as tablets.

■ Steroids may be prescribed to reduce both acute and chronic inflammation. Corticosteroids are used routinely for serious cases of ulcerative colitis, especially if sulfa medications and other therapies are not effective. Oral prednisone (Deltasone) may be used for generalized colitis. Cortisone enemas are commonly used for localized treatment of the rectum and sigmoid colon.

■ Serious disease of the colon may necessitate surgery Either partial or complete removal of the colon may be necessary to solve a chronic, persistent, and/or life-threatening problem. This means dealing with one or more surgeries and, possibly, with an ileostomy, which means having one's excrement come out of an abdominal outlet into a bag. With better medical intervention and more advanced surgical options, ileostomies and colostomies are more rare today than they used to be and, in many cases, are only temporary. When the condition clears, it may be possible to reconnect the intestines and do away with the bag.

DIETARY GUIDELINES

■ While you are in the midst of an attack of ulcerative colitis, eat a soft, more liquid, high-nutrient diet to help resolve irritation. Fresh juices, water, and soups containing vegetables (and fish or chicken) will provide nutrients helpful for healing.

■ Steamed and cooked vegetables and soups are usually well tolerated. Follow a soft, more liquid, high-nutrient diet to help resolve irritation.

■ Foods containing chlorophyll are rich in nutrients and are easy on the digestive tract. Maximize your intake of cooked leafy greens, such as spinach and kale (which provide iron, important if you are experiencing bloody diarrhea), and sea vegetables such as nori, nijiki, and arame, or kombu, which may be added to soups. Spinach and kale are also good sources of iron, which is important if you are experiencing bloody diarrhea.

■ Eliminate from your diet refined sugar, processed foods, caffeine, and alcohol. Caffeine and alcohol are particularly irritating to a stressed digestive tract.

■ Food allergies and hypersensitivities contribute to ulcerative colitis. The most common culprits are cow's milk, wheat, and soy protein, although any food can add to the problem in susceptible individuals. Eliminate suspect foods for a month or so to see if your condition improves, or try a three- or four-day rotation diet (see ROTATION DIET in Part Three). Ask your doctor about radioallergosorbent (RAST) testing, which measures antibody responses to possible food allergens. This may be helpful in designing the right diet for you.

■ Avoid all dairy products, pickled foods, and all products made with yeast, and see if your symptoms improve. These foods are high in histamines, and many people with inflammatory bowel disease are histamine-intolerant. Many may also be allergic to milk. In addition, certain dairy products (some ice creams and commercial yogurts) are stabilized with carrageenan, a substance extracted from seaweed. In large quantities, this normally benign substance has been shown to cause ulcerative colitis in laboratory animals.

NUTRITIONAL SUPPLEMENTS

■ Key nutrients that are often deficient in people with ulcerative colitis include vitamins A and E, folic acid, pantothenic acid, zinc, calcium, vitamin D, and iron, especially if there is bloody diarrhea. For necessary nutritional support, take a good multivitamin and mineral supplement two or three times daily. Select a powder or capsule form; these are easier to digest and assimilate than hard tablets.

Note: Excessive amounts of iron are associated with a variety of health problems, including an increased risk of cardiovascular disease. Do not take supplemental iron unless a deficiency has been diagnosed by your healthcare provider, and do not take the supplement in higher amounts or for a longer period of time than he or she prescribes. If you are pregnant, or intend to get pregnant, or if you have liver disease, consult your doctor before taking supplemental vitamin A.

■ In addition to your multivitamin, take a good antioxidant formula providing 5,000 international units of vitamin A, 15,000 international units of beta-carotene, 3,000 milligrams of vitamin C, 1,500 milligrams of bioflavonoids, and 200 micrograms of selenium, and 15 to 50 milligrams of zinc once or twice daily.

Note: If you are pregnant or have liver disease, consult your doctor before taking supplemental vitamin A.

■ Butyric acid is particularly helpful for the health of the cells lining the colon. Butyric acid is commonly available as calcium and/or magnesium butyrate. Take 500 to 1,000 milligrams two to three times daily.

■ Take additional calcium, up to 500 to 750 milligrams daily, plus 400 to 600 international units of vitamin D. If you are deficient in magnesium, take 200 to 400 milligrams. Select magnesium glycinate, which does not stimulate bowel activity and which will not add to diarrhea.

■ Glutamine is an amino acid that is both nourishing and healing to the entire lining of the gastrointestinal tract. Take 1,000 to 2,000 milligrams of L-glutamine three times daily, after meals, for up to three weeks at a time.

■ The omega-3 essential fatty acids, found in fish oil, and the omega-6 essential fatty acids, found in black currant seed and evening primrose oil, have anti-inflammatory effects and help heal the intestinal lining. Take 500 to 1,000 milligrams of fish oil and an equal amount of black currant seed or evening primrose oil twice daily.

■ Pancreatin aids digestion. Take 350 milligrams three times daily, with meals.

Note: Long-term supplementation with pancreatin is not advised, as it can cause your pancreas to reduce its own production of this important enzyme. Overuse also has the potential to cause nausea or diarrhea. After two months on pancreatin, discontinue use and monitor your reaction. If you find that your problems recur, discuss pancreatin supplementation with your health-care provider.

■ Take a probiotic supplement containing acidophilus, colostrum, or bifidobacteria. The friendly bacteria not only fight candida overgrowth, a common complication of ulcerative colitis, but they are required to resolve any condition involving the gastrointestinal tract. Take a probiotic supplement twice daily, once before breakfast and in the evening, at least an hour away from food. If you are allergic to milk, be sure to select a dairy-free product.

■ Take a vitamin-B complex supplement that supplies 25 to 50 milligrams of each of the primary B vitamins as well as at least 800 micrograms of folic acid and 200 micrograms of vitamin B_{12} daily.

■ Take an additional 500 milligrams of vitamin C with bioflavonoids three times daily. Quercetin, a bioflavonoid, is helpful in healing the gastrointestinal tract, and helps reduce allergic reactions to food as well.

■ Your intake of zinc from all supplements should total at least 30 to 50 milligrams daily. If the above supplements do not supply this amount, take additional zinc to make up the difference.

Note: Take zinc with food to prevent stomach upset. If you take over 30 milligrams of zinc on a daily basis for more than one or two months, you should also take 1 to 2 milligrams of copper each day to maintain a proper mineral balance.

HERBAL TREATMENT

■ Chamomile and peppermint tea can help reduce intes-

tinal gas and cramping. Take a cup of either (or a combination) as needed.

■ The demulcent herbs, including licorice, marshmallow, and slippery elm, are soothing to a stressed gastrointestinal tract. Brew a tea from any or all of these herbs and sip up to three cups daily.

Note: Do not take licorice on a daily basis for more than five days in a row, as it can elevate blood pressure. If you have high blood pressure, omit the licorice entirely.

■ St. John's wort relaxes the nervous system and combats depression. Choose a product containing 0.3 percent hypericin and take 300 milligrams three times daily.

HOMEOPATHY

It is best to treat colitis by seeing a homeopathic physican for a constitutional remedy. However, the following remedies may provide symptomatic relief. Select the remedy that most closely fits your symptoms.

■ *Arsenicum album* is the remedy for an acute attack with burning pain in the abdomen, possibly accompanied by vomiting. You feel worse in the early morning hours and are restless and anxious. Take one dose of *Arsenicum album* 30x or 15c, as directed on the product label, four times daily for up to two days. Discontinue the remedy when your symptoms subside.

■ Choose *Mercurius corrosivus* if you have loose stools and diarrhea with a very strong odor. There is constant abdominal pain and rectal spasms that are unrelieved by passing stool. The stool has a strong odor and contains mucus. You tend to feel worse at night and worse with acidic foods, such as orange juice and tomatoes. Take one dose of *Mercurius corrosivus* 12x or 6c four times a day for up to two days. Discontinue the remedy when your symptoms subside.

■ *Phosphorus* will help if you have blood in the stool and pain that is relieved after the stool is passed. Take one dose of *Phosphorus* 30x or 15c four times daily for up to two days. Discontinue the remedy when your symptoms subside.

■ *Podophyllum* is good if you have long-standing diarrhea, commonly in the early morning; a distended abdomen; and a sensation of weakness in the stomach. You may grind your teeth at night. Take one dose of *Podophyllum* 12x or 6c three times a day, up to a total of ten doses. Discontinue the remedy when your symptoms subside.

BACH FLOWER REMEDIES

Select the remedy that most closely fits your emotional tendencies and concerns, and take it as needed, following the directions on the product label.

■ Holly is helpful for anger, insecurity, fits of bad temper, and, possibly, a tendency toward jealousy.

■ Hornbeam will help relieve the kind of fatigue that is so pervasive it prevents you from enjoying fun times.

■ Impatiens is the remedy for hyperactivity, nervous tension, and irritability.

ACUPRESSURE

For the locations of acupressure points on the body, *see* ADMINISTERING AN ACUPRESSURE TREATMENT in Part Three.

Bladder 23, 25, 27, and 28 relax the nerves that stimulate the intestine, and improve circulation to the area.

Large Intestine 4, 10, and 11 remove energy blocks in the large intestine, promoting a healthier lower abdomen. These points also relax the nervous system.

■ Liver 3 helps tone the digestive tract and relax the nervous system.

Pericardium 6 relaxes the chest and upper digestive tract.

Stomach 36 harmonizes and tones the digestive system, and helps improve digestion.

GENERAL RECOMMENDATIONS

■ Investigate the possibility that you may be allergic or hypersensitive to certain foods. Allergies can contribute to the development of colitis, and can also worsen symptoms.

As much as possible, avoid stress. Stress contributes to all forms of gastrointestinal distress, including ulcerative colitis. You may find it helpful to work with someone who specializes in stress-management techniques to learn better ways of dealing with stress that cannot be avoided.

■ Exercise. All forms of exercise help reduce stress. Yoga postures in particular can be helpful for digestive problems. You might want to consider taking a yoga class. *See* STARTING AN EXERCISE PROGRAM in Part Three.

See your doctor for regular evaluations, which should include examination with a fiber-optic scope to make sure no polyps or precancerous lesions are present in the colon. People with ulcerative colitis have an increased risk of developing colon cancer.

If intestinal parasites or amoebic dysentery is a complication, *see* PARASITES, INTESTINAL.

PREVENTION

■ A high-fiber whole-foods diet helps to prevent the development of gastrointestinal problems, including ulcerative colitis. Avoid refined sugar, processed foods, caffeine, and alcohol.

■ If you are prone to digestive problems, consider consulting a health practitioner who will do a digestive analysis and intestinal permeability test to investigate the function and ecology of your gastrointestinal tract.

Common Cold

The common cold is a viral infection of the upper respiratory tract, caused by one of the many contagious viruses that intrude into the nose, throat, sinuses, or ears. The virus travels either from hand to mouth and nose, or through the air on minute droplets carrying infected secretions from one sneezing, wheezing, coughing person to another. On arrival, the virus settles in and multiplies, causing a multiplicity of problems.

Average, healthy adults usually have no more than two colds a year. Children have many more because their immune systems are still in the process of developing. Children under six years of age have an average of seven colds a year, and older children tend to have an average of four or five colds a year.

You can catch a cold at any time of the year, but most colds occur during the winter months, from October through February. The well-known symptoms include a stuffy and/or runny nose, sneezing, headache, sore throat, coughing, loss of appetite, watery or burning eyes, ear congestion or infection, low-grade fever, and aching muscles and joints. When you have a cold, you may suffer one, some, or all of these annoying symptoms.

As the cold virus multiplies in the body, the mucous membranes in the respiratory tract swell. Mucus production increases. The swelling causes the air passages to narrow, making breathing difficult. The sinuses become congested. The nose runs. Sneezing, a sense of fullness or achiness in the head, and tearing or burning eyes are all part of the process.

The initial phase of a cold, with nasal congestion, low-grade fever, and sore throat, usually lasts for two to five days. At the most contagious phase of a cold, the nasal secretions are thin, watery mucus that is almost entirely composed of viral discharge. When the secretions turn thick and yellowish or greenish, that means the discharge is full of dead white blood cells, dead viral particles, and dead bacteria. This is a sign of healing and the least contagious stage of a cold.

From start to finish, a common cold, if uncomplicated, lasts about five to ten days. If you are sick for more than fourteen days in a row, chances are that you have contracted a series of viruses. While your immune system is busy fighting the first virus, another can settle in more easily. If you have significant fever, it is likely that you are suffering from a flu, not a cold. A person with the flu is also likely to feel worse all over than someone with a cold. (*See* FLU.)

Most colds can be treated successfully at home. However, if you develop a chronic stuffy nose with a thick, greenish nasal discharge, you should consult your physician. During the final stage of a cold this indicates healing, but if it doesn't go away, it may be a sign of a chronic infection, such as a sinus infection. Similarly, if you have a fever that persists, or returns after three days, you may have developed a bacterial infection, such as an ear or sinus infection. By themselves, colds do not ususally cause significant fever. If your cold does not clear up within a week, or if you develop a rash or a honking cough, you may have a different viral illness. The early symptoms of many viral diseases often resemble those of the common cold.

CONVENTIONAL TREATMENT

■ As we all know, there is no cure for the common cold. Antibiotics are ineffective against viruses, and therefore useless in treating colds. Unless you develop another infection, like an ear or sinus infection, in addition to your cold, you should not take antibiotics. In fact, antibiotics can actually inhibit the body in its fight against the common cold. Antibiotics destroy the bacteria normally present in the respiratory tract, giving the cold virus more room to multiply.

■ Treatment of colds is aimed at providing symptomatic relief. Over-the-counter painkillers such as acetaminophen (found in Tylenol, Datril, and many other products), aspirin (Bayer, Ecotrin, and others), or ibuprofen (Advil, Motrin, Nuprin, and others) helps to bring down fever and relieve the aches and pains of the common cold.

■ Decongestants, such as oxymetazoline (found in Dristan), phenylephrine (Neo-Synephrine), phenylpropanolamine (Congespirin, Triaminic), and pseudoephedrine (Sudafed), help decrease swelling and inflammation in the nasal cavity. As the term implies, they can provide relief from a stuffy and runny nose. Decongestants are available in pill and liquid form and as nose drops and sprays. However, if the spray forms are used for more than three days, they become irritating to nasal membranes, resulting in "rebound congestion" that can be worse than the initial symptoms. These drugs can also cause restlessness, insomnia, and an increased heart rate.

■ Because the sneezing and discomfort of a cold can resemble the symptoms of an allergic reaction, many people try using antihistamines, such as brompheniramine (Dimetane), chlorpheniramine (Chlor-Trimeton), pyrilamine (Triaminic), and diphenhydramine (Benadryl), for colds. These medications do dry up secretions in the respiratory tract. However, they have not been shown to be effective for the relief of cold symptoms. They are designed to counteract allergic responses, not viruses, and they are best reserved for their intended purpose. Antihistamines also commonly cause side effects, including drowsiness and dry mouth.

■ There are many over-the-counter medicines that promise relief of the common cold. Most of these are combinations of some of the drugs listed above. In general, they are not the most effective treatment. It usually works best to take medications individually, as called for by your symptoms. Before taking any medication, talk to your doctor about it, read the label, and consider the side effects. Always follow label directions carefully.

■ If at any time during the course of a cold you experience symptoms of respiratory distress, such as rapid breathing, gasping, wheezing, nasal flaring, or a pale or bluish skin color, or if you develop a high fever or unusual lethargy, consult your physician promptly. You may be coming down with a more serious infection, such as pneumonia.

DIETARY GUIDELINES

■ If you don't feel like eating, it's best not to force yourself. Try juice, applesauce, broth, soups (especially vegetable or chicken soup), and herbal teas.

■ If you have a cold, especially if it is accompanied by fever, you can become dehydrated and constipated more easily than usual. Flush your body with as much fluid as you can tolerate, at least eight 8-ounce glasses of water a day. If you become constipated, this condition will most likely correct itself once you begin to feel better and resume eating normally.

■ All fluids, including soups, help alleviate respiratory illnesses. Fluids help to thin secretions, making it easier for the body to clear them. If the secretions are thick and dry, they are more difficult to expel. Take diluted fruit juices, homemade sugarless lemonade (use a bit of honey for sweetening, and drink it either warm or cold), chamomile tea, and lots of nourishing broth and homemade soup. Chicken soup and soup made with astragalus and vegetables (see THERAPEUTIC RECIPES in Part Three) are particularly good.

■ Limit your intake of refined sugars. Sweets can make you feel first energized, then agitated and irritable. They also create acids in the body that can cause a cold to linger. If you crave sugar, take a little honey or a *small* bite of something sweet.

■ Avoid dairy foods, which have a tendency to increase and thicken mucus.

■ Avoid saturated fats, hydrogenated and partially hydrogenated oils, and all fatty or fried foods. These fats are difficult to digest under normal circumstances, and are even harder to digest when the digestive system is weakened by the low-grade infection of a cold. Undigested fats contribute to an increase in mucus and a toxic internal environment.

NUTRITIONAL SUPPLEMENTS

■ The amino acid lysine has antiviral properties. Take 500 milligrams of L-lysine three to four times daily for up to one week.

■ Pantothenic acid supports adrenal function, which is often compromised when you have a cold. It also helps to minimize nasal congestion and fatigue. Take 250 milligrams three times daily for up to one week.

■ We become more susceptible to infections such as the common cold as we age. As we age, the thymus—a key element of the immune system—gradually becomes less active. Taking thymus glandular extract can boost the immune system by increasing the number and activity of infection-fighting white blood cells. Take 250 to 500 milligrams twice a day.

■ Vitamin C and the bioflavonoids have anti-inflammatory properties and help to ease the course of a cold. Take 500 to 1,000 milligrams of each every hour for up to eight hours at the first sign of a cold. If you develop loose stools, reduce the amount to the largest dose you can tolerate. After the first eight hours, take 1,000 milligrams of vitamin C and an equal amount of bioflavonoids three times daily for three days.

■ To help boost your immune system and soothe your throat, take 5 to 10 milligrams of zinc in lozenge form every two to three hours, up to a total of 50 milligrams daily, for three days.

HERBAL TREATMENT

■ Yin Qiao is a Chinese botanical formula that is best taken at the very first sign of a cold and continued for the first forty-eight hours. This remedy usually is not helpful after the third day of symptoms. Take three tablets three times a day during the acute phase of the cold. After the symptoms start to ease, reduce the dosage to one tablet three times daily for one week.

■ Aloe vera has both anti-inflammatory and anti-infective properties. Take $^1/_4$ cup of aloe vera juice three times daily. If you develop diarrhea, reduce the dosage.

■ Boneset and sage help to break up congestion and bring down a fever. Take a cup of sage and boneset tea up to three times daily for three to five days.

■ To help yourself rest and relax, take a cup of chamomile tea twice daily, as needed.

■ If you are restless and irritable, take a soothing herbal bath with chamomile, calendula, rosemary, and/or lavender. Keep the water comfortably warm and treat yourself to a long, lazy soak.

■ Echinacea and goldenseal both stimulate the immune system. Echinacea is antibacterial and antiviral; goldenseal is an antibacterial noted for healing irritated mucous membranes. Take one dose of an echinacea and goldenseal combination formula supplying 250 to 500 milligrams of echinacea and 150 to 300 milligrams of goldenseal three times a day for five days to one week.

■ Elderberry may help to reduce both the severity and the duration of colds. Choose an extract standardized to contain 5 percent total flavonoids and take 500 milligrams three times daily.

■ Garlic has antibacterial properties and helps detoxify the body. Take 500 milligrams three or four times a day for one week. You can substitute one clove of fresh garlic for each capsule, but most people seem to prefer the odorless capsules.

■ Hot ginger tea increases perspiration. This helps to cleanse the body and reduce the intensity of a cold. Take a cup of ginger tea every four hours during the acute phase of a cold.

■ Grape-seed extract is an antioxidant and improves circulation. Choose a standardized extract containing 90 percent proanthocyanidins (PCOs) and take 500 milligrams twice a day.

HOMEOPATHY

At the very first sign of a cold, take $^1/_3$ tube of *Anas barbariae* (sold under various brand names, including Oscillococcinum), as directed on the product label, three times daily for one day. Then, during the acute phase of the cold, take one dose of one of the symptom-specific homeopathic remedies below three to four times daily for three days. If there is no improvement at all after three doses of a remedy, it is unlikely that it will do anything more. Switch to another that matches your symptoms and temperament. If you feel better before three days have passed, stop taking the remedy.

■ If you have a very runny nose and a great deal of irritating, watery nasal secretions that cause inflammation, as well as teary (but not burning) eyes and a lot of sneezing, take *Allium cepa* 12x or 6c. This is homeopathic red onion. It is recommended if your cold makes you feel even worse than you do when you are chopping a strong onion.

■ If you feel chilly, restless, and weak, take *Arsenicum album* 30x or 9c. This remedy is for the individual who, paradoxically, feels worse in a cold room but wants something cold to drink. You probably have a red nose and runny nasal secretions that burn the nose and upper lip. When you are ill, resting in bed with books, magazines, and a television is ideal. You generally want to be left alone, but like a bit of attention every once in a while.

■ If your eyes are the main focus of the cold, take *Euphrasia* 12x. This is for symptoms that are the opposite of those calling for Allium cepa. The nose runs a lot, especially in the morning, but without irritation. You complain of burning eyes and stinging tears, wink frequently, and wipe and rub your eyes. You also yawn a lot and prefer to be inside, away from sunlight and bright lights.

■ *Eupatorium* 12x or 6c is helpful for a severe aching deep in the bones and a feeling of being sore all over.

■ If you have heavy, droopy eyes; feel weak and tired, with aches and chills up and down your back; and want to be alone, take *Gelsemium* 30x or 9c.

If the cold is accompanied by a sore throat that resists treatment, take *Mercurius solubilis* 12x or 6c three times daily until the symptoms are resolved.

If you have a stuffy nose and thick yellow discharge, take *Pulsatilla* 30x or 9c. You feel worse at night, prefer to be outdoors, and want comfort and attention.

ACUPRESSURE

For the locations of acupressure points on the body, *see* ADMINISTERING AN ACUPRESSURE TREATMENT in Part Three.

Bladder 11, 12, 13, and 14 clear and balance a distressed respiratory system.

Large Intestine 4 relieves congestion and headaches.

Lung 7 clears upper respiratory tract infections.

Points along either side of the spine improve circulation, relax the nervous system, and balance the respiratory system.

GENERAL RECOMMENDATIONS

■ Begin treating the cold as soon as you notice the first symptom.

Most people instinctively want to sleep and rest when suffering through a cold, thus conserving energy to fight the virus. If your busy schedule will allow the necessary time off, a cozy bed in a room with an open window to bring in fresh air (weather permitting) usually helps. Make sure not to get chilled.

Use a cool mist humidifier. Humidified air may help to thin secretions, helping to break up a cold and easing the discomfort of a congested head. To avoid having a lot of particles in the air, use distilled, demineralized water. Be sure the humidifier is very clean, so that bacteria do not collect and spread through it into the air.

A nasal saline irrigation, followed by the suctioning out of mucus with a bulb syringe, can be very effective for loosening and removing thick mucus. (*See* NASAL SALINE FLUSH in Part Three).

■ *See also* COUGH; FEVER; SINUSITIS; or SORE THROAT if your cold is accompanied by any of these symptoms.

PREVENTION

■ Because there are so many different viruses that cause colds, it is unlikely that medical science will ever develop a vaccine that can protect against all of them. There are, however, measures that you can take to strengthen your resistance to illness. Although a cold can strike at any time, colds are most common during early fall, midwinter, and early spring, so these are the times it makes the most sense to work actively to boost immunity. Try one or several of the following suggestions:

• American ginseng helps to build the immune system and strengthens the body. Take 200 milligrams twice weekly during the winter months.

   Note: Do not take American ginseng if you have a fever or any other signs of acute infecton, or if you have high blood pressure, heart disease, or hypoglycemia. If you are sensitive to the effects of caffeine and other stimulants, you may want to consult with a qualified herbalist before using ginseng.

• Astragalus strengthens the immune system and upper respiratory tract, and improves energy. Take 500 milligrams of astragalus daily for two weeks out of every month during the cold and flu season. Do not take it if you have a fever or other sign of acute infection, however.

• Take 10,000 international units of beta-carotene and 25 milligrams of zinc daily during the cold and flu season.

• Echinacea and goldenseal stimulate the immune system and help keep the body clear of infections. Take one dose of an echinacea and goldenseal combination formula supplying 500 milligrams of echinacea and 200 milligrams of goldenseal twice weekly during the cold and flu season.

• Siberian ginseng helps to strengthen immune function. Choose a standardized extract containing 0.5 percent eleutheroside E and take 100 milligrams in the morning and again in the afternoon.

• Vitamin C and bioflavonoids make an effective preventive combination. If you don't always eat as many fruits and vegetables as you should, supplement your diet with 500 milligrams of each twice daily during the cold season.

• Take one dose of homeopathic *Anas barbariae* once a week during the cold and flu season.

■ Make it a rule to eat a low-sweets diet with no fried foods. During the cold season, prepare soups of chicken and vegetables, and add the herb astragalus to the soup to help boost your immune system.

■ If you are experiencing emotional distress, you will fall ill more easily. Emotional upset may be caused by stress at work, home, school, or anywhere else. Try to be aware of and work through your problems. Seek support during emotional crises. (*See* STRESS.)

■ Physical stress can create a bodily imbalance that makes you more vulnerable to illness. Exposure to dust and chemicals, too much sugar and fat in the diet, even the kind of sudden and extreme temperature change that occurs when you leave a sunny beach and enter an air-conditioned room, all can potentially make you more susceptible to illness.

■ Practice good hygiene, especially careful and frequent hand-washing. This is particularly important if one member of the household already has a cold. Many viruses are spread via the hands.

Concussion (Head Injury)

Any injury to the head, no matter what the cause, may result in concussion. At some point, we all experience a hard knock on the head from one cause or another. The severity of the symptoms will depend on the extent of injury to the brain.

After a simple concussion, you may seem disoriented or lose consciousness briefly. You may have no memory of events just prior to and immediately following the injury. Headaches, dizziness, and drowsiness are all common immediately after awakening. Such symptoms usually disappear within a few weeks, but can last as long as several months, or even longer, in some cases.

If you suffer a head injury, monitor yourself closely afterward. If any of the following symptoms occurs, even as much as four weeks after a seemingly mild bang on the head, seek medical attention immediately:

- Diminished consciousness.
- Unusually widened pupils.
- Severe headache.
- Drowsiness.
- Personality changes.
- Confusion; loss of memory; speech difficulties.
- Loss of coordination; paralysis.

These symptoms can be signs of bleeding in the brain.

CONVENTIONAL TREATMENT

■ Anytime you suffer a blow to the head, seek medical help immediately. The doctor will examine you and possibly order an x-ray of the skull to check for fracture, or a magnetic resonance imaging (MRI) scan to look for bleeding or swelling in the brain. Be prepared to answer questions about your memories of the accident and its immediate aftermath. The doctor will evaluate your condition and provide appropriate treatment.

■ Your doctor will probably recommend that someone keep a close watch on you for a minimum of twenty-four hours after returning home. Or you may be admitted to the hospital for observation.

■ You will probably be told not to take any medication during that twenty-four-hour observation period. Any change in your mental status is significant, and you don't want to muddy the waters by using medication that might affect your mental functioning.

HOMEOPATHY

■ If you are fully conscious and able to swallow, take one dose of *Aconite* 200x immediately after an accident to alleviate some of the initial shock. Wait ten minutes. Then take one dose of *Arnica* 30x, 200x, 15c, or 30c. *Arnica* helps to decrease bruising and aching. Continue taking one dose of *Arnica* three times a day for two days following an accident.

■ On the third day after an injury, take one dose of *Natrum muriaticum* 30x or 9c as needed to help resolve dizziness, forehead pain, throbbing pain in the temples, or a headache at the base of the skull. Take this remedy three times daily until the pain is alleviated. If there is no improvement after forty-eight hours, discontinue the remedy.

PREVENTION

■ Wear protective headgear whenever you engage in such activities as bicycle or motorcycle riding, roller-blading, skateboarding, boxing, or playing football or hockey.

■ When in a car, always wear your seat belt, whether you are a driver or a passenger. In airplanes, keep your seat belt fastened at all times, except when you must leave your seat.

Conjunctivitis

Conjunctivitis, also known by the descriptive name pink-eye, is an inflammation of the conjunctiva, which is the transparent membrane that covers the eyeball and lines the eyelid. Conjunctivitis can be caused by a viral or bacterial infection, an injury to the eye, or a reaction to fumes, smoke, or pollution. Though the causes may be different, the symptoms are identical. Allergic conjunctivitis is most often caused by pollen, and is therefore usually a seasonal reaction (unless it is the result of exposure to a pet, dust, mold, or some other nonseasonal allergen).

The overwhelming majority of cases of conjunctivitis are caused by viruses, although in rare cases a bacterial infection may be responsible. Viruses and bacteria may be rubbed into the eye, or may travel from an infection in the nose up through a tear duct and into the eye. The infection can be transmitted from one person to another.

Suspect conjunctivitis if the white of your eye shows bright pink or red coloration. In the early stages, your eyes may burn or itch, and may feel as if there is something in them. The eyelid may be swollen, and there can be a sticky yellowish discharge from the eye. The eye may be "glued" shut when you wake up in the morning.

Most cases of simple conjunctivitis last from five to seven days. If you are treating conjunctivitis at home and notice no improvement in that time, or if the infection is painful, draining heavily, interfering with vision, or seems to be affecting the tissues around your eyes, see a doctor for a professional evaluation.

CONVENTIONAL TREATMENT

■ Warm-water compresses are the treatment of choice. Many of the microorganisms that cause conjunctivitis are exquisitely heat sensitive. The heat also loosens up debris and increases blood flow through the area, which helps the body's natural defense mechanisms. You can use either a clean cloth or a cotton ball as a compress. Your doctor is likely to recommend that compresses be applied for ten minutes, four to six times daily. Clean your eyes with warm water after applying the compresses, and wash your hands both before and after the treatment. If you use a cotton ball, throw it away after removing the compress; if you use cloth, wash the compress in detergent and hot water (with chlorine bleach added if possible), separately from all other laundry, before using it again. Always be very cautious when using warm liquids around your eyes. The skin of the eyelid is thin and tender and can burn easily.

■ If you can see no improvement in the condition in four to five days, or if the infection seems to be growing worse, consult a doctor to determine if it might be bacterial in origin. You may need to consult an eye specialist. If conjunctivitis is caused by bacteria, a prescription for antibiotic eye ointment or eye drops may be appropriate (antibiotics are useless against viral or allergic conjunctivitis). Many people are irritated by the stinging sensation caused by some medications, so if your doctor determines that an antibiotic is in order, ask for a formula that is nonirritating, like Polysporin (which contains polymyxin), Tobrex (tobramycin), Ciloxan (ciprofloxacin), or Ilotycin (erythromycin).

■ If you have a diagnosed case of allergic conjunctivitis, your doctor may prescribe steroid drops to help decrease inflammation and relieve itching.

Caution: If there is even a suspicion of a herpes infection, steroid drops should not be used. This can be very dangerous, as the combination of steroids and a herpes infection can result in ulceration through the surface of the eye.

■ Your doctor may recommend a topical antihistamine and decongestant, such as phenylephrine, in a form specifically designed for use in the eyes, to help reduce itching, swelling, and redness in cases of allergic conjunctivitis. Cool compresses may also be comforting in this situation.

■ If at any time the infection seems to be getting worse; if there is a thick, green discharge from your eye; if your eye looks cloudy; if your eye continues swelling or shutting; or if you are becoming increasingly sensitive to light, call your doctor. These are all signs of a worsening infection, or a possible herpes infection. A herpes infection in the eye is a serious, potentially sight-threatening infection that should be treated by an ophthalmologist.

DIETARY GUIDELINES

■ Eliminate all refined sugars from your diet. Sugar makes the body more acidic, which inhibits healing. In addition, bacterial infections thrive in the presence of sugar.

■ Eat plenty of green and yellow vegetables and fruits, which are high in fiber and rich in vitamins A and C. Both of these vitamins support the immune system. In addition, vitamin A protects and heals mucous membranes, and vitamin C fosters healing and is mildly anti-inflammatory.

NUTRITIONAL SUPPLEMENTS

■ Take 25,000 international units of beta-carotene twice a day for five to seven days.

■ Take 500 to 1,000 milligrams of vitamin C with bioflavonoids three times a day for five to seven days.

■ Take 25 milligrams of zinc three times a day for seven days. Take zinc with food to prevent stomach upset.

HERBAL TREATMENT

■ Bilberry is high in bioflavonoids that act to reduce inflammation and irritation. It is especially good for the eyes. Choose a product containing 25 percent anthocyanidins (also called PCOs) and take 80 milligrams twice daily. To ensure ocular health, continue taking bilberry for an additional one to two months after the condition has been resolved.

■ Echinacea and goldenseal stimulate the immune system, so they are important in clearing any infection. Echinacea fights viral infections; goldenseal fights bacteria and soothes mucous membranes. Take 500 milligrams of echinacea and 250 milligrams of goldenseal every two hours, for a total of five doses, during the first day. After that, take one dose three times daily until your condition improves, for up to one week.

■ A warm eyebright compress will help to increase the blood flow to the eye and wash discharge away. Eyebright, a most appropriately named herb, helps relieve redness and swelling of the eye, and can help clear an eye infection. Bring 3 ounces of sterile saline solution to a boil, and pour it over 1 tablespoon of dried cut herb (or one eyebright teabag). Allow it to steep for fifteen minutes, then strain out the herb. When the liquid has cooled to a comfortable temperature, moisten a thin white cotton cloth with the warm eyebright tea and place it over your eyes. The compress should remain in place for fifteen minutes. Then moisten a fresh sterile cloth in the tea and gently wipe away any crusts or scales. Throw away (or sterilize) each cloth after one use. Never reuse the cloth after contact with the eye. To do so is to invite reinfection. Wash your hands before and after the treatment, and either throw away the compress after using it or wash it separately in detergent and hot water with chlorine bleach added before using it again. Always be very cautious when using warm liquids around your eyes. The skin of the eyelid is thin and tender and can burn easily.

■ If you are unable to find eyebright, you can use goldenseal root or simply a compress made with warm spring water, as described under Conventional Treatment, in this entry.

HOMEOPATHY

■ *Euphrasia* is a homeopathic preparation made from eyebright. When your eyes are burning, itching, and tearing, take one dose of *Euphrasia* 12x or 6c, as directed on the product label, three times daily for seven days.

■ If you have a thick yellowish discharge from your eyes and they are matted tightly closed in the morning, take one dose of *Pulsatilla* 12x, 30x, 6c, or 9c three times daily for five days. This is good if you experience such intense burning and itching that you have a constant urge to rub your eyes.

ACUPRESSURE

For the locations of acupressure points on the body, *see* ADMINISTERING AN ACUPRESSURE TREATMENT in Part Three.

■ In Chinese medicine, the liver rules the eyes. Pressure on Liver 3 will help to take the "heat" out of the eyes.

■ Gallbladder 20 improves circulation to the head.

■ Gallbladder 21 takes excessive energy away and down from the infection.

■ Spleen 10 removes "heat" from the blood.

GENERAL RECOMMENDATIONS

■ So that you do not continually reinfect your eyes, do not touch them. If you cannot stop yourself, make sure you keep your hands very clean.

■ If your symptoms do not respond within four to five days, see your doctor.

■ If the conjunctivitis is related to exposure to chemicals, such as sprays, fumes, smoke, or pollution, gently wash your eyes with warm water. If the condition worsens, call your physician.

■ If you are diagnosed as having bacterial conjunctivitis, do not go swimming until the infection clears.

PREVENTION

■ Do not share items such as washcloths, towels, and pillows, even with family members.

■ Be diligent about careful hand-washing, and avoid scratching or rubbing your eyes.

■ Avoid exposure to known eye irritants, such as cigarette smoke, dust, fumes, sprays, pollution, household cleaning products, and excessively chlorinated swimming pools.

■ Include in your daily diet lots of green and yellow vegetables and fruits, which are high in vitamins A and C.

Consciousness, Loss of

See ANAPHYLACTIC SHOCK; FAINTING; SEIZURE; STROKE.

Constipation

The term *constipation* refers to a change in daily bowel habits, particularly a decrease in the number or consistency of bowel movements, or pain or difficulty passing stools. If you are usually regular but go two or more days without a bowel movement, and then have pain or difficulty passing a large, hard stool, you are constipated. If you have a good appetite and are not uncomfortable, there is no need to worry. However, if you lose your appetite, are vomiting, or have discomfort, you should consult a physician without delay.

Constipation is commonly caused by insufficient fluids and too little fiber in the diet. Without enough fluids and bulk, stool becomes hard and develops rough edges. These rough edges can cause a rectal fissure, a painful microscopic tear in the rectum. Too much fat in the diet may contribute to constipation, as can a lack of proper exercise.

People sometimes become constipated as a result of holding back stool. A person who is busy may be reluctant to interrupt whatever he or she is doing to have a bowel movement. When that happens, the retained stool becomes dehydrated and hard and is painful to pass.

The most important factor in determining whether you are constipated is your level of comfort when passing a stool. Even if you have a bowel movement every day, a hard-to-pass stool may indicate constipation. Other indications include abdominal discomfort and a stomach that is unusually firm and tender to the touch.

Most cases of constipation respond to simple at-home treatments. However, if you experience severe pain when passing a stool; if there is blood in the stools; if you notice a cut or tear near your rectum; or if you develop chronic or persistent constipation, you should be examined by a doctor. In some cases, constipation may be a sign of an internal problem, such as an intestinal obstruction. Certain serious health problems, including diverticulitis and hypothyroidism, can also cause chronic constipation. Even if unrelated to an underlying problem, chronic constipation should be taken seriously because it can lead to a loss of muscle tone in the bowel, setting the stage for a lifelong problem.

CONVENTIONAL TREATMENT

■ Increasing the amount of fiber and fluid in your diet is the best place to start when treating constipation (*see under* Dietary Guidelines in this entry).

■ A stool softener, such as docusate sodium (Colace and others), may be prescribed to soften the stool and help it pass through the intestines more easily.

■ If you feel you must take a laxative on occasion, we recommend that you use a bulk-forming type such as Maltsupex or psyllium powder. These work by increasing the amount of bulk in the intestines, softening the stool to make it easier to pass, and initiating peristalsis (the wavelike contractions of the intestines that push waste along). Either of these products should be taken with plenty of water.

■ Magnesium hydroxide (found in milk of magnesia), citrate of magnesia (Evac-Q-Kwik), and phosphosoda (Phospho-soda, Sal-Hepatica) are bulk-forming laxatives that work by drawing fluids from the body into the intestine, increasing the contents of the intestines, and thereby initiating a bowel movement. Use these products with care, as they can sometimes be more effective than anticipated.

■ Stimulant laxatives, such as bisacodyl (found in Dulcolax), castor oil, phenolphthalein (Modane), and senna leaf extract, work by irritating the intestinal wall, thus stimulating peristalsis. Stimulant laxatives are harsh and can cause cramping. If you use these medications at all, do so sparingly. Bulk-forming laxatives are preferable to stimulant types. No laxative should be used on a regular basis, as dependency can develop.

■ Lubricants, such as glycerin and mineral oil, coat the stool and help it slip more easily through the rectum, but they cannot be recommended. Prolonged use of mineral oil can cause inflammation of the liver, spleen, and abdominal lymph nodes, and can interfere with the body's absorption of vitamins A and D. Also, a lubricant can be dangerous if it accidentally goes down the windpipe and enters the lungs.

DIETARY GUIDELINES

■ Every day, upon arising, stir 2 tablespoons of lemon juice into 8 ounces of hot water and drink it. This old folk remedy promotes the production of bile.

■ Because dehydration can lead to constipation, increase the amount of fluids in your diet. Have spring water, herbal teas, juices, and soups readily available, and take them often.

■ Increase the amount of fiber in your diet. Fruits, vegetables, and whole grains are rich sources of fiber. Simply eating a piece of fruit, such as an apple or orange, may help to resolve constipation. The whole fruit provides the most fiber. Take a piece of fruit one-half to one hour before a meal or about one hour after a meal.

■ Prunes are a time-honored remedy for constipation. Stewed prunes or prunes that have been soaked overnight in water may be easier to digest than the dry variety.

■ Taking warm liquids or hot cereal such as oatmeal every morning acts gently to stimulate the intestinal tract, in addition to providing fiber.

■ Foods high in magnesium, such as dark-green leafy vegetables, are very helpful.

■ For overnight relief of constipation, mix $1/2$ cup of prune juice and 1 tablespoon of lemon juice with 1 cup of spring water. Drink this before bedtime.

■ The digestive process begins in your mouth. Enzymes in saliva start breaking down food before you swallow. Remember that your stomach has no teeth. Chew your food completely, and don't overeat.

■ Be aware that stimulants like coffee and alcoholic drinks dehydrate the system and add to the risk of constipation. If you consume these beverages, do so in moderation only.

NUTRITIONAL SUPPLEMENTS

■ Acidophilus and bifidobacteria help to establish favorable intestinal flora, which is very helpful in relieving constipation. If you have chronic or recurrent constipation, probiotic bacteria are strongly indicated. Take a probiotic supplement as recommended on the product label. If you are allergic to milk, select a dairy-free product.

■ If the stool has an exceptionally foul odor, take chlorophyll supplements. This natural deodorizer is high in trace minerals, especially magnesium, and has natural antibacterial properties. Follow the dosage directions on the product label.

■ Organic flaxseed oil or olive oil will help ease the discomfort of passing hard stool. Take 1 tablespoon of either two to three times daily until the problem is resolved.

■ Fructooligosaccharides (FOS) nourish the beneficial intestinal bacteria, and can be very effective in correcting constipation. Take 1 or two capsules, or 1 scant teaspoon of powder, three times daily.

■ The B vitamins are important for digestion and also contribute to the health of the colon. Take a good vitamin-B complex supplying at least 50 milligrams of each of the major B vitamins twice daily. Also take 500 micrograms of vitamin B_{12} twice daily for three days, then once daily for one week, then once a week for ten weeks.

HERBAL TREATMENT

■ Liquid food-grade aloe vera juice is quite helpful in resolving constipation. Make sure you purchase the edible form of aloe vera juice. Take $1/4$ cup two to three times daily until the stool is soft and easy to pass.

■ For overnight relief, consider an herbal formula that includes *Cascara sagrada*. Follow the directions on the product label.

■ Licorice is soothing to irritated intestinal walls and helps relieve chronic constipation. Take a cup of licorice tea or 500 milligrams in capsule form once or twice daily for three or four days.

Note: Do not take licorice on a daily basis for more than five days in a row, as it can elevate blood pressure. Do not take it at all if you have high blood pressure.

■ If you experience constipation alternating with diarrhea, oatmeal cooked in flaxseed tea can be very helpful. It soothes irritated intestines and relieves constipation. Prepare flaxseed tea by adding 1 teaspoon of flaxseeds to 1 quart of spring water; simmer for fifteen minutes. Use the resulting liquid instead of water to cook oatmeal. Or add one cup of the tea to 8 ounces of juice and take one dose daily. Constipation should be relieved within forty-eight hours.

■ Psyllium, available in capsules or powder, is an excellent stool softener with mild laxative properties. Take it as directed on the product label.

■ Slippery elm is invaluable for irritated intestines. It soothes and helps resolve inflammation. Take a cup of slippery elm tea, 500 milligrams in capsule form, or 1 to 2 teaspoons of powder dissolved in a cup of hot water three times a day, as needed.

HOMEOPATHY

If you are chronically constipated, visit a homeopathic physician for a constitutional remedy prescribed specifically for you. For an occasional constipation problem, select a remedy that matches your symptoms from the list that follows.

■ Use *Alumina* if you have stools that are small hard, dry pellets, often covered with mucus, and elimination is very difficult. Take one dose of *Alumina* 30x or 9c, as directed on the product label, two or three times daily for two or three days.

■ *Calcarea carbonica* is often used for constipation in persons with digestive disorders. If you have a hard, distended stomach, but feel fine otherwise, take one dose of *Calcarea carbonica* 30x or 9c twice daily for two or three days.

■ If you have hard, dry stools and experience pain right before a bowel movement, take one dose of *Lycopodium* 30x or 9c two or three times daily for two or three days. This remedy is also recommended if you have lower intestinal gas that smells like rotten eggs.

■ *Natrum muriaticum* is the remedy for the person who loves salt—who sucks salt off pretzels and crackers—and is on the thin side, especially around the neck. If you fit this description and are usually thirsty yet have hard, dry stools, you should benefit from one dose of *Natrum muriaticum* 30x or 9c twice daily for two or three days.

■ *Nux vomica* is helpful if you have a tendency to overeat and become constipated or gassy. You probably also are impatient and agitated; crave rich, greasy, and/or spicy foods; and pass small, dark, hard stools after trying many times to have a bowel movement. Take one dose of *Nux vomica* 30x or 9c twice daily for two or three days.

■ For stubborn constipation, take one dose of *Plumbum metallicum* three times a day for two or three days.

■ Choose *Sulfur* if you often experience anal itching and irritation, typically have an unsuccessful urge to have a bowel movement, and pass stool that is very odorous. Take one dose of *Sulfur* 30x or 9c twice daily for two or three days.

ACUPRESSURE

For the locations of acupressure points on the body, *see* ADMINISTERING AN ACUPRESSURE TREATMENT in Part Three.

■ Massaging Bladder 20 to 25 along the lower back relaxes the nerves that stimulate the intestine.

■ Large Intestine 11 helps relax the large intestine.

■ Stomach 36 tones the digestive tract.

AROMATHERAPY

For specific instructions on how to use aromatherapy, *see* PREPARING AROMATHERAPY TREATMENTS in Part Three.

■ Essential oils of basil, lavender, myrrh, and rose strengthen the digestive system and help to counteract constipation. You can use any or all of them in an aromatherapy bath or add a few drops to massage oil and use it in conjunction with massage (*see under* General Recommendations, below).

GENERAL RECOMMENDATIONS

■ An Epsom salts bath is relaxing and increases circulation. Epsom salts contain magnesium sulfate. An hour or two after an Epsom salts bath, a bowel movement will often occur.

■ Massaging the lower abdomen is comforting and helps to get things moving. Gently massage the abdomen, following the natural movement of the intestines. Start in the lower right "corner," move up toward the ribs, over to the left side, and then down toward the pelvis.

■ Avoid using aluminum cookware. It is possible that taking in minute traces of aluminum can exacerbate constipation.

PREVENTION

■ Drink plenty of spring water and other fluids, and eat a high-fiber diet that includes plenty of fruits, vegetables, and whole grains.

■ Be physically active. You don't need an elaborate exercise regimen. Walking is an effective mode of exercise and most people can do it with little difficulty.

■ Take acidophilus and bifidus on an alternating basis for one month to maintain friendly flora in the intestines and bowels. Also take supplemental fructooligosaccharides (FOS), which supply a special form of carbohydrate that can be digested by friendly bacteria but not by yeast. Start by taking $1/4$ teaspoon of FOS twice a day and work up to 1 teaspoon twice a day over a period of one to two weeks.

■ Respond promptly to your bodily needs, even if you must excuse yourself from an important activity to do so. Holding back causes a difficult and painful bowel movement, and increases the risk that constipation will become a way of life.

Contact Dermatitis

See under DERMATITIS.

Contact-Lens Problems

Contact lenses, those tiny disks that float on a layer of tears in front of the iris to correct vision, have attained a great deal of popularity. Many people wear them regularly with no problems at all, and remain completely satisfied. However, wearing contacts does increase the risk of certain eye problems, most commonly irritation and infection. Less than adequate hygiene is the primary cause of both irritation and infection. Wearing contact lenses can also lead to corneal problems in some cases (*see* CORNEAL PROBLEMS).

Not everyone is a good candidate for contact lenses. If you suffer from hay fever and allergies, or are subject to bouts of conjunctivitis, or if you have arthritis or hand tremors that make inserting and removing the lenses difficult, wearing contact lenses may cause problems for you.

CONVENTIONAL TREATMENT

■ You have only one set of eyes. They are worth at least a phone call to your vision specialist any time you notice a possible problem.

■ If you have an eye infection of any type, do not wear contact lenses until cleared to do so by your doctor. A contact of any type is a foreign body in the eye and lessens the amount of oxygen that reaches the surface of the eye.

DIETARY GUIDELINES

■ Maximize your intake of fresh fruits and vegetables. These healthy foods contain antioxidant phytochemicals that protect all the cells of the body, including those of the eyes, from free-radical damage.

■ Eat clean, lean protein, such as that found in chicken and fish. Both protein and vitamin A are needed to maintain healthy eyes.

■ Limit your intake of sugar and caffeine. These substances contribute to eye irritation and worsen the symptoms caused by many eye problems.

NUTRITIONAL SUPPLEMENTS

■ Beta-carotene is a strong antioxidant that prevents free-radical damage. It is related to vitamin A and has many of the same properties, but it does not become toxic in large doses. Take 10,000 to 25,000 international units of beta-carotene daily.

■ The essential fatty acids (EFAs), found in black currant seed oil, borage oil, evening primrose oil, and flaxseed oil, are required by every cell in the body. They have been shown to reduce pain, inflammation, and swelling. EFAs also help counteract the hardening effects of cholesterol on cell membranes. Take 500 to 1,000 milligrams of black currant seed, borage, evening primrose, or flaxseed oil twice daily.

■ Selenium is an excellent antioxidant that helps prevent free-radical damage throughout the body, including the eyes. While symptoms are acute, take 100 micrograms twice daily. When symptoms improve, reduce the dosage to 100 micrograms once daily.

■ Vitamin A protects against free-radical damage and is especially important to the eyes. Take 10,000 international units of vitamin A three times a day for two months. Then cut back to a maintenance dosage of 5,000 international units twice daily.

Note: If you are pregnant, or intend to get pregnant, or if you have liver disease, consult your doctor before taking supplemental vitamin A. Pregnant women should not ingest a total of more than 25,000 international units of supplemental vitamin A *per week* from all sources.

■ The B vitamins are required for intracellular metabolism in the tissues of the eyes. Inadequate intake of the B-complex vitamins can result in itching, burning, bloodshot eyes that water excessively. Combined with vitamins C and E, the B-complex vitamins are especially beneficial to the eyes. While symptoms are acute, take a B-complex supplement that supplies 50 milligrams of each of the primary B vitamins twice daily. When symptoms improve, reduce the dosage to 25 milligrams twice daily.

■ Vitamin C helps to lower ocular pressure and prevent and clear up infections. It also helps strengthen capillaries, maintain collagen, and prevent tissue hemorrhaging, and is notable for speeding healing. Select a vitamin-C formula that includes bioflavonoids, especially rutin; these nutrients work best together. While symptoms are acute, take 1,000 to 2,000 milligrams of a vitamin-C complex three to four times daily. When symptoms improve, reduce the dosage to 500 to 1,000 milligrams three to four times daily.

■ Vitamin E is an antioxidant and is essential in cellular respiration. Choose a product containing mixed tocopherols and start by taking 200 international units daily, then gradually increase the dosage until you are taking 400 international units twice daily. Maintain that dosage while symptoms are acute. When symptoms improve, reduce the dosage to 200 international units twice daily.

Note: If you have high blood pressure, limit your intake of supplemental vitamin E to a total of 400 international units daily. If you are taking an anticoagulant (blood thinner), consult your physician before taking supplemental vitamin E.

■ Zinc supports the immune system and aids the healing process. While symptoms are acute, take 25 to 50 milligrams of zinc daily. When symptoms improve, reduce the dosage to 15 to 20 milligrams daily.

Note: Take zinc with food to prevent stomach upset. If you take over 30 milligrams of zinc on a daily basis for more than one or two months, you should also take 1 to 2 milligrams of copper each day to maintain a proper mineral balance.

HERBAL TREATMENT

■ Bilberry provides important nutrients that nourish the eyes and enhance visual function. Phytochemicals called anthocyanidins in this herb also help prevent damage to the structures of the eyes. Select a preparation containing 25 percent anthocyanidins (also called PCOs) and take 20 to 40 milligrams three times daily.

■ Eyebright is rich in vitamin A and vitamin C. It also contains moderate amounts of the B-complex vitamins, vitamin D, and traces of vitamin E. Eyebright has been used for centuries both as an eyewash and in tea form as a tonic for the eyes. Taken internally, it helps maintain healthy eyes and good vision. Take 250 to 500 milligrams three times daily. Used as an eyewash, it helps relieve the discomfort arising from eyestrain, inflammation, and minor irritation. To make an eyebright eyewash, bring 3 ounces of sterile saline solution to a boil, and pour it over 1 tablespoon of dried cut herb (or one eyebright teabag). Allow it to steep for fifteen minutes, then strain out the herb. When the liquid has cooled to a comfortable temperature, use it as an eyewash. Bathe your eyes with the eyewash and/or prepare a compress by moistening a sterile cloth in the warm infusion. Place the compress over the closed eye, pressing down gently to achieve contact with the affected area. Relax for at least ten minutes. Then moisten a fresh sterile cloth in the eyewash tea and gently wipe away any crusts or scales. Throw away (or sterilize) each cloth after one use. Never reuse the cloth after contact with the eye. To do so is to invite reinfection.

■ Ginkgo biloba extract contains flavonoids with an affinity for organs that are rich in connective tissue, including the eyes. Ginkgo protects cellular membranes and has notable antioxidant properties. It also enhances the use of oxygen and glucose by the cells, and works to normalize circulation. Select ginkgo leaf extract containing 24 percent ginkgo heterosides (sometimes also called flavoglycosides) and take 40 milligrams three times daily.

HOMEOPATHY

■ *Conium* is for inflamed eyes that are intensely sensitive to light. Take one dose of *Conium* 12x or 6c three times daily, as needed, for up to three days.

■ *Hepar sulfuris calcareum* is for eyes that are sensitive both to the touch and to air passing over them. The eyelids may be red and inflamed. Take one dose of *Hepar sulfuris calcareum* 12x or 6c three times daily, as needed, for up to three days.

■ *Pulsatilla* is for overly sensitive eyes that are red, itching, and burning, with inflamed eyelids. Take one dose of *Pulsatilla* 12x or 6c three times daily, as needed, for up to three days.

GENERAL RECOMMENDATIONS

■ Keep a backup pair of prescription eyeglasses on hand. Wearing contact lenses for too long leads to irritation. If your eyes feel scratchy and irritated, switch to glasses.

■ Replace your lenses as often as required. Soft lenses should be replaced at least ever two years, hard lenses every five to six years. Replace disposable lenses according to the manufacturer's recommendations.

■ Clean and soak your lenses according to the directions given by the manufacturer.

■ Be sure to wash your hands well before taking out your lenses and before inserting them. A quick rinse won't do it. Soap your hands and work the lather for at least ten full seconds before rinsing off the soap. It is very easy to transfer skin oils, dirt, dust, and bacteria from imperfectly cleaned hands to clean lenses.

■ Avoid hot, dry, and smoky environments. These factors contribute to and worsen the irritation often suffered by contact lens wearers.

Convulsion

See under SEIZURE.

Corneal Problems

The cornea is a thin, transparent membrane that covers the center front portion of the eye, where the iris and pupil are. It is curved into a domelike shape (although the dome tends to flatten with age), and is dense and even in thickness.

There are a number of different disorders that can affect the cornea, but the most common are abrasion, infection, and ulceration. An abrasion can occur as a result of falling asleep wearing hard contact lenses, a scratch from a fingernail, or a foreign object getting into the eye. Abrasions typically produce inflammation, increased tearing, and the sensation that something is in the eye, even if the damage was caused by a scratch. Because the cornea is richly endowed with nerve endings, the pain is often disproportionate to the size of the injury.

If an abrasion is not properly tended, infection can result. An untreated corneal infection can lead to an ulcer, or eroding sore. Corneal ulcers may also be caused by bacterial, viral, or fungal infection, or by trauma, and can result in impaired vision. In severe cases, a permanent loss of vision may result. Xerophthalmia is a condition associated with vitamin-A deficiency that can lead to corneal infection and ulceration (*see* DRY EYES).

CONVENTIONAL TREATMENT

■ In the case of corneal abrasion, see an ophthalmologist. He or she will remove any foreign object, irrigate the affected eye with saline solution, and prescribe antibiotic eye drops, which are typically used four times a day for seven to ten days.

■ You may be fitted with an eye patch to rest the eye and prevent further irritation. You can remove the eye patch after the corneal epithelium (the surface layer of cells) heals, usually within twenty-four to forty-eight hours.

■ If you have eye pain and redness, an intolerance to light, watering or a thicker discharge from the eye, and impaired vision, seek medical attention at once. You may have a corneal infection, which is considered an ophthalmic emergency. Improper or inadequate treatment can lead to scarring of the cornea, which directly affects vision, or even ulceration through the surface. A culture of scrapings from the cornea may be necessary to discover the specific cause of the infection. Treatment involves antibiotics to kill the invading organism. Often, topical agents are inadequate, so oral antibiotics may be required. Your doctor may also prescribe topical steroids to reduce inflammation. The use of steroids in the eye should be closely monitored by an ophthalmologist. These drugs can cause dependence, and they are potentially quite dangerous if used in the presence of herpes viruses.

■ Corneal ulceration can admit infectious organisms to deeper structures within the eye and allow permanent scarring. In addition to aggressive antibiotic therapy to combat infection, it may be necessary to graft corneal tissue over the injured area.

DIETARY GUIDELINES

■ Eat plenty of fresh fruits and vegetables. These healthy foods provide valuable vitamins and minerals and contain antioxidant phytochemicals that protect all the cells of the body, including those of the eyes, from free-radical damage.

■ Eat clean, lean protein foods such as chicken and fish. Both protein and vitamin A are needed for healthy eyes.

■ Limit your consumption of sugar and caffeine. These substances contribute to eye irritation and worsen the symptoms caused by many eye problems.

NUTRITIONAL SUPPLEMENTS

■ Beta-carotene is a strong antioxidant that prevents free-radical damage. It is related to vitamin A and has many of the same properties, but it does not become toxic in large doses. Take 10,000 to 25,000 international units of beta-carotene daily.

■ The essential fatty acids (EFAs), found in black currant seed oil, borage oil, evening primrose oil, and flaxseed oil, are required by every cell in the body. They have been shown to reduce pain, inflammation, and swelling. Take 500 to 1,000 milligrams of any of these oils twice daily.

■ Selenium is an excellent antioxidant that helps prevent free-radical damage throughout the body, including the eyes. While symptoms are acute, take 100 micrograms twice daily.

■ Vitamin A protects against free-radical damage and is especially important to the eyes. Without sufficient vitamin A, the eyes are more susceptible to infection, ulcerations, and even blindness. Take 10,000 international units of vitamin A three times a day for two months. Then reduce to a maintenance dosage of 5,000 international units twice daily.

Note: If you are pregnant, or intend to get pregnant, or if you have liver disease, consult your doctor before taking supplemental vitamin A. Pregnant women should not ingest a total of more than 25,000 international units of supplemental vitamin A *per week* from all sources.

■ The B vitamins are required for intracellular metabolism in the tissues of the eyes. Combined with vitamins C and E, the B-complex vitamins are especially beneficial to the eyes. While symptoms are acute, take a B-complex supplement that supplies 50 milligrams of each of the primary B vitamins twice daily. When symptoms improve, reduce the dosage to 25 milligrams twice daily.

■ Vitamin C helps to prevent and clear up infections. It also helps to strengthen capillaries, maintain collagen, and prevent tissue hemorrhaging, and is notable for speeding healing. Select a vitamin-C formula that includes bioflavonoids, especially rutin; these nutrients work best together. While symptoms are acute, take 1,000 to 3,000 milligrams of a vitamin-C complex three times daily. When symptoms improve, reduce the dosage to 500 to 1,000 milligrams three times daily.

■ Vitamin E is an antioxidant and is essential in cellular respiration. Choose a product containing mixed tocopherols and start by taking 200 international units daily, then gradually increase the dosage until you are taking 400 international units twice daily. Maintain that dosage as long as symptoms are acute. When symptoms improve, reduce the dosage to 200 international units twice daily.

Note: If you have high blood pressure, limit your intake of supplemental vitamin E to a total of 400 international units daily. If you are taking an anticoagulant (blood thinner), consult your physician before taking supplemental vitamin E.

■ Zinc supports the immune system and aids in the healing process. While symptoms are acute, take 25 to 50 milligrams of zinc daily. When symptoms improve, reduce the dosage to 15 to 20 milligrams daily.

Note: Take zinc with food to prevent stomach upset. If you take over 30 milligrams of zinc on a daily basis for more than one or two months, you should also take 1 to 2 milligrams of copper each day to maintain a proper mineral balance.

HERBAL TREATMENT

■ Bilberry provides important nutrients that nourish the eyes and enhance visual function. Phytochemicals called anthocyanidins in this herb also help prevent damage to the structures of the eyes. Select a preparation containing 25 percent anthocyanidins (also called PCOs) and take 40 to 80 milligrams three times daily.

■ Echinacea and goldenseal support the immune system and speed healing. Take one dose of an echinacea and goldenseal combination supplying 250 to 500 milligrams of echinacea and 150 to 350 milligrams of goldenseal three to four times daily for three to four days.

■ Eyebright is rich in vitamin A and vitamin C. It also contains moderate amounts of the B-complex vitamins, vitamin D, and traces of vitamin E. Eyebright has been used for centuries both as an eyewash and in tea form as a tonic for the eyes. Take a cup of eyebright tea two to three times daily.

■ Ginkgo biloba extract contains flavonoids with an affinity for organs that are rich in connective tissue, including the eyes. Ginkgo protects cellular membranes and has notable antioxidant properties. It also enhances the use of oxygen and glucose by the cells, and improves circulation. Select a preparation of ginkgo leaf extract containing at least 24 percent ginkgo heterosides (also called flavoglycosides) and take 40 milligrams three times daily.

■ Pine-bark and grape-seed extracts have powerful anti-inflammatory action. Take 25 to 50 milligrams of either three times daily.

HOMEOPATHY

■ *Hepar sulfuris calcareum* is for eyes that are sensitive both to the touch and to air passing over them. The eyelids may be red and inflamed. Take one dose of *Hepar sulfuris calcareum* 12x or 6c three times daily, as needed.

■ *Ipecac* is for an infected eye accompanied by a feeling of nausea when you look at moving objects. Take one dose of *Ipecac* 12x or 6c three times daily, as needed, for up to three days.

Caution: Do not confuse homeopathic *Ipecac* with conventional syrup of ipecac. That is an entirely different product, and it should never be used except at the direction of a doctor or Poison Control Center.

■ *Kali hydriodicum* will prove helpful if you have a red, infected eye that tears profusely. Take one dose of *Kali hydriodicum* 6x or 3c three times daily, as needed, for up to three days.

■ *Pulsatilla* will help if you have a thick yellow or greenish discharge coming from the affected eye. Take one dose of *Pulsatilla* 12x or 6c three times daily, as needed, for up to three days.

GENERAL RECOMMENDATIONS

■ Never neglect an eye abrasion or infection, especially if you suspect you may be developing a sore on the cornea. See an ophthalmologist promptly.

Corns and Calluses

Calluses are thickenings of the stratum corneum, the outermost layer of the skin, in response to constant friction. They are common on the hands and feet. Corns are similar to calluses but are more localized, usually appearing on the sides of toes that are compressed under constant restrictive pressure. The mass of a corn forms an inverted cone of thickened tissue extending deep enough into the skin to cause considerable pain. Unlike plantar warts, which are virally induced masses that have visible blood capillary systems at their base, the deeper tissue of corns and calluses is glassy, like a very heavy wax.

CONVENTIONAL TREATMENT

■ The most important consideration in getting rid of corns and calluses is eliminating the source of friction. Otherwise, they will almost certainly recur. Tight and high-heeled shoes are discouraged. You may even need orthopedically designed shoes or shoe inserts to reduce the friction.

■ Corns and calluses can be soaked in water or a 3 percent acetic acid solution to soften the tissue, then either shaved down with an instrument designed for that purpose or sanded down using a pumice stone.

■ Very thick and bothersome calluses, such as those often found on the heels, may be soaked in a 20-percent urea lotion (Ureacin-20) overnight, then sanded down with a pumice stone.

DIETARY GUIDELINES

■ To reduce inflammation, increase your intake of fresh organic vegetables and fruits.

■ Avoid refined sugar, greasy fried foods, and food additives and preservatives, all of which make the system more acidic.

NUTRITIONAL SUPPLEMENTS

■ Applying vitamin E topically helps to soften corns. Simply pierce a capsule and squeeze the liquid oil onto the affected area. Do this three or four times daily.

HERBAL TREATMENT

■ Applications of calendula and/or chamomile soothe irritated skin and promote healing. Mix 40 drops of liquid calendula or chamomile extract (or a combination of both) with $1/2$ teaspoon of olive oil and apply the mixture to the area several times a day.

HOMEOPATHY

■ *Antimonium crudum* is helpful for painful, inflamed corns. Take one dose of *Antimonium crudum* 12x or 6c three or four times daily for up to one week.

PREVENTION

■ Wear well-made shoes that fit well and that conform to the normal contour of your feet. If you wear high heels and/or shoes with pointy toes, save them for special occasions only—and occasions when you will not be spending many hours on your feet.

Cough

Coughing is a natural protective mechanism designed to clear bacteria, viruses, dust, and pollen out of the body. Coughing clears the lungs and throat of irritants and fluids. A productive cough forces sputum from the breathing tract, thereby clearing the air passages and allowing oxygen to reach the lungs.

A cough is a common symptom of diseases of the ear, nose, and throat. Coughing may be related to a bacterial or viral infection of the respiratory tract, such as bronchitis, laryngitis, pneumonia, or croup. A cough can also be caused by inhaling irritating substances, such as dust, chemical fumes, or cigarette smoke. Food sensitivities and environmental allergies can cause a cough, as can inhaling very cold or very hot air. If you have a persistent cough, emotional stress is another important factor to consider. Some people develop a chronic cough as a result of acid reflux, which occurs when digestive acids are regurgitated from the stomach into the esophagus. (*See* INDIGESTION.) Certain medications can cause a chronic cough as well.

Depending on the cause, a cough may be loud and gasping, harsh and high-pitched, or barking. It may be dry and rasping, or moist with mucus. If asthma is involved, you may wheeze with every inhalation or exhalation.

Although coughing is a necessary and helpful physical response, it can be distressing and very tiring. Continuous, uncontrollable coughing makes sleeping difficult, and it can cause you to feel as if you ache all over. The chest and abdominal muscles can be pulled or strained by continual coughing. Coughing may also cause further irritation to an inflamed respiratory tract.

A sudden coughing fit may signal the presence of a foreign body in the airway. If other signs indicate a blocking of the airway—if you become unable to speak or begin gasping for breath—turn to CHOKING on page 000.

In some cases, a cough may indicate the onset of a more serious or chronic illness. If a cough comes on rapidly and is accompanied by wheezing, a feeling of tightness in the chest, and difficulty breathing, you may be suffering from asthma, and should consult a doctor at once or have someone take you to the emergency room of the nearest hospital. A persistent, lingering cough can be caused by bronchitis; a harsh cough that comes on after a cold and is accompanied by fever, fatigue, and difficulty breathing can be a sign of developing pneumonia. Blood in the sputum can be a symptom of an infection such as bronchitis or tuberculosis, or a more serious problem, such as a tumor.

In general, any cough that persists for a week or longer should be evaluated by a physician. Persistent coughing can have many causes, including allergies, chronic bronchitis, cancer, gastroesophageal reflux, heart disease, or tuberculosis. Your doctor's examination and testing should uncover the cause and point the way to appropriate treatment. Even an ordinary cough should never be ignored. An untreated cough can lead to pneumonia, and the constant irritation coughing causes may result in damage to the respiratory tract.

CONVENTIONAL TREATMENT

■ If you have a stubborn cough and are taking blood pressure medication, see your doctor. Certain blood-pressure medications, such as enalapril (Vasotec) and captopril (Capoten) can cause chronic coughing. A change in prescription may be warranted. *Do not* stop taking any prescription medication on your own, however. Always consult with your doctor first.

■ There are several different types of conventional cough medicines available, some by prescription and others over the counter:

• Codeine is a narcotic cough suppressant that may be prescribed for a cough in severe cases. It works by "turning off" the part of the brain that controls the coughing response. Codeine is a powerful drug and can have side effects, including nausea, sleepiness, and constipation. It can also be highly addictive.

• Dextromethorphan is a common cough suppressant found in many popular over-the-counter medications, usually signified by the initials DM on the label. It is almost as effective as codeine, but is nonnarcotic and reportedly has few side effects. Follow label directions carefully when using this drug.

• Benzonatate (Tessalon) is a prescription cough suppressant that works by anesthetizing the respiratory tract. Unlike other cough medicines, it comes in capsule rather than liquid form, and is a safer alternative to codeine. The capsules should be swallowed whole, never chewed, as they can adversely affect the ability to swallow.

■ Expectorants are medications that work by increasing the production of fluids in the respiratory tract, helping to thin and loosen mucus so that it is easier to cough out. Guaifenesin is an expectorant found in many over-the-counter cough formulas. It can cause drowsiness, so follow label directions carefully.

■ Throat lozenges, such as Chloraseptic lozenges, coat and soothe a sore, irritated throat, and may give temporary relief. Be aware that some lozenges contain an ingredient called phenol, which is a numbing agent that inhibits healing at the same time. Many over-the-counter lozenges also contain food colorings and sugar. Read the ingredients list and label directions carefully before purchasing throat lozenges.

DIETARY GUIDELINES

■ When you have a cough, or any other respiratory condition, eliminate potentially mucus-forming foods, especially dairy products and fried foods.

■ Drink plenty of fluids, preferably at room temperature or warmer. Fluids help to thin mucus and make it easier to cough up. Hot soups and broths are particularly good.

NUTRITIONAL SUPPLEMENTS

■ Persons with low-functioning adrenal glands are more susceptible than most to developing a chronic cough. To boost adrenal function, take 250 milligrams of pantothenic acid three times daily for up to ten days.

■ Take sugar-free lozenges boosted with vitamin C. Vitamin C has anti-inflammatory properties, combats infection, and is soothing and healing to an irritated throat. Take one lozenge an hour, as needed.

■ Take zinc-based lozenges to improve immune response

and help reduce infection and inflammation. Choose sugar-free zinc-based lozenges. Take one lozenge, one to three times daily, as needed. If zinc upsets your stomach, select a capsule or table form and take it with food.

HERBAL TREATMENT

For specific instructions on how to make herbal remedies, *see* PREPARING HERBAL TREATMENTS in Part Three.

Licorice has antibacterial properties, soothes the throat and respiratory tract, and tastes sweet. For a cough, licorice works best when taken in warm tea form. Take one cup three times daily for up to five days.

Note: Do not take licorice on a daily basis for more than five days in a row, as it can elevate blood pressure. Do not take it at all if you have high blood pressure.

Marshmallow root and slippery elm are soothing to the throat and respiratory tract. These are the herbs to use with a dry cough. Make a combination tea and take one cup three times daily for up to five days. Or take 500 milligrams of each in capsule form three times daily for up to five days.

Menthol lozenges contain a purified and refined form of peppermint oil, which is recognized by the U.S. Food and Drug Administration as an effective cough suppressant. Menthol lozenges made without sugar are preferable. Take one lozenge each hour or two, as needed, up to a total of four lozenges a day for up to five days.

When you first begin to cough, take mullein tea. This is a very effective herb known to be highly beneficial to the throat and lungs. It is particularly good in the early stages of a cough, before an expectorant is needed. Take one cup two to three times daily for two to three days. You can add honey and lemon to the tea for flavor.

Osha root is highly aromatic and helps to clear the lungs. It is especially good for a dry cough. Take one cup of osha-root tea three times a day for three to four days.

A tea made from sage and thyme helps to clear mucus out of the lungs. Take one cup three times daily for two days.

For a cough complicated by constipation, take $\frac{1}{4}$ cup of aloe vera juice three times daily until the situation is resolved.

If the cough is accompanied by diarrhea, lungwort is the herbal medicine of choice. Lungwort is high in vitamin C, has astringent properties, and is known for its ability to help clear a cough. Take 500 milligrams or a cup of lungwort tea two to three times daily for two to three days.

HOMEOPATHY

Choose an appropriate symptom-specific homeopathic remedy from the list below. Please note that if you are also using an aromatic herbal treatment (such as menthol lozenges, osha-root tea, or an herbal rub with eucalyptus and/or peppermint), you should allow one hour between it and the homeopathic remedy. Otherwise, the strong smell of the herbal treatment may interfere with the action of the homeopathic remedy.

■ Use *Antimonium tartaricum* if you are pale and tired, have a tight, burning sensation in your chest, and feel breathless. You probably have a rattling cough due to a respiratory tract filled with thick mucus that is difficult to cough up. To loosen the congestion, take one dose of *Antimonium tartaricum* 30x or 9c, as directed on the product label, three times daily for twenty-four to thirty-six hours.

Note: Do not use *Antimonium tartaricum* if you have a fever. If you have a fever, select a different remedy.

■ If you have a cough accompanied by a high fever and are sweating copiously, take one dose of *Belladonna* 30x or 9c three times daily for one day.

■ If you have a dry, painful cough and feel better resting and worse with activity, take one dose of *Bryonia* 30x or 9c three times daily for two days.

■ For a dry, spasmodic cough that is worse at night and when you are lying down, choose *Drosera* 12x or 6c. Take one dose three times daily for two days.

■ If you have a loose, rattling cough with a yellow-green nasal discharge, take one dose of *Pulsatilla* 30x or 9c three times a day for two days.

■ *Spongia tosta* is for the person with a dry, barking cough, who feels better sipping a hot drink. One dose of *Spongia tosta* 12x or 6c, taken three times daily for two days, will help.

■ If none of the remedies above seems suitable, a homeopathic combination cough remedy, available in homeopathic pharmacies, health-food stores, and some drugstores, may be helpful.

AROMATHERAPY

For specific instructions on how to use aromatherapy, *see* PREPARING AROMATHERAPY TREATMENTS in Part Three.

■ Try an aromatherapy rub. Take 4 tablespoons of olive oil and add 2 drops of one or all of the following: eucalyptus, sage, rosemary, and peppermint oil. To ease coughing and soothe the respiratory tract, rub this mixture over your chest.

■ Prepare an aromatherapy bath by putting a few drops of eucalyptus, sage, or thyme oil into a tubful of warm water. Besides being very pleasant, breathing in the aromatic vapors will soothe an irritated throat.

GENERAL RECOMMENDATIONS

■ Avoid exposure to cold winds and changes in temperature, which can aggravate a cough.

■ To help moisten your respiratory tract and thin mucus, use a cool mist humidifier. Be sure to keep this equipment scrupulously clean so that bacteria do not collect in it.

■ *See also* FEVER and/or SORE THROAT if the cough is accompanied by either of these symptoms.

PREVENTION

■ Avoid respiratory irritants and allergens, including environmental pollutants and foods to which you are sensitive. Wood-burning fireplaces and stoves can also be a source of lung irritation.

■ Do not smoke and avoid secondhand smoke. Tobacco smoke greatly irritates the bronchial passages and entire respiratory tract. Exposure to cigarette smoke contributes not only to coughing but to other diseases.

Cravings, Food

See under FOOD ALLERGIES; OBESITY.

Cryptosporidiosis

See under PARASITES, INTESTINAL.

Crohn's Disease

Crohn's disease is a chronic disorder characterized by severe inflammation leading to ulceration of the interior of the intestines. It most often affects the lower part of the small intestine, but it can involve the entire digestive tract, from the mouth to the anus. Unlike ulcerative colitis, which affects the top two layers of tissue lining the intestines, the ulceration in Crohn's disease involves all four layers of the intestinal wall. When affected areas heal, scar tissue often narrows the passageway. In some cases, the bowel becomes partially or completely obstructed. When an area closes, one or more fistulas—abnormal passageways—may develop that join one part of the intestine to another, or even to another organ.

Symptoms produced by Crohn's disease include cramps, abdominal and stomach pain, nausea, diarrhea, weakness, rectal bleeding, a lack of energy, and an overall feeling of tiredness. Recurrent bleeding can lead to iron-deficiency anemia. Fever, chills, and loss of appetite, with accompanying weight loss, are common. An inability to absorb fatty acids may result in steatorrhea (pale, bulky stools that float).

The onset of the disease typically occurs between the mid-teens and age thirty. Attacks may occur every few months or every few years. In about 25 percent of cases, symptoms appear once or twice, and never return. If the disease becomes chronic, however, bowel function deteriorates markedly. Ulcerated intestinal walls may leak, and peritonitis (inflammation of the membrane that lines the entire abdominal cavity) becomes a possibility. The absorption of nutrients is compromised and malnutrition can result. Deficiencies of vitamins C and E are common. Left untreated, Crohn's disease can become life-threatening in some cases.

Once rare, Crohn's disease is becoming more and more common. There are about twice as many cases today as there were thirty years ago, and as many as 500,000 cases are diagnosed annually. This disorder is four times more common in Caucasians and Jews than in people of other races and ethnic backgrounds. Although it is not contagious and no genetic markers have been identified, it does tend to run in families. Statistics show that 20 to 40 percent of people with this disorder have relatives who also have either Crohn's disease or ulcerative colitis.

Although the cause of the disease has not been established, free-radical damage is believed to play a part. In addition, it has been noted that food allergies are more common in those with the disease than in the general population. People with Crohn's disease who adopt allergen-free diets often experience remission, but the disease returns if they go back to their usual diets.

Crohn's disease is diagnosed by means of an x-ray of the digestive tract, usually aided by a barium enema and barium "milkshake." The x-ray is used to track the movement of the barium through the gastrointestinal tract, allowing the doctor to determine what parts of the tract are affected. An endoscopic examination may also be necessary. An endoscope is a tubular device with a light on the end that allows the doctor to examine the inside of the gastrointestinal tract directly to view the nature and extent of the problem.

CONVENTIONAL TREATMENT

■ If you are diagnosed with Crohn's disease, it is wise to seek out and work closely with a gastroenterologist, internist, or other physician who specializes, or at the very least has considerable experience, in the treatment of this condition.

■ There is no medical treatment that can cure Crohn's disease. Treatment is aimed at easing the symptoms and slowing the progression of the disease. Diarrhea may be treated with medications like loperamide (found in Imodium AD and other over-the-counter products) or diphenoxylate and atropine (Lomotil), a prescription medication. Both of these work by slowing peristalsis, the rhythmic movement of the intestines that moves food and wastes along. In some cases, an agent such as cholestyramine (LoCholest, Questran), which binds with bile salts so that they are excreted, may be effective.

■ For cramping, an anticholinergic drug may be prescribed. These drugs work by interfering with the transmission of nerve impulses that cause muscle spasms in the gastrointestinal tract. Examples of this type of medication include dicyclomine (Bentyl) and hyoscyamine, which may be prescribed either on its own (under the brand names Cystospaz, Levbid, Levsin, and Levsinex) or in a combination formula that includes a mild tranquilizer (Arco-Lase, Donnatal).

■ To attempt to control the inflammation of Crohn's disease, a doctor may prescribe a nonsteroidal anti-inflammatory drug (NSAID). The drug most often used is sulfasalazine (Azulfidine), though mesalamine (Asacol, Pentasa, Rowasa), a derivative of sulfasalazine, is also used. Potential side effects of mesalamine include headache, abdominal pain, nausea, sore throat, dizziness, weakness, fatigue, and belching. The side effects of sulfasalazine are similar, plus loss of appetite, vomiting, and, for men, a low sperm count. For an acute attack, a steroid such as prednisone (Deltasone) may be necessary to control inflammation quickly. If such a drug is used, its use should be tapered off as quickly as possible to avoid adverse effects on the adrenal gland and immune system.

■ Really serious disease may be treated with mercaptopurine (Purinethol). This drug depresses the body's immune response, but it takes three to six months before any benefits may be noticeable. Also, this is a drug normally used for cancer chemotherapy, so it is potentially quite toxic.

■ Since none of these drugs used for Crohn's disease can cure the disorder or prevent recurrences, over half of the people with this problem end up having surgery to remove badly affected portions of the intestine. If large portions of the intestine are removed, problems with nutrient absorption may result, necessitating a special low-fat diet and supplementation with medium-chain triglycerides (MCTs) to help maintain a healthy weight.

■ If the disease results in severe malnutrition, intravenous feeding may be necessary. This is the administration of nutrients through a vein instead of by mouth. This is not a real solution—obviously, only known nutrients can be administered this way, and "new" nutrients are being discovered all the time—but if you are unable to get enough nutrition from foods, it may be necessary.

DIETARY GUIDELINES

■ Eat slowly, and chew your food thoroughly.

■ Avoid trans-fatty acids, found in hydrogenated and partially hydrogenated fats and oils.

■ In general, a diet that is low in fiber is best. Usually, fiber is helpful in normalizing bowel function, but too much fiber can worsen Crohn's disease, especially if there is enough intestinal scarring to cause obstruction.

■ Eat plenty of clean, lean protein foods such as chicken and fish. Try to eat four servings of fish a week or, if you dislike fish, take a fish-oil supplement (*See under* Nutritional Supplements, below). Tofu and other soy foods are good protein sources also, though some people with Crohn's disease have trouble digesting them. People with inflammatory bowel diseases need as much as 30 percent more protein than normal.

■ Include in your diet alkaline vegetables such as carrots, celery, kale, zucchini, and other summer squashes.

■ Cook your food simply. Steam or bake vegetables, and steam, poach, or bake chicken and fish. Do not fry foods or eat too many of them raw.

■ Maximize your intake of liquids, including water, herbal teas, and fresh juices. Because of its ability to soothe and help heal, cabbage juice should be your first choice. In addition, make sure to drink eight glasses of pure water daily. A high intake of liquids helps to ensure soft, easy-to-pass stools, and also counteracts dehydration caused by diarrhea.

■ Avoid refined foods, including dry processed cereals and anything made with refined sugar and flour. An excess of refined carbohydrates is associated with the development of Crohn's disease.

■ Avoid substances that are irritating to the digestive tract, including alcohol, anything containing caffeine, carbonated beverages, fried and greasy foods, and spicy foods.

■ Avoid all dairy products, pickled foods, and all products made with yeast, and see if your symptoms improve. These foods are high in histamines, and many people with Crohn's disease are histamine-intolerant. Many may also be allergic to milk. In addition, certain dairy products (some ice creams and commercial yogurts) are stabilized with carrageenan, a substance extracted from seaweed. In large quantities, this normally benign substance has been shown to cause ulcerative colitis in laboratory animals.

■ Since food allergies and sensitivities can have an effect on this disease, avoiding potentially allergenic foods is a good idea. Cravings may be a sign that you have a problem with a particular food. *See* ELIMINATION DIET in Part Three for ways to track down food allergies and sensitivities.

NUTRITIONAL SUPPLEMENTS

■ The drugs commonly prescribed for Crohn's disease interfere with normal metabolism and increase the likelihood of multiple nutritional deficiencies. People with Crohn's disease are often lacking in calcium, magnesium, potassium, vitamin B$_6$ (pyridoxine), folic acid, vitamins C and D, and zinc. Take a good multivitamin and mineral formula that supplies at least the minimum daily requirement of these important nutrients.

■ Antioxidant nutrients scavenge free radicals and have been shown to lower the risk of developing Crohn's disease. Take a good antioxidant formula that supplies 5,000 international units of vitamin A, 25,000 international units of beta-carotene, 250 milligrams of vitamin C, 1,500 milligrams of bioflavonoids, 400 international units of vitamin E, 200 micrograms of selenium, 500 to 1,000 milligrams of N-acetylcysteine (NAC), and 100 milligrams of lipoic acid daily.

Note: If you are pregnant, or intend to get pregnant, or if you have liver disease, consult your doctor before taking supplemental vitamin A. If you are taking an anticoagulant (blood thinner), consult your physician before taking vitamin E.

■ Bromelain, an enzyme derived from pineapple, helps reduce inflammation and aids in the digestion of protein. Take 500 milligrams three times daily, twice between meals and once with the largest meal of the day.

■ In a year-long double-blind Italian study, over 50 percent of people with Crohn's disease who took fish-oil supplements stayed symptom-free, while only 25 percent of those given a placebo remained in remission. Start by taking 1,000 milligrams three times daily. After two weeks, increase the dosage to 2,000 milligrams three times daily, and continue at that dosage for six weeks. Choose an enteric-coated supplement that supplies approximately 800 milligrams of the omega-3 fatty acids per 2,000 milligrams. Enteric coating serves to delay the dissolution of the capsule until it passes through the stomach and into the intestines, thereby protecting the sensitive omega-3 oils from degradation.

Note: If you develop nausea as a result of difficulty digesting fish oil, stop taking the supplement for three days, then resume at half the dosage.

■ The amino acid glutamine helps to soothe an inflamed gastrointestinal tract. Take 3,000 milligrams of L-glutamine three times daily for two weeks, then decrease to 3,000 milligrams twice daily for two weeks. Then take 3,000 milligrams daily for two months.

■ Take a probiotic supplement containing acidophilus, bifidobacteria, or colostrum. The friendly bacteria are necessary for a healthy intestinal tract. Studies show probiotics can help the body overcome Crohn's disease. Take a probiotic supplement as recommended on the product label. If you are allergic to milk, select a dairy-free product.

■ Pine-bark and grape-seed extracts are excellent natural anti-inflammatory agents. Take 25 to 50 milligrams of either twice a day.

HERBAL TREATMENT

■ Aloe vera soothes and heals while it helps ensure soft stools. Select food-grade aloe vera juice and take $\frac{1}{4}$ cup twice daily.

■ Cat's claw has known anti-inflammatory effects, as well as antifungal, antiviral, and antibacterial properties. Take 500 milligrams of standardized extract three times a day.

Note: Do not use cat's claw if you are pregnant or nursing, or if you are an organ-transplant recipient. Use it with caution if you are taking an anticoagulant (blood thinner).

■ Licorice has been shown to have therapeutic effects against long-term ulcers, indicating that it may prove valuable against the ulcerative effects of Crohn's disease. The effective dosage was 760 milligrams taken three times daily. This herb also has anti-inflammatory and antiallergic properties. Select deglycyrrhizinated (DGL) chewable tablets.

Note: Ordinary licorice can elevate blood pressure, and should not be taken on a daily basis for more than five days in a row. DGL should not have this effect, however.

■ Reishi mushroom is an excellent natural anti-inflammatory that is useful for a variety of autoimmune disorders. It often helps to reduce and initiate the healing of ulcers in people with Crohn's disease. Take 500 milligrams three times daily.

HOMEOPATHY

When dealing with Crohn's disease, it is best to consult a homeopathic practitioner for a constitutional remedy. If that is not possible, select among the symptom-specific remedies listed below.

■ *Argentum nitricum* is good if you are anxious, suffer from flatulence and diarrhea, and like sweet foods, even though they are not well tolerated. Take one dose of *Argentum nitricum* 30x or 9c, as directed on the product label, twice a day for four or five days.

■ *China* is the remedy for painless diarrhea accompanied by a swollen abdomen and, probably, flatulence, often occuring after you have eaten too much milk, fruit, or foods containing gluten. Take one dose of *China* 30x or 9c three to four times daily for one or two days.

■ Choose *Ignatia* if your bowels are hypersensitive during periods of emotional distress. Take one dose of *Ignatia* 30x or 9c twice a day for four or five days.

■ *Podophyllum peltatum* is for abdominal pain that is better with heat and better when lying down, and for explosive diarrhea that is watery and yellow, preceded by pain. Take one dose of *Podophyllum peltatum* 30x or 9c three to four times daily for one or two days.

■ *Raphanus niger* 9c or 30x is helpful if you have a distended abdomen but are unable to pass intestinal gas. You may have constipation with bloating, with pain predominantly on the left side. Take one dose of *Raphanus niger* 30x or 9c twice a day for four to five days.

BACH FLOWER REMEDIES

Select the remedy that most closely fits your emotional tendencies and concerns, and take it as needed, following the directions on the product label.

Hornbeam is the best Bach remedy for people who suffer from Crohn's disease. This remedy helps ease the extreme fatigue that often prevents you from enjoying pleasurable activities.

Mimulus is good for fearfulness and dread of specific things.

Mustard helps to relieve feelings of sorrow and depression.

ACUPRESSURE

For the locations of acupressure points on the body, *see* ADMINISTERING AN ACUPRESSURE TREATMENT in Part Three.

■ Large Intestine 4 removes energy blocks in the large intestine, thus promoting a healthier lower abdomen.

Liver 3 helps tone the digestive tract, calm the nerves, and ease muscle cramps and spasms.

Pericardium 6 relaxes the chest and upper digestive tract.

Stomach 36 improves digestion and the absorption of nutrients, helps tone the digestive tract, and strengthens overall well-being.

GENERAL RECOMMENDATIONS

Make sure you have a bowel movement every day.

If you suffer from diarrhea, make certain to take supplements supplying both the major minerals and trace minerals (*see* DIET AND NUTRITION in Part One). Fatigue is often caused by chronic sodium-potassium imbalance. You may find that supplementing your diet with potassium lifts your mood as well as your energy level.

■ Try to avoid stress. Stress worsens an attack. Consider learning biofeedback or yoga or meditation. These disciplines can help immeasurably. When you are in the midst of an acute attack, rest and relax as much as possible.

Avoid all medications possible.

Cuts and Scrapes

Cuts and scrapes are an inevitable part of life. An accident in the kitchen, a mishap in the workshop or garden, or an unexpected fall can result in an open wound. Because any break in the skin, no matter how small, can become infected, even minor injuries should be treated fairly aggressively.

A cut on the head, face, hand, mouth, or foot can bleed profusely, because there are many blood vessels close to the surface of the skin in these areas. To avoid scarring, treat a cut on the face especially carefully. Cuts on the face, fingers, and hands are particularly vulnerable to infection because these parts of the body are not covered with clothing.

You can treat minor cuts and scrapes at home with basic first aid. However, occasions may arise when medical care is essential. If you have any doubt about your ability to care for an injury properly, consult your doctor.

EMERGENCY TREATMENT

■ To stop bleeding, apply firm pressure to the wound with a piece of sterile gauze or a clean cloth. Putting ice on the cut will also stop bleeding, because cold constricts blood vessels and slows blood flow. If you cut your mouth or tongue, use ice or a fruit-juice popsicle.

■ Cleanse and disinfect the site. For a minor cut or scrape, you can do this at home. Wash the wound with generous amounts of water. Thoroughly clean out any particles of dirt or foreign matter that may have gotten into the cut by holding the wound under running water. Hydrogen peroxide can be used as a disinfectant. Once the injury has been cleansed and the bleeding stopped, cover it with an adhesive bandage. A wound that is covered is less likely to become infected.

■ If the bleeding does not stop within ten to fifteen minutes; if the edges of the skin are separated and the wound is open; if the wound is deep or extensive, and/or was caused by a dirty or rusty object; if there is foreign material embedded in the wound; or if the injury affects particularly sensitive parts of the body, such as the lips, see your doctor or go to the emergency room of the nearest hospital. You may require professional treatment including, possibly, stitches, which can help prevent infection, hasten healing, and make any scar that results smaller and less noticeable. Some doctors now use a gluing technique in place of stitches. Your doctor may also administer a tetanus shot, especially if it has been more than five years since you last had one.

CONVENTIONAL TREATMENT

■ Once the injury has been cleansed and the bleeding

stopped, keep the area clean and covered with a bandage until it has healed, usually for a week to ten days, depending on the severity of the cut. To prevent infection, you may wish to apply an over-the-counter antibiotic ointment such as Neosporin, Betadine, or bacitracin before bandaging. Replace the bandage with a clean one daily. You should also replace it if it becomes wet or dirty.

DIETARY GUIDELINES

Eliminate refined sugars from your diet. Sugar makes the body more acidic, which slows healing. When the body is working to repair itself, avoiding sugar helps create a more balanced, alkaline internal environment.

NUTRITIONAL SUPPLEMENTS

If you have a tendency to develop infections, take the following supplements for five days to one week following an injury that breaks the skin. These supplements help to heal skin tissue and support the immune system.

- 15,000 international units of beta-carotene and 5,000 international units of vitamin A twice a day. (If you are pregnant, or intend to get pregnant, or if you have liver disease, consult your doctor before taking supplemental vitamin A.)
- 500 to 2,000 milligrams of mineral ascorbate vitamin C or esterified vitamin C (Ester-C) with an equal amount of bioflavonoids three times daily.
- 200 to 400 international units of vitamin E (mixed tocopherols) three times daily. (If you have high blood pressure, limit your intake of supplemental vitamin E to a total of 400 international units daily, and if you are taking an anticoagulant (blood thinner), consult your physician before taking vitamin E.)
- 25 to 50 milligrams of zinc twice a day. If taking zinc causes stomach upset, take it with food.

HERBAL TREATMENT

After cleansing the wound, apply collagen extract or an herbal or homeopathic calendula gel or ointment topically. Calendula has antibacterial properties and helps to speed healing. It is exceptionally soothing to skin tissue.

Aloe vera gel has skin-soothing and calming properties.

Apply sage or calendula ointment to the wound for its antiseptic properties.

To be on the safe side, whether infection is present or not, take an echinacea and goldenseal herbal combination. These herbs have natural antiviral and antibiotic properties, and can be taken along with any prescribed antibiotics. Take one dose of a combination formula supplying 250 to 500 milligrams of echinacea and 150 to 300 milligrams of goldenseal three times daily for five days.

Goldenseal powder, applied topically, will work

overnight to prevent infection and encourage scabbing. Break open a capsule and add just enough water to make a paste, apply it to the wound, and cover with an adhesive bandage.

HOMEOPATHY

■ Once the wound is fully closed, apply homeopathic *Hypericum* ointment to relieve pain following injury to the fingers or toes. Apply twice a day for three days.

BACH FLOWER REMEDIES

■ Following any injury or crisis, take a dose of Rescue Remedy to calm and stabilize anxiety, shock, or fright. (*See* BACH FLOWER REMEDIES in Part One.)

AROMATHERAPY

For specific instructions on how to use aromatherapy, *see* PREPARING AROMATHERAPY TREATMENTS in Part Three.

■ Tea tree oil (essential oil of *Melaleuca alternifolia*) is an effective antiseptic that can help prevent infection. Dab the injury with undiluted tea tree oil before bandaging.

GENERAL RECOMMENDATIONS

■ Cleanliness is the cornerstone of treatment for any break in the skin. Be sure the wound is cleaned well immediately after the injury, and keep the area scrupulously clean while it is still open and healing. If the cut is deeper than a scratch, cover it with gauze or an adhesive bandage. A superficial scratch can be left open to the air.

■ Keep the wound dry for at least two days, then cover it with the ointment of your choice to speed healing. Raw, unprocessed honey is a natural antiseptic that can be applied directly to a wound. It is especially helpful when no other treatments are readily available. In a pinch, plain (unsweetened) yogurt can be applied to a cut or scrape. It is soothing, prevents infection, and helps to speed healing.

■ The latest innovation in wound care is the use of collagen powder or gel, applied topically to the injury. Collagen extract has antibiotic properties and creates a protective barrier. This treatment can increase the speed of healing by as much as 50 percent.

PREVENTION

■ It is said that no one is ever cut with a sharp knife. Although that isn't strictly true, struggling to cut vegetables with a dull knife causes you to exert more pressure than necessary and, often, a dull knife can slip and result in a cut to the hand. Keep kitchen knives in good repair.

■ If you have a workshop, follow established safety procedures. Keep your fingers well away from equipment while it is in operation (for example, use another piece of wood, not your fingers, to guide a small board through a saw). Always wear safety glasses when operating power machinery, including lawnmowers.

■ Always buckle your seat belt, whether you are the driver or a passenger.

Cystitis

See under URINARY TRACT INFECTION.

Cytomegalovirus Infection

Cytomegalovirus (CMV) is an extremely common virus that is a member of the herpes family. If a healthy adult contracts it, it is not likely to cause any illness, although it does sometimes result in a flulike syndrome with muscle aches, fever, and, possibly, some short-term liver stress. In fact, many people carry CMV in their bodies without knowing it or experiencing any problems. It is usually transmitted sexually, from mother to child during pregnancy, or through blood transfusions or organ transplantation, though presumably it may be spread by coughing and sneezing as well.

While CMV poses little danger to a healthy adult, it can be more serious if it is transmitted to a fetus during pregnancy. Such a child may be born with jaundice, an enlarged liver, mental and physical disabilities, and hearing loss. In people with compromised immune systems, such as people with AIDS, those undergoing cancer chemotherapy, and organ-transplant recipients, CMV can also be quite serious. It can occur anywhere along the gastrointestinal (GI) tract, causing inflammation, ulcers, diarrhea, pain, fever, weight loss, and intestinal bleeding. Up to 15 percent of bone marrow transplant recipients develop a form of the disease that affects the lungs, and an estimated 90 percent of them do not survive. Unique to people with AIDS who contract CMV is an inflammation of the retina that can damage vision. Laboratory tests to detect the presence of the virus and/or antibodies to it are used to confirm a diagnosis of CMV.

CONVENTIONAL TREATMENT

■ Mild cases in otherwise healthy individuals usually require no treatment, but go away on their own.

■ More serious cases may be treated with the antiviral ganciclovir (Cytovene), which may be administered either intravenously or orally. This drug can have many serious side effects—a lowered white blood cell count, red cell count, and platelet count, plus nausea, vomiting, diarrhea, fever, chills, rashes, itching, headaches, and liver problems—and is expensive, though it seems to be effective in stopping progression of the retinal damage. Another drug that may be used to keep eye damage from worsening is foscarnet (Foscavir). This must be administered intravenously and it, too, has potentially serious side effects. It is toxic to the kidneys and can cause ulcerations in the genital area, in addition to altering calcium levels in the body.

DIETARY GUIDELINES

■ Eat plenty of lean, clean protein foods such as chicken, fish, and soy products.

■ Include in your diet steamed leafy green vegetables, which contain many vitamins and minerals required for healing.

■ Investigate the possibility that food allergies and sensitivites may be contributing to the problem. (*See* ELMINA-TION DIET in Part Three.)

NUTRITIONAL SUPPLEMENTS

■ Take a good multivitamin and mineral supplement daily to ensure an adequate supply of all basic nutrients, especially vitamin B_{12}, folic acid, and manganese.

■ Blue-green algae can help to improve energy levels. Take 300 milligrams two or three times daily. If you are having difficulty sleeping, take the last dose at least eight hours before bedtime.

■ Lipoic acid is an antioxidant with some antiviral properties. It helps the liver to function more efficiently, aids in the regulation of blood-sugar levels, and is useful against fatigue. Take 50 milligrams three times daily.

■ The combination of magnesium and malic acid helps to initiate the Krebs cycle, a series of enzyme reactions that results in the conversion of nutrients into energy at the cellular level. Take 100 milligrams of magnesium and 300 milligrams of malic acid one hour before breakfast and again at bedtime until you recover.

■ Nicotinamide adenine dinucleotide hydrogen (NADH) is an antioxidant enzyme that occurs in all living cells. It facilitates the production of neurotransmitters such as dopamine and noradrenaline. Low levels of neurotransmitters are often associated with fibromyalgia. Taking 10 milligrams one-half hour before breakfast often improves concentration, stamina, and energy.

■ Vitamin C boosts the immune response and promotes healing. Take 500 to 1,000 milligrams three times daily.

■ Vitamin E is an antioxidant and anti-inflammatory, and helps to speed healing. Choose a product containing mixed tocopherols and take 400 international units at bedtime.

HERBAL TREATMENT

■ Isatis is a Chinese herb that can be very effective against active viruses. It is most often found in combination formulas with other antimicrobial herbs. Take one dose of such a formula, as directed on the product label, three times daily for two weeks.

Note: Do not use this herb if you have a sensitive stomach.

■ Pine-bark and grape-seed extracts have antioxidant and anti-inflammatory properties. Take 50 milligrams of either three times daily.

■ St. John's wort has antiviral as well as antidepressant effects. Choose a standardized extract containing 0.3-percent hypericin and take 300 milligrams twice a day.

■ If CMV is accompanied by liver dysfunction, as demonstrated by blood tests, milk thistle can help. This herb actually helps the liver to repair itself. Choose a standardized extract containing 80 percent flavonoids (silymarin) and take 100 to 200 milligrams two or three times daily.

■ If you are having difficulty sleeping or experiencing muscle spasms, try passionflower. Choose a standardized extract containing 0.7 percent flavonoids and take 250 to 300 milligrams before bedtime.

HOMEOPATHY

■ *Chininum arsenicosum* is helpful for symptoms of weakness and tiredness, accompanied by poor appetite, sleeplessness, and an inability to tolerate bright light. Your feet and hands may be cold. Take one dose of *Chininum arsenicosum* 30x or 15c three times daily for two days.

■ Choose *Nux vomica* if you are feeling chilly, with a nose that is stuffed during the day but runny at night, and suffer from indigestion. Your symptoms are worse in the morning and with movement, and better after a nap. Take one dose of *Nux vomica* 30x or 15c three times daily for up to two days.

■ *Rhus toxicodendron* is for stiff, painful muscles accompanied by restlessness. Symptoms are worse in rainy weather. Take one dose of *Rhus toxicodendron* 30x or 15c three times daily for up to three days.

BACH FLOWER REMEDIES

Select the remedy that most closely fits your emotional tendencies and concerns, and take it as needed, following the directions on the product label.

■ Choose Agrimony if you tend to maintain a smiling appearance despite inner feelings of anguish.

■ Beech helps to relax a tendency to be perfectionistic and impatient.

■ Choose Holly if you are feeling irritable and angry.

■ Hornbeam is for feelings of complete and utter exhaustion.

■ Mustard helps to ease depression.

ACUPRESSURE

For the locations of acupressure points on the body, *see* ADMINISTERING AN ACUPRESSURE TREATMENT in Part Three.

■ Stomach 36 is a tonic point that improves the body's utilization of nutrients to increase strength and energy.

GENERAL RECOMMENDATIONS

■ Try to reduce your schedule to a level you can handle, and be sure to get adequate rest.

■ Even though you may be feeling very fatigued, it is important to exercise. Gentle stretching, breathing exercises, and light walking are all good choices. Don't overdo, but do be sure to get some type of exercise—no matter how minimal—every day.

PREVENTION

■ There is no vaccine for CMV, but administering an immune globulin injection to transplant patients who have no sign of current infection may help with prevention. Using specially filtered blood products and limiting transfusions as much as possible can also be helpful.

Dandruff

Dandruff is a condition that causes itchy, greasy flakes and scales of dried sebum (an oily skin-lubricating fluid secreted by the sebaceous glands) and dead skin to appear on the scalp and in the hair, and, as the flakes fall, on the shoulders. It is commonly caused by seborrheic dermatitis, a disorder of the sebaceous glands.

The sebaceous glands are tiny glands in the skin that open into hair follicles. These glands are especially numerous in the areas of the scalp, the face, the anus, the nose, the mouth, and the external ear. If they produce too much sebum, it dries into flakes and plugs up the ducts. The sebaceous glands respond by putting forth even more sebum in an attempt to force out the obstructions and open a passageway to the surface of the skin. Scaling, flaking, and itching occur.

Dandruff may be complicated by the presence of a persistent yeast called *Pityrosporum ovale* that normally lives in hair follicles. In severe cases, the face, eyebrows, and ears may be affected.

CONVENTIONAL TREATMENT

■ Antidandruff shampoos available over the counter are effective for many people. The active ingredients in these shampoos may include one or more of the following: salicylic acid, selenium sulfide, menthol, and zinc pyrithione (ZPT). If a particular medicated shampoo seems to be losing its effectiveness after a few uses, select another shampoo with a different active ingredient and switch back and forth between formulas. Medicated shampoos are very drying. For that reason, it is best not to use them more often than necessary.

■ Shampoos containing coal tar are effective against dandruff. Be aware, however, that they can leave a dulling residue behind that darkens light-colored hair.

■ If you do not get satisfactory results with over-the-counter remedies, consult your doctor or dermatologist for a diagnosis. If the condition is complicated by a yeast infection, for example, he or she may prescribe a shampoo containing ketoconazole (Nizoral), an antifungal agent, or a cream containing an antifungal such as miconazole (in Micatin-Derm and Monistat-Derm) or clotrimazole (Lotrimin, Mycelex, and others).

■ Selenium sulfide suspension can be applied directly to the scalp once a week. It is nontoxic, but it can irritate the scalp in some cases, and there have been reports of oiliness, dryness, darkening of very light hair, and changes in the rate of hair loss. Its safety for use by pregnant women has not been tested.

■ In severe, difficult cases, the intermittent use of topical corticosteroids may be recommended. However, it is best to avoid these agents unless they are absolutely necessary, as they may be absorbed into the body through the scalp. In addition, the body gets used to their effects quickly, so that increased doses can become necessary to achieve the same effect.

DIETARY GUIDELINES

■ Eat a high-fiber whole-foods diet.

■ Avoid saturated animal fats and hydrogenated and partially hydrogenated fats and oils.

■ Avoid refined sugars and processed foods. Both bacteria and yeasts thrive on sugar.

■ Yogurt and other fermented foods containing active cultures of probiotic bacteria can help clear a yeast infection. Enjoy them often.

NUTRITIONAL SUPPLEMENTS

■ Essential fatty acids decrease dryness of the skin, which can contribute to dandruff. For their content of the essential fatty acids, take 500 to 1,000 milligrams of black currant seed, borage, evening primrose, or flaxseed oil twice daily.

■ Probiotics (*Lactobacillus acidophilus* and *Bifidobacterium bifidum*) are cleansing to the body. They foster healthy flora and help fight yeast infection. Take a probiotic supplement as recommended on the product label. If you are allergic to milk, select a dairy-free product.

■ Selenium is an antioxidant that fights free radicals and is cleansing to the body. It also tends to have beneficial effects specifically for dandruff. Take 100 micrograms twice daily.

■ Vitamin A and beta-carotene are necessary for healthy skin. Take up to 10,000 international units of vitamin A and 20,000 international units of beta-carotene daily for two weeks.

Note: If you are pregnant, or intend to get pregnant, or if you have liver disease, consult your doctor before taking supplemental vitamin A. Pregnant women should not ingest a total of more than 25,000 international units of supplemental vitamin A *per week* from all sources.

■ Vitamin-E oil can be used topically to soften scales and nourish the scalp. Simply massage it into the affected areas and leave it in place overnight (or for at least thirty minutes), then shampoo.

HERBAL TREATMENT

■ Kelp is rich in the healing trace minerals needed for healthy hair and scalp. Take 300 milligrams in the morning and 150 milligrams with lunch daily.

■ For a dry and flaky scalp, massage alternately with calendula lotion, vitamin-E oil, and almond oil before shampooing. Allow the oil to remain on the scalp for fifteen minutes, shampoo, then gently comb away the loosened scales with a fine-toothed comb. These oils are helpful for all skin irritations and can help lessen itching.

HOMEOPATHY

■ *Sulfur* is a general homeopathic remedy useful for all skin conditions. It is especially helpful if you are the type of person who kicks off the bedcovers and who prefers to sleep without pajamas. Take one dose of *Sulfur* 30x or 9c twice daily for two to three days.

■ *Thuja* is good for the person who is cooler and calmer, and who likes settling down under a thick comforter. If *Sulfur* doesn't clear the condition, take one dose of *Thuja* 30x or 9c twice daily for two days.

■ If neither of the above homeopathic remedies seems to

fit, consult a homeopathic physician for a constitutional remedy.

BACH FLOWER REMEDIES

Select the remedy that most closely fits your emotional tendencies and concerns, and take it as needed, following the directions on the product label.

☐ Red Chestnut is helpful if you are prone to excessive worrying.

■ White Chestnut is the remedy of choice if you have excessive energy and are troubled by obsessive thoughts.

ACUPRESSURE

For the location of acupressure points on the body, *see* ADMINISTERING AN ACUPRESSURE TREATMENT in Part Three.

☐ Gallbladder 20 and 34 improve circulation to the head.

☐ Large Intestine 4 has a beneficial effect on the head and face.

■ Large Intestine 11 relieves itching.

AROMATHERAPY

For specific instructions on how to use aromatherapy, *see* PREPARING AROMATHERAPY TREATMENTS in Part Three.

☐ Tea tree oil fights fungal infection; pine oil soothes itching and inflammation. Add a total of 5 drops of either or both to an ounce of shampoo and massage it well into your scalp, then rinse and repeat. Or simply rub several drops of tea tree oil and grapefruit seed extract into your scalp each night for three weeks.

GENERAL RECOMMENDATIONS

☐ Do not pick at the scales. Doing so may cause an infection.

☐ Applying apple-cider vinegar to the affected areas is an old home remedy that has been helpful to many. Use two parts apple-cider vinegar to one part water. Heat the mixture to a comfortably warm temperature and apply it to your scalp. Wrap a towel around your head and wait thirty minutes, then rinse out the vinegar.

☐ Shampoo thoroughly when you wash your hair. Some people find that using a regular nonmedicated shampoo formulated without oil is more helpful than antidandruff formulas.

PREVENTION

■ To avoid an accumulation of dead skin cells and flakes, gently but thoroughly brush or comb your hair at least twice a day.

■ If your scalp is dry, before shampooing, try massaging your scalp with one of the oils mentioned in this entry at least once a week.

Deafness

See HEARING LOSS.

Decompression Sickness

Decompression sickness, also known as "the bends," is a painful and sometimes life-threatening condition that is caused by a sudden drop in environmental pressure. If the pressure around the body drops rapidly—as can happen if you surface too quickly while scuba diving or climb too rapidly in an unpressurized aircraft—nitrogen and other gases that had been dissolved in the blood collect in bubbles in the blood vessels, blocking them and depriving the body of essential blood nutrients.

Symptoms can include mild to severe joint pain, especially in the shoulders, elbows, hips, and knees; chest pain; shortness of breath; a burning sensation behind the breastbone; difficulty breathing; coughing; weakness; itching; rash; fatigue; numbness and tingling and, possibly, paralysis in an arm or leg; and even loss of consciousness, an inability to speak, and difficulty urinating. Symptoms can begin anytime up to twenty-four hours after a serious change in pressure, and may gradually continue to get worse after that.

The risk of developing decompression sickness is greatest among scuba divers who perform more than one dive in a day, those who fly certain high-performance aircraft, and people who work in compressed-air environments, such as tunnel workers. The risk is increased by a medical history of lung conditions such as asthma, as well as by obesity, heart disease, chronic sinusitis, and alcoholism. Women appear to be somewhat more prone to developing this disorder than are men.

EMERGENCY TREATMENT

■ Decompression sickness is considered a medical emergency. If you have been subjected to a change in pressure and develop any of the symptoms discussed above, seek emergency medical help. You should do this even if initial symptoms seem relatively mild, as they can worsen fairly quickly and the syndrome can progress to the point where it becomes life-threatening. If you have decompression sickness, you will have to be hospitalized and placed in a high-pressure oxygen chamber. This will force the gas bubbles to once again dissolve in the blood. You will then be brought back to normal pressure gradually, under controlled conditions. While you are undergoing treatment, your fluid levels will be closely monitored, and you may be given steroids to decrease inflammation. Even before you receive hyperbaric oxygen therapy, medical personnel should administer continuous standard oxygen treatment, even if you are showing no obvious signs of oxygen deprivation.

CONVENTIONAL TREATMENT

■ For pain, aspirin is usually the only medication recommended. Doctors generally avoid prescribing stronger painkillers because they can distort observable responses to recompression.

DIETARY GUIDELINES

■ As long as you have any residual symptoms, avoid alcohol. Alcohol dehydrates the body and has a sedating effect, which can cause complications if you have any difficulty breathing.

NUTRITIONAL SUPPLEMENTS

The following nutritional supplements are intended to support recovery from decompression sickness, rather than to treat an acute episode. If you suspect decompression sickness, seek immediate medical treatment. When choosing supplements, look for liquid or powder forms, which are more easily assimilated by the digestive tract.

■ The B vitamins support the nervous system and are necessary for the proper transmission of nerve impulses. Take a B-complex supplement that supplies 50 milligrams of each of the major B vitamins three times daily for six weeks.

■ Green-foods supplements, available in health-food stores, supply valuable trace minerals. Take a green-foods supplement twice a day, as directed on the product label.

HERBAL TREATMENT

Herbal treatment is intended to support recovery from decompression sickness, rather than to treat an acute episode. If you suspect decompression sickness, seek immediate medical treatment.

■ Tea made with ginger and turmeric helps to improve circulation and reenergize the body. Add 1 teaspoon each of turmeric and ginger root to 12 ounces of water and bring it to a boil. Reduce the heat and allow the tea to simmer for ten to fifteen minutes, then strain and drink it. Do this twice daily.

HOMEOPATHY

The following homeopathic remedies are intended to support recovery from decompression sickness, rather than to treat an acute episode. If you suspect decompression sickness, seek immediate medical treatment.

■ Once emergency personnel say it is all right to take something by mouth, take one dose of *Arnica* 200x or 200c every hour for three to four hours. This remedy helps to relieve pain in the back and limbs that makes you feel bruised, beaten, and/or sore. Your joints may have a sprained and/or dislocated feeling.

■ *Bellis perennis* is for muscular soreness with a sore, bruised feeling in the abdomen. Take one dose of *Bellis perennis* 6x or 3c four times daily, up to a total of ten doses.

■ *Hydrocyanicum acidum* is good if decompression sickness caused you to suffer collapse, pain and tightness in the chest, a sensation of spasmodic constriction in the larynx, and a spasmodic, dry cough, accompanied by severe fright and agitated breathing. Take one dose of *Hydrocyanicum acidum* 12x or 6c three times daily for up to three days.

BACH FLOWER REMEDIES

■ Take one dose of Rescue Remedy every half hour for the first three hours to ease panic and anxiety.

ACUPRESSURE

■ Gallbladder 20 increases circulation to the head.

■ Gallbladder 34 and Stomach 36 improve circulation to the lower half of the body.

■ Pericardium 6 relaxes the chest.

PREVENTION

■ To become a diver, you must receive training from a licensed instructor. Always remember and practice proper technique, especially when ascending. Always dive with a buddy so that, should one of you need it, a helper will be available. You should also know the location of the nearest appropriate treatment center in any area where you go diving. The National Diver Assistance Network (telephone 919–684–8111) may be able to assist you in this.

Dehydration

Water accounts for approximately two-thirds of the average adult's body weight. It is more important to life than any other substance we know of. Water is involved in virtually every bodily function—the transport and utilization of other nutrients, the removal of toxins, and the maintenance of blood pressure and body temperature, among others. A person is said to be dehydrated if his or her body does not have as much water as it needs to function properly.

Dehydration can have a variety of causes. The most common include vomiting, diarrhea, and profuse sweating, which cause the body to lose fluids rapidly. Dehydration can also result from kidney failure, overuse of diuretics, diabetes, and diseases of the adrenal glands. In most cases, the loss of water is not the only problem. Sodium, potassium, and other minerals are usually lost along with the water, resulting in electrolyte imbalances also.

The first symptom of dehydration is usually significant thirst and dry mouth. The urine may be dark or scanty. More severe dehydration can cause overall weakness, lethargy, and an increased heart rate, sometimes over 100 beats per minute. If not corrected, it can progress to signs of disorientation and even loss of consciousness.

It is also possible to suffer from chronic, low-level dehydration, in which you are not dehydrated enough to have the classic symptoms, but your body is still kept from functioning as well as it should. This problem most often results from the simple failure to consume enough water, and is most common in older adults. Chronic dehydration can lead to chronic constipation, weight gain, elevated cholesterol levels, a decreased threshold of pain, and a decreased ability to clear toxins from the body.

A quick way to assess your state of hydration is to look for a sign called "tenting." To do this, pinch the skin on the back of your hand. If the skin remains standing in the shape of a tent for several seconds before returning to its flattened state, this is a sign of dehydration.

CONVENTIONAL TREATMENT

■ For simple, mild to moderate dehydration, consuming an oral hydrating product such as Gatorade or Power Ade, along with plenty of water, is usually sufficient to correct the problem.

■ If taking fluids orally does not correct the situation, intravenous treatments with fluid solutions that include mineral salts may be necessary.

■ If dehydration is the result of illness, measures should be taken to determine and eliminate the cause, or at least to interrupt the loss of fluids with antidiarrheal or antinausea drugs, as appropriate.

■ An examination of any medications you are taking is important. Medications, especially diuretics, can contribute to dehydration, especially if you are not in the habit of drinking enough fluids in the first place.

DIETARY GUIDELINES

■ After an acute episode, consume as much liquid as you can. Even once the episode is over, increase your water intake for several days to one week to restore depleted fluid reserves. Thereafter, be sure to drink eight 8-ounce glasses of water daily.

■ Avoid alcoholic beverages and beverages containing caffeine. Both alcohol and caffeine act as diuretics, increasing your body's excretion of necessary fluids and electrolytes.

NUTRITIONAL SUPPLEMENTS

■ Take a multivitamin, mineral, and trace-mineral complex daily. All of these valuable nutrients help to carry water successfully through the body.

■ Potassium is necessary to keep water distributed throughout the body, and is involved in the regulation of the heart and kidneys. Take 99 milligrams daily.

HERBAL TREATMENT

■ Licorice helps to strengthen adrenal function. Strong adrenal function is associated with the effective transport of water in the body. Siberian ginseng helps the body to adapt to stress. On days when you will be engaging in strenuous physical activity, whether an athletic event or a physical chore, take 500 milligrams of a licorice and Siberian ginseng combination three times daily. Obviously, this is to be done in combination with sufficient fluid intake, not in place of it.

Note: Do not take licorice on a daily basis for more than five days at a time, as it can elevate blood pressure. Do not take it at all if you have high blood pressure.

GENERAL RECOMMENDATIONS

■ Prolonged diarrhea and vomiting can cause serious dehydration, as can profuse sweating as a result of physical exertion and/or spending time in a hot climate. If you suspect you are becoming dehydrated, with signs such as excessive thirst, dry mouth, decreased urination, weakness, or feelings of lethargy or lightheadedness, you can take an oral electrolyte formula such as Gatorade. Or you can make the following mixtures:

First glass: 8 ounces of orange or apple juice, $1/2$ teaspoon honey or corn syrup, and a pinch of salt.

Second glass: 8 ounces of water and $1/4$ teaspoon of baking soda.

Take small sips of each, alternating between the two glasses. Stay out of direct sunlight, rest, and continue to take fluids until you feel better.

PREVENTION

■ The key to preventing dehydration is water, water, and more water. Do not wait until you are thirsty to drink.

Thirst is not a sensitive indicator of your fluid needs (see the table below) or hydration status. Drink before you are thirsty. Drink when you are thirsty. Drink when you are not thirsty. And drink in between. Increase your water intake even more if you are ill or if you are exercising or spending time in warm temperatures.

Daily Water Requirements for Adults

Body Weight	Activity Level		
	LIGHT	MODERATE	STRENUOUS
100 lbs.	10 cups	11 cups	12 cups
125 lbs.	$10^{1}/_{2}$ cups	$11^{1}/_{2}$ cups	$12^{1}/_{2}$ cups
150 lbs.	11 cups	12 cups	13 cups
175 lbs.	$11^{1}/_{2}$ cups	$12^{1}/_{2}$ cups	$13^{1}/_{2}$ cups
200 lbs.	12 cups	13 cups	14 cups

Dementia

See ALZHEIMER'S DISEASE. See also under HIV DISEASE.

Dental Problems

See PERIODONTAL DISEASE; TOOTH, BROKEN OR KNOCKED OUT; TOOTH DECAY.

Depression

Everyone feels deep sadness from time to time—in response to a death in the family, for example, or an inexplicable tragedy, or losing a job. This is a common and normal reaction to a life situation, and is called *reactive depression*. With the passage of time, the depression lifts, the mood lightens, and life goes on. *Clinical depression*, on the other hand, is persistent depression that is out of proportion to a person's life situation or, in many cases, occurs for no apparent reason.

A person who is depressed is under enormous emotional stress. He or she may experience extreme feelings of sadness, dejection, despair, worthlessness, hopelessness, and emptiness. Early signs of depression include a lack of motivation and an inability to concentrate. A person who is entering a depressed state may exhibit mood swings and may even have crying fits for no obvious reason. If the episode continues, symptoms can include loss of appetite,

erratic sleeping patterns, and a complete loss of interest in normal daily activities, even ones that were previously a source of great pleasure. A seriously depressed person may become completely withdrawn from life and eventually may even refuse—or be unable—to get out of bed. Severely depressed people often have feelings of complete worthlessness and/or guilt over some imagined situation. Thoughts of death and suicide may be uppermost in their minds.

Depression is the most common of the serious psychiatric illnesses. An estimated 10 to 15 percent of all people suffer an episode of depression at some time in their lives. Most often, it is relatively mild and short-lived. More women than men are diagnosed with depression. About one in six women will seek help for depression at some time in their lives, while only one in nine men will do so. However, this disparity may reflect the fact that, in general, women are more willing than men to admit to feelings of hopelessness and depression.

The incidence of depression increases with age. This may be because older people living on their own may be socially isolated and often worry over becoming a burden to their families. In addition, they have often lost many friends and loved ones to death, and may require multiple medications for different medical conditions (many medications can affect mood). Add to this increasing physical frailty and slowing mental faculties, and the scene is set for a depressive episode.

There is no single cause of depression. Many cases appear to be linked to abnormalities in brain chemistry. For example, it has been determined that persons at high risk of suicide have lower than normal levels of serotonin, a neurotransmitter in the brain that controls inhibitions and is closely related to mood. People with reduced levels of serotonin are therefore more likely to act on feelings such as a desire to take their own life. Conversely, increasing the level of serotonin in the brain improves mood in many cases.

Some cases of depression can be traced to inadequate nutrition. Deficiencies of certain vitamins, for example, can result in symptoms of mental and emotional disorders. Food allergies can also result in a depressed state. Hypoglycemia (low blood sugar) can cause mood swings, irrational behavior, and may set the scene for episodes of depression. One type of depression, known as seasonal affective disorder (SAD), appears to be related to insufficient exposure to sunlight. When days are short and skies are gray and overcast, exposure to sunlight is reduced or nonexistent. This causes the retina of the eye to fail to send proper messages to the hypothalamus, which is responsible for transmitting signals that maintain the body in its properly regulated state. The end result may be a form of depression. SAD most often affects those living in northern climes during the cold months of the year.

Postpartum depression (PPD, also called the "baby blues"), is a type of depression that many women experience after the birth of a child. It is caused by an imbalance in hormones that often occurs after delivery. This situation is usually short-lived; new mothers tend to regain their equilibrium as their hormones stabilize. Holiday depression is a common phenomenon suffered by many people. Many people who tend to feel blue during special seasons of the year feel pressured to make everything "perfect," and when they cannot, they end up feeling sad and depressed.

Some women who take oral contraceptives, which affect the body's hormonal balance, fall into a depressed state without knowing why. Over time, hormone deficiencies and imbalances can lead to some forms of depression. A dysfunctional thyroid gland is also a possible source of trouble, as is heavy metal poisoning. Virtually any chronic illness can be accompanied by depression as well.

Manic-depressive disorder (medically termed bipolar mood disorder) is a variant of depression in which periods of deep depression alternate with periods of irrational elation and hyperactivity. (See MANIC-DEPRESSIVE DISORDER.)

CONVENTIONAL TREATMENT

■ If you are suffering from symptoms of depression, see your doctor. The first step in diagnosis is to rule out the possibility that a physical disorder is causing your symptoms. Your doctor will probably do blood tests to check your hormone levels, thyroid function, and other indicators of possible problems.

■ If the depressed state persists and deepens, especially if there is no obvious cause, seek help from a mental-health professional. The prognosis is good for most people with clinical depression. A knowledgeable mental-health professional will tailor his or her treatment approach to your individual situation.

■ If depression is a reaction to a specific event, counseling, psychotherapy, cognitive-behavioral therapy, and/or the simple passage of time will most likely resolve the problem.

■ If there is no obvious cause for the depression, or if reactive depression persists longer than might be expected, or if you are having suicidal thoughts, more aggressive therapy is needed. This means drug therapy and, possibly, hospitalization. The mainstay of drug treatment has long been a group of medications called tricyclic antidepressants, including amoxapine (Asendin), clomipramine (Anafranil), desipramine (Norpramin), imipramine (Tofranil), and nortriptyline (Aventyl, Pamelor). These drugs do not take effect immediately, so a test period of at least two weeks is necessary to determine whether they are working. Toxicity is a problem with these drugs, and therapeutic

levels are close to toxic levels, so repeated blood tests to check the level of the drug in the body are necessary. Possible side effects include delirium, seizures, heart-rhythm problems, dry mouth, low blood pressure, reduced sex drive, depression, drowsiness or agitation, rashes, nausea, vomiting, diarrhea, cramping, and blood problems. For obvious reasons, newer, less potentially toxic medications are now considered more desirable. Fluoxetine (Prozac) is the best known of these. Others include bupropion (Wellbutrin, Zyban), fluvoxamine (Luvox), nefazodone (Serzone), paroxetine (Paxil), sertraline (Zoloft), and venlafaxine (Effexor). Though these drugs are less likely to cause side effects, they still can—effects including sexual problems, nausea, diarrhea, stomach pains, dizziness, tremors, insomnia, dry mouth, and excessive sweating. These drugs should not be mixed with many other classes of drugs. Make sure your doctor knows about everything you are taking.

■ Another type of drug used to treat depression is the monoamine oxidase (MAO) inhibitor. These are usually resorted to only when the others have failed. Phenelzine (Nardil) and tranylcypromine (Parnate) are in this class. These drugs can cause high (sometimes extremely high) or low blood pressure, headaches, liver stress, seizures, nausea, vomiting, diarrhea, stomach pain, rashes, sensitivity to light, and sexual dysfunction. There are also important dietary restrictions that must be adhered to. You must avoid cheeses, chocolate, wine, beer, liver, and more. Eating any of these forbidden foods while on an MAO inhibitor can result in a dangerous spike in blood pressure. Also to be avoided are certain medications, including many over-the-counter cough and cold preparations, eye drops used for glaucoma, and drugs used to treat asthma and emphysema. If you must take an MAO inhibitor, consult your doctor before taking any other medication, whether prescription or over the counter.

■ Though no one understands why, serious depression may respond—and very well—to electroconvulsive therapy (ECT). Most people wince when they hear this. However, it is not quite as barbaric as it may sound, as the patient is unconscious for the brief procedure. Negative reactions are mostly related to heart rhythm, and are remarkably infrequent, but there is a period of amnesia after treatment that can be very disturbing.

■ Seasonal affective disorder may be treated with phototherapy. In this treatment, a person is exposed to full-spectrum light by means of special light fixtures, giving a daily dose of the light frequencies that would be available on a bright sunny day.

■ Most cases of postpartum depression resolve on their own. Participation in a support group with other new mothers can be immensely helpful. In severe cases, antidepressant medication may be prescribed.

■ Holiday blues usually disappear as the season passes. Treatment is seldom necessary.

DIETARY GUIDELINES

■ Follow a healthy diet plan that provides a good balance of all the important nutrients and an adequate amount of fiber. Be sure to include clean, lean protein foods such as fish, chicken, tofu, and plenty of fresh vegetables, especially greens.

It is important to keep your blood-sugar levels in balance. Eat five or six small meals a day rather than three large ones, and eat healthy snacks when you feel hungry.

Include in your diet low-fat dairy products, bananas, soy-based foods, and turkey. These foods are natural sources of tryptophan, which is necessary for the formation of serotonin.

Avoid the artificial stimulation produced by alcohol and caffeine. While both of these substances are stimulating initially, the stimulation is ultimately followed by a depressed state.

NUTRITIONAL SUPPLEMENTS

Many depressed people, including those who are just "on edge," neglect themselves and eat poorly. Take a good multivitamin and mineral formula daily to make sure your body has all the basic nutrients it requires.

Calcium and magnesium are essential to the central nervous system. They work best when taken together. Take a calcium and magnesium combination formula that supplies 500 milligrams of calcium and 250 to 500 milligrams of magnesium twice daily.

Chromium helps keep blood-sugar levels in balance. Take 200 micrograms twice a day for one month, then reduce to 200 micrograms daily.

DL-phenylalanine (DLPA) can be very helpful for a short period of time, if taken correctly. Take 500 to 1,000 milligrams twice a day, between meals, with water or juice only. Do not take it with protein foods. Take it for up to three weeks.

■ Levels of folic acid are often significantly lower than normal in people who are depressed. Take 800 micrograms of folic acid twice a day for one month. Thereafter, take 800 micrograms once daily. If you take any of the B vitamins individually, you should also take a B-complex supplement at a different time of day.

■ Inositol is a B vitamin required for the activity of several important neurotransmitters, including serotonin. Levels of inositol are often low in depressed people. In one study, subjects given 1 gram of inositol per day had therapeutic results similar to common antidepressant drugs,

but with no unwanted side effects. The same results were confirmed in additional studies. Further, Chinese medicine teaches that stagnation of the liver contributes to many problems, including depression. Inositol promotes the export of fat from the liver, thus helping relieve stagnation of this important organ. Take 500 milligrams of inositol three times daily for one week. If you note no improvement after that time, discontinue use; otherwise, continue taking 500 milligrams three times daily as needed. This dosage of inositol should be used under the supervision of a physician.

■ Melatonin may be helpful for some cases of seasonal affective disorder. Some experts believe the body's melatonin mechanism is involved in this form of depression. Melatonin can also be helpful if you are having problems with insomnia. Take 3 milligrams each evening, between one-half hour and two hours before retiring for the night.

■ An excellent supplement for depression is s-adenosyl-L-methionine (SAM or SAM-e). This amino-acid derivative has been compared to prescription medication, but without the side effects. Initial recommended doses are in the range of 400 to 500 milligrams three times daily, followed by a maintenance dose of 400 milligrams a day. Unfortunately, SAM is not easy to obtain, and it is expensive. It can be ordered by mail from the Life Extension Foundation (see the Resources section at the end of the book). Research has found that trimethylglycine (TMG), which is less expensive, is converted into SAM in the body. The initial recommended dose of TMG is 3,000 milligrams a day, followed by a maintenance dose of 1,000 milligrams a day for up to three weeks.

■ Tyrosine is an important amino acid that stimulates the production of norepinephrine, a hormone that is essential to the central nervous system. This nutrient is especially important for the depressed individual who is feeling excessive fatigue. Take 250 to 500 milligrams twice a day for up to three weeks.

Note: If you are taking a monoamine oxidase (MAO) inhibitor drug, *do not* take supplemental tyrosine, as a dangerous elevation in blood pressure may result.

■ A deficiency of vitamin B_6 (pyridoxine) usually accompanies depression. Take 50 milligrams of vitamin B_6 twice a day for two weeks, between meals. Then take 50 milligrams once daily for three weeks, between meals. Thereafter, take a good B-complex formula or a multivitamin and mineral supplement to maintain healthy levels of this vitamin.

■ Vitamin B_{12} can help to increase energy and improve mood. Take 300 to 500 micrograms twice a day. If you take any of the B vitamins individually, you should also take a B-complex supplement at a different time of day.

HERBAL TREATMENT

■ Bupleurum and dong quai make up a Chinese herbal formula that helps reduce anxiety, irritability, and depression. Take 1,000 milligrams of a bupleurum and dong quai combination formula two or three times daily for two weeks out of every month (if you are a woman, take it for the two weeks prior to the anticipated onset of your menstrual period).

■ Ginkgo biloba increases the flow of oxygenated blood to the brain and can significantly reduce the symptoms of depression. This herb must be taken for at least three months before you can assess its effectiveness. Choose a product containing at least 24 percent ginkgo heterosides (sometimes called flavoglycosides) and take 40 to 60 milligrams two or three times a day. This is an especially important supplement if you are over fifty years of age.

■ Kava kava eases mental anguish and anxiety. Choose a product containing 30 percent kavalactones and take 150 milligrams three times a day.

Note: In excess amounts, this herb can cause drowsiness. Do not exceed the recommended dose. Do not use kava kava if you are pregnant or nursing, if you have Parkinson's disease, or if you are taking a prescription medication for depression or anxiety.

■ Oat straw is high in silica, which helps support and strengthen the central nervous system. Take 500 milligrams twice a day.

■ St. John's wort gently alters brain chemistry in such a way as to improve mood and ease depression. Start by taking one 300-milligram capsule of standardized extract containing 0.3 percent hypericin daily. At two-week intervals, you can add another 300-milligram capsule, taken at a different time of day (up to a total of three to four capsules a day), until you achieve the desired effect.

■ Siberian ginseng improves the balance of important neurotransmitters (including serotonin, dopamine, norepinephrine, and epinephrine) in the brain. Select an extract standardized to contain 0.5 percent eleutheroside E and take 100 milligrams first thing in the morning and again before lunch.

■ If sleeplessness is a problem, take 200 to 300 milligrams of standardized valerian extract containing 0.5 percent isovalerenic acids one hour before bedtime and another 200 to 300 milligrams just before going to bed. Do not use this herb on an ongoing basis, but take a week off every four to six weeks.

HOMEOPATHY

■ *Aurum muriaticum* is especially recommended if you are feeling extreme anxiety and suffering almost insupportable distress. This remedy should be applied promptly.

Take *Aurum muriaticum* 30x or 15c three times daily for up to three days.

■ If you are depressed, you will benefit greatly from a constitutional remedy. See a homeopathic physician.

BACH FLOWER REMEDIES

Select the remedy that most closely fits your emotional tendencies and concerns, and take it as needed, following the directions on the product label.

■ Rescue Remedy is the first choice to ease acute anxiety.

■ Choose Agrimony if you tend to maintain a smiling appearance while suffering inner anguish and despair.

■ Centaury is helpful for depression accompanied by feelings of intimidation.

■ Cherry Plum relieves feelings of fearfulness, whether of things real or imagined.

■ Mustard is the remedy for sadness and feelings of ineffectuality.

ACUPRESSURE/MASSAGE

For the location of acupressure points on the body, *see* ADMINISTERING AN ACUPRESSURE TREATMENT in Part Three.

■ Bladder 23 and 60 increase circulation and help clarify thinking.

■ Gallbladder 20 improves circulation to the head.

■ Gallbladder 41 regulates hormonal function.

■ Large Intestine 4 relaxes tension in the head and promotes calm.

■ Liver 3 relaxes the nervous system.

■ Stomach 36 improves digestion, tones the digestive tract, is useful for improving appetite, energizes the immune system, and strengthens overall well-being.

■ Massaging the head, feet, and hands is often helpful.

AROMATHERAPY

For specific instructions on how to use aromatherapy, *see* PREPARING AROMATHERAPY TREATMENTS in Part Three.

■ Many essential oils can lift the spirits. Some of the best known for this purpose include geranium, jasmine, lavender, neroli, rose, and ylang. Use any or all of them as inhalants or in baths, diffuse them into the air, add them to massage oil, or use them in any other way you choose.

GENERAL RECOMMENDATIONS

■ See your physician to rule out any underlying problem that could be causing a depressed state.

■ Exercise. Regular physical activity eases depression,

reduces nervous tension and feelings of anxiety, and is an aid to restful sleep. Studies have shown that exercise is a fast-acting mood elevator that increases feelings of well-being. (*See* STARTING AN EXERCISE PROGRAM in Part Three.)

■ Insomnia often accompanies depression. If insomnia is a problem, try taking hot baths. Soaking in a tub of hot (102°F) water two hours before going to bed can help you to fall asleep faster, sleep more soundly, and awaken more refreshed in the morning. You should allow two hours to pass between the hot bath and retiring, however, for this to be effective.

PREVENTION

■ If possible, make sure your hands and face get adequate exposure to sunlight, at least thirty minutes a day.

Dermatitis

Dermatitis is a general term meaning "inflammation of the skin." There are many different types of dermatitis. *Contact dermatitis*, probably the most common type, is caused by physical contact with an irritant of some type, which can be anything from a mild detergent (or even water) to strong acids or alkalis. If the irritant is comparatively mild, it may take a great deal of contact to cause a problem; strong irritants can create effects in seconds. However, different people can have remarkably different degrees of sensitivity to different irritants. Contact dermatitis is characterized by a reddening of the skin, usually only in the area where the contact actually occurred, so there is often a marked outline. There may be a slight reddening only, or there may be blisters, swelling, itching, pain, weeping areas, or even abscesses.

Allergic contact dermatitis is a variant of contact dermatitis caused by an allergic reaction rather than simple physical irritation. It can take days (as in the case of poison ivy) to years (as with dust mites) to occur, and the severity depends on the individual's sensitivity. Virtually anything—from plants to metals to chemicals in shoes, clothing, and carpeting—can cause allergic contact dermatitis in susceptible individuals. *Photoallergic contact dermatitis* is a form of the disorder in which the combination of exposure to an allergen plus exposure to light results in a reaction.

Atopic dermatitis is an itching skin problem whose cause is unknown. Most doctors believe it to be limited to genetically predisposed individuals, such as those with a family history of allergies. The severity is highly variable, but atopic dermatitis usually causes enough itching to make it difficult to avoid scratching the area, which can lead to sec-

ondary problems. The condition may spread to wide areas of the body, and breaks in the skin caused by scratching can pave the way for bacterial or fungal infection.

Less common forms of dermatitis include neurodermatitis, nummular dermatitis, exfoliative dermatitis, and stasis dermatitis. *Neurodermatitis* appears to have a strong psychological component. In this syndrome, itching leads to scratching, which in turn causes the development of lesions and more itching. The scratching may even be unconscious. *Nummular dermatitis* is most common in middle-aged people, especially during dry winter months. It is characterized by the appearance of coin-shaped itching, scaling, or crusting areas that can come and go maddeningly. *Exfoliative dermatitis* (also known as general dermatitis) can cover wide areas of the body, and often no cause is found, though some cases may be caused by reactions to medication. The skin can be severely affected, to the point that whole areas can slough off. This can occur quickly or slowly, with varying degrees of itching and/or pain. It is important to try to identify the cause of the problem, as the scaling and peeling of the skin can be severe enough to be life-threatening. In severe cases, an underlying illness such as lymphoma can be involved. *Stasis dermatitis* is a problem of the lower legs in which the return of blood to the heart is impaired. This causes swelling around the ankle(s), and the skin becomes thickened to the point of being taut and leathery. Eventually, the lack of blood flow can allow infections and, in many cases, open ulceration to develop. Varicose veins may be involved, but this disorder can occur without them.

Eczema, psoriasis, and seborrhea also are considered types of dermatitis, but these disorders are discussed separately (*see* ECZEMA; PSORIASIS; and/or SEBORRHEA).

CONVENTIONAL TREATMENT

■ Treatment begins with the search for the cause. This can be difficult, but it is worth the effort. If fungal, bacterial, or parasitic infection is involved, for example, it is difficult to clear a dermatitis problem without addressing the cause.

■ Steroids, whether oral or topical, are a mainstay of treatment for most types of dermatitis. Examples include cortisone, fluocinolone, prednisone, and triamcinolone. The use of these drugs must be carefully monitored. Because they can be dramatically effective, it can be tempting to continue them for long periods, but this can lead to a breakdown of normal skin defenses over time, with resulting changes in skin texture and color. Also, cortisone is absorbed into the body even with topical use, which can cause problems resulting from suppression of adrenal function over time. Steroid use is also associated with an increased risk of glaucoma.

■ If steroids alone are not adequate, an antifungal and/or

antibacterial drug may be tried. These can be taken topically or orally.

■ Antihistamines such as diphenhydramine (Benadryl) or hydroxyzine (Atarax, Vistaril) may be effective in controlling the itching of many forms of dermatitis. These too may be taken orally or applied topically. The oral forms can cause drowsiness. However, that side effect may be useful if you are having difficulty sleeping due to severe itching.

■ For some types of dermatitis (*not* the photoallergic variety), exposure to ultraviolet light may help the skin clear considerably, especially on the hands and feet.

■ In severe cases, the drug isotretinoin (Accutane) may be tried. This drug can have serious side effects, however, including increased cholesterol and blood-sugar levels, liver damage, kidney damage, and blood-chemistry changes. It must never be taken by a woman who is pregnant, or who might become pregnant, as it is extremely damaging to a developing fetus and can cause birth defects.

■ For stasis dermatitis, treatment includes elevation of the affected extremity *above the level of the heart* to assist in returning fluids to the heart.

DIETARY GUIDELINES

■ Use an elimination diet to investigate whether food allergies or sensitivities may be contributing to the problem. Food allergies and sensitivities can aggravate many skin conditions. Among the most commonly allergenic foods are dairy products and foods containing gluten, a protein found in wheat, rye, barley, and oats.

■ A deficiency of biotin, one of the B vitamins, is associated with dry, scaly skin. Include in your diet foods that are good sources of biotin, such as soy foods, garlic, sesame, and barley (if you are not sensitive to gluten).

NUTRITIONAL SUPPLEMENTS

■ The B vitamins are important for healthy skin. Take a B-complex supplement that supplies 50 milligrams of each of the major B vitamins three times a day for one month. Then cut back to two doses daily.

■ Cod liver oil is an effective natural anti-inflammatory. Take 1 teaspoon twice a day.

■ Evening primrose oil and flaxseed oil contain essential fatty acids that are useful for moisturizing the skin and reducing inflammation. Take 1 teaspoon (or 500 to 1,000 milligrams in capsule form) of either three times daily.

■ Vitamin A and the carotenes are very important for the health of the skin. Take 10,000 international units of vitamin A two or three times daily for two weeks, then cut back to 10,000 international units daily. Also take a mixed carotene complex containing alpha-, beta-, and gamma-carotene, as well as lycopene. Take 5 milligrams three times daily.

Note: If you are pregnant, or intend to get pregnant, or if you have liver disease, consult your doctor before taking supplemental vitamin A. Pregnant women should not ingest a total of more than 25,000 international units of supplemental vitamin A *per week* from all sources.

■ Zinc promotes healing. Take 15 milligrams three times daily, before meals. If you take over 30 milligrams of zinc on a daily basis for more than one or two months, you should also take 1 to 2 milligrams of copper each day to maintain a proper mineral balance.

HERBAL TREATMENT

■ The following herbal program is very helpful for dermatitis. These herbs have an antibacterial effect and contain valuable nutrients.

Week 1: Take 500 milligrams of goldenseal three times daily, with meals.

Week 2: Take 500 milligrams of red clover three times daily.

Week 3: Take 500 milligrams of burdock root three times dail, with meals.

Week 4: Take 500 milligrams of pau d'arco three times daily, with meals.

Week 5: Take 500 milligrams of quercetin three to four times daily. Then repeat the entire sequence.

HOMEOPATHY

■ *Psorinum* is good for dermatitis behind the ears, scalp, and/or in the bends of the joints. Your skin is worse if you drink coffee, and you may have a tendency toward respiratory problems such as asthma. Take one dose of *Psorinum* 200x or 200c weekly for three weeks.

■ *Sulfur* is good for skin that is dry and scaly, and feels worse with warmth and in springtime and damp weather. Take one dose of *Sulfur* 30x or 15c three times daily for up to three days.

■ *Vinca minor* is helpful for skin that is very sensitive, red, and sore, with intense itching. Take one dose of *Vinca minor* 6x or 3c three times daily for up to three days.

BACH FLOWER REMEDIES

Select the remedy that most closely fits your disposition and emotional tendencies and concerns, and take it as needed, following the directions on the product label.

■ Chicory helps to counteract a lack of self-confidence.

■ Crabapple is good if you feel "dirty" as a result of your skin problem.

■ Holly helps to tame anger.

■ Impatiens calms impatience and irritability.

■ White Chestnut relieves a tendency toward obsessive thinking.

AROMATHERAPY

For specific instructions on how to use aromatherapy, *see* PREPARING AROMATHERAPY TREATMENTS in Part Three.

■ To reduce inflammation and ease itching, use aromatherapy baths or compresses prepared with one to three of the following essential oils: elemi, geranium, lavender, myrrh, neroli, and rose. You can also add a few drops of one to three of these oils to a small quantity of jojoba oil to make a healing body oil.

Note: Be careful not to use too much essential oil in these treatments, and never apply essential oil directly to your skin. Always dilute it in water or a carrier oil. If irritation results, discontinue use of the suspect oil.

GENERAL RECOMMENDATIONS

■ Keep your skin clean, but treat it gently. Avoid harsh soaps and greasy lotions. Use only hypoallergenic skincare products. Keep your bath or shower water warm, not hot; hot water dries out the skin and makes it more vulnerable.

■ Wear loose, comfortable clothing made of natural fibers that breathe, and try to avoid becoming overheated. Perspiration can aggravate the problem.

■ It can be hard to do, but strictly avoid picking at or scratching your skin. This only makes dermatitis worse. It also increases the possibility of infection.

PREVENTION

■ It may not be possible to prevent dermatitis from developing, but it goes without saying that you should avoid contact with anything that has triggered an outbreak in the past.

Diabetes

Diabetes mellitus is a chronic disorder characterized by insufficient or defective production of insulin, a hormone produced by the pancreas. Insulin plays an essential role in the metabolism of carbohydrates. As carbohydrates go through the digestive system, they are broken down further and further into their basic components. Glucose, a simple sugar, is one of the final breakdown products of carbohydrates. Every cell in the body needs and uses glucose as its fuel; glucose gives our cells the energy to perform their tasks. Insulin functions as a "key" that opens the "doors" of the cells to let the glucose in. Thus, even though the body may have an abundant supply of glucose, without insulin, it cannot get into the cells, and without glucose, the cells do not have the energy they need to function properly.

The first symptoms of diabetes include increased frequency of urination, increased and often extreme thirst, increased appetite, weight loss (often despite increased consumption of food), irritability, and fatigue. These symptoms usually appear over a period of about three weeks.

The short-term complications of diabetes include episodes of both very low and very high blood sugar. When blood sugar is abnormally low, you may feel dizzy, lethargic, and irritable; be pale and sweaty; have a headache; and experience a loss of coordination. Such a mild hypoglycemic episode is treated by consuming a quick-acting sugar, such as in the form of orange juice, raisins, or honey. A more severe episode may require hospitalization and an intravenous infusion of glucose. A high blood sugar episode can lead to a condition known as diabetic ketoacidosis, which, if untreated, can be life-threatening. Initial symptoms of developing ketoacidosis include increased thirst, frequent urination, nausea and vomiting, and a peculiar smell on the breath. Diabetic ketoacidosis is treated in the hospital with intravenous infusions of insulin, fluids, glucose, and electrolytes.

Diabetes can also lead to serious long-term complications. These include vision problems, kidney disease, cardiovascular disease, and nerve problems. Diabetes can also complicate pregnancy. The good news is that maintaining close control over blood sugar, allowing fewer and less dramatic rises in blood glucose, helps to delay the onset and slow the progression of the common complications of the disease. The downside of this is that it increases the risk of reducing your blood-sugar level too far and increases the chances of weight gain, but if you work with your physician, you can usually achieve a successful compromise.

There are two types of diabetes mellitus, type I and type II. Type I diabetes, also sometimes called *insulin-dependent diabetes* or *juvenile-onset diabetes*, is usually diagnosed in childhood and involves such a severe lack of insulin that it must be taken by injection every day. Type II diabetes, also known as *noninsulin-dependent diabetes* or *adult-onset diabetes*, most often occurs in obese people who are age forty or older. These individuals typically have higher than normal amounts of insulin in their blood, but their bodies resist its blood-sugar-regulating action. This type of diabetes can sometimes be managed with diet and oral medication rather than insulin injections.

The most reliable method of diagnosing diabetes involves a glucose tolerance test. This test measures the concentration of glucose in the blood after an overnight fast.

The normal range is between 70 and 100 milligrams per deciliter (mg/dL). A blood concentration of 140 mg/dL or higher is considered an indication of diabetes.

In addition to diabetes mellitus, there is a condition known as *diabetes insipidus*. This is a problem caused by the failure of the hypothalamus to release sufficient anti-diuretic hormone. The kidneys become unable to conserve water, resulting in the passage of large amounts of urine. This condition is often accompanied by a voracious appetite, loss of strength, and emaciation. Diabetes insipidus is less common than diabetes mellitus, which affects more than 10 million people in the United States.

Treatment of diabetes is based on maintaining a normal blood-glucose level so that the body will have enough energy to function properly. Diabetes is a lifelong challenge that must be carefully taken care of in order to avoid long-term complications. Because of the complexity and intricacies of treatment, a person who has diabetes should work with a physician and nurse who specialize in the treatment of this illness. A regional hospital or a diabetes center is a good place to start looking for information and references. In addition to conventional medical treatment and dietary modifications, herbs, homeopathy, acupressure, and nutritional supplements can be used to support the endocrine system. Because each person responds differently to this disease, it is best to work closely with qualified professionals. We advise that you choose a medical doctor who is willing to work with a natural health care practitioner (and vice versa). Each of these professionals needs to know what the other is doing, as the interventions of one can affect the treatments of the other.

CONVENTIONAL TREATMENT

Conventional treatment for diabetes involves three key components: insulin, diet, and exercise. These work together to help regulate blood-glucose levels.

■ If you have type I diabetes, your body is not producing adequate amounts of insulin and you will need either oral supplements or injections to get this essential hormone. If you need to give yourself insulin injections, you must learn this important skill from a clinic or hospital nurse. Within a few weeks or months of beginning insulin treatment, your insulin needs may decrease significantly. In fact, you may not need insulin at all at this point. You should be aware, however, that while this "honeymoon period" can last for up to two years, eventually you will need to go back to taking insulin. There are many intricacies involved in dealing with insulin injections. For example, it is important to take the injection in a different spot each day. You should learn about the different types of insulin, as well as the blood and urine tests that are used

---

Might I Have Diabetes?

The American Diabetes Association estimates that there are 8 million Americans who are unaware they have diabetes. Early diagnosis means that treatment can begin before the disease causes damage to the eyes, heart, kidneys, and nerves. The association has therefore issued a new set of guidelines for diabetes testing. They recommend that all adults be tested for diabetes every three years, starting at age forty-five. Those who have high readings should have the test repeated another day. People considered at higher than normal risk should be tested earlier and more often. This group includes anyone who is overweight or has high blood pressure, high cholesterol, or a family history of the disease. People of African, Asian, Latino, and Native American descent are considered to be at higher risk that people of other backgrounds. To assess your personal risk of developing diabetes, take the following test, prepared by the American Diabetes Association, and add up the results:

1. *I weigh at least 20 percent more than is recommended for a medium-framed person of my height.*   True = 5 points   False = 0 points

2. *I am under 65, and I get little or no exercise during a usual day.*   True = 5 points   False = 0 points

3. *I am a woman who has had a baby weighing more than 9 pounds at birth.*   True = 1 point   False = 0 points

4. *I have a sister or brother with diabetes.*   True = 1 point   False = 0 points

5. *I have a parent with diabetes.*   True = 1 point   False = 0 points

If your score adds up to between 3 and 9 points, your risk of diabetes is low.
If your score is 10 or more, you are at high risk. See your health-care provider.   _____ TOTAL SCORE

to monitor sugar and insulin levels. These are some of the many areas you will explore as you learn to live with diabetes.

■ Attention to diet is important. Too many carbohydrates can increase blood sugar; too few will lower it. People with diabetes have the same nutritional and caloric requirements as other people, but they need a diet that is carefully designed to give them the correct balance of carbohydrates, protein, and fats. Simply cutting out sugar is not enough. A successful diet plan includes all types of foods. Once you are taking insulin, it is important to eat appropriately so that your blood sugar doesn't fall too low and cause a hypoglycemic reaction. Also, you will need to eat at the same times each day. You need to eat a snack at midmorning and midafternoon, and you must eat the same number of calories from one day to the next. Five small meals a day are better than three large ones.

■ Exercise is important because it helps to lower blood-glucose levels, strengthen the body, and improve glucose and insulin management. Your doctor may recommend that you eat a snack before exercise so that your blood-sugar level is stable throughout the activity.

■ If you have type II diabetes and are overweight, the treatment of choice is weight loss. If this is not successful, the next step is to try hypoglycemic (blood-sugar-reducing) medicines that are taken orally. These drugs act primarily by stimulating the pancreas to secrete additional insulin. In many cases, however, even this is not enough and insulin, given either orally or by injections, is necessary. As with type I diabetes, appropriate diet and adequate exercise are essential.

■ For years, the sulfonylureas have been the oral medications of choice for type II diabetes. These drugs work by forcing the pancreas to secrete more insulin. Examples include tolbutamide (Orinase), tolazamide (Tolinase), acetohexamide (Dymelor), chlorpropamide (Diabinese), and the newer glyburide (Diaβeta, Glynase, Micronase), glipizide (Glucotrol), and glymeperide (Amaryl), which tend to be stronger and more expensive. While all these drugs work in a similar way, their strength and duration of action vary. Potential side effects also are similar, and include liver problems, low blood sugar, nausea, and an increased risk of heart disease.

■ Metformin (Glucophage), another oral diabetes agent, seems to stabilize both fasting and postprandial (after-meal) levels of blood sugar in adults, though how it works is not understood. It does not cause low blood sugar problems, and is more widely used for obese individuals than the sulfonylureas are. However, side effects of nausea, vomiting, diarrhea, and abdominal pain are common. Cardiovascular problems can be a problem with this drug, too.

■ Acarbose (Precose) is an oral agent that lowers blood sugar by competing with carbohydrates for absorption in the intestional tract rather than by stimulating the release of insulin. Because of this, it can cause a significant increase in bowel gas, diarrhea, and abdominal pain, especially when carbohydrates are ingested. It can be combined with drugs of other types used for blood-sugar control.

■ The U.S. Food and Drug Administration (FDA) recently approved a drug called troglitazone (sold under the brand name Rezulin) that can resensitize the body to insulin. About 15 percent of patients involved in the testing of this drug no longer needed insulin shots once they started taking it. Most patients in the study still needed insulin, but required fewer injections. If you have type II diabetes, you may wish to consult your doctor about the possibility of trying this drug.

■ No matter what type of diabetes you have, it is important that you get regular eye examinations as well as special periodic blood and urine tests to screen for cholesterol and kidney changes. (*See* CHOLESTEROL, HIGH; KIDNEY DISEASE; RETINOPATHY, DIABETIC/VASCULAR.)

DIETARY GUIDELINES

■ Most meal plans for people with diabetes begin by estimating the number of calories you need to maintain a realistic weight. Then 50 to 65 percent of the total daily calories are allocated for complex carbohydrates (grains, vegetables, legumes), 20 to 30 percent for protein, and 15 to 30 (or less) percent for fats.

■ To prevent the development of heart disease, it is important to limit your intake of saturated animal fats and hydrogenated and partially hydrogenated oils. Don't fry foods; use low-fat or skim-milk dairy products; purchase canned foods packed in water rather than in oil; remove the skin from turkey, chicken, and fish; and limit or eliminate red meat.

■ Artichokes, cabbage, and fresh greens are very beneficial. These foods are high in minerals and exert a regulatory effect on liver and gallbladder function, especially important in the digestion of fats.

■ Eat a diet high in fiber, especially soluble fiber. Eat plenty of fresh vegetables, whole-grain cereals, brown rice, barley, millet, and oats. Oat bran seems to be particularly helpful for maintaining a steady blood-sugar level.

■ Include garlic and onions in your diet whenever possible. These foods also help control blood-sugar levels.

■ Include in your diet blueberries, bilberries, blackberries, cranberries, grapes, huckleberries, plums, and raspberries. All of these fruits contain phytochemicals that have a protective effect on the eyes, a source of major concern for people with diabetes.

■ To maintain even blood-sugar levels, eat five small meals a day rather than the usual three. Eating less food at one time places less stress on the pancreas.

■ Avoid alcohol and refined sugar. These substances cause a rapid rise in blood sugar, followed by an equally rapid drop. This roller-coaster effect can be dangerous.

■ Avoid caffeine, which stimulates the release of insulin, causing a drop in blood sugar.

■ Drink plenty of water, but avoid soft water. It has been shown that the incidence of diabetes is higher in soft-water areas. Drink natural, noncarbonated mineral or spring water that contains a good supply of naturally occurring trace minerals.

NUTRITIONAL SUPPLEMENTS

■ In general, a good multivitamin and mineral supplement is useful for people with diabetes. Choose a formula that provides at least the recommended daily allowance (RDA) of all the major vitamins and minerals, and follow the dosage directions on the product label.

■ Beta-carotene and vitamin D can be helpful for people with diabetes. Take 10,000 international units of beta-carotene twice a day and 200 to 400 international units of vitamin D daily.

■ Chromium helps to stabilize blood sugar. Take 100 micrograms of chromium twice a day. If you are battling diabetic retinopathy, take 200 micrograms twice daily for three months, then reduce to 100 micrograms daily. Though GTF chromium is probably the best absorbed form of this mineral, most of the studies that have been done on the use of chromium have used chromium chloride, the cheapest form, which seems to be adequately effective. Recent studies have shown that doses up to 1,000 micrograms (1 milligram) can be very effective for managing type II diabetes, and if you are considering taking chromium in such doses, the economy of using chromium chloride may become significant. Chromium does not appear to be toxic even in very high doses, but you should discuss this approach with your doctor before taking megadoses.

■ Coenzyme Q_{10} is an antioxidant that fights free-radical damage and is a blood oxygenator. Because the eye is so richly supplied with tiny blood vessels, this is another nutrient that can help in cases of retinopathy. Take 50 milligrams of coenzyme Q_{10} twice daily for up to three months, then reduce the dosage to 30 milligrams daily.

■ Gamma-linolenic acid (GLA), found in black currant seed oil, borage oil, and evening primrose oil, has been shown to be helpful for improving damaged nerve function, which is common in diabetes. Take 500 to 1,000 milligrams of any of these oils twice daily.

■ Germanium and selenium are antioxidant minerals. Take 10 milligrams of germanium and 200 micrograms of selenium daily.

Note: Do not take germanium if you have, or have a history of, any kidney disorder.

■ Green-foods supplements are full of trace minerals and help to energize the blood. Take a green-foods supplement as directed on the product label.

■ Lipoic acid has shown considerable promise in protecting the cells in the pancreas that manufacture insulin. It seems to be helpful for both type I and type II diabetes, which is unusual. Take 100 to 500 milligrams daily.

■ People with diabetes have a tendency to lose excessive amounts of minerals in their urine. Take a multimineral formula that includes 1,200 milligrams of calcium, 600 to 800 milligrams of magnesium, 5 milligrams of manganese, and 15 to 50 milligrams of zinc daily.

■ Take an additional 300 milligrams of magnesium daily. This mineral is especially important for anyone who has a family history of cardiovascular disease.

■ Selenium is a valuable antioxidant mineral. Take 200 micrograms daily.

■ Vanadium, or vanadyl sulfate, may reduce the need for insulin. What is unique about this nutrient is that its effects may persist even after you stop taking it. Take 250 micrograms two or three times daily.

■ Take a good vitamin-B complex supplement daily. The B vitamins are necessary for the processes that convert glucose into energy and for a healthy nervous system.

■ Vitamin C and the bioflavonoids may be useful for preventing damage to the nerves caused by excessively elevated blood sugar. Take 500 to 1,000 milligrams of vitamin C and 500 milligrams of mixed bioflavonoids two to three times daily.

■ People with diabetes have a higher than usual need for vitamin E, which improves insulin activity and acts as an antioxidant and a blood oxygenator. The most impressive study on vitamin E and diabetes used a total of 1,350 international units of d-alpha-tocopheryl acetate daily, divided into three doses. Begin by taking 400 international units each morning. After two weeks, add another dose of 400 international units in the evening. After two more weeks, add another 400 international units in the afternoon.

Note: If you have high blood pressure, limit your intake of supplemental vitamin E to a total of 400 international units daily. If you are taking an anticoagulant (blood thinner), consult your physician before taking supplemental vitamin E.

■ Zinc is helpful in regulating insulin metabolism. Take up to 50 milligrams of zinc daily from all sources, including your multivitamin and mineral supplement.

Note: Take zinc with food to prevent stomach upset. If you take over 30 milligrams of zinc on a daily basis for more than one or two months, you should also take 1 to 2 milligrams of copper each day to maintain a proper mineral balance.

HERBAL TREATMENT

■ Blueberry leaf tea has been used historically for insulin regulation. This herb also contains anthocyanidins, which help to protect the eyes. Take a cup of blueberry leaf tea two or three times daily. With repeated use, your need for insulin may be reduced.

■ Bilberry, a botanical relative of blueberry, increases natural insulin production in the body. You can take it instead of (or on an alternating basis with) blueberry leaf tea. Select a product containing 25 percent anthocyanidins (also called PCOs) and take 80 milligrams two or three times daily.

■ Bitter melon aids in the regulation of blood sugar. Take 200 milligrams of standardized bitter melon extract three times a day.

■ Garlic can be helpful in regulating blood sugar. Take at least 1 fresh clove or 1,000 milligrams of dried extract daily.

■ *Gymnema sylvestre*, an herb also known as gurmar, decreases cravings for sweets and helps to control blood sugar. Take 500 milligrams of standardized extract three times a day.

■ Siberian ginseng is an energizer and may help to stabilize blood sugar. Choose a product containing 0.5 percent eleutheroside E and take it according to following program:

Weeks 1–3: Take 100 milligrams in the morning, preferably one-half hour before breakfast.

Weeks 4–7: Add a second 100-milligram dose in the afternoon (but before 2:00 PM).

Weeks 8–12: Take 100 milligrams one-half hour before breakfast, another dose three hours later, and a third dose three hours after that.

After twelve weeks, switch to another herb, such as milk thistle, which strengthens liver function. Choose an extract standardized to contain 80 percent flavonoids (silymarin) and take 200 to 300 milligrams twice daily for one to two months. Another useful herb to consider is fenugreek, which can be taken in tea or capsule form. It has been shown to assist in blood-sugar regulation as well as to increase HDL, the so-called "good cholesterol." Take a cup of fenugreek tea, or 500 milligrams in capsule form, two or three times daily for one to two months. After two months off Siberian ginseng, you can begin the entire rotation over again.

GENERAL RECOMMENDATIONS

■ Glucose-meter readings show your body's response to meals, snacks, exercise, stress, illness, and general habits. In addition to monitoring your insulin levels, keep a diet diary that includes careful notations on everything you consume and the energy you expend. You may find that if you eat a large evening meal and then spend several hours sitting and watching television, your insulin levels skyrocket. Chances are that the same meal followed by a brisk twenty-minute walk might not cause a rise in your insulin level. On examination of your diet diary, you and your physician can work together to devise a diet suited to your tastes and lifestyle.

■ Monitor your blood-sugar level carefully. Insulin requirements can change over time.

■ Keep your weight down. Excess fat actually decreases the number of insulin receptors present in the body, aggravating diabetes. If you are already overweight, slim down. Avoid overeating and emphasize healthy whole foods. In addition to managing your blood-sugar levels appropriately, follow your doctor's recommendations for a weight-reducing diet.

■ Exercise. Both types of diabetes can be greatly improved with a regular moderate exercise program. Aerobic activities such as brisk walking, running, cycling, and swimming have a proven beneficial effect on blood-sugar levels. The utilization of glucose by the exercising muscles improves, and the improvement can last for up to seventy-two hours. Exercise also improves the blood-lipid (fat) profile and helps control blood pressure. Remember, however, that you must carefully monitor your blood sugar during exercise in order to avoid possible overdoses of insulin.

■ Appropriate support for your family is an essential part of successful treatment and a long and happy life. Dealing with a chronic illness is not easy, and it affects many aspects of a family's life. The American Diabetes Association has chapters throughout the country and can help you find needed support for everyone in your family. (See the Resources section at the end of the book.)

PREVENTION

■ Avoid consuming excessive amounts of refined carbohydrates, and keep your weight down. While there is no sure way to prevent diabetes, these measures may help.

Diarrhea

Diarrhea, or frequent and watery stools, is the body's way of ridding itself of toxins and foreign substances. Most cases of simple diarrhea should not be suppressed too quickly. It may be healthier to allow your body to flush itself clean, as long as you can support it with adequate fluids.

There are many microorganisms that can cause diarrhea, including viruses, bacteria, fungi, and protozoa. You can pick up viruses, bacteria, or protozoa from other people or from contaminated food and water. Food poisoning causes diarrhea very quickly. Food allergies and sensitivities can also cause diarrhea.

Less common causes of diarrhea include reactions to drugs, including alcohol; inflammatory bowel disease; hepatitis; cystic fibrosis; and pancreatitis. An anatomical deformity, such as a fistula, or a congenital defect, such as Hirschsprung's disease or short bowel syndrome, can also cause diarrhea. If your diarrhea arises from any of these conditions, you require medical attention.

Most cases of simple diarrhea are caused by viruses. Viruses invade the intestinal tract, causing irritation and inflammation of the intestinal walls. Viruses also induce the cells lining the intestines to secrete fluids. The increase in fluid volume in turn increases peristalsis, the wavelike contractions of the intestines. The result is cramping and the loose, watery, frequent stools characteristic of diarrhea.

Vomiting and stomachache often accompany diarrhea, and abdominal cramps usually come and go, often occurring right before a bowel movement. Depending on the cause of the diarrhea, you may or may not have a fever. When you are suffering from diarrhea, dehydration is always a concern, especially if your temperature is elevated.

If you are alert and are not experiencing cramping between episodes, it's safe to assume your body has the situation under control. But if diarrhea lasts for longer than forty-eight hours or comes and goes over a period of two weeks or longer, or if you feel weak, have cramping that is not relieved between episodes, experience severe or persistent abdominal pain with diarrhea, or have blood in the stool, call your doctor.

CONVENTIONAL TREATMENT

■ Loperamide (sold as Imodium AD and other products) is the most commonly used antidiarrheal. It works by slowing the movement of the intestinal muscle. You should not use this drug if you have a fever over 101°F, or if you have bloody stools.

■ Kaolin-pectin (Donnagel, Kaopectate, Parapectolin), an over-the-counter drug, binds with excess water, thereby solidifying and drying diarrheal stools. This makes it appear as if you are having less diarrhea and more formed stools, but you are actually still losing the same amount of water as you would be if untreated. It just looks different. Kaolin medications give a false sense of reassurance. Moreover, kaolin contains aluminum, which has been implicated as a toxic mineral in the body.

■ Bismuth subsalicylate (Pepto-Bismol) is an over-the-counter drug that works by attaching to the toxin or bacteria that is causing the problem in the intestines. This deactivates the foreign substance and it loses its ability to hurt the body. This medication can turn the stools black.

■ Antibiotics can help, but only if the diarrhea is due to a parasitic or bacterial infection. They should be prescribed only after a stool analysis or culture confirms this.

■ Antidiarrheal medications that contain narcotics, such as paregoric and diphenoxylate (Lomotil), are sometimes prescribed. Like loperamide, these drugs work by slowing down intestinal action and halting bowel movements. These are powerful drugs and they can have significant side effects.

■ If severe diarrhea results in dehydration, rehydration may be necessary. In most cases, this can be accomplished through the diet (see under Dietary Guidelines, below). However, in rare cases, it may be necessary to use intravenous fluids.

DIETARY GUIDELINES

■ Your primary concern when dealing with diarrhea is to prevent dehydration. During the acute phase of diarrhea, when the stools are frequent and watery, make sure you take in enough fluids. Take frequent small sips or drinks of water. You may wish to use an oral electrolyte drink such as Gatorade. Or you can use a homemade formula containing $1/2$ to 1 teaspoon salt, 1 teaspoon baking soda, 4 teaspoons table sugar, and 1 pint of fruit juice added to 1 pint of good spring water. However, it is not well established that using an electrolyte formula is much more effective than sipping broth, or even good spring water, and allowing lost minerals to be replaced in foods once the appetite returns.

■ As long as you are acutely sick with diarrhea, you probably will not want to eat very much. It is better not to force yourself to eat solid foods until your body responds with a renewed interest in food. Sip clear liquids, such as spring water, broths, diluted apple juice, and herbal teas. Avoid filling your stomach, so that your stomach and intestines will have time to rest and heal. An upset digestive tract is like any other injury. Do not expect it to heal overnight.

■ If you have repeated episodes of diarrhea, rest your gastrointestinal tract as much as possible. To avoid dehydration, take repeated small sips of water, miso soup, or diluted fruit juices.

■ If you are vomiting in addition to having diarrhea, even a small sip of water may cause another upset. If vomiting occurs after you drink water, wait one hour and then suck on small chips of ice. If the vomiting reflex is not triggered by the ice, after an hour of calm has passed, take more chips of ice or small sips of water. As an alternative, try taking a teaspoon of Emetrol syrup or raw honey to settle your stomach.

■ As you start to feel better, eat a simple diet so that your digestive tract can easily process and absorb nutrients. Start by drinking barley or rice water in small sips throughout the day. Carrot soup and cooked carrots are also good. (*See* THERAPEUTIC RECIPES in Part Three.)

As improvement continues, eat foods that are easily digested and absorbed, such as puréed rice, bananas, dry cereal, crackers, toast, mashed potatoes (without butter), well-cooked vegetables, and grains.

To give your intestines time to settle and heal, avoid dairy products during an episode of diarrhea and for two weeks after it is resolved.

Eliminate foods that are difficult to digest. Protein foods should be avoided for about forty-eight hours. Fats should be eliminated from the diet during any illness. They are difficult even for a healthy body to digest, and having a distressed intestinal tract makes it even harder. Undigested fats contribute to a toxic internal environment.

■ Eliminate refined sugars, especially if the diarrhea is bacterial in origin. Bacteria thrive in the presence of sugar. Sugar also makes the body more acidic. An overly acidic internal environment slows healing.

■ Avoid stimulants such as coffee, tea, and alcohol, as they stress the intestinal tract.

NUTRITIONAL SUPPLEMENTS

The amino acid glutamine helps to soothe an irritated and inflamed gastrointestinal tract. Take 500 milligrams of L-glutamine three times daily until the diarrhea resolves.

Bifidobacterium bifidum restores healthy flora to the intestines and is very helpful in resolving diarrhea. Select a product with a count of 5 to 10 billion viable (live) bacteria per capsule or half-teaspoon of powder, guaranteed through a printed expiration date, and take it, as recommended on the product labels, twice daily for five days.

Pectin is available in the canning sections of grocery stores and in health-food stores. Take 300 milligrams up to three times daily, as needed.

HERBAL TREATMENT

Curing Pills, a Chinese herbal formula, help to resolve a wide variety of digestive problems, including diarrhea. Take ²/₃ to 1 tube or 2 droppersful three times daily.

■ Goldenseal helps to control diarrhea that is caused by a bacterial infection. Take 20 to 40 drops of liquid goldenseal extract three times daily for two days. Or take 300 milligrams in capsule form three times daily for two days.

A cream made from kuzu root and umeboshi (salt)

plum paste is helpful for easing intestinal upset (*see* THERAPEUTIC RECIPES in Part Three).

■ Powdered slippery elm bark is healing and comforting to intestines in distress. Slippery elm has little taste. Make the powder with just enough water, apple juice, or applesauce to make a paste, and take 1 tablespoon two to three times daily. You can also take 500 milligrams of slippery elm in capsule in place of 1 tablespoon of paste.

HOMEOPATHY

Select a symptom-specific remedy from the suggestions below. Unless otherwise directed, take one dose, as directed on the product label, three to four times a day until symptoms are relieved. The right remedy should work within forty-eight hours. If symptoms are not relieved in forty-eight hours, try another remedy.

■ If you developed diarrhea after eating too much sugar, take *Argentum nitricum* 30x or 9c.

■ *Arsenicum album* 30x or 9c helps to resolve diarrhea related to food poisoning, anxiety, or stress.

■ If the diarrhea occured after you ate dairy products, take *Calcarea carbonica* 30x or 9c.

■ If abdominal bloating and diarrhea are caused by eating too much fruit, take *China* 30x or 9c.

■ *Colocynthis* 12x or 6c is very effective against the twisting and cramping abdominal pain that often accompanies diarrhea.

■ *Magnesia phosphorica* 12x or 6c helps relax the bowel and ease cramping.

■ For any kind of abdominal pain, alternating *Colocynthis* with *Magnesia phosphorica* is excellent. You should not need to take these remedies for more than twenty-four hours.

■ If you have greenish, foul-smelling diarrhea, use *Mercurius solubilis* 30x or 9c.

■ If you have a tendency toward recurrent diarrhea and crave salt, take *Natrum muriaticum* 30x or 9c.

■ If diarrhea is a result of eating fatty foods, take *Pulsatilla* 30x or 9c.

■ If none of the above remedies seems right, a homeopathic combination diarrhea remedy may be helpful.

BACH FLOWER REMEDIES

■ If you suspect that the diarrhea is emotionally based, try Mimulus. It helps to balance emotions. Take it as needed, following the directions on the product label.

ACUPRESSURE

For the location of acupressure points on the body, *see* ADMINISTERING AN ACUPRESSURE TREATMENT in Part Three.

Large Intestine 11 helps to regulate the large intestine.

■ Stomach 36 tones the digestive system.

AROMATHERAPY

For specific instructions on how to use aromatherapy, *see* PREPARING AROMATHERAPY TREATMENTS in Part Three.

Essential oil of chamomile, lavender, and peppermint can help relieve stomach spasms and cramping. Use any or all of these oils in an aromatherapy bath or add a few drops to massage oil.

GENERAL RECOMMENDATIONS

If you suffer repeated bouts of diarrhea, you may have a lactose intolerance. (*See* LACTOSE INTOLERANCE.)

PREVENTION

Always wash your hands properly after going to the bathroom, when working in the kitchen, and before eating.

Many episodes of diarrhea are triggered by ingesting contaminated food or water. Mild cases of food poisoning are often mistaken for the flu. *See* FOOD POISONING for effective preventive measures you can take to guard against food poisoning,

Try to eliminate any food allergies or sensitivities as a cause of diarrhea. Common allergens include citrus fruits, wheat, sugar, and dairy products.

Acidophilus and bifidobacteria restore the friendly bacteria required to keep the intestinal tract free of many organisms that can cause diarrhea. These probiotic supplements qualify as true preventive medicine.

Digestive Problems

See CELIAC DISEASE; COLITIS, ULCERATIVE; CONSTIPATION; CROHN'S DISEASE; DIARRHEA; DIVERTICULAR DISEASE; FOOD POISONING; GAS, INTESTINAL; GASTRITIS; HERNIA, HIATAL; INDIGESTION; IRRITABLE BOWEL SYNDROME; LACTOSE INTOLERANCE; MALABSORPTION/MALNUTRITION; MOTION SICKNESS; NAUSEA AND VOMITING; PARASITES, INTESTINAL.

Discoid Lupus Erythematosus

See under LUPUS.

Diverticular Disease

Diverticuli are small saclike protrusions that develop in the lower part of the large intestine, or colon, and project into the abdominal cavity. The presence of diverticuli is called *diverticulosis.* Although diverticuli can occur anywhere in the gastrointestinal tract, the most common site is in the lower left side of the abdomen, the area where the colon meets the rectum.

The development of diverticuli is generally attributed to a low-fiber diet of refined and processed foods. Insufficient amounts of fiber and water in the diet lead to the formation of small hard, dry stools that are difficult to pass. Straining during bowel movements then causes pressure on the intestinal walls. Portions of the walls that have been weakened by constant straining can develop diverticuli.

Symptoms of diverticulosis can include chronic constipation alternating with diarrhea, and excessive flatulence. Cramping pain may occur in the the affected part of the gastrointestinal tract, and the area may be tender to the touch. Pain is usually relieved by passing gas or having a bowel movement. If the diverticuli bleed, bright red blood may occur in some stools. Surprisingly, however, fully 80 percent of people with diverticulosis have no symptoms at all, and many others mistake its recurring symptoms for occasional bouts of indigestion. In some cases, the condition is discovered during examination for another complaint.

Diverticulosis is rare in people under twenty. It is estimated that more than 50 percent of Americans over the age of sixty have this condition, and the incidence increases with age.

A small percentage of people with diverticulosis go on to develop *diverticulitis,* or inflammation of the diverticuli. Diverticulitis develops when bits of fecal matter become trapped in the diverticuli and cause infection. This condition can cause cramping and severe abdominal pain, primarily in the lower left part of the abdomen. Pressure increases the pain, and nausea and fever are not uncommon. In some people, diverticulitis can flare up and cause disabling pain within a few hours. Others experience mild discomfort over a period of several days, followed by severe pain and more serious symptoms.

If diverticulitis is ignored and remains untreated, complications can occur. For example, a stricture can develop, narrowing the intestines at the site of the inflammation, or a fistula may occur. A fistula is an abnormal opening that connects one part of the intestine to another. Or an abscess may form in or around the colon, and peritonitis can develop. Peritonitis is an inflammation of the peritoneum, the membrane that forms the protective lining of the abdominal cavity. Symptoms of peritonitis include swelling and severe abdominal pain that increases with movement and may be accompanied by nausea, vomiting, chills and fever, and a rapid heartbeat. Dehydration is a common complication, and shock may occur, causing the heart rate and breathing to become faster, but making blood pressure and body temperature fall dangerously, resulting in pale skin, cold sweats, and obvious weakness. If there is even a suspicion that shock is developing, you should call for emergency medical assistance right away.

Risk factors for diverticular disease include poor dietary habits, stress, gallbladder disease, obesity, and cardiovascular disease. Chronic food sensitivities or allergies aggravate diverticulitis, and may contribute to it. Inconsistent eating habits, such as skipping breakfast and/or lunch and overeating at dinner and late in the day, can also contribute to this disease. The processes of the gastrointestinal tract slow down as the body prepares for sleep, which increases the possibility of infection. Diverticular disease seems to run in families. However, the tendency to diverticular disease is probably more related to family eating habits than heredity. Smoking is another a contributing factor.

Diagnosis of diverticulitis may involve a barium enema. In this procedure, a tube is inserted into the rectum to introduce a fluid agent that shows up on x-rays. The x-rays taken after the barium enema show any existing diverticuli, strictures, or fistulas. The bowel must be completely empty beforehand, so usually a plain enema is administered first. Sigmoidoscopy or colonoscopy may be performed as well. In these techniques, the physician uses a narrow, flexible tube with a light at the end to view the affected parts of the colon directly, and, if necessary, to remove tissue samples for biopsy. Either or both of these procedures may be repeated at intervals to judge the effectiveness of treatment.

CONVENTIONAL MEDICINE

■ Uncomplicated diverticulitis is usually treated with multiple antibiotics, such as metronidazole (Flagyl, Metric, Protostat) and ciprofloxacin (Cipro), or sulfamethoxazole plus trimethoprim (Bactrim, Co-trimoxazole, Septra), depending on your individual tolerance to these drugs. Be aware that if you must take antibiotics, you should take a probiotic supplement to reestablish normal bowel flora (see under Nutritional Supplements, below).

■ If the disease becomes acutely painful, hospitalization and treatment with intravenous (IV) fluids and antibiotics may be required. If the bowel is obstructed, it may be necessary to insert a tube that runs from the nose down to the stomach to suction out fluids so they do not accumulate at the site of the obstruction.

■ If divericulitis does not respond to antibiotic treatment, surgery may be required. An estimated 20 to 30 percent of people hospitalized for diverticulitis require surgery to remove the diseased section of the colon. The remaining sections of the colon are then joined together. In some cases, a temporary colostomy may be necessary. If peritonitis develops, emergency surgery to remove the diseased section of the intestine is required, followed by aggressive antibiotic therapy.

■ If diverticular disease is not well developed, you may be able to avoid surgery by increasing the amount of fiber and water in your diet. Bulking agents, such as psyllium and oat bran, may be recommended. Because ingesting too much fiber all at once can cause gas and bloating, your physician will probably tell you to start with a small amount and gradually increase your intake over a period of three to four weeks.

DIETARY GUIDELINES

■ While inflammation is acute and symptoms are severe, eat only bland, easily digested soft foods. Organic baby food is best. If you have diarrhea, eating cooked carrots or carrot soup (see THERAPEUTIC RECIPES in Part Three) can help arrest it.

■ Limit your consumption of the raw grains, fruits, and vegetables. People with diverticular disease often have difficulty completely digesting uncooked complex carbohydrates. Carbohydrates that are not fully digested can ferment, causing more inflammation.

■ Once the diarrhea subsides, maximize your intake of the type of quality protein found in vegetables, fish, chicken, and eggs, which are comparatively easy to digest.

■ Avoid processed foods, greasy or fatty foods, spicy foods, carbonated drinks, alcohol, and red meat. All these items will aggravate symptoms and make you even more uncomfortable.

■ Drink eight 8-ounce glasses of pure water every day. Water is essential for the formation of soft, easily passed stools, and also helps flush toxins from the intestinal tract.

■ Avoid eating seeds, nuts, and other foods with small, hard particles that can become lodged in the diverticuli.

■ Once the condition is under control, eat a diet that is low in fat and high in protein and fiber. A lack of fiber in the diet contributes to diverticulitis. To make sure you get the optimum amount of fiber, maximize your intake of fruits and vegetables, rice, whole grains, and cereals. Thirty grams of fiber per day is the recommended amount.

■ Avoid refined and processed foods, which foster the formation of hard, dry stools.

NUTRITIONAL SUPPLEMENTS

■ If you are suffering from acute inflammation, take 500 milligrams of bromelain three times a day, between meals.

■ To insure full digestion, take a full-spectrum digestive-enzyme supplement containing 5,000 international units of lipase, 2,500 international units of amylase, 300 international units of protease, plus 500 to 1,000 milligrams of pancreatin, with each meal.

Note: Long-term supplementation with pancreatin is not advised, as it can cause your pancreas to reduce its own production of this important enzyme. Overuse also has the potential to cause nausea or diarrhea. After two months on pancreatin, discontinue use and monitor your reaction. If you find that your digestive problems recur, discuss pancreatin supplementation with your health-care provider.

■ The essential fatty acids present in borage oil, evening primrose oil, and flaxseed oil help reduce inflammation and ease the passage of stools by providing lubrication. Use all three, on a rotating basis. Take 1 tablespoon twice a day until the condition is resolved.

■ Probiotic supplements are essential for a healthy intestinal tract, especially if you must take antibiotics. Take supplemental acidophilus and bifidus (either on a rotating basis or in combination) two to three times a day, between meals. If you are allergic to milk, select dairy-free formulas.

■ If your diet does not provide sufficient fiber, take psyllium powder or oat bran. When adding a fiber supplement to your diet, begin slowly and gradually increase to the desired amount. Take the fiber supplement with a full 8-ounce glass of spring water, and at least one hour away from food, other supplements, and any medications.

■ To reduce inflammation and help heal the mucous membranes of the colon, take an antioxidant formula that contains 400 international units of vitamin E daily.

Note: If you are taking an anticoagulant (blood thinner), consult your physician before taking supplemental vitamin E.

HERBAL TREATMENT

■ Aloe vera resolves constipation, and will help heal the mucous membranes of the colon. Select a food-grade product and take $^1/_4$ cup twice a day.

■ If the condition is stress related, resulting in a nervous bowel, take a cup of chamomile or linden tea two or three times daily. Both of these herbs are very soothing to the nervous system. It is best to alternate them with oat straw tea.

■ Garlic is a time-honored remedy with strong antibacterial properties. Take 500 milligrams two or three times daily.

■ Goldenseal is an antibacterial herb that is valuable in all cases of acute infection. Take 250 to 300 milligrams two or three times daily for one week.

■ Marshmallow root is soothing to the bowel. Take a cup of marshmallow root tea, or take 500 milligrams in capsule form, three times daily for two weeks.

■ Pau d'arco is an ancient South American remedy with noteworthy antibacterial and anti-inflammatory activity. The bark of the tree is the part used medicinally. Select a whole extract and take 500 milligrams three times daily for six weeks. Or brew a decoction from the bark (*see* PREPARING HERBAL TRATMENTS in Part Three) and take one cup three times daily.

■ Schizandra is a Chinese herb that is very effective in regulating the digestive tract. Take 100 milligrams twice daily for one month.

HOMEOPATHY

■ *Bryonia* is the remedy for irritability, constipation, and severe abdominal pain. Take one dose of *Bryonia* 30x or 15c, as directed on the product label, three times daily as long as you have symptoms.

■ *Colocynthis* will help if you are suffering from painful spasms. Take one dose of *Colocynthis* 12x or 6c three times daily as long as you have symptoms.

■ *Magnesia phosphorica* is good for abdominal cramping that is eased by the application of heat. Take one dose of *Magnesia phosphorica* 12x or 6c three times daily as long as you have symptoms.

BACH FLOWER REMEDIES

Select the remedy that most closely fits your emotional tendencies and concerns, and take it as needed, following the directions on the product label.

■ Holly helps to calm anger, agitation, and fits of temper.

■ Hornbeam helps to ease fatigue.

■ Impatiens is for the impatient individual with a type-A personality.

■ Mimulus calms fear.

■ Red Chestnut helps relieve chronic worry.

■ White Chestnut is the remedy for obsessive thinking and a tendency to dwell on the same issues endlessly.

ACUPRESSURE

For the location of acupressure points on the body, *see* ADMINISTERING AN ACUPRESSURE TREATMENT in Part Three.

■ The lower Bladder points increase circulation to the large intestine.

■ Large Intestine 4 removes energy blocks in the large intestine, thus promoting a healthier lower abdomen.

■ Stomach 36 and 40 harmonize and tone the digestive system, improve digestion, and strengthen overall well-being.

AROMATHERAPY

For specific instructions on how to use aromatherapy, *see* PREPARING AROMATHERAPY TREATMENTS in Part Three.

■ Essential oils of basil, lavender, myrrh, and rose strengthen the digestive system and help to counteract constipation. Add one or more of them to a bath or massage oil.

■ Chamomile, lavender, and peppermint oils can help relieve stomach spasms and cramping. Use any or all of these oils in an aromatherapy bath or add a few drops to massage oil.

■ Many essential oils can be used to reduce stress, a contributing factor in diverticular disease. The oils best known for this property include bergamot, elemi, frankincense, lavender, neroli, thyme, and ylang ylang. You can use one to three of these as an inhalant, diffuse them into the air, or add them to a bath or massage oil.

PREVENTION

■ Taking in sufficient fiber and water every day is the best preventive measure against constipation, which leads to the development of diverticuli.

■ Because stress is a contributing factor, learning ways to diffuse it and minimize its impact on your nervous system can be helpful. *See* RELAXATION TECHNIQUES in Part Three.

Dizziness

See under VERTIGO.

Dog Bite

See BITES, ANIMAL AND HUMAN.

Drug Abuse

Drug abuse is the ingestion of a substance, whether legal or illegal, to excess. Whether the substance is sniffed, swal-

lowed, inhaled, or injected, the user takes it for its mind-altering effects. Drug addiction is characterized by an overwhelming physical and/or psychological need to take the drug. A person who is addicted to a drug eventually centers his or her entire life around the substance. Nothing matters except the next "fix." Drug dependence is reinforced by the fact that the user knows, perhaps from past experience, that being without the substance will result in intolerable symptoms, whether physical or psychological (or both). This gives rise to feelings of intense panic if the drug is not readily available.

People begin abusing drugs for many reasons, primarily because a substance seems to the user to improve performance, produces a changed outlook, relieves feelings of anxiety or depression, or brings oblivion. Because the most commonly abused drugs are illegal (with the exception of tobacco and alcohol), it is impossible to arrive at a reliable count of drug abusers in the United States. However, it has been estimated that more than 4 million people use cocaine regularly and at least 2 million people have experimented with heroin. One of the most insidious characteristics of most abused drugs is that the user builds up a tolerance to their effects. This means that as time goes by, the user requires ever-increasing amounts to produce the desired effect—or to prevent the unpleasant effects that occur when the addict's physical and psychological needs are not fully met.

Everyone knows of the dangers of drug overdose. However, many people are unaware of other dangers associated with recreational drug use. Cocaine and heroin can cause life-threatening damage to the heart. The long-term use of marijuana can reduce the protective abilities of the immune system by as much as 40 percent. This is because it destroys white blood cells, the body's first line of defense against infection. Most other drugs of abuse weaken the immune system as well. Intravenous drug use, which commonly includes the sharing of needles among several users, is a documented risk factor for HIV disease and hepatitis.

Women who abuse drugs—including cocaine, heroin, methadone, diazepam (Valium), phenobarbital, and alcohol—while pregnant are at high risk of having children with birth defects, including subnormal intelligence. Their babies may also be born drug-addicted. An infant born addicted to drugs suffers horrendous withdrawal symptoms, including breathing distress, excessive sweating, high fever, vomiting, diarrhea, and dehydration. Dehydration can be life-threatening, and convulsions are common. These babies are pale, cry shrilly, sneeze, and suck desperately on their fists but eat poorly. They yawn, but have difficulty falling asleep. Some of these infants are actually born with nose and knee abrasions, caused by thrashing around in the womb under the influence of the drug.

One variation within the realm of drug abuse includes the intentional infliction of mind-altering drugs on other people. This problem has come to light in recent years with the case of Rohypnol (sometimes referred to as "roofies"), the so-called "date-rape drug." Illegal in the United States but accessible south of the border, this agent, when mixed with alcohol, not only can knock a person out, but can affect the memory of recent events to the point of amnesia. There have been numerous reports of this drug being used, especially on college campuses, to render women unable to resist—or even remember—a sexual attack, often multiple assaults. A second compound, gamma-hydroxy-butyrate (GHB) has also been used for these purposes. GHB is a natural chemical, manufactured by the body, that is useful as a relaxant. Though it can promote sleep and enhance the effects of alcohol, it is non-toxic (unlike Rohypnol, or the alcohol it is mixed with).

Many different kinds of drugs are commonly abused. The potential for physical addiction varies. Drugs that depress the central nervous system are the most likely to cause physiological dependence. These agents include alcohol; antianxiety agents such as diazepam (Valium) and oxazepam (Serax); barbiturates, such as phenobarbital, pentobarbital (Nembutal), and secobarbital (Seconal); methaqualone (Quaalude); the opiates, principally heroin; and synthetic narcotics such as codeine, hydromorphone (Dilaudid), meperidine (Demerol), and oxycodone (in Percocet, Percodan, Tylox, and other medications). Other drugs, though they are very difficult to give up and do result in tolerance, do not technically cause physiological dependence. Examples include marijuana, mescaline (peyote), cocaine, amphetamine, methamphetamine, and lysergic acid diethylamide, better known as LSD. Other commonly abused substances include phencyclidine (PCP or angel dust), solvents, and amyl nitrite ("poppers"). For a summary of the signs of abuse and addiction to various drugs, see the inset on page 252.

This entry focuses on what you can do to minimize withdrawal symptoms and restore health to your body once you decide to stop abusing drugs. Although medical treatment is mandatory for true cases of addiction, alternative therapies—including strong nutritional support—are immensely valuable. Many drugs deplete the body of essential nutrients. The understanding and help of concerned family and friends play an important part as well.

CONVENTIONAL TREATMENT

■ Treatment of drug abuse is difficult, as people who engage in it may not, whether overtly or deep down, really want to recover. If you have determined that you truly do desire to recover, you must accept the fact that you cannot use the formerly abused drug again. Then you must withdraw from the drug. The appropriate way of doing this depends on the particular drug you have been using. If you have been using central nervous system depressants such as heroin, barbiturates, or antianxiety agents, you will have to taper off gradually under the supervision of a health-care professional, possibly in a hospital setting. The days of locking an addicted patient in a room and letting nature take its course are over. Sudden withdrawal can be extremely dangerous. It can take anywhere from one to two months (or longer) of gradually weaning the body from the substance to achieve complete remission.

■ If you are addicted to heroin, methadone therapy may be prescribed. Methadone is a less addictive narcotic that can ease the stress and depression caused by withdrawal. Without methadone, these symptoms can be so severe they drive a user back to the drug. Methadone is used only under a doctor's supervision, and it is meant to be used for a limited period of time. Methadone itself is addictive, and withdrawal of methadone must be done slowly over a period of six to seven weeks to avoid unpleasant withdrawal symptoms. It should not be taken by anyone with liver disease, or by pregnant women or nursing mothers. Mothers addicted to methadone can give birth to addicted babies.

■ Lithium may be prescribed to relieve depression, but it tends to be most effective for bipolar, or manic, depression. This trace mineral is available only by prescription.

■ Stopping the use of drugs such as marijuana, cocaine, or amphetamines can result in depression and fatigue, but there is generally no need for physiological support. Withdrawing from hallucinogens often requires considerable reassurance that the bizarre thoughts that can accompany withdrawal will pass.

■ Withdrawal from phencyclidine (PCP) can cause seizure activity, and a tranquilizer such as diazepam may be required to interrupt them. Treatment for high—sometimes extremely high—blood pressure may be necessary as well.

■ Solvent-fume addiction can cause a multiplicity of problems. Most of these substances are very toxic, particularly to the liver, so complications affecting that organ are not uncommon. The specific treatment necessary depends on the particular agent involved and focuses on trying to control the damage.

■ Amyl nitrite causes no withdrawal requiring medical intervention other than controlling symptoms. However, there is some question as to whether this drug can depress the immune system.

■ Once you are physically "clean," appropriate support in the form of an outpatient maintenance program, psychotherapy, a self-help group such as Narcotics Anonymous or Cocaine Anonymous, a halfway house, or some other proven approach to dealing with substance abuse is recommended to help you deal with cravings and psy-

Warning Signs of Drug Abuse and Addiction

Different drugs have different effects on the body and mind. The table below outlines common signs of abuse and addiction that occur with different classes of drugs.

Type of Drug	Signs of Abuse	Signs of Addiction
Amphetamines ("uppers" or "speed")	Abnormally high energy level, dilated pupils, weight loss, insomnia.	Rapid speech, anxiety, agitation; inability to sleep without drugs; hallucinations; possible suicide attempts. Pattern of highs followed by lows. Amphetamine users often become addicted to antianxiety drugs or tranquilizers, taken to bring them down off a high or help them go to sleep.
Antianxiety drugs, tranquilizers, sleeping pills ("downers")	Lack of interest, slurred speech, poor balance, constricted pupils, excessive need for sleep.	Excessive drowsiness, lack of coordination, inability to concentrate, impaired memory, tremors, paranoia.
Cocaine, crack	Inhaled: Ulcerated nostrils. Injected: Needle tracks. Smoked: Runny nose, sniffles.	Excitement alternating with depression; nausea vomiting, stomach cramps; dizziness; tremors; chills; fever; possible drug-induced coma. Crack cocaine has been associated with violent, even criminal, behavior.
Hallucinogens (lysergic acid dimethylide [LSD], mescaline [peyote], some "designer" drugs	Unpredictable hallucinations, sometimes pleasant, sometimes frightening; dilated pupils; irregular heart rate.	Sweating, trembling, fever, chills; erratic behavior. Long-term psychological problems may occur from one-time use.
Inhalants (volatile fumes from glue or cleaning fluids)	Unpredictable hallucinations, euphoria, silliness, dilated pupils.	Confusion, flushed face, unconsciousness. Suffocation is possible. High risk of serious brain, liver, or kidney damage.
Marijuana (pot), hashish (hash)	Red eyes, dilated pupils, excessive "goofiness," mood swings, abnormally slow reflexes and sense of time, increased appetite.	Lethargy, dizziness, inability to think or move quickly, loss of short-term memory, lack of motivation. These "entry-level" drugs often lead to "hard drugs," such as cocaine.
Opiates (heroin, opium, morphine)	Mood swings, sweating, slurred speech, drowsiness, weight loss, lethargy.	Nausea; vomiting; dizziness; constipation. The user may become more sensitive to pain after the drug has worn off. Euphoria is temporary.

chological dependence, and stay away from drugs. Staying clean requires that you make substantial lifestyle changes, which is always difficult.

■ An important premise of drug treatment is that loved ones must learn how to stop "enabling" the abuser. This is necessary if he or she is to be cut free of anything that protects against having to meet the situation head-on. To this end, friends and family members can receive invaluable education through the services of Nar-Anon or Al-Anon, which are designed to help other people in the life of a drug abuser realize how they may have been involved in the behavior. Even though they may be completely unaware of it, they may have been making the situation worse.

■ Have your thyroid checked. If your addiction centers on stimulants, such as amphetamines, it is possible that you may have subclinical or even clearly diagnosable hypothyroidism. You are likely to be more successful in

withdrawing from a stimulant if your thyroid is functioning normally.

DIETARY GUIDELINES

■ A wholesome, well-balanced diet is especially important for recovering drug abusers. Almost without exception, former substance abusers suffer from varying degrees of malnutrition. Three meals per day that incorporate a good balance of clean, lean protein, vegetables, fruits, whole grains, and complex carbohydrates can help provide the nutrients needed for bodywide repair.

■ Many abusers substitute their drug of choice for food, which causes the stomach to shrink. If you find it difficult to take in much food at one sitting, eat smaller, more frequent meals, plus healthy snacks. Stabilizing your blood-sugar level is very important. Eat nutrient-dense foods every three or four hours.

■ First thing in the morning, dilute 2 tablespoons of

lemon juice in 8 ounces of spring water and drink it. This is an age-old "prescription" that helps to gently cleanse the liver.

■ For fast detoxification, once any acute withdrawal symptoms have resolved, consider undertaking a two- or three-day juice fast—but discuss this with your health-care practitioner first. If fasting seems too extreme, two days per week, eat only steamed vegetables, broths, and herbal teas, and drink plenty of pure water.

Avoid refined sugar. Sugar makes blood-sugar levels rise abruptly, followed by an equally rapid crash. Low blood sugar contributes to shakiness and wild mood swings. If a craving for sweets proves irresistible, try taking a *little* honey, barley malt, or rice syrup instead.

To help flush toxins from your body, drink six to eight 8-ounce glasses of pure water every day.

NUTRITIONAL SUPPLEMENTS

All nutrients are needed in maximum concentration. Take a high-potency multivitamin and mineral formula daily.

If fatigue is a significant problem, adrenal glandular extract may be useful. To strengthen the adrenal glands, take 250 milligrams of supplemental adrenal extract three times daily, in morning and afternoon (but before 2:00 PM).

■ Amino acids supply the protein required to nourish and strengthen a body stressed by drug abuse. Take a free-form amino-acid complex supplement as directed on the product label.

Calcium and magnesium are essential to the central nervous system. Three times daily, take 500 milligrams of calcium and 400 milligrams of magnesium. Many symptoms associated with withdrawal, including tremors, can be eased with consistent amounts of calcium and magnesium. If you develop loose stools, reduce the dosage of magnesium to the largest amount you can tolerate.

Glutamine helps to improve mental clarity. If you are feeling "fuzzy," a not-uncommon symptom of withdrawal, take 500 milligrams of L-glutamine three to four times daily for two to four weeks.

Glutathione can help detoxify the body and helps reduce the harmful residual effects of drugs. It also reduces the desire for drugs, including alcohol. Take 500 milligrams twice a day.

■ If fatigue and depression are predominant, tyrosine can elevate mood and increase energy levels. Take 500 milligrams of tyrosine with breakfast and another 500 milligrams at lunch for two to four weeks.

Note: If you are taking a monoamine oxidase (MAO) inhibitor drug, do not take supplemental tyrosine, as a sudden and dangerous rise in blood pressure may result.

■ The B-complex vitamins ease stress and help to nourish and strengthen the liver. Because the liver is responsible for detoxifying drugs and ridding the body of poisons, this organ is badly affected by substance abuse. Talk to your doctor about injections of the the full B complex, plus extra vitamin B_{12} and pantothenic acid. If your doctor feels injections are not indicated, take a B-complex supplement supplying 50 to 100 milligrams of each of the major B vitamins daily, plus an additional 1,000 micrograms of vitamin B_{12} and 250 milligrams of pantothenic acid.

■ Vitamin C helps detoxify the body and may reduce cravings. Take 1,000 milligrams of a buffered vitamin-C formula that includes the bioflavonoids three times daily.

HERBAL TREATMENT

■ When withdrawing from any substance, it is important to simultaneously detoxify the liver and relax the nervous system. A tea made from the following herbs can enhance liver function and calm the nerves. Use 2 parts oat straw; 1 part dandelion root; 1 part passionflower; 1 part Siberian ginseng; and $1/2$ part skullcap. (*See* PREPARING HERBAL TREATMENTS in Part Three.)

■ Dandelion root is one of the finest liver remedies. It enhances the flow of bile, which has a beneficial effect on the liver. It is also a mild diuretic, which can speed the release of toxins from the body. Select dandelion capsules or tablets and take 250 milligrams three times daily for six weeks. Stop for one month, then repeat.

■ Hsiao Yao Wan is a remarkable 2,000-year-old Chinese formula that helps relax the nervous system and improve liver function. This remedy is very effective in easing the mental and physical tension associated with withdrawal. Take the equivalent of 500 milligrams three times daily.

■ Kava kava induces a very comfortable, non-threatening relaxed state. If you suffer mental anxiety during withdrawal, choose a product containing 30 percent kavalactones and take 200 to 250 milligrams two or three times a day.

Note: In excess amounts, this herb can cause drowsiness. Do not exceed the recommended dose. Do not use kava kava if you are pregnant or nursing, if you have Parkinson's disease, or if you are taking a prescription medication for depression or anxiety.

■ Milk thistle is one of the most effective herbs for liver detoxification. It contains silymarin, which has been shown in clinical studies to protect against liver damage and enhance liver function. It can actually stimulate the production of new liver cells to replace damaged ones. Choose an extract standardized to contain 80 percent flavonoids (silymarin) and start by taking 200 to 300 milligrams daily. After one week, increase to 200 to 300 milligrams twice daily; after another week, add another 200 to 300 milligrams daily. Do not take a tincture, which is alcohol based.

St. John's wort is very helpful for mental depression and mood swings. It also has immune-stimulating benefits and antiviral properties. It is not uncommon to have herpes outbreaks, skin rashes, or other symptoms of depressed immunity when using or withdrawing from drugs. If taken for three to four months, St. John's wort can help stabilize both mood and the immune system. Choose a product containing 0.3 percent hypericin and take 300 milligrams three times daily.

Valerian can be very valuable if withdrawal has caused a sleep disorder. This herb is very relaxing, especially when taken with calcium and magnesium. It helps people fall asleep faster and also helps prevent restless sleep. Select an extract standardized to contain 0.5 percent isovalerenic acids and take 100 milligrams in the morning and 200 to 400 milligrams in the evening, one to one-half hour before bedtime.

HOMEOPATHY

Lycopodium is homeopathic club moss, a plant that has been the first choice of Chinese physicians for liver detoxification for millennia. Former substance abusers usually have compromised liver function. Take one dose of *Lycopodium* 30x or 15c, as directed on the product label, three times daily for up to three days.

Nux vomica detoxifies the body and helps to reduce cravings. Take one dose of *Nux vomica* 30x or 15c twice a day for up to one week.

BACH FLOWER REMEDIES

Select the remedy that most closely fits your emotional tendencies and concerns, and take it as needed, following the directions on the product label.

Holly is good for feelings of anger and insecurity, especially if you somehow seem to feel better after indulging in a fit of bad temper.

Impatiens can ease nervousness, tension, hyperactivity, and irritability.

Larch can help build self-confidence and restore self-esteem.

■ Olive can help relieve a feeling of being exhausted to the very core and being beset by inner demons.

Rock Water is helpful for the person who finds it difficult to forgive his or her past transgressions.

Sweet Chestnut is for feelings of anguish and alienation.

ACUPRESSURE

For the location of acupressure points on the body, see **ADMINISTERING AN ACUPRESSURE TREATMENT** in Part Three.

■ Four Gates relaxes the body.

■ Gallbladder 20 and 34 improve circulation to the head. Gallbladder 20 is also associated with freeing up blocked energy that goes to the head. Many modern acupuncturists use this point when treating disorders such as chronic fatigue and fatigue associated with drug withdrawal.

■ Pericardium 6 relaxes the mind and eases nausea.

■ Spleen 10 detoxifies the blood.

■ Stomach 36 tones the digestive system and strengthens overall well-being.

GENERAL RECOMMENDATIONS

■ Consult a licensed acupuncturist. Acupuncture has been found to be very effective in diminishing cravings and restoring balance to the body. Ask your physician for a referral, or consult an organization such as the American Association of Oriental Medicine (see the Resources section at the end of the book).

■ Be aware of the signs of abuse. If you suspect you are losing control over your behavior, or if a loved one exhibits signs of trouble, don't wait to see what's going to happen. Remember, the earlier you recognize a problem, the less serious it is likely to become. For substantial help, contact a local chapter of Narcotics Anonymous, listed in the white pages of most local telephone directories.

■ Until an addict recognizes and admits that a problem exists, there is no chance for recovery. An intervention, wherein the substance abuser is confronted by loved ones and encouraged to look at the problems his or her addiction have caused, is sometimes helpful, sometimes not. This is not something that should be attempted by a layperson. If you are contemplating an intervention, seek professional help.

■ It is important for family and friends of substance abusers to seek out appropriate support. They need to learn that "tough love" is the best way to help. Meeting the needs of an addict, whether it is with emotional or financial support, enables the addiction to continue.

■ If you consume alcohol, be aware of the possibility that people may attempt to add things to your drink. At social gatherings, always keep your drink within your sight, preferably in your hand, especially if people you do not know well and absolutely trust are present.

PREVENTION

■ It has been established that the children of drug users and alcoholic parents are 400 times more likely to become substance abusers than those whose parents and family members abstain, or take only an occasional drink. Whether the tendency to abuse is inherited or is learned behavior remains controversial. However, if you know that other family members have had a tendency toward substance abuse, use this knowledge to your benefit. Act as you would with any other hereditary condition. If you have inherited an allergy to penicillin, you would obviously avoid that drug. Do the same with recreational drugs, including alcohol.

■ If you don't want your children to use drugs, don't demonstrate how by using them yourself. And never tell a child that medicine is "candy" in an attempt to persuade him or her to take it. That can pave the way for a careless attitude toward drugs. You should also make children aware of the dangers of drugs. You can't start too early. Although most drug use begins in adolescence, even children in elementary school are in danger of experimenting. Peer pressure is very strong. Parents must be stronger.

Dry Eyes

If the tear ducts fail to produce enough fluid to keep the eyes moist, the result is dryness of the eyes and irritation that causes itching and a burning sensation. This condition is more common in women, particularly after menopause, and the incidence increases with age in both sexes.

Dry eyes can also be a symptom of other conditions, such as rheumatoid arthritis and lupus, and they can be a side effect of certain drugs, including common antidepressants, beta-blockers, and marijuana. Dry eyes are often a problem for people who wear contact lenses.

Xerophthalmia is the medical term for dryness of the surface of the eye resulting from vitamin-A deficiency. In this condition, the cornea becomes dry, hazy, and, if the condition is severe enough, the cornea and/or the conjunctiva, the transparent membrane adjacent to the cornea, begin to disintegrate. Foamy white patches on the surface of the eye, called Bitot's spots, may develop.

CONVENTIONAL TREATMENT

■ See your physician. Dry eyes can be a symptom of a more serious condition. In addition, the constant irritation caused by dry eyes can damage your vision over the long term.

■ If you are taking antidepressants or beta-blockers, ask your physician if one of the side effects of the drugs you are taking is dry eyes. You may need a change in prescription.

■ Artificial tears are available over the counter. These products are helpful in the short term, but provide only symptomatic relief. The preservatives in these drops can cause irritation in some people. If inflammation develops or seems to be becoming worse, discontinue using them.

■ In severe cases, an ophthalmologist may recommend surgery to close the internal tear ducts, which funnel a portion of the tears from your eyes into your nose, and redirect the flow onto the surface of your eyes to provide greater lubrication.

■ Xerophthalmia is treated with therapeutic doses of vitamin A.

DIETARY GUIDELINES

■ Maximize your intake of fresh fruits and vegetables. These healthy foods contain antioxidant phytochemicals that protect all the cells of the body, including those of the eyes, from free-radical damage.

■ Eat clean, lean protein, such as that found in chicken and fish. Both protein and vitamin A are needed to maintain healthy eyes.

■ Limit your intake of sugar, caffeine, and alcohol. These substances contribute to eye irritation and worsen the symptoms caused by many eye problems. Alcohol can also cause dehydration.

NUTRITIONAL SUPPLEMENTS

■ Beta-carotene is a strong antioxidant that prevents free-radical damage. It is related to vitamin A and has many of the same properties, but it does not become toxic in large doses. Take 10,000 to 25,000 international units of beta-carotene daily.

■ The essential fatty acids (EFAs), found in black currant seed oil, borage oil, evening primrose oil, and flaxseed oil, are required by every cell in the body. They have been shown to reduce pain, inflammation, and swelling. Take 500 to 1,000 milligrams of any of these oils two or three times daily.

■ Selenium is an excellent antioxidant that helps prevent free-radical damage throughout the body, including the eyes. While symptoms are acute, take 100 micrograms twice daily. When symptoms improve, reduce the dosage to 100 micrograms once daily.

■ Vitamin A protects against free-radical damage and is especially important to the eyes. Without sufficient vitamin A, the eyes are more susceptible to infection, ulcerations, and even blindness. Take 10,000 international units of vitamin A three times a day for two months. Then cut back to a maintenance dosage of 5,000 international units twice daily.

Note: If you are pregnant, or intend to get pregnant, or if you have liver disease, consult your doctor before taking supplemental vitamin A. Pregnant women should not ingest a total of more than 25,000 international units of supplemental vitamin A *per week* from all sources.

■ Combined with vitamins C and E, the B-complex vitamins are especially beneficial to the eyes. While symptoms are acute, take a B-complex supplement that supplies 50 milligrams of each of the primary B vitamins twice daily. When symptoms improve, reduce the dosage to 25 milligrams twice daily.

■ Vitamin C helps to prevent and clear up infections. It also helps strengthen capillaries, maintains collagen, and prevents tissue hemorrhaging, and is notable for speeding healing. Select a vitamin-C formula that includes bioflavonoids, especially rutin; these nutrients work best together. While symptoms are acute, take 1,000 to 3,000 milligrams of a vitamin-C complex three times daily. When symptoms improve, reduce the dosage to 500 to 1,000 milligrams three times daily.

■ Vitamin E is an antioxidant and is essential in cellular respiration. It has been shown to improve eyesight in clinical studies. Choose a product containing mixed tocopherols and begin by taking 200 international units, then gradually increase the dosage until you are taking 400 international units of vitamin E twice daily. Maintain this dosage as long as symptoms are acute. When symptoms improve, cut back to 200 international units twice daily.

Note: If you have high blood pressure, limit your intake of supplemental vitamin E to a total of 400 international units daily. If you are taking an anticoagulant (blood thinner), consult your physician before taking supplemental vitamin E.

■ Zinc supports the immune system and aids in the healing process. While symptoms are acute, take 25 to 50 milligrams of zinc daily. When symptoms improve, reduce the dosage to 15 to 20 milligrams daily.

Note: Take zinc with food to prevent stomach upset. If you take over 30 milligrams of zinc on a daily basis for more than one or two months, you should also take 1 to 2 milligrams of copper each day to maintain a proper mineral balance.

HERBAL TREATMENT

■ Bilberry provides important nutrients that nourish the eyes and enhance visual function. Phytochemicals called anthocyanidins in this herb also help prevent damage to the structures of the eyes. Select a preparation containing 25 percent anthocyanidins (also called PCOs) and take 40 to 60 milligrams three times daily.

■ Eyebright is rich in vitamin A and vitamin C. It also contains moderate amounts of the B-complex vitamins and vitamin D, and traces of vitamin E. Eyebright has been used for centuries both as an eyewash and in tea form as a tonic for the eyes. Taken internally, it helps maintain healthy eyes and good vision. Take 500 milligrams three times daily. Used as an eye bath, it can provide welcome relief from dry eyes. Bring 3 ounces of sterile saline solution to a boil, and pour it over 1 tablespoon of dried cut herb (or one eyebright teabag). Allow it to steep for fifteen minutes, then strain out the herb. When the liquid has cooled to a comfortable temperature, use it as an eyewash. Or moisten a thin white cotton cloth with the warm eyebright tea and place it over your eyes. Leave the compress in place for fifteen minutes. Then moisten a fresh sterile cloth in the tea and gently wipe away any crusts or scales. Throw away (or sterilize) each cloth after one use. Wash your hands before and after the treatment. Always be very cautious when using warm liquids around your eyes. The skin of the eyelid is thin and tender and can burn easily.

■ Ginkgo biloba extract contains flavonoids with an affinity for organs that are rich in connective tissue, including the eyes. Ginkgo protects cellular membranes and has notable antioxidant properties. It also enhances the use of oxygen and glucose by the cells, and works to normalize circulation. Select a ginkgo leaf extract containing at least 24 percent ginkgo heterosides (sometimes called flavoglycosides) and take 40 milligrams three times daily.

GENERAL RECOMMENDATIONS

■ If you have dry eyes, you will probably feel a strong temptation to rub them. Don't. Normal eyes respond to rubbing by tearing, but dry eyes cannot. Rubbing only adds to the irritation.

■ If your inside environment is dry, use a humidifier to add moisture to the air.

■ Protect your eyes from breezes, which can worsen symptoms. Wear wraparound sunglasses.

■ Shield your eyes as much as possible when using a hair dryer, or let your hair dry naturally. Hot air coming from a hair dryer can dry the surface of your eyes very quickly.

■ Avoid anything that can irritate your eyes, especially smoke. Whether it comes from a cigarette or a sweet-smelling wood fire, smoke is very hard on the eyes and worsens symptoms.

Ear Infection

The ear is a complex structure that consists of three sections: the outer, middle, and inner ears. The outer ear is the part we see. It is the external canal that picks up the vibrations from sound and transmits them through the eardrum to the middle ear. The middle ear contains three small bones that take these vibrations into the inner ear, which contains the nerve endings that make hearing possible. The inner ear is also involved in maintaining balance.

Ear infections are most common in young children, but they can occur at any age. Any portion of the ear may be affected, but the outer and middle ears are the most common sites. An outer-ear infection can develop if you get water or other substances in your ear, particularly if the irritant is then trapped by earwax, or if the ear canal is subjected to trauma, such as cleaning with a cotton swab. These situations set the stage for bacteria to multiply. The skin of the outer ear canal becomes red and swollen, and pus may develop as the body attempts to fight the infection. Symptoms include pain (especially when you touch or pull on the ear), itching, and, possibly, discharge from the ear. In addition to a generalized infection, it is also possible to develop boils in the ear canal or on the outer ear (see BOILS).

The middle ear is another possible site of infection. This part of the ear is connected to the nasal cavity and the throat by means of a passageway called the eustachian tube. This path allows excess secretions from the middle ear to drain away from the ear and into the nose and throat. If the eustachian tube is not draining properly, secretions build up in the middle ear, with the result that pressure in the ear rises and the ear becomes painful and, often, infected.

Ear infections are often a complication of a common cold or other upper respiratory infection, such as infection of the adenoids, tonsils, or sinuses. They are sometimes accompanied by coughing, a runny nose, sore throat, and, occasionally, vomiting and diarrhea. Depending on the cause of the infection, a fever may be present. The defining symptom of a middle ear infection is pain, which is constant and can be severe. Another common symptom is a feeling of fullness and pressure. This is caused by the excess fluid pushing against the eardrum. You may also experience a slight hearing loss in the affected ear. Sometimes the pressure is strong enough to rupture the eardrum. If you experience sharp, severe pain, followed by a sudden drainage of blood and/or pus from your ear, you may have a perforated eardrum. When the buildup of pressure finally causes the drum to rupture, the relief from pressure can actually cause a dramatic lessening of the pain. Even if you seem to be feeling better, consult your physician right away.

CONVENTIONAL TREATMENT

■ Antibiotics, such as amoxicillin (sold under the brand names Amoxil and Augmentin, among others), cefaclor (Ceclor), cefixme (Suprax), erythromycin (ERYC, Ilotycin), and sulfamethoxazole plus trimethoprim (Bactrim, Co-trimoxazole, Septra), are commonly prescribed for ear infection. Most people begin to feel significantly better within forty-eight to seventy-two hours after starting a course of antibiotics, but it is important to continue taking the medication for the full course to be certain all infection is gone.

Your health-care provider will want to see you once the full course of antibiotics is completed to make sure the infection has cleared.

■ Some ear infections do not respond to the first medication prescribed. If your symptoms do not seem to be improving after four or five days, talk with your doctor. Another office visit and evaluation, and possibly a change of medication, may be required.

■ An analgesic, such as acetaminophen (Tylenol, Datril, and others), aspirin (Bayer, Ecotrin, and others), or ibuprofen (Advil, Motrin, Nuprin, and others) can help relieve the pain of an ear infection and also bring down a fever. If these over-the-counter products are not sufficient to relieve pain, your doctor may prescribe a stronger painkiller such as codeine, which is sold under many different brand names, often combined with acetaminophen, aspirin, or ibuprofen.

Note: In excessive amounts, acetaminophen can cause liver damage. If the recommended amount does not give the relief you want, do not increase the dosage, but try a different medication. Take aspirin or ibuprofen with food to prevent possible stomach upset.

■ If your ear infection is related to sinus or nasal congestion, an antihistamine and/or a decongestant may be prescribed. Antihistamines often cause drowsiness, so if you are having difficulty sleeping because of the discomfort, your doctor may recommend one. Research has not shown these medications to be helpful in actually curing ear infections, however.

■ If you have an ear infection and develop a fever, chills, dizziness, or serious hearing loss, or experience a severe headache, a stiff neck, lethargy, or changes in consciousness, contact your physician immediately These can be signs of serious complications, such as meningitis or an infection that has traveled to the inner ear.

DIETARY GUIDELINES

■ Drink plenty of liquids to make sure you stay well hydrated.

■ Eliminate dairy foods from your diet. Dairy foods thicken and increase the production of mucus, making it more difficult for an infected ear to drain.

NUTRITIONAL SUPPLEMENTS

■ If you must take antibiotics, take an acidophilus or bifidus supplement to replace the necessary friendly bacteria stripped from the intestinal tract by those drugs. Take it as recommended on the product label. If you are allergic to milk, select a dairy-free formula.

■ Vitamin C and bioflavonoids are helpful for an ear infection. They are both mildly anti-inflammatory. Take 500 to 1,000 milligrams of each four or five times daily until the infection clears. Select a product that contains mineral-ascorbate-buffered vitamin C but no sugar.

■ Zinc boosts the immune response and helps reduce infection. Take 15 milligrams three times daily, before meals. If you take over 30 milligrams of zinc on a daily basis for more than one or two months, you should also take 1 to 2 milligrams of copper each day to maintain a proper mineral balance.

HERBAL TREATMENT

■ Cat's claw enhances the immune response and has antibacterial properties. Take 500 milligrams of standardized extract three times a day until the infection clears.

Note: Do not use cat's claw if you are pregnant or nursing, or if you are an organ-transplant recipient. Use it with caution if you are taking an anticoagulant (blood thinner).

■ Echinacea and goldenseal are important for clearing any type of infection. Echinacea is antiviral; goldenseal is antibacterial and soothes irritated mucous membranes. Both herbs stimulate the immune system. Take one dose of an echinacea and goldenseal combination formula supplying 250 to 500 milligrams of echinacea and 150 to 300 milligrams of goldenseal every two hours while the infection is acute, up to a total of four doses. Then continue taking one dose three times daily for five days.

■ Garlic is an antibacterial that can help heal an ear infection. Take 500 milligrams three or four times daily. You can also heat a fresh garlic clove in 1 to 2 tablespoons of olive oil and, lying on your side, put one or two drops of warm (not hot) oil into the affected ear.

■ Mullein oil, available in health-food and herb shops, is a traditional Native American remedy used to reduce swelling and inflammation. Gently heat mullein oil to slightly above body temperature and, lying on your side, put one or two drops into the affected ear. The heat feels comforting, while the mullein goes to work on the problem.

■ Oregano has antibacterial properties and helps to fight infection. Take 75 to 150 milligrams of standardized extract three times a day.

HOMEOPATHY

The symptom-specific remedies listed here should work quickly. If the pain does not subside within twenty-four hours, call your physician.

■ If you have a throbbing earache that is relieved by resting with your head elevated, accompanied by a fever, a flushed face, dilated pupils, and hot and moist skin, take one dose of *Belladonna* 30x or 9c two to three times daily for one day.

■ For an earache that causes intolerable pain and is accompanied by irritability and feelings of anger, choose *Chamomilla*. You may have one red cheek and one pale cheek, with hot, moist skin. Take one dose of *Chamomilla* 12x, 30x, 6c, or 9c three times daily for one to two days.

■ If you have a fever along with an ear infection, take *Ferrum phosphoricum*. This homeopathic preparation can be taken together with another symptom-specific remedy. Take a dose of *Ferrum phosphoricum* 12x or 6c every thirty minutes, up to a total of four doses.

■ *Kali muriaticum* helps relieve nasal congestion and swollen glands. It will help if you have a blocked eustachian tube that has affected your hearing. Take one dose of *Kali muriaticum* 12x or 6c three times daily for one to two days.

■ If you have a moderate fever and an earache that came on gradually, use *Pulsatilla*. An important symptom that distinguishes the *Pulsatilla* person is the desire for cold; you want to be in fresh air—near a window or outdoors—and feel better with a cold compress. Take one dose of *Pulsatilla* 30x or 9c three times daily for one to two days.

■ *Mercurius dulcis* often works if other remedies have failed. Take one dose of *Mercurius dulcis* 12x or 6c three times daily for two days.

■ If none of the above remedies seems right for you, a homeopathic combination earache remedy may be helpful.

GENERAL RECOMMENDATIONS

■ The pain of an earache is caused by pressure as the congested middle ear pushes on the eardrum. To promote drainage, when you lie down, do not position yourself flat on your back, but lie on the unaffected side and prop your head up with several pillows.

■ Try applying warm compresses. If the warmth is comforting, use that knowledge to guide you in choosing an appropriate symptom-specific homeopathic remedy. Some people feel better with a cold compress. Experiment with hot and cold to see what helps.

■ If you have an ear infection, avoid air travel. Traveling by air can be very uncomfortable for a person with an ear infection. Air travel does not necessarily injure the ear or increase your risk of developing an ear infection, but the change of air pressure in the cabin on takeoff and landing can greatly increase the pain. If you must fly, it may be worthwhile to take nasal decongestant drops, along with a painkiller, before takeoff. A product called Ear Planes may help as well, by maintaining an even air pressure within the ears. The same effect may be achieved by holding foam drinking cups very tightly over each ear. If you ask a flight attendant for two foam cups for your ears, she or he will understand. Some attendants will even wet paper towels with very hot water, wring them out well, and insert them in the bottom of the cups for you. The warmth is comforting, but this small addition is unnecessary.

PREVENTION

■ Avoid cigarette smoke. People who are exposed to tobacco smoke are more likely to develop ear infections.

■ Massaging your ear can help keep the eustachian tube open. Using gentle pressure, draw a line along the back of the ear and down the back of the jawbone. Gently push and release the flap of skin in front of the ear several times. You can also massage your ear by placing the fleshy part of your palm, just below your thumb, over your ear and rotating the ear in all directions.

■ Use an elimination diet to determine if food allergies are contributing to the problem. Dairy products top the list of the most common troublemakers. Other common allergens worth deleting include eggs, wheat, corn, oranges, and nuts.

■ Avoid exposure to common irritating allergens such as pet dander. Down comforters and pillows are another possible source of trouble. Items like carpets and draperies can collect dust as well.

Earache

See EAR INFECTION; MENIERE'S DISEASE.

Eating Disorders

See ANOREXIA NERVOSA; BULIMIA.

Eczema

Eczema is an inflammatory skin disorder characterized by patches of red, dry, flaking skin and areas that are inflamed, moist, and oozing. If the condition becomes chronic, the affected skin cells may become thick and scaly and the skin may change color. Itching can be so severe that scratching is virtually inevitable. A person with eczema may scratch until the skin cracks and bleeds, preferring the hurt caused by rubbing the skin raw to the intolerable itching.

The condition can affect any part of the body, but is most common on the face and scalp, behind the ears, and in the creases of the elbows, knees, and groin. It can be short-lived (acute) or last for several years with periods of remission and exacerbation (chronic). It is not contagious. People who have eczema usually have very dry, itchy skin that doesn't hold moisture well.

Eczema can be a result of either atopic dermatitis or contact dermatitis. Atopic dermatitis is an inherited form of hypersensitivity that usually first appears in infancy or early childhood. People with atopic dermatitis often have other family members with allergies and a history of eczema. It can become worse after you eat certain foods or are exposed to an allergen like dust or pollen. Atopic eczema can be a long-term condition.

Contact dermatitis is the more common form of the condition. This type of eczema is often an allergic response to something a person has touched, including topical medicines. Eczema can also be caused by many irritants that come in contact with the skin, such as soaps, bubble bath, fabric dyes, feathers, cosmetics, wool, plants, and environmental pollutants.

Both types of eczema are considered allergic responses. If you have eczema, you may have other allergies as well, such as food sensitivities, asthma, or hay fever.

Emotional stress can exacerbate a case of eczema. Also, even though eczema is not caused by a virus or bacteria, the open lesions can become infected. When dealing with eczema, watch for signs of infection, and if infection develops, call your doctor.

CONVENTIONAL TREATMENT

■ Topical anti-inflammatory ointments containing corticosteroids such as hydrocortisone (in Hytone, LactiCare HC, Vytone, and others), triamcinolone (Aristocort, Triacet, and others), or betamethasone (Beta-Val, Diprolene) are the medications most commonly prescribed for eczema. Your doctor will direct you to rub a small amount into the affected area, taking care not to apply it to open lesions. In more severe cases, you may be instructed to wrap the area with an occlusive dressing, such as Saran Wrap, to increase the medication's effectiveness. Because long-term use of steroids often creates side effects, such as thin, fragile dry skin and even suppression of the adrenal glands over time, these medications should be used only for short periods.

■ To counter the allergic response and help decrease the awful itching, an antihistamine such as diphenhydramine (found in Benadryl and other over-the-counter medications), hydroxyzine (Atarax, Vistaril), or chlorpheniramine (Chlor-Trimeton) may be recommended. Antihistamines can cause sleepiness, but this can be very helpful at bedtime, when itching is often at its worst, making it difficult to fall asleep.

■ If the lesions are weeping, Burow's solution may be recommended. This soothing powder is available over the counter at many drugstores. Be aware that it contains aluminum.

■ Coal-tar cream (Fototar) may contain the flaking and itching, but it can stain clothing, irritate skin, and cause sensitivity to sunlight.

DIETARY GUIDELINES

■ Very often, allergies to citrus fruits, eggs, wheat, cow's milk, shellfish, and/or chocolate are related to eczema. Suspect an allergy to any food that you have cravings for or eat every day. Use an elimination diet to check for any possible food allergies (see ELIMINATION DIET in Part Three).

■ Include foods high in potassium and vitamin A or beta-carotene in your diet. Lightly steamed carrots and leafy greens such as kale and dandelion leaves are excellent choices.

■ Eat at least 1 tablespoon of olive oil, flaxseed oil, or walnut oil daily to increase the moisture-holding potential of your skin.

■ Make a nourishing vegetable soup. You can use the recipe for Astragalus and Vegetable Soup found under THERAPEUTIC RECIPES in Part Three, with the following modifications: Eliminate the astragalus root and add parsley and garlic to taste, plus 4 ounces of fresh burdock root. Garlic and onions contain sulfur and amino acids beneficial to the skin; burdock helps to cleanse the blood. If you don't care for the taste of the whole herbs and/or vegetables, you can strain the soup to remove them and add noodles, rice, or barley to the soup just before serving it. That way, you can still ingest all the beneficial vitamins and minerals.

NUTRITIONAL SUPPLEMENTS

You may want to try adding the nutritional supplements that follow one at a time. See how you respond to the first nutrient introduced and add another after a week or so.

■ A good multivitamin and mineral supplement should be the first supplement you try, to ensure you are getting adequate amounts of all the major vitamins and minerals.

■ Beta-carotene and vitamin A promote tissue healing. Take 10,000 international units of each twice a day for one month.

Note: If you are pregnant, or intend to get pregnant, or if you have liver disease, consult your doctor before taking supplemental vitamin A. Pregnant women should not ingest a total of more than 25,000 international units of supplemental vitamin A *per week* from all sources.

■ Many people with eczema are low in digestive enzymes. Taking a pancreatic-enzyme supplement with meals may not only enhance digestion, but also improve the condition of your skin within weeks. Some formulations contain betaine hydrochloride, which increases the level of stomach acid. This may be beneficial if you do not produce enough stomach acid on your own, as long as it does not cause a burning sensation.

■ Evening primrose oil can be taken internally (500 to 1,000 milligrams two to three times daily) or applied topically to help reduce inflammation. You should not take evening primrose oil if you have a fever.

■ Mineral ascorbate vitamin C and bioflavonoids have a mild anti-inflammatory action and are helpful for eczema. Vitamin C also helps in the formation of collagen, the number-one repair protein in the body. Take 500 to 1,000 milligrams of each at least twice daily for one to two months.

■ Vitamin E is good for the skin and aids tissue healing. It can be applied topically, taken internally, or both. Choose a product containing mixed tocopherols or d-alpha-tocopherol (avoid dl-tocopherol forms) and start by taking 400 international units each morning. After two weeks, add another 400 international units in the evening, and after another two weeks, add 400 more, in the middle of the day.

Note: If you have high blood pressure, limit your intake of supplemental vitamin E to a total of 400 international units daily. If you are taking an anticoagulant (blood thinner), consult your physician before taking supplemental vitamin E.

■ Selenium helps the body use vitamin E effectively and supports the healthy functioning of cell membranes. Take 50 to 100 micrograms daily for up to one month.

■ Zinc promotes the healing of wounds. Take 15 to 25 milligrams two to three times daily for one month. Take zinc with food to prevent stomach upset. If you take over 30 milligrams of zinc on a daily basis for more than one or two months, you should also take 1 to 2 milligrams of copper (either on its own or as part of a multivitamin and mineral supplement) each day to maintain a proper mineral balance.

HERBAL TREATMENT

■ A four-week herbal regimen can help resolve eczema. Take each herb for a period of seven days, in the order given, as follows.

Week 1: Burdock root acts to detoxify the blood and helps to heal the skin. Take one cup of burdock tea, or 500 milligrams in capsule form, two to three times daily.

Week 2: Echinacea and goldenseal help detoxify the blood. Take one dose of an echinacea and goldenseal combination remedy supplying 250 to 350 milligrams of echinacea and 100 to 250 milligrams of goldenseal two to three times daily.

Week 3: Red clover is a cleansing and blood-purifying herb useful in treating skin conditions. Take 500 milligrams or one cup of tea two to three times daily.

Week 4: Licorice is a natural anti-inflammatory. Take 250 milligrams of deglycyrrhizinated licorice (DGL) twice a day.

Note: Ordinary licorice can elevate blood pressure, and should not be taken on a daily basis for more than five days in a row. DGL should not have this effect, however.

■ Balsam of Peru cream, available at health-food stores, can be useful against eczema. It can be applied to the skin alone, or diluted with oil.

■ An herbal cream made from comfrey and licorice, such as Simicort or Alticort, or a high-potency chamomile cream such as CamoCare, can have a very soothing and anti-inflammatory effect. Follow the directions on the product label.

■ Dry eczema can benefit from the application of calendula ointment. Follow the directions on the product label.

■ Pine-bark and grape-seed extracts are high in bioflavonoids and are excellent anti-inflammatory agents. Take 40 to 50 milligrams of either twice daily for one month.

HOMEOPATHY

When treating eczema with a symptom-specific homeopathic remedy, continue taking the remedy until you notice an improvement. Once your skin begins to improve, discontinue the remedy. If the eczema gets worse after you take a remedy, stop using it.

■ Take *Graphites* if the patches of eczema are moist and oozing, with a clear or slightly yellow discharge. The eczema may be anywhere on the body, but it is most likely to be on the palms of your hands, behind your ears, and on your scalp. Take one dose of *Graphites* 30x or 9c, as directed on the product label, three times a day for up to five days.

■ If your eczema is infected, oozing, and particularly bad on your scalp, take one dose of *Mezereum* 30x or 9c three times daily for up to five days.

■ If the eczema is worse on your legs, try using *Psorinum* 30x or 9c three times a day for up to three days.

■ If you have dry, red, itchy areas in the folds of your joints, possibly with small blisters on the surface of your skin, use *Rhus toxicodendron*. This remedy is for the person who feels better with warmth, likes to snuggle under the covers, and who enjoys warm oatmeal baths (see below). Take one dose of *Rhus toxicodendron* 30x or 9c three times daily for up to five days.

■ If you are sweaty, dislike bathing, throw off the covers, and feel better with your skin exposed to the air, choose

Sulfur. This is for the person who feels warm and has very red, dry, hot-looking patches of skin. Take one dose of *Sulfur* 30x or 9c once daily for three days.

■ If the eczema is wet and weeping, apply homeopathic *Calendula* cream directly to the area two to three times a day.

■ If the eczema is dry and scaly, apply *Urtica urens* ointment or gel two to three times a day until the dryness is relieved.

■ If none of the above remedies seems right, a homeopathic combination eczema remedy may be helpful.

BACH FLOWER REMEDIES

■ Rescue Remedy is available in an ointment form that is soothing and helpful for dry eczema. Follow the directions on the product label.

ACUPRESSURE

For the locations of acupressure points on the body, *see* ADMINISTERING AN ACUPRESSURE TREATMENT in Part Three.

■ Liver 3 and Large Intestine 4 relax the nervous system.

■ Spleen 10 helps improve circulation to the skin and take "heat" out of the blood.

■ Stomach 36 improves the body's utilization of nutrients.

AROMATHERAPY

For specific instructions on how to use aromatherapy, *see* PREPARING AROMATHERAPY TREATMENTS in Part Three.

■ To reduce inflammation and ease itching, use aromatherapy baths or compresses prepared with one to three of the following essential oils: elemi, geranium, lavender, myrrh, neroli, and rose. You can also add a few drops of one to three of these oils to a small quantity of jojoba oil to make a healing body oil.

Note: Be careful not to use too much essential oil in these treatments, and never apply essential oil directly to your skin. Always dilute it in water or a carrier oil. If irritation results, discontinue use of the suspect oil.

GENERAL RECOMMENDATIONS

■ Do anything and everything you can to reduce the itching. If you scratch, skin cells will reproduce rapidly and the patches of eczema will spread, making the condition difficult to control. A cool, wet compress applied to the area may help decrease itching quickly. An Aveeno or oatmeal bath is also good. Wrap a cup of oatmeal in a clean cloth or washcloth. Put this bag under the running faucet and swish it through the bath water. Squeeze and rub the wet bag over your skin. Oatmeal is very soothing to dry and inflamed skin.

■ Avoid anything that dries out your skin. Do not linger too long in the bath or shower, as this strips natural oils from the skin. After bathing, apply a very mild, nonallergenic lotion all over your body to lock in moisture and prevent further drying.

■ Expose the affected skin to fresh air and moderate amounts of sunshine. A thirty-minute exposure to ultraviolet rays will reduce inflammation. Monitor your exposure carefully, however, and don't stay out in the sun too long. Lengthy exposure to the sun can worsen eczema.

■ Wear soft, gentle cotton clothing. Avoid skin-irritating substances, such as soap residue in just-washed clothes, and other allergens that can exacerbate the condition. Make sure that clothes, towels, and washcloths are free of soap. A second rinse cycle may be helpful.

■ Consider possible food and environmental allergies.

■ To decrease the stress associated with this condition, learn relaxation and visualization techniques (*see* RELAXATION TECHNIQUES in Part Three).

Edema

See under CARDIOVASCULAR DISEASE; LYMPHEDEMA.

Ehrlichiosis

See under LYME AND OTHER TICKBORNE DISEASES.

Emphysema

Emphysema is a form of chronic obstructive pulmonary disease (COPD) that occurs when the alveoli, the tiny air sacs in the lungs, become damaged. A healthy lung contains millions of alveoli, which are connected to bronchioles (air passages). It has an elastic, spongy texture, and is able to contract and expand. In a lung affected by emphysema, the walls of some of the tiny air sacs break, and they merge with neighboring sacs, forming fewer and larger air sacs than normal. This reduces the total surface area of the alveolar walls. It is through the very thin walls of the alveoli that oxygen passes into the bloodstream and carbon dioxide passes out of the bloodstream to leave the body

with each exhalation. With less surface area for the exchange of oxygen and carbon dioxide to take place, air becomes trapped in the lungs with each inhalation, and less carbon dioxide can be removed with each exhalation. The result is a kind of slow suffocation.

Emphysema develops slowly, and there may be no outward symptoms in the beginning stages. The first symptoms of emphysema are shortness of breath and coughing. The shortness of breath becomes more severe as the disease progresses. Eventually, it becomes difficult to take in enough oxygen even when at rest. Other possible symptoms include fast and shallow breathing and a barrel-chested appearance. Some people with emphysema breathe rapidly to take in sufficient oxygen and retain a normal skin color. Others turn a bluish color due to oxygen deprivation, and swell because of fluid trapped in the tissues. High levels of carbon dioxide that accumulate in the blood cause anxiety, confusion, and weakness. Fluid in the lungs, congestive heart failure, and lung failure are common in advanced cases.

People whose occupations require repeated use of forceful lung power, such as glass blowers and those who play wind instruments, have a higher risk than others of developing emphysema. This is because subjecting the lungs to higher than normal pressures can weaken and ultimately damage the walls of the tiny air sacs. Hard efforts at breathing, such as may occur in asthma, bronchopneumonia, chronic bronchitis, near-suffocation, tuberculosis, whooping cough, and even during prolonged labor, can damage the alveoli as well. However, the vast majority of cases of emphysema are caused by cigarette smoking. Tobacco smoke not only irritates lung tissue directly, but appears to cause the release of chemicals within the alveoli that injure their walls, accelerating emphysema. Aging also has an effect. As the body ages, the lungs become less and less elastic, which further reduces the efficiency of the oxygen-carbon dioxide exchange.

Another factor in the development of emphysema is antitrypsin, a protein normally present in the bloodstream. Antitrypsin helps to protect against the release of damaging chemicals in the lungs prompted by exposure to tobacco smoke and other pollutants. People who have low levels of antitrypsin are more likely to develop emphysema than those with normal levels. In rare cases, an individual may have a hereditary condition that results in a deficiency of this hormone. Such a person is at high risk for COPD.

Emphysema is diagnosed by means of a chest x-ray, spirometry (tests that measure breathing capacity), and blood tests that reveal the ratio of oxygen and carbon dioxide in the bloodstream.

CONVENTIONAL TREATMENT

■ If you suffer from emphysema, it is wise to seek out and work closely with a pulmonary specialist or other physician who specializes, or at the very least has considerable experience, in the treatment of this condition.

■ There is no cure for emphysema. Treatment is directed at relieving the symptoms, managing complications, and slowing the progression of the disease. This starts with education about the things that make the disease worse, especially smoking. Quitting smoking is paramount. Nicotine patches may help some people to get free of the habit (see NICOTINE ADDICTION).

■ Bronchodilators, medications that open the airways, are a mainstay of treatment. Examples include albuterol (Proventil, Ventolin) and metaproterenol (Alupent). They are usually used in aerosol inhaler form, but the same types of drugs can be taken orally. Another oral bronchodilator is theophylline (Theo-dur, Slo-Bid), which is an oral bronchodilator. These drugs can cause a wide variety of side effects, including high blood pressure, rapid heart rate, nervousness, and tremors (unfortunately, drugs that relax lung tissue tend to have the opposite effect elsewhere in the body). Other possible effects include headaches, nausea, vomiting, rashes, and abdominal discomfort. If your doctor prescribes theophylline, the dosage level will have to be carefully monitored, as overdoses can cause serious heart-rhythm disturbances, convulsions, and even death.

■ Another inhaled bronchodilator, ipratropium bromide (Atrovent), is reserved for later stages of the disease and may enhance the effect of other medications to some degree. Potential side effects of this drug include worsening of the symptoms being treated, cough, nervousness, dizziness, headache, nausea, gastrointestinal discomfort, and dry mouth. This medication should not be used by people who also have glaucoma, prostate enlargement, or problems with urinary outflow.

■ Controlling the production of mucus and sputum is important for preventing infection. This may be done by increasing your fluid intake or with a technique such as postural drainage or chest percussion. In postural drainage, gravity is used to attempt to remove sputum from the lungs; chest percussion is an attempt to break it loose by means of vibratory pounding on the chest. Sometimes an expectorant such as guaifenesin (Duratuss, Humibid, Organidin, and others), a decongestant such as pseudoephedrine (Sudafed and others)—or a combination of the two, like Entex or Guaifed—may be tried, but medication is not commonly believed to be very helpful for this purpose. If infection does occur, a broad-spectrum antibiotic will likely be prescribed.

■ As with asthma, a steroid such as beclomethasone (Beclovent, Vanceril, and others) or triamcinolone (Azmacort, Nasacort) may be prescribed to cut down on inflammation and sensitivity to stimuli that can cause acute

worsening of symptoms. Since steroids have an adverse effect on the immune system as well as on the beneficial bacteria in the intestines, it is best to use these drugs as little as possible.

■ Anxiety caused by serious shortness of breath may be treated with a codeine-type medication or an antianxiety drug such as diazepam (Valium).

■ In advanced emphysema, supplemental oxygen therapy may be necessary.

■ A surgical procedure in which the worst areas of diseased tissue are removed has been reported to yield a modest improvement in symptoms. For very severe emphysema, the only hope is a lung transplant, usually done as part of a heart and lung transplant procedure. Transplantable organs are in short supply, however, and this surgery is extremely expensive. Moreover, the antirejection drugs that must be taken after organ transplantation destroy the immune system. Nevertheless, people who survive the operation and the immediate postoperative period can usually expect an improvement in lung function.

DIETARY GUIDELINES

■ Because most people with emphysema have a history of smoking (or exposure to secondhand smoke), their digestion is usually poor. Chinese medicine teaches that smoking not only causes damage to the lungs, but also increases stomach acidity and impairs digestion. It is important to eat high-quality nutrient-rich foods. Refinement, processing, microwaving, and long cooking should be kept to an absolute minimum.

■ Eat a diet high in fiber. Stress fresh vegetables, especially leafy greens. Maximize your intake of fresh fruits, whole grains, and the clean, lean protein found in chicken and fish.

■ Because they increase the production of mucus, avoid fried, greasy, and fatty foods and keep your intake of dairy products and refined sugars to a minimum.

■ To aid digestion, eat slowly and chew your food thoroughly. Take the time to enjoy what you eat, and don't swallow large particles of food. If chewing is a problem, purée your foods when possible.

■ Investigate the possibility of food allergies. For at least seven days, avoid any food you have cravings for or normally eat every day. Then reintroduce the food and be alert for changes in symptoms. If they worsen, avoid that food. To uncover a sensitivity to dairy foods, unfortunately, it may take up to three weeks of abstinence.

NUTRITIONAL SUPPLEMENTS

■ To counteract nutritional deficiencies, take a multivitamin and mineral supplement that contains more than the recommended daily allowances (RDAs) of all major nutrients except for iron and copper, which should be at or below the RDAs.

■ Chinese medicine teaches that when the lungs are impaired, the kidneys cannot "catch" energy. Strengthening the adrenal glands can help reduce breathlessness associated with weak kidneys and poor adrenal function. Take 150 milligrams adrenal glandular extract twice daily.

■ The antioxidants fight free radicals. Many of the symptoms of emphysema are associated with the impaired use of oxygen due to free-radical damage. Take a good antioxidant combination formula that provides 10,000 international units of vitamin A, 15,000 international units of beta-carotene, 3,000 milligrams of vitamin C, 1,500 milligrams of bioflavonoids, and 200 mcg of selenium daily.

■ L-carnitine is a nutrient that allows the energy "factories" of the body to burn fat for energy, which helps to improve exercise tolerance in people with lung disease. Take 500 milligrams two to three times daily.

■ Coenzyme Q_{10} has been shown in treadmill tests of patients with pulmonary disease to help with energy production when taken in doses of 90 to 100 milligrams a day. If your antioxidant formula does not contain this much, you may wish to consider augmenting it with an additional supplement.

■ To help ensure full digestion of nutrients, take a full-spectrum digestive-enzyme supplement containing 5,000 international units of lipase, 2,500 international units of amylase, and 300 international units of protease, plus 500 to 1,000 milligrams of pancreatin, with each meal. The fatigue associated with emphysema is sometimes related to incomplete utilization of nutrients.

Note: Long-term supplementation with pancreatin is not advised, as it can cause your pancreas to reduce its own production of this important enzyme. Overuse also has the potential to cause nausea or diarrhea. After two months on pancreatin, discontinue use and monitor your reaction. If you find that your problems recur, discuss pancreatin supplementation with your health-care provider.

■ Green-foods supplements contain important trace minerals that are essential for the repair of lung tissue. They also provide chlorophyll, a valuable antioxidant. Take a green-foods supplement as directed on the product label.

■ Magnesium helps to relax bronchial tissue. Even if you are not deficient in this mineral, it can be helpful. Take 500 milligrams three times daily. If you develop loose stools, reduce the dosage to the greatest amount that does not cause diarrhea.

■ N-acetylcysteine (NAC) helps to loosen mucus and boosts the production of glutathione, a powerful free-rad-

ical quencher in lung tissue. It has been used in Europe for years, and has an excellent track record for improving lung function when taken in doses of 1,000 to 2,000 milligrams a day.

■ Proteolytic enzymes act as natural anti-inflammatories. Take a proteolytic-enzyme formula two to three times daily between meals.

■ Vitamin A helps heal the mucous membranes of the lungs. Take 25,000 international units of emulsified vitamin A three times daily for one month. Then reduce your intake to 25,000 international units twice a day for a month. During the third month, reduce your intake to 25,000 international units once a day.

Note: If you are pregnant, or intend to get pregnant, or if you have liver disease, consult your doctor before taking supplemental vitamin A. Pregnant women should not ingest a total of more than 25,000 international units of supplemental vitamin A *per week* from all sources.

■ Vitamin C is not only an antioxidant, but also an important element in the production of collagen, the number-one repair protein in the body. Take 1,000 milligrams twice a day.

HERBAL TREATMENT

■ Chinese (Korean) ginseng is a whole-body tonic herb that helps to relieve shortness of breath and ease stress. This revitalizing and energizing herb also supports adrenal function. Select a standardized extract containing 7 percent ginsenosides and take 100 milligrams one-half hour before breakfast. This is a powerful herb. If you are interested in taking it on a regular basis, you should do so under the supervision of a health-care professional.

Note: Do not use Chinese ginseng if you have high blood pressure, heart disease, or hypoglycemia. If you are sensitive to the effects of caffeine and other stimulants, you may want to consult with a qualified herbalist before using ginseng.

■ Cordyceps is a tonic herb that increases the oxygen supply to body systems, enhances immunity, and acts as an antioxidant. Take 1,000 milligrams of standardized extract twice a day.

■ Licorice supports adrenal function. This herb is a good anti-inflammatory and expectorant that is traditionally used in Chinese medicine against asthma. It is particularly valuable against respiratory problems and also enhances the immune system. Select deglycyrrhizinated licorice and take 250 milligrams twice a day.

Note: Ordinary licorice can elevate blood pressure, and should not be taken on a daily basis for more than five days a row. DGL should not have this effect, however.

■ Loquat is a Chinese herb that is an anti-inflammatory

for the lungs and is used to expel phlegm. Take 250 milligrams twice a day.

■ Marshmallow root can help ease the dryness and inflammation of the lungs associated with emphysema. Take a cup of marshmallow root tea, or 500 milligrams in capsule form, twice daily.

■ Mullein helps to loosen phlegm, relieve muscle spasms, and reduce inflammation. Take a cup of mullein tea three times a day.

■ Slippery elm is soothing to the respiratory system. It has been used for centuries to treat coughs and a wide variety of lung problems. Take 250 to 500 milligrams or a cup of slippery elm tea up to three times a day, as needed.

HOMEOPATHY

Emphysema is best treated with a constitutional remedy. See a homeopathic physician who can prescribe one for you. For relief of acute symptoms, select one of the following symptom-specific remedies.

■ *Bryonia* is good if you have a dry cough, with a dry throat, and mucus that is difficult to dislodge but that ultimately loosens after a lot of coughing. You may also be irritable and suffer from constipation. Take one dose of *Bryonia* 12x or 6c, as directed on the product label, three or four times a day, as needed, for up to three days.

■ *Hepar sulfuris calcareum* will help if you have a dry, hoarse cough made worse by exposure to cold or by eating anything cold. You may lose your voice from time to time. Take one dose of *Hepar sulfuris calcareum* 12x or 6c three times a day, as needed, for up to three days.

■ *Spongia tosta* 12x or 6c is for a barking, "croupy" cough with a hoarse voice and a larynx that may be sensitive to the touch. You may have a tendency toward heart palpitations as well. Take one dose of *Spongia tosta* 12x or 6c three or four times a day, as needed, for up to three days.

■ *Stannum* is for a violent dry cough that is worse in the evening and is made worse by laughing, singing, and talking. You are probably hoarse and expel greenish mucus during the day. Take one dose of *Stannum* 12x or 6c three or four times a day, as needed, for up to three days.

BACH FLOWER REMEDIES

Select the remedy that most closely fits your emotional tendencies and concerns, and take it as needed, following the directions on the product label.

■ Holly helps to ease anger and fits of bad temper.

■ Choose Hornbeam if you are so exhausted and fatigued that you cannot participate in everyday activities.

■ Impatiens calms nervousness, irritability, and hyperactivity.

■ Mimulus is for fearfulness and shyness. You may talk of being afraid, and are well able to name your fears.

ACUPRESSURE

For the locations of acupressure points on the body, *see* ADMINISTERING AN ACUPRESSURE TREATMENT in Part Three.

■ Bladder 13, 14, 15, 16, 17, and 23 relax the chest.

■ Heart 3 increases circulation in the chest.

■ Kidney 7 is an important point for strengthening kidney function. In Chinese medicine, the kidneys support the flow of energy to the lungs. If the kidneys are strong, the lungs will heal more easily.

■ Lung 7 helps to clear the lungs.

■ Pericardium 3 improves circulation in the chest.

■ Pericardium 6 relaxes the chest.

■ Stomach 36 improves the utilization of nutrients, thereby enhancing overall well-being.

AROMATHERAPY

For specific instructions on how to use aromatherapy, *see* PREPARING AROMATHERAPY TREATMENTS in Part Three.

■ A steam inhalation treatment made with basil, pine, and/or tea tree oil can help to clear mucus and ease breathing. Rubbing a massage oil prepared with any or all of these oils over the chest may also be helpful.

GENERAL RECOMMENDATIONS

■ If you are a smoker, stop immediately. Cigarette smoking is far and away the number-one cause of emphysema.

■ Avoid environments with polluted air, including areas where you are subject to occupational chemicals and/or secondhand smoke. Air pollution worsens emphysema.

■ Try to avoid any type of respiratory infection, including the common cold. Stay out of crowds, if possible, and wash your hands frequently. Having a respiratory infection in addition to emphysema can worsen symptoms and will place an additional burden on your already damaged lungs.

■ Exercise can slow the progress of this disease. However, too little exercise and too much exercise are equally dangerous. A program of simple, gradually escalating exercises has proven helpful in many cases. Both swimming and bicycling help open the lungs, and yoga helps with breathing. Discuss this with your doctor to determine what exercises are safe for you.

■ Physical therapy that includes breathing retraining can be extremely helpful. Discuss the possibility with your doctor.

PREVENTION

■ Don't smoke, and avoid secondhand smoke. The overwhelming majority of cases of emphysema are a direct result of cigarette smoking.

Endocarditis

See under NAIL PROBLEMS AND INJURIES; VASCULITIS.

Endometriosis

Endometriosis is a condition in which cells of the endometrium (the lining of the uterus) are found growing in other parts of the pelvic cavity. Even though these cells are not located in the uterine lining, they continue to act as if they were, following the regular monthly cycle of becoming engorged with blood and then bleeding during the menstrual period. Since this extraneous blood has no way to leave the body, cysts form within the pelvic cavity. As the cysts grow, they may form adhesions that bind together tissues and organs that are not meant to be bound together. Adhesions can become very painful.

Symptoms of endometriosis include severe abdominal, uterine, and/or lower-back pain, usually just prior to and/or during menstruation, and abnormal or heavy bleeding. The passage of clots and small pieces of tissue during menstruation is not uncommon. Nausea, vomiting, and constipation may occur. Sexual intercourse may become extremely painful. Interestingly, the severity of the pain is not necessarily an indicator of how extensive or severe the disease is.

Endometriosis occurs most often in women between the ages of twenty-five and forty. In the United States alone, more than 12 million women are affected. This condition has a close association with infertility, although the nature of the association is not clearly understood. It has long been known that moderate to severe endometriosis can cause infertility, usually by blocking the fallopian tubes. However, more recent research shows that even mild cases can lead to infertility, even in women who are ovulating normally. All in all, an estimated 30 to 40 percent of women who have endometriosis are unable to conceive. Fortunately, this can sometimes be reversed by surgical removal or destruction of the abnormal growths.

The cause or causes of endometriosis are not known, but there are several theories that have been advanced within the medical community. One theory holds that it occurs because fragments of endometrial tissue shed during menstruation fail to leave the body during the menstrual flow, but instead travel back through the fallopian tubes and enter into the pelvic cavity, where they adhere to various structures and grow. Known as the *reflux menstruation theory,* this idea was first postulated in 1920. Another theory attempts to explain the condition by saying that endometrial cells travel to other parts of the body through the bloodstream and lymphatic system. A more recent explanation holds that endometriosis is the consequence of a defect that occurs during fetal development. According to this theory, endometrial cells fail to reach their proper place in the cluster of cells that are destined to become the uterus, and instead become embedded in the peritoneum (the membrane that lines the entire abdominal cavity) and other sites within the pelvic cavity.

Endometriosis is diagnosed on the basis of symptoms, a pelvic examination to check for signs of masses adhering to internal organs, and, possibly, direct examination by laparoscopy, a procedure in which a small lighted instrument is used to directly examine the interior of the abdominal cavity.

CONVENTIONAL TREATMENT

■ If the pain during menstrual periods is not too severe, it can usually be managed with nonsteroidal anti-inflammatory drugs (NSAIDs) such as aspirin (in Bayer, Ecotrin, and other medications), ibuprofen (Advil, Motrin, Nuprin, and others), or naproxen (Aleve). Take these drugs with food to prevent possible stomach upset. More severe pain may require prescription medication.

■ Treatment for endometriosis focuses on controlling symptoms without adversely affecting a woman's fertility. There are two principal approaches: drug therapy to suppress ovulation for up to nine months, to keep the cysts from growing and allow them to heal, or surgery to remove or destroy the lesions. There is some controversy within the medical community as to which approach should be preferred.

■ A primary drug for stopping ovulation is danazol (Danocrine), which works by blocking the receptor sites for female sex hormones, so that a woman no longer experiences monthly cycles. Potential side effects include masculinizing changes (such as smaller breasts, a lowered voice, and abnormal hair growth) as well as cramping, swelling, liver problems, drying of the vagina, and mood swings.

■ Another class of drugs used to suppress ovulation include nafarelin (Synarel) and leuprolide (Lupron). With repeated use, these drugs "empty" the pituitary gland of the hormones that stimulate release of the sex hormones. As a result, tissues that rely on such stimulation (like the uterus and ovaries) are not signaled to function, so they become dormant. Possible problems with these drugs include joint pains and decreased bone density, headaches, changes in sex drive, nausea, vomiting, hot flashes, vaginal drying, and mood swings.

■ Oral contraceptives are sometimes prescribed for endometriosis, to be taken continuously, without a break each month, for up to six months. Potential side effects include irregular vaginal bleeding, bloating, nausea, depression, headaches, thinning of the hair, and darkening of the skin, as well as more serious problems such as blood clots, heart attack, and stroke. Oral contraceptives should not be taken by women who smoke or who have a known history of cardiovascular disease or gynecological cancer.

■ Surgical procedures employed to treat endometriosis include laparoscopy with either electric cautery (burning) or laser excision of the abnormal tissue. Adhesions can be a problem following any type of surgery. Many doctors believe that removing only the dark-colored "chocolate" cysts considered characteristic of endometriosis is sufficient. However, doctors who believe that endometriosis results from an inborn defect say that endometrial cysts come in many colors, and often change color as they develop. They maintain that removing only the dark cysts leaves seeds of the disease behind, and they claim greater than usual success from removing both the typical dark-colored cysts and atypical cysts, which range in color from very pale to very dark.

■ The only permanent means of stopping all signs of the disease is complete removal of both ovaries. Obviously, this kind of surgery is reserved for the most severe cases and/or women who have completed childbearing.

DIETARY GUIDELINES

■ The right diet is very important. Eat a diet containing plenty of fiber, with an emphasis on lightly steamed green vegetables. Eating easily digested foods helps to reduce the formation of gas and can make the lower abdomen more comfortable.

■ Avoid refined sugar, greasy foods, fat, caffeine, and alcohol. These substances promote an acidic environment that impairs digestion.

■ To flush toxins from your body and promote good digestion, drink six to eight glasses of pure water daily.

NUTRITIONAL SUPPLEMENTS

■ Calcium and magnesium calm the nervous system; magnesium also prevents constipation, which can make the pain of endometriosis worse. Take 500 milligrams of calcium three times daily and 500 milligrams of magnesium twice a day.

Note: If you develop loose stools, decrease the dosage to the highest level that does not result in diarrhea.

■ To help relieve abdominal gases and reduce abdominal stress and discomfort, take a full-spectrum digestive-enzyme supplement providing 5,000 international units of lipase, 2,500 international units of amylase, and 300 international units of protease, plus 500 to 1,000 milligrams of pancreatin, with each meal. Digestive enzymes are essential for complete digestion.

Note: Long-term supplementation with pancreatin is not advised, as it can cause your pancreas to reduce its own production of this important enzyme. Overuse also has the potential to cause nausea or diarrhea. After two months on pancreatin, discontinue use and monitor your reaction. If you find that your problems recur, discuss pancreatin supplementation with your health-care provider.

■ Green-foods supplements are high in important trace minerals that strengthen the blood, and they also have antioxidant action. In addition, they provide chlorophyll and vitamin K, essential for normal blood clotting. These nutrients are especially important if you experience heavy bleeding. Take a green-foods supplement as directed on the product label.

■ If hypothyroidism is a problem, take 150 milligrams of kelp three times daily. This sea vegetable is high in iodine, which strengthens thyroid function. It is also high in iron, which is an important nutrient for the woman with heavy menstrual bleeding. Many women with endometriosis are deficient in iron.

■ Selenium is an antioxidant that helps defuse free radicals and reduce inflammation. Take 200 micrograms twice a day for two weeks, then cut back to 200 micrograms daily.

■ The B vitamins are essential for hormonal balance and neurotransmission. Take a B-complex supplement that supplies 25 milligrams of each of the primary B vitamins two to three times daily. In addition, take an extra 50 milligrams of pantothenic acid and 25 milligrams of vitamin B_6 (pyridoxine) three times daily, between meals. Pantothenic acid assists adrenal function and vitamin B_6 is important for the synthesis of many hormones.

■ Vitamin C and bioflavonoids have anti-inflammatory properties, act to strengthen tissue, detoxify the blood, and promote healing. Three times a day, take 500 to 1,000 milligrams of a vitamin-C formula that contains bioflavonoids, particularly rutin.

■ Vitamin E helps to maintain proper hormonal balance. Choose a product containing mixed tocopherols and start by taking 200 international units daily, then gradually increase the dosage until you are taking 400 international units in the morning and another 400 international units in the afternoon or evening.

Note: If you have high blood pressure, limit your intake of supplemental vitamin E to a total of 400 international units daily. If you are taking an anticoagulant (blood thinner), consult your physician before taking supplemental vitamin E.

HERBAL TREATMENT

■ Butiao is the premier herbal remedy for endometriosis. This is a Chinese formula has been used for over 3,000 years to help resolve excessive uterine bleeding and ease abdominal cramping and menstrual pain. For six months, take the equivalent of 500 milligrams three times daily during the two weeks before the anticipated onset of your period.

■ Bupleurum and dong quai have been used for millennia by the Chinese to regulate female hormones and relax a stressed nervous system. Take 1,000 milligrams of a bupleurum and dong quai combination formula three times daily for the two weeks prior to the anticipated onset of your menstrual period for up to three months.

■ Carthamus and persica is another excellent herbal combination used in Chinese medicine to decrease inflammation in the lower abdomen and ease discomfort. Take 500 milligrams three times daily for up to two months.

■ Nettle is a excellent blood-building tonic herb that is rich in trace minerals that are often missing in the diet. To help revitalize the blood, take 250 to 500 milligrams three times daily for one to two weeks following menstruation.

■ Pine-bark and grape-seed extracts have natural anti-inflammatory properties. Take 50 milligrams of either three times daily for the two weeks prior to the anticipated onset of your menstrual period. Consistency is important—generally, there is a noticeable improvement after six complete menstrual cycles.

■ Red raspberry leaf has historically been used to ease menstrual cramps. One study demonstrated that it helps to relax the uterus. It also contains oligomeric proanthocyanadins, or PCOs, which have a natural anti-inflammatory action. Take a cup of red raspberry leaf tea two to three times daily, as needed.

■ Siberian ginseng can help to revitalize hormonal function and restore energy. To relieve fatigue, choose a standardized extract containing 0.5 percent eleutheroside E and take 100 milligrams twice daily, first thing in the morning and at lunchtime.

HOMEOPATHY

Endometriosis responds best to a constitutional remedy; it is best to see a homeopathic practitioner who can prescribe one for you. The following remedies can be used to provide short-term relief of symptoms.

■ *Colocynthis* is the remedy for intense, agonizing pain in the lower abdomen, especially around the ovaries, that feels better when your knees are drawn up close to your chest. The pain is accompanied by irritablity and restlessness. Take one dose of *Colocynthis* 12x or 6c, as recommended on the product label, three times daily, as needed.

■ Choose *Cupurum metallicum* if your abdomen is tense, hot, and tender to the touch, and you feel better after drinking cold water. Your periods may tend to be late, and cramping pain may radiate into the chest area. You may suffer cramps before, during, or after a menstrual period. Take one dose of *Cupurum metallicum* 12x or 6c three times daily, as needed.

■ *Dioscorea villosa* is for pain that radiates from the uterus throughout the abdominal area. There may be lot of abdominal gas and flatulence as well. Take one dose of *Dioscorea villosa* 6x or 3c three times daily, as needed.

■ *Magnesia phosphorica* is very effective for cramps, menstrual pain, and bloating. If your abdomen is distended and you are experiencing spasms in your lower abdomen, and particularly if the pain improves with the application of heat, try this remedy. Take one dose of *Magnesia phosphorica* 12x or 6c three times daily, as needed.

BACH FLOWER REMEDIES

Select the remedy that most closely fits your emotional tendencies and concerns, and take it as needed, following the directions on the product label.

■ Holly calms feelings of anger and jealousy that burst out into fits of bad temper.

■ Hornbeam can help ease fatigue and exhaustion that render you so tired you miss out on normal daily activities.

■ Scleranthus helps to overcome uncertainty and difficulty making decisions.

■ White Chestnut counteracts a tendency to obsess on ideas or events long after they should have been forgotten.

ACUPRESSURE

For the locations of acupressure points on the body, *see* ADMINISTERING AN ACUPRESSURE TREATMENT in Part Three.

■ Gallbladder 41 regulates hormonal function.

■ Kidney 3 and 7 increase circulation to the reproductive organs.

■ Large Intestine 10 improves the functioning of the large intestine. Traditional Chinese medicine maintains that if the lower abdomen is "comfortable"—if digestion is good and there is a minimum of abdominal gas—menstrual cramps will be minimized.

■ Spleen 6 reduces uterine cramping.

AROMATHERAPY

For specific instructions on how to use aromatherapy, *see* PREPARING AROMATHERAPY TREATMENTS in Part Three.

■ Essential oils of chamomile, rose, and ylang-ylang can help to ease cramping and pain, and lift the spirits. Use either or both of these oils in an aromatherapy bath or to make a hot or cold compress, or add a few drops to massage oil.

GENERAL RECOMMENDATIONS

■ Regular daily exercise helps ease symptoms. Moderate low-impact exercise, such as walking and stretching, have been shown to be beneficial.

■ Use sanitary pads, not tampons, which can contribute to pain and cramping. Tampons also may add to the risk of reflux menstruation.

■ Orian Truss, MD, and William Crook, MD, who have extensive experience with systemic yeast infection, have found a relationship between yeast in the body and endometriosis. In his book *The Yeast Connection and the Woman* (Professional Books, 1995), Dr. Crook states that there is very significant association between chronic candidiasis and endometriosis. *See* CANDIDA INFECTION for additional dietary and nutritional-supplement recommendations.

■ The use of topical natural progesterone cream can be helpful for some women with endometriosis. Discuss this possibility with your gynecologist.

PREVENTION

■ Get regular exercise. Regular strenuous aerobic exercise lowers the level of estrogen circulating in the body, which helps lower the risk of developing endometriosis. A study conducted by the Harvard Medical School determined that young women who exercised more than seven hours a week had one-fifth the risk of developing this condition as compared with women who did not exercise. Unfortunately, this finding applied only to young women who began exercising before the age of twenty-six.

■ The incidence of endometriosis has been increasing in recent years. Once a medical curiosity, it is now a common condition. Interestingly, this has occurred since the introduction of birth-control pills. No one has yet researched the possibility of a connection here, but since hormones are used in the control of this disease, it seems reasonable to consider the possibility that hormones may be involved in causing it. Avoiding oral contraceptives, especially at a young age, seems a worthwhile precaution, particularly for women with family history of endometriosis.

Epilepsy

See under SEIZURE.

Epididymitis

Epididymitis is an inflammation of the epididymis, a structure located along the back of the testicle. Newly formed sperm cells pass from the testis, where they are produced, into the epididymis, where they spend ten to twenty days, continuing to grow and mature. When the sperm cells are capable of fertilizing an egg, they travel from the epididymis through the vas deferens (sperm duct) to the seminal vesicles, where they are held until ejaculation. The epididymis is a long but tightly coiled tube. If one of these tiny tubes were stretched out straight, it would measure from about thirteen to twenty feet in length.

The earliest symptom of epididymitis is swelling that occurs on the back of one or both testicles, where the epididymides are situated. The affected area becomes hot, tender, and very painful. As the swelling continues to build over a period of a few hours, the scrotum may swell and stiffen. A man suffering from epididymitis may waddle when he walks. This awkward posture is an attempt to protect the affected area. If the testis also becomes inflamed and infected, the condition is called epididymoorchitis.

Epididymitis can result from several causes. A urinary tract infection can spread through the sperm ducts to the epididymis. This disorder can also be a result of prostatitis (infection of the prostate gland), and it can occur after prostatectomy (surgical removal of the prostate). Organisms that commonly infect the region this way include staphylococci, streptococci, and *Escherichia coli*. Epididymitis is also a common complication of sexually transmitted diseases, primarily chlamydia, but also gonorrhea and syphilis. In some cases, epididymitis develops as a complication of long-term use of an indwelling catheter.

If you think you have epididymitis, contact your physician immediately. Diagnosis is made by analysis of a urine sample and, sometimes, prostate secretions, to identify the source of the infection. In sexually active men with multiple partners, epididymitis is very often the result of urethritis (infection of the urethra) caused by chlamydia (*see* CHLAMYDIA). If it is determined that the disorder was sexually transmitted, both partners should be treated to prevent them from passing the infection back and forth. It is important that the infection be adequately treated. If it becomes chronic, it can cause formation of pus pockets, or abscesses, and may lead to sterility.

CONVENTIONAL MEDICINE

While the inflammation is acute, keep movement to an absolute minimum. Elevation of the scrotum may be recommended to avoid any pressure on the area.

If the condition was contracted as a result of sexual contact, both partners should receive antibiotics. The usual approach is dual-drug treatment with an injection of a cephalosporin antibiotic such as ceftriaxone (Rocephin) followed by a ten-day course of an oral tetracycline antibiotic such as doxycycline (Doryx, Vibramycin, and others).

If the condition was not sexually transmitted but a result of a urinary tract infection or an infection of the prostate, three to four weeks of oral antibiotic therapy will probably be prescribed.

In especially severe or chronic cases, surgery may be recommended to drain the infection and allow the area to heal.

DIETARY GUIDELINES

Eat a diet that is high in unrefined complex carbohydrates and includes plenty of lean, clean protein foods such as soy products, chicken, and fish.

Maximize your intake of steamed green vegetables. Include plentiful amounts of parsley (leaf and root), burdock root, and daikon radish. These healthy vegetables can now be found in almost every supermarket. They help to detoxify the liver and genitourinary tract.

Drink cranberry and pineapple juices. Cranberry is a noted antibacterial, and pineapple has anti-inflammatory properties.

During the acute stage of the infection, avoid spicy, greasy, and rich foods, including red meat. Also avoid alcohol, caffeine, and soft drinks. All these foods aggravate symptoms.

Drink eight glasses of pure water daily. Water flushes toxins from the body and helps cleanse the genitourinary tract.

Once the condition has been resolved, include pumpkin seeds in your diet. Pumpkin seeds are naturally high in zinc, which is required for a healthy prostate.

NUTRITIONAL SUPPLEMENTS

If you must take antibiotics, you should take a probiotic supplement to replace the friendly bacteria destroyed by antibiotics. Take it as recommended on the product label three times daily for two weeks after completing a course of antibiotics. If you are allergic to milk, select a dairy-free formula.

■ Vitamin A has strong antioxidant properties, fights free-radical damage, and has anti-inflammatory action. Take 25,000 international units twice daily for one week.

Note: If you have liver disease, consult your doctor before taking supplemental vitamin A.

■ Vitamin C is a natural antibacterial that fights infection and inflammation. It also stimulates immune function. Take 1,000 milligrams of mineral ascorbate or esterified vitamin C (Ester-C) with bioflavonoids four to five times daily during the acute phase of the condition. Then reduce the dosage to 1,000 milligrams two to three times daily for three to four weeks after the infection has been resolved. If at any point you develop diarrhea, cut the dosage back moderately until you no longer have loose stools.

■ Vitamin E is an antioxidant nutrient and helps stimulate the immune system. Choose a product containing mixed tocopherols and start by taking 200 international units daily, then gradually increase the dosage until you are taking 400 international units twice a day.

Note: If you have high blood pressure, limit your intake of supplemental vitamin E to a total of 400 international units daily. If you are taking an anticoagulant (blood thinner), consult your physician before taking supplemental vitamin E.

■ A deficiency of zinc is associated with prostate problems, as well as urinary tract infections. This necessary mineral also supports the immune system. Take 15 milligrams of zinc three times daily.

Note: Take zinc with food to prevent stomach upset. If you take over 30 milligrams of zinc on a daily basis for more than one or two months, you should also take 1 to 2 milligrams of copper each day to maintain a proper mineral balance.

■ The essential fatty acids in borage, evening primrose, or flaxseed oil help to regulate hormonal function, which becomes unbalanced during an episode of epididymitis and/or urinary tract infection. Once the infection has cleared, take 1 tablespoon (or 500 to 1,000 milligrams in capsule form) of any of these oils twice daily.

HERBAL TREATMENT

■ Cat's claw enhances the immune response and has antibacterial properties. Take 500 milligrams of standardized extract three times a day until your condition improves.

Note: Do not use cat's claw if you are pregnant or nursing, or if you are an organ-transplant recipient. Use it with caution if you are taking an anticoagulant (blood thinner).

■ Corn silk is a mild natural diuretic that can help cleanse the urinary tract of infection. Juniper berry has antiseptic properties that are helpful to the genitourinary tract. Marshmallow root is soothing to the mucous membranes of the genitourinary tract. Uva ursi is a natural antibacterial agent. You can use these herbs singly or in any combination. Take them brewed as a tea (*see* PREPARING HERBAL TREATMENTS in Part Three) or take them in capsule form, a total of 500 to 1,000 milligrams three to four times daily.

■ Echinacea and goldenseal are natural antibacterials that help to resolve infection. During the acute phase of the infection, take one dose of an echinacea and goldenseal combination formula supplying 250 to 500 milligrams of echinacea and 150 to 350 milligrams of goldenseal three to four times daily for five to seven days.

■ Oregano has antibacterial properties and helps to fight infection. Take 75 milligrams of standardized extract three times a day.

■ Pine-bark and grape-seed extracts are excellent anti-inflammatories. Take 50 milligrams of either three times daily.

HOMEOPATHY

■ *Belladonna* is for intensely hot, red, and swollen testicles that cause a lot of pain and make you very sensitive to the slightest motion. Wearing pants is an ordeal. Take one dose of *Belladonna* 30x or 15c, as directed on the product label, three to four times daily, as long as you have symptoms. When the heat subsides, discontinue the remedy.

■ *Cantharis* is the remedy for epididymitis accompanied by a urinary tract infection and burning on urination. To resolve the burning, take one dose of *Cantharis* 30x or 15c four times daily, as needed.

■ *Hamamelis* is for a hot, swollen testicle complicated by pain shooting up to the bladder. You may also have varicose veins in your legs. Take one dose of *Hamamelis* 12x or 6c four times daily, as long as symptoms persist.

■ If none of the above remedies seems suitable or proves successful, try *Sulfur*. This remedy is for the person who feels hot and may sleep with his feet outside the covers. The epididymitis may be accompanied by a skin rash. Take one dose of *Sulfur* 30x or 15c, while you have symptoms.

BACH FLOWER REMEDIES

Select the remedy that most closely fits your emotional tendencies and concerns, and take it as needed, following the directions on the product label.

■ Holly helps to tame anger and fits of temper, especially if they are really an expression of insecurity and jealousy.

■ Impatiens helps to calm impatience, hyperactivity, and nervous tension.

■ Mimulus eases fears that you can articulate. You may be naturally shy and may even blush on occasion.

■ White Chestnut helps to counteract a tendency to obsess on events, even those that may be long past.

ACUPRESSURE

For the locations of acupressure points on the body, *see* ADMINISTERING AN ACUPRESSURE TREATMENT in Part Three.

■ Pressure on the back Bladder points increases circulation throughout the body, with an emphasis on the genitourinary tract.

■ Bladder 60 and 62 increase circulation to the reproductive organs.

■ Kidney 3 and 7 are considered strategic in resolving many genitourinary problems.

■ Spleen 10 detoxifies the body.

■ Stomach 36 aids in strengthening the entire system.

GENERAL RECOMMENDATIONS

■ If the testes are swollen and very painful, bed rest is best. Applying an ice pack can help ease the pain, reduce inflammation, and bring down the swelling.

■ If you are mobile, reduce the strain on the affected area by supporting the scrotum with a jockstrap until the condition is resolved.

■ Once the infection is resolved, walk regularly every day. Walking stimulates and helps strengthen the musculature involved. If you are a bike rider, avoid bicycling for at least two months after the episode is over.

PREVENTION

■ Water, cranberry juice, and pineapple juice should be prominently featured on your menu.

■ The herbs listed under Herbal Treatment, above, all support the genitourinary tract and can be used preventively. Enjoy them as teas.

■ Saw palmetto supports the male genitourinary tract. This herb has achieved notable success in treating benign prostate enlargement, and also stimulates the functioning of the testes. Because of this effect, saw palmetto should not be used during the acute phase of infection. However, it may be used as an effective preventive. Choose a standardized extract containing 90 percent essential fatty acids and sterols, and take 200 to 400 milligrams twice a day.

Eye Problems

See BLEPHARITIS; CATARACTS; CONJUNCTIVITIS; CONTACT-

LENS PROBLEMS; CORNEAL PROBLEMS; DRY EYES; EYE-STRAIN; FLOATERS; GLAUCOMA; MACULAR DEGENERATION; NIGHT BLINDNESS; PHOTOPHOBIA; PRESBYOPIA; RETINA, DETACHED; RETINITIS PIGMENTOSA; RETINOPATHY, DIABET-IC/VASCULAR; STYE; UVEITIS. *Also see under* CYTOMEGALO-VIRUS.

Eyelid, Twitching

See under EYESTRAIN.

Eyestrain

Eyestrain is a condition that develops as a result of over-using your eyes, usually during activities that require close, precise focus. Eyestrain can cause eye pain and head pain ranging from a dull ache to a full-blown headache, and can even lead to a generalized feeling of exhaustion. Eye fatigue can also cause an involuntary twitching of the eyelids—a rhythmic twitch or tic that occurs in the small muscle groups of one eyelid. The most common symptom, however, is simply "tired" eyes.

Reading and needlework are common causes of eye-strain. People in particularly demanding occupations that require close continuous focus, such as computer opera-tors and jewelers, often strain their eyes by continuing past the point of comfort. Another possible cause of eye-strain is the wearing of corrective lenses (glasses or contact lenses) that are either the wrong prescription or not adjust-ed properly. If you find it becoming difficult to focus and you are blinking excessively, you may be suffering from eyestrain.

CONVENTIONAL TREATMENT

■ Correcting simple eyestrain is as simple as resting your eyes. One useful technique involves sitting in a comfort-able position, perhaps with your elbows resting on a table-top, and cupping your hands and placing them over your eyes so that you are not able to see any light. Do not press on your eyelids. Remain in this position for ten minutes or longer.

■ If you wear corrective lenses and have a problem with eyestrain after getting a new pair of glasses or contact lens-es, call your eye doctor. There may be a problem with the lenses.

■ If you suffer disturbed vision and sudden eye pain accompanied by nausea and/or vomiting, see a physician promptly or go to the emergency room of the nearest hos-

pital. These symptoms may be a sign of an acute attack of glaucoma, a serious eye disorder (*see* GLAUCOMA).

DIETARY GUIDELINES

■ Maximize your intake of fresh fruits and vegetables. These healthy foods contain valuable vitamins and min-erals as well as antioxidants that protect the eyes.

■ Eat clean, lean protein, such as that found in chicken and fish. Both protein and vitamin A are needed to main-tain healthy eyes.

■ Limit your intake of sugar and caffeine. These sub-stances contribute to eye irritation and worsen the symp-toms caused by many eye problems.

NUTRITIONAL SUPPLEMENTS

■ Beta-carotene is a strong antioxidant that prevents free-radical damage. It is related to vitamin A and has many of the same properties, but it does not become toxic in large doses. Take 10,000 to 25,000 international units of beta-carotene daily.

■ The essential fatty acids (EFAs), found in black currant seed oil, borage oil, evening primrose oil, and flaxseed oil, are required by every cell in the body. They have been shown to reduce pain, inflammation, and swelling. Take 500 to 1,000 milligrams of any of these oils twice daily.

■ Vitamin A protects against free-radical damage and is especially important to the eyes. Even a slight deficiency can contribute to eyestrain and cause the eyes to tire easi-ly. Take 10,000 international units of vitamin A three times a day for two months. Then reduce to a maintenance dosage of 5,000 international units twice daily.

Note: If you are pregnant, or intend to get pregnant, or if you have liver disease, consult your doctor before tak-ing supplemental vitamin A. Pregnant women should not ingest a total of more than 25,000 international units of supplemental vitamin A *per week* from all sources.

■ The B vitamins are required for intracellular metabo-lism in the tissues of the eyes. Inadequate intake of the B-complex vitamins can result in itching, burning, blood-shot eyes that water excessively. Vitamin B_2, in particu-lar, has been shown to reduce the incidence of floaters and "halos" around lights or objects. Combined with vitamins C and E, the B-complex vitamins are especially beneficial to the eyes. While symptoms are acute, take a B-complex supplement that supplies 50 milligrams of each of the primary B vitamins twice a day. When symp-toms improve, reduce the dosage to 25 milligrams twice daily.

■ Vitamin C helps to lower ocular pressure and protect and strengthen mucous membranes, including those of the eyes. Select a vitamin-C formula that includes bioflavonoids, especially rutin; these nutrients work best together. While symptoms are acute, take 1,000 to 3,000 milligrams of a vitamin-C complex three times daily. When symptoms improve, reduce the dosage to 500 to 1,000 milligrams three times daily.

■ Vitamin E is an antioxidant and is essential in cellular respiration. It has been shown to improve eyesight in clinical studies. The use of vitamin E has been shown to help relieve blurred and double vision. Choose a product containing mixed tocopherols and start by taking 200 international units daily, then gradually increase the dosage until you are taking 400 international units twice daily. Maintain this dosage as long as symptoms are acute. When symptoms improve, reduce the dosage to 200 international units twice daily.

Note: If you have high blood pressure, limit your intake of supplemental vitamin E to a total of 400 international units daily. If you are taking an anticoagulant (blood thinner), consult your physician before taking supplemental vitamin E.

HERBAL TREATMENT

■ Bilberry provides important nutrients that nourish the eyes and enhance visual function. Phytochemicals called anthocyanidins in this herb also help prevent damage to the structures of the eyes. Select a preparation containing 25 percent anthocyanidins (or PCOs) and take 40 to 80 milligrams three times daily.

■ Eyebright is rich in vitamin A and vitamin C. It also contains moderate amounts of the B-complex vitamins, vitamin D, and traces of vitamin E. Eyebright has been used for centuries both as an eyewash and in tea form as a tonic for the eyes. Taken internally, it helps maintain healthy eyes and good vision. Take 500 milligrams twice daily. Used as an eyewash, it helps relieve the discomfort of eyestrain. To make an eyebright eyewash, bring 3 ounces of sterile saline solution to a boil, and pour it over 1 tablespoon of dried cut herb (or one eyebright teabag). Allow it to steep for fifteen minutes, then strain out the herb. When the liquid has cooled to a comfortable temperature, bathe your eyes with the eyewash and/or prepare a compress by moistening a sterile cloth in the infusion. Place the compress over the closed eye, pressing down gently to achieve contact with the affected area. Relax for at least ten minutes. Then moisten a fresh sterile cloth in the eyewash tea and gently wipe the edges of your eyelids with it. Throw away (or sterilize) each cloth after one use.

■ Ginkgo biloba extract contains flavonoids with an affinity for organs that are rich in connective tissue, including the eyes. It enhances the use of oxygen and glucose by the cells, and works to normalize circulation. Select a preparation of ginkgo leaf extract containing at least 24 percent ginkgo heterosides (sometimes called flavoglycosides) and take 40 milligrams three times daily.

HOMEOPATHY

■ *Arnica* is the first remedy to try for tired eyes. Take one dose of *Arnica* 12x or 6c four times daily, as needed, for up to three days.

■ *Agaricus* helps a persistent eyelid tic that makes reading difficult, possibly accompanied by double vision. Take one dose of *Agaricus* 12x or 6c four times daily, as needed, for up to two days.

■ *Argentum nitricum* is for eyestrain with symptoms including redness, blurred vision, and possibly spots before the eyes. You may find it difficult to focus and have a poor sense of balance. The eye fatigue may be accompanied by insomnia. Take one dose of *Argentum nitricum* 12x or 6c four times daily, as needed, for up to three days.

■ *Euphrasia* is helpful for red, tired eyes that water all the time. Take one dose of *Euphrasia* 12x or 6c four times daily, as needed, for up to three days.

■ *Gelsemium* helps to calm twitching of the eyelids associated with eyes that are very heavy and droopy, with a tendency to close. One pupil may be more dilated than the other. Take one dose of *Gelsemium* 12x or 6c four times daily, as needed, for up to two days.

■ *Phosphorus* is for eyestrain accompanied by nervousness, anxiety, or fear. Take one dose of *Phosphorus* 12x or 6c four times daily, as needed, for up to three days.

■ *Pulsatilla* helps calm twitching of the eyelid that is accompanied by inflammation. Take one dose of *Pulsatilla* 12x or 6c four times daily, as needed, for up to two days.

■ *Ruta graveolens* is for tired eyes that are red, hot, and painful, and worse with close work, such as sewing a fine seam or concentrating on fine print. Eyestrain is usually followed by a headache. Take one dose of *Ruta graveolens* 12x or 6c four times daily, as needed, for up to three days.

■ If none of the above remedies seems right, see a homeopathic physician for a constitutional remedy tailored to your particular set of symptoms.

GENERAL RECOMMENDATIONS

■ To refresh tired eyes and relieve the strain, lie down and relax for at least fifteen minutes with a cold compress over your eyes.

■ For twitching of the eyelid, gentle pressure often quiets the muscles involved and banishes a twitch quickly.

PREVENTION

■ Avoid straining your eyes. If your occupation (or a hobby) requires close focus for long periods of time, take periodic breaks. Every twenty or thirty minutes, look away from what you are doing and rest your eyes by focusing on something in the distance for a minute or two. If you don't have a window with a view, look as far as possible across the room and zero in on a picture or a clock (or a coworker).

Fainting

Fainting—medically termed syncope (sing´-ka-pee)—is a sudden and temporary loss of consciousness that occurs as a result of a lack of sufficient blood flow to the brain. There are a number of things that can cause this to happen, including a sudden drop in blood pressure, anemia, an irregular heartbeat, seizures, extreme heat, hyperventilation, hunger, and hypoglycemia. Standing for a long time in a hot, stuffy room, exhaustion, emotional upset, fear, or fever may also cause a person to faint. People who have cardiovascular problems and those who take certain drugs may be more prone to fainting than the average person.

In the moments before a fainting episode, you may experience dizziness, weakness, nausea, sweating, blurred vision, and/or a feeling of numbness in your hands or feet; you may suddenly turn pale and your skin may feel cold. Upon awakening, you may feel tired and develop a headache.

If you lose consciousness apparently due to one of the factors listed above, and make a complete recovery within fifteen minutes, it is likely that you have experienced a fainting episode. A person who has fainted will usually awaken fairly readily, especially if smelling salts are used, and will be aware and oriented upon awakening. If you regain consciousness with difficulty and are disoriented, you may have a more serious problem.

EMERGENCY TREATMENT

See the inset on page 275.

CONVENTIONAL TREATMENT

■ If you see someone faint, follow the procedure outlined under Emergency Treatment for Fainting (see inset, page 275).

■ If you have fainted, once you regain consciousness and your condition is stable, call your doctor and explain the situation. Your doctor will want to examine you so that the cause of the problem can be determined and, if appropriate, treated. Your doctor may order blood tests, a chest x-ray, an electrocardiogram (ECG), an electroencephalogram (EEG), or other tests to see if there is any underlying health problem that may have caused you to faint. Treat-

ment recommendations, if any, will depend on the results of your doctor's evaluation.

DIETARY GUIDELINES

■ If you suspect hypoglycemia (low blood sugar) as the cause of fainting, take a glass of fruit juice or sweetened tea as soon as you can swallow. Turn to HYPOGLYCEMIA for additional recommendations for ways to manage this problem.

HERBAL TREATMENT

■ Once you recover and your condition is stable, take a cup of ginger and/or licorice tea to increase circulation.

HOMEOPATHY

Take one dose of *Aconite* 30x or 9c as soon as possible to help ease the shock from fainting. Follow the *Aconite* with one dose of the following symptom-specific remedies, as directed on the product label, every ten minutes until you feel better, up to a total of three doses.

■ If the fainting was related to exhaustion and weakness, choose *China* 30x or 9c.

■ If the fainting was due to emotional upset or fear, perhaps even bordering on hysteria, choose *Ignatia* 30x or 9c.

■ If the fainting occurred as a result of extreme pain, choose *Chamomilla* 30x or 9c.

■ For fainting that occurred indoors in a stuffy room, use *Pulsatilla* 30x or 9c.

BACH FLOWER REMEDIES

■ After a fainting episode, put a few drops of Rescue Remedy in a glass of water and sip it throughout the day.

■ If fainting was related to fear, take one dose of Mimulus three times daily for three days.

ACUPRESSURE

For the locations of acupressure points on the body, *see* ADMINISTERING AN ACUPRESSURE TREATMENT in Part Three.

■ If you awaken with a headache, apply pressure to Large Intestine 4. This acupressure point relaxes tension in the head.

■ Four Gates helps to relax and reestablish equlibrium throughout the body.

GENERAL RECOMMENDATIONS

■ If you feel faint and have recently started taking a new medication, call your doctor and explain the situation. You may need a change in prescription. Do not stop taking or reduce the dosage of a prescribed medication on your own, however. Always consult with your physician first.

Emergency Treatment for Fainting

■ If you see someone lose consciousness, take the following measures immediately:

1. Check for pulse and breathing. *If pulse and/or breathing is absent, or if either stops at any time during the episode, turn to* CARDIOPULMONARY RESUSCITATION *on page 000.* Begin taking the appropriate measures at once.

2. If the person is breathing and his or her heart rate seems to be fine, check for signs of injury. If the person is unknown to you, look to see if he or she is wearing a Medic Alert bracelet that offers an explanation for the episode, such as a history of diabetes or seizures.

3. If there are no signs of injury, try the following, in order, to provoke a response:
   - Call the person's name.
   - Pat his or her face gently.
   - Wave smelling salts under his or her nose. If smelling salts are not readily available, try using an open bottle of perfume or essential oil.
   - Apply acupressure to Gallbladder 21 (see illustration, page 589).

4. If the person is still limp and unresponsive, lay him or her down flat with the feet elevated, or the head lowered, to a 45-degree angle if possible. This will increase the flow of blood to the brain. Loosen the person's clothing and place him or her in the recovery position, as follows: Roll the body as a unit (without twisting the torso) onto one side. Place the lower arm behind the person's back and pull the top knee up and forward slightly so that it rests on the ground. Place the upper arm under the head, which should be turned to the side (see illustration, below). This position ensures that if vomiting occurs, the airway will not be obstructed. Cover the person with a blanket and stay with him or her to monitor pulse and breathing.

5. If the person does not regain consciousness within two or three minutes, or if his or her pulse or breathing becomes weaker, call for emergency help.

■ Once the person regains consciousness, help him or her into a sitting position, leaning forward, with the head between the knees to increase circulation to the brain.

■ Have the person sit still for an additional ten to fifteen minutes after the episode, to be sure he or she is stable enough to walk.

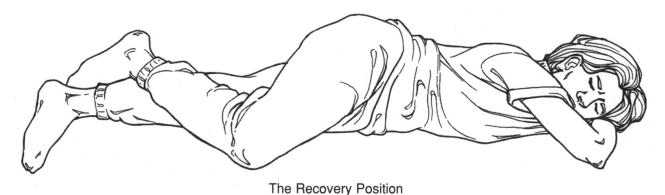

The Recovery Position

PREVENTION

■ If you start to feel dizzy or faint, or experience any other signs that a fainting episode may be coming on, immediately sit down, lean forward, and lower your head between your legs. Give a few deep coughs. This will increase the blood flow to the brain. Applying presssure to the acupressure point called Governing Vessel 21, located directly under the nose, can prevent a faint if done immediately.

■ Avoid standing up abruptly. Go from lying down to sitting to standing slowly and gradually.

■ Avoid situations and circumstances that are conducive to fainting, such as warm, stuffy rooms, standing for too long, overexertion and exhaustion, going for too long without eating, or anything else that has been associated with fainting in the past. If you become faint in response to powerful emotions, learn relaxation or visualization techniques. Sometimes just learning to breathe regularly, deeply, and consciously is all you need to keep your emotions from overpowering your body. (*See* RELAXATION TECHNIQUES in Part Three.)

Farsightedness

See PRESBYOPIA.

Fatigue

Each of us develops a sleep-wake cycle that supplies the energy needed to participate in life's necessary activities. Fatigue that makes you unable to handle your daily activities or causes you to begin sleeping more than usual deserves attention. While all people get run down from time to time, any fatigue that lasts longer than two or three weeks indicates a problem. That problem may be an unhealthy lifestyle, emotional distress, or an underlying illness. Fatigue can be the earliest sign of many illnesses and may appear before other symptoms, or even before a blood test or other diagnostic tool indicates that something is wrong.

Excessive fatigue can be a symptom of acute illnesses, such as viral or bacterial infections, as well as more serious chronic conditions, including anemia, cardiovascular disease, thyroid problems, and certain types of cancer. Chronic fatigue syndrome is another possibility. Fatigue can also be a sign of depression. People on the edge of depression often "escape" into sleep.

Because of the possibility that fatigue may be caused by an underlying illness, if you are feeling unusually tired, you should be examined by a doctor. Your doctor will perform a physical examination and may order blood tests to rule out hypothyroidism, diabetes, anemia, allergies, leukemia, athritis, medication reactions, or a viral or bacterial infection. Medical science is often unable to identify the cause of fatigue, however. If a serious underlying condition is ruled out, this is the perfect time to use natural remedies.

CONVENTIONAL TREATMENT

■ Assuming all standard laboratory test results are normal, current conventional "treatment" usually consists of reassurance and encouragement to participate in whatever activities you can. A person who consults his or her doctor for symptoms of serious fatigue for which no physical cause can be found may be referred for psychiatric evaluation. Occasionally, antidepressants are prescribed. Unfortunately, fatigue and its symptoms often do not fit neatly into any of conventional medicine's strictly defined categories. As a result, many medical doctors are disconcerted by it and uncomfortable treating it.

■ If you have access to a nutritionally oriented physician, it can be worthwhile to ask for an injection of vitamin B_{12}, possibly with the addition of folic acid, even if blood tests do not show a clinical deficiency of these nutrients. This kind of treatment is very safe and inexpensive, and many people find them helpful for fatigue. The shots can be repeated weekly until they cease to cause additional improvement.

DIETARY GUIDELINES

■ Excessive fatigue can often be traced to diet. Eat a wholesome, whole-foods diet based on fresh vegetables, fruits, grains, and lean proteins. Limit saturated, hydrogenated, and partially hydrogenated fats. Be sure you eat adequate amounts of lean protein.

■ Avoid processed foods and sugar. Eliminate from your diet all alcohol, caffeine, and soft drinks.

■ Do not smoke, and avoid secondhand smoke.

■ Use an elimination diet or diet diary to check for food allergies and sensitivities. Unsuspected food allergies can be a drain on the system. (*See* ELIMINATION DIET in Part Three.)

NUTRITIONAL SUPPLEMENTS

■ Take a multivitamin and mineral supplement each day to help resolve any possible deficiencies that may be contributing to your fatigue.

■ Adrenal glandular extract can be helpful for fatigue due to compromised adrenal-hormone production. Take 150 milligrams two or three times daily.

■ Carnitine, a substance related to the B vitamins but often grouped with the amino acids, can help to enhance energy as well as physical performance. People who take carnitine demonstrate stronger muscle performance and better energy metabolism within muscle tissue. Take 500 milligrams of L-carnitine three times daily.

■ Chlorophyll contains magnesium and other micronutrients that help to build up the blood. Take a chlorophyll supplement, following the dosage directions on the product label, for one month. Then discontinue the supplement for one month. Repeat this cycle three times (a total of six months).

■ Green-drink products such as Green Magma, Green Vibrance, and Green Essence, available in health-food stores, provide many enzymes, proteins, vitamins, minerals, and other nutrients that may be helpful in eliminating fatigue related to nutritional deficiency. Take a green-drink supplement, as directed on the product label, for one to two months.

■ Lipoic acid aids in the process of converting carbohydrates to energy. An excellent antioxidant, it improves energy metabolism, especially if fatigue is due to liver problems, diabetes, and/or cardiovascular disease. Take 100 milligrams three times daily.

■ Magnesium jump-starts the process that generates energy at the cellular level. Take 100 milligrams of magnesium with 300 milligrams of malic acid twenty to thirty minutes before breakfast.

The B vitamins, especially vitamin B_{12}, may be helpful for fatigue that is caused by poor diet. Take a balanced B-complex supplement supplying 25 to 50 milligrams of each of the major B vitamins, plus an additional 500 to 1,000 micrograms of vitamin B_{12} daily for three weeks to one month.

Vitamin C can help with fatigue, especially if it is related to iron deficiency, because vitamin C enhances the absorption of iron. Take an antioxidant formula containing 20,000 international units of beta-carotene, 1,000 milligrams of vitamin C, 400 international units of vitamin E, and 100 micrograms of selenium every day for one month.

Note: If you are taking an anticoagulant (blood thinner), consult your physician before taking vitamin E.

Dehydroepiandrosterone (DHEA) has received a great deal of attention as a treatment of severe chronic fatigue. DHEA is a hormone, not a nutrient, and the long-term effects of swallowing it (instead of using only the amount your body makes) are not well established. Nevertheless, many people claim that a daily dose of 25 to 50 milligrams has given them almost a new life. Even doses as low as 5 milligrams daily, taken in the morning, may be helpful, especially if taken in conjunction with Siberian ginseng. If you are interested in trying DHEA, we recommend that you consult a health-care professional experienced in its use who can do periodic testing of your blood and urine to ensure that you are using the amount that is right for you (the lowest dose that boosts your level to that of a twenty-five- to thirty- year-old). DHEA is not recommended for people under forty.

HERBAL TREATMENT

The Chinese believe that astragalus raises chi, or energy. Take 300 to 500 milligrams two or three times daily. Take the last dose at least six hours before bedtime.

Bee propolis, available in liquid ampules, is very useful for enhancing energy and athletic performance. Use one vial two or three times daily.

Cordyceps is a tonic herb that increases the oxygen supply to body systems, enhances immunity, and acts as an antioxidant. Take 1,000 milligrams of standardized extract twice a day.

Echinacea and goldenseal help to treat lingering infection that can cause fatigue. Take one dose of an echinacea and goldenseal combination formula supplying 250 to 500 milligrams of echinacea and 150 to 300 milligrams of goldenseal three times a day for five days.

■ All ginsengs contain micronutrients and trace minerals that help strengthen the constitution and act as energizers. Russian studies have shown that Siberian ginseng is very effective for many problems, including fatigue. If you have recently been ill, are over age sixty-five, or suffer from hypersensitivity to cold, you may be helped by Chinese or Korean red ginseng. American ginseng is preferred by many because it is not one of the "hot" ginsengs. That is, it is easy to tolerate and seldom provokes a reaction. It is an adaptogenic herb that improves metabolism and strengthens the endocrine system. Select an appropriate form of ginseng and take one dose, as recommended on the product label, in the morning, half an hour before breakfast, for six weeks. If you are troubled by afternoon fatigue, add a second dose before lunch. After six weeks on ginseng, stop for one week. Then resume taking it as before for another six weeks.

Note: Do not use American or Chinese (Korean) ginseng if you have high blood pressure, heart disease, or hypoglycemia. If you are sensitive to the effects of caffeine and other stimulants, you may want to consult with a qualified herbalist before using ginseng.

AROMATHERAPY

For specific instructions on how to use aromatherapy, *see* PREPARING AROMATHERAPY TREATMENTS in Part Three.

■ Essential oil of basil, elemi, geranium, lavender, patchouli, peppermint, pine, thyme, and vetiver have energizing and stimulating properties. Add one or more (up to three different ones) of these essential oils to bath water or massage oil, use them as inhalants, or diffuse them into the air in your home.

GENERAL RECOMMENDATIONS

■ Maintain a regular sleep-wake cycle. Try to awaken around the same time every day, and maintain a regular bedtime. If you feel tired and cranky, take a rest, or treat yourself to a thirty-minute "power nap." Sleep requirements vary from one person to another. Go to bed early enough to give your body time to store up energy for the day ahead. Ideally, you should awaken, feeling refreshed, around the same time every morning without the need for an alarm clock.

■ Get regular exercise. Exercise promotes sound, refreshing sleep, increases the body's oxygen supply, and improves energy all around. You may have to start very slowly and gently, but even mild exercise should yield results, and you will be able to increase your activity level as you become stronger. (*See* STARTING AN EXERCISE PROGRAM in Part Three.)

■ Consider seeing a physician who uses a hyperbaric oxygen chamber. Often, taking sixty to ninety minutes of hyperbaric oxygen therapy (HBOT) two to three times weekly for one month can make an enormous difference.

PREVENTION

■ The best way to prevent fatigue from developing is to ensure that your diet includes healthy, whole foods that provide a full range of necessary nutrients; that you follow a consistent sleep schedule; and that you get regular exercise. Make exceptions in your dietary and sleep regimen only on special occasions. Allow enough time to unwind before going to bed.

■ Stress and anxiety can cause fatigue. When you are under stress, try to address your problems calmly. Relaxation techniques can help relieve stress as well (see RELAXATION TECHNIQUES in Part Three). Biofeedback and yoga can also be very beneficial.

Fever

Fever has been defined as a body temperature elevated to at least 1°F above 98.6°F (37.0°C). Actually, body temperature normally varies by as much as 2°F, depending on the level of activity, emotional stress, the amount of clothing worn, the time of day, and the temperature of the environment, among other factors. When taken by mouth, body temperature is usually between 96.8°F and 99.4°F.

A fever can be caused by a wide variety of things, including dehydration, overexertion, allergic or toxic reactions, certain types of cancer, HIV disease, and, of course, viral or bacterial infection. Fever of unknown origin (FUO) is a condition defined as an elevated temperature lasting for three weeks after investigation lasting a week or more fails to identify a cause.

In most cases, a fever is the body's reaction to an acute viral or bacterial infection. It is not necessarily a dangerous condition. Rather, it is a sign that the body is defending itself against the infectious invader. Since viruses and bacteria do not survive as well in a body with an elevated temperature, fever is actually an ally in fighting infection. It is one of the ways in which the body defends and heals itself. An elevated temperature also increases the production of infection-fighting white blood cells and even increases their speed of response and enhances their killing capacity.

If you have a slight fever, no intervention may be necessary. For temperatures up to 102°F, fever-reducing medication usually is not needed. However, an elevated temperature may make you feel very uncomfortable, causing

you to lose your appetite and making your whole body ache. A fever raises the body's overall metabolic rate. With your metabolism racing, you can easily lose weight and body fluids. Gently bringing a fever down can not only help you feel better, but can also help to prevent complications, such as dehydration.

Bringing down a fever can also help indicate the severity of your illness and aid in diagnosis. If you have a temperature of 103°F or more, you will look and feel terrible, whether the fever is caused by a minor infection such as a cold or a more serious problem. If you have a minor infection, you will look and feel noticeably better after the fever is brought down—a strong indication that it was the fever itself that was causing you to look and feel ill. If you have a more serious problem, you will probably continue to look and feel sick, even with a lower temperature. In addition, fever caused by serious illness is generally more difficult to bring down with over-the-counter medication.

CONVENTIONAL TREATMENT

■ Aspirin (in Bayer, Ecotrin, and other over-the-counter products) is the old standby for bringing down fever and reducing pain and inflammation. If it causes stomach upset, try a buffered form and take it with food.

Note: Do not take aspirin during the last three months of pregnancy unless directed to do so by a physician.

■ Acetaminophen (Tylenol, Datril, and others) is a drug that helps to lower fever. Acetaminophen is also an analgesic, so it eases the discomfort and body aches that accompany a fever.

Note: In excessive amounts, this drug can cause liver damage. Do not exceed the recommended dosage.

■ Ibuprofen (Advil, Motrin, Nuprin, and others) is another fever-reducing medication that relieves mild to moderate aches and pains.

Note: Take ibuprofren with food to prevent an upset stomach.

DIETARY GUIDELINES

■ Be sure to get plenty of fluids to keep yourself well hydrated. The increased metabolic rate that results from a fever causes the body to lose fluids rapidly. Drink spring water, herbal teas, soups, and diluted fruit juices. Frozen fruit-juice popsicles are good as well.

NUTRITIONAL SUPPLEMENTS

■ A deficiency of vitamin A reduces the body's ability to fight infection. Take 5,000 international units daily for one week.

Note: If you are pregnant, or intend to get pregnant, or if you have liver disease, consult your doctor before taking supplemental vitamin A. Pregnant women should not ingest a total of more than 25,000 international units of supplemental vitamin A *per week* from all sources.

■ Vitamin C has anti-inflammatory properties and is helpful in resolving a fever associated with a minor infection. Select mineral ascorbate vitamin C or esterified vitamin C (Ester-C) with bioflavonoids. Take 500 to 1,000 milligrams of each every two hours, up to a total of four to five doses.

■ Zinc improves immune function by improving the functioning of the thymus, the site where T-lymphocytes (T-cells) mature. T-cells are white blood cells that are a key component of the immune system. Zinc also has an antiviral effect. Take 15 milligrams three times a day for five days, then reduce to 15 milligrams twice daily until you are better. Take zinc with food to prevent stomach upset. If you take over 30 milligrams of zinc on a daily basis for more than one or two months, you should also take 1 to 2 milligrams of copper each day to maintain a proper mineral balance.

HERBAL TREATMENT

■ To help clear a possible underlying infection, take echinacea and goldenseal. The immune-boosting effects of these herbs are well documented, and both of them have infection-fighting properties as well. Take one dose of an echinacea and goldenseal combination supplying 350 to 500 milligrams of echinacea and 250 to 350 milligrams of goldenseal every two hours, up to a total of four or five doses in the first twenty-four hours. Then take one dose three times daily for one week.

■ Brew a fever-reducing herbal tea to decrease chills and increase perspiration. Use equal parts of some or all of the following: chamomile flower, elder flower, lemon balm leaf, licorice root, and peppermint leaf (*see* **PREPARING HERBAL TREATMENTS** in Part Three). Chamomile calms and relaxes; elder flower and lemon balm are soothing and promote perspiration; licorice sweetens the tea and enhances the effects of the other herbs; and peppermint cools a fever. To improve the flavor, you can sweeten the tea with a bit of honey. Take a cup of tea three or four times daily, as needed. If you are using peppermint in the tea and also taking a homeopathic preparation, allow one hour both before and after taking the homeopathic preparation and drinking this tea.

Note: Do not take licorice on a daily basis for more than five days in a row, as it can elevate blood pressure. Do not take it at all if you have high blood pressure.

■ Garlic has documented antibacterial properties. It can help resolve an infection associated with fever. This pungent herb may be easier to take in odorless capsule form. Take 500 milligrams five times daily until the fever sub-

sides. Then cut back to 500 milligrams four times daily for three days, then three times daily for one week.

■ Ginger tea is especially effective against fever associated with a cold, flu, or stomach upset. It is most helpful if you are the type of person who tends to feel cold, especially in the hands and feet. To decrease chills and increase perspiration, get into bed under light covers after drinking the tea. Take one cup four times daily for one day. If you find the taste too pungent, mix the tea with fruit juice or dilute it with water, or add a bit of honey to sweeten the tea.

■ Yarrow promotes sweating and helps to lower fever. Take 500 milligrams three times a day, as needed, for one or two days.

HOMEOPATHY

When you have a fever, select the most appropriate symptom-specific homeopathic remedy and begin taking it as soon as possible. You should notice some response within thirty minutes. After one or two doses, the temperature will usually start coming down. If the fever does not respond, try a different remedy. If you try two remedies without a response, call your doctor.

■ *Aconite* is useful at the very beginning of a fever and for a fever of sudden onset. This homeopathic is most often used during winter, when people are often exposed to cold wind. It is recommended for the person who is restless, moving around and tossing and turning in bed. Take one dose of *Aconite* 30x or 9c, as directed on the product label, every two hours, for a total of two doses. After the second dose of *Aconite*, switch to another remedy.

■ *Arsenicum album* 30x or 9c is for a fever that increases between midnight and 2:00 AM, accompanied by anxiety, restlessness, and pain in the legs. The *Arsenicum* person feels better with a cold compress on the head and blankets on the legs. Take one dose of *Arsenicum album* 30x or 9c every two hours, up to a total of four doses.

■ *Belladonna* also is used for a sudden fever accompanied by chills and a flushed and heated face and body. The pupils are typically dilated, and noise and light are disturbing. Take one dose of *Belladonna* 30x, 200x, 15c, or 30c every hour, up to a total of four doses.

■ *Bryonia* 30x or 9c is for fever with irritability, strong thirst, and, possibly, constipation. This person prefers to be left alone. Take one dose of *Bryonia* 30x or 9c every two hours, up to a total of four doses.

■ *Ferrum phosphoricum* treats a moderate fever, including a previously high fever that has been lowered by *Aconite* or *Belladonna*. *Ferrum phosphoricum* is also useful for a fever that is not sudden, high, or rapid in onset. It is good for the person who is pale and feels weak. Take one dose of *Ferrum phosphoricum* 6x, 12x, 6c, or 9c every two hours, up to a total of six doses.

■ *Gelsemium* is for a fever with an all-over achy, flushed feeling. The eyelids are heavy and droopy, and there is no thirst. Take one dose of *Gelsemium* 30x or 9c every two hours, up to a total of four doses.

Mercurius solubilis is recommended for a fever with offensive-smelling breath, body odor, stool, and/or urine. Take one dose of *Mercurius solubilis* 12x or 6c every two hours, up to a total of four doses.

Phosphorus is useful for a cough or respiratory infection with fever, especially for the person who craves ice-cold drinks (which, unfortunately, may not stay down for very long). Take one dose of *Phosphorus* 30x or 9c every two hours, up to a total of four doses.

If none of the above remedies seems right, a homeopathic combination fever remedy may be helpful. Follow the dosage directions on the product label.

ACUPRESSURE

For the locations of acupressure points on the body, *see* ADMINISTERING AN ACUPRESSURE TREATMENT in Part Three.

Four Gates helps to relax the body.

Large Intestine 4 clears heat in the body and promotes calm.

AROMATHERAPY

For specific instructions on how to use aromatherapy, *see* PREPARING AROMATHERAPY TREATMENTS in Part Three.

A lukewarm bath prepared with elemi, myrrh, pine, and/or tea tree oil can help to ease a fever and the achiness that comes with it.

GENERAL RECOMMENDATIONS

If you have a low-grade temperature, rest in cool pajamas under a light sheet. Avoid becoming chilled. A chill brings on shivering, which can increase the metabolic rate and cause the fever to escalate.

Do not sponge yourself off with cold water or rubbing alcohol or take a cold bath. Cold and alcohol cause the blood vessels in the skin to constrict, making it more difficult for heat to escape from the body.

Fever Blisters

See under HERPES.

Fibrocystic Breast Disease

Fibrocystic breast disease is a condition characterized by the presence of lumps in the breast that are round, firm, and rubbery, and that can be moved around under the skin. One or both breasts typically become lumpy and tender, even painful, in the week or so before menstruation begins. These symptoms are related to hormonal changes, dietary choices, and intestinal health.

The condition often progresses through three stages. In the first stage, which occurs when a woman is in her late teens and early twenties, there may be a few lumps in the breasts. Typically, the breasts are tender during the week before the onset of menstruation. In the second stage, between the ages of thirty and forty, tenderness intensifies and pain may occur. The breasts become more nodular and the lumps are more noticeable during the week or so before the menstrual period begins. Finally, when a woman is in her late forties and fifties, her periods become irregular as menopause approaches, and symptoms of fibrocystic breasts become correspondingly erratic. The discomfort may come and go, pain may appear quite suddenly, and the breasts may become hypersensitive.

Fibrocystic breast disease is extremely common—about half of all American women have it to some extent—and it has been associated with a somewhat increased risk of breast cancer. Although at least 80 percent of all breast lumps are noncancerous, any mass, cyst, or swelling that can be felt in the breast tissue needs medical evaluation. An experienced physician can make an educated guess by examining the breasts manually, but physical examination does not always reveal whether a growth is cancerous or benign. A mammogram and/or a biopsy may be required for a firm diagnosis.

CONVENTIONAL TREATMENT

■ For minor, intermittent pain, your doctor is likely to recommend a nonsteroidal anti-inflammatory drug such as aspirin (Bayer, Ecotrin, and others), ibuprofen (Advil, Motrin, Nuprin, and others), ketoprofen (Orudis, Oruvail), or naproxen (Aleve, Anaprox, Naprelan, Naprosyn). Some of these are available over the counter, others by prescription. They are best taken with food to prevent stomach irritation.

■ If fibrocystic lumps cause serious discomfort, they can be drained of fluid in a simple outpatient procedure, or they can be surgically removed.

■ If pain is severe, or the condition is widely disseminated, a synthetic androgen (male sex hormone) called danazol (Danocrine) may be effective. However, this drug has masculinizing side effects that many women find objectionable. It is generally reserved for cases that respond to nothing else.

DIETARY GUIDELINES

■ Avoid chocolate and anything containing caffeine. These foods contain compounds known as methylxanthines, which have been linked with benign breast lumps.

■ Adopt a high-fiber diet regimen with an emphasis on fresh raw fruits and vegetables. Avoid saturated animal fats and hydrogenated and partially hydrogenated fats. Reducing the amount of these fats in your diet can diminish discomfort.

■ Eat smaller, more frequent meals rather than two or three large meals daily. In Chinese medicine, the root cause of fibrocystic breast disease is poor digestion, and eating too much at one time overwhelms the digestive system. Also try eliminating from your diet any foods you may have difficulty digesting.

NUTRITIONAL SUPPLEMENTS

■ Borage oil and evening primrose oil provide essential fatty acids that help to regulate hormone production. Take 500 to 1,000 milligrams of either twice daily.

■ Although the relationship is not entirely clear, chronic constipation has been linked to benign breast lumps. To prevent constipation, take 1,200 milligrams of calcium and 800 milligrams of magnesium daily. If you develop loose stools, cut the dosage in half.

■ Impaired fat digestion is a factor in fibrocystic breast disease. Choline, methionine, and inositol are very effective in helping the body metabolize fats. Take a lipotropic combination supplement supplying approximately 350 milligrams of choline, 250 milligrams of methionine, and 200 milligrams of inositol per dose, and take one dose with each of the two largest meals of the day.

■ Quercetin, a flavonoid, is an excellent anti-inflammatory. It is most commonly used for allergies, but it is also useful in reducing the discomfort of fibrocystic breasts. Take 300 milligrams three times daily, one-half hour before eating.

■ Selenium is a valuable antioxidant that helps prevent free-radical damage. Take 200 micrograms daily.

■ Vitamin C and bioflavonoids have anti-inflammatory properties. Take 500 milligrams of each three times daily.

■ Vitamin E is an antioxidant that has been shown to reduce inflammation and breast tenderness. A six-month course of high-dose vitamin-E therapy can be very effective in minimizing symptoms. Choose a product containing mixed tocopherols and take it as follows:

Weeks 1–3: Take 400 international units each morning.

Weeks 4–7: Take 400 international units each morning and another 400 international units in the evening.

Weeks 8–12: Take 400 international units in the morning, again in the afternoon, and again in the evening.

Weeks 13–24: Continue taking 400 international units in the morning, afternoon, and evening, and add a fourth dose at dinnertime.

Note: Before beginning this type of therapy, consult with your gynecologist or other health-care practitioner. If you have high blood pressure, you should limit your intake of supplemental vitamin E to 400 international units daily from all sources. If you are on anticoagulants (blood thinners), consult your physician before taking any vitamin E.

HERBAL TREATMENT

■ Applying warm castor-oil packs to the area over the liver can help improve liver function, which ultimately helps reduce inflammation. Chinese medicine teaches that liver stagnation contributes to breast problems. Prepare a warm castor-oil pack by saturating several layers of clean white cloth with the oil. Either warm the oil on the stove before preparing the pack, or prepare the pack, place it on a clean plate, and warm it in a microwave oven for twenty to thirty seconds. The pack should be warm but not hot. Place the warm pack over the upper right quadrant of your abdomen and leave it in place for fifteen to twenty minutes. Apply the warm pack a total of three times during the week before the anticipated onset of your period.

■ Chaste tree berry, also called *Vitex agnus-castus*, is a little-known herb that helps regulate hormones. It inhibits the release of follicle-stimulating hormone (FSH) and increases the production of luteinizing hormone (LH). This leads to a shift in the estrogen-progesterone balance, resulting in less estrogen to stimulate breast tissue and aggravate symptoms. Take 125 milligrams of standardized chaste tree berry extract twice daily for the ten days preceding the anticipated onset of your menstrual period.

■ To help detoxify your body, one week before the anticipated onset of your menstrual period, take one dose of an echinacea and goldenseal formula supplying 350 to 500 milligrams of echinacea and 250 to 350 milligrams of goldenseal twice daily for seven days.

■ Milk thistle helps quickly rid the body of toxins and hormonal metabolites. Choose an extract standardized to contain 80 percent flavonoids (silymarin) and take 100 to 200 milligrams twice daily for seven days, starting one week before the anticipated onset of menstruation.

■ Pine-bark and grape-seed extracts have powerful natural anti-inflammatory properties. Take 50 milligrams of either two or three times a day.

HOMEOPATHY

If your breasts are hard and lumpy, with acute pain that spreads all over the chest, use *Phytolacca*. Take one dose of *Phytolacca* 12x or 6c, as directed on the product label, three times daily while symptoms are present. When your symptoms abate, stop the treatment.

ACUPRESSURE

For the locations of acupressure points on the body, *see* ADMINISTERING AN ACUPRESSURE TREATMENT in Part Three.

The back Bladder points increase circulation.

Bladder 60 increases circulation to the reproductive organs.

Gallbladder 21 improves circulation in the upper body.

Liver 3 brings blocked energy down from the head.

Pericardium 6 relaxes the chest, increases circulation, and quiets the mind.

Spleen 6 and Stomach 36 are used together to regulate female energy.

GENERAL RECOMMENDATIONS

■ Become familiar with the way your breasts normally feel, and examine them regularly (*see* BREAST SELF-EXAMINATION in Part Three). If you detect anything out of the ordinary, see your doctor.

PREVENTION

Women who have irregular bowel habits and who are often constipated are more than four times more likely to develop fibrocystic breast disease than women who have a bowel movement every day. *See* CONSTIPATION for ways to prevent or overcome that condition.

Fibroids, Uterine

Fibroid is the common name given to a noncancerous tumor of the smooth muscle. These growths are not actually fibrous in origin, but consist of slow-growing bundles of smooth muscle and connective tissue. Multiple benign tumors of this type often develop in the wall of the uterus. They are firm and round and, usually, grayish-white in color. As a fibroid enlarges, it may grow within the muscle so that the uterus becomes distorted, or it may protrude from the uterine wall into the uterine cavity, remaining attached to the wall by a stalk. Fibroids range from pea-sized to the size a grapefruit, and several of them may develop simultaneously.

In about half of the women who have them, fibroids cause no symptoms, especially if they are small in size. However, if a fibroid erodes the lining of the uterine cavity, there may be heavy bleeding during menstrual periods. Over time, this can lead to anemia. Other problems fibroids can cause include increased vaginal discharge and pain during and bleeding after sexual intercourse. Very large fibroids can exert pressure on the bladder, causing discomfort during urination, or on the bowel, resulting in constipation and/or backache, or even, in severe cases, kidney obstruction. Occasionally, a large fibroid attached to the uterine wall will cause pain in the lower abdomen. Fibroids that distort the uterus can cause miscarriage. If the fallopian tubes are affected, infertility may result.

Fibroids are one of the most common of all tumors, occurring in from 20 to 30 percent of women over the age of thirty. They are most common between the ages of thirty-five and fifty, and seldom occur before age twenty. Although medical science cannot explain why, these tumors are more prevalent among women of African ancestry who have never been pregnant. Fibroids tend to shrink and often disappear after menopause.

CONVENTIONAL MEDICINE

■ Small fibroids that cause no symptoms are not usually treated, but regular pelvic examinations may be recommended to determine whether they are growing.

■ If fibroids cause very heavy menstrual periods with subsequent loss of blood, a synthetic form of the hormone progesterone or a synthetic androgen such as danazol (Danocrine) may be prescribed. These drugs stop the menstrual cycles and, therefore, the bleeding, making it possible to correct any anemia before undertaking other treatments to remove the fibroids. Both of these drugs can cause acne, increased hair growth, liver damage, and nausea, among other side effects.

■ Surgical options to remove fibroids include hysterectomy (removal of the uterus). This is likely to be recommended if there are many large fibroids. A woman who wishes to retain her ability to have children may opt for myomectomy (removal of the fibroids from the uterine wall) instead. There is no guarantee that a woman who undergoes myomectomy will subsequently be able to bear children, but this surgical procedure does leave the uterus intact.

■ A newer technique for treating fibroids, pioneered by the University of California–Los Angeles Medical Center, involves making a very small (one-quarter inch) incision in the groin, then guiding a catheter through an artery and into the uterus with the aid of x-ray imaging. Small plastic particles are then inserted through the catheter into the blood vessels that feed the tumor. This cuts off the tumor's blood supply, which ultimately causes it to die. Performed under local anesthesia, the entire procedure takes about an hour, and recuperation is almost immediate. While long-term success is not yet known, this procedure appears to be effective, and is safer than more extensive surgery.

DIETARY GUIDELINES

■ Eat a high-fiber whole-foods diet with plenty of raw and cooked fresh vegetables. Make certain you eat five servings of both vegetables and fruits daily.

■ Maximize your intake of green vegetables, such as spinach, kale, and broccoli. Also include sea vegetables such as kelp in your diet. Sea vegetables contain iodine, required for healthy thyroid function. Thyroid insufficiency is sometimes associated with the development of fibroids.

Include in your diet soy foods such as tofu, tempeh, and miso. Soy-based foods exert a natural and positive estrogenic effect that helps even out hormonal irregularities associated with fibroids.

To assist your body in cleansing itself, drink at least six 8-ounce glasses of pure water daily.

■ Avoid fried, greasy, and high-fat foods, especially saturated animal fats and hydrogenated and partially hydrogenated fats and oils, which are difficult to digest. Chinese medicine teaches that when your abdomen is "happy," fibroids may resolve more quickly.

■ Avoid refined sugars, processed foods, gas-producing foods, caffeine, and alcohol. These foods are difficult to metabolize. Chinese medicine teaches that fibroids are fostered by stagnation of the digestive system.

NUTRITIONAL SUPPLEMENTS

Bromelain, an enzyme derived from pineapple, helps reduce inflammation. Take 500 milligrams of bromelain three to four times daily, between meals.

Choline assists in strengthening liver function. It is necessary for exporting fat from the liver. In Chinese medicine, relieving stagnation of the liver is an essential part of treating fibroids. Take 500 milligrams of choline twice daily, with meals.

■ In Chinese medicine, it is believed that when the abdomen is comfortable, the fibroids cannot grow larger. To relieve stagnation, take a full-spectrum digestive-enzyme supplement providing 5,000 international units of lipase, 2,500 international units of amylase, and 300 international units of protease, plus 500 to 1,000 milligrams of pancreatin, with each meal. Digestive enzymes are especially important for those who experience bloating in the lower abdomen.

Note: Long-term supplementation with pancreatin is not advised, as it can cause your pancreas to reduce its own production of this important enzyme. Overuse also has the potential to cause nausea or diarrhea. After two months on pancreatin, discontinue use and monitor your reaction. If you find that your digestive problems recur, discuss pancreatin supplementation with your health-care provider.

■ Flaxseed oil provides essential fatty acids, has anti-inflammatory properties, and also helps regulate steroid production and hormone synthesis. Take 1 tablespoon (or 500 to 1,000 milligrams) twice daily.

■ Vitamin C and bioflavonoids have a measurable anti-inflammatory effect and also combat free radicals. Take 500 milligrams of each three times daily.

■ Vitamin E is a natural anti-inflammatory that also helps with hormone regulation. Studies show that taking vitamin E with evening primrose oil can help reduce the size of fibroids. Choose a vitamin-E supplement containing mixed tocopherols, and start by taking 200 international units daily, then gradually increase the dosage until you are taking 400 international units twice daily. Also take 500 milligrams of evening primrose oil twice daily.

Note: If you have high blood pressure, limit your intake of supplemental vitamin E to a total of 400 international units daily. If you are taking an anticoagulant (blood thinner), consult your physician before taking supplemental vitamin E.

HERBAL TREATMENT

■ If the fibroids are causing heavy bleeding during menstruation, take 2 to 3 tablets (or 2 droppersful of the liquid formula) of Butiao, a Chinese herbal medicine, three times a day for two weeks prior to the anticipated onset of your menstrual period.

■ Carthamus and persica, a Chinese herbal combination, acts to relieve stagnation, gas, and abdominal bloating. Take 350 to 500 milligrams three times daily for three months.

■ Squawvine has been used for centuries by native Americans to fight inflammation in the genitourinary tract. Take 350 to 500 milligrams twice daily for three months.

■ Wild yam progesterone cream, used topically, can be very helpful if fibroids are associated with excess estrogen and low levels of progesterone. Apply 1/4 teaspoon to soft skin, such as that of the forearm, hands, or inner thigh twice daily on days five through twenty-eight of the menstrual cycle. Rotate application sites and continue for three months.

Note: Before using progesterone cream, you should discuss this treatment with your gynecologist or other health-care professional.

■ Chinese herbal medicine often utilizes a combination

formula for fibroids, taken as a tea, that contains the following: 6 parts each *Dictamnus dasycarpus, Potentilla chinensis,* and *Rehmannia glutinosa;* 4 parts each *Ledebouriella seseloides, Lophatherum gracile, Paeonia lactiflora,* and *Tribulus terrestris;* 3 parts *Clematis armandii;* and 2 parts each *Glycyrrhiza uralensis* and *Schizonepeta tenuifolia.* A Chinese herbal pharmacy should be able to prepare this formula for you. If there is no Chinese herbal pharmacy in your area, you should be able to locate a number of them on the Internet.

HOMEOPATHY

The best approach to treating fibroids homeopathically is to see a homeopathic physician for a constitutional remedy. If that is not possible, select among the following symptom-specific homeopathic remedies.

■ *Aurum muriaticum* will help if your uterus feels full and painful. You may experience lower abdominal and vaginal contractions, and be in a "bad mood" and/or the throes of an exaggerated depression. Take one dose of *Aurum muriaticum* 30x or 15c three times daily every other week for three weeks.

■ *Hydrastis* is the remedy to choose if there is a strong-smelling vaginal discharge that occurs after the menstrual period. Take one dose of *Hydrastis* 30x or 15c three times daily, as needed.

■ *Lachesis* is good if you are in great pain, but feel better after menstruation begins. The menstrual flow is usually scanty, and you may be approaching menopause. You have a strong dislike of tight clothing around your abdomen. Take one dose of *Lachesis* 30x or 15c, as directed on the label.

■ *Lapis albus* is good for strong, burning pain in the abdomen accompanied by breast discomfort and heavy bleeding. You may have an increased appetite. Take one dose of *Lapis albus* 12x or 6c three times daily, as needed.

■ *Thlaspi bursa pastoris* is for continuous vaginal bleeding. Take one dose of *Thlaspi bursa pastoris* 12x or 6c four times daily until the bleeding stops.

■ *Phosphorus* is the remedy of choice if the menstrual blood is bright red. Take one dose of *Phosphorus* 12x or 6c three times daily for the three days preceding the anticipated onset of your period, or when menstruation begins.

■ Choose *Silicea* if you feel cold, tired, and weak. You may experience bleeding between periods and find your menstrual flow is heavier than normal. Take one dose of *Silicea* 30x or 15c three times daily for three days before the anticipated onset of menstruation.

■ *Trillium* helps relax the pelvis area to relieve the cramping pain associated with fibroids. This remedy is also useful for heavy bleeding. Take one dose of *Trillium* 12x or 6c three times daily, as needed.

■ *Calcarea fluorica* is very valuable after fibroid surgery, especially if you have a tendency to develop adhesions. Take *Calcarea fluorica* 12x or 6c three times daily for five days out of the month for three to four months after surgery.

BACH FLOWER REMEDIES

Select the remedy that most closely fits your emotional tendencies and concerns, and take it as needed, following the directions on the product label.

■ Rescue Remedy may be taken as needed. This gentle remedy helps to ease anxiety and apprehension, and relieve tension.

■ Aspen is the remedy for fears that you cannot (or cannot bear to) explain. You may also suffer from nightmares.

■ Holly soothes anger, insecurity, and fits of temper.

■ Impatiens calms nervousness, tension, impatience, and irritability.

■ Mimulus eases timidity and shyness. It is the remedy for the person who has many well-articulated fears.

■ White Chestnut helps to counteract a tendency to obsess on both past and upcoming events.

ACUPRESSURE

For the locations of acupressure points on the body, *see* ADMINISTERING AN ACUPRESSURE TREATMENT in Part Three.

■ The lower Bladder points (Bladder 23 and those below it) increase circulation throughout the genitourinary tract.

■ Gallbladder 34 helps to relax muscles.

■ Gallbladder 41 regulates hormones.

■ Large Intestine 4 promotes a healthier lower abdomen and relaxes the nervous system.

■ Liver 3 relieves muscle cramps and spasms.

■ Pericardium 6 relaxes the nervous system.

■ Spleen 6 reduces uterine cramping.

■ Stomach 36 is helpful for improving digestion, especially when used in combination with Spleen 6.

GENERAL RECOMMENDATIONS

■ Exercise daily. Exercise helps recovery from virtually any health problem, and is particularly important for this disorder. Modest exercise, taken on a daily basis, is the key. Yoga is especially helpful.

■ Practice visualization therapy. (*See* RELAXATION AND VISUALIZATION TECHNIQUES in Part Three.)

PREVENTION

■ Western medicine has not yet come up with any preventive measures against uterine fibroids. According to the teachings of Chinese medicine, however, preventing stagnation of the liver and digestive system is a worthwhile objective. Eat a clean diet of whole foods, including plenty of green vegetables and soy-based foods, and exercise daily. This is a helpful preventive "prescription" against many different diseases.

Fibromyalgia

Fibromyalgia is a relatively new term used to describe an age-old problem: muscle and joint pain that persists for no discernible reason. *Fibro* refers to fibrous connective tissue that cushions joints; *myalgia* refers to pain in the muscles. The primary symptoms include stiff, aching muscles and burning or throbbing pain, with certain distinct points on the body being tender to the touch. These areas include the muscles at the base of the skull, the base of the neck, the upper back, the mid-back, the second rib, the side of the elbow, the upper and outer muscles of the buttocks, the upper part of the thigh, and the middle of the knee. These symptoms are typically worse in the morning, and lessen somewhat as the day wears on. Some people with fibromyalgia also complain of headaches, sleep disorders, heart palpitations, dizziness, upsets in balance, feelings of anxiety and/or depression, and a degree of memory loss. Women with fibromyalgia may have premenstrual syndrome (PMS) and menstrual cramps.

Doctors believe that although fibromyalgia involves joint pain, it is not a form of arthritis but rather an inflammatory condition akin to rheumatism. This condition has also been known variously as arthralgia (pain in the joints), myalgia (pain in the muscles), fibromyositis and fibrositis (which signify accompanying inflammation), nonarticular rheumatism, chronic muscle-contraction syndrome, psychogenic rheumatism, and psychophysiological musculoskeletal pain. All of these labels really don't matter, but they do show how many attempts have been made to describe this disorder over the years.

The cause of fibromyalgia is not well understood. Some experts believe it may be due to a malfunction of the immune system. Others cite a disturbance in the brain. Still others say that a pervasive candida (yeast) infection may contribute to the condition. Other theories as to the cause include mercury poisoning (primarily from amalgam dental fillings), food or chemical allergies, heavy metal poisoning, intestinal parasites, hypoglycemia, hypothyroidism, anemia, viral infection, and chronic fatigue syndrome, which causes similar symptoms. In fact, fibromyalgia is so closely associated with chronic fatigue syndrome that many doctors simply assume that anyone suffering from chronic fatigue syndrome also has fibromyalgia.

Fibromyalgia affects more women than men, and usually arises first in early adulthood. The symptoms begin slowly and gradually increase over the years. In many cases, people with this condition eventually find it difficult to carry on their daily activities. Some are completely disabled by the disease.

Hepatitis, Lyme disease, anemia, chronic fatigue syndrome, and even depression cause similar symptoms. If you have been suffering from unexplained fatigue and/or muscle aches and pains that last longer than two weeks, see your health-care provider. Once any underlying conditions have been ruled out, a diagnosis of fibromyalgia may be made on the basis of your clinical history.

CONVENTIONAL MEDICINE

■ Before any treatment is tried for fibromyalgia, your doctor will want to make sure that there is no other explanation for your symptoms. This may take some time, as there are many possibilities to rule out, but it is important if you are to get the treatment you need.

■ In some cases, people with fibromyalgia get better on their own, without any kind of treatment. Reassurance from a medical professional may help. Anxiety and stress are believed to play a part in this condition, and are known to exacerbate symptoms. If these factors can be reduced, symptoms may improve.

■ Over-the-counter pain medications are not helpful in the majority of cases, but some people find they give relief, so they may be worth trying. Gentle massage, heat therapy, moderate exercise, and additional sleep may also be helpful.

■ Some doctors prescribe very low doses of an antidepressant such as amitriptyline (Elavil) or nortriptyline (Aventyl, Pamelor) for people with fibromyalgia. The lower the dose used, the better, as these drugs can cause side effects including dry mouth, confusion, high or low blood pressure, heart palpitations, rashes, numbness, tingling, tremors, blood abnormalities, nausea, vomiting, diarrhea, abdominal pain, and liver damage.

DIETARY GUIDELINES

■ Eat a high-fiber diet that includes plentiful servings of raw and steamed vegetables. Maximize your intake of greens.

■ Make sure your diet includes ample servings of clean, lean protein, such as that found in fish, poultry, and fresh raw nuts and seeds.

■ To keep a steady supply of nutrients available for proper muscle function, eat four to five small meals daily rather than three larger ones.

■ Avoid processed foods and all foods that are high in saturated or hydrogenated fats, such as dairy products, meat, and margarine. Saturated fats interfere with circulation, increasing inflammation and pain.

Avoid caffeine, alcohol, and sugar. These substances enhance fatigue, increase muscle pain, and can interfere with normal sleep patterns.

Drink eight glasses of pure water daily. Fresh juices and herbal teas are also good choices. A plentiful intake of liquids is important for flushing out toxins.

Investigate the possibility that food allergies and/or sensitivities may be contributing to the problem. (*See* ELIMINATION DIET in Part Three.)

NUTRITIONAL SUPPLEMENTS

Antioxidants help reduce free-radical damage and fight inflammation. Take a good antioxidant formula that provides 5,000 to 10,000 international units of vitamin A; 400 to 800 international units of vitamin E; up to 10,000 milligrams of buffered vitamin C; and 200 micrograms of selenium daily.

Note: If you are pregnant, or intend to get pregnant, or if you have liver disease, consult your doctor before taking supplemental vitamin A. If you have high blood pressure, limit your intake of supplemental vitamin E to a total of 400 international units daily, and if you are taking an anticoagulant (blood thinner), consult your physician before taking supplemental vitamin E.

■ Bromelain helps reduce inflammation. Take 400 milligrams three times daily, between meals.

Coenzyme Q$_{10}$ is also an antioxidant and helps deliver oxygen to cells. Take 60 milligrams twice daily, between meals.

Lipoic acid is very useful for enhancing the body's utilization of carbohydrates and enhancing energy. Take 100 milligrams three times daily.

The combination of magnesium and malic acid helps to increase energy. These nutrients are precursors to the Krebs cycle, a series of enzyme reactions that are a key part of the production of energy on the cellular level. Take 100 to 200 milligrams of magnesium and 400 to 800 milligrams of malic acid three times a day, twenty minutes before each meal.

Nicotinamide adenine dinucleotide hydrogen (NADH) is an antioxidant enzyme that occurs in all living cells. It facilitates the production of neurotransmitters such as dopamine and noradrenaline. Low levels of neurotransmitters are often associated with fibromyalgia. Taking 15 milligrams one-half hour before breakfast and dinner often improves concentration, stamina, and energy.

Phosphatidylserine, a type of lipid, can be helpful if memory problems accompany fibromyalgia. It often yields rapid and impressive improvement in memory and mental alertness. Unfortunately, it is relatively expensive. Take 75 to 100 milligrams three times daily.

■ S-adenosylmethionine (SAM or SAM-e) is an amino-acid derivative that has been shown in clinical trials to reduce the number of trigger points and areas of pain, lessen pain and fatigue, and improve mood. Take 400 milligrams two or three times daily. Be patient—it can take up to six weeks to see results.

HERBAL TREATMENT

■ Pine-bark and grape-seed extracts are natural anti-inflammatories that help to ease pain. Take 50 milligrams of either two to three times daily.

■ St. John's wort has both antiviral and antidepressant properties. If you are not taking a conventional antidepressant and your mood is not what it used to be, this herb can help. Choose a standardized extract containing 0.3 percent hypericin and take 300 milligrams three times daily.

■ Siberian ginseng is an energizing herb that can help resolve the fatigue associated with fibromyalgia. Choose a standardized extract containing 0.5 percent eleutheroside E and take 100 milligrams twice daily, one-half hour before breakfast and lunch. After two weeks, you can gradually increase the dosage as needed. After six weeks, take one week off, then take the herb for another six weeks.

■ Turmeric contains curcumin, which helps to reduce pain and inflammation. Take 400 to 500 milligrams three times daily.

HOMEOPATHY

■ Homeopathic *Arnica* is the first remedy to consider for pain, tenderness, stiffness, and a "bruised" feeling. Take one dose of *Arnica* 30x or 15c, as directed on the product label, three times daily for up to three days. *Arnica* cream or gel can also be used topically. Follow the directions on the product label.

■ *Bryonia* helps ease pain that increases with movement and is better when resting. You may also have a tendency to become constipated. Take one dose of *Bryonia* 30x or 15c three times daily for up to three days.

■ *Hypericum* is for unbearable prickly pain that radiates along nerve pathways, is worse with movement, and worse when touched. This remedy is especially effective for pain in the extremities. Take one dose of *Hypericum* 12x, 6x, 6c, or 3c three times daily for up to three days.

■ *Rhus toxicodendron* is for the individual who feels better after moving around. Take one dose of *Rhus toxicodendron* 30x or 9c three times daily for up to three days.

BACH FLOWER REMEDIES

Select the remedy that most closely fits your emotional

tendencies and concerns, and take it as needed, following the directions on the product label.

 Aspen is the remedy for fears that you cannot (or cannot bear to) explain. You may have trouble falling asleep and also be subject to nightmares.

■ Gorse is good for those times when you feel as if you will never get better.

■ Holly helps to tame a feeling of being mad at the world that comes out in fits of temper.

 Impatiens eases feelings of impatience and helps resolve nervous tension.

 Mimulus eases timidity and shyness. It is the remedy for the person who has many well-articulated fears.

ACUPRESSURE

For the locations of acupressure points on the body, *see* ADMINISTERING AN ACUPRESSURE TREATMENT in Part Three.

 Gallbladder 20, 30, 31, and 34 are instrumental in strengthening and enhancing circulation to the muscles and tendons.

 Liver 3 quiets the nervous system and relaxes muscle cramps and spasms.

 Pericardium 6 relaxes the chest and upper digestive tract, and helps relax the mind.

■ The combination of Spleen 6 and Stomach 36 enhances the absorption and transport of nutrients.

AROMATHERAPY

For specific instructions on how to use aromatherapy, *see* PREPARING AROMATHERAPY TREATMENTS in Part Three.

 Soothing aromatherapy baths and massages can help to ease muscle and joint pain. Choose one or more of the following essential oils to add to bath water or massage oil: basil, black pepper, elemi, eucalyptus, myrrh, peppermint, and pine.

 Many essential oils help to reduce stress, a major factor in this condition. Some of the best known for this purpose are elemi, frankincense, geranium, jasmine, lavender, myrrh, and neroli. Choose the one (or the combination) you like best and use it as an inhalant or diffuse it into the air in your home.

GENERAL RECOMMENDATIONS

 To help relieve morning stiffness, take a hot shower or bath upon awakening to stimulate circulation and loosen up stiff muscles. Recent research suggests that alternating hot and cold water in the shower may help relieve the pain associated with fibromyalgia.

 Exercise. Mild daily exercise can be immensely helpful

in reducing symptoms of this condition. Walking and easy stretching are good choices for getting started, especially if you are accustomed to a sedentary lifestyle.

■ Many people with fibromyalgia also suffer from restless legs syndrome, which can aggravate fibromyalgia by making it difficult to get adequate sleep. *See* RESTLESS LEGS SYNDROME for suggestions that can help.

PREVENTION

■ There is no known way of preventing fibromyalgia. However, because nutritional deficiencies are common in people with this problem, it would be wise to make sure your diet provides optimum nutrition. To make absolutely sure you are giving your body what it needs, add appropriate supplements to your daily regimen.

Flatulence

See GAS, INTESTINAL.

Floaters

Floaters are tiny bits of cellular debris floating within the vitreous humor, the gel-like fluid that fills the inside of the eyeball and keeps it round in shape. These bits of flotsam occur when the vitreous humor begins to break down. As it does so, specks of protein become trapped in the fluid and cast shadows on the retina. The result is tiny spots that seem to float before your eyes. They are particularly obvious when you look into the light or at a solid light-colored surface.

People with diabetes or hypoglycemia seem to be particularly prone to floaters, as are nearsighted and elderly people. In Chinese medicine, floaters are considered to be a symptom of poor liver or gallbladder function. In most cases, they are merely a common result of the aging process. They are sometimes a nuisance, but are not usually considered dangerous. However, a sudden cascade of floaters can be symptom of a more serious problem, such as a tear in the retina or retinal detachment.

CONVENTIONAL MEDICINE

■ If you suddenly become aware of a great many floating specks in one eye, or if floaters you have been experiencing suddenly increase in size, see an ophthalmologist immediately. This may be a sign that you are developing a retinal problem and need professional treatment to preserve your sight.

DIETARY GUIDELINES

Maximize your intake of fresh fruits and vegetables, especially green, yellow, and orange types. These healthy foods contain antioxidant phytochemicals that protect all the cells of the body, including those of the eyes, from free-radical damage.

■ Eat clean, lean protein, such as that found in chicken and fish. Both protein and vitamin A are needed to maintain healthy eyes.

NUTRITIONAL SUPPLEMENTS

Beta-carotene is a strong antioxidant that prevents free-radical damage. It is related to vitamin A and has many of the same properties, but it does not become toxic in large doses. Take 10,000 to 25,000 international units of beta-carotene daily.

The essential fatty acids (EFAs), found in black currant seed oil, borage oil, evening primrose oil, flaxseed oil, and fish oils are required by every cell in the body. Select one of the above oils and take 1 tablespoon (or 500 to 1,000 milligrams) twice daily.

Selenium is an excellent antioxidant that helps prevent free-radical damage throughout the body, including the eyes. Take 100 micrograms daily.

Vitamin A protects against free-radical damage and is especially important to the eyes. Even a slight deficiency can contribute to eye problems. Take 10,000 international units of vitamin A three times a day for two months. Then reduce to a maintenance dosage of 5,000 international units twice daily.

Note: If you are pregnant, or intend to get pregnant, or if you have liver disease, consult your doctor before taking supplemental vitamin A. Pregnant women should not ingest a total of more than 25,000 international units of supplemental vitamin A *per week* from all sources.

The B vitamins are required for intracellular metabolism in the tissues of the eyes. Combined with vitamins C and E, the B-complex vitamins are especially beneficial to the eyes. Vitamin B_2 in particular has been shown to reduce the incidence of floaters and "halos" around lights or objects. Take a B-complex supplement that supplies 50 milligrams of each of the primary B vitamins twice a day for two months, then reduce the dosage to 25 milligrams twice daily.

Vitamin C helps to lower ocular pressure and prevent and clear up infections. It also helps strengthen capillaries, maintains collagen, and prevents tissue hemorrhaging, and is notable for speeding healing. Select a vitamin-C formula that includes bioflavonoids, especially rutin; these nutrients work best together. Take 500 to 1,000 milligrams of a vitamin-C complex three times daily.

■ Vitamin E is an antioxidant and is essential in cellular respiration. It has been shown to improve eyesight in clinical studies. Choose a product containing mixed tocopherols and take 200 international units daily for two weeks, then increase the dosage to 200 international units twice daily.

Note: If you are taking an anticoagulant (blood thinner), consult your physician before taking supplemental vitamin E.

■ Zinc supports the immune system and aids in the healing process. A deficiency of zinc is believed to be a contributing factor in retinal detachment. Take 25 to 50 milligrams daily.

Note: Take zinc with food to prevent stomach upset. If you take over 30 milligrams of zinc on a daily basis for more than one or two months, you should also take 1 to 2 milligrams of copper each day to maintain a proper mineral balance.

HERBAL TREATMENT

■ Bilberry provides important nutrients that nourish the eyes and enhance visual function. Phytochemicals called anthocyanidins in this herb also help prevent damage to the structures of the eyes. Select a preparation containing 25 percent anthocyanidins (also called PCOs) and take 40 to 80 milligrams three times daily.

■ Eyebright is rich in vitamin A and vitamin C. It also contains moderate amounts of the B-complex vitamins and vitamin D, and traces of vitamin E. Eyebright has been used for centuries both as an eyewash and in tea form as a tonic for the eyes. Taken internally, it helps maintain healthy eyes and good vision. Take 500 milligrams three times daily for up to three months.

■ Ginkgo biloba extract contains flavonoids with an affinity for organs that are rich in connective tissue, including the eyes. Ginkgo protects cellular membranes and has notable antioxidant properties. Select a preparation of ginkgo leaf extract containing at least 24 percent ginkgo heterosides (sometimes called flavoglycosides) and take 40 milligrams three times daily, or follow the recommendations on the product label.

HOMEOPATHY

■ *Arnica* 12x or 6c is the remedy for floaters that develop following an accident or trauma. Take one dose of *Arnica* 12x or 6c, as directed on the product label, three times daily for up to three days, while symptoms persist.

■ *Nux vomica* is for floaters associated with excessive alcohol and/or tobacco use. You may also suffer from intense discomfort in bright light. Take one dose of *Nux vomica* 30x or 15c three times daily for up to three days, while symptoms persist.

■ *Phosphorus* is helpful for black flecks that seem to float before the eyes. The *Phosphorus* person tends to be nervous, anxious and fearful, and seems to see better when shading the eyes with his or her hands. Take one dose of *Phosphorus* 30x or 15c three times daily, for up to three days with symptoms.

GENERAL RECOMMENDATIONS

■ Floaters may be annoying, but they are generally harmless. It may help to remember that they often become less noticeable over time.

Flu

Influenza—better known as "the flu"—is a viral infection of the respiratory tract. It can occur in epidemic proportions during the winter. Because the structure of the virus may change every two or three years, the population will periodically be confronted with a virus it has never been exposed to before. This creates the possibility of an epidemic outbreak of influenza every two to three years. Between epidemics, smaller outbreaks may occur as people not exposed in the previous round are infected.

The flu is very contagious and is spread by contact with an infected person. A person is contagious from about two days before symptoms occur until about the fifth day of the illness. Symptoms often develop suddenly, in a matter of hours, and include chills, fever, headache, chest discomfort, sore throat, cough, body-wide aches and pains, fatigue and weakness progressing to exhaustion, and lack of appetite.

The acute illness generally runs its course in three to four days, but weakness and fatigue can persist for up to three weeks. Treatment is generally directed at alleviating symptoms, which can make you truly miserable. However, if you begin experiencing signs of respiratory distress, such as rapid breathing, shortness of breath, a feeling of tightness in the chest, or wheezing, call your doctor. Pneumonia is a relatively common complication of influenza and it can become quite serious, especially in the young, the old, and those with compromised immune systems. Also, if your symptoms do not start to improve within three days, or if new symptoms appear, you should consult your physician. Other possible complications include bronchitis and even, in some cases, seizures or encephalitis. These conditions require immediate medical attention.

CONVENTIONAL TREATMENT

■ Because influenza is caused by a virus, antibiotics have no effectiveness and are not used.

■ A drug containing amantadine hydrochloride (Symmetrel) is sometimes used in epidemics known to be caused by influenza type A. This drug is effective only if started in the first two days after the onset of symptoms. Potential side effects include nausea, diarrhea, constipation, dizziness, fatigue, irritability, heart failure, and hallucinations. In rare cases, a condition called neuroleptic malignant syndrome, characterized by high fever and a confusional state, among other symptoms, may occur when this drug is discontinued.

■ The cornerstones of treatment for influenza are fever control, rest, and fluids. Acetaminophen (in Tylenol, Datril, and other medications), aspirin (Bayer, Ecotrin, and others), or ibuprofen (Advil, Nuprin, and others) can be used to reduce fever and alleviate achiness.

Note: In excessive amounts, acetaminophen can cause liver damage. Do not exceed the recommended dosage. Take aspirin or ibuprofen with food to prevent possible stomach upset. Do not take aspirin during the last three months of pregnancy unless directed to do so by a physician.

DIETARY GUIDELINES

■ If you don't feel like eating, it's best not to force yourself. When you do feel hungry, choose easily digested foods such as juices, lemonade (hot or cold), herbal teas, applesauce, and lots of nourishing broth and homemade soups. Miso and chicken soup are good choices.

■ Getting plenty of fluids, including soups, is particularly important. Fluids help to thin secretions, making it easier for the body to clear them, and also help to prevent constipation and flush toxins from the body.

■ Avoid dairy products, which have a tendency to increase and thicken mucus.

NUTRITIONAL SUPPLEMENTS

■ Thymus glandular extract boosts immune function by increasing the number and activity of infection-fighting white blood cells. Take 250 to 500 milligrams twice a day. This is especially important for people over forty, as thymus function declines with age.

■ Vitamin C has anti-inflammatory properties and helps to ease the course of a respiratory illness. Bioflavonoids have potent antiviral properties and can be useful at any stage of an infection. Take 500 to 1,000 milligrams of each five times a day for five days to one week.

■ To help boost your immune system, take 5 to 10 milligrams of zinc five times daily for five days to one week. Take zinc with food to prevent stomach upset.

HERBAL TREATMENT

■ At the first sign of the flu, begin taking the Chinese

botanical formula Yin Qiao. This remedy usually is not helpful after the third day of symptoms. Take two or three tablets three times a day, up to twelve tablets in a twenty-four-hour period, during the acute phase of the flu. After the symptoms start to ease, reduce the dosage to one tablet three times daily for one week.

■ To help yourself rest and relax, take a cup of chamomile tea twice a day.

☐ Echinacea and goldenseal stimulate the immune system. Goldenseal also helps to soothe mucous membranes. Take one dose of an echinacea and goldenseal combination remedy supplying 250 to 500 milligrams of echinacea and 150 to 300 milligrams of goldenseal three times daily for five days.

☐ In a 1995 Israeli study, elderberry extract was found to reduce both the severity of symptoms and the duration of flu (two to three days in the treated group versus six days in the placebo group). Choose an extract standardized to contain 5 percent total flavonoids and take 500 milligrams twice daily.

☐ Garlic helps to detoxify the body. Take 500 milligrams (or one clove) three times a day for up to five days.

☐ Ginger tea is excellent if the stomach is affected. Take a cup as needed.

HOMEOPATHY

☐ At the very first sign that flu is developing, take ½ tube of *Anas barbariae* (marketed under various brand names, including Oscillococcinum) every two hours, for a total of five doses.

☐ If you are feeling chilly, restless, and weak, choose *Arsenicum album*. This is for the person who feels worse in a cold room, but wants something cold to drink. You probably have a red nose with runny nasal secretions that burn the nose and upper lip. When ill, you prefer to sit in bed with books, magazines, and a television, and be left alone for the most part, but like a bit of attention every once in a while. Take one dose of *Arsenicum album* 30x or 9c, as directed on the product label, three to four times a day for up to eight doses.

☐ *Bryonia* is good if symptoms include a headache, cough, constipation, thirst, and irritability. Take one dose of *Bryonia* 30x or 9c three to four times a day for up to three days.

☐ *Eupatorium* is helpful for severe aching deep in the bones that makes you feel sore all over. Take one dose of *Eupatorium* 12x or 6c three to four times a day for up to ten doses.

■ Take *Gelsemium* if you have heavy, droopy eyes; feel weak and tired, with aches and chills up and down your back; and want to be alone. Take one dose of *Gelsemium* 12x or 6c three to four times a day for up to eight doses.

■ *Mercurius solubilis* is for a lingering flu that just doesn't seem to go away. You may have a sore throat, bad breath, and tender, swollen glands. Take one dose of *Mercurius solubilis* 12x or 6c three times a day for up to three days.

■ *Rhus toxicodendron* is good if you are feeling restless and complain of achy, stiff muscles. Take one dose of *Rhus toxicodendron* 30x or 9c three times a day for up to three days.

BACH FLOWER REMEDIES

■ Impatiens will help if you are feeling impatient and tired of being sick. Take this remedy three times a day for three days (*see* BACH FLOWER REMEDIES in Part One).

ACUPRESSURE

For the locations of acupressure points on the body, *see* ADMINISTERING AN ACUPRESSURE TREATMENT in Part Three.

■ Bladder 11, 12, 13, and 14 clear and balance the respiratory system.

■ Large Intestine 4 controls the head. This acupressure point relieves congestion and headaches.

■ Lung 7 helps to clear upper respiratory tract infections.

■ Massaging the feet is comforting and helps to bring energy down from the head to aid healing.

AROMATHERAPY

For specific instructions on how to use aromatherapy, *see* PREPARING AROMATHERAPY TREATMENTS in Part Three.

■ Essential oils of basil, eucalyptus, peppermint, and pine help to ease nasal congestion. Choose one to three of these oils and use them as inhalants or in steam inhalation treatments. For chest congestion, a steam inhalation treatment made with basil, pine, and/or tea tree oil can help to clear mucus and ease breathing. Rubbing a massage oil prepared with these oils over the chest may also be helpful.

■ An aromatherapy bath prepared with elemi, myrrh, pine, and/or tea tree oil can help to soothe that all-over achy feeling. Use a lukewarm bath for fever, a hot bath for chills.

GENERAL RECOMMENDATIONS

■ Begin treating the flu as soon as symptoms appear.

■ Most people suffering through the flu naturally want to sleep and rest, sparing body energy to fight the virus. A comfortable bed and an open window bringing in fresh air (if weather permits) will help. Avoid becoming chilled, however.

■ *See also* COUGH; FEVER; SINUSITIS; and/or SORE THROAT if the flu is accompanied by these symptoms.

PREVENTION

■ Flu vaccines are offered yearly. These are sometimes recommended by family physicians for people who are most likely to be exposed to or endangered by the illness, such as health-care workers, elderly people, and people with chronic heart, lung, or kidney diseases. The flu shot itself may cause mild flulike symptoms. Also, since flu vaccines are formulated based on viruses that have caused outbreaks in the past, they may or may not be effective in preventing flu caused by this year's virus.

■ Astragalus helps to build the immune system, and thus make you less vulnerable to the flu. Take 250 to 500 milligrams in the morning three times a week during the flu season.

Note: Do not take this herb if you have a fever.

■ American ginseng helps to boost the immune system and strengthen the body. Take 200 milligrams one-half hour before breakfast once or twice a week during the winter months.

Note: Do not use ginseng if you have high blood pressure, heart disease, or hypoglycemia. If you are sensitive to the effects of caffeine and other stimulants, you may want to consult with a qualified herbalist before using ginseng.

■ Echinacea and goldenseal stimulate the immune system and help keep the body clear of infections. Take one dose of an echinacea and goldenseal combination formula supplying 500 milligrams of echinacea and 350 milligrams of goldenseal twice weekly during the flu season.

■ Take one dose of homeopathic *Anas barbariae* each week or every other week during the flu season.

■ Make it a rule to eat a low-sweet diet and no fried foods. During the flu season, prepare lots of vegetable and astragalus soup to help boost your immune system (*see* THERAPEUTIC RECIPES in Part Three).

■ People under stress may fall ill more easily. Both physical and emotional stress can create imbalances that make the body more vulnerable to illness. Learn to deal with unavoidable stress in a constructive manner. Avoid exposure to dust and chemicals, too much sugar and/or fat in the diet, and even sudden and extreme temperature changes.

■ Vitamin C and bioflavonoids, taken daily, help to prevent colds and flu. Take 300 milligrams of each daily during the cold season.

Food Allergies

An allergy is a hypersensitive reaction to a normally harmless substance. There are a variety of substances, termed allergens, that may prove troublesome to susceptible individuals. Common allergens include pollen, animal dander, house dust, feathers, mites, chemicals, and a variety of foods. This section is devoted to food-related allergies.

Allergic reactions to food can occur immediately, or they can be delayed and take days to surface. A delayed allergic reaction can make it more difficult to pinpoint the allergen. Common symptoms of an allergic reaction include respiratory congestion, eye inflammation, dark circles and/or puffiness under the eyes, swelling, itching, hives, unexplained fluid retention, and stomach upset and vomiting. Food allergies can also contribute to chronic health problems, such as acne, asthma, anxiety, bladder infections, swollen glands, sinusitis, diarrhea, ear infections, eczema, fatigue, hay fever, headache, irritability, joint pain, chronic runny nose, mood swings, sleep disturbances, feelings of disorientation, and even difficulty maintaining concentration. In addition, food allergies can cause intestinal irritation and swelling that interferes with the absorption of vitamins and minerals. Even if you are eating a wholesome, nutritious diet, if you are consuming foods to which you are allergic, the food may not be absorbed properly and you may not be getting the full benefit of many essential nutrients.

The most common foods that cause allergic reactions are wheat, milk and other dairy products, eggs, fish and seafood, chocolate, citrus fruits, soy products, corn, nuts, and berries. Many people also are allergic to sulfites, which are found in some frozen foods and dried fruits, as well as in medications.

It has been observed that some people actively dislike the foods that produce an allergic reaction. They seem to know instinctively that certain foods will cause a problem. Paradoxically, however, some people seem to be particularly drawn to the very foods they are allergic to. People who enthusiastically eat lots of wheat bread, wheat crackers, and wheat cereals, or who crave milk, ice cream, and other dairy products, may actually be exhibiting allergies to those foods. Some people seem to be genetically predisposed to food allergies. If one or both of your parents have food allergies, there is a greater chance that you will have the same difficulties.

Sometimes, if all the irritating foods are eliminated from the diet for several months, the body will have a chance to rest and heal, after which it will be able to handle small amounts of these foods without reacting. Sometimes, too, there is an underlying issue such as a parasitic or yeast infection in the intestine that is contributing to the allergic response. If these underlying problems are cleared up, the body may be less reactive to certain substances.

"Food allergy" is a term that is often used loosely to describe any adverse reaction to eating certain foods.

There is a difference between food allergies and food sensitivities and intolerances, however. True food allergies are caused by an inappropriate response by the immune system to a normally benign component (often a protein molecule) in a certain food. Someone with a sensitivity to certain substances—monosodium glutamate (MSG), for example—may suffer a severe headache after eating foods containing this well-known flavor enhancer, but the immune system is not involved. A person who is lactose intolerant does not have an allergic reaction to milk and dairy products, but rather fails to produce enough of the enzyme lactase to digest these foods, leading to symptoms of diarrhea, gas, and bloating (*see* LACTOSE INTOLERANCE).

EMERGENCY TREATMENT

■ Occasionally, an allergic reaction is so severe it can be life-threatening. If you develop rapidly spreading hives or if there is any sign that you are developing difficulty breathing due to a severe allergic reaction—especially if you have a history of severe reactions—have someone take you immediately to the emergency room of the nearest hospital. If this is not possible, call for emergency help and stress the urgency of the situation. Every second counts. If an emergency adrenaline kit, such as the Ana-Kit or EpiPen, is available, administer it immediately, followed by 25 to 50 milligrams of an antihistamine such as diphenhydramine (Benadryl). Do not eat or drink anything if you are having difficulty breathing. Even if you respond quickly to the administration of the emergency adrenaline kit, you should go to the emergency room for professional evaluation and treatment. Trust hospital personnel to take appropriate measures to stabilize your condition and bring the reaction under control.

CONVENTIONAL TREATMENT

■ The most important part of treating food allergies, obviously, is to identify—and then avoid—the foods that are causing the reaction. There are two techniques, the elimination diet and the rotation diet, that enable you to do this (*see* ELIMINATION DIET and ROTATION DIET in Part Three).

■ In cases of severe multiple food allergies, oral cromolyn sodium (Gastrocrom) may be prescribed as a preventive measure. This is the same drug that is used in inhaled form to prevent asthma attacks. It is a patented form of a bioflavonoid, and side effects and toxicity are low.

■ If you suffer from recurrent allergic reactions, an antihistamine may be recommended.

■ Some doctors recommend desensitization therapy for people with allergies. This involves repeated injections of a dilution of the offending food. Desensitization has vary-

ing degrees of success. In general, it tends to work better for airborne or chemical allergies than food allergies.

DIETARY GUIDELINES

■ Use an elimination or rotation diet to determine which foods are causing the symptoms. Some of the foods that most commonly cause a reaction are dairy products, wheat, citrus fruits, nuts (including peanut butter), corn, soy products, cane sugar, and eggs. You may wish to try eliminating these first.

■ Once you have identified the foods or classes of foods that cause symptoms, remember to read the labels on all the processed food products you buy. Many food products contain surprising "hidden" ingredients—especially additives such as artificial flavorings and colorings—that can cause allergic reactions. It's better to base your diet on whole foods that you prepare yourself.

NUTRITIONAL SUPPLEMENTS

■ Take a good hypoallergenic multivitamin and mineral complex daily to ensure a supply of all the major nutrients. It is not uncommon for people with food allergies to absorb and utilize nutrients from food poorly.

■ Acidophilus and bifidobacteria improve immune function within the intestines. Take either or both twice a day as recommended on the product label. If you are allergic to milk, be sure to choose dairy-free formulas.

■ A low-functioning adrenal or thyroid gland can be a contributing factor to food allergies. Ask your doctor to check your adrenal and thryoid function. If you register in the low or low-normal range, you may benefit from taking adrenal and/or thyroid glandular extract. Adrenal extract is particularly effective if you suffer from both allergies and fatigue.

■ The antioxidants support the immune system and help to moderate the inflammatory response. Take 5,000 international units of vitamin A, 25,000 international units of beta-carotene, 200 international units of vitamin E, and 100 micrograms of selenium twice daily.

Note: If you are pregnant, or intend to get pregnant, or if you have liver disease, consult your doctor before taking supplemental vitamin A. If you are taking an anticoagulant (blood thinner), consult your physician before taking supplemental vitamin E.

■ Calcium and magnesium help to reduce sensitivity and nervousness associated with allergies. Take a combination formula containing 500 milligrams of calcium and 250 to 300 milligrams of magnesium twice a day for two to three months.

■ Some food allergies are exacerbated by imperfect digestion. To insure full digestion, take a full-spectrum digestive-enzyme supplement providing 5,000 international units of lipase, 2,500 international units of amylase, 300 international units of protease, plus 500 to 1,000 milligrams of pancreatin, with each meal.

Note: Long-term supplementation with pancreatin is not advised, as it can cause your pancreas to reduce its own production of this important enzyme. Overuse also has the potential to cause nausea or diarrhea. After two months on pancreatin, discontinue use and monitor your reaction. If you find that your digestive problems recur, discuss pancreatin supplementation with your health-care provider.

■ Fish oil and flaxseed oil contain essential fatty acids that moderate the inflammatory response, and that are lacking in most foods. Take 1 tablespoonful of flaxseed oil daily or 900 milligrams of fish oil twice a day.

■ Glutamine is an amino acid that improves the integrity of cells in the gastrointestinal tract and also acts to diminish the inflammatory response. Take 500 to 1,000 milligrams of L-glutamine three times a day.

■ Methylsulfonylmethane (MSM) is a good source of sulfur, a trace mineral that may help to reduce the severity of the allergic response. Take 500 milligrams three or four times daily, with meals.

■ The B vitamins help support adrenal function. Take a vitamin-B complex supplement supplying 25 to 50 milligrams of each of the major B vitamins twice a day for two to three months, plus an additional 250 milligrams of pantothenic acid twice daily for one month. Additional vitamin B_{12}, especially if administered in injections, is often very effective for people with food allergies. Ask your health-care provider if he or she is willing to provide this treatment twice a week for three to four weeks. If not, take 500 micrograms of vitamin B_{12} orally in the morning every other day for three weeks.

■ Thymus glandular extract helps to improve immune function. It can be particularly helpful if you have a history of diminished immunity and are prone to developing infections, or if you are over forty-five and only recently developed food allergies or sensitivities. Take 200 to 300 milligrams twice daily.

■ Vitamin C helps to stimulate immune function. Bioflavonoids have potent anti-allergy and anti-inflammatory properties. Take 1,000 milligrams of vitamin C, in mineral ascorbate form with bioflavonoids, twice a day for two to three months. Taking additional bioflavonoids, up to 1,000 milligrams two or three times daily, can provide additional benefits.

HERBAL TREATMENT

■ If the food allergy is complicated by chronic upper res-

piratory problems, take 500 milligrams of astragalus once or twice daily, with breakfast and/or lunch, for two to three months.

■ Cat's claw slowly helps regulate immune function and has anti-inflammatory benefits. Take 250 to 500 milligrams of standardized extract two or three times daily.

Note: Do not take cat's claw if you are pregnant or nursing, or if you are an organ transplant recipient. Use it with caution if you are taking an anticoagulant (blood thinner).

■ Milk thistle contains silymarin, which helps to detoxify the liver and is especially beneficial for food allergies. Choose an extract standardized to contain 80 percent flavonoids (silymarin) and take 100 to 150 milligrams three times daily for one week out of each month.

■ Pine-bark and grape-seed extracts are natural anti-inflammatories that are high in bioflavonoids. Take 50 milligrams of either three times daily.

■ Siberian ginseng is a tonic herb that helps strengthen the whole body. Choose a standardized extract containing 0.5 percent eleutheroside E and take 100 to 200 milligrams twice daily, one-half hour before breakfast and again one-half hour before lunch.

HOMEOPATHY

There are no magic remedies for reversing allergic reactions, but some homeopathic remedies are useful for treating symptoms.

■ For acid indigestion and/or pain in the upper abdomen region, take one dose of *Carbo vegetabilis* 30x or 15c as needed.

■ *Nux vomica* is helpful if you have become more hypersensitive to certain foods as a result of taking a lot of medication, or if you have a propensity to take sugar, fat, and alcohol to excess. Take one dose of *Nux vomica* 30x or 15c as needed.

■ See a homeopathic physician for a constitutional remedy. *Medhorrinum*, available only by prescription, is often helpful for people who suffer from a wide variety of allergies.

GENERAL RECOMMENDATIONS

■ Because allergic reactions can take numerous forms, from headaches to fatigue, you may want to consult other entries in this book that correspond to your particular symptoms.

PREVENTION

■ Eat a varied diet. Eating particular foods too much or too frequently can foster the development of food allergies.

Food Poisoning

Food poisoning is most commonly a reaction to toxins produced by bacteria. These organisms thrive in food that is not prepared hygienically, that is kept out of refrigeration for too long, or that is not thoroughly cooked.

Most cases of food poisoning come about as a result of food being handled by unclean hands or meat not being cooked long enough and at a high enough temperature to kill microorganisms. For example, if a cook shapes hamburger patties and then cuts raw vegetables, without washing his or her hands in between, bacteria from the meat can migrate via the hands to contaminate the vegetables. Foods with mayonnaise-type dressings that have been left out of refrigeration for too long can also cause problems, as can cooked foods (such as pizza) that have been removed from heat and then left at room temperature for too long. Some cases of food poisoning occur as a result of toxic reactions to poisonous plants, certain types of mushrooms, or contaminated shellfish. Eating raw fish or shellfish, foods containing raw eggs (such as homemade eggnog or Caesar salad dressing), food that was canned improperly, or food from damaged cans can also lead to food poisoning. Another possible cause is exposure to chemical contaminants such as heavy metals or pesticides.

Common symptoms of food poisoning include nausea, vomiting, diarrhea, abdominal pain and cramping, fever, and general malaise. Symptoms usually come on suddenly, sometimes within hours of eating the contaminated food. Because the symptoms can persist for several days, however, food poisoning is often mistaken for a case of the flu. If you experience a sudden bout of nausea, vomiting, and/or diarrhea a couple of hours after eating, you may be suffering from food poisoning.

Minor food poisoning episodes can usually be treated at home with the remedies outlined in this entry. However, you should contact your health-care provider for advice if you suspect food poisoning and you develop any of the following symptoms: fever above 102°F; severe vomiting; severe diarrhea, especially if it continues for more than twenty-four hours or contains blood; difficulty breathing or speaking; changes in vision; localized abdominal pain. Any of these symptoms should be evaluated by a professional.

CONVENTIONAL TREATMENT

■ At the beginning, nausea and vomiting may indicate that your body is trying to expel toxins from the stomach before they become absorbed through the lower intestinal tract. It is often wiser to allow the body to perform this natural protective function at the outset, as it may help you avoid a longer illness later. If you vomit more than three or four times, or if the vomit becomes bitter (a result of bile being brought up), you may wish to take action to stop it.

■ Emetrol is a gentle over-the-counter product that is useful for relieving nausea and vomiting. Follow the dosage directions on the product label.

■ For frequent, watery diarrhea, loperamide (found in Imodium AD and other over-the-counter products) may be helpful. This medication works by slowing the movement of the intestinal muscle. Follow the dosage directions on the product label. You should not use this drug if you have a fever over 101°F, or if you have bloody stools.

■ If the vomiting is severe and you are unable to keep anything down, your doctor may prescribe an antiemetic in suppository form. Prochlorperazine (sold under the brand name Compazine), promethazine (Phenergan), and trimethobenzamide (Tigan) are prescription drugs that are sometimes used for this purpose. Occasionally these are given in injectable form as well.

■ Dimenhydrinate (Dramamine) is sometimes useful for milder vomiting. Follow the dosage directions on the product label.

■ Activated charcoal, which can be taken in capsule form or mixed with water, may be recommended, particularly if a drug or chemical toxin is suspected.

DIETARY GUIDELINES

■ The most important thing to remember in treating food poisoning is that an inflamed stomach tends to go into spasm when stretched, resulting in vomiting. Consequently, if you are vomiting and take anything by mouth, it should be in very small quantities (1 teaspoon or less) at frequent intervals.

■ Rest quietly and take frequent small sips of fluids. Barley and/or rice water make good choices. (*See* THERAPEUTIC RECIPES in Part Three.)

■ Do not eat anything until you really want to. Once you feel ready to eat, start slowly, with easily digested foods such as toast, broth, applesauce, mashed bananas, and diluted juices.

■ Do not consume any milk or any other dairy products during and for at least seventy-two hours after an episode of food poisoning.

NUTRITIONAL SUPPLEMENTS

■ Acidophilus and bifidus supplements will reintroduce beneficial flora to the intestinal tract. Starting twenty-four hours after an episode of food poisoning, take one dose of each, as directed on the product label, three times daily for one week. Then take one dose daily for at least one month. If you are allergic to milk, select dairy-free formulas.

■ Take 100 milligrams of potassium twice daily for two days to restore your body's electrolyte balance. This is especially important if you had a lot of diarrhea or watery stools.

HERBAL TREATMENT

■ Cat's claw fights inflammation and infection. Take 500 milligrams three times daily until your symptoms have resolved.

■ Curing Pill formula, a Chinese herbal combination, helps to resolve diarrhea, nausea, and stomach pain. Take one dose, as directed on the product label, three or four times a day for the first day or two following an episode of food poisoning.

■ After taking Curing Pill formula, take Huang Lian Su, a Chinese patent medicine that is particularly useful if the stool continues to be loose and has a foul odor. Take two tablets two or three times daily for two to three days.

■ Ginger tea helps to stop nausea and cleanse the digestive tract, as well as providing fluids. Take a cup of ginger tea or 250 milligrams of standardized extract three times a day for the first twenty-four hours.

■ Goldenseal is useful as an antibacterial for resolving diarrhea. It has a bitter taste, however. If you can tolerate it, take a cup of goldenseal tea three times a day for the first twenty-four hours. If you prefer, you can substitute 250 to 500 milligrams of goldenseal extract for each cup of tea.

■ Peppermint may help to restore appetite following a bout of food poisoning. Try taking one cup of peppermint tea, or 500 milligrams in capsule form, three times a day for two days.

Note: If you are using peppermint and also taking a homeopathic preparation, allow one hour between the two. Otherwise, the strong smell of the mint may interfere with the action of the homeopathic remedy.

■ A paste made from the Japanese umeboshi plum is gentle and very settling for an upset stomach (see THERAPEUTIC RECIPES in Part Three). This can be diluted in warm water and taken as a tea, or you can put a small dab (about $1/4$ teaspoon) on your tongue and let it dissolve. It has a pleasing taste and is very gentle, so it can be repeated as needed.

HOMEOPATHY

Choose the appropriate homeopathic remedy from the list below, and take one dose every hour, up to a total of five doses.

■ *Arsenicum album* 30x or 9c is the premier homeopathic for food poisoning. This is for the person who has diarrhea and chills, feels anxious, and feels worse between midnight and 2:00 AM.

■ *Carbo vegetabilis* is good for pain in the center of the stomach. Take one dose of *Carbo vegetabilis* 30x or 9c three times a day, up to a total of eight doses.

■ *China* 30x or 9c is good if you are feeling exhausted and weak, with a lower abdomen that is very gaseous and sensitive to touch or pressure. It is a good remedy to use once the initial phase of food poisoning has been addressed because it helps the digestive tract to repair itself.

■ *Colocynthis* 12x or 6c helps to relieve stabbing pains in the lower abdomen. The food poisoning episode may have occurred after you experienced overwhelming anger.

■ *Nux vomica* 30x or 9c is for food poisoning that occurs after excessive consumption of rich foods. It is helpful if you are feeling irritable, and your abdominal pain is improved by the passing of stool.

■ *Phosphorus* 30x or 9c is useful for vomiting and diarrhea, with burning anal pain as stool passes. You may crave ice and iced drinks but be unable to keep them down.

■ Choose *Podophyllum* 12x or 9c if you have greenish-colored diarrhea that is worse in the morning and that is accompanied by abdominal cramping.

■ *Pulsatilla* 30x or 9c will help if your stools are quite varied and consuming any fatty foods in the seventy-two hours after the initial food poisoning episode makes the diarrhea worse. The *Pulsatilla* person is sensitive and emotionally vulnerable.

GENERAL RECOMMENDATIONS

■ Prolonged diarrhea and vomiting can cause serious dehydration. If you suspect you are becoming dehydrated, you can take an oral electrolyte formula (see DEHYDRATION).

■ See also DIARRHEA and/or NAUSEA AND VOMITING for additional suggestions.

PREVENTION

■ Keep all hot foods hot and cold foods cold. Bacteria do not grow at temperatures below 40°F or above 150°F.

■ Keep the temperature in your refrigerator at 40°F or below and that in your freezer at 0°F or below. You can use a refrigerator thermometer to monitor temperature.

■ Thaw all frozen foods in the refrigerator rather than at room temperature. If you use a microwave oven to defrost food, make sure to finish cooking it right away.

■ Keep uncooked meats, fish, and poultry in the refrigerator as briefly as possible. In any case, use red meat within three to five days, poultry within two days, and fish within twenty-four hours.

Types of Food Poisoning

Different infectious organisms cause different kinds of foodborne illness. The most common types of food poisoning include campylobacteriosis (*Campylobacter* infection) salmonellosis (*Salmonella* poisoning), botulism, *Escherichia coli* (*E. coli*) poisoning, staphylococcal food poisoning, clostridial poisoning, and listeriosis.

Campylobacteriosis is probably the most common type of food poisoning in the United States. It most often results from eating improperly cooked infected poultry (birds can carry the bacteria with no signs of illness), though it can also be contracted from drinking contaminated water or unpasteurized milk. Symptoms can begin anywhere from two to five days after exposure, and include diarrhea, cramping, fever, nausea, and vomiting. There is often abdominal pain right in the center of the stomach, and there may be blood in the stools. Most people recover on their own in a matter of a week or so, but people with compromised immune systems may require antibiotic treatment to prevent the illness from spreading to the bloodstream and becoming a dangerous systemic infection.

The incidence of salmonellosis has been increasing in recent years. It is the possibility of *Salmonella* contamination that has led to recommendations against eating any foods containing raw eggs. Symptoms of *Salmonella* poisoning include stomach cramps, diarrhea, chills, high fever, headache, and nausea and vomiting. They usually come on fairly soon after contact with the contaminated food and run their course in twenty-four hours or so.

In contrast, botulism is a potentially life-threatening form of food poisoning. Symptoms usually begin sometime between sixteen hours and five days after the ingestion of contaminated food, and include headache and dizziness, double vision, muscle paralysis, vomiting, and difficulty breathing and swallowing. If you develop symptoms of botulism, it is vital that you seek medical attention immediately.

Escherichia coli (*E. coli*) is a normally benign intestinal bacteria that is present in all animals, including humans. However, one strain of this bacteria, known as 0157:H7, can be deadly. The major sources of this bacteria are undercooked ground beef and unpasteurized milk. The presence of *E. coli* in food or water indicates fecal contamination. Symptoms of *E. coli* poisoning include stomach cramps that progress to extremely painful abdominal cramping; unremitting diarrhea that progresses to bloody diarrhea; and fever and/or chills. Symptoms manifest themselves quickly, and most cases subside in five to ten days. However, in rare cases there can be complications including urinary tract infection, kidney failure, seizures, and stroke. Children, elderly people, and people with compromised immune systems are at highest risk of developing complications. Prompt diagnosis and aggressive treatment are mandatory.

Staphylococcal food poisoning is a rapidly developing syndrome caused by a toxin rather than by the bacteria itself. Within a few hours of eating contaminated food, a sudden attack of nausea, vomiting, and cramping is common. Fever and diarrhea are also possible. Most attacks last only a few hours and resolve themselves without any further consequences, although severe cases can occur, particularly in very young or elderly people. The most common suspect foods are creamy items like custard or pastry, along with fish and processed meats left out at room temperature.

Clostridium perfringens food poisoning is also caused by a toxin the bacteria produce. It usually causes nausea, vomiting, and diarrhea that clear up relatively quickly. However, there are some strains of the bacteria that can cause serious diarrhea, abdominal pain and distention, and even the destruction of portions of the intestines.

Listeria bacteria infect shellfish and mammals, including cows. They are transmitted to humans by direct contact with infected animals. Any secretion from an infected animal or person may contain the organism. The symptoms caused by listeriosis include a dark red rash over the trunk and legs, inflammation of the heart that may be experienced as sharp, stabbing chest pain and, possibly, difficulty breathing. Enlargement of the liver and spleen are also possible, and may cause a bloated feeling in the upper abdomen and difficulty breathing deeply, in addition to making it possible to feel the organs from the outside. This infection can also lead to shock. Signs and symptoms vary, depending on the severity of the infection and age and prior condition of the affected individual. This is a potentially serious disease that requires aggressive treatment with intravenous antibiotics.

■ Keep two cutting boards in your kitchen, one for cutting meat and the other for fruits and vegetables. Contrary to what some believe, a recent study showed that wooden cutting boards are easier to clean and keep free of bacteria than plastic ones are. Wash your cutting boards with a solution of bleach and water after each use.

■ Always wash your hands thoroughly before handling food, and make sure to keep them clean by washing as often as necessary during food preparation. Antibacterial soaps are helpful, but they cannot replace proper attention to hygiene. Any soap will remove dirt and bacteria. Whatever kind of soap you use, it takes both soap and friction to get rid of bacteria. You must lather up and rub your hands together for at least ten seconds before rinsing well with warm water. Ten seconds may be longer than you think. In order to judge the length of time required, watch the second hand on your kitchen clock or set the timer on your microwave for ten seconds while you are soaping your hands a couple of times, until you get a feeling for how long ten seconds really is.

■ After you wash your hands for ten seconds with soap and hot water, dry your hands with a clean towel reserved just for that purpose, not a dish towel. Wash all kitchen towels daily in hot water, preferably with chlorine bleach added.

■ Kitchen sponges can spread bacterial contamination over hand-washed dishes, counters, and stove tops. As soon as a sponge or dishcloth gets wet, the bacteria are reactivated. For complete protection, microwave kitchen sponges for thirty to sixty seconds on high before every use.

■ Cook all red meat, fish, and poultry thoroughly. Meats should be cooked to an internal temperature of at least 165°F, poultry to 180°F, and fish to 140°F. Do not serve any meat (especially pork) raw, rare, or even medium-rare. If meat is even a little pink, it may harbor live bacteria.

■ Be careful when cooking with a microwave. If you cook meat in your microwave, always use a thermometer to verify that the internal temperature is high enough. When cooking red meat in a microwave, precook the meat on the high setting for thirty to ninety seconds and discard the juices. Then continue cooking the meat immediately.

■ Do not cook stuffing inside turkeys or other poultry. Instead, bake stuffing separately in the oven or prepare it on top of the stove.

■ Always cook eggs for at least three minutes. Never use raw eggs that are cracked.

■ Use different utensils for handling raw and cooked foods.

■ Clean any dishes and utensils that have come into contact with raw meat, poultry, eggs, or seafood. Do not put cooked foods into dishes that held them when they were raw without washing the dishes first.

■ Never eat foods containing raw meat, poultry, eggs, fish, or shellfish, either before or during cooking. (This means no nibbling on raw cookie dough!)

■ Never use food from any can that is bulging, rusted, bent, or sticky, or that has a loose lid.

■ After meals, refrigerate any leftovers as soon as possible. Do not refrigerate foods in the same pots or bowls you used for cooking or serving; if you transfer them to different containers before refrigerating, the food will take less time to cool. Use any stored leftovers within five days.

■ When reheating soups, stews, sauces, and gravies, bring them to a rapid boil, if possible, and cook for at least four minutes. Be aware that microwave ovens, while convenient, do not necessarily kill bacteria when they are used to reheat food.

■ Be careful when eating out. Do not eat foods that smell odd or taste spoiled, even if you are eating in a "nice" restaurant. Avoid salad bars that do not look fresh and clean. If you are traveling in a developing country, you may want to completely avoid foods that can spoil or become contaminated easily, such as mayonnaise and dairy products.

■ Drink green tea with meals. Catechin, a flavonoid found in green tea, has effective antibacterial properties. In the laboratory, many of the organisms commonly involved in food poisoning have been shown to be unable to grow in the presence of concentrations of catechin comparable to those found in green tea.

Foot Problems

See ATHLETE'S FOOT; BLISTERS; BUNION; CORNS AND CALLUSES; NAIL PROBLEMS AND INJURIES; WARTS.

Forgetfulness

See MEMORY PROBLEMS.

Fracture

See BONE, BROKEN.

Frostbite

When tissues are exposed to too much cold for too long, blood flow to the area decreases and ice crystals form in the tissues, with the result that cells are damaged and die. This type of injury is called frostbite.

Mild freezing of the tissues can involve only the skin and shallower structures, but more severe injury can involve deeper tissues. Early symptoms include numbness, tingling, and, usually, a "prickly" feeling. The skin also loses its normal elasticity. If the condition is not alleviated, the area may become immobile, with swelling, blisters, and destruction of tissue, and eventually may become gangrenous as a result of the lack of adequate blood flow to the tissues to keep them alive. Rewarming causes a burning sensation.

The hands and feet are the areas of the body most likely to suffer frostbite, since they are most likely to be exposed to cold for long periods. People with circulatory problems such as arteriosclerosis or Raynaud's syndrome and people who smoke are more likely than others to develop frostbite. Taking beta-blockers (a type of drug often prescribed for high blood pressure) may increase the risk as well.

CONVENTIONAL TREATMENT

■ As soon as possible, the entire body should be warmed, and the frostbitten part dried, covered, and warmed as fast as possible to above body temperature. This is usually done in a warm-water bath to allow for better temperature control. However, it is not usually done until no further exposure to extreme cold is likely, as freezing, thawing, and refreezing can worsen the damage.

■ The injured tissues should not be rubbed. In fact, anything that comes into contact with the skin should be removed, if possible, to avoid damage from friction in the early stages of treatment.

■ The affected area should be evaluated for possible infection, and antibiotic therapy, if necessary, started as soon as possible.

■ Blisters may be treated with topical dressings and applications of silver sulfadiazine (Silvadene) or aloe vera.

■ Depending on the severity of the exposure, pain medication may be necessary. Nonsteroidal anti-inflammatory drugs (NSAIDs) such as ibuprofen (Advil, Motrin, Nuprin, and others) or naproxen (Aleve, Anaprox, Naprelan, Naprosyn) are often used, but stronger drugs may be necessary in some cases.

■ With proper treatment, mild cases of frostbite can heal completely. In severe cases, surgery may ultimately be required to remove necrotic (dead) tissue. If gangrene develops, amputation may even be necessary. However, surgery is usually delayed as long as possible to allow the injury time to heal. A radiographic technique called scintigraphy, in which a radioisotope is administered intravenously and its progress through the circulatory system tracked by a special scanner, can be used to determine which tissues are viable and which are not going to survive, requiring removal.

DIETARY GUIDELINES

■ Drink plenty of fluids to rehydrate your body. Use warm drinks like herbal teas and vegetable soups.

■ *Avoid* alcoholic beverages. While alcohol may feel as if it has a warming effect, in fact it cools the body down by dilating the blood vessels near the surface of the skin. If you have suffered frostbite, your body shut down circulation to those blood vessels because your core temperature was in danger of becoming too low. Thus, alcohol thwarts the body's effort to protect itself.

NUTRITIONAL SUPPLEMENTS

■ The B vitamins are required for healthy circulation. Take a B-complex supplement supplying 25 to 50 milligrams of each of the major B vitamins twice daily. Choose a liquid formula for easier absorption.

HERBAL TREATMENT

■ Cayenne (capsicum), applied topically, improves circulation. Apply a cayenne or capsaicin cream to the affected area as directed on the product label.

■ Ginger is warming and also improves circulation. Take a cup of ginger tea three times a day for up to five days.

■ Pine-bark and grape-seed extracts help to reduce inflammation. Take 25 to 50 milligrams of either three times daily.

HOMEOPATHY

■ *Aconite* helps to relieve numbness, tingling, shooting pains, icy coldness, and lack of sensation in the hands and feet. Take one dose of *Aconite* 6x or 3c four times over the course of the first twenty-four hours.

■ *Abrotanum* is good for pricking sensations and coldness associated with frostbite of the fingers, feet, and arms. After finishing the *Aconite*, take one dose of *Abrotanum* 30x or 15c four times daily, up to a total of ten doses.

BACH FLOWER REMEDIES

■ Rescue Remedy can help relieve anxiety. Take one dose hourly for the first four hours after the injury.

AROMATHERAPY

■ Use essential oils of lavender, orange, and rosemary to enhance circulation and relieve anxiety. Add three drops of each to a tubful of warm water and enjoy a soothing aromatherapy bath.

GENERAL RECOMMENDATIONS

■ Serious frostbite requires medical attention. However, while you are waiting for help to arrive, you can do the following:

- Remove all wet clothing and put on dry clothing and plenty of blankets, leaving the frostbitten area or areas accessible.
- Fill a large container with warm (104° to 108°F [40° to 42°C]) water, and add ¹/₂ teaspoon cayenne powder. Cayenne helps to increase circulation.
- Soak the affected body part in the water until the area flushes pink and becomes sensitive. You may need to add water to keep the bath properly warm.
- After the skin becomes pink, dry the area. A hair dryer set on low is better for this purpose than a towel, as frostbitten areas should not be rubbed. Loosely wrap the area with cotton bandages.

■ Do not smoke, and avoid secondhand smoke. The nicotine in tobacco smoke impairs circulation.

PREVENTION

■ Dress in layers. Wearing several layers of loose, warm clothing not only helps to keep you from getting too cold, but from getting too warm. If you start sweating, take off a layer. Otherwise, your sweat will cool you down too much, and blood will be drawn away from the extremities in an effort to conserve body heat.

■ Before going outdoors in cold weather, make certain your head, neck, face, and ears are well covered. Use any combination of hats, scarves, earmuffs, ski masks, and whatever other articles of clothing you find comfortable. This is particularly important on windy days.

■ When you will be spending time outdoors, take along extra socks and long underwear. Exchanging partially damp clothes for dry ones is the best way to maintain body temperature and reduce the risk of frostbite.

■ Wear at least two pairs of socks and mittens rather than gloves—or, better yet, a pair of mittens over a pair of gloves. Make sure socks and gloves or mittens are not too tight. It is the layer of air trapped next to your skin and between layers of clothing that preserves your body heat.

■ Before spending time outdoors, eat a nutritious meal or snack. Eating will make you feel warmer within ten to fifteen minutes.

■ If you feel your hands and/or feet becoming cold,

move your shoulders in a circular motion, wiggle your toes, and hop up and down to increase the circulation to your extremities.

■ When you get tired, seek warm shelter. A fatigued body has more difficulty staying warm.

■ Avoid alcohol and tobacco if you will be spending time outdoors.

Fungal Infection

See ATHLETE'S FOOT; CANDIDA INFECTION; JOCK ITCH; RINGWORM; YEAST INFECTION.

Gallbladder Problems

The gallbladder is a small pear-shaped organ situated underneath the liver. Its function is to store bile, which is produced by the liver, and release it as needed for digestion. During the digestive process, bile released by the gallbladder travels through the common bile duct into the duodenum (the upper part of the small intestine). This process is triggered by the passage of food from the stomach into the small intestine; when partially digested food matter arrives, gastrointestinal hormones cause the gallbladder to contract and expel bile into the duodenum. Bile is greenish-yellow in color and contains cholesterol, lecithin, bile salts, and other substances. It emulsifies the fats in food, breaking them into small fragments so they can be further digested and absorbed in the small intestine. If the gallbladder is not working as it should, the digestion of fats can be seriously impaired.

The most common type of gallbladder problem is *gallstones*. Every year, about one million Americans develop them. Although there are three different types of gallstones, the great majority are made up of crystallized cholesterol combined with bile salts. In some people, gallstones produce no symptoms at all. Others suffer severe pain centered on the right side of the abdomen as the gallbladder tries to expel the stones into the intestine.

If a stone becomes lodged in the bile duct, trapped bile can irritate and inflame the walls of the gallbladder. This condition, called *acute cholecystitis,* causes excruciating colic-like pain in the region, fever, and abdominal tenderness. Nausea and vomiting are not uncommon. Cholecystitis can become chronic. In the chronic form of the disease, the gallbladder can cease to function altogether. If the inflammation occurs in the absence of gallstones, it is known as acalculous cholecystitis.

Rarely, cholecystitis is followed by a condition called *empyema*. In this condition, the gallbladder fills with pus, resulting in high fever and severe abdominal pain. In addition, if the gallbladder happens to be empty of bile when a stone blocks the outlet, it may fill with mucus secreted from the gallbladder walls. A distended mucus-filled gallbladder is known as a *mucocele*. It is also possible to develop cancer of the gallbladder in conjunction with gallstones, although this cancer is extremely unusual. Only three people in 100,000 are diagnosed with this condition each year.

Gallbladder problems seldom occur before the age of forty. However, from that point on, gallstones are increasingly common. Women are affected four times as often as men. Obesity, elevated cholesterol levels, diabetes, a low-functioning thyroid gland, and inflammation of the gallbladder all foster the formation of gallstones.

CONVENTIONAL TREATMENT

■ If the gallbladder is unable to expel the stones and send them into the small intestine, the stones can be fragmented with sound waves or surgically removed. However, conventional therapy for most problems with the gallbladder remains cholecystectomy, or surgical removal of the gallbladder. With the advent of laparoscopic surgical techniques, which involve operating through a small "hose" with tiny tools, this operation has become less traumatic and less disfiguring than in the past, requiring a small incision only an inch or so in length. About 20 percent of people with gallstones have symptoms so serious that this is the best option. The digestive system can function without the gallbladder, so removing it seldom causes serious adverse aftereffects.

■ If the gallbladder or pancreas becomes inflamed as a result of gallstone blockage (the pancreas is located nearby and can become affected), this acute problem must be dealt with first before the gallbladder can be removed. Stopping eating and resorting to intravenous feeding, using general antibiotics, and controlling symptoms with appropriate medication are usually sufficient to calm the situation.

■ For cancer of the gallbladder, surgery can effect a complete cure if the tumor is fully contained within the gallbladder itself.

■ Occasionally, removal of the gallbladder can result in scarring of the remaining bile duct, which may require dilation and placement of a tube to keep the duct open.

DIETARY GUIDELINES

■ Eat a low-fat diet. Avoid all fatty and fried foods. A compromised gallbladder is placed under additional stress when fat is ingested.

■ To rest the gallbladder, eat only small amounts of food five or six times a day rather than eating two or three large meals. Avoid eating large amounts of food at any one time, especially at bedtime.

■ Olive oil, beets, and beet greens contain phytochemicals that help to thin bile. Enjoy these foods often.

■ Avoid carbonated beverages. If you have gallstones, the carbonation can trigger movement of the stones, resulting in additional pain.

NUTRITIONAL SUPPLEMENTS

■ Carnitine improves the digestion of fats and helps lower elevated cholesterol, which is common in people with gallbladder problems. This compound is responsible for the conversion of long-chain fatty acids into energy, and is required whenever you eat fats or are under stress. Stress is often a factor in gallbladder problems. Take 500 milligrams of L-carnitine twice daily.

■ As an aid to complete digestion, take a full-spectrum digestive-enzyme supplement providing 5,000 international units of lipase, 2,500 international units of amylase, and 300 international units of protease, plus 500 to 1,000 milligrams of pancreatin, with each meal. Be aware, however, that many digestive enzyme supplements contain hydrochloric acid (HCl). HCl can irritate the stomach, and should be avoided if you have a peptic ulcer or a tendency to stomach inflammation. If you experience irritation, either discontinue the supplement or choose a different formula without HCl.

Note: Long-term supplementation with pancreatin is not advised, as it can cause your pancreas to reduce its own production of this important enzyme. Overuse also has the potential to cause nausea or diarrhea. After two months on pancreatin, discontinue use and monitor your reaction. If you find that your problems recur, discuss pancreatin supplementation with your health-care provider.

■ Lecithin helps improve digestion and aids the transport of fats. Take 1,200 milligrams in capsule form or 1 to 2 teaspoons of liquid with each meal.

■ Magnesium helps relax the bile duct, eases stress, and is important for the entire central nervous system. Take 350 milligrams of chelated magnesium twice daily.

■ Vitamin E is a powerful antioxidant that scavenges free radicals. Choose a product containing mixed tocopherols and begin by taking 100 or 200 international units at bedtime, then gradually increase the dosage until you are taking 400 international units daily.

Note: If you are taking an anticoagulant (blood thinner), consult your physician before taking supplemental vitamin E.

HERBAL TREATMENT

Artichoke leaf helps to improve bile production and decrease stone formation. Take 250 to 500 milligrams of standardized extract two or three times daily.

■ Dandelion root has been used for centuries to improve the functioning of the gallbladder and liver. Take 250 milligrams three times daily for six weeks. Stop taking it for one month, then repeat.

■ Ginger helps to reduce inflammation and aids in the digestion of fats by improving bile secretion. Choose a product containing 5 percent gingeoles and take 200 milligrams twice daily, with food.

In one study of 225 patients with chronic gallstones, symptoms disappeared within forty-eight hours of beginning treatment with goldenseal. Take 125 to 250 milligrams of goldenseal three times daily, before meals.

Milk thistle contains silymarin, which helps to rejuvenate and repair liver function. Choose an extract standardized to contain 80 percent flavonoids (silymarin) and take 100 to 200 milligrams three times daily for one month. Stop for one month, then repeat.

Turmeric has anti-inflammatory properties, enhances the flow of bile, and protects the liver. It also has been shown in studies to inhibit the growth of most organisms that cause inflammation of the gallbladder. Take 250 to 500 milligrams three times daily.

HOMEOPATHY

Berberis vulgaris is the remedy for pain in the gallbladder area that is worse with pressure. The pain may extend throughout the whole region, from the kidneys to the liver to the stomach. You probably feel tired and may have a headache that feels as if you are wearing a too-tight cap on your head, and your symptoms can change rapidly, with hunger switching quickly to a lack of appetite. Take one dose of *Berberis vulgaris* 12x or 6c three times daily for one week. Stop for one week. Repeat the dosage for one week, then stop entirely.

Chelidonium is for liver and gallbladder problems that cause pain in the right shoulder, possibly accompanied by abdominal distension and constipation. The pain usually feels worse in the morning. Other possible symptoms include mild discomfort on breathing and itchy skin. Take one dose of *Chelidonium* 12x or 6c three times daily for one week. Stop for one week. Repeat the dosage for one week, then stop entirely.

Taraxacum is the remedy for liver and gallbladder dysfunction accompanied by a sour stomach and flatulence. You may also have night sweats. Take one dose of *Taraxacum* 12x or 6c three times daily for one week. Stop for one week. Repeat for one week, then stop entirely.

BACH FLOWER REMEDIES

Select the remedy that most closely fits your emotional tendencies and concerns, and take it as needed, following the directions on the product label.

■ Holly helps to ease anger and fits of temper.

■ Red Chestnut tames a tendency to worry constantly.

■ Scleranthus is the remedy for feelings of uncertainty and difficulty making decisions.

■ White Chestnut is very helpful for counteracting a tendency to become fixated on a particular idea and obsess on it constantly.

ACUPRESSURE

For the locations of acupressure points on the body, *see* ADMINISTERING AN ACUPRESSURE TREATMENT in Part Three.

■ Bladder 18, 19, 20, and 23 improve circulation in the digestive tract.

■ Gallbladder 21, 34, and 41 improve gallbladder function.

■ Liver 3 relaxes the nervous system, and is helpful if gallbladder spasms are a problem.

■ Spleen 6 and Stomach 36 improve digestion.

GENERAL RECOMMENDATIONS

■ To encourage gallstones to pass, take three tablespoons of olive oil with the juice of one lemon before bed and before breakfast. Many people have rid themselves of gallstones with this method.

■ As much as possible, avoid stress. Stress adds to the distress experienced by those with gallbladder problems.

PREVENTION

■ Eat clean and lean. Excessive fat consumption is at the heart of most gallbladder problems.

■ If you are overweight, slim down. Obesity increases the risk of gallbladder problems.

■ Exercise. Regular exercise helps tone the entire body, including the gallbladder and liver. Studies show that exercise may reduce the risk of developing gallstones by 20 to 40 percent, possibly because it reduces cholesterol and triglyceride levels, which have been linked to gallstones. (*See* STARTING AN EXERCISE PROGRAM in Part Three.)

Gas, Intestinal

Gases are produced in the intestinal tract during the digestion of carbohydrates and amino acids. The gas is a combination of hydrogen, carbon dioxide, and methane. Considerable quantities of gas are produced every day. A large portion of it is absorbed into the bloodstream through the intestinal wall; the rest is expelled through the rectum. The average person discharges nearly a quart of intestinal gas every day, usually without being aware of it.

Swallowing air with food or water is another source of discomfort and is often mistaken for gas. When the body is in a upright position, most swallowed air passes back up the esophagus and is expelled through the mouth. However, when the body is in a prone position—or even if you bend over a water fountain to take a drink—air may pass into your stomach and enter your intestines, where it has the same effect as true gas.

Symptoms of both gas and swallowed air range from flatulence to a mild discomfort that can be relieved by burping, to bloating and pressure, to severe pain and abdominal cramping.

CONVENTIONAL TREATMENT

■ Simethicone (available in Mylicon) is a compound that acts on the surface of gas bubbles to break them up, thus relieving gas pain and pressure. If large gas bubbles are the primary problem, this can be an effective treatment. Simethicone is available over the counter.

■ Other drugs, including sedatives such as phenobarbital and antispasmodics like dicyclomine (Bentyl), are sometimes prescribed and occasionally offer limited relief, but in most cases they are of little benefit. In addition, they can have serious side effects. Ask your doctor to explain all of the pros and cons of any prescription medications before taking them.

DIETARY GUIDELINES

■ Excessive production of intestinal gas may signal a food allergy or sensitivity. The most common offenders are dairy products, beans, chocolate, caffeine, melons, cucumbers, peppers, citrus fruits and juices, and spicy foods. To track down food allergies, try an elimination or rotation diet (see ELIMINATION DIET and ROTATION DIET in Part Three). Following these diets may seem like an overwhelming task, but the results can be very worthwhile. An alternative is to keep an ongoing food diary to help you identify a possible relationship between the foods you eat and your symptoms. If you discover a hidden sensitivity that you hadn't suspected, simply avoiding that food will likely help you feel better and alleviate your gas attacks.

■ Limit your intake of gas-forming foods. These include cauliflower, broccoli, Brussels sprouts, cucumbers, red and green peppers, onions, beans, and legumes. Other foods that can contribute to gas include cow's milk, bananas, berries, and anything that contains caffeine.

■ Limit the amount of raw foods in your diet. Eat a diet composed of 70 to 80 percent cooked foods, and only 20 to 30 percent raw foods. Keep your diet simple.

NUTRITIONAL SUPPLEMENTS

■ It is not uncommon to suffer gas attacks while taking antibiotics. Antibiotics kill off the friendly bacteria that contribute to the digestive processes. *Lactobacillus acidophilus*, friendly bacteria specific to the small intestine, can help to ease digestion and resolve gas. *Bifidobacterium bifidum*, a type of friendly bacteria specific to the large intestine, also helps improve digestion. Some experts believe bifidobacteria may be more effective than acidophilus in normalizing the digestive tract and preventing gas attacks. Take them as recommended on the product labels. If you are allergic to milk, select dairy-free formulas.

■ For acute discomfort, activated charcoal is very effective. Take a 500-milligram capsule tablet three times daily, after meals. Charcoal should not be used for a long period of time, however, because it may alter the absorption of nutrients.

HERBAL TREATMENT

■ Chamomile and oat-straw teas are both well-known soothers and relaxants. Take one cup of either three times daily, as needed.

■ Fennel can also be helpful in relieving gas. Take a cup of fennel tea three to four times a day, as needed.

■ Ginger tea is a known digestive aid. Take a cup of tea as needed.

■ Peppermint tea helps to speed the emptying time of the stomach, enhances digestion, and acts as an antiflatulent. Take a cup of peppermint tea four to five times a day, as needed.

Note: If you are taking peppermint tea as well as a homeopathic preparation, allow one hour between the two. Otherwise, the strong smell of the mint may interfere with the action of the homeopathic remedy.

■ Try a combination herbal tea. Israeli researchers found that a daily dose of $1/2$ cup of a tea made from chamomile, licorice, fennel, and balm-mint was effective in easing the symptoms of intestinal gas in babies. Adults can take a cup three to four times daily, as needed.

Note: Do not take licorice on a daily basis for more than five days at a time, as it can elevate blood pressure. Omit it entirely if you have high blood pressure.

HOMEOPATHY

Like most homeopathic formulas, the remedies listed here are symptom-specific. Select a suitable remedy.

■ *Colocynthis* and *Magnesia phosphorica*, two abdominal

relaxants, are the most commonly prescribed homeopathics for intestinal gas. They are especially effective when used together. Take one dose of a combination formula three times daily, as needed. This remedy should bring quick relief. If the gas has not eased after two days, stop taking the remedy. It is unlikely that it will be helpful.

■ *Carbo vegetabilis* is for gas accompanied by a distended upper abdomen and a pale face. Your legs may be cold from the foot to the knee, and you likely feel restless and burp a lot after eating. Take one dose of *Carbo vegetabilis* 12x, 30x, or 9c three times daily for two days or until symptoms improve.

If you are flushed and have a red face that feels hot, take *Chamomilla* 12x, 30x, 9c, or 15c three times a day for two days or until symptoms improve.

Homeopathic combination formulas are available that may offer relief of intestinal gas.

ACUPRESSURE

For the locations of acupressure points on the body, *see* ADMINISTERING AN ACUPRESSURE TREATMENT in Part Three.

Stomach 36 helps to activate the digestive system.

Massaging the points along either side of the spine improves circulation and relaxes the nervous system.

GENERAL RECOMMENDATIONS

■ Keep a record of your gas attacks and look for a common denominator. Try to determine whether certain foods or activities trigger an episode. Should you discover a link, eliminate the food or activity that you think may be responsible.

Stress and tension can contribute to a gas attack and make the problem worse. Try to avoid upsets.

Massage your stomach with a non-alcohol-based lotion or oil. Following the natural path of the intestines, gently rub from the lower right "corner" of the abdomen up across the bottom of the rib cage, down to the lower left "corner," and around again.

PREVENTION

To get rid of the gas-promoting agents found in dried beans, soak them for at least twelve hours. Discard the water and rinse well. Add fresh cold water to the rinsed beans and cook them until they are very tender.

■ A product called Beano is said to help reduce the formation of gas that builds up while eating troublesome foods. Follow the dosage directions of the product label.

When eating, stay in an upright position to avoid swallowing air. Don't rush through your meals, and don't overeat.

Gastritis

Gastritis is a general term meaning "inflammation of the stomach." In most cases, it involves erosion (if not perforation) and bleeding of the stomach lining. The most common causes are alcohol and certain drugs. Ironically, medications used to control inflammation in other parts of the body are among the most serious offenders. The nonsteroidal anti-inflammatory drugs (NSAIDs) have a long history of irritating the stomach and parts of the gastrointestinal (GI) tract. Drugs in this class include aspirin (Bayer, Ecotrin, and others), ibuprofen (Advil, Motrin, Nuprin, and others), naproxen (Aleve, Anaprox, Naprelan, Naprosyn), and many others, some available by prescription and others over the counter. Alcoholics are well known to have stomach trouble, including bleeding, from their excessive intake.

Another type of gastritis is "stress" gastritis, which occurs in surgical patients and people with serious medical problems, such as burns, trauma, massive infection, organ failure, cirrhosis of the liver, and acute local infections caused by a variety of bacteria, viruses, fungi, and even parasites. Exposure to radiation or caustic substances such as acids and drain cleaners can also cause this type of gastritis.

While most forms of this disorder disrupt the mucosa (surface layer) of the stomach lining, there are exceptions to every rule. *Helicobacter pylori* (*H. pylori*), a bacterium, can cause inflammation underneath the mucous layer that coats the stomach, and has been implicated in stomach ulcers (*see* PEPTIC ULCER). Another form of gastritis in which the surface remains intact is gastritis associated with pernicious anemia. This is a disorder of the immune system in which vitamin B_{12} fails to be absorbed properly because of inadequate production of stomach acid and a substance called *intrinsic factor* (*see under* ANEMIA).

Gastritis can be painless even if there is considerable disruption of the stomach lining. If there are symptoms, they can include a loss of appetite, nausea, vomiting, indigestion, bloating, or outright abdominal pain. Pain may be made worse by eating. The primary diagnostic technique used to examine the stomach lining is endoscopic examination—either gastroscopy, which is used to examine the stomach, or a procedure with the daunting name of esophagogastroduodenoscopy (EGD), in which both the stomach and the duodenum, the first section of the small intestine, are examined. Either procedure involves inserting a flexible fiber-optic tube through the mouth and guiding it down the throat into (and possibly through) the stomach. The doctor can then look directly at the stomach lining and determine the presence and extent of bleeding or eroded areas. This is not usually done, however, unless there is some question as to whether there is a more serious condition, such as an ulcer, or unless gastritis has become a chronic problem.

CONVENTIONAL TREATMENT

■ Over-the-counter antacids such as Mylanta, Maalox, or Rolaids are usually tried first. These agents have a short span of action, but with repeated use, they may inhibit stomach acid enough to disrupt digestion and interfere with the absorption of nutrients.

■ A popular treatment (and preventive) is sucralfate (Carafate). This drug, primarily used for ulcers farther down in the gastrointestinal tract, is used for gastritis because it seems to act as a protectant against acid, bile, and pepsin. Possible side effects of this drug include constipation, and minor incidents of diarrhea, dry mouth, gas, itching, rash, and insomnia. Not much is absorbed into the bloodstream, but sucralfate does contain a significant amount of aluminum, which has been implicated as a possible cause of disease, and which has no known beneficial effect in the human body. Sucralfate can also interfere with the absorption of many other types of drugs, including some antibiotics, epilepsy medications, antifungal drugs, ulcer drugs, asthma drugs, and heart medications, so it should be taken separately from other drugs. Read package inserts carefully, and discuss your situation with your doctor.

■ Acid-blockers may be used for variable lengths of time. Examples include cimetidine (Tagamet), famotidine (Pepcid), nizatidine (Axid), and ranitidine (Zantac). These drugs block acid secretion to lower stress on irritated stomach tissues. Possible side effects include constipation, diarrhea, nausea, vomiting, rash, occasional heart-rhythm changes, and blood-count changes. The drugs can pass into breast milk, so nursing mothers should avoid them.

■ A more recent type of medication used for gastritis is the proton pump inhibitor. Omeprazole (Prilosec) and lansoprazole (Prevacid) are two examples. These drugs also inhibit the production of stomach acid, but by a different mechanism than the one the acid-blockers use. Possible side effects include headache, diarrhea, nausea, abdominal pain, pancreatic and liver stress, and rashes.

■ Gastritis due to infection may be treated with antibiotics. Inflammation due to chemical or toxic insults may require gastric lavage (stomach pumping) or treatment with activated charcoal.

■ *Avoid* all nonsteroidal anti-inflammatories unless specifically directed to take them by your doctor.

DIETARY GUIDELINES

■ Eliminate dairy products from your diet until the digestive tract is healed.

■ Drink at least eight 8-ounce glasses of pure water daily.

NUTRITIONAL SUPPLEMENTS

■ Take a good multivitamin and mineral supplement daily to protect against (or correct) deficiencies of the major nutrients. A soft gel or liquid formula is best.

■ Duodenal extract is often helpful for reducing the pain of stomach inflammation. Take 350 milligrams three to four times daily for two weeks.

■ Probiotics replenish the natural intestinal flora and are soothing to the gastrointestinal tract. If you must take antibiotics, once antibiotic therapy is finished, take an acidophilus supplement, as directed on the product label, two to three times daily.

■ Vitamin E is a natural mild anti-inflammatory. Choose a product containing mixed tocopherols and take 400 international units at bedtime.

Note: If you are taking an anticoagulant (blood thinner), consult your physician before taking vitamin E.

■ If anemia is a problem, consider taking supplemental chlorophyll. Chlorophyll is high in trace minerals and minute amounts of bioavailable, easily digested iron. Take 2 capsules three times daily.

HERBAL TREATMENT

■ Licorice is very effective for healing an ulcerated gastrointestinal tract. Be sure to select deglycyrrhizinated licorice (DGL), and chew 350 to 600 milligrams twenty to thirty minutes before each meal.

Note: Ordinary licorice can elevate blood pressure, and should not be taken on a daily basis for more than ten days in a row. DGL should not have this effect, however.

■ Slippery elm soothes the entire gastrointestinal tract. Take 500 milligrams three times daily.

HOMEOPATHY

As with any chronic disorder, an integrated health program along with a possible constitutional homeopathic may be the best solution. However, the following homeopathics can bring relief for symptoms in the short term.

■ *Carbo vegetabilis* helps to relieve a burning sensation in the stomach. Take one dose of *Carbo vegetabilis* 30x or 15c three times daily for up to three days.

■ *Nux vomica* is for nausea accompanied by colicky pain and shortness of breath. You may feel you want to vomit but cannot, and your abdomen may feel bruised. Take one dose of *Nux vomica* 30x or 15c three times daily for up to three days.

BACH FLOWER REMEDIES

Holly helps to calm anger that bursts out in fits of bad temper.

Impatiens eases impatience and irritability.

■ White Chestnut helps to counteract a tendency toward obsessive thoughts.

ACUPRESSURE

For the locations of acupressure points on the body, *see* ADMINISTERING AN ACUPRESSURE TREATMENT in Part Three.

■ Pericardium 6 relaxes the upper digestive tract.

Stomach 36 tones the digestive system and strengthens overall well-being.

AROMATHERAPY

For specific instructions on how to use aromatherapy, *see* PREPARING AROMATHERAPY TREATMENTS in Part Three.

Orange oil helps to relieve nausea; lavender calms the nerves. Use either or both as inhalants, add them to bath water, diffuse them into the air, or add them to massage oil and use them in conjunction with massage.

GENERAL RECOMMENDATIONS

Do not smoke, and avoid secondhand smoke. Tobacco smoke irritates the stomach lining and increases stomach acidity.

As much as possible, avoid stress, and learn ways to manage the stress you cannot avoid. (*See* RELAXATION TECHNIQUES in Part Three.)

PREVENTION

It may not be possible to prevent gastritis. However, regular supplementation with probiotic bacteria is an excellent way to protect the health of the entire gastrointestinal tract.

Gastroesophageal Reflux

See under INDIGESTION.

Gingivitis

See under PERIODONTAL DISEASE.

Glaucoma

Glaucoma is a condition in which the pressure within the eye becomes so strong that it causes damage to the optic nerve. The pressure results when fluid in the eye fails to drain properly and builds up in the front part of the eye.

In addition to tears, which wash the surface of the eye, the eyes produce a fluid called the aqueous humor, which circulates from behind the iris, through the pupil, and into a chamber between the iris and the cornea (see illustration). As it does so, it nourishes all these tissues with a mixture of oxygen and vital nutrients. While tears leave the body through external tear ducts, the aqueous humor stays within the body. In a healthy eye, it drains out through a structure called the trabecular meshwork, which is located in the area where the iris and cornea meet. This area is called the *drainage angle*. From the angle, the fluid enters a channel that funnels it into a network of small veins.

In a normal eye, the rate at which the aqueous humor drains is equivalent to the rate at which it is produced, resulting in an even level of pressure in the eye. However, if the trabecular meshwork does not work properly or is obstructed, the aqueous humor either flows too slowly or fails to drain at all, causing pressure to build up against the outer wall of the eyeball. A certain amount of pressure is required to maintain the shape of the eyeball, but too much compresses the small internal blood vessels and fibers of the optic nerve. The end result is nerve-fiber destruction and, with it, a progressive loss of vision. Glaucoma is one of the leading causes of blindness.

There are two general categories of glaucoma: open-angle and closed-angle. In chronic open-angle glaucoma, the most common form, the drainage angle looks normal but gradually becomes blocked by minute bits of debris. This process usually takes place over a period of years, causing a slow rise in intraocular pressure. Chronic glaucoma tends to run in families. In the early stages, it usually causes no symptoms at all, although some people experience a frequent need for changes in eyeglass prescription or a tendency to see "halos" around electric lights. As a result, many people have it without knowing it—until it is advanced enough to cause vision loss. Even the vision loss can be easy to overlook at first, because it occurs gradually, with the development of tiny blind spots in the field of vision, usually in the periphery. Only when a substantial amount of vision is lost is a person likely to become aware of it.

Closed-angle glaucoma occurs when the drainage angle is blocked by one of the structures of the eye itself, usually the iris. In some cases, the iris may actually become stuck to the drainage angle, causing a permanent obstruction. Unlike chronic open-angle glaucoma, this condition often affects only one eye. Symptoms include blurred vision, pain, a bloodshot appearance, and the appearance of halos around lights. A preliminary episode of this type usually occurs in the evening, and lasts as long as the drainage angle is blocked. As the condition progresses, the same symptoms recur, but in more severe form. Peripheral vision may be lost. Pain may be felt in the head, as well as the eye, and the cornea may appear hazy. The eyeball may feel hard to the touch. Nausea and vomiting may accompany the other symptoms.

As many as 2 million Americans have glaucoma. It is rare in people under age forty, but nearly 2 percent of people over that age have the chronic form of this condition. Glaucoma affects men and women equally, and the incidence rises with age. People with diabetes, high blood pressure, and/or severe myopia are at higher than normal risk of glaucoma. The use of certain drugs, such as steroids, antihistamines, and some antidepressants, increases the risk of developing this condition. If early treatment is undertaken, glaucoma can usually be controlled. However, if the optic nerve has been damaged, some loss of vision is inevitable. If glaucoma is ignored, blindness is the ultimate result.

CONVENTIONAL TREATMENT

■ If you suffer from glaucoma, it is wise to seek out and work closely with an ophthalmologist or other eye doctor who specializes, or at the very least has considerable experience, in the treatment of this condition.

■ With closed-angle glaucoma, prompt treatment is required to bring down the pressure in the eye. Generally, drug therapy is used first. Once the acute attack is brought under control, a surgical procedure called iridotomy is performed. In this operation, the ophthalmologist uses a laser to create a tiny channel through the iris to allow drainage of the aqueous humor. This usually prevents further attacks.

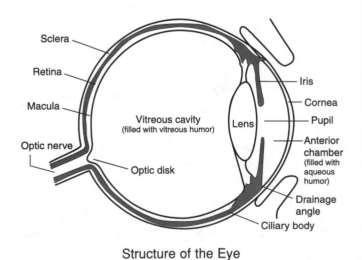

Structure of the Eye

■ Chronic open-angle glaucoma can usually be controlled with either a drying agent, eyedrops that stimulate better fluid outflow from the eyes, and/or drops, tablets, or injections that reduce the production of aqueous humor. Regular checkups to make sure the pressure is under control are essential. In most cases, these medications must be taken for life. Beta-blockers, a type of drug used in eyedrop form to reduce the production of aqueous humor, can have undesirable side effects, including a loss of HDL ("good" cholesterol) and an increase in LDL ("bad" cholesterol). You may wish to discuss this finding with your doctor. Many people experience the onset of asthma after they start using eyedrops to treat glaucoma, even if they have never had asthma before. If this happens, see your doctor immediately. The symptoms are not likely to subside without a change in medication.

■ If medication fails to reduce the intraocular pressure sufficiently, iridotomy or a more complex procedure called a trabeculoplasty may be necessary. In this procedure, a laser is used to make multiple minute holes in the tissue of the angle, which helps facilitate drainage of the aqueous humor.

DIETARY GUIDELINES

■ Eat a healthy high-fiber diet, with an emphasis on whole foods.

■ Maximize your intake of vegetables and fruits rich in carotenes. Carotenoids are precursors of vitamin A, the "eye vitamin." Yellow and orange vegetables and fruits, plus green leafy vegetables (including beet greens, spinach, and broccoli), are all rich sources of these important phytochemicals.

■ To avoid adding to the production of aqueous humor, do not drink large amounts of liquids at any one time.

■ Avoid alcohol. Alcohol makes the body overly acidic. In excess, it impairs liver function, which can adversely affect the eyes.

■ Lutein, a carotenoid usually extracted from the marigold, has been shown to be very useful in restoring and maintaining ocular health. Take 5 milligrams of a carotene complex with lutein three or four times daily.

NUTRITIONAL SUPPLEMENTS

■ Chinese medicine teaches that the eyes and liver are related. When liver function is enhanced, there is a general improvement in the eyes. Choline is required for the proper metabolism of fats in the liver, and aids in the transmission of nerve impulses. Take 350 milligrams of choline twice a day.

■ Flaxseed oil provides essential fatty acids that are missing in most people's diets. Take 1 tablespoon, or 500 to 1,000 milligrams in capsule form, twice daily.

■ Lipoic acid is a strong antioxidant that scavenges free radicals. Take 50 milligrams two to three times daily.

■ Vitamin C and bioflavonoids have anti-inflammatory properties, and vitamin C is also important in the manufacture of collagen, which helps stabilize the eye. Take 500 to 1,000 milligrams of vitamin C with bioflavonoids three to four times daily.

■ Vitamin A is required by the eyes. To keep the eye tissue healthy, take 5,000 international units of vitamin A twice a day.

Note: If you are pregnant, or intend to get pregnant, or if you have liver disease, consult your doctor before taking supplemental vitamin A. Pregnant women should not ingest a total of more than 25,000 international units of supplemental vitamin A *per week* from all sources.

HERBAL TREATMENT

■ Bilberry is beneficial for all conditions affecting the eyes. Select a product containing 25 percent anthocyanidins (also called PCOs) and take 80 milligrams two to three times daily.

■ Coleus contains forskolin, which has antioxidant properties and has also been shown to be beneficial to the eyes. Take 250 milligrams of 1-percent extract twice a day.

■ Pine-bark and grape-seed extracts are strong anti-inflammatories with antioxidant action. Take 50 milligrams of either three times daily.

■ Herbs that dilate the pupils, such as ma huang (ephedra) and belladonna, should be *avoided.* Also avoid licorice. This herb can contribute to a rise in blood pressure, which is a factor in glaucoma.

HOMEOPATHY

■ *Euphrasia* is helpful for reducing the sensation of pressure associated with glaucoma. Take one dose of *Euphrasia* 12x or 6c, as directed on the product label, three times daily for up to three days. Do this twice monthly for three months.

■ *Naphthalinum* has a clear affinity for the eye. It is commonly used for cataracts and detached retina, but is also useful in reducing the pain associated with glaucoma. Take one dose of *Naphthalinum* 12x or 6c three times daily for up to three days. Do this twice monthly for three months.

BACH FLOWER REMEDIES

Select the remedy that most closely fits your emotional tendencies and concerns, and take it as needed, following the directions on the product label.

■ Mustard eases sadness and depression that may be related to a loss of some kind.

■ Vervain helps to counteract perfectionist tendencies, nervousness, and tension that may lead to insomnia.

ACUPRESSURE

For the locations of acupressure points on the body, *see* ADMINISTERING AN ACUPRESSURE TREATMENT in Part Three.

■ Gallbladder 21 improves circulation in the head.

■ Large Intestine 4 relaxes tension in the head.

■ Liver 3 relaxes the nervous system and is beneficial for the eyes.

■ Pericardium 6 relaxes the nervous system.

■ Stomach 36 improves the body's utilization of nutrients.

GENERAL RECOMMENDATIONS

■ If you are using medication, including eyedrops, for glaucoma, follow your ophthalmologist's instructions exactly. Be sure to keep all follow-up appointments.

■ Avoid stressing your eyes. Activities that require a steady focus for a long period of time—whether watching television, reading, doing needlework, or using a computer—put added stress on the eyes. To rest and refresh your eyes, look away two or three times an hour. Spend ten seconds or so focusing on an object in the middle distance, then an object further away.

■ Don't smoke, and avoid secondhand smoke. Whether it comes from a fireplace or a cigarette, smoke is very irritating to the eyes.

PREVENTION

■ There is no known way to prevent glaucoma, but early detection and early treatment can prevent the damage to the optic nerve that leads to blindness. Have your eyes checked regularly, especially if you are over forty.

Goiter

See under HYPERTHYROIDISM; HYPOTHYROIDISM.

Gonorrhea

Gonorrhea is one of the most common sexually transmitted infectious diseases in the world. Caused by the bacteria *Neisseria gonorrhoeae,* it is passed from partner to partner during sexual intercourse, including oral and anal sex, and by contact with body fluids containing the organism. Not surprisingly, gonorrhea is most common among those who have multiple sex partners.

The incubation period for this disease differs between men and women. In men, symptoms arise between two and fourteen days after infection. In women, it takes a little longer, from seven to twenty-one days. Men usually develop a thick yellowish discharge from the penis and experience pain and difficulty urinating. Although some women have a cloudy vaginal discharge and feel a hot, burning sensation on urination, more than half of infected women have no symptoms at all in the early stages. As the disease progresses, an infected woman may go on to experience abnormal menstrual bleeding, rectal itching, and acute inflammation in the pelvic area. At this stage, a woman is usually diagnosed as suffering from pelvic inflammatory disease, or PID, caused by the gonococcal bacteria.

Gonorrhea that is not properly treated can spread to other parts of the body. In men, it can cause an inflamed prostate or inflammation of the testes, and may affect fertility. A woman who develops PID can suffer damage to the ovaries and/or fallopian tubes, resulting in infertility. The bacteria can also cause gonococcal arthritis, which results in pain and swelling of the joints around the body. This condition may be misdiagnosed as simple arthritis.

Gonorrhea contracted through oral sex can cause gonococcal pharyngitis, or inflammation of the throat. This can result in a very sore throat, although many infected people have no symptoms. If the infection affects the eyes, it is called gonococcal conjunctivitis, and it can lead to scarring and even blindness. Anal sex with an infected partner can cause gonococcal proctitis, resulting in inflammation of the rectum and anus. This form of the disease causes symptoms, such as pain and discharge from the anus, in only about 10 percent of those infected.

A woman who is infected—whether she knows it or not—can transmit the disease to her baby during childbirth. During passage through the birth canal, an infant may contract gonococcal ophthalmia, a severe inflammation that can affect one or both eyes. *Neisseria gonorrhoeae* organisms in the bloodstream can cause blood poisoning, with symptoms that include fever and exhaustion. If the bacteria reach the brain or heart, the infection can be life-threatening.

Because many disorders cause a vaginal or penile discharge, a definitive diagnosis of gonorrhea must be made by laboratory testing. If a laboratory culture confirms the diagnosis, prompt, effective treatment is important.

CONVENTIONAL MEDICINE

■ Gonorrhea is treated with antibiotics. Penicillin was once universally effective against this disease. However, some strains of *Neisseria gonorrhoeae* have now developed a resistance to both penicillin and tetracycline. Other antibiotics, such as ceftriaxone (Rocephin) or cefixime (Suprax) are now commonly prescribed. Both partners must be treated. If multiple partners are involved, all of them should be traced and treated. As with any antibiotic treatment, it is important to continue taking the medication for the full course prescribed by your physician.

■ After one or two weeks of treatment, a follow-up visit is necessary to be sure the infection has been cured. It is also not uncommon for syphilis to "tag along" with a gonorrheal infection, necessitating further treatment once the gonorrhea has been cured.

■ Burning on urination or other symptoms after the end of treatment for gonorrhea may indicate a simultaneous infection with chlamydia, which does not respond to the same antibiotics as the gonococcal bacteria. For this reason, your doctor may add other antibiotics to the original regimen.

DIETARY GUIDELINES

■ Eat a high-fiber diet of whole foods that contain no chemicals that add stress to the body. Maximize your intake of fresh vegetables and fruits. Include in your diet clean, lean protein foods such as chicken and fish.

■ Add seaweed to your diet. Besides improving thyroid function, the high iodine content of sea vegetables enhances circulation and helps detoxify the blood.

■ Avoid refined sugar, alcohol, and caffeine. These substances increase the acidity of the body, which adds to inflammation and worsens symptoms.

NUTRITIONAL SUPPLEMENTS

■ Digestion is often compromised with an infection as serious as gonorrhea, especially if the diet is less than complete. Take a good multivitamin and mineral supplement daily to guard against any nutritional deficiencies.

■ Green-foods supplements supply cleansing chlorophyll and trace minerals that may be missing in the diet. Take a green-foods supplement as directed on the product label.

■ Anytime you must take antibiotics, probiotic supplements (acidophilus and bifidus) are extremely important. Antibiotics kill the friendly bacteria your body needs right along with the dangerous organisms. These bacteria are especially important to the female genital tract. Take them as recommended on the product label. If you are allergic to milk, be sure to select dairy-free formulas.

■ Proteolytic enzymes act to reduce inflammation and help repair damaged tissue. Take proteolytic enzymes with each main meal of the day, and also twice a day between meals.

Vitamin A helps heal mucous membranes and is necessary for the repair of injured tissue. Take 25,000 international units twice a day for three weeks.

Note: If you are pregnant, or intend to get pregnant, or if you have liver disease, consult your doctor before taking supplemental vitamin A. Pregnant women should not ingest a total of more than 25,000 international units of supplemental vitamin A *per week* from all sources.

Vitamin C and bioflavonoids have anti-inflammatory action and stimulate healing. They are also antioxidants that fight free-radical damage. For three weeks, take 1,000 milligrams of a vitamin-C formula that contains rutin and other bioflavonoids four to five times daily.

Vitamin E improves circulation, stimulates healing, and is required for tissue repair. It also has antioxidant properties and scavenges free radicals. Choose a product containing mixed tocopherols and start by taking 200 international units daily, then gradually increase the dosage until you are taking 400 international units once or twice daily.

Note: If you have high blood pressure, limit your intake of supplemental vitamin E to a total of 400 international units daily. If you are taking an anticoagulant (blood thinner), consult your physician before taking supplemental vitamin E.

HERBAL TREATMENT

Bayberry and barberry have traditionally been used to combat urinary tract symptoms associated with gonorrhea. Take 250 milligrams of each three or four times daily for a week to ten days.

Echinacea and goldenseal make a powerful combination that supports the immune system and offers antibacterial, antifungal, and antiviral action. They are also useful if there are any lingering symptoms of infection after antibiotic therapy. Take one dose of an echinacea and goldenseal combination formula supplying 500 milligrams of echinacea and 350 milligrams of goldenseal three times daily for one week.

Reishi mushroom is helpful for easing fatigue and improving both stamina and resistance to infection. If fatigue lingers once the infection is gone, take 500 to 1,000 milligrams three or four times daily.

HOMEOPATHY

Gonorrhea is best treated constitutionally. See a homeopathic physician for a constitutional remedy. The following remedies can provide symptomatic relief during the acute phase of the infection.

Cantharis is the remedy for burning and stinging of the genitals, with intense pain on urination. Take one dose of *Cantharis* 12x or 6c three times a day, as needed, for up to three days.

■ *Rhus toxicodendron* is for itching and burning of the genitals that feels worse with cold and damp. Take one dose of *Rhus toxicodendron* 12x or 6c three times a day, as needed, for up to three days.

■ *Sempervivum tectorum* is for the person whose whole genital area is very tender and very painful, especially at night. Take one dose of *Sempervivum tectorum* 12x or 6c three times a day, as needed, for up to three days.

■ If the preceding remedies do not match your symptoms or fail to bring relief, try *Sulfur*. Indications for this remedy include urethral burning and frequent urination, with mucus and pus in the urine. In women, there is much itching and burning in the vaginal area; in men, there is spasmodic pain in the penis. Take one dose of *Sulfur* 30x or 15c three times a day, as needed, for up to three days.

BACH FLOWER REMEDIES

Select the remedy that most closely fits your emotional tendencies and concerns, and take it as needed, following the directions on the product label.

■ Holly helps to tame anger and fits of bad temper that may reflect underlying feelings of jealousy and insecurity.

■ Hornbeam helps to lift exhaustion so extreme that it makes you miss out on interesting activities.

■ Impatiens calms hyperactivity, impatience, and tension.

■ White Chestnut helps to counteract a tendency to obsess on ideas or events long after the subject should have been forgotten.

ACUPRESSURE

For the locations of acupressure points on the body, *see* ADMINISTERING AN ACUPRESSURE TREATMENT in Part Three.

■ Conception Vessel 4 and 12 improve circulation in the genitourinary area.

■ Kidney 3 and 7 increase circulation in the genitourinary tract.

■ Liver 3 relaxes the nervous system.

■ The combination of Spleen 6 and Stomach 36 improves immune function.

GENERAL RECOMMENDATIONS

■ Take the entire course of antibiotics. Even if your symptoms seem to disappear, do not fail to take your medication on schedule. Only the weaker bacteria succumb early; the stronger and more powerful organisms may survive to create future problems. Always take all your prescribed antibiotics.

■ Be sure to see your doctor at the appointed time for a follow-up visit to make sure your treatment is working.

PREVENTION

■ Abstinence (or a monogamous relationship with a partner who is known to be healthy) is the only sure way to avoid contracting a sexually transmitted disease. Using a latex (not animal-skin) condom is your next best choice. Be aware, however, that the use of a condom is not an absolute guarantee of protection against STDs.

Gout

Gout is a metabolic disorder that causes extremely painful attacks of arthritis, usually in a single joint, most notably the joint at the base of the big toe. However, it can affect other joints, including the knees, ankles, wrists, feet, and the small joints of the hands. Gout afflicts ten times more men than women; 90 percent of the people who have it are men over the age of thirty. In men, this condition can occur at any time after puberty; in women, it usually occurs only after menopause.

Gout occurs when uric acid in the body migrates into the tissue surrounding a joint. As the excess uric acid accumulates, needle-shaped crystals form that become lodged within the joint. The surrounding tissue becomes inflamed and the nerve endings become severely irritated, resulting in extreme pain.

Uric acid is a byproduct of the metabolism of proteins and substances called purines. Some purines are produced by the body; others are ingested in certain foods. Uric acid cannot be absorbed by the body and must be excreted in urine. If the kidneys are not filtering as they should, the blood becomes saturated with uric acid, which may then start to crystallize in various parts of the body, especially the joints.

CONVENTIONAL TREATMENT

■ The over-the-counter painkillers ibuprofen (in Advil, Motrin, Nuprin, and other products), ketoprofen (Orudis), and naproxen (Aleve) relieve both pain and inflammation, and can be effective for relieving symptoms. Acetaminophen (Tylenol, Datril, and others) can also be used, but it tends to be less effective for this condition. *Do not use any product that contains aspirin.* Aspirin inhibits the excretion of uric acid.

■ If over-the-counter painkillers are not effective, your doctor will likely give you a prescription nonsteroidal anti-

inflammatory drug (NSAID). Medications in this category include a higher-potency version of ibuprofen (Motrin) as well as indomethacin (Indocin) and naproxen (Naprosyn). Any drug in this class can cause stomach upset, ulcers, and intestinal bleeding, among other side effects.

■ If prescription NSAIDs are not sufficient to relieve the pain, your doctor may resort to stronger medications such as codeine (sold under different brand names, often combined with acetaminophen, aspirin, or ibuprofen) or meperidine (Demerol). These are powerful narcotics that block the perception of pain. Possible side effects include sedation, slowed breathing, low blood pressure, stomach upset, and constipation.

■ If you are unable to tolerate NSAIDs, colchicine (a compound derived from the autumn crocus) may be prescribed. Though no one knows exactly how, this drug helps relieve the pain of an acute gout attack. It can be dramatically effective, but it causes adverse side effects in four out of five people treated with it, so it is avoided if possible. These problems include nausea, vomiting, diarrhea, abdominal pain, muscle weakness, blood abnormalities, and skin problems. Given intravenously, it is even more potentially toxic.

■ Steroids such as hydrocortisone and triamcinolone, taken by mouth or administered intravenously, and/or locally by direct injection, are often very effective for resolving an attack of gout. Because these drugs depress the immune system and place stress on the adrenal glands, they should be used in the lowest effective dose and for the shortest time possible. They must be tapered off gradually, as symptoms permit, rather than discontinued suddenly.

■ Once the acute attack has subsided, you must take care to *avoid* certain medications, including aspirin and diuretics, as well as certain foods that can increase the level of uric acid in the blood (*see* Dietary Guidelines, below). If your doctor deems repeat attacks very likely, he or she may recommend medications to ward them off. One possibility is a daily low dose of colchicine. Other choices include drugs to increase excretion of uric acid in the urine, such as probenicid (Benemid), or to inhibit the production of uric acid, such as allopurinol (Zyloprim). Probenicid requires good kidney function and good fluid intake to work, and side effects including rash, nausea, vomiting and diarrhea are possible. Allopurinol, paradoxically, can cause the kind of attack it is meant to prevent, and can also cause serious skin reactions, liver damage, and gastrointestinal problems, among other side effects. It also interacts with other drugs, such as theophylline, oral medications for diabetes, and some cancer chemotherapy agents.

DIETARY GUIDELINES

■ Avoid foods that contain high levels of purines, including shellfish, red meat, organ meats, poultry, sardines, anchovies, and legumes. Alcoholic beverages also are a source of purines.

■ Avoid saturated and hydrogenated fats, refined sugars, and foods and beverages containing caffeine. These promote inflammation, which increases the pain.

■ Emphasize fruits and vegetables. Fruits and vegetables act to reduce the body's acidity, and they do not contribute to uric-acid buildup.

Increase your consumption of foods such as citrus fruits, berries, tomatoes, green peppers, and leafy greens, which are high in natural vitamin C and the bioflavonoids that reduce inflammation.

■ Enjoy cherries and cherry juice often. Cherries are an old nutritional remedy known to help reduce uric-acid levels.

Drink at least eight 8-ounce glasses of pure water daily to help flush toxins from your body.

NUTRITIONAL SUPPLEMENTS

Take a good multivitamin and mineral supplement daily, but read the label first to be sure it contains no more than 5,000 international units of vitamin A and that the form of vitamin B_3 it contains is niacinamide rather than niacin. In amounts greater than this, vitamin A can worsen gout. Beta-carotene, which the body uses to produce vitamin A, is a better choice. Niacin raises uric-acid levels and increases heat and inflammation. Niacinamide, a mild derivative of niacin, won't add to your misery.

Flaxseed oil contains essential fatty acids that act as natural anti-inflammatories. Take 1 teaspoon (or 500 to 1,000 milligrams) two or three times daily.

Glucosamine sulfate helps to relieve pain. Take 300 milligrams twice daily.

Green-foods supplements such as chlorella, spirulina, and green barley are among the most densely packed bioavailable whole-food sources of cleansing chlorophyll. They are also a source of gamma-linolenic acid (GLA), have antioxidant properties, and are high in beta-carotene and vitamin E, which are helpful for gout because they reduce acidity in the body. These supplements are also good sources of needed trace minerals. Take a green-foods supplement as directed on the product label.

■ Vitamin C and the bioflavonoids work together to reduce inflammation, which helps ease the pain. Select a formula that provides both vitamin C and the bioflavonoids and take up to 1,000 milligrams daily.

HERBAL TREATMENT

Bilberry contains compounds called anthocyanidins that have proven valuable against gout. These substances reduce uric-acid levels and inhibit tissue destruction. Choose a product containing 25 percent anthocyanidins (also called PCOs) and take 80 milligrams three times daily.

■ Hawthorn offers some of the same properties as bilberry. Choose a standardized extract containing 1.8 vitexin-2 rhamnosides and take 100 to 200 milligrams two or three times a day.

■ Juniper berry is a diuretic herb that helps reduce uric acid. Take 350 to 500 milligrams in capsule form or 1 cup of tea twice daily.

■ Nettle root increases the excretion of uric acid from the kidneys. Take 250 milligrams three times a day.

■ Pine-bark and grape-seed extracts act to reduce inflammation, thus easing pain. Take 50 to 100 milligrams of either two to three times daily.

■ Turmeric has powerful anti-inflammatory action. It is used in both Chinese and Ayurvedic medicine against gout, arthritis, and other inflammatory conditions. Take 250 to 500 milligrams three times a day.

HOMEOPATHY

■ *Berberis vulgaris* is especially good for gout accompanied by low back pain. A short course of this remedy helps detoxify the kidneys. Take one dose of *Berberis vulgaris* 6x or 3c three times daily for up to three days. You can use *Berberis vulgaris* either before or after *Colchicum* (see below).

■ *Bryonia* is for wandering pain accompanied by irritability. Take one dose of *Bryonia* 30x or 15c three times daily for up to three days.

■ *Colchicum* is the remedy of choice if the pain is concentrated in your big toes and you are feeling irritable. Take one dose of *Colchicum* 12x or 6c three times daily for up to three days.

■ Choose *Pulsatilla* if the pain wanders from toe to toe, and you are feeling sorry for yourself. Take one dose of *Pulsatilla* 30x or 15c three times daily for up to three days.

■ If none of these remedies matches your symptoms, see a homeopathic physician for a constitutional remedy.

BACH FLOWER REMEDIES

Select the remedy that most closely fits your emotional tendencies and concerns, and take it as needed, following the directions on the product label.

■ Beech helps ease restlessness and impatience.

■ Holly is good if you are filled with anger and given to fits of temper.

■ Vervain helps to ease you out of "overdrive" and reduce feelings of tension.

ACUPRESSURE

For the locations of acupressure points on the body, *see* ADMINISTERING AN ACUPRESSURE TREATMENT in Part Three.

■ Bladder 23 increases circulation in the genitourinary tract.

■ Gallbladder 20, 21, 34, and 41 increase the efficiency of digestion.

■ Large Intestine 4, 10, and 11 detoxify the large intestine.

■ Stomach 36 improves digestion.

GENERAL RECOMMENDATIONS

■ Don't be afraid to exercise, but avoid heavy-duty exercise that causes pain. Instead, do stretching exercises, low-impact aerobics, or—best of all—water aerobics. Exercise increases circulation and can help your body eliminate toxins faster.

Graves' Disease

See under HYPERTHYROIDISM.

Hair Loss

Individual hairs do not grow continuously. Rather, each hair follicle (the tiny cavity from which a hair emerges) goes through an anagen, or growth, phase, followed by a telogen, or resting, phase. After the telogen phase, the hair is shed and the process begins again. It is normal to lose up to fifty scalp hairs a day as the follicles go through their cycles. However, if enough follicles fail to produce new hairs after the old ones have been shed, or if the hair produced is weak and brittle, noticeable thinning and/or loss of hair can result.

Doctors usually divide types of hair loss—medically termed *alopecia*—into two categories: scarring and non-scarring forms. The scarring forms tend to be less reversible. They usually result from infection that causes inflammation around hair follicles, which eventually leads to the follicles being replaced by scar tissue. Deep bacterial and fungal infection (such as ringworm) can lead to this type of hair loss, as can infection with the herpes zoster virus. A culture of scalp tissue, usually taken at the border of the problem area, and examination of other damaged skin areas may be done to track down the organism responsible for infection and guide in treatment. Scarring

alopecia can also result from physical trauma such as abrasive, chemical, or thermal burns.

It is also possible for hair follicles to atrophy (waste away). In many cases, the reason for this is not understood. Other possible causes of scarring alopecia can include lupus, syphilis, tuberculosis, and sarcoidosis, a mysterious disorder characterized by the appearance of multiple small benign lesions on skin and, often, lung tissue. Some tumors can cause scarring of the scalp, but this is very uncommon. Slightly more common, unfortunately, is scarring due to radiation treatment for brain tumors.

Nonscarring alopecia is the more common form of hair loss. In this category, *androgenic alopecia*—better known as male pattern baldness—predominates. In this condition, the hair begins to thin and recede back from the forehead, over the top, and down the sides. This process often takes many years, usually beginning in a man's late thirties or early forties, although it may begin as early as the mid-twenties or even the late teens, in some cases. The exact mechanism that causes this is not completely understood, but it is known that both hereditary factors and sex hormones are involved. In particular, this kind of hair loss is linked to high levels of the hormone testosterone. Some geneticists say that though this is a male problem, it is in fact passed on by the mother. To predict the extent to which you will experience it, they say, look at your maternal grandfather's hair.

Women also can develop hormone-related hair loss. Usually this takes place after menopause, but it can occur during and after pregnancy—all times when hormone levels are shifting significantly. However, women generally experience this kind of hair loss primarily as a thinning of the hair, and hair loss is not as extensive as it is for men.

Some people suffer temporary hair loss as a consequence of severe illness, usually illness that is accompanied by high fever. The same type of hair loss can be caused by certain medications, most notably drugs used for cancer chemotherapy. This occurs because chemotherapy drugs kill cells and tissues that are actively growing. This is what enables them to kill cancer cells, but it also accounts for their toxic effects on other parts of the body, such as the hair and the lining of the gastrointestinal tract.

The effects of cancer chemotherapy agents on hair can be dramatic, but these are not the only drugs that can cause or accelerate hair loss. Birth control pills, hormones, anticoagulants, allopurinol (Zyloprim, a drug used in the treatment of gout), some anti-inflammatory drugs, and some blood-pressure medications can all have this effect in susceptible individuals. Paradoxically, although vitamin A is necessary for healthy skin and hair, taking very high doses of vitamin A can do the same thing, but this kind of toxicity develops only at far higher doses than most people would consider taking. Other kinds of bodily stress that can cause temporary hair loss include glandular problems, particularly hypothyroidism; mineral deficiencies; ill-conceived weight loss methods such as crash dieting or single-food plans; malnutrition; and surgery.

Another type of nonscarring hair loss is *alopecia areata*. This condition is characterized by the rapid loss of patches of hair, usually coin-sized, while the surrounding areas of hair appear normal. The cause of this disorder is unknown, though scientists theorize it may be related to an immune-system problem. The hair tends to return at intervals, but recurring hair loss is common. Some people ultimately lose all of their hair—not only the hair on their heads, but eyebrows, eyelashes, and body hair as well.

Some cases of hair loss can be described as fashion-related. Hair that is repeatedly pulled into tight braids or ponytails, or subjected to strong dyes, permanent-wave solutions, and bleaches can suffer a considerable amount of damage, resulting in hair loss. The chemical effects of repeated swimming in chlorinated or brominated pool water, or lounging in hot tubs that have heavily treated water, can also have an adverse effect. Some people seem to develop cyclical patterns in which they lose hair either at the same time every year or every several years. Though the reason for this is not understood, it may simply be normal for some people.

Whatever the cause, hair loss can be distressing.

CONVENTIONAL TREATMENT

■ Medical treatment of hair loss first requires identification of any underlying cause. Careful medical evaluation may uncover a treatable problem that can mean a return of hair growth. Among the disorders that should be ruled out are hypothyroidism, parasitic infestation, protein deficiency, mineral deficiency, hormonal changes, ringworm, side effects of drugs, and stress. Sometimes hair loss can be a delayed reaction to one or more of these factors, coming as much as several months afterward, so your doctor should thoroughly review your recent history with you. A scalp biopsy may also be performed to track down the cause of the problem. If an underlying medical problem is identified, it will be treated accordingly.

■ Scarring types of alopecia may or may not be reversible, depending on the extent of damage to the hair follicles. Once true scarring has occurred, hair loss cannot be reversed; however, if an infection is treated early, some or all follicular activity may return.

■ Most of the medical treatments for hair loss are designed to address male pattern baldness. The drug minoxidil (Rogaine), originally a blood-pressure regulator, was found to cause hair growth as a side effect (often undesirable) in certain individuals, and so was adapted for topical use to treat male pattern baldness. Unfortunately, it rarely results in a significant regrowth of hair, and it must be used on an ongoing basis.

■ The latest drug therapy for male pattern baldness is finasteride (Propecia). This is actually the same drug marketed under the brand name Proscar and used for benign prostate enlargement, but at a lower dosage. The drug converts dihydrotestosterone, a strongly androgenic (masculinizing) hormone, into testosterone, which is somewhat less androgenic. This reduces the hormonal contribution to hair loss. Reports of hair growth with this drug have been less than spectacular, but the effect varies from person to person. Possible side effects include decreased sex drive, rash, and breast tenderness. Finasteride is not suitable for use by women. In fact, women who are pregnant, or who may become pregnant, should not even touch a broken tablet, as this can lead to malformation of sex organs in a developing male fetus.

■ If the blood flow to the scalp is still good, hair transplants may be a rewarding solution for male pattern baldness. In this technique, plugs of healthy hair are taken from areas of prominent growth, such as the back of the neck, and "punched" into the scalp areas with poor hair growth. Results vary, but the technique is continually being improved. If you are interested in trying this, seek the advice of an experienced specialist. The results of transplantation tend to be disappointing in cases of scarring alopecia, as the scar tissue can be thick enough to considerably diminish the flow of blood to the surface of the scalp.

■ Hair loss that occurs in response to physical stress such as treatment with cancer chemotherapy drugs is usually temporary; the hair starts to grow back once the stress is removed.

■ Alopecia areata may be treated with steroids, either injected into the bald patches or applied topically. Results vary. In some cases, the application of skin irritants, such as dinitrochlorobenzene (DNCB) or squaric acid dibutyl ester, to the affected sites can cause the body to start growing hair again. As with the use of steroids, the results are highly variable, and long-term safety considerations are unknown. In general, the earlier the condition starts, the longer the episodes, and the larger the area affected, the more severe and resistant to treatment it is likely to be.

DIETARY GUIDELINES

■ Eat a nourishing and well-balanced diet that includes plenty of good-quality lean protein, such as that found in fish, grains, and legumes. If your cholesterol level is not too high, include moderate amounts of cheese and eggs in your diet. Also eat lots of mineral-rich foods like vegetables, grains and legumes, plus some nuts and seeds and sea vegetables. This type of diet will supply ample protein and minerals and best support hair growth. Deficiencies of protein and minerals may be factors in hair loss.

Chinese medicine teaches that the kidneys influence the scalp and hair. Avoid eating excessive amounts of meat, which stresses the kidneys. A diet based on meat seems to speed up hair loss.

■ Avoid consuming excessive amounts of animal fats, animal proteins, and salt. This may help delay hair loss in men prone to male pattern baldness.

NUTRITIONAL SUPPLEMENTS

To address possible deficiencies, take a good multivitamin and mineral supplement daily.

If your skin is dry and flaky, take 500 milligrams of flaxseed oil two or three times daily.

To assure proper assimilation of nutrients, take a full-spectrum digestive enzyme supplement providing 5,000 international units of lipase, 2,500 international units of amylase, and 300 international units of protease, plus 500 to 1,000 milligrams of pancreatin, with each meal.

Note: Long-term supplementation with pancreatin is not advised, as it can cause your pancreas to reduce its own production of this important enzyme. Overuse also has the potential to cause nausea or diarrhea. After two months on pancreatin, discontinue use and monitor your reaction. If you find that your problems recur, discuss pancreatin supplementation with your health-care provider.

High doses of inositol can stimulate hair growth in some individuals with nonscarring types of hair loss, even after long-term loss. Take 200 milligrams twice a day.

Choline acts together with inositol. If you take inositol, take an equal amount of choline.

Vitamin E is necessary for skin and scalp health, including the health of the hair follicles. Choose a product containing mixed tocopherols or d-alpha-tocopherol (avoid the dl-alpha-tocopherol form) and start by taking 200 international units daily. After two weeks, increase the dosage to 400 international units daily.

Note: If you are taking an anticoagulant (blood thinner), consult your physician before taking supplemental vitamin E.

Selenium assists in the utilization of vitamin E. Take 100 to 200 micrograms daily.

Try the following supplement program:

• Take 1,000 to 3,000 milligrams (1 to 3 grams) of a free-form amino-acid formula, in capsule or powder form, two or three times daily, either before or after meals.

• Take 1,000 to 3,000 milligrams (1 to 3 grams) of a mixed chelated mineral formula at lunchtime and 2,000 milligrams at night.

• Silica and zinc are important for hair growth and strength. Take 100 to 250 milligrams of silica once or twice daily, plus 15 milligrams of zinc twice daily. Take zinc with food to prevent stomach upset. If you take over 30 milligrams of zinc on a daily basis for more than one or two months, you should also take 1 to 2 milligrams of copper each day to maintain a proper mineral balance.

• Take a vitamin-B-complex supplement that supplies 25 to 50 milligrams of the major B vitamins two or three times daily.

• Take an additional 500 micrograms to 2 milligrams of biotin daily.

• Take 500 to 1,000 milligrams of vitamin C twice daily. Vitamin C supports hair formation and helps with the structural support of the hair follicles.

HERBAL TREATMENT

■ Saw palmetto has been reported to cause some reversal of male pattern baldness in some cases. Choose a standardized extract containing 90 percent essential fatty acids and sterols, and take 160 milligrams twice daily.

■ There are a number of herbal formulas that are intended to reduce hair loss and support hair growth. Perhaps the best known is a patent medicine called Alopecia Areata. It is a formula designed specifically for hair loss in women, and has been reported to yield impressive results. Fo-ti (*Polygonum multiflorum*) is a Chinese herb that many men have used in tea form to arrest hair loss and slow graying. It is available in Shou Wu Shih, an inexpensive product available in many Chinese markets that sell herbal remedies. Take any of these formulas as directed on the product label.

HOMEOPATHY

■ *Alumina* 200x or 200c is for hair that falls out and a scalp that is itchy and dry. The skin and mucous membranes also are dry, and you may have throbbing headaches accompanied by constipation. Take one dose of *Alumina* 200x or 200c three times a week. Stop for two weeks, then repeat.

■ *Natrum muriaticum* is for hair loss accompanied by a craving for salt. You may have blinding headaches in the morning that feel as if a thousand little hammers were knocking on your brain. If you are a woman, menstrual periods are likely to be profuse and irregular. Take one dose of *Natrum muriaticum* 200x or 200c twice a week. Stop for one week, then repeat.

■ *Phosphoricum acidum* helps with thinning of hair, often accompanied by debility and fatigue that are worse with exertion. Your hair probably grayed relatively early in life. Take one dose of *Phosphoricum acidum* 30x or 15c three times daily for three days. Stop for two weeks, then repeat.

ACUPRESSURE/MASSAGE

For the locations of acupressure points on the body, *see* ADMINISTERING AN ACUPRESSURE TREATMENT in Part Three.

■ Massaging the scalp can help to stimulate hair growth.

AROMATHERAPY

For specific instructions on how to use aromatherapy, *see* PREPARING AROMATHERAPY TREATMENTS in Part Three.

■ Essential oil of rosemary and cayenne can be stimulating to hair growth. Make a massage oil with rosemary oil and add one or two drops of cayenne oil, and use the oil to massage your entire scalp. You can also add rosemary oil to your shampoo. Use 5 drops of essential oil to 1 ounce of shampoo.

GENERAL RECOMMENDATIONS

■ Take good care of your hair. Keep it clean, but avoid excessive washing and harsh chemicals. Use gentle and nourishing hair-care products. Avoid doing or using anything that pulls on the hair.

■ If you are experiencing hair loss, have a hair analysis done to uncover any nutritional deficiencies or toxic metal contamination. As hair is formed, available minerals and amino acids circulating in the blood are laid down in the hair. A hair analysis can therefore provide a picture of your mineral status and pick up any exposure to toxic metals. You should also consult your physician to check for an underlying health problem, such as hypothyroidism or infection.

■ Consider topical applications of polysorbate 60 or polysorbate 80, which have been shown to break up impacted sebum that can choke off new hair growth. There are many products available along this line. One of the best is Advanced Hair Regrowth Formula, available from the Life Extension Foundation (see the Resources section at the end of the book).

■ There are cosmetic hair systems available that increase the presence of visible hair by weaving strands of hair into currently existing hair and extending the pattern across balding areas with knotting techniques. Consumer satisfaction with these approaches varies.

PREVENTION

■ The best way to prevent hair loss is to choose parents and grandparents with great hair. Unfortunately, choosing one's genes is not (yet) an option. Consequently, hair loss cannot be considered preventable. It goes without saying, however, that you should take good care of your hair and consult a physician should you suspect you are developing any kind of infection on your scalp.

Halitosis

See BAD BREATH.

Hay Fever

Hay fever is a type of allergy that can, at certain times of the year, lead to a fairly miserable existence. The mucous membranes lining the nasal passages swell, and the nose, throat, and roof of the mouth itch. The eyes also itch and redden, and there may be considerable tearing. As the allergic reaction progresses, it causes sneezing and, possibly, coughing (even wheezing), with a clear or thin nasal discharge. The medical term for this type of condition is *allergic rhinitis*.

In addition to suffering the local symptoms of allergic reaction, a person with hay fever may feel fatigued and experience vague feelings of unease. Loss of appetite, inability to sleep, and even depression are not uncommon. Over time, polyps can develop and block the nasal passages.

All allergies are inappropriate immune-system responses to normally harmless substances. When confronted with a substance to which a person is sensitive, the immune system releases chemicals called histamines, which trigger the uncomfortable itching, sneezing, and tearing in an attempt to expel what it perceives as a foreign invader. Hay fever is a seasonal allergy because it is a reaction to pollens in the air. Symptoms recur at about the same time every year, usually when the offending plant is in bloom. Spring hay fever is most often due to pollens from grass and trees, while hay fever in later summer and early fall is usually caused by sensitivity to ragweed pollen and molds. Unfortunately, it is possible to be allergic to more than one type of pollen, resulting in hay fever that persists for many months out of the year.

Though it is not usually considered a serious disorder, hay fever can be a maddening nuisance. Tracking down the cause or causes can be equally trying. The most common type of allergy testing is skin, or "scratch" testing. In this technique, suspected allergens are introduced in dilute doses under the skin. If a red bump forms at the site, you are considered allergic to that substance. Another type of allergy testing is the radioallergosorbent test (RAST). This is a blood test that measures antibodies produced by the immune system in response to certain substances.

Why certain people suffer allergic reactions, including

hay fever, is not known. However, allergies do tend to run in families. Other factors that may contribute to the development of hay fever or a worsening of symptoms include your general state of health, underlying food allergies, intestinal yeast or parasites, exposure to smoke and/or chemicals, nutritional deficiencies, low thyroid function, and physical or emotional stress.

CONVENTIONAL TREATMENT

■ The first treatment your doctor is likely to recommend is the use of an over-the-counter antihistamine such as diphenhydramine (found in Benadryl and other products), chlorpheniramine (Chlor-Trimeton and others), or brompheniramine (Allerhist, Dimetane, and others). If the over-the-counter varieties fail to relieve symptoms, a prescription antihistamine such as hydroxyzine (Atarax, Vistaril) or cetirizine (Zyrtec) may be tried. These drugs work by blocking the effect of histamine, thus reducing the itching, swelling, redness, and discharge that result from histamine release. All of these drugs, whether prescription or over-the-counter, can cause side effects, most commonly drowsiness, fatigue, and dry mouth. The drowsiness may be helpful, though, if hay fever symptoms make it difficult to sleep. In some cases, these medications may cause dizziness, tremor, nervousness, and other effects as well.

■ A number of newer antihistamines have been developed that are less likely to cause drowsiness. One example is astemizole (Hismanal). However, these drugs can still cause side effects, including heart palpitations, nervousness, and dry mouth, and if they are taken in combination with certain other drugs, serious heart problems can result. Loratadine (Claritin) and fexofenadine (Allegra) are two newer antihistamines that seem to cause less drowsiness than others do, and without interacting with other drugs to cause heart problems, but they can still cause headache, dry mouth, drowsiness, blood-pressure changes, heart-rhythm changes, nausea, vomiting, diarrhea, and/or agitation. These drugs also pass into breast milk.

■ Decongestants such as pseudoephedrine (Sudafed) are often used to relieve nasal symptoms without causing drowsiness or fatigue. These drugs also can cause side effects. They are stimulating to the heart, and may cause high blood pressure, headache, dizziness, palpitations, nervousness, and other unpleasant symptoms.

■ Another approach to treating hay fever is the use of cromolyn sodium (Intal, Nasalcrom), applied directly to the nasal tissues to stabilize the mast cells, the cells that release histamine. This drug is better at preventing recurrences rather than stopping acute attacks. A close relative of the bioflavonoids, it has virtually no side effects or toxicity. It is, however, somewhat more expensive than other treatments.

■ Inhaled steroids may be recommended for more stubborn cases. This class of drugs includes beclomethasone (Beclovent, Beconase, Vanceril, Vancenase), dexamethasone (Dexacort), fluticasone (Flonase), and flunisolide (Nasarel). Possible side effects include nasal discomfort, nosebleeds, nausea, an altered sense of smell, impaired healing, and others. These drugs also tend to depress the functioning of the adrenal glands, and should be used judiciously.

■ For more severe, systemic symptoms, oral steroids such as cortisone or prednisone (Deltasone) may be used to suppress the immune system. These are stronger than the topical steroids and cause more serious side effects, so they should be reserved for the very worst cases.

■ Some doctors recommend desensitization therapy for people with hay fever. This involves injecting dilute doses of allergen in gradually increased strengths to "train" the body to handle the offending agent. This process is expensive and time-consuming, and not always successful.

DIETARY GUIDELINES

■ A balanced, nutrient-rich, noncongesting diet is best. Eat plenty of fresh fruits and vegetables; whole grains like rice, millet, and oats; legumes, both cooked and sprouted; some raw seeds and nuts (but not peanuts); and some lean, clean fish and poultry proteins. Avoid foods that tend to promote congestion. These include breads and baked goods, cheese and dairy foods, sugar and refined flours, and most packaged or processed foods.

■ Eliminate any potentially allergenic food from your diet for at least two weeks (three for dairy products) to see whether your symptoms improve. Common allergenic foods include dairy products, eggs, wheat, sugar, soy products, yeasts, peanuts, and citrus fruits. However, eating any food regularly may lead to allergies.

■ Include in your diet cold-water fish such as flounder, mackerel, and salmon, at least three times a week if possible. The oils these fish contain have an anti-inflammatory effect.

■ Avoid sugar, caffeine, alcohol and nicotine. All of these substances place added stress on an already stressed immune system.

NUTRITIONAL SUPPLEMENTS

■ Take a good multivitamin and mineral supplement daily.

■ Acidophilus and other probiotics support healthy intestinal bacteria and gastrointestinal function. This assists digestion, which is important because incompletely digested and absorbed foods can trigger an allergic response. Take a probiotic supplement as recommended on the product label. If you are allergic to milk, select a dairy-free formula.

■ To support adrenal function, increase energy, and reduce allergic symptoms, take 50 to 150 milligrams of adrenal glandular extract twice daily.

■ Black currant seed oil, borage oil, evening primrose oil, and flaxseed oil contain gamma-linolenic acid (GLA), which has anti-inflammatory and anti-allergenic effects. Take a dose of black currant seed, borage, evening primrose, or flaxseed oil that supplies 250 milligrams of gamma-linolenic acid (GLA) three times a day.

■ Magnesium has a relaxing effect on smooth muscle, including the muscle of the bronchial passages, which can make breathing easier. It is especially useful if hay fever symptoms are sometimes a prelude to an asthmatic episode. Take 250 milligrams twice a day.

■ N-acetylcysteine (NAC) protects the liver and can help to minimize allergic-type reactions. Take 500 to 600 milligrams once or twice a day.

■ Sulfur, in the form of methylsulfonylmethane (MSM), may help decrease an allergic reaction. Take 500 milligrams two or three times daily.

■ The B-complex vitamins, especially vitamin B_6 (pyridoxine) and pantothenic acid, aid in the processing of foods and amino acids. They also support the function of the adrenal glands, which is important in the control of allergies. Take a B-complex supplement supplying 25 milligrams of each of the major B vitamins two or three times daily. In addition, you can take 250 milligrams of pantothenic acid three times daily and 100 milligrams of vitamin B_6 (pyridoxine) twice a day, between meals, for up to five days in a row as needed for symptoms.

■ Taking 1,000 milligrams of vitamin C, plus an equal amount of bioflavonoids, at least three times daily may have a beneficial effect, especially if started approximately six weeks before the hay-fever season arrives.

■ Bioflavonoids enhance the effect of vitamin C and help to stabilize the mast cells, which secrete histamine. Take 1,000 milligrams of citrus bioflavonoids three times daily.

HERBAL TREATMENT

■ Echinacea and goldenseal support the immune system and aid in liver detoxification. Echinacea has been used for years as an allergy treatment. Take one dose of an echinacea and goldenseal combination formula supplying 350 to 500 milligrams of echinacea and 200 to 350 milligrams of goldenseal three times daily for up to five days.

■ Garlic can help cleanse the blood and reduce allergies. Take the equivalent of 500 milligrams of fresh garlic three times daily.

■ Licorice supports adrenal function. Choose deglycyrrhizinated licorice (DGL) and take 300 milligrams three times daily.

Note: Ordinary licorice can elevate blood pressure, and should not be taken on a daily basis for more than ten days in a row. DGL should not have this effect, however.

■ Nettle leaf is a natural diuretic and is useful for reducing tissue swelling associated with hay fever. Take 150 to 300 milligrams three or four times daily, as needed for symptoms.

■ Turmeric is a natural anti-inflammatory. Take 250 to 350 milligrams three or four times daily, as needed for symptoms.

HOMEOPATHY

■ *Arsenicum album* is good if you are anxious and restless and have a thin, watery nasal discharge and a stopped-up nose. You feel better indoors and worse in the open air. Take one dose of *Arsenicum album* 12x or 6c three to four times a day, as needed, for up to two days.

■ *Dulcamara* is for the person who sneezes constantly and has swollen and watery eyes. You feel worse in damp weather and outdoors, and tend to become chilled after exertion. Take one dose of *Dulcamara* 12x or 6c three to four times a day, as needed, for up to two days.

■ *Euphrasia* is for a bland discharge from the nose and a burning sensation in the eyes. You feel worse indoors but better outdoors. Take one dose of *Euphrasia* 12x or 6c three to four times a day, as needed, for up to two days.

■ *Gelsemium* is for constant sneezing accompanied by heavy, puffy eyes and a listless, dizzy, and shaky feeling. Take one dose of *Gelsemium* 12x or 6c three to four times a day, as needed, for up to two days.

■ *Hepar sulfuris calcareum* is for a thick nasal discharge, though your nose stops up and you sneeze every time you are exposed to cold, dry air. You probably have a tendency to develop cold sores. Take one dose of *Hepar sulfuris calcareum* 12x or 6c three to four times a day, as needed, for up to two days.

■ *Sabadilla* is for a runny nose and a watery nasal discharge accompanied by sneezing, sinus pain, and red eyes. Take one dose of *Sabadilla* 12x or 6c three to four times a day, as needed, for up to two days.

■ *Sanguinaria* is the remedy for chronic rhinitis with dry nasal membranes and a congested nose. You have a tendency to develop nasal polyps and a mucous discharge, and may have diarrhea often. Take one dose of *Sanguinaria* 12x or 6c three to four times a day, as needed, for up to two days.

■ There are many homeopathic combination remedies

available for allergies. You may want to experiment with these. Follow the dosage directions on the product label.

BACH FLOWER REMEDIES

Select the remedy that most closely fits your emotional tendencies and concerns, and take it as needed, following the directions on the product label.

Chicory is the remedy to choose if your feelings are easily hurt and you tend to be insecure, sometimes selfish, and want constant attention.

Gentian helps to combat a tendency to become discouraged easily.

Impatiens is for the hyperactive "type-A" person who is tense, nervous, and impatient.

Choose Larch if you lack self confidence and prefer not to call attention to yourself.

ACUPRESSURE

For the locations of acupressure points on the body, see ADMINISTERING AN ACUPRESSURE TREATMENT in Part Three.

Gallbladder 20 and Large Intestine 4 help to relieve head congestion.

AROMATHERAPY

For specific instructions on how to use aromatherapy, see PREPARING AROMATHERAPY TREATMENTS in Part Three.

Essential oils of basil, peppermint, and pine help to ease congestion. Choose one and use it as an inhalant, diffuse it into the air, or make a steam inhalation treatment with it.

Lavender oil relaxes the nervous system; rosemary helps to clear the head. Use either or both as inhalants or diffuse them into the air.

GENERAL RECOMMENDATIONS

Seek an environment as free of allergens as possible. Some people need to cover pillows and mattresses, and carefully clean dusty, moldy areas or remove the more serious dust-collecting items.

■ An air purifier may help. These devices use an electrostatic charge to cause allergens to settle out of the air. Some include filters to aid with the removal of tiny particles.

Get regular exercise. This is important for maintaining overall health and cleansing the body of toxins that can add to the allergen load your body must deal with.

■ Embarking on a seven- to ten-day juice fast just before spring can rid the body of toxins and help prevent allergic reactions.

■ Strive to keep your immune system as unstressed as possible. Avoid tobacco smoke and other environmental pollutants. Also avoid emotional stress and extremes as much as possible. All of these factors affect the immune system and make you more prone to allergic reactions. Be sure to get regular, adequate sleep.

■ We recommend that you try natural therapies first before resorting to drugs. However, many people find a combination of therapies to yield the best results with a minimum of side effects.

■ Allergies usually cause a clear, thin nasal discharge. If you develop a discharge that is thick and yellowish or greenish in color and that does not seem to go away, you may have a different problem, such as a sinus infection. Consult your physician.

Headache

Headaches can be caused by muscle tension, an underlying illness or infection, or disturbances in the blood vessels in the head. The latter scenario produces migraine headaches. These typically recur periodically and are characterized by severe pain that is aggravated by light, may be preceded by disturbances in vision, and are often associated with nausea and vomiting. Often, the pain is concentrated on one side of the head.

An attack of migraine can last for days; sleep may or may not be helpful in easing the pain. You may not even be aware of head pain, but rather of nausea, vomiting, and stomachache. Migraines can be triggered by a number of different factors, including emotional stress, low blood sugar, food allergies, head injuries, oral contraceptives, or hormonal changes related to the menstrual cycle, which may be why girls and women are more likely to suffer from them. The disorder also tends to run in families.

Headaches can sometimes be related to disorders that warrant further investigation, such as infections of the scalp, ears, sinuses, or spinal fluid. They can also be caused by allergies, sensitivities to certain substances, fever, high blood pressure, epilepsy, brain tumors, severe cavities or oral infections, temporomandibular joint (TMJ) syndrome, certain drugs, or an injury to the head.

Different people develop different kinds of headaches. Some come down with a "sick headache" after spending time in a heavily perfumed environment or around people who wear certain scents. Others develop a headache after eating foods containing monosodium glutamate (MSG). Still others are sensitive to organic compounds called amines, which are found naturally in many foods. Such an individual may develop a headache after consuming tomatoes, potatoes, eggplant, bananas, pineapple, some cheeses, yeast, beer, or wine. The amine headache is similar to a migraine; the pain is caused by constriction of the blood vessels in the scalp. In sensitive individuals, amines first dilate the vessels, which then respond with a rebound effect, resulting in pinching and constriction.

Most often, headaches are related to muscle tension. A tension headache often feels like a tight band around the head. The pain may be throbbing or dull, mild or severe. Sudden movements often seem to make a tension headache worse. A headache may develop suddenly, or come on gradually. Tension headaches most often occur during the day, worsen as the day goes on, and may be relieved with sleep. If you awaken with a headache in the middle of the night, the cause is most likely something other than tension.

Most headaches can be treated at home with the remedies discussed in this entry. However, if your headaches are so severe that they interfere with normal activities, or if they are frequent rather than isolated occurrences, you should consult with a physician. If you get an extremely severe headache that comes on quickly, especially if you have never had a similar type of pain before; or if you have a headache in combination with a high fever, severe vomiting, a stiff neck, confusion, disorientation, or extreme fatigue, see a doctor or go to the emergency room without delay, as these can be signs of serious problems requiring immediate intervention.

CONVENTIONAL TREATMENT

■ A mild pain reliever, such as ibuprofen (found in Advil, Nuprin, and other medications), aspirin (Bayer, Ecotrin, and others), or acetaminophen (Tylenol, Tempra, and others) can relieve a headache. These drugs are most effective when taken early; headache pain becomes increasingly difficult to relieve as it becomes more severe. Ibuprofen generally works better for headaches, especially migraine headaches, than aspirin or acetaminophen does.

Note: Take aspirin or ibuprofen with food to avoid possible stomach upset. Do not take aspirin or any other nonsteroidal anti-inflammatory drug (NSAID) in the last three months of pregnancy, as it can damage the developing fetus and cause complications during delivery. Acetaminophen can cause liver damage if taken in excessive amounts. Do not exceed the recommended dosage.

■ For extremely severe headaches, a combination of acetaminophen and codeine may be prescribed. Codeine is a powerful narcotic painkiller that works by blocking the brain's perception of pain. It can also cause serious side effects, including nausea, sleepiness, and constipation, and it can be highly addictive.

■ If you suffer from migraines, ibuprofen or acetaminophen is likely to be suggested first, and may be all that is needed to ease the pain. The antihistamine diphenhydramine (Benadryl) may also be suggested. The reason it works is not well understood, but it may offer relief.

■ If you suffer from migraines that are not relieved by ordinary painkillers, an ergotamine preparation may be prescribed. These drugs work by constricting blood vessels. They are available in forms that can be taken orally, rectally, as a nasal spray, or placed under the tongue; some formulations contain caffeine. Ergotamine works best if it is taken as soon as the pain begins, but it should be used with care because it is possible to become dependent on it. Possible side effects include stomach and/or muscle cramps, dizziness, nausea, vomiting, and diarrhea.

■ Another drug, sumatriptan (sold under the brand name Imitrex), appears to be very effective in alleviating a severe attack of migraine. It works by increasing the amount of serotonin in the brain. Serotonin is involved in vasoconstriction (the constriction of blood vessels); since migraine is in part a result of a disturbance in circulation in the brain, increasing serotonin levels may help to restore balance in the tension of blood vessels. This treatment is expensive, however, and can also produce unpleasant side effects, including increased heart rate, elevated blood pressure, and a feeling of tightness in the chest, jaw, or neck.

■ There is some evidence that a daily low dose of the beta-blocker propranolol (Inderal) may help prevent recurrent, incapacitating migraine headaches. Side effects can include fatigue, depression, shortness of breath, and cold hands and feet. This drug should not be taken by anyone with asthma or diabetes.

■ Butorphanol (Stadol) is a potent pain reliever similar in action to narcotic painkillers. It is available in injection form and as a nasal spray. It can be very effective—many migraine sufferers have hailed it as a "miracle" pain reliever—but it has the potential to cause dependence with repeated use, and has been linked to a number of deaths associated with addiction. The U.S. Drug Enforcement Administration (DEA) is now regulating it as a controlled substance.

■ If headaches are chronic and debilitating, it may be helpful to consult a neurologist to investigate the possibility of an underlying problem.

DIETARY GUIDELINES

■ Because low blood sugar can provoke a headache, make sure to eat three whole-foods meals and several healthful snacks each day. Do not eat sugary foods. Sugar causes blood-sugar levels to soar, then crash, making a headache worse.

■ Limit your intake of saturated fats and hydrogenated and partially hydrogenated fats and oils. These are difficult to digest and can lead to stomach upset and headache. Avoid greasy and fried foods.

■ Chocolate, monosodium glutamate (MSG), and the preservatives in hot dogs and other processed meats have been found to cause headaches, especially migraines. If you typically get a headache after eating one of these foods, banish the offender from the menu. Be aware of hidden MSG in processed food products. For example, if the label lists an additive called hydrolyzed protein, the product contains MSG. Other additives that contain MSG include autolyzed yeast, sodium caseinate, and calcium caseinate. Read labels carefully.

■ A food allergy or sensitivity can provoke headaches. Use an elimination diet or a diet diary to uncover hidden food allergies (*see* ELIMINATION DIET in Part Three).

NUTRITIONAL SUPPLEMENTS

■ If a headache (whether tension or migraine) is centered in the front of the head—especially if you suspect it may be related to something you ate—try taking an acidophilus supplement, as directed on the product label, every four hours until the headache is gone. If you are allergic to milk, select a dairy-free product.

■ Calcium and magnesium help to calm muscles and relax blood vessels. A transitory deficit of magnesium especially has been associated with the onset of migraine. Twice a day, take one dose of a combination supplement supplying 500 milligrams of calcium and 250 milligrams of magnesium.

■ Chromium helps control blood-sugar levels. This mineral maintains a healthy blood-sugar balance and may enable you to go longer between meals without snacks. Take 200 micrograms once or twice daily.

HERBAL TREATMENT

■ When used as a rub, an herbal tincture of arnica can be effective in resolving a headache. Simply rub arnica tincture into your temples and/or forehead. Be very careful to keep tinctures away from your eyes, and do not use them on broken skin.

■ Chamomile and passionflower relax the nervous system and can bring relief for a tension headache. Take a cup of chamomile and/or passionflower tea as needed. You can also prepare a herbal bath and take a long, relaxing soak. The beneficial effects of the herbs will be absorbed through the skin.

■ Feverfew inhibits the release of inflammatory prostaglandins implicated in migraine. Taken regularly, this herb can ward off migraines. Feverfew is a documented preventive, but its effects are cumulative. Don't expect immediate relief. Take 150 milligrams of freeze-dried feverfew-leaf extract or 200 to 400 milligrams of the herb two to three times daily. Allow sufficient time for the effects to build.

Note: Do not use this herb if you are allergic to plants in the daisy family.

■ Ginger and/or peppermint tea is helpful for either a tension or a migraine headache that is located in the front of the head. These herbs are also helpful for a congested and full headache, and can help relieve a headache caused by overeating as well. Take a cup of tea as needed.

■ Skullcap is excellent for headaches due to nervous tension. Take a cup of tea as needed.

■ White willow bark contains salicin, an aspirinlike compound, and has been used for centuries for headaches and a variety of other aches and pains. For relief of headache, take a dose of standardized extract supplying 80 to 120 milligrams of salicin. If you wish to use it as a preventive, take a dose equal to 20 to 40 milligrams of salicin daily.

Note: Do not use this herb if you are allergic to aspirin.

HOMEOPATHY

■ For tension headaches, choose the homeopathic remedy most suited to your symptoms and take it as follows: Take one dose of the remedy. Wait twenty minutes. If there is no relief after twenty minutes, take a second dose and wait another twenty minutes. If you still feel no relief, wait thirty minutes and select another remedy that suits your symptoms and temperament.

- *Bryonia* 30x or 9c is recommended for a headache in combination with constipation and much eye pain.
- Choose *Ferrum phosphoricum* 12x or 5c if you have a headache and your face is pale and cold or red and flushed, and generally alternates between the two. Your hands and feet are probably cold, and you may get a headache when you are fatigued.
- *Gelsemium* 12x or 6c is useful if you experience visual disturbances, such as blurring, and for the type of tension headache that is associated with performance anxiety before a big event.
- Take *Natrum muriaticum* 30x or 9c if you develop a headache after any kind of intense mental work, such as a project that has a raise or promotion riding on it. The *Natrum muriaticum* person is very ambitious, hard on him- or herself, and eager to achieve. He or she may also have a craving for salt.

■ If you have a migraine, choose one of the following and take one dose four times a day for up to two days:

- *Iris* 30x or 9c is recommended if you complain of impaired or blurred vision. You may also be vomiting and the pain may recur periodically—you may have a headache every Monday, for example.
- Use *Lachesis* 30x or 9c if the pain begins or is worse on the left side of the head.
- If the migraine begins or is worse on the right side of the head, choose *Lycopodium* 30x or 9c.

- *Silica* 30x or 9c is for a migraine that starts at the base of the back of the head and travels into one eye.

■ Whichever remedy you choose, if you are using any form of peppermint or Tiger Balm in addition to one of the homeopathic remedies recommended here, you should take the homeopathic remedies at least half an hour before or after. Otherwise, the strong odors of these herbal preparations may interfere with the action of the remedy.

If headaches are chronic, and an underlying illness has been ruled out, it may be helpful to consult a homeopathic physician for a constitutional remedy.

ACUPRESSURE/MASSAGE

For the locations of acupressure points on the body, *see* ADMINISTERING AN ACUPRESSURE TREATMENT in Part Three.

Large Intestine 4 relaxes tension in the head. It is especially comforting for a frontal headache.

■ Liver 3 quiets the nervous system and relaxes tense muscles.

Neck and Shoulder Release unkinks and relaxes the muscles most often tight and tense during a headache.

To help yourself relax, have someone rub the two muscles that run along your spine.

■ A back rub or foot rub can help release tension and help you feel cared for and nurtured when you are tense or upset.

AROMATHERAPY

For specific instructions on how to use aromatherapy, *see* PREPARING AROMATHERAPY TREATMENTS in Part Three.

Peppermint oil can help relieve headache pain. Add a few drops of peppermint oil to massage oil and gently massage the mixture into your temples. Be sure to keep the oil away from your eyes, and do not use it on broken skin. Or add peppermint oil to cold water and use it to make a compress. Apply the compress to your forehead (avoiding your eyes) or the back of your neck and relax for at least ten minutes.

GENERAL RECOMMENDATIONS

Lie down and rest in a darkened, quiet room.

■ Put a cool washcloth on your forehead.

A tension headache may get better on its own if you give yourself permission to express your worries to a loving and supportive friend or family member.

■ A French study done at the University of Dijon found a correlation between hypothyroidism and chronic headaches. Further, they found that headaches associated with hypothyroidism responded very well to thyroid hormone therapy. If you have begun to suffer from headaches for no apparent reason, you may want to ask your physician to check your thyroid function.

■ People who suffer from cluster headaches often have abnormal fluctuations in their melatonin levels surrounding the attacks. Some naturopathic physicians test people who have cluster headaches to see if they are losing unusually high levels of this hormone through urination; if they are, melatonin therapy may be in order. Abnormal excretion of melatonin may be associated with dysfunction of the hypothalamus, a portion of the brain that controls hunger, thirst, body temperature, and other aspects of the body's metabolic balance. Hypothalamic dysfunction can be related to perimenopause and menopausal symptoms. If you are a menopausal or perimenopausal woman who has recently begun suffering from cluster headaches, you may wish to discuss this possibility with your physician.

■ Relaxation techniques, including yoga, meditation, progressive relaxation, guided imagery, and autogenic training can be helpful. Biofeedback training, which involves reprogramming the body to respond to stressors with relaxation rather than the "fight-or-flight" stress response, has been found to be effective for up to 75 percent of migraine sufferers who have tried it. Exactly how these techniques work is not understood, but research consistently confirms their effectiveness.

■ Consider consulting a licensed acupuncturist. Acupuncture helps to release energy blockages within the body, leading to increased relaxation.

■ If headaches are due to structural stress, chiropractic is often very effective in relieving musculoskeletal pain and restoring function and mobility.

■ Psychologists and psychiatrists agree that making adjustments in one's relationships may be important in getting rid of chronic headaches. This includes setting limits on the demands of others and learning to say no without feeling guilty. Cognitive restructuring is another popular psychiatric tool. In this technique, you learn to identify unconscious irrational beliefs—such as "My headaches are my punishment for things I've done wrong," or "If I were a better person, I wouldn't have these headaches"—that may be contributing to the problem, and then to replace them with simple positive commands, such as "Headaches are manageable, and I need to learn how," or "I deserve to be healthy and feel good."

■ Electrotherapy, a combination of pulsating mechanical messages and deep-tissue electrical stimulation (usually of specific acupuncture points) has been shown to deeply relax muscles and trigger the release of endorphins, the body's natural pain-blocking chemicals. Sessions usually last from fifteen to thirty minutes and can help reduce both immediate pain and recurrences.

■ For a headache related to constipation, take an Epsom salts bath. The salts will increase circulation and help relax tension. A bowel movement will usually occur an hour or two after the bath.

■ Tiger Balm liniment works very well for tension headaches. Rub the ointment into the temple area.

PREVENTION

Some people tend to get tense, depressed, or overwhelmed. By carefully observing and responding to your needs, you can help yourself deal with emotional and physical stresses and perhaps avert tension headaches.

To help release the tensions of the day, prepare a warm herbal bath before bed. If possible, exchange a comforting massage with a loved one. Talk about the day, express concerns or anxieties, and ask for help or support if you need it. If this is not possible, keep a journal. Sometimes just writing out your worries can relieve tension and help you to see things in a new light.

Eat three good meals every day and have healthy snacks on hand. Avoid sugar, fried foods, and heavy fats. Eliminate from your diet any foods that you know from experience can trigger a headache.

Go to bed and awaken at the same time each day.

Exercise at least four times each week.

■ Avoid foods and beverages, such as diet sodas, that contain the artificial sweetener aspartame (NutraSweet). This chemical can trigger headaches in susceptible individuals.

Do not smoke. Avoid secondhand smoke and other environmental pollutants.

■ Explore meditation or relaxation techniques (*see* RELAXATION TECHNIQUES in Part Three). Massage or chiropractic adjustment may also help.

Try to resolve interpersonal disputes in a positive way, and learn to forgive, to accept the forgiveness of others, and, most important, to accept human imperfections. Psychologists have found a distinct correlation between tension headaches and an inability (or unwillingness) to accept human imperfection.

A variety of different drugs may be recommended as preventives for people who suffer recurring migraines. These include beta-blockers (propranolol [Inderal] is one of the most popular of these), calcium-channel blockers, and low doses of antidepressants, among others. All of these are powerful medications that can have serious side effects, and should be used with caution, if at all.

■ If you suffer from migraines, keep a diary that records the circumstances surrounding each attack, such as foods recently eaten, exposure to pollutants and possible allergens, activities, emotional factors, your physical environment, and so on. Try to be as observant as possible. Notice the obviously unhealthy things, such as cigarette smoke or car exhaust, but don't overlook things that seem harmless or even pleasant, such as perfumes or the smell of new fabrics. Once you do this, a pattern may emerge pointing to certain factors that could be triggering the headaches. You can then make appropriate alterations in your diet and/or lifestyle.

■ Acupuncture and biofeedback have both been used to good effect against chronic headaches, whether from migraine or tension. If frequent headaches are making you miserable, it may be worthwhile to consult a qualified acupuncturist or a practitioner skilled in biofeedback techniques.

Hearing Loss

Hearing is essentially a three-step process. First, the ear concentrates sound waves and converts them into magnified mechanical pulses. This is known as the *conduction phase*. The mechanical pulses are then converted into a nerve stimulation (a process described as the *sensory phase*) for transmission to the brain (the *neural phase*) to be translated into what we think of as sound. Anything that interferes with any step in this progression can result in hearing loss.

The most common type of hearing loss is conductive hearing loss. To focus sound waves, the ear canal is shaped like a tapered cone. This leaves it susceptible to being blocked by foreign bodies of all sorts. Often, the culprit is an accumulation of cerumen (earwax). Cerumen is produced to lubricate the ear canal, but if too much is produced, or if it is not transported properly through the canal, it can build up.

Conductive hearing loss can also occur if something interferes with the conversion of sound waves from the outer ear to mechanical pulses in the middle ear, behind the eardrum. Trauma to the outer ear or pressure from an infection behind the eardrum can cause the drum to tear, decreasing sound transmission. In addition, there are three tiny, mobile bones called ossicles that transport the vibration of sound waves to the inner ear, where the auditory nerve is stimulated. If fluid builds up around the ossicles as a result of a middle-ear infection, the ossicles can be muffled. They can also become immobile due to a condition called otosclerosis, which is similar to arthritis, or they can become detached from each other, disrupting the transmission of sound impulses.

Another cause of hearing loss is damage to the organ of Corti, the hearing sensor in the inner ear. This can be a result of exposure to an extremely high volume of noise, head trauma, or drugs that can destroy parts of the organ. It can also be involved in *presbycusis,* or age-related hearing loss. Drugs known for causing this type of damage, called *ototoxicity,* include a class of antibiotics called the aminoglycosides. This group includes gentamicin (Garamycin), tobramycin (Nebcin), and amikacin (Amikin). Because of this, these drugs are reserved for only the most serious infections. Other drugs that can have this effect include the loop diuretics, such as furosemide (Lasix), bumetanide (Bumex), and ethacrynic acid (Edecrin); several anticancer drugs, most notably cisplatin (Platinol); and even high doses of plain aspirin.

Sensory hearing loss can be inherited, or it can be a result of other disorders, including diabetes, kidney failure, hypothyroidism, infections such as measles or mumps, and lupus. Exposure to loud noises can also result in sensory hearing loss.

Neural hearing loss is the least common form. Damage to the auditory nerve can occur due to causes like tumors, blood clots in or ruptures of blood vessels feeding the nerve, and multiple sclerosis.

Hearing is evaluated by means of audiometric testing. In this procedure, tones at specific pitches are presented to each ear at different volumes to determine the exact nature of hearing loss, if any. This is because the degree of hearing loss may not be the same across all frequencies. Audiometric testing determines both the range and degree of loss so that the most effective types of treatment may be prescribed.

CONVENTIONAL TREATMENT

■ Foreign bodies and impacted earwax may be removed by means of lavage, in which high-pressure water flow is used to clean out the ear canal. Other alternatives include the use of a specialized suction device or direct manual removal in the doctor's office. Hydrogen peroxide or carbamide peroxide may be used first to help loosen hard wax. It is unwise to attempt to remove impacted earwax on your own, as it is easy to end up further impacting the wax or even perforating the eardrum. If you do attempt to wash out your own ear, you should completely dry out the ear afterwards using either isopropyl alcohol or a hair dryer on the lowest setting.

■ If there is a buildup of fluid behind the eardrum, it may be watery or it may contain pus. Watery, or serous, otitis may be treated with a decongestant such as pseudoephedrine (Sudafed and others) or phenylpropanolamine (Entex and others); a steroid such as cortisone or prednisone (Deltasone); or an antibiotic such as amoxicillin (Amoxil) or erythromycin (ERYC, Ilotycin, and others). The fact that such a variety of treatments may be used implies that none is accepted as a complete solution. If there is pus

behind the eardrum, or acute otitis media, it is presumed to be a bacterial infection and treated with an antibiotic like amoxicillin, erythromycin, or cefaclor (Ceclor). A buildup of fluid behind the eardrum can cause pain and pressure. If the pain is extreme, the drum may be deliberately perforated to allow the fluid to drain. The eardrum may also perforate by itself. A perforated eardrum, whatever the cause, usually heals by itself, though occasionally surgical intervention is required.

■ Hearing aids designed to augment the sound entering the ear canal have become highly sophisticated, and in many cases can now be hidden completely within the ear. Some are digitally programmable, and are adjusted to the results of audiometric testing.

■ If the ossicles are dislocated or scarred together, surgery may be recommended to repair the problem. The results of such procedures vary, depending on the extent of the problem and the skill of the surgeon.

■ In some cases of otosclerosis, sodium fluoride tablets may stop the progression of hearing loss if used for extended periods. Current evidence on the effectiveness of this treatment is not conclusive, but you may want to discuss this with an ear specialist.

■ Cochlear implants—electronic devices that can be surgically placed within the inner ear to stimulate the auditory nerve—can permit about 50 percent of adults with profound hearing loss to understand some speech without resorting to visual cues.

■ There are many assistive aids available to help people with irreversible hearing loss in using the telephone and understanding radio and television broadcasts. Some magnify sound; others add visible captions.

DIETARY GUIDELINES

■ Include sea vegetables such as dulse, hijiki, and kombu in your diet. Sea vegetables are high in iodine, which helps to initiate healthy thyroid function, in turn enhancing metabolism. Add sea vegetables to soups or enjoy them as side dishes.

■ Eat fresh pineapple. Fresh pineapple contains bromelain, which is excellent for reducing inflammation.

■ Avoid deep-fried foods and cooked saturated fats, which slow digestion and increase the production of earwax.

■ Investigate the possibility of food allergies. (*See* ELIMINATION DIET in Part Three.)

NUTRITIONAL SUPPLEMENTS

■ Take a good multivitamin and mineral supplement that includes the trace minerals. Choose powdered or capsule forms, which are more easily absorbed by the body.

■ Take a full-spectrum digestive-enzyme supplement providing 5,000 international units of lipase, 2,500 international units of amylase, and 300 international units of protease with each meal. Digestive enzymes improve the body's utilization of nutrition, which can in turn decrease inflammation.

■ Proteolytic enzymes help reduce inflammation. Take 500 milligrams twice a day, between meals.

■ Vitamin E improves circulation, an important factor in some types of hearing loss. Choose a product containing mixed tocopherols and start by taking 200 international units daily, then gradually increase the dosage until you are taking 400 international units in the morning and another 400 international units in the evening.

HERBAL TREATMENT

■ Ginkgo biloba is valuable in the treatment cochlear deafness caused by insufficient oxygen and/or sound trauma. This herb has been shown to increase the oxygen supply to the tissues and improve neural transmission. Select a standardized extract containing at least 24 percent ginkgo heterosides (sometimes called flavoglycosides) and take 40 to 60 milligrams three times daily.

HOMEOPATHY

■ The best approach to treating hearing loss homeopathically is to consult a qualified homeopath who can prescribe a constitutional remedy tailored to your specific needs.

■ *Lycopodium* is the remedy for hardness of hearing accompanied by humming and roaring sounds in the ear. Every noise may cause a peculiar echo in the ear. Take one dose of *Lycopodium* 30x or 15c three times daily for up to three days. Wait two weeks, then repeat.

■ Take *Phosphorous* if you experience re-echoing of sounds and have particular difficulty hearing the human voice. Take one dose of *Phosphorous* 30x or 15c three times daily for up to three days.

■ *Silicea* is for roaring in the ears and a heightened sensitivity to noise. You also tend to be somewhat nervous and excitable. Take one dose of *Silicea* 200x or 200c once daily for up to three days. Wait three weeks, then repeat.

BACH FLOWER REMEDIES

Select the remedy that most closely fits your disposition and emotional tendencies and concerns, and take it as needed, following the directions on the product label.

■ Mimulus eases fearfulness and shyness. It is the remedy for the person who has many well-articulated fears.

■ Choose Scleranthus if you are feeling uncertain and have trouble making decisions and sticking with them.

■ Water violet gently helps to counteract a tendency to be alone, asocial, and removed from friends.

ACUPRESSURE

For the locations of acupressure points on the body, *see* ADMINISTERING AN ACUPRESSURE TREATMENT in Part Three.

■ Triple Warmer 5 and Gallbladder 20 together help to stimulate hearing.

AROMATHERAPY

For specific instructions on how to use aromatherapy, *see* PREPARING AROMATHERAPY TREATMENTS in Part Three.

■ Essential oil of rosemary is stimulating to circulation in the head. You can use it as an inhalant, diffuse it into the room, or use it in a steam inhalation treatment.

GENERAL RECOMMENDATIONS

■ If you experience a noticeable loss or diminishment of hearing that lasts for more than seventy-two hours, you should consult an audiologist for a professional evaluation. Consult your physician for a referral.

PREVENTION

■ Protect your ears from loud noises. An assault of high decibels is known to cause hearing loss. If you are going to be exposed to a high noise level, wear earplugs. This applies whether you are operating a power mower or heavy equipment, or attending a rock concert or a symphony. The acoustics in some halls are so good that the music becomes loud enough to cause damage. Damage to the ear caused by loud noise cannot be remedied; it must be prevented.

Heart Attack/ Heart Disease

See under CARDIOVASCULAR DISEASE.

Heartburn

See under INDIGESTION.

Heat Exhaustion/ Heatstroke

If you engage in prolonged vigorous activity in a hot environment without taking in adequate amounts of fluid and, possibly, electrolytes, you may develop heat exhaustion. This problem is not uncommon among amateur athletes, who may tackle events for which they are not really prepared, but they are not the only ones who develop heat exhaustion.

In a hot environment, the blood vessels dilate to allow more blood to come close to the skin's surface for cooling (the skin's surface is cooler than the body's core areas). At the same time, a loss of fluid from exertion and sweating lowers blood volume even further. The result can be heat exhaustion. The first symptoms are usually thirst, fatigue, weakness, and heavy sweating, with possible changes in pulse rate and blood pressure. If fluids are not replaced and/or the body is not allowed to rest, symptoms can progress to anxiety, changes in mental status, and even a loss of consciousness.

Heatstroke is not the same thing as heat exhaustion, although it can occur as a progression of that condition. Heatstroke represents a serious malfunction of the body's heat-regulating mechanism. It is more likely to occur in the very old and very young. Other risk factors include chronic alcohol use, obesity, the use of medications such as antihistamines and major tranquilizers, and also cocaine use, all of which interfere with the body's normal heat-dissipating mechanism.

In heatstroke, sweating ceases, allowing the body's core temperature to rise precipitously. The skin is usually dry, and headache and dizziness are common. A person suffering from heatstroke may become quite disoriented, and may even experience convulsions or lose consciousness. He or she will likely feel quite hot to the touch; body temperature can go as high as 104° to 106°F. This is a true medical emergency.

EMERGENCY TREATMENT FOR HEATSTROKE

■ If you suspect heatstroke, call for emergency medical assistance right away. While waiting for help, clothing should be removed and the person sprayed with water while others actively fan him or her. Snow or ice may be used, but complete immersion is not recommended, as it is possible to lower the temperature too far too fast that way.

CONVENTIONAL TREATMENT

■ A person with heat exhaustion should lie down flat or, if possible, with the head lower than the feet in a shaded environment. Cool liquids, slightly salty if possible, should be taken at intervals. It is not necessary to consume very large amounts of salt or liquids, and in most cases oral fluid and electrolyte replacement is adequate. A day's rest is recommended after an episode of heat exhaustion.

■ In case of heatstroke, once emergency personnel arrive

to take over, rely on them to take appropriate measures and arrange for transport to the hospital. The goal in treating heatstroke is to get body temperature down to about 101°F (but not lower) within an hour. At the hospital, body temperature will be monitored. If necessary, medication may be administered to control convulsions. Since body temperature can be erratic for some time even once the crisis is past, it may be necessary to be hospitalized briefly for observation. After release from the hospital, several days of bed rest will likely be recommended.

DIETARY GUIDELINES

■ Get plenty of fluids. Fresh vegetable and fruit juices are good choices because they are rich in minerals and vitamins that help to revive the body and restore its normal electrolyte balance.

■ Eat simply, eat slowly, and chew your food thoroughly before swallowing. Your body is recovering from overwhelming stress, so you should avoid placing undue demands on your digestive system.

■ To help restore your body's normal mineral balance, salt your food for several days following the episode.

NUTRITIONAL SUPPLEMENTS

■ Green-drink supplements, available in health-food stores, are good sources of minerals and trace elements. These are generally sold in powder form, and can be mixed with either water or juice. Take a green-drink supplement, as directed on the product label, two or three times daily.

■ To normalize your digestive system, take a probiotic supplement such as acidophilus or bifidobacteria as recommended on the product label. If you are allergic to milk, be sure to select a dairy-free formula.

HERBAL TREATMENT

■ Linden and passionflower, taken in tea form, help to gently relieve stress and anxiety following an episode of heat exhaustion. Take a cup of either three times daily for a day or two.

BACH FLOWER REMEDIES

■ To speed recovery, take a dose of Rescue Remedy three times over the course of the first twenty-four hours.

AROMATHERAPY

For specific instructions on how to use aromatherapy, see PREPARING AROMATHERAPY TREATMENTS in Part Three.

■ Essential oil of pine is stimulating and energizing. Once your condition has stabilized and you are feeling better, enjoy a soak in a bath prepared with a few drops of pine oil.

PREVENTION

■ Avoid overly strenuous activity in hot weather. If you exercise on hot summer days, try to do so in either morning or evening, not in the middle of the day, and be sure to take in adequate fluids while exercising. If you become overheated, stop.

Hematoma

See under BRUISE.

Hemorrhage

See BLEEDING, SEVERE.

Hemophilia

Hemophilia is a bleeding disorder in which blood does not coagulate (clot) as it should. Blood clotting is a complex process involving a chain of reactions among different substances in the blood and blood vessels. In people with hemophilia, there is some degree of deficiency of one of these substances. There are two types of the disease, classified according to which of two different clotting factors is deficient. The more common form is hemophilia A, which involves a deficiency of what is called factor VIII. Hemophilia B involves inadequate levels of factor IX. The symptoms of the two forms of hemophilia are the same, but the specific treatments are different.

People with mild hemophilia may experience prolonged bleeding after surgery or a serious injury, but may not be much affected otherwise. For people with a significant degree of hemophilia, it is not so much external as internal bleeding that poses a problem. Internal bleeding can occur at any site in the body, but the locations most commonly affected are the joints such as the ankle, elbow, or knee; the gastrointestinal (GI) tract; and the muscles. Usually, a mild trauma—a small bump that might cause a bruise, if anything, in a healthy individual—sets off the problem, but if the degree of clotting-factor deficiency is severe, bleeding can start spontaneously. Over time, bleeding into the joints can cause progressive disability.

Hemophilia is caused by a defect in a single gene. For the most part, it is a sex-linked inherited disease of males, but a female could be affected if her father has the disease and her mother is a carrier. One particularly tragic side of the disease is that transfusions of blood products are frequently required, and many hemophiliacs contracted HIV (the virus that causes AIDS) before donated blood was adequately screened for its presence (or before the virus was even identified). Now, not only do many people with hemophilia also have AIDS, but AIDS often increases the severity of the bleeding problem. Hepatitis B and C also figure prominently as risks of transfusion.

CONVENTIONAL TREATMENT

■ Because of the complexity and intricacies of treatment, a person who has hemophilia should work closely with a hematologist or other physician who specializes in the treatment of this illness.

■ Transfusions of clotting-factor concentrates derived from donated plasma are the primary treatment. These are now heat-treated to kill the HIV virus. Specific dosages and regimens for administering these depend on the severity of the bleeding problem and other factors. Blood tests are used to monitor the effectiveness of treatment, and the treatment regimen may have to be adjusted periodically. It is possible to become immune to the transfused factors. In this case, the dosage may have to be increased, or it may be necessary to use drugs to decrease the immune response. Type B hemophilia poses the additional problem that factor IX concentrate is more likely than factor VIII concentrate to cause clotting. This makes decisions of when to administer transfusions more difficult.

■ If you have type A hemophilia, the drug desmopressin (DDAVP) may be used if you need to have a minor surgical procedure or dental work performed. Desmopressin is a synthetic version of vasopressin, a hormone secreted by the pituitary gland, and it has the effect of stimulating factor VIII levels. This treatment does not work for people with type B hemophilia, however.

■ *Avoid* aspirin and all other nonsteroidal anti-inflammatory drugs (NSAIDs) unless they are specifically prescribed by your physician. These drugs interfere with blood clotting. Many over-the-counter remedies include NSAIDs, so you should always read labels. When in doubt, check with your doctor or pharmacist.

■ Because of the risk of hepatitis associated with transfused blood products, vaccination against hepatitis B is often advised.

DIETARY GUIDELINES

■ Include in your diet plenty of green vegetables, such as broccoli, kale, and all leafy greens. These foods are good sources of vitamin K, which is needed for proper blood clotting.

NUTRITIONAL SUPPLEMENTS

■ To ensure an adequate supply of basic nutrients, take a good multivitamin and mineral supplement daily. Choose a powdered or capsule form for best absorption.

■ Green-foods supplements such as barley greens, spirulina, and blue-green algae are good sources of vitamin K and trace minerals. Take a green-foods supplement as directed on the product label.

■ Vitamin C and bioflavonoids help to maintain the strength and integrity of blood-vessel walls, which is important in preventing excessive bleeding. Take 500 to 1,000 milligrams of each two or three times daily.

■ Vitamin K, which is vital for blood clotting, is available in supplement form. Take 150 micrograms twice a day.

HERBAL TREATMENT

■ Bilberry and grape-seed extracts are rich sources of bioflavonoids that decrease the fragility of the capillaries. Choose standardized bilberry extract containing 25 percent anthocyanidins (also called PCOs) and take 80 milligrams three times a day. Or take 50 to 100 milligrams of standardized grape-seed extract containing 90 percent PCOs three times a day.

GENERAL RECOMMENDATIONS

■ Avoid anything that creates a risk of bleeding, external or internal.

■ Meticulous oral hygiene is important. This helps to prevent the need for invasive dental procedures.

■ Get regular exercise, but avoid activities such as football, wrestling, and skiing, which pose a high risk of injury. Non-contact activities such as swimming, walking, running, and cycling are good choices.

■ Do not take any drug, whether prescription or over-the-counter, without discussing it with your doctor or pharmacist to be sure it is safe.

■ If you bruise yourself, clean any wound and apply firm pressure. If bleeding continues, go to the emergency room of the nearest hospital. If you injure a joint, apply an ice pack, bandage the joint firmly, and go to the hospital immediately.

■ Obtain a Medic Alert bracelet or pendant and wear it at all times so that others will be alerted to your condition, if necessary (see the Resources section at the back of the book for more information).

PREVENTION

■ Hemophilia is genetic in origin, and there is no known way to prevent it. However, if you are a woman with a family history of the disease and are considering having children, you should seek genetic counseling to learn about your individual risks and options.

Hemorrhoids

Hemorrhoids are enlarged veins that develop in the lower rectum and/or anus when a vein becomes blocked. External hemorrhoids appear outside the anal opening. They are seldom painful, and there is no bleeding unless the hemorrhoidal vein breaks. Internal hemorrhoids begin above the opening of the anus. If they remain small, they may never be noticed unless they bleed during a bowel movement. If they do bleed, the blood is fresh and bright red. An internal hemorrhoid can become large enough to protrude from the anus, in which case it is known as a prolapsed hemorrhoid. Prolapsed hemorrhoids can become extremely painful. Additional symptoms include burning and itching sensations.

Hemorrhoids are very common. An estimated 50 to 70 percent of the population develop hemorrhoids at some time in their lives. Many people are unaware they have them. Hemorrhoids can occur in anyone at any time, but become more common with age. Women tend to develop hemorrhoids during pregnancy. They usually disappear a few months after the baby is born and the body is no longer under the stress of carrying a child.

In general, hemorrhoids are the result of increased pressure on the veins of the rectum and anus. This can occur as a result of constipation with consequent straining to expel hard feces that are difficult to pass. Hemorrhoids can also result from sitting or standing for long periods, or from lifting heavy or awkward objects incorrectly. Obesity, lack of exercise, too little fiber in the diet, and food allergies can be contributing factors.

CONVENTIONAL TREATMENT

■ Conservative treatment for hemorrhoids includes measures to minimize constipation and straining, such as increasing fluid intake and using stool softeners and/or supplementary fiber. Psyllium seed, Metamucil, and Fiberall are often recommended.

■ Though topical creams do not seem to offer great relief, suppositories that shrink and anesthetize, such as Anusol, may offer relief in the case of larger, protruding hemorrhoids, once they have been manually (gently!) worked back into place.

■ Warm sitz baths can help to relieve pain and itching.

■ If conservative measures are ineffective, injection sclerotherapy may be tried. This technique involves injecting the hemorrhoid with a chemical that shrinks and scars the inside of the mass. This can be effective in stopping bleeding.

■ If sclerotherapy fails, your doctor may recommend banding, or ligation, in which a tiny rubber band is placed around the base of the hemorrhoid, "strangling" it. The hemorrhoid then dies and is sloughed off.

■ Very large, painful hemorrhoids may require surgical opening and removal of some of the stretched tissue. A surgeon performing this procedure has to be careful not to remove too much tissue and not to allow infection, or scarring and narrowing of the rectum or anus may occur.

DIETARY GUIDELINES

Because constipation is a major factor in the development of hemorrhoids, it is essential to follow a high-fiber diet plan. Whole grains, fruits, and vegetables—both raw and cooked—should form the foundation of the diet.

Drink at least six 8-ounce glasses of pure water daily. Hard, dry feces that cause straining contribute to the occurrence of hemorrhoids. Water not only helps flush toxins from the body, but is essential to the formation of easily passed stool.

NUTRITIONAL SUPPLEMENTS

■ To reduce the discomfort of acute inflammation, take 500 milligrams of bromelain two to three times daily, as needed.

Flaxseed and olive oils provide much-needed lubrication and can help ease the pain associated with a bowel movement. Take one tablespoon of olive or flaxseed oil daily.

Magnesium helps prevent constipation and also improves liver and gallbladder function, which indirectly affect hemorrhoids. Take 350 milligrams of chelated magnesium twice daily.

Take a good probiotic supplement containing acidophilus or bifidobacteria. These friendly bacteria are essential for a healthy intestinal tract. Take it as recommended on the product label. If you are allergic to milk, select a dairy-free formula.

Vitamin C and bioflavonoids have anti-inflammatory action, are necessary for the manufacture of collagen, and help heal and strengthen tissue. Take 500 milligrams of vitamin C with bioflavonoids two to three times daily.

Vitamin E is a strong antioxidant that guards against free-radical damage. It also helps speed healing. Choose a product containing mixed tocopherols and start by taking 200 international units at bedtime, then gradually increase the dosage until you are taking 400 international units daily.

Note: If you are taking an anticoagulant (blood thin-ner), consult your physician before taking supplemental vitamin E.

HERBAL TREATMENT

■ Butcher's broom is commonly used against varicose veins, which are a close relative of hemorrhoids. It is very effective in helping to resolve hemorrhoids. Take 300 to 500 milligrams three times daily.

■ Carthamus and persica is an herbal combination that has been used in China for over 2,000 years to help hemorrhoids heal more quickly. It is especially effective if you have abdominal swelling and discomfort accompanied by flatulence. Take 500 milligrams three times daily.

■ Collinsonia, also known as stone root, is a mildly astringent herb that can be very effective in helping to shrink hemorrhoids. Take 500 milligrams three times daily for six to eight weeks.

■ Fargelin is an ancient herbal formula that is the first choice for hemorrhoids in the Chinese pharmacy. It helps shrink swollen tissue and reduces inflammation quickly. Follow the dosage directions on the product label.

■ Witch hazel leaves, brewed as a tea, can be applied topically. This soothing botanical helps reduce local inflammation, and also helps shrink swollen tissue. Apply it as needed.

HOMEOPATHY

■ *Aesculus hippocastanum* is the remedy for acute hemorrhoid pain and discomfort. You typically have a lot of pain after passing stool, and the pain can be so intense that it seems to run up your back. This remedy relieves the burning sensation in the anus, and eases bleeding hemorrhoids. It is also helpful for menopausal women with hemorrhoids. Take one dose of *Aesculus hippocastanum* 12x or 6c three times daily, as needed.

■ *Calcarea fluorica* is for bleeding hemorrhoids, with intolerable itching of the anus, accompanied by lower back pain and abdominal gas. You feel worse during changes in the weather, but better with the application of warmth. Take one dose of *Calcarea fluorica* 12x or 6c three times daily, as needed.

■ *Collinsonia* is good if you are constipated and have a frequent desire to pass stool, accompanied by lower abdominal gas. You have a lot of itching, a sense of constriction, and, possibly, bleeding. The stool may be dry and the hemorrhoids may be prolapsed (protruding). Take one dose of *Collinsonia* 12x or 6c three times daily, as needed.

■ *Hamamelis virginica* is the remedy of choice if the anus is raw, bruised, and bleeding. You may be uncomfortably conscious of a pulsing sensation in the area. Take one dose of *Hamamelis virginica* 12x or 6c three times daily, as needed.

■ *Nux vomica* is for hemorrhoids that are large and inflamed. You are usually sedentary; love rich, spicy foods; and may have a history of excessive alcohol consumption. You may also have a classic type-A personality. Take one dose of *Nux vomica* 12x or 6c three times daily, as needed.

■ *Sulfur* is the remedy if you have no bleeding, but the area around the anus is very red and inflamed. You feel worse with heat and dampness, prefer airy clothes, and often go without underwear. Take one dose of *Sulfur* 12x or 6c three times daily, as needed.

BACH FLOWER REMEDIES

Select the remedy that most closely fits your emotional tendencies and concerns, and take it as needed, following the directions on the product label.

Beech tames a tendency to be impatient, intolerant, and greatly upset by anything that disrupts your schedule.

Cherry plum eases fearfulness, particularly if you are the kind of person who avoids situations over which you have no control. For example, you may hate to fly and avoid air travel as much as possible.

Crabapple is the remedy to choose if you are compulsively neat and hate disorder and untidiness.

■ Choose Rock Water if you are always striving for perfection and are very hard on yourself. You may have a somewhat rigid and unforgiving nature.

ACUPRESSURE

For the locations of acupressure points on the body, *see* ADMINISTERING AN ACUPRESSURE TREATMENT in Part Three.

Bladder 25, 27, and 60 increase circulation in the lower digestive tract.

Kidney 1 improves circulation in the lower part of the body.

Liver 3 relaxes the nervous system.

Stomach 36 improves the utilization of nutrients.

AROMATHERAPY

For specific instructions on how to use aromatherapy, *see* PREPARING AROMATHERAPY TREATMENTS in Part Three.

You can enhance the effectiveness of sitz baths by incorporating aromatherapy into the treatment. Add a dozen or so drops of myrrh and/or tea tree oil to the bath water.

GENERAL RECOMMENDATIONS

■ Take measures to correct constipation. (*See* CONSTIPATION.)

■ Obesity is a contributing factor to hemorrhoids. If you are overweight, slim down. Adopt a sensible weight-loss program that includes exercise (*see* OBESITY).

■ People with very painful prolapsed hemorrhoids often find relief by sitting on a "doughnut." This is a foam-rubber pillow with a hole in the middle that prevents hemorrhoids from being crushed when you sit down, which adds to the pain.

PREVENTION

■ The best way to prevent hemorrhoids is to make sure your intestinal tract is in good working order. A healthy low-fat, fiber-rich diet is your first line of defense against constipation, which is the primary cause of hemorrhoids.

■ Consistent regular exercise tones the whole body, including the intestinal tract. People who exercise regularly are less likely to be troubled by hemorrhoids than those who do not.

Hepatitis

Hepatitis is a general term that means inflammation of the liver. Located just under the breastbone and extending to just under the bottom of the rib cage on the right side, the liver is the body's largest internal organ. Its functions include the production and metabolism of bile, which is necessary to metabolize fats, and the detoxification of harmful substances that find their way into the body. When the liver isn't working at top efficiency, as occurs during hepatitis, it cannot excrete bile efficiently. Bilirubin, an orange-red pigment normally excreted in bile, then builds up in the liver and can escape into the bloodstream. If it does, some accumulates in the skin, giving it the typical yellowish cast of jaundice, and some is excreted by the kidneys, making the urine dark. In severe hepatitis, the liver may become enlarged. Other symptoms include nausea, vomiting, loss of appetite, fever, malaise, flulike symptoms, clay-colored stools, and diarrhea.

Hepatitis can be caused by a wide range of viruses. In addition to the hepatitis A, B, and C viruses, Epstein-Barr virus (also responsible for infectious mononucleosis) and cytomegalovirus (CMV) can cause hepatitis. The diagnosis of which virus is involved is made based on the history of the illness and on blood tests. There are also drugs, toxins, and allergic reactions that can cause the liver to become inflamed.

There are three basic classifications of the disease. Hepatitis A, once called infectious hepatitis because of its highly contagious nature, is spread by direct contact with an infected person or through fecal-infected food or water.

It has a one-month incubation period—that is, it can take one month for the illness to appear after the virus enters the body—but illness can then come on very rapidly.

Hepatitis B has a two- to four-month incubation period. The onset is slow, the course may be longer, and the illness is more serious. Hepatitis B is not highly contagious. It can be transmitted by the transfusion of infected blood, by the use of unsterile needles and instruments, or through sexual contact. In addition to the standard symptoms, a person with hepatitis B may also have arthritis, rashes, and very itchy skin.

The hepatitis C virus is the one responsible for most cases of hepatitis related to blood transfusions, plasma, needles, or other instruments. The incubation period varies from six weeks to six months. This type of hepatitis is marked by the sudden onset of headache, fever, chills, general weakness, nausea, vomiting, abdominal pain, exhaustion, jaundice, and itching, and results in an enlarged and very tender liver.

There is no cure for hepatitis, but most people recover on their own without suffering permanent consequences. Recovery may take one to three months, however. A small percentage of people may develop chronic hepatitis, which lasts for six months or longer. The good news is that chronic hepatitis too may clear up without inflicting permanent harm, even if the sufferer has carried the virus for years. However, like cirrhosis, chronic hepatitis is associated with an increased risk of developing liver cancer.

CONVENTIONAL TREATMENT

■ Medical treatment for hepatitis consists primarily of observation to make sure the illness resolves and that complications do not develop. Hospitalization is reserved for the most serious cases, in which nitrogen builds up in the blood because the liver cannot process it normally. This can create complications in the brain. A low-protein, low-fat diet; intravenous infusions of potassium; laxatives; and medication to bring down blood-nitrogen levels may be used to correct this problem.

■ If you are diagnosed with hepatitis, your doctor may prescribe certain dietary modifications. Follow your doctor's instructions.

■ If nausea keeps you from eating an adequately nutritious diet, your doctor may prescribe an antiemetic (a drug that inhibits vomiting) such as prochlorperazine (Compazine), promethazine (Phenergan), or trimethobenzamide (Tigan).

■ During the acute and recovery phases of hepatitis, it is important to keep follow-up appointments with your physician to make certain the inflammation clears and does not become chronic.

■ *Avoid* any product that contains acetaminophen, such

as Tylenol, until your liver is healed. Acetaminophen is irritating to the liver, especially during the period of acute infection.

■ Interferon alfa is a drug that appears to have some effectiveness against chronic hepatitis B, as well as limited effectiveness against chronic hepatitis C.

■ If you are diagnosed with hepatitis A or B, close contacts of yours should be treated with immune globulin, which may prevent them from contracting the disease.

DIETARY GUIDELINES

■ Proper nutrition is essential for a full and timely recovery from hepatitis. When rested and supplied with the proper nutrients, the liver can actually regenerate itself. To rest the liver and allow it to heal, eliminate fats from your diet.

■ Most people with hepatitis have a poor appetite, yet supplying the body with the proper nutrients is essential. To support the body in the healing process, eat multiple very small, nutrient-dense meals daily.

■ Fruits are usually well tolerated. Try grapes, applesauce, and fruit juices diluted with spring water. Frozen fruit-juice popsicles are also good.

■ Lightly steamed greens, such as artichokes, collards, and endive, support the body during the healing process.

■ Keeping yourself well hydrated is very important. Keep a glass of fresh water by your bed and take frequent sips.

NUTRITIONAL SUPPLEMENTS

■ To ensure a supply of all the most vital nutrients, take a multivitamin and mineral complex supplying 25 milligrams of each of the major B vitamins three times daily. To help to restore energy, take an additional 100 micrograms of vitamin B_{12} three times daily as well.

■ Acidophilus and bifidobacteria help to maintain friendly flora in the gastrointestinal tract. Take bifidobacteria during the acute phase of the illness, acidophilus during the recovery period, as directed on the product label. If you are allergic to milk, be sure to select dairy-free formulas.

■ Catechin, a bioflavonoid, pine-bark extract, and grape-seed extract have been shown to be very helpful in treating the symptoms of hepatitis. Take 500 milligrams of catechin two to three times daily or 50 milligrams of pine-bark or grape-seed extract twice a day until recovery is complete.

■ Chlorophyll is high in vitamins and minerals, especially magnesium. It helps to restore and detoxify the blood. Take 500 milligrams two or three times daily. Or take a green-foods supplement, such as spirulina or chlorella, that supplies an equivalent amount of chlorophyll.

■ Choline, a component of lecithin, is beneficial to the liver. Take 250 milligrams of phosphatidylcholine or choline citrate twice daily until recovery is complete.

■ Coenzyme Q_{10} increases tissue oxygenation at the cellular level, and is helpful in fighting viral infection. Take 25 milligrams two or three times daily.

■ Selenium, vitamin E, and lipoic acid fight free radicals that can damage the liver. Take 100 to 200 micrograms of selenium and 400 international units of vitamin E daily. Also take 25 milligrams of lipoic acid two to three times daily.

   Note: If you are taking an anticoagulant (blood thinner), consult your physician before taking vitamin E.

   Vitamin C and bioflavonoids have an anti-inflammatory effect. Take 500 to 1,000 milligrams of each three times a day during the acute phase. Then take 500 to 1,000 milligrams of each a day for one month.

   Avoid any supplements containing iron during the acute phase of the infection. A stressed liver cannot process iron effectively.

HERBAL TREATMENT

■ Castor-oil packs reduce acute inflammation and help restore proper liver function. Prepare a warm castor-oil pack by saturating several layers of clean white cloth with the oil. You can either warm the oil before preparing the pack or prepare the pack, place it on a clean plate, and warm it in a microwave oven for twenty to thirty seconds. Make sure the pack is warm, not hot. Place the warm pack over the upper right quadrant of your abdomen and leave it in place for fifteen to twenty minutes. Do this once a day for five to seven days.

   Dandelion root, taken in tea or extract form, is noted for its strengthening effect on the liver. Take 500 milligrams or one cup of tea three times a day for up to one month.

   To support your immune system and give it a boost, take echinacea and goldenseal. This herbal combination is both antibacterial and antiviral. Take one dose of an echinacea and goldenseal combination formula supplying 350 to 500 milligrams of echinacea and 200 to 350 milligrams of goldenseal twice a day for one week. Then discontinue for one week. Repeat this cycle for up to six weeks.

■ Gentian strengthens the liver and helps normalize the flow of bile. When used in conjunction with goldenseal and dandelion, it helps stimulate the appetite. Take 250 to 500 milligrams twice daily, with the two largest meals of the day.

■ Milk thistle is good for any type of liver inflammation. Choose an extract standardized to contain 80 percent flavonoids (silymarin) and take 100 to 200 milligrams three times daily during the acute phase, and twice a day for one month during recovery.

■ Schizandra is a Chinese herb that has been sucessfully used for thousands of years for liver complaints. It reduces inflammation and promotes healing. Take 250 milligrams of schizandra upon arising and again at bedtime. There are also many Chinese patent medicines and liver-related formulas that combine schizandra with bupleurum, which strengthens the immune system and is especially helpful to the liver. These remedies are excellent for the recovery stage, once fever and all other signs of acute infection are gone. Choose such a formula and take it as directed on the product label twice daily for one to two months.

HOMEOPATHY

■ *Phosphorus* is the first homeopathic remedy to try for hepatitis. Take one dose of *Phosphorus* 30x or 9c, as recommended on the product label, twice daily for three days. Stop for three days. Then take one dose twice daily for another three days. Then choose one of the symptom-specific remedies that follow.

■ *Chelidonium* helps to relieve pain in the upper right quadrant of the abdomen, over the liver, as well as in the right shoulder. Take one dose of *Chelidonium* 12x or 6c three times a day until the pain lessens.

■ If you are having difficulty sleeping, try *Coffea cruda*. This remedy can help even an anxious person drift off to sleep. Take one dose of *Coffea cruda* 12x or 6c one hour before dinner, and another dose half an hour before bedtime.

■ *Lycopodium* is the remedy to select if you are suffering from flatulence and discomfort due to bowel gases. This remedy is also excellent if you are feeling anxious, especially if you are worrying about personal responsibilities that may be neglected during the recovery period. *Lycopodium* promotes mental relaxation. Take one dose of *Lycopodium* 30x or 15c three times daily for up to three days. Stop for one week, then repeat.

■ *Nux vomica* is useful for nausea. Take one dose of *Nux vomica* 30x or 9c three times a day, up to a total of six doses.

■ *Taraxacum* helps relieve bitter burping and nausea. It is also helpful for pain on the left side of the abdomen. Take one dose of *Taraxacum* 12x or 6c three times a day for up to four days.

ACUPRESSURE

For the locations of acupressure points on the body, *see* ADMINISTERING AN ACUPRESSURE TREATMENT in Part Three.

■ Four Gates is calming and soothing if you are feeling restless and uncomfortable.

GENERAL RECOMMENDATIONS

■ Get plenty of rest. This is of primary importance in the treatment of hepatitis.

■ Ask your doctor about the need for isolation from other household members. Some doctors recommend that an individual with hepatitis not have contact with others for at least three weeks from the beginning of the illness.

■ If you do not have a dishwasher, wash your dishes and tableware with hot water and antibacterial soap, separately from those used by other members of the household.

■ Wash your bed linens separately in hot water liberally laced with a disinfectant such as chlorine bleach. Do not mix contaminated bed linen with other family wash.

■ You are no longer considered contagious seven to ten days after the onset of jaundice. Be sure to check with your doctor first, but if you are feeling well, you may be able to return to work around this time.

PREVENTION

■ If you learn that someone you have close contact with has, or has been exposed to, hepatitis, contact your physician immediately. Immune globulin increases the immune response to a variety of viruses, including hepatitis A. To prevent or reduce the symptoms of hepatitis, it must be given within two weeks of exposure. Some doctors recommend this treatment prior to foreign travel as well. Possible side effects include allergic reaction, and pain and swelling at the site of the injection. If you are exposed to a person with a known case of hepatitis B, your doctor may administer hepatitis B immune globulin (HBIG). This is given not to cure hepatitis, but rather to protect a person who has been exposed to hepatitis from getting the illness. Some people, unfortunately, have allergic reactions to this drug.

■ A vaccine that protects against hepatitis B is available. Medical doctors now recommend that all infants and children, as well as people considered to be at high risk of the disease, receive a series of vaccinations against hepatitis B. A vaccine for hepatitis A was recently approved by the U.S. Food and Drug Administration (FDA). It can be administered two weeks before anticipated exposure to the virus (if you will be traveling to a part of the world where exposure is likely, for example).

Hernia, Hiatal

Hiatal hernia is the name given to a defect that allows a portion of the stomach to pass through the opening (hiatus) in the diaphragm and slip into the chest. There are three types of hiatal hernias. In persons with a *sliding hiatal hernia*, a small portion of the stomach slides into and out of place. With a *paraesophageal rolling hernia*, a portion of the stomach protrudes up and out of the diaphragm and remains there, beside the esophagus. Some people have *mixed hernias*, which include features of both.

Sliding hernias are much more common than the esophageal type, and in many cases cause no symptoms at all. If there are symptoms, they generally include a feeling of fullness in the chest, a sensation similar to angina pain, and pain resulting from spasms in the chest. If the symptoms are severe, they can be mistaken for those of a heart attack. Most sliding hernias are a result of muscle weakness that often accompanies aging. This condition is more common in women than in men, and the incidence rises with age.

Acid reflux is the most common complaint associated with esophageal hernias. This occurs when a backup of stomach acid enters the esophagus, causing pain in the lower part of the esophagus and heartburn, or a burning sensation in the chest and upper abdomen. These symptoms can sometimes be mistaken for those of a heart attack in progress. It should be noted, however, that not all people who suffer from acid reflux have hiatal hernias, and not all people with hiatal hernias are troubled by acid reflux.

Regardless of the type of hernia, symptoms can occur anywhere from one to four hours after eating. Heartburn, burping, regurgitation of acid into the throat, vomiting, pain, and muscle spasms in the chest may all be experienced to some degree. Symptoms tend to be worse if you have overeaten or are bending or stooping, and are usually much worse when you lie down.

Hiatal hernias are very common, especially among older people who are overweight. It is estimated that almost half of all people over forty years of age have them. By themselves, hiatal hernias are not considered dangerous. However, continuing acid reflux can lead to inflammation, even ulceration, of the esophagus, and should be treated. If your symptoms are severe, tests may be recommended to make sure your esophagus is healthy, to measure the buildup of acid, and to check on the extent of a hiatal hernia.

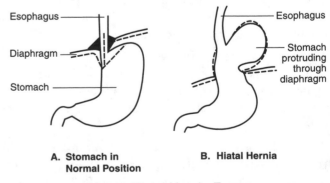

A. Stomach in Normal Position **B. Hiatal Hernia**

How a Hiatal Hernia Forms

CONVENTIONAL TREATMENT

■ If a hiatal hernia causes no symptoms, no treatment is required.

■ If there is burning and pain, over-the-counter antacids are likely to be recommended first. Be sure to choose a product that does *not* contain aluminum. A calcium-based formula is best.

■ If antacids are not effective, an acid-blocker may be recommended. These drugs decrease the amount of acid produced by the stomach. Some are available by prescription, others over the counter. Examples include cimetidine (Tagamet), famotidine (Pepcid), nizatidine (Axid), and ranitidine (Zantac). Side effects can include nausea, vomiting, changes in bowel habits (diarrhea or constipation), abdominal pain, liver damage, blood abnormalities, and rashes. Joint pains and heart-rhythm changes, while rare, can occur as well.

■ Some doctors prescribe drugs that enhance peristalsis, the wavelike movements of the gastrointestinal tract that move food through the system. Speeding peristalsis can tighten the valve, or sphincter, that separates the stomach from the esophagus. Examples of this kind of drug include cisapride (Propulsid), bethanechol (Urecholine), and metoclopramide (Reglan). Side effects of cisapride can include headache, abdominal pain, runny nose, infections, and abnormal vision. Rarely, there can be serious heart arrhythmias. Bethanechol can cause low blood pressure, nausea, vomiting, diarrhea, cramps, asthma, headache, flushing, and involuntary bowel movements. Metoclopramide can be responsible for dizziness, stomach upset, jerking movements reminiscent of Parkinson's disease, and considerable fatigue. All of these drugs interact with a number of other medications, and may be secreted into a nursing mother's milk, so if you must take them, follow your doctor's instructions carefully.

■ If more aggressive treatment is needed—for instance, if reflux is causing damage to the esophagus—a type of drug called a proton-pump inhibitor may be prescribed. These drugs too interfere with the secretion of stomach acid, but are more potent than ordinary acid blockers. Examples include omeprazole (Prilosec) and lansoprazole (Prevacid). Possible side effects include headache, diarrhea, and abdominal pain. Though people who take these drugs often need to use them on an ongoing basis, only omeprazole is intended for that purpose.

■ If necessary, surgery can be performed to repair damaged tissue. This procedure often can be performed through a laparoscope, which requires only a tiny incision and is less traumatic than older surgical techniques.

DIETARY GUIDELINES

■ Modify your diet. Fried foods, spicy foods, and very hot or very cold foods can all make symptoms worse. Avoid dietary extremes.

■ An overly full stomach worsens symptoms. Do not eat large meals. Instead, eat only small amounts of food at any one time. Eat slowly and chew each bite well.

■ Drink 1 to 2 ounces of cabbage juice two to three times daily for two weeks. This common cruciferous vegetable contains phytochemicals that help soothe the gastric lining. Cabbage juice has been used for centuries for ulcers. It can provide exceptional relief for acid reflux.

■ Papaya is an excellent source of digestive enzymes. Enjoy it often.

■ Avoid citrus fruit juices and coffee. These common beverages contribute to additional acid in the stomach.

■ Do not eat anything for at least two hours before going to bed. You may be able to avoid problems simply by giving your stomach time to empty out before you lie down.

NUTRITIONAL SUPPLEMENTS

■ To counteract acidity, take 1 tablespoon of a liquid calcium and magnesium combination formula twice a day. This is often more effective than prescription or over-the-counter antacid formulas.

■ Green clay, available in health-food stores, neutralizes excess acid. Stir 1 tablespoon of green clay into a glass of spring water, and allow it to sit overnight. Take frequent sips of the treated water throughout the following day. Green clay has excellent antacid properties.

■ To ease digestive problems that may contribute to symptoms, take a digestive-enzyme formula that includes bromelain and/or papain with each meal. Choose a formula *without* hydrochloric acid (HCl). HCl is part of the normal digestive juices, but if you have a hiatal hernia, adding more acid can worsen symptoms rather than alleviating them.

■ Magnesium is essential to the central nervous system and can help relax the upper abdomen. Take 250 milligrams of chelated magnesium twice daily. If you develop loose stools, stop taking it for three days, then try it again at one-quarter the previous dose.

■ Take a good multivitamin and mineral supplement daily. While excess stomach acid can make you uncomfortable, your body makes acid for a reason. Long-term inhibition of acid production can hinder the absorption of nutrients, leading to deficiencies.

■ For overall gastrointestinal health, take a probiotic supplement containing acidophilus and bifidobacteria as recommended on the product label. Acidophilus can also calm acid symptoms.

■ If you have hard stools and are constantly constipated,

take a tablespoon of flaxseed or olive oil twice a day and increase your consumption of water. This will soften stools and prevent straining. Straining the lower abdomen can worsen symptoms.

■ If you follow a vegetarian diet, or have problems with constipation, ask your doctor about injections of vitamin B$_{12}$. This essential element of the B complex is found only in foods of animal origin, so deficiency is common among vegetarians.

HERBAL TREATMENT

■ Aloe vera has a healing and cooling effect on the digestive tract. Select a food-grade product and start by taking $^1/_8$ cup once or twice daily, then gradually increase to $^1/_4$ cup once or twice daily.

■ Fare You is a Chinese patent medicine whose chief ingredient is cabbage. It is especially good if you have upper abdominal pain or a history of peptic ulcer. Take it as directed on the product label.

■ Slippery elm is very soothing to the entire digestive tract. Take 500 milligrams two or three times a day, as needed.

HOMEOPATHY

■ *Argentum nitricum* is the remedy for frequent burping. You may have a history of peptic ulcer and you probably crave sweet foods, although you have difficulty digesting them. Take one dose of *Argentum nitricum* 30x or 15c three times daily for up to three days.

■ Try *Arsenicum album* if you awaken between 1:00 and 4:00 AM with gnawing pain and indigestion. You may feel very thirsty, but usually drink only a little bit. You may also have feelings of anxiety that register in the pit of your stomach, and crave acidic foods, including coffee, citrus juices, and vinegar dressings—all of which contribute to acid reflux and heartburn pain. Take one dose of *Arsenicum album* 200x or 200c daily for up to two days. Stop for one week. If your symptoms have improved, but not to your satisfaction, repeat the regimen and consult with your health-care provider. In addition to taking *Arsenicum album*, you should avoid eating too many raw vegetables and too much melon.

■ *Carbo vegetabilis* is for a too-full feeling with an upper abdomen that is swollen and painful to the touch. You may feel sleepy and have a burning feeling in your stomach about thirty minutes after you eat, and you probably burp a lot. Your digestion is so sluggish that foods can putrefy before digestion is accomplished. Take one dose of *Carbo vegetabilis* 30x or 15c three times daily for up to three days. Stop for one week. If your symptoms have improved, but not to your satisfaction, repeat the regimen and consult with your health-care provider.

■ Choose *Lycopodium* if you have a lot of stomach gas and a swollen abdomen. You find yourself easily and openly irritated at home, but force yourself to stay pleasant at work. Take one dose of *Lycopodium* 30x or 15c three times daily for up to three days.

■ *Nux vomica* is for heartburn caused by an acid stomach that occurs soon after a meal. This remedy is recommended if you enjoy indulging in rich, spicy foods; possibly consume alcohol to excess; and are generally a workaholic with a type-A personality. Take one dose of *Nux vomica* 30x or 15c three times a day for up to three days. Stop for one week. If your symptoms have improved, but not to your satisfaction, repeat the regimen and consult with your health-care provider.

ACUPRESSURE

For the locations of acupressure points on the body, *see* ADMINISTERING AN ACUPRESSURE TREATMENT in Part Three.

■ Bladder 14, 15, 16, 17, 18, 19, and 20 improve circulation in the gastrointestinal tract.

■ Gallbladder 21 improves circulation in the upper part of the body.

■ Pericardium 6 relaxes the chest and upper digestive tract.

■ Stomach 36 harmonizes and tones the digestive system, and strengthens overall well-being.

AROMATHERAPY

For specific instructions on how to use aromatherapy, *see* PREPARING AROMATHERAPY TREATMENTS in Part Three.

■ There are a number of essential oils that can help improve digestion, among them bergamot, frankincense, lavender, neroli, peppermint, and thyme. Add any one to three of these oils to massage oil and gently massage your abdomen and back as needed.

GENERAL RECOMMENDATIONS

■ Avoid activities that increase abdominal pressure, such as straining during bowel movements. Do not wear tight clothing that constricts the area.

■ If you have a cough, take measures to suppress it (*see* COUGH). Coughing can trigger a sliding hiatal hernia and worsen symptoms.

■ See a chiropractor. You may require several adjustments to bring the stomach into its correct position, but chiropractic treatment can yield excellent results.

■ Do not smoke. Smoking stimulates the production of stomach acids and can worsen symptoms.

PREVENTION

■ Because weakened muscles are a primary cause of

hiatal hernia, exercises such as sit-ups, which strengthen the upper chest and abdominal muscles, may help prevent this condition.

Herpes

Herpes viruses are a family of viruses that cause skin eruptions or blisters. The herpes simplex virus 1 (HSV1) usually causes cold sores (also known as fever blisters). Herpes simplex virus 2 (HSV2) involves the genitals and is usually, although not always, passed through sexual contact. The varicella-zoster virus causes chickenpox and shingles. Zoster oticus involves facial nerves. The Epstein-Barr virus causes mononucleosis.

This entry addresses the problems caused by HSV1 and HSV2. Once these viruses enter the body, they can remain dormant in the nervous system for varying amounts of time. They can then be reactivated by fever, physical or emotional stress, excessive exposure to sunlight, and some foods or drugs. Herpes outbreaks can recur for life, but they generally taper off after age fifty.

Herpes simplex produces small, irritating fluid-filled blisters and red, burning, itchy sores on the skin and mucous membranes. It also affects the nervous system. Symptoms of HSV generally make themselves known within one or two weeks after contraction of the virus.

The initial symptoms of HSV1 include a burning, tingling, or itching sensation around the edges of the lips or nose as a cold sore begins to form. Small red pimples develop within a few hours, followed by the formation of small fever blisters filled with fluid. The blisters itch and hurt and are very annoying. You may run a mild fever, and the lymph nodes in your neck may become enlarged. After about seven days, the blisters form thin yellow crusts, indicating that the virus has run its course and healing has begun.

In both men and women, initial symptoms of HSV2 include a burning, tingling, or itching sensation in the genital area, progressing to painful blisters on the skin and moist linings of the sex organs. The fluid-filled blisters turn into red and painful surface sores that itch and burn and can easily become infected. Fever and swelling of the lymph nodes in the groin are common. Members of both sexes may experience pain when urinating.

Both HSV1 and HSV2 infections are extremely common. According to some estimates, over 90 percent of the American population will soon be infected with the herpes virus. A herpes outbreak can be extremely irritating and uncomfortable. For those who have had herpes before, the early burning and tingling sensation signals an imminent outbreak. Knowing what's coming can add to the stress, which in turn may increase the severity of the outbreak. Once the blisters form into sores, healing usually occurs within seven to ten days.

An HSV2 infection in a pregnant woman poses a serious danger to the fetus. The virus can travel from the infected genitals to the fetus, or a newborn can contract the illness from contact with the lesions during the birth process. The herpes virus can then attack the baby's nervous system, leading to seizures, mental retardation, or developmental disabilities. To avoid infecting a baby with this serious illness, it is recommended that infants be delivered by cesarean section if the mother has a herpes outbreak within three weeks of delivery.

CONVENTIONAL TREATMENT

■ The treatment of cold sores caused by HSV is aimed at relieving symptoms. To reduce the risk of secondary infection, you can gently wash the sores with soap and water. Ointments that inhibit the herpes virus (see below) may be helpful in speeding healing.

■ A viscous solution of lidocaine (Xylocaine) is a topical anesthetic that can be prescribed to decrease the pain of a herpes sore in the mouth.

Note: It is extremely important not to exceed the recommended dosage of this drug because of its potential toxicity.

■ To ease discomfort, you can take acetaminophen (in Tylenol, Datril, and other products) or ibuprofen (Advil, Motrin, Nuprin, and others).

Note: In excessive amounts, acetaminophen can cause liver damage. Do not exceed the recommended dosage.

■ An astringent such as Campho-Phenique can help relieve symptoms and speed healing, although it may sting when first applied.

■ The antiviral acyclovir (Zovirax) is a common treatment for genital and oral herpes. It is a relatively safe and well-tolerated drug, and some people have taken it for years. The course of treatment requires that the drug be taken every four hours for up to ten days. If you take acyclovir on a regular basis as a preventive measure, exercise caution. When the drug is stopped, outbreaks sometimes become more severe. However, studies show that this drug does prevent outbreaks in over 90 percent of patients. Acyclovir is also available in ointment form. When applied at the beginning of an outbreak, it can minimize the severity of the attack, but it is not as effective as the oral form of the drug.

DIETARY GUIDELINES

■ To help cleanse your system, keep yourself well hydrated. Drink at least six to eight 8-ounce glasses of pure water every day. Herbal teas (without caffeine) also are highly recommended, as are vegetable soups and juices.

■ Maintain a nutritious diet of healthy whole foods, including plenty of vegetables.

■ Avoid processed foods, soft drinks, alcohol, sugar, refined carbohydrates, and any beverages that contain caffeine. All of these contribute to a buildup of toxins in the body.

■ During an outbreak, or when one is imminent, reduce (or eliminate) foods containing the amino acid L-arginine, which can promote the growth of the virus. Foods containing L-arginine include whole-wheat products, brown rice, raw cereals (including oatmeal), chocolate, carob, corn (including popcorn), dairy products, raisins, nuts, and seeds.

■ While the virus is active, eliminate from your diet acidic citrus fruits and juices, such as orange and grapefruit juice. An overly acidic internal environment can slow healing.

■ Eating soft, cool foods may cause less discomfort to a sore mouth.

NUTRITIONAL SUPPLEMENTS

■ An outbreak of herpes is a sign that the body is under stress, and stress increases your requirements for all nutrients. Take a good multivitamin and mineral supplement daily.

■ Folic acid and vitamin B_{12} help to heal mucous membranes and are helpful for oral herpes. Chew a 400- or 800-microgram tablet of folic acid three times a day for one week or until the outbreak subsides. Also take 250 micrograms of vitamin B_{12} each day for one week. If you take any of the B vitamins individually, you should also take a B-complex supplement at a different time of day.

■ *Lactobacillus acidophilus* helps to balance the acidity of the body and thus speed healing. Take an acidophilus supplement for two weeks, following the dosage directions on the product label. If you are allergic to milk, choose a dairy-free formula.

■ The amino acid lysine fights the herpes virus. Take 250 milligrams of L-lysine four times a day (on an empty stomach) for one to two weeks. Then take the same dose twice a week for three months. L-lysine is also available in a cream form. The application of this over-the-counter cream can help minimize an outbreak.

■ Selenium and vitamin E have antioxidant properties and activate the immune system. Vitamin E is also an anti-inflammatory that is helpful in treating all skin conditions. Take 200 micrograms of selenium and 400 international units of vitamin E (in mixed-tocopherol form) once or twice daily for the duration of the outbreak.

Note: If you have high blood pressure, limit your intake of supplemental vitamin E to a total of 400 international units daily. If you are taking an anticoagulant (blood thinner), consult your physician before taking supplemental vitamin E.

■ Mineral ascorbate vitamin C and bioflavonoids have anti-inflammatory properties. Take 500 to 1,000 milligrams of each three times daily for three days. Then take one dose a day for four days, followed by one-half dose a day for one week.

HERBAL TREATMENT

■ Echinacea and goldenseal have antiviral and astringent properties. They also stimulate the immune system, help detoxify the blood, and soothe irritated mucous membranes. Take one dose of an echinacea and goldenseal combination formula supplying 350 to 500 milligrams of echinacea and 250 to 350 milligrams of goldenseal three times daily during a herpes outbreak. A liquid formula is preferred because it is more bioavailable, meaning that it is more readily used by the body. You can also use this remedy topically to help dry out the lesions.

■ Garlic has antiviral properties helpful in treating herpes. Take 500 milligrams three times a day for one week. Then take the same dose once a day for one week.

■ Glycyrrhizic-acid ointment, formulated from licorice root, speeds healing.

■ Goldenseal powder can be made into a paste and applied topically to dry out the lesions.

■ A topical solution of grapefruit-seed extract and tea tree oil, available in health-food stores, fights bacterial and viral infection and can shorten the length of an outbreak. Follow the directions on the product label.

■ Licorice root has antibiotic properties that are helpful in clearing an infection and detoxifying the blood. Take 300 to 500 milligrams two to three times daily for up to three days during an outbreak.

Note: Do not use licorice on a daily basis for more than five days at a time, as it can elevate blood pressure. Do not use it at all if you have high blood pressure.

■ Topical melissa is an excellent healing salve for herpes. Follow the label directions.

HOMEOPATHY

The following homeopathic remedies are recommended for oral herpes. They are also helpful for genital herpes if the penis or testes are swollen, or if there is inflammation of the vulva. Use these remedies if a genital herpes outbreak is accompanied by a sore throat.

■ If your tongue and the inside of your mouth are swollen, red, and dry, and pushing the tongue against the floor of the mouth causes pain, take *Mercurius corrosivus* or *Mercurius solubilis* 12x, 30x, 6c, or 9c. You probably are feeling subdued, with a depressed spirit. Take one dose three times daily for up to three days.

■ *Natrum muriaticum* is for mouth sores accompanied by an increased desire for salt. Take one dose of *Natrum muriaticum* 12x, 30x, 6c, or 9c three times daily for up to three days.

■ If neither of the above remedies seems right, a combination homeopathic herpes remedy may be helpful.

ACUPRESSURE

For the locations of acupressure points on the body, *see* ADMINISTERING AN ACUPRESSURE TREATMENT in Part Three.

■ Four Gates relaxes the nervous system.

■ Spleen 10 detoxifies the blood.

GENERAL RECOMMENDATIONS

■ Stress can add to the possibility and severity of an outbreak. Take measures to learn to manage stressful situations. Allow yourself to talk about your feelings and concerns, and accept the support of others. Learn and practice relaxation techniques. Get plenty of rest.

■ Practice scrupulous hygiene. Keep the genital area clean.

■ To encourage air circulation, if you have genital herpes, wear loose-fitting cotton underwear. Males should wear boxer shorts, not briefs. Briefs hold the genitals close to the body, creating a warm, moist environment that fosters the growth of the virus. For both sexes, bikinis are out, especially the nylon ones, which don't breathe.

PREVENTION

■ Cold sores are highly contagious. Try to minimize contact with anyone who is infected.

■ Although genital herpes is not always contracted through sexual contact with an infected partner, this is the primary method of transmission. The best way to avoid this disorder is to have a monogamous relationship with a partner you know to be healthy. If you have multiple partners, and/or if you engage in sex with anyone whose health status is unknown to you, *always* use a latex (not animal-skin) condom. Be aware, however, that even a latex condom is not a 100-percent guarantee against sexually transmitted disease.

Hiccups

Hiccups are sudden, involuntary spasms of the diaphragm, the muscular structure that separates the abdomen from the chest. They are usually harmless and most go away on their own within a few minutes. Everyone gets hiccups from time to time. Even babies in utero can have hiccups.

Hiccups have a variety of causes, most often indigestion and too-rapid eating. If you eat too fast, you will sometimes swallow air. With no place to go, the swallowed air can attempt to come out as hiccups. Prolonged bouts of hiccups result from irritation of the nerve that serves the diaphragm. Long-lasting cases usually have identifiable causes, such as pneumonia, pleurisy, abdominal surgery, tumors, bowel disease, pancreatic disease, or other conditions that can continuously irritate the diaphragm.

CONVENTIONAL TREATMENT

■ In very extreme and rare cases, a sedative may be prescribed, or carbon dioxide may be administered with oxygen (raising the level of carbon dioxide in the blood tends to inhibit the spasms). Other methods that have been tried for severe and long-lasting hiccups include placing tubes in the esophagus to dilate it, administering nerve blocks, and even surgery to cut nerves. For the overwhelming majority of cases, however, your doctor is likely to make suggestions similar to the ones listed under General Recommendations, below.

HOMEOPATHY

■ Follow these five steps to get rid of hiccups:

1. Begin with one dose of *Aconite* 30x, 200x, 9c, or 30c. Wait five minutes.

2. If the hiccups are still occurring, take one dose of *Arnica* 30x or 9c. Wait another five minutes.

3. If you are still hiccupping, take one dose of *Ignatia* 30x or 9c and wait five minutes

4. If you are *still* hiccupping, take one dose of *Magnesia phosphorica* 30x or 9c. Wait five minutes.

5. Finally, you can try a dose of *Lycopodium* 30x or 9c. This remedy is especially helpful if you have a history of low bowel gas and repeated hiccups.

ACUPRESSURE

For the locations of acupressure points on the body, *see* ADMINISTERING AN ACUPRESSURE TREATMENT in Part Three.

■ Pericardium 6 helps to relax the chest.

GENERAL RECOMMENDATIONS

Everyone has a favorite way of getting rid of hiccups. Many people have found the following measures helpful.

■ Slowly sip several glasses of cold water.

■ Take a deep breath and hold it for as long as possible. It may help if you tip your head far backward while doing this.

- Breathe into a paper bag.

- Slowly sip cold water while holding your breath.

- Gargle with water for a minute or two.

- Lean over and sip cold water from the opposite rim of the glass.

- Have someone close your ears with his or her thumbs and slowly sip water while holding your breath.

- Try pulling on your tongue, pressing gently on your eyeballs, or rapidly swallowing cold water or ice. These measures stimulate the vagus nerve, which can help stop hiccups.

PREVENTION

- Eating slowly is probably the best way to prevent hiccups. To avoid swallowing air, eat at a leisurely pace. Avoid overeating.

- If you are prone to hiccups, avoiding overly spicy foods, alcohol, carbonated beverages, and other dietary irritants may help to prevent a problem.

High Blood Pressure

Blood pressure, the force exerted by the blood against arterial walls, is what keeps blood circulating. If the level of pressure in the blood vessels is inadequate, circulation is impaired and may even stop. However, if the pressure is too high, it places a strain on the arteries that can lead to serious problems throughout the body. Of all the risk factors for cardiovascular disease, high blood pressure is one of the greatest. This is especially true for people over sixty-five, the age group most likely to suffer from heart disease.

A blood-pressure reading consists of two numbers, which represent the pressure within the blood vessels at two different phases of the heart's cycle. The first number, the systolic pressure, is the highest amount of pressure against the arterial walls, which occurs when the heart contracts to pump out blood. The second number, the diastolic pressure, is the pressure between heartbeats, when the heart is relaxed.

There is no single blood-pressure reading that is normal for everyone. Most newborns have systolic readings between 20 and 60, and that number generally rises progressively throughout life. For healthy adults, however, a reading of 120/80 (120 over 80) is widely considered the norm. Even so, blood pressure varies throughout the day in response to your level of activity, stress, and other factors. Blood pressure also normally rises somewhat with age. Tense or excitable individuals often experience a rise

in blood pressure simply as a result of having their blood pressure read, which results in a false reading. Some doctors take a second reading after giving a nervous patient time to calm down.

High blood pressure, known to doctors as *hypertension,* is one of the liabilities of modern life. Factors common to this day and age that foster an unhealthy rise in blood pressure include poor dietary choices—excessive consumption of alcoholic and caffeine-containing beverages, for example—a lack of exercise, and the multiplicity of stresses we are all subjected to.

About 90 percent of all people diagnosed with elevated blood pressure suffer from essential, or primary, hypertension. This is simply high blood pressure that has no obvious underlying cause. The remaining 10 percent have high blood pressure as a result of some other condition or disorder, such as kidney disease or adrenal or thyroid problems. Sometimes high blood pressure is a side effect of certain medications. Nearly one in five Americans, around 50 million people, have high blood pressure. The incidence is twice as high among African-Americans as it is among people of other ethnic backgrounds, and it affects more men than women.

It is possible to have high blood pressure and not know it. While some people with the condition suffer headaches, sweating, episodes of dizziness, and even nosebleeds that send them to the doctor, most experience no symptoms at all. High blood pressure may go undiscovered until detected during a routine physical or an examination for another health problem.

Essential hypertension seems to run in families. Although it usually doesn't surface until middle age, some people seem to be more prone to develop high blood pressure than others. Whether this is a result of genetics or lifestyle choices passed down within families is not known, however. High blood pressure has been linked to diet, alcohol consumption, smoking, the use of stimulants, drug abuse, excessive consumption of sodium and caffeine, and obesity. In some cases, women on birth control pills develop hypertension, and a rise in blood pressure is not uncommon during pregnancy.

A small percentage of people with high blood pressure have what is known as *malignant hypertension.* This does not refer to cancer, but rather signifies that it is a form of high blood pressure that is dangerous and difficult to control. Diabetes, kidney disease, certain disorders of the adrenal glands, or coarctation (narrowing) of the aorta can all lead to malignant hypertension. Although rare, this condition comes on suddenly and causes the blood pressure to shoot up dangerously. If left untreated, malignant hypertension becomes life-threatening in a very short time.

CONVENTIONAL MEDICINE

- If lifestyle changes such as losing excess weight and

restricting your salt intake do not bring your blood pressure down to 160/100 or below, your doctor will probably prescribe medication to lower the pressure. There is a long list of antihypertensive medications, but there is no single ideal drug for this job. You should work closely with your health-care practitioner to find the regimen that is appropriate for you. Your doctor may suggest that you purchase a blood-pressure monitor so that you can take periodic readings and report back to him or her.

■ A diuretic is often the first drug prescribed for high blood pressure. Diuretics promote the excretion of fluids through the kidneys, thus lowering the amount of fluid circulating in the bloodstream. This reduces the pressure. The so-called thiazide diuretics are the type most commonly prescribed. Examples of these include chlorothiazide (Diuril) and hydrochlorothiazide (HydroDiuril). These drugs can cause side effects including abnormally low potassium levels, low blood pressure (enough to cause lightheadedness) on standing, high blood sugar, high blood uric acid (see GOUT), nausea, and unfavorable changes in the levels of fats in the blood. There are other classes of diuretics and some medications that combine different types, but these are less commonly used.

■ Beta-blockers are drugs that inhibit the transmission of certain nerve impulses, causing the heart to slow its rate and lower its output of blood. This in turn lowers blood pressure. The generic names of these drugs usually end in the syllables *olol;* examples include atenolol (Tenormin), metoprolol (Lopressor), and propranolol (Inderal). These drugs can cause a wide variety of side effects, including an abnormally slow heart rate, asthmatic attacks, dizziness, depression, fatigue, nausea, and heart failure. They also lower the level of high-density lipoproteins (HDL, the so-called "good" cholesterol) in the blood. Beta-blockers should not be taken by anyone who has asthma.

■ Angiotensin-converting enzyme (ACE) inhibitors are a more recent entrant in the field of blood-pressure medication. These drugs inhibit the production of an enzyme that causes the formation of angiotensin, a hormone that is a potent blood-vessel constrictor, thus relaxing the vessels and lowering blood pressure. They also have other mechanisms of action that are not understood. Examples include captopril (Capoten), enalapril (Vasotec), and ramipril (Altace). Possible side effects include headaches, dizziness, nausea, fatigue, a nagging cough, low blood pressure on standing, and low potassium levels. However, side effects tend to be less of a problem with ACE inhibitors than with other types of drugs used for high blood pressure.

■ Calcium-channel blockers block the transfer of calcium ions into smooth-muscle cells. This has the effect of relaxing blood vessels and lowering blood pressure. Members of this class of drug include diltiazem (Cardizem), nifedip-

ine (Adalat, Procardia), and verapamil (Calan). They can cause a range of side effects including fatigue, nausea, swelling, shortness of breath, heart failure, and liver damage. They are not generally suitable for use by people with heart-rhythm problems, and should be used with great caution by people with heart failure or liver or kidney disease.

■ Alpha-blockers lower blood pressure by dilating blood vessels. They may also lower total blood cholesterol and triglyceride levels. Doxazosin (Cardura), prazosin (Minipress), and terazosin (Hytrin) are examples of this kind of drug. Possible side effects include dizziness, fatigue, headache, fainting, and nasal congestion. These drugs should be used with caution by pregnant women and nursing mothers.

■ Central alpha agonists such as clonidine (Catapres), methyldopa (Aldomet), and guanfacine (Tenex) lower blood pressure by reducing constriction of blood vessels. These drugs can cause drowsiness, rashes, constipation, and joint pain, and should be used with caution in the presence of liver disease.

■ If an individual drug proves to be inadequate, two or more different medications may be combined for greater effect. Unfortunately, this can result in a combination of side effects as well.

■ People with high blood pressure usually have high triglyceride and/or cholesterol levels. Unfortunately, many (if not all) of the drugs used to lower blood pressure tend to raise triglycerides and/or cholesterol. If you must take medication for high blood pressure, it is important to maintain regular, close communication with your health-care provider and undergo periodic testing to monitor the situation.

DIETARY GUIDELINES

■ It is important to eat a healthy high-fiber diet. High-fiber foods include whole grains, beans, fruits, and vegetables. Oat fiber is considered the best source. In fact, oats have been shown to be so beneficial that the U.S. Food and Drug Administration (FDA) permits food companies to make health claims for products that contain them.

■ Onions and garlic contain compounds that help to bring down blood pressure and lower cholesterol levels. Enjoy them often.

■ Avoid saturated animal fats and hydrogenated and partially hydrogenated fats and oils, found in most types of margarine and many processed food products. Blood pressure is considerably lower, on average, among those who follow a vegetarian diet than among those who do not.

■ Excessive salt consumption has long been linked to hypertension because salt contains sodium, which causes the body to retain fluid. This in turn makes the heart work harder. Recently, however, evidence has surfaced that for most people, the role of sodium in heart disease may not be as great as was once thought. Nevertheless, most Americans consume a great deal more sodium than they need. It makes sense to practice moderation. Avoid heavy salt use. Be aware that processed food products and fast-food offerings are often loaded with alarming amounts of sodium. Especially avoid foods processed with a large amount of salt, such as canned meats, smoked meats, and smoked cheeses. Use herbs instead of salt to season your foods. Garlic, onions, and parsley are all good choices. In addition to adding flavor, these foods all have properties that are beneficial for the cardiovascular system. There are also many different salt-free seasoning mixtures available that make excellent alternatives to table salt.

■ Heavy consumption of caffeine can contribute to an elevated blood pressure. Limit your consumption of beverages that contain caffeine, including coffee, black tea, colas, and some sodas.

■ Practice great moderation in your use of alcohol (no more than one drink daily), or avoid it entirely. High blood pressure has been linked to excessive alcohol consumption.

NUTRITIONAL SUPPLEMENTS

■ The antioxidant nutrients—vitamin A, beta-carotene, selenium, and vitamin E—improve blood oxygenation, which helps guard the heart from the strain of high blood pressure. Take a good antioxidant formula that supplies 5,000 international units of vitamin A, 25,000 international units of beta-carotene, 200 micrograms of selenium, and 400 international units of vitamin E daily.

Note: If you are pregnant, or intend to get pregnant, or if you have liver disease, consult your doctor before taking supplemental vitamin A. If you are taking an anticoagulant (blood thinner), consult your physician before taking vitamin E.

■ Calcium and magnesium are important for maintaining proper muscle tone, including that of the heart and blood vessels. Calcium has been shown to lower blood pressure, and magnesium has been recommended for hypertension for over thirty years. Take 500 to 600 milligrams of calcium and 300 to 350 milligrams of magnesium twice daily.

■ Carnitine has a proven track record for protecting the heart, a particularly important consideration if you are taking beta-blockers, which work by interfering with the nerve and muscle actions of that organ. Take 500 milligrams of L-carnitine once or twice daily.

■ Coenzyme Q_{10} increases tissue oxygenation and has been shown to help bring down high blood pressure. It is also an excellent antioxidant. Take at least 100 milligrams daily.

■ The essential fatty acids (EFAs) found in black currant seed oil, borage oil, evening primrose oil, and flaxseed oil help reduce blood pressure levels. Choose any of these oils and take 500 to 1,000 milligrams two or three times daily.

■ Lecithin helps emulsify fat, and can be effective if you have a history of alcohol consumption. Take 1,200 milligrams two or three times daily, with meals.

■ Excessive consumption of salt coupled with low levels of potassium can lead to elevated blood pressure. Unless you are taking a potassium-sparing diuretic (examples include amiloride [Midamor], dyrenium [Triamterene], and spironolactone [Aldactone]) or a combination diuretic that contains a potassium-sparing element, such as Maxzide, Dyazide, or Aldactazide, take 99 milligrams of potassium twice daily. If you are unsure about the type of blood-pressure medication you are taking, ask your doctor or pharmacist before taking potassium supplements.

■ People who are deficient in vitamin C are more likely to have high blood pressure than are those who maintain an adequate intake of this important vitamin. Take 1,000 milligrams twice daily.

HERBAL TREATMENT

■ Garlic can help to bring down blood pressure. This ancient herb also helps to decrease excessive levels of cholesterol and triglycerides, which protects the heart. Take 500 milligrams three times daily.

■ Hawthorn berry is one of the most broadly prescribed herbal medicines in Europe. This herb brings down high blood pressure, lowers blood cholesterol, and helps regulate heart function. Choose a standardized extract containing 1.8 percent vitexin-2 rhamnosides and take 100 to 200 milligrams two or three times a day.

■ Parsley is a natural diuretic and is also high in potassium, which is known to reduce elevated blood pressure. Take 500 milligrams twice a day for one week out of each month. Continue this program for six months.

■ Siberian ginseng is especially helpful if you have high blood pressure and also suffer from fatigue. Choose a standardized extract containing 0.5 percent eleutheroside E and take 100 milligrams daily, in the morning.

Note: Do not substitute Chinese (Korean) or American ginseng for Siberian ginseng. You should not use Chinese or American ginseng if you have high blood pressure.

ACUPRESSURE

For the locations of acupressure points on the body, *see* ADMINISTERING AN ACUPRESSURE TREATMENT in Part Three.

- Liver 3 helps relax the nervous system.

- Massaging the inner and outer Bladder points relaxes the entire nervous system.

AROMATHERAPY

For specific instructions on how to use aromatherapy, *see* PREPARING AROMATHERAPY TREATMENTS in Part Three.

- Essential oils of lavender, neroli, and ylang-ylang have calming and stress-reducing properties. Use any of them individually or combine up to three different oils in relaxing baths or massage oil. Or simply inhale from the bottle as the need arises.

GENERAL RECOMMENDATIONS

- If you are overweight, consult your doctor about a diet and exercise program that will enable you to lose weight safely and effectively.

- Do not smoke, and avoid secondhand smoke. Nicotine causes the blood vessels to constrict, increasing the blood pressure.

- As much as possible, avoid stress. Consider learning stress-management techniques to help you deal with the unavoidable stresses in your life. (*See* RELAXATION TECHNIQUES in Part Three.)

- Get regular moderate exercise. Exercise has been proven to actually reduce blood pressure. *See* STARTING AN EXERCISE PROGRAM in Part Three for suggestions.

Note: Before beginning any exercise program, discuss it with your physician.

PREVENTION

- It may not be possible to prevent high blood pressure. However, you can minimize your risk by making intelligent lifestyle choices that include a healthy, nutritionally complete diet; daily exercise; and avoidance of stress and such habits as smoking and excessive alcohol consumption. It is also wise to monitor your blood pressure periodically, particularly if you are over thirty, so that if you do develop hypertension, you can begin treatment in a timely fashion.

HIV Disease

The human immunodeficiency virus (HIV) is known to have been present in the United States since 1978, though some people believe it may have arrived as much as two decades earlier. It is a type of virus known as a retrovirus. All viruses can multiply only after entering the cells of a living being, but retroviruses actually take over the genetic material of the cells they invade, causing the cells to create additional copies of the virus.

In the case of HIV, the particular cells the virus invades are called T-lymphocytes (T-cells), a type of white blood cell that is a key component of the immune system. T-cells recognize infectious invaders and mobilize the immune response against them. As HIV uses T-cells to manufacture copies of itself, the copies invade other T-cells. This process is repeated over and over, destroying more and more T-cells and seriously weakening the body's ability to fight off infection and disease.

A healthy person has a T-cell count of between 1,000 and 1,500 per microliter of blood (1,000 to 1,500 μL). After infection with HIV, the T-cell count begins to fall, usually in a slow, steady decline punctuated by occasional sudden, sharp drops. People with acquired immunodeficiency syndrome (AIDS), the severest stage of HIV disease, generally have a T-cell count of 200 or less.

The incubation period for this illness is both long and variable. Some people experience a brief flulike illness soon after infection, but most feel perfectly healthy and are likely to be unaware they have contracted HIV. After a period of several weeks (or even longer, in some cases), the body begins to make antibodies to the virus. Unfortunately, because of the way retroviruses operate, these antibodies cannot protect the body against HIV and its effects, but they are useful for diagnosis. If a person is found to have HIV antibodies in his or her blood, this is proof that he or she has been infected. Such a person is said to be *HIV-positive.*

At some point after becoming HIV-positive, the infected individual may begin to suffer such symptoms as chronically enlarged lymph nodes, weight loss, fatigue, diarrhea, unexplained fevers, and night sweats. This phase of the disease is called AIDS-related complex (ARC), although the term is being used less frequently than in the past since the symptoms are so variable and it does not assist with treatment. ARC may develop anywhere from several months to many years after the initial infection.

As the person's T-cell count continues to fall, he or she becomes susceptible to a wide array of infections and other illnesses, many of which are otherwise quite rare. These include, but are hardly limited to, *Pneumocystis carinii* pneumonia (PCP), persistent and systemic candida (yeast) infection, Kaposi's sarcoma, toxoplasmic encephalitis, and cytomegalovirus (CMV) infection. PCP is a kind of fungal pneumonia. A systemic candida infection may be manifested in many different ways. Oral thrush and persistent vaginitis are two of the most common. Kaposi's sarcoma is a form of skin cancer that once affected primarily older men of Mediterranean ancestry, but has now become closely associated with AIDS. It is characterized by the appearance on the body of spots or nodules that may be pink, red, purple, or brown in color. Toxoplasmic encephalitis is an infection of the brain caused by the parasite *Toxoplasma gondii*. This disease can result in severe headache, partial paralysis, seizures, confusion, and other symptoms. CMV is a common virus that many people carry in their systems without knowing it, but in persons with HIV it can infect the kidneys, the central nervous system, and, especially, the eyes, leading to blindness.

Virtually all infectious diseases are more common, and more dangerous, in people who have HIV. For example, tuberculosis is both more common and more difficult to treat in people with HIV. Chronic fever, diarrhea, anemia, fatigue, severe weight loss, and other symptoms may develop and/or worsen as the body becomes unable to defend itself against the effects of organisms that normally are relatively harmless. If HIV infects the brain, it can cause dementia, a deterioration in mental functioning. If a person's T-cell count falls below 200 or certain characteristic infections or cancer develop, he or she is diagnosed with AIDS.

The time between infection with HIV and the development of AIDS varies greatly. Today, it is generally believed that an otherwise healthy person who contracts HIV can expect eight to twelve years of continuing health before the onset of AIDS. This is just a statistic, however. Every person is an individual, and there are many different factors that affect an individual's experience. Your overall state of health when you become infected, how well you care for yourself, the level of stress in your life, how early you begin treatment and how well you respond to it—all of these are important considerations in determining how well your immune system will continue to function despite the presence of HIV. Then, too, there are some people who show no signs of impaired immunity and remain healthy for many years after contracting the virus. These individuals, known as *long-term nonprogressors*, are naturally the subject of considerable interest among those involved in HIV and AIDS research.

HIV is contracted principally through sexual or blood-to-blood contact, such as occurs during blood transfusions or the sharing of needles by intravenous drug users. Women who are HIV-positive can transmit the virus to a developing fetus during pregnancy or to an infant during childbirth or through breastfeeding. HIV *cannot* be transmitted from one person to another through coughing and sneezing, as colds can, nor through normal everyday interactions at home or work, including hugs and dry kisses. Similarly, you should understand that it is not possible to contract the virus by donating blood. It is also important to know that exposure to HIV does not always result in infection, but, in general, the greater and more frequent the exposure, the more likely it is that a person will become infected. Persons with one or more other sexually transmitted diseases appear to be more likely to contract HIV through sexual contact.

In the early years of the AIDS epidemic in the United States, HIV primarily affected men who had sex with other men. This has changed over time, however. The number of people acquiring HIV through heterosexual sex is rising, as is the incidence of infection among women. The largest number of new cases currently can be attributed to intravenous drug use with sharing of syringes and/or needles. A very small percentage of cases occurs among health-care workers who are exposed to infected body fluids through accidental needlesticks and similar incidents. One alarming trend is that the infection rate among young people is rising. An estimated one out of every four new cases of HIV infection occurs in a person under the age of twenty-one.

HIV has had a devastating impact on the portion of the population who have hemophilia, an inherited blood-clotting disorder. Treatment for hemophilia involves the use of blood products and transfusions. Donated blood is now screened for HIV, and the clotting factors used by hemophiliacs are heat-treated as a preventive, but for close to a decade, there were no such precautions and many hemophiliacs contracted the virus through the very treatments they depended on to remain healthy.

If you are HIV-positive, whether you have AIDS or not, your goal should be to avoid secondary infections, if possible; to treat any health problems promptly and aggressively; and to do everything you can to support your immune system.

CONVENTIONAL TREATMENT

■ The first step in treating HIV disease is getting a correct diagnosis. A simple blood test to detect HIV antibodies, known as the ELISA test, can be done at a testing site, a doctor's office, or a clinic. If the initial result is positive, the blood is retested to verify the result. If the result of that test, too, is positive, a more sophisticated test, the Western blot test, is done to confirm the findings of the ELISA.

Experts recommend that anyone in a group considered to be at high risk of HIV infection be tested for the disease so that treatment, if necessary, can be begun promptly. Those at high risk include males who have had unprotected sex with other males; individuals who have shared needles or syringes to inject drugs or steroids; anyone who has had unprotected sex with a partner without knowing his or her history and risk behavior; anyone who has had unprotected sex with multiple partners within the last ten years; anyone who has had any sexually transmitted disease within the last ten years; anyone who received a blood transfusion or blood-clotting factor between 1978 and 1985 (the screening of donated blood for HIV did not begin until 1985); and anyone who has had unprotected sex with anyone who might fit the categories outlined above. They also recommend testing for women who are, or who plan to become, pregnant.

■ If you are diagnosed with HIV, it is important to find and work closely with a physician who specializes, or at the very least has considerable experience, in treating this condition. Treatment of HIV disease is extremely complicated, and new information and treatment approaches surface virtually on a daily basis. Working with a practitioner you can count on to know the latest developments and findings is vital. Studies suggest that the length of survival and the quality of life for a person with HIV disease may be related more to the expertise of his or her physician than to any other factor. It is also important to find a doctor with whom you feel comfortable, since yours will be a long-term relationship.

■ If you are found to be HIV-positive, your CD4 (white-cell) count should be monitored at least every six months. Antiviral treatment is usually started when the count falls below 500 or when symptoms begin.

■ Treatment of HIV infection itself is aimed at inhibiting the virus and keeping it from reproducing. There is a long list of drugs that are used for this purpose. Delavirdine (Rescriptor), didanosine (Videx, known colloquially as ddI), lamivudine (Epivir, or 3TC), nevirapine (Viramune, or NVP), stavudine (Zerit, or d4T), zalcitabine (Hivid, or ddC), and zidovudine (Retrovir, still generally referred to by its former name, azidothymidine, or AZT) do this by inhibiting the action of the enzyme reverse transcriptase, which plays a necessary role in the reproduction of the virus. Indinavir (Crixivan), nelfinavir (Viracept), ritonavir (Norvir), and saquinavir (Invirase) are drugs that block the action of another viral enzyme, protease. One problem with all of the drugs used to suppress HIV is that the virus has the ability to develop resistance to them, often within a relatively short period of time. For this reason, combination therapy using two or three different drugs at once has become the preferred approach. It may be necessary to experiment with different drug combinations to find the regimen that works best for you. All of the agents used against HIV can cause significant side effects, ranging from nausea, headaches, mouth ulcers, and skin rashes to disorders of fat metabolism to blood abnormalities, liver damage, and pancreatitis. Though they can be unpleasant, side effects must be weighed against the seriousness of the condition you are trying to fight.

■ Another general approach to treating HIV involves efforts to "jump-start" the hematopoietic (blood-building) system, boosting the production of red or white blood cells to compensate for those destroyed by the virus. The drugs used for this purpose are expensive, and include epoetin alfa (Epogen, Procrit), filgrastim (Neupogen, or G-CSF), and sargramostim (Leukine, or GM-CSF). These therapies are generally reserved for the later stages of the disease.

■ Specific infections and complications should be treated promptly and aggressively, as they occur:

• *Pneumocystis carinii,* the most common opportunistic infection, is treated with powerful combination antibiotics, such as trimethoprim plus sulfamethoxazole (Bactrim, Co-trimoxazole, Septra; also known as TMP/SMX). Unfortunately, many people have allergic reactions to the sulfa component of this drug. If you cannot tolerate TMP/SMX, or if it proves ineffective, other drugs may be tried, including dapsone (a drug originally used to treat leprosy) and pentamidine (Pentam). Potential side effects of dapsone include blood problems, muscle weakness, nausea, vomiting, abdominal pain, dizziness, and serious skin reactions. Pentamidine must be used with caution, as it can cause severely low blood pressure, low blood sugar, and heart and pancreatic problems. In addition to antibiotics, steroids may be prescribed for a brief period to decrease inflammation. Aggressive oxygen and respiratory therapy may be needed in severe cases. Pneumocystis pneumonia also carries a risk of pneumothorax, in which air gets trapped outside the lung but inside the chest cavity. This can become an ongoing problem. The evacuation tube inserted surgically through the chest wall to treat the situation tends to heal poorly, sometimes requiring the application of an irritant such as talc or bleomycin to induce the opening to scar itself closed. Otherwise, the area may have to be stapled closed or further surgical intervention may be required.

• Viral infections such as CMV may be treated with antiviral medication such as foscarnet (Foscavir) or ganciclovir (Cytovene). These drugs are potentially quite toxic, and may only slow the progression of a viral disease rather than curing it altogether.

• For fungal (yeast) infections, such as oral thrush or yeast vaginitis, a doctor may prescribe an oral antifungal agent such as fluconazole (Diflucan) or itraconazole (Sporanox).

• Parasitic infections, such as giardiasis and cryptosporidiosis, along with viral, bacterial, and amoebic infection, are all potential causes of enterocolitis, a common problem. This is an inflammation of the colon that results in potentially serious diarrhea, along with high fever and abdominal pain. This problem can affect anyone, whether HIV-positive or not, but it tends to be both more severe and more chronic in people with HIV. Treatment starts with stool cultures and microscopic examination to track down the offending organism. This is of paramount importance, as different organisms are treated with different antibiotics. For some organisms, unfortunately, such as cryptosporidia, there is still no universally effective treatment, so a variety of different drugs may be tried. Both bacterial and parasitic infections are treated aggressively with antibiotics, possibly administered intravenously. Whenever you must take antibiotics, be sure to take them for the full course prescribed by your physician.

- Nausea, a common problem for people with HIV disease, is often a result of a yeast outbreak in the throat, so it is often treated with an oral antifungal medication. If that fails, an antiemetic such as prochlorperazine (Compazine) or metoclopramide (Reglan) may be prescribed. These drugs can cause drowsiness, restlessness, unusual involuntary movements, and other side effects, but it is important to treat nausea to keep weight loss at a minimum.

- Loss of appetite and resulting weight loss are real dangers for people with AIDS. Besides nutritional counseling and the use of high-calorie dietary supplements, a variety of drugs may be used for this, including megestrol (Megace), a synthetic derivative of the hormone progesterone that stimulates the appetite; dronabinol (Marinol), a compound extracted from marijuana that both stimulates the appetite and combats nausea; and growth hormone (Genotropin). All of these treatments have downsides, unfortunately. Megestrol can cause blood clots, heart failure, mood changes, and increases in blood sugar and blood pressure. Marinol can cause drowsiness, behavioral changes, altered gait, and anxiety. It also has significant abuse potential. Growth hormone is expensive, costing over $150.00 a day, and can cause muscle aches, swelling, and other side effects. Anabolic steroids, administered by injection or skin patch, may be used to combat weight loss as well, but they are normally reserved for those who are willing and able to do weight training. Possible side effects include stroke, breast tenderness and/or enlargement, urinary tract infections, prostate inflammation, and others.

- Fever is a common problem. If no underlying infection can be found, standard antipyretics (fever-reducing drugs) are used. Ibuprofen (Advil, Motrin, Nuprin, and others) and naproxen (Aleve, Anaprox, Naprelan, Naprosyn) are considered more effective than either aspirin or acetaminophen (Tylenol) for this purpose.

- There is little that can be done for unexplained sweats, which are also common in people with AIDS, even in the absence of fever. This symptom usually causes renewed examination for hidden infections, however.

- Diarrhea is usually treated with standard therapies (see DIARRHEA), but more aggressively than in healthy individuals because the complications of weight loss make it a more serious symptom for people with HIV disease.

- If you have a history of opportunistic bacterial or yeast infection, a lower dose, longer term regimen of antibiotics may be prescribed as a preventive. This kind of treatment must be closely monitored by a physician.

- Blood transfusions are not uncommon in advanced cases to increase the presence of infection-fighting white blood cells. Epoetin alfa, a very expensive drug, may be used in an attempt to lessen the number of transfusions required.

DIETARY GUIDELINES

■ Be sure to take in adequate amounts of clean, lean protein, at least one gram of protein for each two pounds of body weight. If you find this difficult, take a whey-protein supplement to bring your consumption to that level.

■ To help flush toxins from your body, drink at least eight 8-ounce glasses of pure water every day. *Do not drink tap water.* Tap water contains various contaminants, including chlorine, which damages red blood cells. Also, many municipal water supplies have been found to contain tiny parasites such as giardia and cryptosporidia that can be devastating to a person with a compromised immune system.

■ Include in your diet generous amounts of the cruciferous vegetables—broccoli, cabbage, cauliflower, Brussels sprouts, and their relatives—which contain cancer-fighting phytochemicals. Also enjoy onions and garlic often. These plants have natural antibiotic properties.

■ If weight loss is a problem, try eating multiple small meals rather than two or three large ones each day, and take protein and carbohydrate supplements between meals.

■ Eliminate all alcohol, caffeine, sugar, fried foods, and junk food from your diet. These substances stress the body and depress the immune system.

■ As much as possible, eat organically grown and raised foods to reduce your exposure to pesticide residues and other toxins. Wash all produce thoroughly before eating it. To minimize your chances of developing foodborne illness, be scrupulously clean in your handling and preparation of food. (*See* FOOD POISONING.)

■ Some people with HIV disease have reported feeling better after switching to a macrobiotic diet, which consists primarily of well-cooked whole grains, fresh vegetables, protein-rich beans and soy foods, and sea vegetables, with limited amounts of fish and other animal protein. If you are interested in trying such a diet, *The Macrobiotic Way* by Michio Kushi (Avery Publishing, 1993) can serve as an excellent introduction.

NUTRITIONAL SUPPLEMENTS

■ To be certain you get all necessary nutrients, take a high-quality multivitamin and mineral supplement daily. Choose a capsule or liquid formula. These are easier to absorb and assimilate than hard, dry pills.

■ Black currant seed oil, borage oil, evening primrose oil, and flaxseed oil provide essential fatty acids (EFAs), which help to regulate endocrine function and also have anti-inflammatory properties. Choose one of these oils and take 500 to 1,000 milligrams twice daily. If diarrhea is a problem, discontinue until the diarrhea improves.

■ Bromelain is a natural anti-inflammatory and is very useful for respiratory complaints such as bronchitis and pneumonia. Take 400 milligrams three times daily, between meals. Goldenseal is also helpful (see under Herbal Treatment, below).

■ Carnitine supplementation can greatly improve the utilization of fat and the conversion of fats into energy, a process that is often compromised in people with HIV. L-carnitine is also useful in preventing toxic overload from such drugs as AZT and, in one study, HIV patients who took 6,000 milligrams (6 grams) of L-carnitine daily were shown to have improved immune function. You may wish to discuss this supplement with a nutritionally oriented physician.

■ All of the carotenes have antioxidant properties that prevent free-radical damage. Take 75,000 to 100,000 international units of a carotene-complex formula daily.

■ To insure full assimilation and utilization of all nutrients, take a full-spectrum digestive enzyme supplement providing 5,000 international units of lipase, 2,500 international units of amylase, and 300 international units of protease, plus 500 to 1,000 milligrams of pancreatin, with each meal.

Note: Long-term supplementation with pancreatin is not advised, as it can cause your pancreas to reduce its own production of this important enzyme. Overuse also has the potential to cause nausea or diarrhea. After two months on pancreatin, discontinue use and monitor your reaction. If you find that your problems recur, discuss pancreatin supplementation with your health-care provider.

■ If mouth sores are a problem, chew on folic-acid tablets. Take 400 micrograms of folic acid up to three times daily this way.

■ Take a green-foods or sea-greens supplement such as Green Magma or spirulina as directed on the product label. Green supplements are rich in natural trace minerals.

■ Lipoic acid fights herpes viruses, helps the liver function more efficiently, and is useful against chronic fatigue. Take 100 milligrams three times daily.

■ To control the proliferation of candida (yeast), take a quality probiotic supplement. Follow the directions on the product label. Most people with HIV take many powerful drugs that wipe out the essential bacteria that keep candida under control in a healthy body. Probiotics are also useful for combating diarrhea. If you are allergic to milk, be sure to select a dairy-free formula.

■ To support immune function, consider taking adrenal, spleen, and/or thymus glandular extracts. Take one dose, as directed on the product label, twice daily.

■ Take a trace-mineral combination formula that provides 5 milligrams of manganese, 200 micrograms of chromium, and 5 milligrams of vanadium daily. These elements are seldom included in common multimineral formulas.

■ Studies suggest that HIV-positive people with sufficient blood levels of vitamin B_{12} may remain symptom-free for about twice as long, on average, as those who are deficient in that vitamin. Cobalamin is an active component of vitamin B_{12}. Take 500 micrograms of cyanocobalamin or methocobalamin twice a day, or ask your physician about injections. If you take any of the B vitamins individually, you should also take a B-complex supplement at a different time of day.

■ Vitamin C is an infection-fighting, anti-inflammatory antioxidant vitamin that supports the immune system and also fights free radicals. Take 3,000 to 10,000 milligrams (3 to 10 grams) of vitamin C daily.

■ Vitamin E is an antioxidant that also plays an essential role in cellular respiration. Choose a product containing mixed tocopherols and start by taking 200 international units daily, then gradually increase the dosage until you are taking 400 international units in the morning and again in the evening.

Note: If you have high blood pressure, limit your intake of supplemental vitamin E to a total of 400 international units daily. If you are taking an anticoagulant (blood thinner), consult your physician before taking supplemental vitamin E.

■ Zinc boosts immune function. Take 15 milligrams three times daily, at the beginning of a meal. To maintain a proper mineral balance in the body, you should also take 1 to 2 milligrams of copper each day.

HERBAL TREATMENT

■ Aloe vera is healing and soothing to mucous membranes. If you suffer from mouth sores, swish a mouthful of aloe vera juice around in your mouth several times daily. Be sure to use a food-grade product for this purpose.

■ Astragalus helps strengthen immune function. It enhances interferon production and helps inhibit viral infection. Take 350 to 500 milligrams twice daily, before breakfast and again before lunch.

Note: Do not take astragalus if you have a fever or any other signs of acute infection.

■ Take ginger or peppermint tea with meals to combat nausea and enhance digestion. Green tea also is an excellent beverage to take with meals. It improves digestion and supplies potent antioxidant bioflavonoids that can help prevent free-radical damage.

■ Goldenseal and the Chinese patent medicine Huang Lian Su contain berberine alkaloids, which have antibiotic effects and can be helpful for diarrhea. Choose a standardized goldenseal root providing 8 to 10 percent berberine and take 500 milligrams three times daily for up to one week. Or take two tablets of Huang Lian Su three times daily for three days to one week. If you take either of these herbs for more than three days, be sure to take a probiotic supplement, such as bifidobacteria, to renew the bowel flora and improve your utilization of nutrients.

Licorice enhances immune function and inhibits viruses, especially those of the herpes group. Take 500 milligrams twice a day for up to one week.

Note: Do not take licorice by itself on a daily basis for more than five days at a time, as it can elevate blood pressure. Do not take it at all if you have high blood pressure.

Pine-bark and grape-seed extracts are rich in powerful natural anti-inflammatory agents. Take 50 milligrams of either three times daily.

St. John's wort helps strengthen immune function and combats depression. Choose a product containing 0.3 percent hypericin and take 300 milligrams two or three times daily.

Siberian ginseng helps to strengthen the endocrine system, and enhances energy and well-being. Choose a standardized extract containing 0.5 percent eleutheroside E and take 200 milligrams twice daily, one-half hour before breakfast and again one-half hour before lunch.

Turmeric contains curcumin, a natural anti-inflammatory. Take 500 milligrams twice a day.

HOMEOPATHY

When treating a condition as complex as HIV disease, it is best to see a homeopathic physician for a constitutional remedy. For individual symptoms such as nausea or diarrhea, consult the appropriate sections in this book for suggestions.

ACUPRESSURE

For the locations of acupressure points on the body, *see* ADMINISTERING AN ACUPRESSURE TREATMENT in Part Three.

All Bladder points relax the nerves and, in combination with Stomach 36, gradually improve the absorption of nutrients. Stomach 36 also improves digestion, tones the digestive tract, is useful for improving appetite, and strengthens overall well-being.

■ Four Gates relaxes the body.

BACH FLOWER REMEDIES

Select the remedy that most closely fits your emotional tendencies and concerns, and take it as needed, following the directions on the product label.

■ Aspen is helpful for fear of the unknown.

■ Mimulus will help tame known fears and a dread of what is coming.

■ Mustard is for sorrow and depression.

■ Olive can help alleviate exhaustion.

■ Rock Rose can help calm feelings of panic.

■ Star of Bethlehem helps to ease the emotional shock that follows a life-changing experience.

GENERAL RECOMMENDATIONS

■ As much as possible, avoid stress. Stress taxes the immune system. Get regular, adequate sleep. Avoid exposure to pollutants and toxins such as automobile exhaust, tobacco smoke, and household chemicals. Also avoid excessive sun exposure and extremes of temperature, either heat or cold. Experiment with meditation and relaxation techniques to help you deal with those stresses you cannot avoid. (*See* RELAXATION TECHNIQUES in Part Three.)

■ If you become pregnant, seek medical treatment immediately. There are drugs that can minimize your risk of passing the infection on to your child. Prenatal care is important for all pregnant women and their future children, but is doubly so for the woman with HIV and her child.

■ As much as possible, avoid coming into contact with people who may have contagious illnesses. For example, phone ahead before visiting friends or family to be sure all household members are healthy. Try to avoid spending time in crowded public environments. Practice careful personal hygiene, especially frequent hand-washing. Many infectious organisms are spread via the hands.

■ Exercise is important for keeping in shape, easing depression, increasing tissue oxygenation, and enhancing immunity. Get regular moderate exercise—within the limits of your capabilities, of course.

■ The psychological aspects of living with HIV can be as daunting as the physical ones. Do not hesitate to seek out sources of support such as counseling or membership in a support group. Participating in a support group can also be an excellent way to learn about new developments in HIV treatment and research. If mobility is a problem, consider connecting with the outside world by means of the Internet. (See the Resources section at the end of the book for organizations that serve as sources of information and support for people with HIV.)

PREVENTION

■ The only sure way to avoid contracting HIV through

sex is to abstain from sex entirely. Obviously, this is not something most people would consider. The next choice is to have a monogamous relationship with a partner you know to be free of the virus. If you have multiple sexual partners, or if you have sexual contact with anyone whose health status or background is not known to you, practice safer sex. Use a latex (not animal-skin) condom *every time,* for oral and anal sex as well as genital-to-genital contact. For added protection, use a spermicide in addition to the condom. Always remember that a person who is HIV-positive may show no signs of the infection and, in fact, may not have any idea he or she is infected.

■ Never share needles or syringes. HIV from an infected person can remain undetected in a needle or syringe and may then be injected directly into the body of the next person who uses it.

■ If you plan to have your ears pierced or get a tattoo, go to a qualified professional who uses new needles for each procedure. Some sterilization procedures are not completely effective.

Hives

Also called *urticaria,* this is a skin disorder that can have a variety of causes, including drug allergies, insect bites, food sensitivities, and contact with irritating or allergenic substances. Itching is normally the first symptom, and it can be intense. This is soon followed by the appearance of patches of red, raised wheals that can grow, disappear, and reappear elsewhere, sometimes clearing in the center to form large ringlike areas.

Hives usually last only a few days to weeks, then clear up on their own. A complete medical history and physical examination are often more valuable than laboratory tests for identifying the cause. Some people develop chronic hives, however, the cause of which can be extremely frustrating to track down.

Angioedema is a problem involving a reaction similar to that of hives, but affecting deeper tissues than just the skin, causing more diffuse swelling of the affected area. If angioedema affects the throat, a disorder known as *laryngeal angioedema,* the swelling can interfere with a person's ability to breathe. This constitutes a medical emergency. Gasping for breath and sudden, acute wheezing can be signs that laryngeal angioedema may be developing.

EMERGENCY TREATMENT

■ If you suspect you may be developing laryngeal angioedema, have someone take you to the emergency room of the nearest hospital or call for emergency medical assistance immediately. Emergency personnel will administer epinephrine, in both injectable and aerosolized forms, along with intravenous antihistamines. Depending on the severity of the problem and the response to treatment, other treatment may be required, including the administration of oxygen, placement of a breathing tube down the airway, or even a tracheostomy, in which an opening is cut in the front part of the throat for the insertion of a breathing tube directly below the problem area.

CONVENTIONAL TREATMENT

■ If the cause can be determined—insects or an offending drug, for example—removing it is the first course of action.

■ An antihistamine may be prescribed to reduce symptoms. Diphenhydramine (Benadryl), hydroxyzine (Atarax, Vistaril), or cyproheptadine (Periactin), taken orally, is usually sufficient. All of these drugs can cause side effects including fatigue, drowsiness, dizziness, dry mouth, and anxiety.

■ For more severe cases, an oral corticosteroid such as prednisone (Deltasone) may be prescribed. These are powerful drugs that depress adrenal function and suppress the immune response, and their use must be carefully monitored, so they are not the first choice for treatment of hives.

■ Topical treatment of hives tends to be unrewarding, and is rarely recommended.

DIETARY GUIDELINES

■ Eliminate allergenic foods from your diet. Hives are often associated with allergies to medications, eggs, dairy products, fruits, and food colorings, preservatives, and other additives.

NUTRITIONAL SUPPLEMENTS

■ Take a good multivitamin and mineral supplement daily. Be sure to choose a hypoallergenic formula.

■ Evening primrose and flaxseed oil contain essential fatty acids that are vital for the health of the skin, and that also act as anti-inflammatories. Take 1,000 milligrams of either twice a day.

■ Pantothenic acid supports adrenal function, which is important for normalizing the body's immune response. During an outbreak, take 250 milligrams three to four times daily. When the hives subside, continue taking 250 milligrams once or twice daily for one week.

■ Quercetin is a flavonoid that has strong anti-inflammatory properties. It is very useful in diminishing itchiness and swelling. Take 300 milligrams three to four times daily.

■ Vitamin C is an antioxidant and has anti-inflammatory properties. Take 500 milligrams three to four times daily.

■ Vitamin E promotes healing and helps to regulate the immune response. Choose a product containing mixed tocopherols and take 200 international units in the morning and again at bedtime.

Note: If you are taking an anticoagulant (blood thinner), consult your physician before taking vitamin E.

HERBAL TREATMENT

■ Bilberry extract has been shown to reduce the permeability of capillaries, thereby helping to counteract the effect of histamines in the body. Select an extract standardized to contain 25 percent anthocyanidins (also called PCOs) and take 60 milligrams three times daily.

HOMEOPATHY

Rhus toxicodendron helps to reduce redness, itching, and swelling. Take one dose of *Rhus toxicodendron* 30x or 15c three to four times daily for up to two days.

If the redness and swelling is not resolved after two days of taking *Rhus toxicodendron,* take one dose of *Bovista* 6x or 3c three times daily for up to three days.

In addition to the remedies mentioned above, there are many homeopathic combination skin remedies available that are useful for the acute symptoms of hives.

BACH FLOWER REMEDIES

Impatiens can help you relax while you are dealing with the annoying symptoms of hives. Take it as needed, following the directions on the product label.

ACUPRESSURE

For the locations of acupressure points on the body, *see* ADMINISTERING AN ACUPRESSURE TREATMENT in Part Three.

The back Bladder points relax the body.

Spleen 10 detoxifies the blood, clearing it of excess histamine.

AROMATHERAPY

For specific instructions on how to use aromatherapy, *see* PREPARING AROMATHERAPY TREATMENTS in Part Three.

The essential oils of chamomile, lavender, and rosemary are soothing and excellent for relieving stress. Aromatherapy baths or compresses prepared with one or more of these oils can help ease inflammation and itching. Start with a small amount, and be careful not to use too much essential oil in these treatments.

Note: Never apply essential oil directly to your skin. Always dilute it in water or a carrier oil first. If irritation results, discontinue use of the suspect oil.

GENERAL RECOMMENDATIONS

■ Avoid exposure to environmental toxins as much as possible, whether in such obvious forms as cigarette smoke or harsh household cleansers, or more subtle forms such as laundry-detergent residue or treated fabrics.

■ Keep your skin clean, but treat it gently. Avoid harsh soaps and greasy lotions. Use only unscented hypoallergenic skin-care products.

PREVENTION

■ It may not be possible to prevent hives from developing. It goes without saying, however, that you should avoid contact with anything that has provoked such a reaction in the past.

Hodgkin's Disease

See under CANCER.

Hyperhidrosis

See PERSPIRATION, EXCESSIVE.

Hypertension

See HIGH BLOOD PRESSURE.

Hyperthyroidism

Hyperthyroidism is a condition in which the thyroid gland becomes overactive and secretes excessive amounts of the hormone thyroxine. The thyroid is a small, somewhat butterfly-shaped structure located at the base of the neck. The hormone it produces, thyroxine (also known as T_4), is converted in the liver into another hormone, triiodothyronine (T_3), which regulates metabolism. If the thyroid produces too much thyroxine, this ultimately throws the body's metabolic processes into overdrive and speeds up many of the functions of the body.

Symptoms can range from mild to severe. One of the primary symptoms of hyperthyroidism is a disturbance in appetite. You may find you have little interest in food, or you may be much hungrier than normal. No matter how much you eat, however, you will likely experience noticeable weight loss. Because the digestive processes are strongly affected by excessive amounts of thyroid hormone, nutrient absorption falters and the body fails to receive the nutrient support required for normal functioning. As a result, you may eat more and more in an attempt to give your body what it needs, but continue to lose weight.

Other symptoms of hyperthyroidism include fine tremors of the hands and fingers; warm, moist palms; fatigue; irritability; nervousness; rapid heartbeat; heart palpitations; elevated blood pressure; sleep disturbances; bulging eyes; breathlessness; frequent bowel movements; stomach and intestinal spasms; muscle weakness; intolerance to heat; profuse perspiration; hair loss; and light, infrequent menstrual periods. As the disease progress, a swollen thyroid gland may become apparent. This is known as a goiter. It usually occurs in people who are deficient in iodine, which the thyroid requires in order to function. Hyperthyroidism can also lead to an enlarged thymus, overgrowth of the lymph nodes, and heart and bone disorders.

There are different types of hyperthyroidism. One of the most common is *Graves' disease.* This is believed to be an autoimmune disorder in which the immune system produces antibodies that stimulate the thyroid to produce excessive amounts of thyroxine. In addition to the classic symptoms of hyperthyroidism, Graves' disease can cause the eyes to bulge visibly and the skin of the legs to become thickened and itchy. Blurred or double vision may also occur.

Another type of hyperthyroidism is *toxic multinodular goiter,* or *Plummer's disease.* For reasons unknown, some of the nodules in the thyroid fail to respond to the normal chemical messages that govern thyroid function, and begin producing excessive amounts of thyroid hormone. *Thyroid storm* is an uncommon but very serious and extreme form of hyperthyroidism that comes on suddenly and causes severe symptoms, including fever, wild mood swings, muscle-wasting with marked muscle weakness, anxiety, confusion, and even overt psychosis or coma. There may also be liver enlargement and jaundice, with the eyes and even the skin turning distinctly yellow. This condition can be a result of infection, trauma, surgery, severe emotional stress, or preeclampsia (toxemia of pregnancy). Because this sudden and extreme speeding up of the metabolism causes great strain on the heart, it can become life-threatening if not treated as an emergency. It is also possible to develop hyperthyroidism as a result of a tumor of the pituitary gland or the ovary.

Hyperthyroidism affects about one percent of the population, is more common among women than men, occurs most often between the ages of twenty and forty, and often arises after an infection or following physical or emotional stress. This condition is diagnosed by measuring the levels of thyroid hormones present in the blood.

CONVENTIONAL MEDICINE

■ Propylthiouracil and methimazole (Tapazole) are drugs that lower the output of thyroid hormone. These are often the first type of treatment used for hyperthyroidism. Once the levels of thyroid hormone have been reduced to within the normal range with these drugs, the dosage is usually reduced until an appropriate maintenance regimen is determined. Unfortunately, the effect of these drugs is not always permanent, and it is possible for the production of thyroid hormone to be reduced too much. One potentially serious complication that can occur with these drugs is agranulocytosis, a condition in which the production of white blood cells is "shut off." Fortunately, this is both uncommon and reversible. More common side effects include itching, rashes, nausea, abdominal discomfort, hair loss, and liver stress.

■ If drugs are ineffective or cause intolerable side effects, your doctor may recommend a procedure to destroy overactive thyroid tissue. This is accomplished by taking radioactive iodine, or I-131. Since most of the iodine that enters the body is taken up by the thyroid, the effect of the radiation is focused there, and some of the gland's cells are destroyed. The idea is to destroy only enough cells to bring the production of thyroid hormone down to a normal level, but very often too much is destroyed and permanent *hypo*thyroidism results, necessitating oral treatment with thyroid hormone for the rest of one's life. Treatment with radioactive iodine is not appropriate during pregnancy, as the radiation can harm a developing fetus.

■ Iopanoic acid (Telepaque), a drug used to aid in visualizing organs in radiologic examinations, has been found to block thyroid hormones, but the body responds less and less to it over several months' time. However, it may be very effective in certain cases. Possible side effects include liver damage, kidney damage, nausea, vomiting, hives, and, paradoxically, hyperthyroidism.

■ Surgery to remove a portion of the thyroid tissue was once a common approach to treating hyperthyroidism, but it is used more rarely today. Possible problems with this technique include accidental removal of the parathyroid glands, which are located at the back of the thyroid gland and control the body's use of calcium and phosphorous, and damage to the nerve to the vocal cords.

■ Symptoms of hyperthyroidism can be controlled by a type of drug called a beta-blocker, which blocks the transmission of certain nerve impulses. The drug most often used for this purpose is propranolol (Inderal). It handles almost all of the symptoms of the condition, even though it has no effect whatsoever on the actual output of thyroid hormone. If hyperthyroidism goes away on its own after a short time, this may be the only treatment necessary, but often more aggressive types of treatment, such as those mentioned above, are necessary. Also, beta-blockers are not suitable for everyone. They should not be taken by anyone with a history of asthma or congestive heart failure, for example.

■ Treatment of thyroid storm is much the same as for ordinary hyperthyroidism, but is undertaken more aggressively. Propylthiouracil or methimazole is used to lower the output of thyroid hormone, and propranolol is prescribed to lower the heart rate and the stress on that organ. Hydrocortisone, a steroid, is used initially to reduce symptoms (the dose is then lowered as quickly as possible to avoid damage to the adrenal glands). For thyroid storm that occurs during pregnancy, the lowest possible doses of propylthiouracil are used and thyroid function is left somewhat elevated, if possible, until after delivery. This drug appears in lower concentrations in breast milk than methimazole, so it is preferred over that drug. Occasionally, if other measures fail, surgery on the thyroid gland is required.

■ If hyperthyroidism is due to a tumor elsewhere in the body, treatment consists of surgical removal of the tumor.

DIETARY GUIDELINES

■ The cruciferous vegetables, including broccoli, cauliflower, and kale, contain a substance that helps suppress thyroxine production. Enjoy these vegetables often. For best effect, eat them raw.

■ Do not rely on iodized salt to obtain the iodine your thyroid gland requires. For their content of natural iodine, which can prevent goiter, include sea vegetables such as dulse, hijiki, and kombu in your diet. Add them to soups or enjoy them as side dishes.

■ Avoid stimulants such as caffeine and alcohol.

NUTRITIONAL SUPPLEMENTS

■ Calcium and magnesium help calm the nervous system. Take 400 milligrams of calcium and 200 to 300 milligrams of magnesium three times daily.

■ The essential fatty acids (EFAs) found in black currant seed oil, borage oil, evening primrose oil, and flaxseed oil assist in the regulation of the immune response. They also help to stimulate steroid production and aid in the transmission of nerve impulses. If you suffer from fatigue, dry skin, dry hair, constipation, depression, and/or frequent colds and flu, you may want to consider taking 500 to 1,000 milligrams of any of these oils twice daily.

■ Gamma-aminobutyric acid (GABA) is an amino acid that acts as a calming neurotransmitter. It can be helpful if nervousness is overwhelming or if you have been diagnosed with hyperthyroidism and are perimenopausal. Take 500 milligrams two to three times daily for one week. Stop for one week, then repeat.

■ A green-foods supplement that contains iodine, such as spirulina or chlorella, can help to improve and regulate metabolic and endocrine gland function. Take a dose that supplies the equivalent of 150 micrograms of iodine daily.

■ The B vitamins help to support and regenerate the nervous system. Take a B-complex vitamin supplement supplying 25 milligrams of each of the major B vitamins twice a day.

HERBAL TREATMENT

■ Bupleurum and dong quai, also known as Hsiao Yao Wan, is a Chinese patent medicine that helps to regulate the endocrine system. Take 500 milligrams three times daily for two months. Stop for one month, then repeat.

■ Dandelion root is noted for its ability to regulate liver function, which in turn benefits the thyroid gland. Take 500 milligrams or one cup of dandelion-root tea twice a day for six weeks. Stop for one month, then repeat.

■ Iceland moss, Irish moss, and kelp are natural sources of the iodine the thyroid gland requires. Take a dose supplying the equivalent of 150 micrograms of iodine daily.

■ Valerian is a noted calmative that is a proven aid to sleep. Choose a standardized extract containing 0.5 percent isovalerenic acids and take 200 to 300 milligrams one-half hour before bedtime.

HOMEOPATHY

When dealing with hyperthyroidism, it is best to see a homeopathic practitioner who can prescribe a constitutional remedy formulated especially for you. However, the following remedies may afford relief of acute symptoms.

■ *Iodium* is good if you have dark hair and brown eyes, often feel very warm, tend to be obsessive about details, and are usually very much in a rush. Take one dose of *Iodium* 200x or 30c twice daily for three consecutive days. Stop for one week, then repeat.

■ *Natrum muriaticum* is the remedy to choose if you have heart palpitations, constipation, and, possibly, a craving for salt. Take one dose of *Natrum muriaticum* 200x or 30c twice daily for three consecutive days. Stop for one week, then repeat.

BACH FLOWER REMEDIES

Select the remedy that most closely fits your emotional tendencies and concerns, and take it as needed, following the directions on the product label.

■ Holly helps to resolve anger and agitation.

- Impatiens eases nervousness, impatience, and irritability.

- White Chestnut is helpful if you find yourself becoming fixated on certain ideas and tend to dwell on them.

ACUPRESSURE

For the locations of acupressure points on the body, *see* ADMINISTERING AN ACUPRESSURE TREATMENT in Part Three.

- Liver 3 and Pericardium 6 relax and regulate the chest and upper body.

- Four Gates helps to calm the nervous system and reestablish equlibrium throughout the body.

AROMATHERAPY

For specific instructions on how to use aromatherapy, *see* PREPARING AROMATHERAPY TREATMENTS in Part Three.

- The combination of lavender and rosemary oil is soothing to the nerves. Use them as an inhalant or diffuse them into the air in your home. Or add a few drops to a relaxing bath or massage oil.

GENERAL RECOMMENDATIONS

- Get some type of exercise daily. Regular exercise benefits the whole body, and can even help stabilize metabolic function.

- Consult a licensed acupuncturist. Acupuncture is very helpful for endocrine disorders because it works to restore balance in the body. Craniosacral therapy, which involves gentle, subtle manipulation of bones in the head, face, and vertebral column, can also be beneficial.

Hypoglycemia

Severe hypoglycemia, or low blood sugar, is a condition that most often occurs in people who use insulin to treat diabetes and those who consume excessive quantities of alcohol. In such individuals, blood sugar can drop to dangerous levels very suddenly, resulting in a syndrome that can progress rapidly from dizziness, anxiety, headache, and sweating to a loss of coordination, seizures, and changes in consciousness, even coma. (*See* DIABETES.) Functional hypoglycemia, on the other hand, is a less extreme low blood sugar problem that is directly related to dietary habits. It is not the result of a serious physiological abnormality. Rather, it can be caused by eating too little, by not eating often enough, or—the most common cause—eating excessive amounts of sugar.

When you consume sugar, your pancreas responds by producing insulin, the hormone that regulates the levels of glucose (sugar) circulating in the blood. If you have hypoglycemia, your pancreas produces more insulin than necessary. The excess insulin that rushes into your bloodstream brings your blood-sugar level down very rapidly. The end result is that an abnormally low level of glucose remains circulating in your bloodstream.

The symptoms of hypoglycemia include mood swings, irritability, chronic fatigue, hunger, food cravings, dizziness, weakness, sweating, cold sweats, tremors, impaired coordination, a lack of mental clarity, problems with vision, and pronounced personality changes that may manifest themselves in feelings of depression and anxiety or that may cause a person to become confrontational and argumentative. These changes come about because the brain relies on a steady supply of glucose to function normally. If not enough glucose is available, the central nervous system responds by releasing the adrenal hormones adrenaline and cortisol to stimulate the liver to release more glucose. These hormones have other effects in the body as well, causing symptoms similar to those of a panic attack. If the hypoglycemic situation is not corrected promptly and blood sugar continues to fall, brain function suffers directly as a result.

A person who does not have hypoglycemia can safely trust his or her pancreas to handle an occasional overdose of sugar. However, consuming sugar can lead to mood swings, irritability, and other symptoms even in people who do not have this problem. Hypoglycemia has become one of those "fashionable" maladies that is popular in some circles. As a result, this is an overdiagnosed condition. Don't assume that you are hypoglycemic just because you feel a surge of energy, followed by a letdown, after eating a high amount of sugar. These effects are perfectly normal, and they soon disappear.

Sometimes low blood sugar is a result of an underlying disorder. Other conditions that can cause hypoglycemia include an overgrowth of candida (yeast) in the body, thyroid and pituitary disorders, kidney and liver problems, pancreatitis, and adrenal insufficiency. The adrenal glands play an important part in regulating the use of nutrients and energy. If these glands are not functioning as they should, blood-sugar levels are affected. Some people develop hypoglycemia after stomach surgery. People with depressed immune systems are often hypoglycemic as well. High stress levels can be a contributing factor.

Because the symptoms of low blood sugar are the same as those of a number of other disorders—including digestive and intestinal problems, allergies, asthma, chronic fatigue syndrome, nutritional deficiencies, and neurological disorders—the first step in diagnosing hypoglycemia is to rule out any possible underlying conditions. A firm diagnosis can be confirmed only by a five-hour glucose-tolerance test, which shows how much insulin your pancreas produces in response to the ingestion of sugar.

CONVENTIONAL MEDICINE

■ For an acute episode of low blood sugar, the quick answer is a dose of sugar stirred into orange juice, which will give the excess insulin coursing through the body enough glucose to stabilize blood-sugar levels.

■ Functional hypoglycemia is best treated with proper dietary management (see Dietary Guidelines, below). Be aware, however, that this is an overdiagnosed condition. A doctor may interpret a glucose-tolerance test as showing oversensitivity to sugar if it yields a positive result and there is no medical reason (a history of stomach surgery, for example) for you to have low blood sugar.

■ Some physicians may prescribe a mild sedative to combat the anxiety and mood swings, but usually this is not necessary.

DIETARY GUIDELINES

■ Plan your meals around fresh vegetables, lean protein foods such as fish and poultry, and high-fiber whole grains.

■ Eat six to eight small, well-balanced meals every day, rather than two or three large ones. If this is impractical, have three small meals plus wholesome snacks in mid-morning, midafternoon, and midevening. A wholesome snack might include some raw vegetables and a bit of cottage cheese. If you wish, enjoy a small serving of un-processed protein-rich cheese, such as Monterey jack, part-skim mozzarella, or Cheddar. Avoid processed cheeses.

■ Limit your consumption of natural sugars, including those present in fruits, honey, maple syrup, and molasses. Although natural sugar is metabolized more slowly than refined sugar, it still provokes the production of insulin. If you feel you absolutely must have something sweet, have half a piece of fruit.

■ Avoid refined sugars. Presweetened cereals, sodas, and refined and processed foods—even foods that don't taste sweet, such as tomato sauce and peanut butter—can contain sugar, sometimes in surprisingly large amounts. If you buy processed foods, be sure to read labels, and be aware of the many ways in which sugar shows up in food products. Brown sugar, corn syrup, dextrose, fructose, glucose, high-fructose corn syrup, honey, invert sugar, lactose, maltose, mannitol, molasses, rice syrup, sorbitol, sucrose, xylitol—these are just some of the words that tell you a product contains sugar.

■ Avoid artificial sweeteners, caffeine-containing beverages, and alcohol.

NUTRITIONAL SUPPLEMENTS

■ Calcium and magnesium assist in the utilization of glu-cose and calm the nervous system. Take 500 milligrams of calcium and 250 milligrams of magnesium twice daily.

■ Carnitine assists in the conversion of fats to energy and helps keep energy levels balanced. Take 500 to 1,000 milligrams of L-carnitine daily.

■ Chromium improves the efficiency of glucose utilization, which is especially important if you have hypoglycemia. Take 100 to 200 micrograms once or twice daily.

■ Cysteine is an important amino acid that helps normalize blood-sugar levels. Take 500 milligrams of N-acetyl-cysteine daily.

■ To ensure full digestion, take a full-spectrum digestive-enzyme supplement providing 5,000 international units of lipase, 2,500 international units of amylase, 300 international units of protease, plus 500 to 1,000 milligrams of pancreatin, immediately before the two largest meals of the day.

Note: Long-term supplementation with pancreatin is not advised, as it can cause your pancreas to reduce its own production of this important enzyme. Overuse also has the potential to cause nausea or diarrhea. After two months on pancreatin, discontinue use and monitor your reaction. If you find that your problems recur, discuss pancreatin supplementation with your health-care provider.

■ Trace minerals assist in the regulation of blood sugar. Take a trace-mineral supplement or a green-foods supplement such as blue-green algae, chlorella, or spirulina as directed on the product label.

■ The B vitamins, especially vitamins B_1 (thiamine), vitamin B_3 (niacin), vitamin B_{12} (cobalamin), and pantothenic acid, are essential for the proper digestion of carbohydrates and help keep energy levels high. Take a B-complex supplement supplying 25 to 50 milligrams of the major B vitamins daily.

■ Most people who suffer from hypoglycemia have low levels of vitamin C and zinc. Take 500 milligrams of vitamin C, 500 milligrams of bioflavonoids, and 15 milligrams of zinc twice daily, immediately before a meal.

Note: If you take 30 or more milligrams of zinc on a daily basis for more than one or two months, you should also take 1 to 2 milligrams of copper each day to maintain a proper mineral balance.

HERBAL TREATMENT

■ Dandelion root and milk thistle can improve liver function, which is often impaired in individuals suffering from hypoglycemia. Take 500 milligrams of dandelion twice a day for six weeks. Stop for one month, then repeat. For milk thistle, choose an extract standardized to contain 80 percent flavonoids (silymarin) and take 100 milligrams twice daily for three months.

■ Because it strengthens adrenal function, licorice root is very effective in regulating blood-sugar levels. Take 300 to 500 milligrams two to three times daily for five days. Stop for two weeks, then repeat.

Note: Do not use licorice on a daily basis for more than five days at a time, as it can elevate blood pressure. Do not use it at all if you have high blood pressure.

HOMEOPATHY

■ Choose *Lycopodium* if you have a blood-sugar problem accompanied by flatulence. Take one dose of *Lycopodium* 30x or 15c twice daily for three days. Stop for ten days, then repeat.

■ *Natrum muriaticum* is the remedy to choose if you have hypoglycemia and crave salty foods. Take one dose of *Natrum muriaticum* 30x or 15c twice daily for three days. Stop for ten days, then repeat.

■ If you are hypoglycemic and crave rich, spicy foods and alcohol, *Nux vomica* is the remedy of choice. Take one dose of *Nux vomica* 30x or 15c twice daily for three days. Stop for ten days, then repeat.

ACUPRESSURE

For the locations of acupressure points on the body, *see* ADMINISTERING AN ACUPRESSURE TREATMENT in Part Three.

■ All inner and outer Bladder points relax the nervous system and improve digestion.

■ Pericardium 6 relaxes the upper stomach.

■ Spleen 6 and Stomach 36 together improve digestion.

GENERAL RECOMMENDATIONS

■ Don't starve yourself, and don't go more than four to six hours without supplying your body with nutrients.

■ Exercise has been shown to be one of the most important factors in regulating blood sugar. Get regular exercise.

PREVENTION

■ Functional hypoglycemia is caused by a diet that contains too much refined sugar. Eating regular, well-balanced meals is your best defense against this disorder.

Hypothermia

Exposure to extreme cold, or even moderately cold temperatures over a long period of time, can cause a lowering of body temperature. If body temperature reaches 95°F or below, a person is said to have systemic hypothermia. Even cool (not cold) temperatures can cause the problem

for people who are already ill; who are on any type of sedating medication, including alcohol; or who are elderly or very young.

Symptoms include fatigue or weakness, later progressing to confusion, then stupor. The pulse slows and breathing becomes shallow, sometimes intermittent. Once a person has developed true hypothermia, he or she is not likely to be shivering. If nothing is done to correct the situation, coma and death result.

Even if hypothermia is properly treated, it is possible to develop organ damage later as a result. Possible complications following an episode of hypothermia include pneumonia, pancreatitis, kidney failure, and gangrene.

CONVENTIONAL TREATMENT

■ Obviously, rewarming is the treatment of choice, but the speed with which normal temperature is regained is important. Specifically, it should not be done at a rate greater than 1°F per hour. For mild to moderate hypothermia, resting while covered with a blanket in a warm (not hot) room, to conserve residual body heat, may be sufficient, though ideally medical assistance should be enlisted to monitor for possible complications.

■ Severe hypothermia requires more active rewarming, including the administration of warm intravenous fluids and heated oxygen. Placement of a breathing tube and assisted breathing are usually necessary, along with close monitoring for complications, which are likely. If there is no pulse, electrical defibrillation is used to attempt to restart the heart.

DIETARY GUIDELINES

■ When recovering from an episode of hypothermia, drink plenty of fluids to rehydrate your body. Warm drinks like soups and herbal teas are good choices.

■ *Avoid* alcoholic beverages. While alcohol may feel as if it has a warming effect, in fact its effect on the body is just the opposite.

NUTRITIONAL SUPPLEMENTS

■ Hypothermia disrupts the body's electrolyte balance. While recovering from an episode of this nature, take a multimineral supplement that includes all the trace minerals.

■ The B vitamins are required for healthy circulation. Take a B-complex supplement supplying 25 to 50 milligrams of each of the major B vitamins twice daily. Choose a liquid formula for easier absorption.

HERBAL TREATMENT

■ Ginger is warming and also improves circulation. Take a cup of warm ginger tea three times a day for up to five days.

HOMEOPATHY

■ *Aconite* helps to relieve icy coldness, numbness, tingling, and shooting pains. Once you are well enough to take something by mouth, take one dose of *Aconite* 6x or 3c four times over the course of twenty-four hours.

■ *Abrotanum* is good for pricking sensations and coldness. After finishing the *Aconite*, take one dose of *Abrotanum* 30x or 15c four times daily, up to a total of ten doses.

BACH FLOWER REMEDIES

■ Rescue Remedy can help relieve anxiety. Once you are well enough to take something by mouth, take one dose hourly for four hours.

AROMATHERAPY

■ Essential oils of lavender, orange, and rosemary enhance circulation and relieve anxiety. After emergency care has been administered and you are home from the hospital, add three drops of each to a tubful of warm water each day and enjoy a soothing aromatherapy bath.

PREVENTION

■ When the weather is cold, dress in layers. Wearing several layers of loose, warm clothing not only helps to keep you from getting too cold, but from getting too warm. If you start sweating, remove a layer. Otherwise, your sweat will cool your body down too much.

■ Before going outdoors in very cold weather, make certain your head, neck, and ears are well covered. Use any combination of hats, scarves, earmuffs, ski masks, and whatever other articles of clothing you find comfortable. This is particularly important on windy days.

■ When you will be spending time outdoors, take along extra socks and long underwear. Exchanging partially damp clothes for dry ones helps to maintain body temperature.

■ Before spending time outdoors, eat a nutritious meal or snack. Eating will make you feel warmer within ten to fifteen minutes.

■ When you get tired, seek warm shelter. A fatigued body has more difficulty staying warm.

■ Avoid alcohol and tobacco if you will be spending time outdoors in cold weather.

Hypothyroidism

Hypothyroidism is caused by low activity of the thyroid gland, which results in the underproduction of thyroid hormones. Because thyroid hormones initiate energy production and are involved in governing metabolism, a deficiency can cause fatigue, followed by apathy and lethargy. You may lose interest in things that formerly brought pleasure. Unexplained weight gain is common, and the heart rate often slows. Muscle weakness and/or cramps are not uncommon. Other symptoms can include a chronically low body temperature and an inability to tolerate cold; slowed heartbeat; dry, flaky skin and a puffy face and eyes; heavy menstrual periods; a dulling of the hair and hair loss, including thinning or loss of the eyebrows; brittle nails; numbness and tingling in the hands and feet; carpal tunnel syndrome; constipation; thickening of the tongue; and a change in the timbre of the voice.

A deficiency of thyroid hormone also leads to an alteration in the levels of other hormones in the body. In women of childbearing age, reproductive function can suffer. A woman with a serious thyroid deficiency may be unable to conceive. If she does become pregnant, she may miscarry or have a premature baby with a low birth weight, or even give birth to a child with his or her own thyroid problems. Fortunately, with proper treatment, fertility can be restored.

The severity of the symptoms of hypothyroidism depends on the degree of hormone deficiency. A mild case may cause no overt symptoms except for a vague feeling of malaise, while a severe deficiency may cause the full range of problems associated with this condition. Moderate deficiency may cause some or all of these symptoms to some degree.

Most cases of hypothyroidism are a result of *Hashimoto's thyroiditis,* an autoimmune disorder in which the body mistakenly develops antibodies that attack the thyroid gland, resulting in inflammation and, ultimately, destruction of thyroid tissue. Hypothyroidism can also result from treatments for the opposite problem, hyperthyroidism, particularly surgery in which part of the gland is removed and also radiation therapy. In some countries, goitrous hypothyroidism, a result of iodine deficiency, causes many cases of hypothyroidism accompanied by goiter, a grossly swollen thyroid gland. This condition has been rare in Western countries since the introduction of iodized salt, but in some parts of the world it is a serious and widespread problem.

Hypothyroidism, sometimes also called *myxedema,* affects five to eight times more women than men. In around half of the cases, the symptoms come on so gradually and progress so slowly that the affected person may not be aware he or she has a real problem. It is all too easy to attribute early symptoms like forgetfulness, slowed reactions, tiredness, and weight gain to other causes.

Hypothyroidism is diagnosed by measuring the level of thyroid hormones in the blood. The diagnosis of overt hypothyroidism with a blood test is a relatively straightforward proposition. Diagnosing subclinical hypothyroidism—hypothyroidism that is severe enough to cause troublesome symptoms, but too mild to be diagnosed by a blood test—is more difficult. Some people with many symptoms continually test in the low-normal range of thyroid function. If that happens, a doctor is likely to tell you that no medication is indicated and no help is available, while you are actually suffering from a nearly undetectable form of the disease.

If you have symptoms of this condition, you can test your thyroid function yourself. This simple procedure has been called a nuisance by some and a godsend by others. Here's what to do: Keep a thermometer beside your bed. When you awaken in the morning, before moving around (yes, even before you make a trip to the bathroom), tuck the thermometer snugly in your armpit and keep it in place for fifteen minutes. Keep as still as possible. Then remove the thermometer, take a reading, and write it down. Follow this procedure for three days, then determine an average reading by adding all three readings together and dividing by three. If your average temperature is below 97.5°F, in all probability you are suffering from subclinical hypothyroidism and should discuss your findings with your doctor. If you are a woman of childbearing age, time your three-day temperature test to avoid the first week of your menstrual cycle and the few days when you are ovulating, which occur in the middle of the cycle. Because of hormonal swings during these times, the readings will not accurately reflect your true temperature and cannot be used to detect subclinical hypothyroidism.

CONVENTIONAL TREATMENT

■ Levothyroxine (also sold under the brand names Levoxyl and Synthroid) is by far the drug of choice in conventional treatment of hypothyroidism. This is a synthetic copy of the hormone thyroxine (T_4), the hormone produced by the thyroid gland. It is then converted by the body to tri-iodothyronine (T_3), which is more active in regulating metabolism. While many doctors have long believed that there is a big difference in effectiveness between generic and brand-name versions of this drug, it has been shown that in fact there is no real difference. If cost is a factor, you may wish to discuss this with your doctor. The brand-name versions typically cost two to three times more than the generic.

■ If you do not respond to levothyroxine, it may be that your body has difficulty converting T_4 to T_3. In that case, liothyronine (Cytomel), which is synthetic T_3, may be tried. The dosage must be monitored carefully, as overdosage can cause hyperthyroid symptoms.

■ Natural thyroid hormone is available by prescription, but is rarely used today as it is considered old-fashioned and harder to tailor the dosage to an individual's needs.

■ In severe hypothyroidism leading to coma, a combination of thyroid medication and other drugs may be given intravenously, as fast action is important.

■ In most cases, hormone therapy must be continued throughout life. Your doctor will likely recommend regular follow-up appointments—every few months at first, then annually—to monitor your blood levels of thyroid hormone. Remember that hormone requirements can fluctuate, and it is important to be sure that you are taking the correct dosage at all times. For example, too much thyroid hormone can increase the risk of osteoporosis and heart disease, while the correct amount helps to lower cholesterol levels. Hypothyroidism is a chronic disorder that cannot be cured, but that can be managed successfully.

DIETARY GUIDELINES

■ Add to your menu foods that are rich sources of natural iodine. Iodine is vital for the functioning of the thyroid gland. Enjoy seafood and sea vegetables, such as kelp, dulse, hijiki, and kombu.

■ When eaten raw, certain foods can contribute to sluggish thyroid action, among them cabbage, Brussels sprouts, and broccoli. Enjoy these healthy foods cooked, not raw.

NUTRITIONAL SUPPLEMENTS

■ Iodine is required for normal thyroid function. Take 150 micrograms daily.

■ Thyroid glandular extract has proven invaluable to many people with hypothyroidism. Take 60 milligrams daily.

■ Tyrosine is an important amino acid that helps stimulate thyroid function. Take 500 milligrams daily, with breakfast, for up to three weeks at a time.

Note: If you are taking a monoamine oxidase (MAO) inhibitor drug, do not take supplemental tyrosine, as a sudden and dangerous rise in blood pressure may result.

■ The B vitamins are necessary for regulation of the endocrine system, including the thyroid. Take a good B-complex formula supplying 25 to 50 milligrams of each of the major B vitamins daily.

■ If you are a perimenopausal woman with hypothyroidism, hypothalamus/pituitary glandular extract may be helpful, especially if you are feeling depressed and having difficulty with your weight. You may wish to discuss this with your health-care practitioner.

HERBAL TREATMENT

■ Exhaustion goes hand in hand with hypothyroidism. American and Siberian ginseng help to reduce fatigue and restore energy. Take 250 milligrams of American ginseng or 100 to 200 milligrams of Siberian ginseng extract standardized to contain 0.5 percent eleutheroside E twice daily, one-half hour before breakfast and again one-half hour before lunch.

Note: Do not use American ginseng if you have high blood pressure, heart disease, or hypoglycemia. If you are sensitive to the effects of caffeine and other stimulants, you may want to consult with a qualified herbalist before using ginseng.

■ For iodine, which supports the thyroid, take a dose of kelp supplying the equivalent of 150 milligrams of iodine daily.

■ Mild depression is common among people with underactive thyroids. St. John's wort acts to gently but effectively restore good spirits. Choose a product containing 0.3 percent hypericin and take 200 to 300 milligrams once or twice daily.

HOMEOPATHY

■ *Calcarea carbonica* helps to stimulate the thyroid. Take one dose of *Calcarea carbonica* 30c or 200x three times a week for three weeks.

■ Take homeopathic thyroid 200x or 30c for one week out of every month. Take one each morning for five days. Stop for three weeks, then repeat. Follow this cycle a total of three times.

BACH FLOWER REMEDIES

Select the remedy that most closely fits your emotional tendencies and concerns, and take it as needed, following the directions on the product label.

■ For exhaustion, take Hornbeam or Olive.

■ Choose Larch if you lack self confidence.

■ Scleranthus helps to counteract feelings of uncertainty and the inability to make decisions.

ACUPRESSURE

For the locations of acupressure points on the body, *see* ADMINISTERING AN ACUPRESSURE TREATMENT in Part Three.

■ All Bladder points relax the nervous system and improve circulation.

■ Pericardium 6 improves energy metabolism.

■ Spleen 6 and Stomach 36 together improve digestion.

GENERAL RECOMMENDATIONS

■ Exercise, exercise, exercise. If you are suffering from hypothyroidism, exercising is the best thing you can do for yourself. Exercise both stimulates and normalizes thyroid function. It also helps increase your energy levels, fight depression, and reduce stress.

Impotence

Impotence is the inability of an adult male to achieve (or sustain) an erection sufficient to copulate successfully. It is a very common problem. Most men experience an episode of impotence at some time in their lives. More than 15 million men in the United States suffer from it on a chronic basis.

Impotence can be physical or psychological in origin. Physical causes include diseases or anatomical defects in the genitalia, poor overall health, diabetes, cancer, prostate surgery, hormonal imbalances, spinal-cord damage, and hardening of the arteries. Impotence can also be a side effect of various drugs, particularly tranquilizers, blood-pressure medications, certain antidepressants, alcohol, marijuana, and nicotine. Excessive alcohol consumption in particular is a major cause of a temporary inability to perform. Most of these factors result in impotence because they interfere with either the flow of blood to the penis or the transmission of nerve impulses to and from the penis. In some cases, impotence may be traced to a deficiency of the sex hormone testosterone, but this is quite rare, as only a very small amount of this hormone is required for successful erections.

This disorder becomes more common as men get older. Studies show that by age sixty, many men find it takes longer to achieve an erection. This does not mean, however, that impotence is a natural consequence of aging. Rather, it points to the fact that as a man gets older, he is increasingly likely to have other conditions or take medications that can result in erectile difficulties. Then, too, older men may feel less need to ejaculate because their bodies produce smaller amounts of semen, which translates into less desire. Nevertheless, many men continue to enjoy satisfying sex lives into their seventies and eighties.

If you are impotent only from time to time, if you have erections during the night, and/or if you can achieve an erection through masturbation, it is likely that the cause of your problem is psychological in nature. Psychological factors that can lead to impotence include anxiety, depression, stress, anger or conflict with one's partner, guilt feelings, fear (of intimacy, failure, disease, or impregnating one's partner), and lack of desire. Any of these can be compounded by fatigue, overwork, certain drugs, and nutritional deficiencies. Sometimes, a combination of physical and psychological factors are involved in this problem.

CONVENTIONAL MEDICINE

■ If you are taking any drugs, for any reason at all, discuss your problems with your doctor. Common suspects here include some hormones, blood-pressure medications, amphetamines, tranquilizers, antidepressants, and sedatives. It may be advisable to discontinue a medication, adjust the dosage, or switch to an alternative that works better for you. *Do not* simply decide to alter your use of a prescription drug on your own, however. Always consult with your physician.

■ If there is no obvious cause for impotence, a complete physical examination, including hormone studies and anatomical evaluation, may be necessary.

■ If a deficiency of testosterone is discovered, hormone therapy may be prescribed.

■ Sometimes the blood vessels that serve the penis can become blocked by clots or atherosclerotic plaques. If a physical exam detects such a problem, surgery may be recommended to reconstruct or bypass the problem areas.

■ If no physical cause can be found and a psychological basis is suspected, counseling may be all that is necessary. There are clinics and practitioners who specialize in this kind of work. Ask your physician for a referral.

■ If all else fails, there are a number of "artificial" strategies to help men achieve erection. These include:

• External vacuum-type devices that draw blood into the penis, supplemented with a constriction ring to keep it there.

• Penile implants.

• Medications that cause blood to be held in the plexus of veins in the penis. These are administered by injection, either with a tiny needle or a plunger-type device, and can result in erections lasting an hour or more. Determining the proper dosage is important, as too much can cause painful, long-lasting erections.

• Yohimbine (Yocon, Yohimex) is a prescription drug that may increase peripheral blood flow, including blood flow to the penis. Depending on the cause of your problem, this may be worth a try. Possible side effects include elevated blood pressure and/or heart rate, irritability, tremor, and nervousness.

■ The latest pharmaceutical offered for the treatment of impotence is sildenafil (Viagra). This drug relaxes blood vessels in the penis, allowing more blood to flow into it to create an erection. Sildenafil requires sexual stimulation to work—you cannot just take the drug and wait for results. Possible side effects include headache, flushing, digestive difficulties, nasal congestion, blurred vision, light sensitivity, and changes in color vision. There is also a risk of too-low blood pressure, heart failure, and cardiac arrest. You should not use sildenafil if you take any medication of the nitrate class for angina pectoris, or chest pain due to an inadequate supply of oxygen to the heart muscle. These drugs include nitroglycerin (Nitro-Bid, Nitro-Dur, Nitro-

stat), isosorbide dinitrate (Isordil, Sorbitrate), and isosorbide mononitrite (Imdur, Monoket).

DIETARY GUIDELINES

■ Follow a high-fiber diet plan that is low in saturated, hydrogenated, and partially hydrogenated fats. A diet high in these fats not only contributes to clogged coronary arteries, but also inhibits blood supply to the penis.

■ Limit your consumption of alcohol and caffeine. Alcohol especially impairs sexual prowess. A glass of wine with dinner is fine, but excessive alcohol consumption can leave you (and therefore your partner) unable to fully enjoy "dessert."

■ A romantic dinner may set the scene, but do not eat a large meal before engaging in sex. If your body is fully occupied with the digestive processes, sexual functioning can suffer.

NUTRITIONAL SUPPLEMENTS

■ Bovine prostate glandular and orchic tissue extract is a formula that has proven helpful to many men troubled by impotence. Take 100 to 300 milligrams twice daily.

■ If you suffer from gas and bloating, take digestive enzymes with meals to ensure full digestion and make your lower abdomen more comfortable. Digestive enzymes can also help with circulatory problems.

■ The essential fatty acids, found in black currant seed oil, borage oil, evening primrose oil, and flaxseed oil, are needed for the health of the prostate gland and are instrumental in maintaining normal levels of hormones. Choose one of these oils and take 1,000 milligrams twice daily.

■ Magnesium helps relax the nervous system and relieve anxiety. It also regulates the bowels and prevents constipation, which is sometimes a factor in impotence. Take 200 milligrams of magnesium twice daily.

■ Vitamin E, often called the "sex vitamin," helps to strengthen hormonal and reproductive function. Choose a product containing mixed tocopherols and begin by taking 200 international units daily, then gradually increase the dosage until you are taking 400 international units in the morning and again in the evening.

Note: If you have high blood pressure, limit your intake of supplemental vitamin E to a total of 400 international units daily. If you are taking an anticoagulant (blood thinner), consult your physician before taking supplemental vitamin E.

■ Zinc is necessary for healthy prostate function and the production of testosterone. Take 25 milligrams daily. Take zinc with food to prevent stomach upset.

HERBAL TREATMENT

■ Chinese (Korean) ginseng contains precursors the body

can use in the production of sex hormones. Select a standardized extract containing 7 percent ginsenosides and begin by taking half the manufacturer's recommended dose, then gradually increase the amount until you are taking it as directed on the product label.

Note: Do not use Chinese ginseng if you have high blood pressure, heart disease, or hypoglycemia. If you are sensitive to the effects of caffeine and other stimulants, you may want to consult with a qualified herbalist before using ginseng.

Damiana, a tonic herb that is helpful to the male hormonal system, is considered an aphrodisiac. Take 250 to 500 milligrams twice a day for up to one month.

The Chinese herb fo-ti (also known as *ho shou wu*) is an effective blood tonic that can be helpful if impotence is accompanied by excessive fatigue. Take 500 to 1,000 milligrams once or twice daily.

Ginkgo biloba has been shown to help restore blood flow to the genitals, even if it has been inhibited by medication such as antidepressants. Choose a product containing at least 24 percent ginkgo heterosides (sometimes called flavoglycosides) and take 40 milligrams three times daily. Be aware that to attain the desired result, you must use this herb for six to eight months.

■ Oat straw has shown beneficial effects in sexual performance and desire for both men and women. Take 500 milligrams two or three times daily.

Saw palmetto has been used for centuries as an aid to the prostate. If impotence originates with a swollen prostate (benign hyperprostatitis), choose a standardized extract containing 90 percent essential fatty acids and sterols, and take 200 to 400 milligrams two or three times daily.

HOMEOPATHY

Choose *Baryta carbonica* if you feel chilly, mentally dull, and physically slow. You may be somewhat overweight and lethargic. Take one dose of *Baryta carbonica* 30x or 15c twice daily for four to five days.

If lower bowel gases interfere with sexual function, *Lycopodium* is the remedy of choice. Take one dose of *Lycopodium* 30x or 15c twice daily for four to five days.

Staphysagria is good if you have a strong sex drive and prefer masturbation to having sex with a partner because of the difficulty in achieving an erection. Take one dose of *Staphysagria* 30x or 15c twice daily for four to five days.

ACUPRESSURE

For the locations of acupressure points on the body, *see* ADMINISTERING AN ACUPRESSURE TREATMENT in Part Three.

■ The back Bladder points relax and tone the nervous system, and increase circulation to the urinary tract and reproductive organs.

■ Gallbladder 20 helps to bring down energy from the head and keep it circulating throughout the body.

■ Kidney 3 increases circulation to the urinary tract and reproductive organs.

■ Liver 3 relaxes the nervous system and brings energy down from the head.

■ Spleen 6 and Stomach 36 together tone the digestive tract and strengthen overall well-being.

AROMATHERAPY

For specific instructions on how to use aromatherapy, *see* PREPARING AROMATHERAPY TREATMENTS in Part Three.

■ There are many essential oils that can help reduce stress and heighten sexual desire. Jasmine, patchouli, rose, sandalwood, and ylang-ylang are among the best known for this purpose. Choose one to three of these oils and prepare a sensual, relaxing aromatherapy bath or massage in preparation for lovemaking.

GENERAL RECOMMENDATIONS

■ If you are overweight, lose the excess pounds. Obesity can compromise sexual function. Sometimes simply losing weight can make a dramatic difference in your sexual ability.

■ Exercise. Satisfying sex involves many muscles. It takes roughly the same amount of energy to have intercourse as it does to climb two flights of stairs. If your body is toned and fit, you will not only be less likely to suffer from impotence, but you (and your partner) will enjoy sex more. This "prescription" applies no matter how old you are.

■ If you consume alcohol, do so in moderation only. Men who consume excessive amounts of alcohol are more likely to suffer from impotence as they get older than are those who abstain or drink only moderately.

■ If you smoke, quit, and avoid secondhand smoke. Nicotine constricts blood vessels, including those that serve the penis. Consequently, smokers are at higher risk for impotence than nonsmokers.

■ If impotence is an occasional problem, remember that sex is not synonymous with intercourse. Engage in play and exploration with your partner to find other ways you can give each other satisfaction and pleasure.

■ Remember that every man has a problem with impotence at least once in his life. Anxiety over performance and fear of failure only make things worse. Try not to become obsessed with the problem.

PREVENTION

■ A healthy lifestyle is the best preventive. Many diseases linked to diet and lifestyle can lead to impotence.

Incontinence

Urinary incontinence, or the uncontrolled leaking of urine, is a relatively common problem among older adults, but it can affect people in other age groups as well. There are four basic types of urinary incontinence:

1. Total incontinence. This condition is characterized by a more or less steady loss of small amounts of urine, regardless of body position. Possible causes include damage to the urinary sphincter as a result of an anatomical abnormality or injury from childbirth or surgery; nerve damage; infiltrating tumors; and the presence of fistulas, or abnormal passages, through which the urine exits the body, bypassing the urethra.

2. Stress incontinence. In this condition, coughing, lifting, sneezing, or anything else that increases pressure within the abdomen forces urine to leak. This is far more common in women than in men, especially women who have had many children, which stretches the muscles of the pelvic floor, or who have had surgery in the pelvic region.

3. Urge incontinence. Urge incontinence involves inflammation of the bladder or neurological problems that can cause sudden, uncontrollable urges to void, leaving no time to make it to the bathroom.

4. Overflow incontinence. In persons with overflow incontinence, the bladder is distended, so no additional urine can enter without some dribbling out. Chronic retention of urine can lead to this problem. It is most common in older adults and in men with enlarged prostates, which restricts the outflow of urine.

Incontinence is not necessarily a permanent problem. Pregnancy, delirium, infection, vaginal irritation, depression, and psychosis can all cause some form of incontinence. Certain medications can be responsible as well, among them diuretics such as furosemide (Lasix); antidepressants such as amitriptyline (Elavil) and desipramine (Norpramin); antipsychotics such as thioridazine (Mellaril) and haloperidol (Haldol); sedatives such as diazepam (Valium) and flurazepam (Dalmane); and many blood-pressure drugs, decongestants, antihistamines, and others. Alcohol also can affect incontinence.

The most common cause of incontinence in elderly people is a condition called *detrusor overactivity,* in which the detrusor muscle, which surrounds the bladder, contracts without warning, resulting in urge incontinence. Often, no underlying cause can be found for this problem. However, tumors, bladder stones, or some other obstruction of the urinary tract can be involved in some cases.

Routine urinalysis and a urine culture are usually per-formed to check for irritating infections or abnormal kidney function. An anatomical abnormality such as a fistula, urine retention, or a bladder neck that has shifted, can be detected by a cystogram, in which a fluid that is visible on x-ray is introduced into the bladder by means of a catheter, and x-ray photographs are taken both while you are at rest and while you are straining. Ultrasound may be useful. A procedure called cystometry may be used to look for nerve damage, drug reactions, inflammation, and other problems. In this technique, carbon dioxide gas or water is put into the bladder and pressures are noted in the presence of different stimuli, such as certain drugs, straining, and so on.

Much less common than urinary incontinence is fecal incontinence. A variety of problems, including nerve damage; diarrhea; local surgery; pressure from an enlarged prostate, tumors, or fecal impaction; and anal tears from childbirth trauma can permit unintended loss of stool.

CONVENTIONAL TREATMENT

■ Stress incontinence may be treated with phenylpropanolamine, a decongestant that can increase resistance in the urethra. If physical examination determines that the bladder neck has descended too low to be effective at holding back urine flow, surgery may be recommended to correct the problem. For menopausal and postmenopausal women, treatment with a topical estrogen cream may help.

■ Urge incontinence usually requires medical intervention to stabilize the detrusor muscle or the urethra. Medications commonly used for this purpose include oxybutinin (Ditropan), a type of drug classified as an antispasmodic; propantheline (Pro-Banthine), an anticholinergic; or the tricyclic antidepressant imipramine (Tofranil). All of these drugs act to relax the bladder muscle. Possible side effects of oxybutinin include decreased sweating, with an increased risk of heatstroke, drowsiness, restlessness, hallucinations, constipation, nausea, dry mouth, and increased heart rate. Pro-Banthine can cause similar side effects. Tofranil can cause high or low blood pressure, increased heart rate, numbness, tremors, blood cell changes, drowsiness, sex drive decrease, and changes in blood-sugar level. A newer drug, tolterodine (Detrol), works for urge incontinence by competing against muscle receptors that make the bladder contract, so that a larger volume of urine may be held. Possible side effects include dry mouth, digestive problems, headache, constipation, dry eyes, high blood pressure, dizziness, and blurred vision. This drug should not to be used if you suffer from urinary or gastric retention, or if you have narrow-angle glaucoma.

■ Overflow incontinence is treated first by inserting a catheter into the bladder to remove retained urine. If an enlarged prostate is at the root of the problem, that may be addressed in various ways (*see* PROSTATE PROBLEMS). If the underlying problem is urethral blockage or stricture, a doctor may correct it by inserting a probe past the area in question to permit easier and earlier urine flow, so that the overflow situation does not recur. In some cases, more invasive types of surgery may be needed to release the obstruction. The medications used for urge incontinence may also be tried.

In cases of total incontinence, surgical reconstruction of the outflow tract may be possible. This may include artificial urinary sphincter placement or the injection of collagen around the urethra for support.

If an anatomical abnormality is causing anal incontinence, surgical repair may be indicated. If examination of the anal sphincter muscle shows it has a poorer than normal ability to contract, biofeedback therapy to train and strengthen the musculature may help.

■ If you regularly take any type of medication, whether prescription or over the counter, you may wish to review it with your doctor, since certain drugs can contribute to incontinence. It may be possible to change your prescription. Do not discontinue any prescription medication or alter the dosage on your own, however. Always consult with your physician first.

DIETARY GUIDELINES

Avoid sweets and anything containing refined sugar. Excessive sugar consumption weakens the proper functioning of the genitourinary tract.

If you are overweight, begin a healthy weight-loss program to help you lose the extra pounds (*see* OBESITY). Overweight can be a significant contributing factor in incontinence.

NUTRITIONAL SUPPLEMENTS

■ To strengthen the kidneys, take 500 milligrams of kidney extract four times a day for one month. Then cut back to 500 milligrams three times a day for one month.

HERBAL TREATMENT

■ There are two Chinese herbal formulas known in English as Support the Right Kidney and Support the Left Kidney. Available at Chinese herbal pharmacies, these remedies have been used for centuries to strengthen genitourinary function and resolve incontinence. Take 500 milligrams of each twice a day.

HOMEOPATHY

■ For chronic incontinence, see a qualified homeopathic practitioner who can prescribe an appropriate constitutional remedy.

■ If incontinence is accompanied by low back pain, weak-

ness, and fatigue, and you feel considerably better physically when your mind is engaged, try *Helonias-Chamaelirium*. Take one dose of *Helonias-Chamaelirium* 6x or 3c three times daily for up to four days. Wait two weeks, then repeat.

BACH FLOWER REMEDIES

Select the remedy that most closely fits your disposition and emotional tendencies and concerns, and take it as needed, following the directions on the product label.

■ Mimulus helps to resolve fear.

■ Wild Oat aids in overcoming difficulty making decisions.

ACUPRESSURE

For the locations of acupressure points on the body, *see* ADMINISTERING AN ACUPRESSURE TREATMENT in Part Three.

■ The combination of Kidney 3 and 7, Spleen 6, and Stomach 36 strengthens genitourinary function.

GENERAL RECOMMENDATIONS

■ A type of pelvic-floor exercise called Kegel exercises retrain and strengthen the muscles and sphincters of the pelvic floor. They are easy to perform, are not time-consuming, and can be done anywhere, as follows: Squeeze the muscles tightly around the front and back passages, as if trying to stop urination. Hold the contraction for two seconds, then release, wait a moment, and repeat. Ten contractions equals one set of exercises. Over time, you should gradually work up to holding each contraction for ten seconds. Often it takes several months to be able to do this, so be patient. You should try to do ten sets of exercises each day. Many people do them while watching television, talking on the phone, or even while stopped at red lights while driving.

Indigestion

Go into any supermarket or drugstore and you will find it awash in antacids. Turn on the television or radio and you will find heartburn, "sour stomach," and the like to be the subject of virtually every other commercial. This is testimony to the fact that indigestion is a pervasive problem in our society.

Actually, indigestion is not a single disorder but a catch-all term that may be used to describe any of a number of minor discomforts associated with eating, including a mild burning sensation, gas, bloating, slow digestion, regurgitation, an acidic taste in the mouth, even nausea. The medical version of this term is *dyspepsia*.

The causes of indigestion are as variable as the symptoms. There are many common medications that can cause digestive upset. Nonsteroidal anti-inflammatory drugs (NSAIDs) such as aspirin and ibuprofen are notorious for this. (In fact, in larger doses, or over long periods of time, they can produce full-blown ulcers.) The presence of parasites, having either too much or too little stomach acid, undiagnosed infection, any of a myriad of toxins, or any combination of these factors may be involved as well. Heartburn is often caused by *gastroesophageal reflux,* better known as *acid reflux*. In this condition, the sphincter muscle that is supposed to provide a one-way valve from the esophagus down into the stomach does not function properly, allowing stomach acid to back up into the esophagus. This irritates the tissues and causes pain.

Nearly everyone can name a food, or list of foods, that does not agree with him or her. Food sensitivities are real, and abstinence from these foods can mean the difference between being comfortable and uncomfortable, if not downright ill. Then, too, emotional disturbances such as nervousness, anxiety, impatience, fear, anger, resentment, or depression, plus the wearing effects of fatigue, can play a large part in how food is digested, as can eating in a hurry. Digestion starts in the mouth, and fast eating or inadequate chewing can set you up for an uncomfortable after-meal episode. Looked at another way, digestion begins even before you start eating, with the "foreplay" of smelling the food and anticipating a really good meal; this causes the stomach to prepare by secreting acid and enzymes necessary for good digestion.

There are certain diseases that can manifest themselves in indigestion. These include gallbladder disease, pancreatitis, thyroid problems, diabetes, cardiovascular disease, even various cancers. However, the majority of cases of indigestion are functional—that is, they are not caused by any underlying disease.

If you suffer from indigestion that is persistent, no matter what solution you try or what you eat, or if the problem seems to be getting worse, a checkup is in order to rule out any potentially serious cause. Otherwise, this is a excellent time to try natural remedies. They can be highly effective and have little or no toxicity, a distinct advantage over most, if not all, conventional drugs. Contrary to what many people believe, indigestion is *not* an unavoidable part of life. Even with today's stressful, hassled lifestyles, a little education and a tiny bit of foresight can probably make your indigestion nothing more than a not-so-fond memory.

CONVENTIONAL TREATMENT

■ For gas symptoms, a product containing simethicone, such as Gas-X, Mylanta Gas, or Phazyme is likely to be recommended. Simethicone breaks up gas bubbles and tends to bring about some relief. These products are available over the counter.

■ For heartburn, antacids are the old standby of conventional treatment. This class of medications includes such well-known products as Tums, Rolaids, and Maalox, which buffer the acid in the stomach and tend to provide some relief (although many physicians feel the action is a placebo effect). If you use these products, read labels carefully. Some utilize aluminum hydroxide, a form of aluminum, and while no firm connection has been established, high levels of aluminum have been linked to Alzheimer's disease. Choose a calcium-based product instead. Because some antacids can actually end up increasing the production of acids in the stomach, or cause constipation or diarrhea, they should not be used indiscriminately.

■ In addition to standard antacids, there is now a variety of acid-blocking agents available over the counter. These include nizatidine (Axid AR), famotidine (Pepcid AC), and cimetidine (Tagamet HB). It should be kept in mind that acid is present in the stomach for a reason, and that digestion and absorption may be adversely affected anytime these medications are used.

■ Drugs to speed the movement of food through the digestive tract can sometimes afford relief of acid-reflux symptoms. Examples of drugs in this class include cisapride (Propulsid) and metoclopramide (Reglan). Possible side effects of cisapride include headaches, visual disturbances, infections, and, paradoxically, gastrointestinal problems; potential problems with metoclopramide include dizziness, high or low blood pressure, the development of tardive dyskinesia (a disorder characterized by odd, involuntary movements), and, again, gastrointestinal problems. These medications can also interact with other drugs, so discuss their use with your doctor before taking them.

DIETARY GUIDELINES

■ Eat in a relaxed environment. Taking the time to actually enjoy a meal can make a big difference. Eat slowly, chew your food well, and try not to swallow air while eating.

■ Try adding steamed cabbage to the menu. It contains glutamine, which can calm an irritated stomach. Fresh cabbage juice also works well. The cabbage should be juiced and the juice taken immediately after preparation.

■ Many foods have a tendency to cause indigestion. If you have a sensitive digestive tract, avoid cucumbers, peppers, tomatoes, onions, cabbage, beans, and refined carbohydrates. You should also stay away from heavily spiced foods, rich foods, fried foods, junk foods, alcohol, caffeine, carbonated beverages, and processed foods full of unpronounceable additives. All these substances have the potential to cause digestive disturbances.

■ To track down specific foods that may be causing problems, eliminate from your diet any food you either have cravings for or eat every day, and see if your symptoms improve. You can also keep a diary of what you eat and any symptoms you have following meals. Once you have identified the offenders, banish them from the menu.

■ Avoid overeating. If you have a sensitive stomach, you may be able to avoid discomfort simply by eating smaller meals. Try eating five or six small meals instead of three large ones.

■ Don't smoke. Smoking increases acidity in the stomach.

NUTRITIONAL SUPPLEMENTS

■ Many people with acid reflux find their symptoms improve if they take supplements containing betaine hydrochloride (HCl). Apparently, if the level of acid in the stomach is too low, the sphincter muscle separating the stomach and the esophagus can loosen, allowing what acid there is to escape up into the esophagus. Betaine HCl increases the acidity of the stomach and helps prevent this problem. It is available in a variety of formulas, both on its own and with additional digestive enzymes. Follow the dosage directions on the product label and take it immediately *after* meals.

■ If your main complaint occurs within thirty minutes of eating, take a full-spectrum digestive-enzyme supplement providing 5,000 international units of lipase, 2,500 international units of amylase, and 300 international units of protease, plus 500 to 1,000 milligrams of pancreatin, immediately after the two largest meals of the day to ensure complete digestion.

Note: Long-term supplementation with pancreatin is not advised, as it can cause your pancreas to reduce its own production of this important enzyme. Overuse also has the potential to cause nausea or diarrhea. After two months on pancreatin, discontinue use and monitor your reaction. If you find that your digestive problems recur, discuss pancreatin supplementation with your health-care provider.

■ Glutamine can help soothe irritation in the gastrointestinal tract. Try taking 500 milligrams of L-glutamine two to three times daily for up to one month.

■ Take probiotic supplements of acidophilus and/or bifidobacteria. For indigestion, powdered or liquid formulas are the best choice; these work in the stomach, while capsules open in the intestines. Tablets are not usually as effective, and must be chewed thoroughly. Acidophilus powder can be taken any time for indigestion—simply take $1/4$ to $1/2$ teaspoon as needed. If you must use capsules, open them and pour the contents onto your tongue rather than swallowing them whole. If you are allergic to milk, select a dairy-free formula.

■ Vitamin E soothes the stomach. Choose the mixed-tocopherol or d-alpha tocopherol form, not dl-alpha-tocopherol. Begin by taking 200 international units daily and gradually increase the dosage until you are taking 400 international units once or twice daily.

Note: If you have high blood pressure, limit your intake of supplemental vitamin E to a total of 400 international units daily. If you are taking an anticoagulant (blood thinner), consult your physician before taking supplemental vitamin E.

HERBAL TREATMENT

■ Aloe vera juice helps to clear and resolve an upset stomach that feels "burning." Make sure to get a food-grade product. Take 1 tablespoon diluted in 6 ounces of water up to three times daily. Use it sparingly; it can be a strong cathartic.

■ Gentian root is a bitter herb that has been used for centuries throughout Europe to enhance digestion, especially of proteins and fats. Take 500 milligrams twice a day, with meals.

■ Ginger is a notable digestive aid. It aids digestion, enhances assimilation, and reduces nausea. Take one or two 500-milligram capsules as needed.

■ Deglycyrrhizinated licorice (DGL) can be amazingly helpful. Chew two 250- to 500-milligram lozenges with a glass of water twenty minutes before each meal.

Note: Ordinary licorice can elevate blood pressure, and should not be taken on a daily basis for more than five days in a row. DGL should not have this effect, however.

■ Peppermint is a time-tested, time-honored herb that is very effective for all forms of indigestion. It enhances digestion, speeds the emptying time of the stomach, and reduces flatulence. Drink peppermint tea with meals.

Note: If you are using peppermint tea and also taking a homeopathic preparation, allow one hour between the two. Otherwise, the strong smell of the mint may interfere with the action of the homeopathic remedy.

HOMEOPATHY

■ *Carbo vegetabilis* is for the individual with a sensitive stomach. You tend to have burning pain in the center of the stomach, burp a lot, and may suffer from nausea in the morning on arising. Take one dose of *Carbo vegetabilis* 30x or 15c twenty minutes after eating up to three or four times a day, as needed, for up to two days.

■ *Nux vomica* is good if you have abdominal gas and flatulence, love fat, and desire stimulants such as strong coffee. Take one dose of *Nux vomica* 30x or 15c twenty minutes after eating up to three or four times a day, as needed, for up to two days.

BACH FLOWER REMEDIES

Select the remedy that most closely fits your emotional tendencies and concerns, and take it as needed, following the directions on the product label.

■ Elm is the remedy for feelings of inadequacy.

■ Holly calms anger and a tendency to indulge in fits of bad temper, possibly due to underlying feelings of jealousy and insecurity.

Impatiens helps to tame the tension, nervousness, and impatience typical of the type-A personality.

Mustard is good for sadness and depression, possibly as a result of a loss of some kind.

Red Chestnut helps relieve chronic worry and excessive concern over the well-being of others.

Scleranthus is helpful if you often feel uncertain and just can't make decisions—you tend to waver between one course of action and another.

White Chestnut is good if you tend to obsess about events that should have been forgotten long ago.

ACUPRESSURE

For the locations of acupressure points on the body, see ADMINISTERING AN ACUPRESSURE TREATMENT in Part Three.

■ Gallbladder 34 improves digestion.

Liver 3 relaxes the nervous system.

■ Spleen 6 and Stomach 36 together tone the digestive system and improve digestion.

AROMATHERAPY

For specific instructions on how to use aromatherapy, see PREPARING AROMATHERAPY TREATMENTS in Part Three.

Essential oil of bergamot helps to relieve flatulence; basil, peppermint, and thyme oils promote overall digestion. Use up to three of them as inhalants or diffuse them into the air. Or add a few drops to massage oil and gently massage the abdominal area.

Note: Do not take essential oils internally. They are suitable for external use only.

GENERAL RECOMMENDATIONS

To lessen stomach acidity and ease nausea, a mixture of baking soda and water is effective. However, this old standby should be used only once. Dissolve $1/4$ teaspoon of baking soda in $1/2$ cup of pure water.

■ Green clay helps to neutralize an acid stomach and relieve nausea. Mix 1 teaspoon of clay in 1 cup of spring water. The mixture can be taken immediately, but most people don't care for the taste. It is usually better to per-mit the mixture to stand overnight to allow the clay to settle out and drink it in the morning.

■ If you have chronic indigestion, or if the problem seems to be getting worse, consult your health-care provider. You may have an underlying condition that requires treatment.

■ If you have significant nausea, are vomiting, or have diarrhea after eating, chances are that you have food poisoning, not indigestion, and should treat it accordingly. (See FOOD POISONING.)

■ Apple-cider vinegar is a digestive aid with proven benefits. Add 1 to 2 teaspoons of apple cider vinegar and honey (to taste) to a small amount of hot water. Sip this mixture twice daily, with meals, for one month.

■ Some people develop a chronic cough as a result of acid reflux. If you have a cough as well as acid reflux, see your doctor.

PREVENTION

■ Eat slowly and chew your food thoroughly. Spend at least thirty leisurely minutes at the table, even if you finish a plateful of food in fifteen minutes. Train yourself to slow down. Drink peppermint tea with meals.

■ Don't overeat. Take only a small amount of food at one sitting. Opt for five or six small meals a day instead of three large ones.

Infertility

A couple who fail to conceive after a year (or more) of unprotected sexual intercourse are said to be infertile. As many as one in every four couples in this country experiences infertility at some point.

Conception depends on the successful completion of an intricate and complex chain of events involving both partners. In the woman, an egg must mature in one of the ovaries, be released into the fallopian tube, be fertilized in the upper reaches of the tube, complete the journey through the fallopian tube to the uterus—the lining of which has, in the meantime, been building up in preparation for receiving the fertilized egg—and be implanted in the uterine wall. In men, the testes must produce sufficient sperm, which then must mature in the epididymides, coiled tubes located behind the testes, over a period of two to four weeks; travel through tubes called the vas deferens to the seminal vesicles, located under the bladder, where they are stored; be ejaculated successfully into the woman's body; and travel through the cervix and uterus to fertilize the egg in the fallopian tube. Anything that interferes with any of these processes can result in infertility. Moreover, since a woman generally ovulates (releases an egg) only once every twenty-six to thirty-five days, the timing of all of these events must be just right for conception to result. In this section, we will examine some of the more common scenarios that lead to infertility.

Conditions Affecting Women

Among women, the most common cause of infertility is that the ovaries fail to release a mature egg. The ovaries are small oval-shaped organs located on each side of the uterus. In an adult, they are from one to two inches long. Beginning at puberty, the ovaries normally release one mature egg cell at the midpoint of each menstrual cycle.

An infant girl is born with anywhere from 40,000 to 300,000 immature egg cells in each ovary. Obviously, only a few hundred of these thousands of eggs will reach maturity during a woman's reproductive years. Hormones from the pituitary gland control the production of female sex hormones and regulate the processes by which eggs mature. A hormonal imbalance that either prevents ovulation or reduces the frequency of ovulation is very often the reason for failure to conceive. Although ovulatory failure can occur spontaneously, for no obvious reason, it can also be the result of a disorder of the ovaries, such as a tumor or cyst, or even stress. Whether from illness, intense physical activity, or emotional or psychological difficulties, stress can cause a drop in hormone production. Age is another consideration. A woman's fertility naturally begins to decline when she reaches her thirties, making it more difficult for her to conceive.

If ovulation is normal but there is a blockage of the fallopian tubes, the sperm and egg can be prevented from reaching each other. This kind of blockage is often a consequence of pelvic inflammatory disease (PID), a complication of sexually transmitted diseases such as chlamydia. Chlamydia infects an estimated 4 million Americans annually and is the cause of many cases of infertility.

Disorders of the uterus, such as fibroids or endometriosis, can also cause infertility. A 1997 article in *The New England Journal of Medicine* stated that from 30 to 40 percent of women with unexplained difficulty conceiving actually have a mild form of endometriosis. (*See* ENDOMETRIOSIS.) The condition may be so slight that there is no evidence of blockage, and ovulation is normal, which makes it very difficult to diagnose the problem.

Some one in fifty to one in twenty women of reproductive age may have *polycystic ovary syndrome,* also called Stein-Leventhal syndrome, which causes chronic anovulation (failure to release an egg each month) and, consequently, infertility. The cause of this problem is unknown, but it is known that women who have this problem do not experience normal monthly fluctuations in hormone levels. Instead, the levels of several hormones remain both constant and high. One of these, luteinizing hormone

(LH), causes changes in the ovary, resulting in the formation of cysts, cessation of ovulation, and excess growth of cells that produce androgens (masculinizing hormones). As a result, many of these women tend to have hirsutism (excessive hair growth) and other masculinized characteristics, as well as either a lack of menstrual bleeding or excessive bleeding. Many of these women are also overweight. They also, unfortunately, have an increased incidence of breast cancer and endometrial cancer (cancer of the lining of the uterus) due to a continually elevated estrogen level.

In rare cases, a chromosomal abnormality known as *testicular feminization* may cause infertility. In this syndrome, a genetically male fetus fails to respond normally to the presence of testosterone, and instead develops physiologically as a female, at least externally. This situation can be confirmed by chromosomal analysis. Other possible causes of infertility include nutritional deficiencies, especially a lack of sufficient protein, iron, and vitamins such as folic acid and biotin; malfunctioning pituitary, thyroid, or adrenal glands; congenital deformities of the cervix, uterus, fallopian tubes, or ovaries; and even unsuspected complications from using douches, lubricants, or vaginal deodorants that can interfere with sperm. Occasionally, the mucus in a woman's genital tract, which normally assists the sperm in their journey, is an abnormal consistency and prevents the sperm from reaching their destination. In some cases it is even "hostile" to partner's sperm—that is, it contains antibodies produced by the woman's immune system that kill or immobilize the sperm. It is also possible, although rare, for a woman to have an autoimmune response in which her immune system mistakenly identifies a fertilized egg as a foreign body and eliminates it. An allergy to a partner's sperm is also a possibility. Problems like these can be very difficult to diagnose.

The first step in diagnosis is a thorough physical examination to rule out underlying disorders that are affecting fertility. This evaluation can start with examination of a woman's cervical mucus to assure that its consistency is acceptable and that it is not hostile to sperm. Hormone levels are checked, along with any factors in the woman's medical history that might be hindering conception, such as infections or chromosomal anomalies. An evaluation of both partners may find antigens between them that will not permit conception to take place.

To check for anatomical abnormalities of the cervix, uterus, and fallopian tubes, a *hysterosalpingogram* may be performed. This involves introducing a dye into the uterus, followed by x-ray study. If a woman has a history of pelvic infection, she will be given an antibiotic along with the test to assure that the dye does not spread any infection. Ultrasound monitoring of maturing egg follicles in the ovary can determine whether they are developing and rupturing properly. A biopsy of endometrial tissue, timed correctly to a woman's cycle, can determine whether the uterine lining is developing properly and at the right time.

If none of these procedures finds the cause of infertility, laparoscopy may be recommended. This is a microsurgical procedure using a fiber-optic instrument to look for obstruction of the fallopian tubes, adhesions, or endometriosis. It may be able to determine whether there is a problem that can be corrected, or whether a woman is a good candidate for in vitro fertilization.

Conditions Affecting Men

For men, the major problem with fertility is a failure to produce enough viable sperm. Unlike women, who are born with all the egg cells they will ever have, a healthy man is constantly producing sperm, and at a rate of 10 to 30 billion each month. *Azoospermia* is a condition in which there is no sperm at all present in the ejaculate, and is usually a result of blockage, a testicular disorder, and/or congenital malformation of some type. *Oligospermia* is the medical term for an abnormally low sperm count.

Infertility can also result if the sperm produced are defective in some way. In some cases, the sperm do not live long enough after ejaculation to travel the distance necessary to reach the egg. The production of defective sperm can be due to a blockage of the spermatic tubes or damage to the spermatic ducts, a situation that can be a consequence of a sexually transmitted disease. It can also be a result of abnormal development of the testes or damage to the testes. If a man or boy after the age of puberty has mumps that causes pain and swelling of the testicles, the disease may interfere with his ability to produce normal sperm. Certain illnesses, such as high fever within the past three months, and certain drugs can also cause fertility problems. Medications that can have this effect include phenytoin (Dilantin), which is used to control seizures; cimetidine (Tagamet), a stomach-acid blocker; sulfasalazine (Azulfidine), a drug used to treat ulcerative colitis and rheumatoid arthritis; and nitrofurantoin (Furadantin, Macrobid, Macrodantin), an antibiotic. Most have the effect of depressing either the development or the motility of sperm. Alcohol and marijuana also affect motility, while androgenic steroids can impair sperm development. Varicocele (varicose veins) in the scrotum may be a factor in infertility as well. In very rare cases, a chromosomal abnormality such as Klinefelter's syndrome or a genetic disease such as cystic fibrosis can cause infertility.

Diagnosis of a fertility problem begins with a thorough physical examination to rule out any physical disorders that may be contributing to the problem. If the general state of your health is satisfactory, a semen analysis is the next step. For two days prior to the test, you will be instructed to refrain from intercourse and masturbation so that the number of sperm in the sample is at its highest level. It is also important that the semen be examined as soon as possible after collection.

A laboratory technician will do an actual count of live sperm present in the sample, closely examine their shape to detect any abnormalities, and evaluate their degree of motility—the power to "swim upstream." A normal sperm count, with good motility and shape, is considered to begin at about 50 million sperm per milliliter (about $1/5$ teaspoon) of semen. A count of 100 million viable sperm per milliliter makes conception likely.

Be aware that sperm count varies. A man found to have a low sperm count one day may have a much higher count a week or a month later. It may be necessary to have a second test to determine if a low count merely represented a temporary fluctuation. Under normal conditions, sperm production is continuous. However, severe illness of any kind, as well as intense exercise and mental stress, may temporarily suspend the production of sperm. Then, too, sperm production is most efficient at about 93°F, or roughly 6°F *below* normal body temperature (this is why the testes are suspended outside the body, in the scrotum). High temperatures prevent new sperm from forming, which can result in temporary infertility. Wearing tight-fitting underwear that holds the scrotum close to the body can raise the temperature of the testes enough to interfere with sperm production.

CONVENTIONAL MEDICINE

For Women

■ If you are found to have an underactive thyroid, treatment with thyroid hormone should reverse the problem. (*See* HYPOTHYROIDISM.) Any infections may have to be eradicated with antibiotics.

■ If you are not ovulating, or if ovulation is sporadic, your doctor may prescribe treatment with clomiphene (Clomid, Serophene) to stimulate ovulation. As long as this is your only problem, this drug can be very effective. However, it has been linked to an increased incidence of ovarian cancer when used for longer than one year, and some women develop ovarian cysts that are painful enough to make them discontinue the drug. Additional prices you may have to pay for the pitter-patter of little feet include abdominal pain, bloating, blurred vision (sometimes permanent eye damage), and depression.

■ If clomiphene fails, bromocriptine (Parlodel) may be tried. Your hormone levels have to be just right for this drug to work, and side effects are more common, including low blood pressure, nausea, headache, dizziness, and fatigue. This drug has also been known to cause seizures, strokes, and heart attacks.

■ If you have fallopian tubes that are blocked due to earlier infection or tubal ligation, microsurgery to reopen the tubes may be recommended. The rates of successful pregnancy after such procedures are variable.

■ Another alternative is in vitro fertilization (IVF). In this technique, a woman is treated with hormones to stimulate the maturation of multiple eggs, which are then removed from her body, fertilized in a laboratory, and reintroduced into her body. Current versions of this practice include gamete intrafallopian transfer (GIFT) and zygote intrafallopian transfer (ZIFT). In these procedures, the egg—either before or after fertilization—is introduced into the fallopian tube instead of the uterus, as in earlier techniques, so it is a bit more invasive, requiring an incision. This allows early development of the embryo to take place in its natural site. However, recent statistics have shown the success rate with this technique to be no better than that of regular IVF, in which the embryo is placed in the uterus.

■ If the cervical mucus is of an abnormal consistency or volume and therefore possibly preventing sperm from passing into the uterus, treatment with female hormones may help the mucus reach the proper volume and consistency. Sperm can also be introduced into the uterus by artificial insemination, thus bypassing mucus that is abnormal or hostile to their passage.

■ If conception remains elusive and there is no clear-cut reason for it, examination by laparoscopy and/or ultrasound—and, if any evidence (however minimal) of endometriosis of fibroids is found, surgery to remove or destroy any growths—may resolve the problem.

■ Women who have polycystic ovary syndrome may benefit from losing weight if they are overweight. This lowers the total amount of estrogen circulating in their bodies, and may permit ovulation. Fertility drugs such as clomiphene (Clomid, Serophene), or the steroid dexamethasone (Decadron), may be effective as well. Surgery on the ovary in which a portion of the ovary is removed, called a *wedge resection*, may also restore ovulation (and fertility), though drug treatment is often tried first.

■ If a woman with polycystic ovary syndrome does not desire to become pregnant, medroxyprogesterone (Provera), a synthetic form of the hormone progesterone, can be used to cause monthly shedding of the uterine lining. Possible side effects include blood-clot formation, swelling, jaundice, depression, nausea, and acne. Oral contraceptives may also be prescribed for this purpose. These drugs can help with hirsutism as well, though they may take months to help. Electrolysis and depilatories (hair-removing chemicals) can also help with the hair problem. In some cases, removal of the uterus and ovaries, followed by oral hormone replacement therapy, may be recommended. The diuretic spironolactone (Aldactone and others) may help

as well. Potential side effects of this drug include blood electrolyte imbalances, headache, nausea, drowsiness, rash, confusion, and gastric ulcers.

For Men

■ If a chronic urinary tract infection is identified, antibiotics may be needed.

■ If your testosterone level is abnormally low, this can be corrected. Low testosterone levels can have a distinct effect on male fertility.

■ In some cases, sperm are produced normally, but ejaculation is poor, actually going in the wrong direction within the man. This condition is known as retrograde ejaculation, and it results in sperm being ejaculated into the bladder. Occasionally, treatment with a medication such as pseudoephedrine (Sudafed) or imipramine (Tofranil) can correct this. If that fails, sperm may be collected from the urine or by electrical stimulation, then artificially introduced into the uterus.

■ If you have an anatomical abnormality such as weakness or an obstruction of the reproductive tract, it may be possible to correct the problem with microsurgery.

■ Some drugs, including common acid-blockers such as cimetidine (Tagamet) and ranitidine (Zantac), can lower the sperm count. If you have a low sperm count and are taking any medications at all, ask your doctor about the possibility that the drugs are causing the difficulty.

■ If your sperm count is very low, artificial insemination combined with techniques to select and concentrate the most viable sperm may be successful in bringing about conception. In vitro fertilization is another possibility.

DIETARY GUIDELINES

■ Eat a healthy high-fiber diet with plenty of clean, lean protein foods such as chicken and fish. Avoid eating large amounts of food at any one time.

■ Avoid gas-producing foods, such as beans and legumes, that cause discomfort in the lower abdomen.

■ To flush toxins from your system, drink eight 8-ounce glasses of pure water daily.

■ Eliminate or reduce your consumption of foods and beverages containing caffeine, including coffee, tea (except for herbal teas), chocolate, and colas.

NUTRITIONAL SUPPLEMENTS

■ Carnitine, a substance related to the B vitamins but often grouped with the amino acids, has been shown to increase the number as well as the motility of sperm. A man should start by taking a dose of 250 to 500 milligrams of L-carnitine with breakfast. After one week, add a second dose, with lunch. After another week, add a third dose, so that you are taking 250 to 500 milligrams with each meal. Continue taking L-carnitine for three to four months.

■ Taking supplemental digestive enzymes ensures full utilization of all nutrients. Take a full-spectrum digestive-enzyme supplement providing 5,000 international units of lipase, 2,500 international units of amylase, and 300 international units of protease, plus 500 to 1,000 milligrams of pancreatin, immediately before each meal.

Note: Long-term supplementation with pancreatin is not advised, as it can cause your pancreas to reduce its own production of this important enzyme. Overuse also has the potential to cause nausea or diarrhea. After two months on pancreatin, discontinue use and monitor your reaction. If you find that your digestive problems recur, discuss pancreatin supplementation with your health-care provider.

■ Essential fatty acids, found in black currant seed oil, borage oil, evening primrose oil, and flaxseed oil, are required for normal glandular activity in both men and women. This supplement is especially important for women who are highly athletic and/or very strict about eating a low-fat diet. Take 500 to 1,000 milligrams of any of these oils two or three times daily.

■ Folic acid is necessary for successful conception and pregnancy. Moreover, low levels of folic acid early in pregnancy have been linked with an increased risk in so-called neural tube defects, such as spina bifida, in the developing fetus. A woman who wishes to become pregnant should take 400 milligrams of supplemental folic acid twice a day.

■ Royal jelly is rich in hormonal factors that help optimize hormone balance in both sexes. In men, it has been found to increase sperm count, and many believe it also enhances sexual performance. Take 20 milligrams of royal jelly daily.

■ Selenium is an antioxidant that prevents free-radical damage, works synergistically with vitamin E, and preserves tissue elasticity. In men, it is essential for sperm production—almost half of the male body's supply of selenium is concentrated in the testicles and the seminal ducts adjacent to the prostate gland. Take 200 micrograms of selenium daily.

■ The B vitamins are required for a healthy nervous system and help maintain muscle tone in the intestinal tract. Take a good B-complex supplement that supplies 25 to 50 milligrams of each of the major B vitamins daily.

■ Vitamin E helps to normalize hormone production by rejuvenating the endocrine system. It is also essential in cellular respiration and the absorption of fat-soluble vitamins. Choose a product containing mixed tocopherols and begin by taking 200 international units daily, then gradually increase the dosage until you are taking 400 international units twice daily.

Note: If you have high blood pressure, limit your intake of supplemental vitamin E to a total of 400 international units daily. If you are taking an anticoagulant (blood thinner), consult your physician before taking supplemental vitamin E.

■ Zinc supports the immune system, aids in the digestive process, and helps speed healing. In men, it is an important component of reproductive fluids and is important for prostate health. Take 15 to 25 milligrams of zinc daily. Take it with food to prevent stomach upset.

HERBAL TREATMENT

For Women

■ A dong quai combination formula, such as dong quai and peony or dong quai and bupleurum, help to strengthen the female hormonal system. Take a dong quai combination formula as directed on the product label.

■ Wild yam contains a phytochemical that is a precursor of progesterone, the hormone that stimulates the uterus to prepare for pregnancy. Use a wild-yam cream as directed on the product label.

For Men

■ Chinese, or Korean, (*Panax*) ginseng has been used for centuries to enhance male potency. In laboratory animals, it has been shown to increase testosterone levels and improve sperm formation. Select a standardized extract containing 7 percent ginsenosides and take 100 milligrams twice daily for two to three weeks. Stop taking the preparation for two weeks, then repeat. If the herb does not have the sought-after effects within this period of time, discontinue using it. It is unlikely that it will do anything further.

Note: Do not use Chinese ginseng if you have high blood pressure, heart disease, or hypoglycemia. If you are sensitive to the effects of caffeine and other stimulants, you may want to consult with a qualified herbalist before using ginseng.

HOMEOPATHY

For Women

■ See a homeopathic physician for a constitutional remedy formulated especially for you.

For Men

■ *Cannabis sativa* will prove valuable if you have a history of marijuana use and a reduced sex drive because of it. You may urinate in a split stream and suffer a burning sensation when urinating. Take one dose of *Cannabis sativa*

30x or 15c three times daily for up to three days. Follow this program once a month for three months.

■ *Lycopodium* is the remedy of choice if you have wrinkles in your forehead and a tendency to balding on the top of the head, the so-called "monk's-pattern" baldness. You may often suffer from abdominal discomfort and indigestion. Take one dose of *Lycopodium* 30x or 15c three times daily for up to three days. Follow this program once a month for three months.

■ *Medorrhinum* is good if you are nervous and sensitive, with a history of on-again, off-again impotence. You may also have occasional pain on urination, as well as a number of allergies. Take one dose of *Medorrhinum* 200x or 200c three times over the course of a week. Stop for two months, then repeat.

BACH FLOWER REMEDIES

Select the remedy that most closely fits your emotional tendencies and concerns, and take it as needed, following the directions on the product label.

For Women

Beech is the remedy to choose if you are full of impatience.

Choose Cherry Plum if you are fearful and feel you have no control over events.

Elm can help if you are burdened by feelings of inadequacy.

■ Holly will ease anger and temper sharp words.

Impatiens is helpful against impatience and nervousness.

Mustard is for sadness and despair.

White Chestnut helps to counteract a tendency to obsesses about the situation.

For Men

Oak is helpful if you have a typical type-A personality and feel relentlessly driven to excel.

White Chestnut is the remedy of choice if you have difficulty forgetting about your work and are constantly dwelling on things undone.

ACUPRESSURE

For the locations of acupressure points on the body, *see* ADMINISTERING AN ACUPRESSURE TREATMENT in Part Three.

For Women

■ Liver 3 relaxes the nervous system.

■ Spleen 6 and Stomach 36 improve circulation.

For Men

■ All Bladder points improve circulation to the genitourinary tract.

■ Kidney 3 increases circulation to the urinary tract and reproductive organs.

■ Liver 3 and Spleen 6 strengthen the blood.

GENERAL RECOMMENDATIONS

■ Don't have intercourse more than three times a week. More frequent intercourse may reduce the number of viable sperm in the male partner's semen.

■ Time intercourse to coincide with ovulation, which usually occurs midway between menstrual periods. Some women can tell when they are ovulating. Signs of ovulation include bloating and breast tenderness and, for some women, a slight cramping pain known as mittelschmerz. Unfortunately, many women experience no telltale signs. There are over-the-counter tests that can help you pinpoint the time of ovulation. These are urine tests that employ a chemically treated dipstick to detect the hormone that triggers the release of an egg.

■ After intercourse, spend ten to fifteen minutes quietly in each other's arms before getting up. If a woman stays in a prone position for fifteen minutes or so following intercourse, this allows the maximum number of sperm the maximum amount of time to reach the egg.

■ A woman should consider seeing a licensed acupuncturist. Acupuncture has proven to be quite effective in helping strengthen the female reproductive system.

■ If it has been determined that the female partner's body is producing antibodies that are damaging or destroying sperm, the male partner should use a condom for six months. With no contact with the antigen—the sperm—the antibodies the woman's body produces may be lulled into inactivity. After this rest period, time intercourse (without a condom) to coincide with ovulation.

■ Exercise regularly but moderately. Maintaining a high level of physical fitness increases the possibility of conception. For both men and women, the ability to reproduce is dependent on a healthy body. If your idea of exercise is getting up from your chair to find the remote control, if your dietary habits are poor, or even if you are on a reducing diet, your fertility can suffer.

■ Infertility itself can be extremely stressful, but as much as possible, do try to avoid stress. Stressing your body with intensive exercise can cause a decrease in fertility. Mental and emotional stress have the same impact. Try to eliminate the stress in your life as much as possible.

■ Avoid tobacco and alcohol. In women, alcohol consumption can actually prevent implantation of a fertilized egg. In men, both smoking and alcohol consumption have been shown to lower sperm count.

■ A man should not wear underwear that holds his testicles close to his body. Sperm require cool temperatures to remain active. Loose-fitting boxer shorts made of a natural, breathable fiber such as cotton permit air to circulate and help keep the temperature within your testicles down. For the same reason, a man wishing to become a father should avoid hot baths, hot tubs, jacuzzis, saunas, and steam baths. These indulgences may reduce stress and create a sensual mood, but they can also reduce your ability to impregnate your partner.

PREVENTION

■ It may not be possible to prevent infertility, but there are measures you can take to minimize the possibility. Whether you are male or female, if you have any suspicion you may have contracted a sexually transmitted disease, see your doctor promptly so that treatment, if necessary, can be begun in a timely fashion. A woman should have regular gynecological examinations starting at age eighteen or within six months of becoming sexually active, whichever comes first, so that any developing problems can be detected and corrected early. Adopt a healthy lifestyle that includes a wholesome diet, regular exercise, avoidance of toxins of all kinds (including recreational drugs), and measures to reduce stress. If you consume alcohol, do so in moderation only.

Influenza

See FLU.

Insect Bite

See BITES AND STINGS, INSECT AND SPIDER.

Insomnia

Insomnia, quite simply, is the inability to sleep. Almost everyone suffers from lost sleep on occasion, usually because of stress, worry over an upcoming event, an irregular work schedule, or consuming alcohol or caffeine too close to bedtime. A deficiency—or excess—of certain vitamins and minerals can also cause insomnia. For many people, however, insomnia is not just an occasional nuisance. Chronic insomnia can have a real impact on your waking life. The National Commission on Sleep Disorders Research (NCSDR), established by the U.S. Congress to study these problems, has concluded that insomnia not only harms economic productivity but also endangers the health and safety of many Americans.

Over 40 million Americans suffer from sleep disorders, including insomnia, restless legs syndrome, and sleep apnea. Insomnia can take the form of an inability to fall asleep, or a tendency to wake in the night and be unable to go back to sleep. Most cases are related to stress and anxiety. Insomnia can also be related to depression, chronic pain, breathing difficulties, jet lag, an irregular schedule, or an undiagnosed infection. If the natural approaches suggested in this section fail to help sufficiently, consult your doctor. He or she may refer you to a sleep disorder clinic for a thorough evaluation.

CONVENTIONAL TREATMENT

■ Antihistamines, such as diphenhydramine (Benadryl), dimenhydrinate (Dramamine), or even hydroxyzine (Atarax or Vistaril, available by prescription only), can be helpful. These drugs are intended to treat the symptoms of an allergic reaction (or, in the case of dimenhydrinate, nausea), but one of their well-known side effects is drowsiness, which can be useful at times. These tend to be the least bothersome of the drugs recommended for sleeplessness. Possible side effects include tremor and dry mouth.

■ In certain cases, a mild tranquilizer of the class known as the benzodiazepines may be prescribed. Examples include diazepam (Valium), flurazepam (Dalmane), and temazepam (Restoril). While they can be effective, these drugs can also be habit-forming and have such possible side effects as confusion, weakness, liver stress, and blood abnormalities. A related drug, triazolam (Halcion), can also bring sleep, but is associated with even more disturbing side effects, including amnesia, anxiety, hallucinations, and depression.

■ A newer drug, zolpidem (Ambien), may be tried. Zolpidem supposedly causes fewer problems than other agents used to induce sleep, but it can leave the user with a drugged feeling while awake, as well as dizziness, diarrhea, and amnesia.

■ An antidepressant such as amitriptyline (Elavil) or imipramine (Tofranil) may be suggested, particularly if sleep problems are related to depression. These should be used only under the supervision of a psychiatrist experienced in their use. Possible side effects include heart attack, stroke, confusion, seizures, hallucinations, urinary retention, involuntary movements, rashes, bone-marrow depression, and decreased libido.

■ There are numerous over-the-counter medications that claim to promote sleep. On the whole, it is best to avoid these. Insomnia is a prime area in which to consider alternatives.

DIETARY GUIDELINES

■ Avoid taking any stimulants, such as foods and beverages containing caffeine, refined sugars, or chocolate, too close to bedtime. Be aware that a caffeine "buzz" lasts from six to eight hours and plan accordingly. (See the table below for an analysis of the caffeine content of selected foods and medicines.)

■ Avoid alcohol within two hours of going to bed. The traditional nightcap may make you feel drowsy at first, but alcohol results in light, unsatisfying sleep and the sedative effect wears off in four hours. This rebound effect may leave you wakeful in the wee hours.

■ Avoid eating and exercising for three hours before bedtime. Food and exercise both boost the metabolism and the heart rate, leaving you wakeful, not sleepy.

■ Make sure your diet includes foods containing the amino acid tryptophan, which helps to stabilize moods and alleviate stress. It is used by the brain to produce serotonin, a chemical that regulates the mechanisms of normal sleep. Foods high in tryptophan include bananas, cottage cheese, fish, dates, milk, peanuts, and turkey. Having complex carbohydrates such as pasta or rice for dinner is a good sleep-inducer, too.

Caffeine Content of Selected Foods and Medicines

Food/Medicine (quantity)	Caffeine Content
Chocolate, milk (1 oz)	1–10 mg
Chocolate, dark (1 oz)	5–35 mg
Chocolate cake (1 slice)	20–30 mg
Cocoa, hot (6 fl oz)	2–20 mg
Coffee, decaffeinated (6 fl oz)	2–7 mg
Coffee, drip/brewed (6 fl oz)	80–175 mg
Coffee, instant (6 fl oz)	60–100 mg
Cola (12 fl oz)	45 mg
Espresso (2 fl oz)	90–110 mg
Tea, black (6 fl oz)	200–100 mg
Anacin or Midol (2 tablets)	64 mg
Excedrin (2 tablets)	130 mg
NoDoz (2 tablets)	200 mg

NUTRITIONAL SUPPLEMENTS

■ Brewer's yeast is high in natural B vitamins as well as other vitamins and minerals that help to calm the nervous system. Take 1 teaspoon (or 1,500 milligrams) one hour before bedtime.

■ Calcium and magnesium act together to calm the nervous system. A calcium and magnesium combination can be very helpful if you experience sleeplessness accompanied by leg cramps. Take one dose of a supplement supplying 500 milligrams of calcium and 250 milligrams of magnesium when you awaken and again at bedtime.

■ Melatonin is a hormone produced by the pineal gland that is vital to the sleep-wake cycle. Depressed melatonin secretion can be at the root of insomnia, a condition most common in people over the age of sixty-five. Take 3 milligrams each evening, between one-half hour and two hours before retiring for the night. Do not take it during the day, as it may interfere with your body's normal rhythms and cause drowsiness.

■ People with low levels of iron very often awaken several times during the night. If your multivitamin supplement does not provide it, take 5 to 10 milligrams once or twice daily, at the beginning of a meal.

Note: Too much iron can be toxic. Do not exceed the recommended dosage from all supplements.

■ Deficiencies of vitamin B_3 (niacin), vitamin B_6 (pyridoxine), pantothenic acid, and trace minerals, including copper, are associated with insomnia. Take a balanced multivitamin and mineral supplement daily. Because an excess of vitamin B_{12} taken late in the day can contribute to wakefulness, it is best to take it in the morning.

HERBAL TREATMENT

■ To help yourself unwind and relax, take a cup of chamomile tea, an herbal relaxant, an hour before bedtime. A combination herbal tea, such as Celestial Seasonings' Sleepytime tea, may also be used.

■ Try brewing a tea combining equal amounts of chamomile, passionflower, skullcap, and valerian, and take a cup at bedtime.

■ Valerian root is an effective sleep-inducer that won't leave you with a drug-induced "hangover" in the morning. Select a standardized extract containing 0.5 percent isovalerenic acids and take 200 to 300 milligrams one-half hour before bedtime.

HOMEOPATHY

■ *Carbo vegetabilis* is helpful if you wake up in the middle of the night with an upset stomach. Take one dose of *Carbo vegetabilis* 30x or 15c when you awaken in the night.

■ *Coffea cruda*, homeopathic coffee, relieves symptoms similar to those you might feel after drinking a strong cup of espresso. This remedy effectively quiets an active mind. It helps relieve the nervous symptoms (mental and physical) that may be interfering with sleeping. If you lie sleepless in bed with racing thoughts, take one dose of *Coffea*

Are You Getting Enough Sleep?

At the beginning of the twentieth century, Americans slept for nine hours a night, on average. That figure has now dropped to seven hours a night. Most experts agree that while some people function very well on six hours of sleep or less, the average adult requires about eight hours of sound sleep every night, and some need as much as ten hours (or more) to feel their best.

When assessing your personal sleep needs, the most important factor to consider is the quality of your sleep. Answer the following questions:

- How long does it take you to fall asleep? People who are healthy sleepers generally take about twenty minutes to fall asleep. If you are not getting enough sleep, you may drop off within five minutes.

- Do you sleep through the night, or toss restlessly and wake up repeatedly? And how rested do you feel upon awakening? If the alarm clock jars you out of a sound sleep, chances are you are building up a sleep deficit. If you have had enough sleep,

you will awaken naturally, without an alarm clock.

- Are you alert and active during the waking hours, or do you find yourself nodding off during the day when you have a little down time? If you have slept long enough to truly restore your body, you should find it almost impossible to nap during the daylight hours.

If you are suffering from a sleep deficit, you may not have enough energy to get up in the morning, or to keep up with the activities of the day. Lack of sleep fogs the memory, reduces alertness, lengthens reaction time, dims the creative spark, and can even twist your tongue. On top of all that, when you force your body to function without enough sleep, your ability to resist illness and disease declines. Long-term sleep deprivation can also have a serious effect on your psychological state, and can even induce psychotic symptoms. No matter how wholesome your diet and regular your exercise routine, it is impossible to be truly healthy and at your best without sufficient, regular good-quality sleep.

---

cruda 12x or 6c one hour before dinner, and another dose half an hour before bedtime.

ACUPRESSURE

For the locations of acupressure points on the body, *see* ADMINISTERING AN ACUPRESSURE TREATMENT in Part Three.

■ Bladder 60 helps to take energy down and away from the head.

■ Gallbladder 21 also brings energy away from the head.

■ Four Gates helps relax the nervous system.

■ Pericardium 6 helps relax the mind and alleviate nervous excitement.

■ Massaging the muscles on either side of the spine will contact a series of points that help to relax the entire system.

AROMATHERAPY

For specific instructions on how to use aromatherapy, *see* PREPARING AROMATHERAPY TREATMENTS in Part Three.

■ There are many essential oils that have a calming effect that can help to promote a sound sleep. The best known for this purpose is probably lavender oil, but neroli and ylang ylang are also good. Add a few drops to your hot

bath or massage oil, inhale directly from the bottle, or diffuse them into the air. You can also put a drop or two in a spray bottle full of distilled water, shake gently, and spray the mixture on your pillow shortly before you go to bed.

GENERAL RECOMMENDATIONS

■ Set a reasonable sleep schedule and stick to it as closely as possible. Be flexible enough to adjust the schedule if it does not match your normal cycle. Some people are "larks" who naturally awaken early, while some are "owls" who prefer to stay up a little later. Initiate a regular bedtime, and try to wake up at the same time every day. Adhere to your schedule even on weekends and during holidays, with only rare exceptions for special occasions.

■ Follow a simple regimen to slow down your metabolic rate and allow time to unwind before retiring. Sip a cup of herbal tea, read something light, listen to soothing music, or practice relaxation techniques. (*See* RELAXATION TECHNIQUES in Part Three.) A back rub or a foot rub can also help you settle down comfortably.

■ Make yourself supremely comfortable. The right mattress, the right pillow, and the right covering will help you sleep soundly throughout the night. Keep your bedroom quiet, dark, and cool.

■ Don't fall asleep in front of the television, even if the

sound is off. The flickering light affects your nervous system and interferes with restorative sleep.

■ Try a hot bath. Soaking in a hot (102°F) bath for thirty minutes before going to bed can help you fall asleep faster, experience less wakefulness during the night, and awaken feeling refreshed. For this to work, you have to allow two hours to pass between the bath and going to bed. A high body temperature contributes to wakefulness, not sleepiness.

■ Get regular aerobic exercise, but do your exercising at least two hours before bedtime. People who exercise regularly generally have less trouble with insomnia.

PREVENTION

■ People who do shift work, especially those who work night shifts, often have problems when trying to readjust to daylight hours once a week. After your last night shift for the week, go home and sleep soundly for two or three hours, but get up by noon and begin your daytime life. You'll be ready to go to sleep again at night, and should awaken the following morning fully refreshed and ready for the day's activities.

Iritis

See under UVEITIS.

Irritable Bowel Syndrome

Irritable bowel syndrome (IBS) is a condition in which the intestines do not function as they should. Normally, rhythmic and predictable muscular contractions move waste from the small intestine to the large intestine to the rectum, where it exits the body. In a person with IBS, the contractions are erratic—either too forceful or not forceful enough, and irregular rather than rhythmic—which results in spasms. Often complicating the situation are greater than normal sensitivity to sensations in the chest, abdomen, intestines, and rectum, and a sensitive gastrointestinal tract that reacts with spasms to certain influences in the diet and environment. The result is a variety of uncomfortable symptoms, including pain, cramping, gas, bloating, and, especially, constipation and/or diarrhea, sometimes alternating. Pain and cramping often begin after eating, and the discomfort is usually relieved by passing gas or having a bowel movement. Whether the stools are loose or hard, bowel movements are often painful, and there may be mucus in the stool. A person with this syndrome may develop a form of malnutrition even if he or she eats well, because IBS can interfere with the absorption of nutrients.

Doctors consider IBS a functional problem, meaning that symptoms result not from observable disease (as in Crohn's disease and ulcerative colitis, for example) but from poor functioning of intestines that otherwise appear to be normal. The fundamental cause of this syndrome is not known, but a number of things are known to trigger and/or worsen acute attacks. Among these are stress, an overgrowth of candida, lactose intolerance, and food sensitivities. Many people with IBS are sensitive to one or more foods. When troublesome foods are avoided, symptoms often abate.

IBS is diagnosed by a process of elimination. More serious problems that can cause similar symptoms—including Crohn's disease, ulcerative colitis, diverticulitis, intestinal parasites, and colorectal cancer—must be ruled out before a firm diagnosis of irritable bowel syndrome can be made. If you are diagnosed with IBS, you may find it reassuring to know that while it can be uncomfortable, even painful, it is not considered a serious disorder. You also have plenty of company. An estimated one in five Americans suffers from IBS, and this syndrome accounts for more than half of all referrals to gastroenterologists. It is twice as common in women as in men, and while people can be affected at any age, most people who have IBS start having symptoms when they are between the ages of twenty-five and forty.

CONVENTIONAL TREATMENT

■ For frequent watery diarrhea, loperamide (found in Imodium AD and many other products) may be recommended. Loperamide slows the movement of the digestive tract, allowing more time for reabsorption of water and electrolytes from the stool. This drug is often prescribed for chronic diarrhea associated with inflammatory bowel disease. However, you should not use it if you have a fever over 101°F, or if you have bloody stools.

■ A drug called hyoscyamine may be prescribed in some cases, either on its own (sold under the brand names Cystospaz, Levbid, Levsin, and Levsinex) or in a combination formula that includes a mild tranquilizer (Arco-Lase, Donnatal). These preparations reduce spasms and cramping by inhibiting the action of the nerves that stimulate the muscles of the stomach and intestines to contract. Other drugs in this class are dicyclomine (Bentyl) and propantheline (Pro-Banthine). All of these agents can cause similar side effects, including dry mouth, drowsiness, nausea, vomiting, constipation, abdomnal pain, dizziness, blurred vision, increased heart rate, shortness of breath, and impotence.

■ Fiber products such as psyllium, bran, or methylcellulose can be used if constipation is a problem. If this is not successful, a gastrointestinal stimulant such as cisapride (Propulsid) may be tried. Possible side effects of this drug include headache, nausea, vomiting, diarrhea, vision changes, and heart-rhythm abnormalities.

■ If your physician feels a psychological disturbance may be involved in your pain, he or she may recommend trying a tricyclic antidepressant such as amitriptyline (Elavil). Potential side effects of this drug include drowsiness, nausea, vomiting, abdominal pain, dry mouth, changes in heart rhythm, anxiety, confusion, blood-pressure changes, and decreased sex drive.

DIETARY GUIDELINES

■ A high-fiber diet based on vegetables and whole grains is of paramount importance. This kind of diet works quickly to reduce the uncomfortable symptoms of IBS. If you are unaccustomed to consuming significant quantities of fiber, increase your intake of fiber-rich foods slowly to avoid gas and bloating. If you find it difficult to get sufficient fiber in your diet, take a fiber supplement.

■ Many people with IBS are sensitive to wheat. Try using brown rice, barley, oats, and oat bran as your whole-grain choices for seven days, and monitor your body's reaction. If your symptoms improve, you are probably sensitive to wheat. This doesn't mean you can never eat wheat or wheat-based products again, however. Following a rotation diet can help you overcome the problem (see ROTATION DIET in Part Three).

■ Avoid all dairy products for seven days and monitor your body's reaction. If your symptoms are relieved, you may be lactose intolerant (see LACTOSE INTOLERANCE).

■ Saturated and hydrogenated fats are the most difficult of all nutrients to digest. Consuming fats also stimulates muscle contractions. Avoid butter, margarine, fried foods, fat-loaded processed foods, and red meat. For protein, eat white-meat poultry, fish, grains, and soy foods.

■ Minimize your intake of gas-producing foods such as beans and legumes, cabbage, Brussels sprouts, broccoli, cauliflower, and onions.

■ Avoid caffeine-containing, carbonated, and alcoholic beverages. These common stimulants are irritating to the digestive tract and they add to stress.

■ People with IBS often have a sensitivity to artificial sweeteners, even in very small amounts, such as that in a stick of sugar-free gum. Avoid all artificial sweeteners.

■ Drink eight 8-ounce glasses of pure water every day. Sufficient water is vital for the functioning of every organ and system in the body, including the gastrointestinal tract.

NUTRITIONAL SUPPLEMENTS

■ People with IBS often suffer from impaired digestion. To help ensure full absorption and assimilation of nutrients, take digestive enzymes with meals.

■ To be sure you are getting all the basic nutrients you need, take a good multivitamin and mineral supplement daily.

■ Any problem involving the intestinal tract calls for supplemental acidophilus and bifidobacteria. The friendly bacteria found in quality probiotics are required for healthy, normal activity in the colon. Probiotic supplements are especially important if you have been taking antibiotics, as these drugs destroy both harmful and friendly bacteria indiscriminately. Take a probiotic supplement as recommended on the product label. If you are allergic to milk, be sure to select a dairy-free formula.

■ Fiber has both a healing and cleansing effect on the intestinal tract, and also promotes efficient bowel action. Choose a fiber supplement such as psyllium seeds (which have a laxative effect), flaxseeds, guar gum, or oat bran (not wheat bran), and take it as directed on the product label. Flaxseeds have the additional advantage of providing the essential fatty acids that help protect the intestinal lining.

■ The amino acid glutamine helps to soothe the digestive tract, and is often beneficial for inflammatory bowel disorders such as IBS. Take 500 milligrams of L-glutamine three times daily for two weeks, then decrease to 500 milligrams twice daily for two weeks. Then take 500 milligrams daily for two months.

■ Magnesium and calcium are important to the central nervous system, and help soothe a nervous stomach and irritated bowel. Take 500 milligrams of calcium and 250 milligrams of magnesium twice a day.

■ The B vitamins are needed for a healthy intestinal tract, including the efficient absorption of proteins, carbohydrates, and fats. Take a good B-vitamin complex that supplies 50 milligrams of each of the major B vitamins, plus an additional 200 micrograms of vitamin B_{12}, twice daily.

HERBAL TREATMENT

■ Aloe vera soothes and helps heal a stressed digestive tract. It also helps slow down metabolism and aids in keeping the intestinal walls clear of excess mucus. Be sure to select a food-grade preparation. Take $1/8$ cup twice a day.

■ Chinese (Korean) ginseng can decrease sensitivity to stress, a common contributing factor in IBS. Select a standardized extract containing 7 percent ginsenosides and take 100 milligrams twice daily for two to three weeks. Stop taking the preparation for two weeks, then repeat.

Note: Do not use ginseng if you have high blood pressure, heart disease, or hypoglycemia. If you are sensitive to the effects of caffeine and other stimulants, you may want to consult with a qualified herbalist before using ginseng.

■ Ginger has beneficial effects on the entire gastrointestinal tract, and is famous for relieving nausea. Take 500 milligrams three times daily.

Milk thistle contains silymarin, which is highly beneficial to the liver. A sluggish liver contributes to digestive disturbances. Choose an extract standardized to contain 80 percent flavonoids (silymarin) and take 200 to 300 milligrams twice daily for three months.

Pau d'arco has been used for centuries for intestinal complaints. It has antibacterial, antiviral, and anti-inflammatory activity. Take 500 milligrams twice a day.

Peppermint is nature's premier digestive aid. Taken as a tea, it relieves nausea, eases flatulence, promotes burping, calms stomach spasms, and relieves an overfull feeling. Taken in capsule form, it helps alleviate intestinal cramps and spasms. Be sure to select enteric-coated peppermint-oil capsules, as the coating ensures that the contents will be released in your intestines, not your stomach. Take them as directed on the product label. If you experience a burning sensation when you move your bowels, reduce the dosage.

Note: If you are using peppermint and also taking a homeopathic preparation, allow one hour between the two. Otherwise, the strong smell of the mint may interfere with the action of the homeopathic remedy.

Turmeric is full of active bioflavonoids that are effective in relieving inflammation. Take 200 to 500 milligrams once or twice daily.

Valerian has the ability to relax intestinal muscles, making it valuable against intestinal cramps. Valerian also reduces agitation, eases stress, and has a gentle normalizing effect on the central nervous system. Choose a standardized extract containing 0.5 percent isovalerenic acids and take 200 to 300 milligrams one-half hour before bedtime.

HOMEOPATHY

Argentum nitricum is the remedy to choose if you are nervous, crave fatty foods, and typically get an upset stomach after eating sweets. Take one dose of *Argentum nitricum* 30x or 15c three times daily for up to three days.

Nux vomica is helpful for indigestion accompanied by irritability. Take one dose of *Nux vomica* 30x or 15c three times daily for up to three days, or as needed.

BACH FLOWER REMEDIES

Select the remedy that most closely fits your emotional tendencies and concerns, and take it as needed, following the directions on the product label.

■ Beech helps to counteract perfectionistic tendencies, impatience with the shortcomings of others, and an inability to tolerate last-minute changes in plans.

■ Impatiens can ease stress, impatience, tension, and a tendency to be irritated by little things.

■ Rescue Remedy calms the nervous system and alleviates stress. This combination remedy is particularly useful in acute situations, such as when the frustrating symptoms of IBS strike.

ACUPRESSURE

For the locations of acupressure points on the body, *see* ADMINISTERING AN ACUPRESSURE TREATMENT in Part Three.

■ Gallbladder 34 helps to relax muscles in the abdomen.

■ Large Intestine 10 reduces inflammation.

■ Liver 3 relieves muscle cramps and spasms.

■ Pericardium 6 relaxes the chest and upper digestive tract, relieves nausea, and calms the mind.

■ Small Intestine 5 reduces inflammation.

■ Stomach 36 harmonizes and tones the digestive system and improves digestion.

GENERAL RECOMMENDATIONS

■ Everyone has stress in his or her life, but some people manage it better than others. Work to reduce the effects of stress, both physically and mentally, by practicing stress-management and relaxation techniques. (*See* RELAXATION TECHNIQUES in Part Three.)

■ Get regular exercise. Exercise works against irritable bowel syndrome in two ways. First, physical activity stimulates intestinal activity in a positive way, and can actually reduce the symptoms of IBS. For example, bent-knee sit-ups exercise the colon and relieve spasms. Second, exercise reduces stress dramatically. Walk away the stresses of the day. Walking for half an hour four or five times a week will work wonders for both your body and your mind.

PREVENTION

■ There is no known way to prevent irritable bowel syndrome. However, eating a healthful diet and getting regular moderate exercise may reduce your chances of developing it. Should you already have IBS, these measures will help to prevent acute flare-ups.

Itching

See SKIN RASH.

Jaundice

Jaundice is a yellowing of the skin and the whites of the eyes caused by an accumulation of a cellular waste product called bilirubin. The discoloration is often, but by no means always, accompanied by itching, which can be intense, as well as by nausea, vomiting, headache, fever, dark-colored urine, abdominal pain, loss of appetite, abdominal swelling, and light-colored stools.

Jaundice is not a disease in and of itself, but a sign that the liver is having a problem handling bilirubin as it should. The liver makes bilirubin from dying red blood cells and other sources. It then converts bilirubin into bile, which has several purposes, among them the digestion of fatty acids and neutralization of stomach acid. If there is too much bilirubin for the liver to deal with, or if the liver's functioning is compromised, jaundice can result.

The specific causes of jaundice are numerous. The major categories of problems that can lead to jaundice include conditions that result in an excessive breakdown of red blood cells; hereditary diseases that impair the liver's ability to convert bilirubin into bile; liver damage from exposure to toxic chemicals, including alcohol, carbon tetrachloride, and others; liver diseases such as hepatitis, bacterial infection, parasitic infestation, or cancer; and obstructions that block the outflow of bile so that it cannot leave the liver as it is supposed to. Newborns often develop some degree of jaundice in the days after birth, as their bodies adjust to life outside the womb, but this is not usually a serious problem.

An extensive medical workup may be required to determine the precise cause of jaundice. A detailed medical history is an important first step. Illnesses you may have been exposed to, medications you take or have taken, possible exposures to toxic compounds or alcohol, travel to places where food and/or water safety might be questionable, possible encounters with infected animals, a family history of blood diseases, liver problems, chromosomal abnormalities, cancer, or HIV disease—all of these are important factors that can help your physician in evaluating the cause of the problem. Laboratory tests are done to examine the levels of enzymes and other body chemicals directly involved in the health of the liver. These can help determine where along the line of processing bilirubin the problem may be. Ultrasound, computerized tomography (CT), and magnetic resonance imaging (MRI) are imaging studies that may be done to detect blocked ducts, tumors, liver enlargement, and changes in blood-vessel size that might lead to an explanation. Though the blood work and some phases of the imaging scans require the insertion of a needle in a vein, these studies are considered minimally invasive.

If an obstruction becomes the likely explanation, one of two other tests may be performed. These are endoscopic retrograde cholangiopancreatography (ERCP) and percutaneous transhepatic cholangiography (PTC). Both involve guiding a catheter to the site of interest, then injecting a dye that can be seen on an x-ray study. In ERCP, the catheter is inserted through the intestinal tract; in PTC, it is inserted through the skin.

If no cause can be found by any other techniques, a percutaneous liver biopsy may be recommended. In this test, a needle is inserted through the skin and into the liver, sometimes with the guidance of ultrasound or a CT scan, and a sample of liver tissue is removed for microscopic examination.

CONVENTIONAL TREATMENT

■ Treatment depends on the underlying cause, and may involve removal of the offending agent; administration of antibiotic, antiviral, antifungal, or antiparasitic drugs; surgery to correct blockage; the use of chemotherapy, anti-inflammatory, or steroid medications; dietary changes; measures to minimize symptoms; or any combination of the above. The need to limit activity depends entirely on the underlying cause of the jaundice, but in general, only serious problems require severe limitations.

DIETARY GUIDELINES

■ Eat vegetable broth, which is replete with minerals and trace minerals, and is easy to digest. Fresh vegetable juices are an excellent dietary supplement as well.

■ Eat a diet of whole, unprocessed foods. Avoid processed food products that contain preservatives, artificial flavorings and colorings, and other additives.

■ Avoid saturated animal fats, fried foods, and large meals, all of which place added stress on the liver.

■ Strictly avoid alcohol, which is toxic to the liver. Also eliminate from your diet refined sugar and anything containing caffeine.

NUTRITIONAL SUPPLEMENTS

■ To ensure an adequate supply of basic nutrients, take a good multivitamin and mineral supplement daily. Choose a capsule or soft gel-cap form for best absorption.

■ Colostrum has been shown to strengthen immune function and improve digestion. Take 500 milligrams three to four times daily.

■ Lipoic acid is an antioxidant that helps to improve liver function. Take 100 milligrams daily.

■ The combination of magnesium and malic acid helps to initiate the Krebs cycle, a series of enzyme reactions that results in the conversion of nutrients into energy at the cellular level. If fatigue is a problem, take 100 milligrams of magnesium and 300 milligrams of malic acid one hour before breakfast.

■ Vitamin C and bioflavonoids have anti-inflammatory properties. Take 500 milligrams five to six times daily. This can reduce the duration of jaundice. If you have a sensitive stomach, choose an esterified form (Ester-C).

Vitamin E is a powerful antioxidant. Choose a product containing mixed tocopherols and take 200 international units in the morning and again at bedtime.

HERBAL TREATMENT

Milk thistle is the premier herbal remedy for the liver. It contains silymarin, which is an excellent antioxidant and has been found to increase the liver's supply of glutathione. Glutathione is an amino acid that protects the liver by binding to toxins and neutralizing them so they cannot attack the cells of this vital organ. Choose an extract standardized to contain 80 percent flavonoids (silymarin) and take 100 milligrams three times daily.

Barberry helps to resolve jaundice, aids digestion, and fights infection. The active ingredients are believed to be compounds called isoquinoline alkaloids, which include berberine, berbamine, and oxyacanthine. Take 500 milligrams three times daily.

Gentian root has traditionally been used for disorders of the liver and organs in the pelvic area. It is very bitter, and is said to stimulate the production of bile, thus aiding digestion. It is also believed to have some antibiotic properties. Take 500 milligrams three times daily.

Note: Do not use this herb if you have diarrhea.

HOMEOPATHY

Chelidonium is for jaundice accompanied by itching skin and pain under the right shoulder blade. Take one dose of *Chelidonium* 12x or 6c three times daily for up to four days. If your symptoms start to improve before that, stop taking the remedy.

Phosphorus is for jaundice accompanied by abdominal pains and a feeling of tightness in the chest. You feel weakness after a bowel movement, and are thirsty for cold water. Take one dose of *Phosphorus* 30x or 15c three times daily for up to three days. If your symptoms start to improve before that, stop taking the remedy.

Choose *Taraxacum* if you are jaundiced and suffer from flatulence and night sweats, and have a bitter taste in your mouth. Your fingertips are often cold as well. Take one dose of *Taraxacum* 12x or 6c three times daily for up to four days. If your symptoms start to improve before that, stop taking the remedy.

Once jaundice has started to lessen, *Lycopodium* is an effective remedy for indigestion and a feeling of bloatedness after eating, even if you eat only a small amount. You may crave sweets, wake in the night feeling hungry, and feel sadness upon awakening in the morning. Take one dose of *Lycopodium* 30x or 15c three times daily for up to three days.

BACH FLOWER REMEDIES

Select the remedy that most closely fits your disposition and emotional tendencies and concerns, and take it as needed, following the directions on the product label.

■ Holly helps to ease anger that bursts out in fits of temper, and that may stem from underlying feelings of insecurity.

■ Impatiens helps to tame impatience, tension, and irritability. It is particularly suitable if you are a type-A personality who finds it nearly impossible to sit still.

■ Wild Oat is good if you have a tendency to be fearful and anxious about the future.

■ Willow helps to counteract a tendency toward resentfulness and an inability to feel pleased or satisfied.

ACUPRESSURE

For the locations of acupressure points on the body, *see* ADMINISTERING AN ACUPRESSURE TREATMENT in Part Three.

■ The back Bladder points enhance digestion and relax the body.

■ Liver 3 and Gallbladder 34 improve liver function.

AROMATHERAPY

For specific instructions on how to use aromatherapy, *see* PREPARING AROMATHERAPY TREATMENTS in Part Three.

■ Essential oils of orange and rosemary can help to improve liver function and strengthen the nervous system. Use them as inhalants or, better, add them to a soothing warm bath and enjoy a leisurely soak.

GENERAL RECOMMENDATIONS

■ Get twenty to thirty minutes of mild exercise, such as walking or yoga, each day.

■ Be sure to get twenty minutes or so of exposure to sunlight each day.

Jock Itch

This irritating problem, known to doctors as *tinea cruris*, is a fungal infection that occurs in the groin area. A close relative of ringworm and athlete's foot, it is far more common in men than in women. It may be caused by any of several different organisms called dermatophytes that live parasitically on skin.

Jock itch typically appears as a reddish, moist, itching area that extends from the inner thigh up to its intersection with the scrotum. The genitals themselves may be minimally affected, if at all. It is not considered a serious infection, but it can be persistent, and recurrences are common. Once the skin becomes susceptible, the organism seems to be able to take advantage of any opportunity. Such chances occur more frequently during the summer months.

Tight clothing can make the situation worse, as friction, lack of air, and sweating tend to favor fungal growth. The itching can set the stage for other problems, such as bacterial infection and candidiasis, to complicate the situation. In addition, reactions to some of the ingredients in the medications used to treat jock itch can sometimes cause local inflammatory skin reactions.

Contact dermatitis, or skin eruptions due to sensitivity to something that comes into contact with the skin, may sometimes be mistaken for jock itch, as can psoriasis. (*See* DERMATITIS and/or PSORIASIS.)

CONVENTIONAL TREATMENT

■ Conventional treatment usually consists of the use of topical antifungal agents, such as miconazole (in Monistat-Derm), clotrimazole (Lotrimin, Mycelex), ketoconazole (Nizoral), terbinafine (Lamisil), ciclopirox (Loprox), or naftifine (Naftin). Side effects tend to be limited, with burning, itching, redness, or stinging the most common.

■ To reduce inflammation while fighting the infection, a medication combining an antifungal with a topical steroid may be prescribed. Lotrisone is one example. Be aware that continued use of steroid creams can cause atrophy (drying, shrinking, and aging) of the skin it touches. Normally, these medications are not necessary for jock itch.

■ Rarely, if the infection is extremely severe and/or persistent, an oral antifungal may be needed. Drugs of this type include fluconazole (Diflucan), ketoconazole (Nizoral), itraconazole (Sporanox), and terbinafine (Lamisil). Most people experience no problems with these drugs, but they can cause side effects such as gastrointestinal disturbances, headache, and rash in some people. In rare cases, they can cause liver stress.

DIETARY GUIDELINES

■ Keep your diet simple, with plenty of green vegetables and good amounts of clean, lean protein foods such as fish, chicken, and tofu.

■ Avoid all refined sugars, soda pop, and processed foods. Fungi thrive on simple sugars.

NUTRITIONAL SUPPLEMENTS

■ A multivitamin and mineral complex that includes trace minerals is important for maintaining general well-being while treating any fungal infection. Take it as directed on the product label.

■ Fungal infection is often associated with low levels of friendly bacteria, which normally keep fungi in check. To replenish the friendly bacteria, take a probiotic supplement such as acidophilus. Select a dairy-free product with a count of 5 to 10 billion viable (live) bacteria per capsule or half-teaspoon of powder, guaranteed through a printed expiration date, and take the dose recommended on the product label three times daily, between meals. If you wish, you can alternate acidophilus with other types of probiotics, such as bifidobacteria, or with fructooligosaccharides (FOS), which nourish the friendly bacteria.

■ Bioflavonoids protect the capillaries, the smallest blood vessels in the body, and have powerful anti-inflammatory effects. Take 500 milligrams of mixed bioflavonoids three to four times daily while the infection lasts. Then take 500 milligrams three times daily for two weeks.

■ Caprylic acid is a fatty acid that aids in restoring the body's good bacteria, and helping to eliminate an overabundance of yeast in the body. Take 200 milligrams twice a day, immediately before meals, for three to four weeks.

■ Methylsulfonylmethane (MSM) is a good source of sulfur, a trace mineral that helps to fight parasites and fungi. It can be applied directly to the affected area in cream or spray form. Follow the directions on the product label.

HERBAL TREATMENT

■ Calendula ointment is soothing. Apply it three times daily.

■ Cat's claw enhances the immune response and has antifungal properties. Take 500 milligrams of standardized extract three times a day until the infection clears.

Note: Do not use cat's claw if you are pregnant or nursing, or if you are an organ-transplant recipient. Use it with caution if you are taking an anticoagulant (blood thinner).

■ Garlic has antifungal properties. Take 500 to 1,000 milligrams three times daily.

■ Grapefruit-seed extract has been shown to have strong antifungal properties. This type of supplement is very concentrated—the recommended dosage is usually in the range of 2 to 6 drops two to three times daily. Follow the directions on the product label.

■ Pau d'arco contains three different antifungal compounds: beta-lapachone, lapachol, and xyloidine. You can use this herb topically and/or orally, in the form of one cup of tea or 500 milligrams in capsule form three times daily. Be patient. Pau d'arco is effective, but it can be slow acting, and may take some time to show effectiveness.

HOMEOPATHY

Sulfur is the remedy for skin that is dry, scaly, itching, and burning. Take one dose of *Sulfur* 30x or 15c three times daily, up to a total of ten doses. As soon as you notice an aggravation or an improvement, stop taking the remedy.

■ *Psorinum* is helpful if symptoms include intolerable itching and profuse perspiration, and are significantly worse if you drink coffee. You may feel somewhat melancholy. Take one dose of *Psorinum* 200x or 200c daily for three days.

A combination skin remedy is often helpful. Follow the directions on the product label.

ACUPRESSURE

For the locations of acupressure points on the body, *see* ADMINISTERING AN ACUPRESSURE TREATMENT in Part Three.

Stomach 36 and Spleen 6 together improve the absorption of nutrients.

Spleen 10 removes "heat" from the skin and is used commonly to address a wide variety of skin infections.

AROMATHERAPY

For specific instructions on how to use aromatherapy, *see* PREPARING AROMATHERAPY TREATMENTS in Part Three.

Essential oil of tea tree has antifungal properties, and can be applied topically to the affected area. Follow the directions for proper dilution on the product label.

GENERAL RECOMMENDATIONS

Wear clean cotton underwear. If possible, wearing loose cotton pants with no underwear for several or more hours per day is recommended, especially when the rash is at its worst.

Excessive moisture tends to worsen the rash. Try not to wear thick, warm clothing that would cause excessive sweating. After showering or bathing, make certain that the area is thoroughly patted dry—and then wash the towel in hot water, with chlorine bleach added if possible, to avoid reinfecting yourself.

PREVENTION

■ Practice meticulous hygiene. Keep the groin area clean, cool, and dry.

■ Don't share towels, washcloths, or anything else that might harbor infectious fungi.

Kaposi's Sarcoma

See under HIV DISEASE; SKIN CANCER.

Keloids

Breaks in the skin, whether from injury or incision, heal better in some people than others. The remaining scars are the result of imperfect healing, apparently due to less than optimal blood flow, and consequently an inadequate supply of oxygen and nutrients, to the injured area. If a scar overgrows into a large, rounded, raised pinkish mass, this is known as a keloid. Sometimes keloids form in areas affected by acne; sometimes they form for no apparent reason at all. People of African ancestry are more likely to develop keloids than those of other ethnic backgrounds. The upper back, shoulders, and chest are the most common sites.

Keloids resulting from cuts and incisions are more common than ones resulting from acne. The latter are more likely to form with deep acne that forms abscesses chronically draining pus. If this happens on the scalp or the back of the neck, permanent hair loss can result in the affected area.

CONVENTIONAL TREATMENT

■ Surgery or laser treatment may be used to remove the tissue. After removal, the area is injected with a steroid such as triamcinolone (Aristospan) to prevent re-scarring in the area. Repeat injections may be deemed necessary in some cases. The benefits of repeat injections have to be weighed against the adverse effects of steroid treatment, which include thinning of the skin, impaired wound healing, stress to the adrenal glands, and depressed immune response, among others. The results of this type of treatment are variable.

■ If keloids are a result of acne, long-term antibiotic therapy may be tried as a preventive to ward off new acne lesions.

NUTRITIONAL SUPPLEMENTS

■ Taking high doses of vitamin E may help. Choose a formula containing mixed tocopherols and start by taking 100 international units daily. Then gradually increase the dosage to 400 to 800 international units twice daily over a period of two to four weeks, making sure you have no problem with an increase in blood pressure. This may help contract the scars over the course of several months.

Note: If you have high blood pressure, limit your intake of supplemental vitamin E to a total of 400 international units daily. If you are taking an anticoagulant (blood thinner), consult your physician before taking vitamin E.

■ Selenium works with vitamin E, and may also have its own role in helping to nourish the skin. Take 100 to 400 micrograms daily.

DIETARY GUIDELINES

■ There is no research showing that any particular dietary measures can resolve (or prevent) keloids, but if you are prone to keloids and have recently injured yourself or are expecting to have a surgical procedure, you are best advised to eat a balanced diet that emphasizes green vegetables, lean protein foods, and whole grains. Avoid refined sugar and anything that contains it.

HERBAL TREATMENT

■ Gotu kola has been shown to encourage wound healing. Choose a standardized extract containing 16 percent triterpenes and take 100 to 200 milligrams three times daily for one month.

HOMEOPATHY

■ *Thiosinaminum-Rhodalin* helps to dissolve scar tissue. Take one dose of *Thiosinaminum-Rhodalin* 3x or 3c three times daily for ten days following an injury or surgical procedure.

BACH FLOWER REMEDIES

Select the remedy that most closely fits your disposition and emotional tendencies and concerns, and take it as needed, following the directions on the product label.

■ Walnut is good if you have a tendency to be easily influenced.

■ White Chestnut eases a tendency to dwell on certain ideas or events without letup.

ACUPRESSURE

For the locations of acupressure points on the body, *see* ADMINISTERING AN ACUPRESSURE TREATMENT in Part Three.

■ Spleen 6 and Stomach 36 are tonic points that help to strengthen and regulate the body.

GENERAL RECOMMENDATIONS

■ Applying vitamin-E oil to the scar, then coating it with a light film of dimethylsulfoxide (DMSO), may help shrink the mass from the outside. DMSO helps draw the vitamin E deeper into the skin. Use a 99.9-percent pure, 50-percent concentration solution. Clean the skin with plain soap before this treatment.

PREVENTION

■ It may not be possible to prevent keloids. However, if you know you are prone to developing them, you should avoid elective surgery and anything else that might lead to a break in the skin.

Kidney Disease

The main functions of the kidneys are to regulate the body's fluid balance and electrolyte levels and to eliminate waste products. They perform these important tasks by filtering the blood and removing unnecessary water and soluble wastes, including excess amounts of minerals, which are excreted in the urine. About twenty times every hour, all of the blood in your body passes through your kidneys. The kidneys are also involved in the regulation of blood pressure. They secrete a hormone called renin, which causes the formation of another hormone, angiotensin, in the blood. Angiotensin is a potent blood-vessel constrictor, and acts to increase blood pressure.

The kidneys are located at the back of the abdominal cavity, just above the waist, on either side of the spinal column. The right kidney is situated under the liver, and the left is under the spleen. In the average adult, the kidneys are about four to five inches long and weigh about six ounces apiece. A renal artery enters each kidney and then branches out into a network of progressively smaller blood vessels, culminating in clusters of tiny capillaries called glomeruli. The term *glomerulus* comes from the Latin *glomus,* which, roughly translated, means "ball of yarn." The glomeruli are the main filtering units of the kidney, and each kidney houses many of them. Membranes in these tiny structures filter nutrients and wastes from the blood. The filtered material then passes into structures called tubules. The tubules are surrounded by blood vessels that absorb essential nutrients (amino acids, glucose, salt, and water) from the liquid. Once that has been accomplished, the material that has been removed from the blood is concentrated to become urine. Urine continually trickles down the tubules, through the ureters, and into the bladder, where it is stored until it is passed. The cleansed and filtered blood, meanwhile, passes into the renal vein and returns to the circulation.

Together, glomeruli and tubules make up nephrons, which are the basic functional units of the kidneys. During the natural aging process, the number of functioning nephrons declines. A baby enters the world with about a million or more working nephrons, but the average forty-year-old has only around 375,000 still functioning. By the age of eighty, that number has been reduced to approximately 150,000. Certain diseases also reduce the number of functioning nephrons.

The term *nephritis* denotes any condition characterized by inflammation of the kidneys. *Glomerulonephritis* is inflammation of the glomeruli, the filtering units of the kidneys. This condition usually develops because of an immune response to infection. For example, infection with *Streptococcus* bacteria can precipitate glomerulonephritis, just as it can lead to rheumatic fever. Symptoms can include fluid retention and bloating, decreased frequency of urination, nausea and vomiting, fever, exhaustion, abdominal and/or lower back pain, elevated blood pressure, and dark or bloody urine. *Pyelonephritis* refers to inflammation of the kidney itself, including the entire kidney and the renal pelvis, the area connecting the kidney to the top of the ureter, the tube that carries urine to the bladder. This condition can cause chills, fever, pain, nausea, and vomiting.

Nephrotic syndrome is not, strictly speaking, a disease, but rather a well-defined collection of symptoms. One of the main symptoms is swelling due to fluid retention. This can be generalized throughout the body, but may also be concentrated in the abdomen, scrotum, knees, ankles, and/or eyelids, and these areas of concentration may shift over the course of the day. If fluid builds up in the chest, it can cause shortness of breath. Other symptoms that are part of this syndrome include abdominal pain, loss of appetite, and urine that appears frothy. Urinalysis and blood tests generally detect other problems, particularly an increase in the level of protein in both the blood and the urine. Because people with this syndrome excrete more nutrients than normal in the urine, they may develop nutritional deficiencies as well. Dehydration and acidosis may also result. Nephrotic syndrome is usually caused by some form of glomerulonephritis, but can also occur as a complication of lupus, diabetes, cancer, HIV disease, severe allergies, or treatment with certain drugs. Sometimes, the cause is unknown.

The causes of the above kidney diseases include infections that migrate upward from the urinary tract and exposure to certain drugs or toxins. Kidney problems are often a complication of other disorders, such as diabetes, lupus, high blood pressure, and liver disease. If kidney function is seriously impaired, toxic wastes cannot be properly eliminated and may accumulate in the bloodstream, resulting in uremic poisoning, a sign of potential kidney failure.

Kidney failure can be acute or chronic. Acute failure can itself be divided into three separate types: prerenal, renal, and postrenal. Prerenal failure is also called *prerenal azotemia*, meaning that there are excess nitrogen waste products left in the bloodstream that the kidney was supposed to have filtered into the urine for removal, but did not. This is a sign of poor filtration due to an inadequate flow of blood reaching the kidney, not disease within the kidney itself. This can be due to dehydration, excessive blood loss, blockage of the artery that serves the kidney, liver disease that inhibits blood flow, heart failure, and the use of certain drugs. The two drugs best known for doing this are angiotensin-converting enzyme (ACE) inhibitors, used to treat high blood pressure, and the type of painkiller known as nonsteroidal anti-inflammatory drugs (NSAIDs). Postrenal failure, or postrenal azotemia, results from blockage of the outflow of urine after the kidney has finished processing it. This can occur in prostate disease in men, in which the outflow tract can be compressed. Other possible causes include stones in the bladder and severe trauma. These conditions are not common, but they are the most treatable, as they tend to be localized and, as long as the problem is caught early, there is no disease in the kidney itself.

Failure within the kidney itself, known as intrinsic failure, takes many different forms, depending on exactly which part of the filtering unit is damaged. Usually it is due to chemical damage or acutely low blood flow to the kidney. Chemical damage can be a result of using certain drugs, the worst of which are the so-called aminoglycoside antibiotics, x-ray contrast material used for visualizing the kidney, and the immune-system suppressant cyclosporine (Neoral, Sandimmune).

Chronic renal failure is kidney failure that lasts for weeks to months, with the azotemia gradually becoming worse, and can be due to many forms of kidney tissue disease. The symptoms can be highly varied and difficult to pin down, and can include fatigue, weakness, itching, easy bruising, shortness of breath, nausea, vomiting, chronic hiccups, leg cramps and numbness, impotence, irritability, and difficulty concentrating.

Some forms of kidney disease are hereditary. In cystic kidney disease, multiple cysts—fluid-filled cavities of different sizes—form within the kidneys, ultimately destroying kidney tissue. This condition tends to be more severe and progress more rapidly in children than in adults, and kidney failure is often the eventual result. Other types of hereditary kidney disease include Bartter's syndrome, Fanconi's syndrome, Hartnup disease, and Liddle syndrome. All of these disorders are characterized by improper functioning of the kidneys that results in metabolic problems, principally electrolyte imbalances, which in turn can lead to nutritional deficiencies and blood-pressure disturbances.

Tests to measure kidney function include urinalysis, in which urine is examined microscopically for blood cells, pus, and infectious agents. Kidney function can also be evaluated by measuring the concentration in the blood of substances, such as urea, that are normally eliminated from the body by healthy kidneys. X-ray and ultrasound scans may also be performed.

CONVENTIONAL MEDICINE

All disorders of the kidney are handled first by treating the underlying condition, if any, that is causing the problem. If no underlying cause is found, the following are the usual treatment approaches.

■ If you have chronic kidney disease, you should seek out and work closely with a urologist or other physician who specializes, or at the very least has considerable experience, in the treatment of your condition.

■ Infection is treated with antibiotics. Depending on the organism involved and the severity of the infection, either oral or intravenous antibiotics may be used.

■ Inflammation of kidney tissues is usually first treated with a corticosteroid such as prednisone (Deltasone). If that is inadequate, stronger immunosuppressant drugs are necessary.

■ If you have kidney failure, your doctor will likely advise you to restrict your intake of protein, minerals, and, possibly, water to reduce the stress on your kidneys. If kidney failure is very severe, or what is called end-stage, dialysis may be necessary. There are two principal types of dialysis. In *hemodialysis,* access to a vein is established, and blood flows from the vein through a filtering machine and is then returned to the body. Hemodialysis is usually performed three times a week, at home or in a clinic, with each session lasting about three hours. In *peritoneal dialysis,* a tube is inserted through the abdominal wall and a special fluid solution is introduced into the abdominal cavity that draws out waste materials from the bloodstream. The fluid is then drained out of the abdominal cavity. Peritoneal dialysis has become more popular among many people with chronic kidney failure because it enables them to handle dialysis on their own, although infections are a common problem with this technique. Another option is a kidney transplant.

DIETARY GUIDELINES

■ Eat a well-balanced, high-fiber diet with adequate amounts of clean, lean protein and plenty of yellow and green vegetables.

■ Asparagus, parsley, watercress, celery, and watermelon are cleansing to the entire urinary tract. Enjoy them often.

■ Cranberry juice acidifies the urine, destroys bacteria, and promotes healing. The natural unsweetened juice is best. If you find it too tart, dilute it with spring water.

■ Avoid excessively rich and spicy foods and minimize your intake of animal proteins. These substances are difficult for kidneys under stress to process.

■ To flush toxins from the body and ease your burdened kidneys, drink eight 8-ounce glasses of pure water daily, unless you suffer from kidney failure, in which case you may have to restrict your water intake.

NUTRITIONAL SUPPLEMENTS

■ To ensure an adequate supply of all basic nutrients, take a good multivitamin and mineral supplement daily.

■ Digestive enzymes help ensure complete digestion of foods, which relieves stressed kidneys, and also ensures better assimilation. This means more nutrients are available to help rebuild the kidneys. Take a full-spectrum digestive-enzyme supplement providing 5,000 international units of lipase, 2,500 international units of amylase, and 300 international units of protease, plus 500 to 1,000 milligrams of pancreatin, with each meal.

Note: Long-term supplementation with pancreatin is not advised, as it can cause your pancreas to reduce its own production of this important enzyme. Overuse also has the potential to cause nausea or diarrhea. After two months on pancreatin, discontinue use and monitor your reaction. If you find that your problems recur, discuss pancreatin supplementation with your health-care provider.

■ Green-drink products such as Green Magma and Green Essence, and green-foods supplements such as chlorella and spirulina, available in health-food stores, are rich in cleansing chlorophyll and important trace minerals, which are often depleted in people with kidney disease. Take a green-drink supplement as recommended on the product label.

■ Most people with kidney disease are deficient in magnesium. Take 300 milligrams of magnesium twice a day.

■ Vitamin B_6 (pyridoxine) deficiency is common in people with kidney disease. This important B vitamin helps reduce fluid retention. Take 50 milligrams twice daily, between meals. If you take any of the B vitamins individually, you should also take a B-complex supplement at a different time of day.

■ High doses of vitamin C can offer excellent "health insurance" for the kidneys. Take 1,000 milligrams at least twice daily.

HERBAL TREATMENT

■ Cranberry acidifies the urine, destroys bacteria, and promotes healing. If you cannot drink enough of the juice (or if you're just plain tired of it), you can take 500 milligrams in capsule form two or three times daily.

■ Dandelion root helps cleanse toxic metabolites from the kidneys. Take 500 milligrams twice a day.

■ Horsetail is high in silica and is especially good for treatment of chronic infections. Take 500 milligrams twice daily.

■ Marshmallow root is soothing to the entire genitourinary tract. Take 500 milligrams twice a day.

■ Oregon grape root has very strong antibacterial properties. Take 500 milligrams twice daily.

■ Parsley helps clear uric acid from the urinary tract. Take 500 milligrams twice a day.

Siberian ginseng has demonstrated the ability to improve kidney function in studies involving acute pyelonephritis. It also helps regulate blood pressure. Choose a standardized extract containing 5 percent eleutheroside E and take 100 milligrams in the morning.

■ Uva ursi is a diuretic herb containing antibiotic factors. It also has mild astringent properties and is very cleansing to the entire urinary tract. This herb has a long history of effective use against both kidney stones and urinary tract infections. Take 500 milligrams twice a day. Or take a cup of uva ursi tea as needed.

HOMEOPATHY

Equisetum is helpful if you experience pain on passing urine, especially if the pain occurs near the end of urination. Take one dose of *Equisetum* 12x or 6c three times a day for up to three days.

Thuja is the remedy for a chronic infection of the genitourinary tract. Take one dose of *Thuja* 30x or 15c two times daily for up to four days.

BACH FLOWER REMEDIES

Select the remedy that most closely fits your emotional tendencies and concerns, and take it as needed, following the directions on the product label.

■ Hornbeam will prove helpful if you are so exhausted you cannot participate in your normal activities.

Impatiens is the remedy to choose if you are nervous, hyperactive, impatient, nervous, and easily irritated.

Mimulus helps to ease fear of known things.

■ Mustard is the remedy for sadness and depression, possibly related to a loss of some kind.

ACUPRESSURE

For the locations of acupressure points on the body, *see* ADMINISTERING AN ACUPRESSURE TREATMENT in Part Three.

Kidney 3 and 7 help to strengthen the kidneys.

Liver 3 brings energy down from the head and helps to speed recovery.

Spleen 6 and Stomach 36 together improve digestion and immune function.

PREVENTION

■ Anytime you you suspect a urinary tract infection, seek treatment promptly. Left untreated, an infection can migrate up through the ureters to the kidneys.

■ If you have a history of kidney infection, consider taking 500 milligrams of cranberry extract daily on an ongoing basis.

Kidney Stones

Kidney stones, medically termed *renal calculi*, are accumulations of mineral salts, such as calcium, uric acid, struvite, and cystine. Human urine normally contains minute particles of minerals and other solid substances suspended in solution. If a certain critical mass is reached, they can begin to crystallize, ultimately forming stones that can lodge anywhere in the urinary tract. About 80 percent of all kidney stones are composed of calcium, and result from excessive absorption of calcium from the intestines that in turn increases calcium in the urine. The excess calcium can crystallize to form stones, which can range in size from an unnoticeable speck to a troublesome half-inch.

There are many factors that can predispose a person to forming stones. High humidity and temperature, high sodium intake, low fluid intake, and low fiber intake are all thought to be risk factors for stone-forming individuals. A lack of dietary fiber in particular can increase the level of calcium in the urine because it slows the passage of food through the intestines, allowing more calcium to be absorbed into the bloodstream, and also because it results in a lack of sufficient fiber to bind to calcium in the gastrointestinal (GI) tract. A sedentary lifestyle seems to increase the possibility of stone formation, too. More important seems to be the degree of concentration and the level of acidity of the urine. Heredity also plays a role. For example, only specific types of individuals, designated *type II hypercalciuric*, seem to benefit at all from lowering their calcium intake to avoid stone formation.

If you ever have a kidney stone, it is likely you will never forget the sensation. The pain is usually severe, beginning suddenly and specifically in the flank region. Nausea and vomiting may follow, as may chills and fever, and there may be pus and blood in the urine. It is usually difficult to stay still, unlike in other acute abdominal problems, which make it hurt to move at all. The pain moves with the stone, and stone size does not seem to have any relationship to the degree of pain. Urinary urgency may occur if the stone lodges at the junction of the bladder and ureter (the tube from the kidney to the bladder).

Your doctor may wish to know the chemical composition of the stone, and ask you to urinate through a screen to catch the stone if it is passed. It may be worthwhile to have a twenty-four-hour urine sample taken to see whether you have some defect in urinary volume or the excretion of calcium, phosphate, uric acid, oxalate, or citrate. A standard urinalysis will usually show the presence of some blood and will determine the relative acidity of the urine, which is an important clue to the type of stone that is causing the problem.

Most stones can be found using standard x-ray films and ultrasound. If any uncertainty remains, a doctor may order an intravenous pyelogram (IVP). In this test, a dye is introduced to the bloodstream using a small intravenous line, and then x-rays are taken to see how the dye flows through the kidney. This test is usually reserved for more severe kidney disease, however, as the dye has been known to cause both allergic reactions and acute kidney failure in some cases.

CONVENTIONAL MEDICINE

■ The treatment for stones in the urinary tract depends on their size and location—whether they are in the kidney, ureter, bladder, or urethra.

■ If the stones are small and cause no symptoms, no treatment is necessary, although they should be monitored.

■ Larger stones that are causing obstruction can sometimes be treated with extracorporeal shock wave lithotripsy (ESWL). In this technique, you are placed in a pool of water and high-frequency sound waves are sent through the water. This fragments the stones so that they can pass out of your body in the urine.

■ If ESWL is unsuccessful, and the urinary tract is obstructed, your doctor may recommend surgery to remove the stones. However, watchful waiting may also be recommended.

DIETARY GUIDELINES

■ To flush toxins from the body, ease your burdened kidneys, and encourage the stones to pass, drink at least eight 8-ounce glasses of pure water daily.

■ Eat a well-balanced high-fiber diet with adequate amounts of clean, lean protein and plenty of green and yellow vegetables.

■ Include asparagus, parsley, watercress, celery, and watermelon in your diet. These foods are cleansing to the entire urinary tract.

■ Avoid rich and spicy foods, and minimize your intake of animal proteins. These substances are difficult for kidneys under stress to process.

■ Avoid chocolate, spinach, and rhubarb. These foods contain oxalic acid, which can ultimately form kidney stones.

■ Avoid eating foods that are very high in calcium, such as dairy products. Most kidney stones are a result of excessive levels of calcium in the urine.

NUTRITIONAL SUPPLEMENTS

■ Digestive enzymes help to ensure complete digestion of foods, which relieves stressed kidneys, as well as better assimilation of nutrients. Take a full-spectrum digestive-enzyme supplement providing 5,000 international units of lipase, 2,500 international units of amylase, and 300 international units of protease, plus 500 to 1,000 milligrams of pancreatin, with each meal.

Note: Long-term supplementation with pancreatin is not advised, as it can cause your pancreas to reduce its own production of this important enzyme. Overuse also has the potential to cause nausea or diarrhea. After two months on pancreatin, discontinue use and monitor your reaction. If you find that your problems recur, discuss pancreatin supplementation with your health-care provider.

■ High doses of vitamin C can offer excellent "health insurance" for the kidneys. Take 500 to 1,000 milligrams at least twice daily.

HERBAL TREATMENT

■ Dandelion root helps cleanse toxic metabolites from the kidneys. Take 500 milligrams twice a day for six weeks. Stop for one month, then repeat.

■ Parsley helps clear uric acid from the urinary tract and is high in potassium. Take 500 milligrams twice daily.

■ Uva ursi is a diuretic herb containing antibiotic factors. It also has mild astringent properties and is very cleansing to the entire urinary tract. This herb has a long history of effective use against kidney stones. Take 500 milligrams twice a day.

HOMEOPATHY

■ *Equisetum* is helpful if you experience pain on passing urine, especially if the pain occurs near the end of urination. Take one dose of *Equisetum* 12x or 6c three times a day for up to three days.

BACH FLOWER REMEDIES

Select the remedy that most closely fits your emotional tendencies and concerns, and take it as needed, following the directions on the product label.

■ Hornbeam will prove helpful if you are so exhausted you cannot participate in normal activities.

■ Choose Impatiens if you are nervous, hyperactive, impatient, and easily irritated.

■ Mimulus is the remedy for fear of known things.

■ Mustard is the remedy for sadness and depression, possibly related to a loss of some kind.

ACUPRESSURE

For the locations of acupressure points on the body, *see* ADMINISTERING AN ACUPRESSURE TREATMENT in Part Three.

■ Kidney 3 and 7 strengthen the kidneys and bladder.

■ Liver 3 brings energy down from the head to speed recovery, and also relieves crampy, colicky pain.

■ Spleen 6 and Stomach 36 together improve the absorption of nutrients and strengthens overall well-being. They are particularly useful if kidney stones are related to a disturbance in the digestive tract.

Labyrinthitis

The inner ear, or labyrinth, contains a series of fluid-filled semicircular canals whose function is to maintain the body's sense of balance. In labyrinthitis, this area becomes inflamed, causing vertigo, which is usually severe. This is a sensation that your surroundings are spinning around you. It is different from mere lightheadedness, or feeling faint. The vertigo is usually accompanied by some degree of hearing loss and tinnitus (a ringing or buzzing sound in the affected ear). Recovery may take up to several weeks, and some hearing loss may remain permanently. Also, rapid head movements may cause mild, transient vertigo for some time afterward. The cause of labyrinthitis is unknown, but it often seems to be associated with an earlier upper respiratory tract illness.

CONVENTIONAL TREATMENT

■ Since the cause of this disorder is unknown, treatment focuses on relieving symptoms. Unfortunately, the drugs that are used for this problem have been found to adversely affect the healing process, so they are normally used for as short a period as possible.

■ Vertigo may be treated first with a drug like meclizine (Antivert, Bonine) or dimenhydrinate (Dramamine), both antihistamines commonly used to treat motion sickness. Possible side effects include dry mouth, sleepiness, and a decreased ability to concentrate.

■ If meclizine or dimenhydrinate proves inadequate, a transdermal patch containing scopolamine (Transderm Scop) may be prescribed. Potential side effects of this drug are more severe, and include dry mouth, blurred vision, and urinary tract obstruction.

■ For the worst vertigo, diazepam (Valium) may be given intravenously. Side effects can include drowsiness, impaired memory, jaundice, and a low white blood cell count. This drug also has considerable abuse potential.

DIETARY GUIDELINES

■ Avoid refined sugar (and any foods that contain it) and greasy fried foods.

NUTRITIONAL SUPPLEMENTS

■ Take a good multivitamin and mineral supplement daily. Choose a powder or capsule form for best absorption.

■ Adrenal glandular extract is useful if labyrinthitis is associated with fatigue. In Chinese medicine, labyrinthitis is related to deficient "kidney *chi*." Adrenal extract helps to restore "kidney *chi*." Take 350 milligrams of adrenal extract before breakfast and another 350 milligrams before lunch.

Note: Do not take this supplement if you have high blood pressure.

■ A deficiency of vitamin B_{12} has been associated with labyrinthitis. Take 500 micrograms of vitamin B_{12} with 400 micrograms of folic acid twice a day for one month. If you take any of the B vitamins individually, you should also take a B-complex supplement at a different time of day.

HERBAL TREATMENT

■ Ginkgo biloba, with its unique ability to improve circulation to the head, has been shown to be helpful for symptoms of dizziness and tinnitus. Select a standardized extract containing at least 24 percent ginkgo heterosides (sometimes called flavoglycosides) and take 60 milligrams two or three times daily, as needed, for one month.

■ Reishi mushroom helps the body cope with stress. It has long been used in Chinese medicine to hasten recovery from illness. Take 500 milligrams three times daily for one month.

HOMEOPATHY

■ *Carboneum sulfuratum* is for labyrinthitis with noises in the head, dizziness, headache, irritability, anxiety, and mental sluggishness. Your mood is likely changeable, and your sight may be affected. Take one dose of *Carboneum sulfuratum* 12x or 6c three times daily for up to four days.

■ *Cocculus* is helpful for vertigo with nausea that is worse when riding in a car, standing up, or lying on the back of the head. Symptoms are also worse after eating or if you don't get sufficient sleep. Take one dose of *Cocculus* 12x or 6c three times daily for up to four days.

BACH FLOWER REMEDIES

Select the remedy that most closely fits your disposition and emotional tendencies and concerns, and take it as needed, following the directions on the product label.

■ Gorse helps to ease feelings of despair.

■ Larch is beneficial if you lack self-confidence.

■ Olive gently lifts exhaustion.

■ Scleranthus is good for feelings of uncertainty.

ACUPRESSURE

For the locations of acupressure points on the body, *see* ADMINISTERING AN ACUPRESSURE TREATMENT in Part Three.

■ Gallbladder 20 and Stomach 36 help to regulate circulation.

■ Kidney 1, 3, and 7 help to strengthen kidney energy. In Chinese medicine, labyrinthitis is associated with a deficiency of energy in the kidneys.

GENERAL RECOMMENDATIONS

■ Don't smoke, and avoid secondhand smoke. All ear disorders are more common in smokers than nonsmokers.

Lactose Intolerance

Milk products contain a type of sugar called lactose. Digesting this sugar requires the enzyme lactase. Babies and young children almost always produce ample amounts of lactase, but by adolescence, lactase production often falls. In some people, it virtually disappears. As a result, consuming milk and most other dairy products can cause symptoms such as bloating, cramping, abdominal gas, and even diarrhea, as the undigested lactose ferments in the digestive system. The severity of symptoms is usually related to how much lactose is consumed.

Lactose intolerance occurs in about 25 percent of Caucasians of northern European descent, but 50 to 95 percent of people with other ethnic backgrounds may be affected. Crohn's disease, gastroenteritis, intestinal parasites, and other disorders affecting the small intestine, where lactase is made, can make the situation worse.

A diagnosis of lactose intolerance is made by family history and a trial of a lactose-free diet. If symptoms improve, it can be assumed that lactose is the problem. A doctor may confirm the diagnosis by giving a dose of milk sugar and then measuring the level of hydrogen released in the breath.

CONVENTIONAL TREATMENT

■ Treatment is usually based on avoiding excessive consumption of dairy products. Most people do not need to give up dairy completely, and can determine the level they can tolerate. Also, some dairy products are more likely to provoke symptoms than others. Milk, cottage cheese, and ice cream are high in lactose, aged cheeses contain far less, and plain, unpasteurized yogurt is formed by bacteria that provide their own lactase enzyme.

■ Lactase tablets (Lactaid) are available over the counter. You can take these before ingesting milk products to pro-vide the required enzyme. The number of tablets needed depends on the individual and the quantity of dairy foods involved.

DIETARY GUIDELINES

■ People who are lactose intolerant are often advised to eliminate all dairy products from the diet at first. After a couple of months, you may try drinking small amounts of milk if you take lactase along with it (*see under* Conventional Treatment, in this entry). As an alternative, milk that is pretreated with lactase is available. If symptoms return, however, you may have to consider avoiding dairy foods entirely.

■ Low-fat dairy products such as yogurt are usually easier to tolerate than milk. In fact, unpasteurized yogurt that contains active yogurt culture can be extremely beneficial for digestion. Goat's milk, buttermilk, and aged cheeses have a lower proportion of lactose than other types of dairy products, so you may be able to consume these even if cow's milk causes a problem.

■ Avoid processed food products that contain lactose as an ingredient.

NUTRITIONAL SUPPLEMENTS

■ Acidophilus aids digestion by replenishing beneficial bacteria in the intestinal tract. Select a dairy-free product and take one dose twice daily and/or when you eat dairy products, as directed on the product label.

■ If you determine that you would like to dramatically reduce or delete dairy products from your diet, consider taking supplemental calcium, magnesium, and vitamin D. A daily dose of 800 to 1,000 milligrams of calcium and 400 to 500 milligrams of magnesium should prevent deficiency. If you do not get at least fifteen minutes of exposure to direct sunlight daily, also take 200 to 400 international units of vitamin D each day.

HERBAL TREATMENT

■ Try drinking ginger tea with meals containing lactose. Ginger is an excellent digestive aid and may often minimize digestive disturbance.

HOMEOPATHY

■ *Aethusa cynapium* is good if you have a marked inability to digest milk accompanied by poor circulation and difficulty focusing your attention. You may have a tendency to become constipated after consuming dairy products. Take one dose of *Aethusa cynapium* 12x or 6c three times daily for up to three days.

■ *Calcarea fluorica* is useful for abdominal gas and acute indigestion with fatigue. Take one dose of *Calcarea fluorica* 30x or 15c after meals.

Carbo vegetabilis is for symptoms of pain in the center of the stomach, accompanied by a distended abdomen, that feel better after you pass gas. Take one dose of *Carbo vegetabilis* 30x or 15c after meals.

ACUPRESSURE

For the locations of acupressure points on the body, *see* ADMINISTERING AN ACUPRESSURE TREATMENT in Part Three.

- Stomach 36 enhances digestion.
- Pericardium relaxes the upper abdomen.

BACH FLOWER REMEDIES

Select the remedy that most closely fits your disposition and emotional tendencies and concerns, and take it as needed, following the directions on the product label.

- Walnut helps to counteract a tendency to be easily influenced that arises from a sensitive nature.
- White Chestnut helps to tame obsessive thinking and a tendency to dwell on certain ideas.

AROMATHERAPY

For specific instructions on how to use aromatherapy, *see* PREPARING AROMATHERAPY TREATMENTS in Part Three.

- Orange oil is known to enhance digestion. Use it as an inhalant or diffuse it into the air at mealtimes.

GENERAL RECOMMENDATIONS

- If eliminating dairy products from your diet brings no results, consult with your doctor to make sure you are not suffering from another digestive condition.

Laryngitis

See under SORE THROAT.

Legionnaire's Disease

Legionnaire's disease is a form of pneumonia that was originally difficult to diagnose because the organism that causes it, *Legionella pneumophila*, cannot be seen on the standard laboratory test done to identify microorganisms in sputum. As a result, doctors refer to it as an "atypical pneumonia," even though it is a common cause of pneumonia acquired in such community settings as hospitals and hotels. It is not usually transmitted from person to person, but spread through such mechanisms as air conditioning and ventilating systems.

The disease is more common in people with compromised immune systems and/or established lung disease, as well as in smokers. The initial symptoms are similar to those of many other illnesses, including fever, fatigue, headache, and muscle aches. These are followed by the development of a cough, chest pain while breathing and/or coughing, and poor production of sputum. People with this illness usually appear and feel quite ill.

If Legionnaire's disease is suspected, tests on sputum, blood, and urine are performed, using special culture techniques to identify the infecting organism. An x-ray may be performed as well. This cannot provide a specific diagnosis, but it can show areas of disease in the lungs.

CONVENTIONAL TREATMENT

■ The antibiotic erythromycin (Eryc, Ery-Tab, PCE, and others) is normally the drug of choice for treating this disease. Initially, antibiotics are often administered intravenously to make sure they are having the desired effect. Other similar drugs, such as azithromycin (Zithromax) and clarithromycin (Biaxin), may also be used, but are more expensive. Possible side effects of these drugs include nausea, vomiting, rash, liver stress, and the appearance of other infections against which they are ineffective.

■ If you are unable to tolerate erythromycin, another type of antibiotic may be used. Possibilities include tetracycline (Achromycin), sulfamethoxazole plus trimethoprim (Bactrim, Septra), and ciprofloxacin (Cipro). Potential side effects of these drugs include liver toxicity, nausea, and vomiting.

■ For severe infections, the tuberculosis drug rifampin (Rifadin) may be added to the regimen. This drug can cause a wide range of side effects, including jaundice, hepatitis, headache, drowsiness, dizziness, confusion, rash, blood cell changes, and others.

DIETARY GUIDELINES

■ Simplify your diet. Try to eat as many raw and lightly steamed vegetables as your digestive system can tolerate. Hot soups are good as well, because they are soothing and may be easier to take than solid foods. Avoid alcohol, dairy products, all fried foods, and anything containing refined sugar until healing is complete.

■ Drink at least eight 8-ounce glasses of pure water each day to prevent dehydration.

NUTRITIONAL SUPPLEMENTS

■ Bromelain, an enzyme derived from pineapple, is a

good anti-inflammatory. Take 400 milligrams twice daily, between meals.

■ Colostrum is a probiotic that helps to regulate and reinvigorate digestion. It also enhances immune function. Take 500 milligrams three times a day.

■ Thymus glandular extract helps to enhance immune function. Take a dose supplying 350 milligrams of crude polypeptide fraction twice a day.

■ Vitamin A is essential for the health and repair of the tissues that line the respiratory passages. Take 10,000 international units three times daily for one month.

Note: If you are pregnant, or intend to get pregnant, or if you have liver disease, consult your doctor before taking supplemental vitamin A. Pregnant women should not ingest a total of more than 25,000 international units of supplemental vitamin A *per week* from all sources.

■ Vitamin C and bioflavonoids reduce inflammation and help the body to fight infection. These nutrients work best if taken together. Take 500 milligrams of vitamin C and 100 milligrams of mixed bioflavonoids three times daily.

HERBAL TREATMENT

■ Cat's claw enhances the immune response and has antibacterial properties. Take 500 milligrams of standardized extract three times a day until your condition improves.

Note: Do not use cat's claw if you are pregnant or nursing, or if you are an organ-transplant recipient. Use it with caution if you are taking an anticoagulant (blood thinner).

■ Cordyceps is a tonic herb that increases the oxygen supply to body systems, enhances immunity, and acts as an antioxidant. Take 1,000 milligrams of standardized extract twice a day.

■ Goldenseal has antibiotic properties and benefits the mucous membranes of the respiratory tract. Choose a standardized extract containing at least 5 percent total alkaloids and take 300 milligrams three times daily for ten days.

■ Licorice contains glycyrrhizin, which has a powerful anti-inflammatory effect. Licorice also eases coughing and is soothing to the mucous membranes of the lungs, and it has antibacterial and antiviral properties. Take 300 to 500 milligrams two or three times daily.

Note: Do not take licorice by itself on a daily basis for more than five days at a time, as it can elevate blood pressure. Do not take it at all if you have high blood pressure.

■ Oregano has antibacterial properties and helps to fight infection. Take 75 milligrams of standardized extract three times a day

■ Schizandra is a Chinese herb that has long been used as a tonic to help the body resist physical, biological, and environmental stresses. It reduces inflammation and promotes healing. Take 250 milligrams of schizandra upon arising and again at bedtime.

HOMEOPATHY

■ In the first stages of the illness, *Gelsemium* can be helpful for flulike symptoms accompanied by dizziness, drowsiness, trembling, a dry cough, and an oppressive feeling in chest. You want quiet and to be left alone. Take one dose of *Gelsemium* 12x or 6c three times daily for up to two days.

■ *Veratrum viride* is good for congestion of the lungs with difficulty breathing and a sensation of a heavy load pressing on the chest. Take one dose of *Veratrum viride* 12x or 6c three times daily for up to three days.

BACH FLOWER REMEDIES

■ Olive helps to relieve exhaustion so profound that you have a sense of being fatigued to the core. Take it as directed on the product label.

ACUPRESSURE

For the locations of acupressure points on the body, *see* ADMINISTERING AN ACUPRESSURE TREATMENT in Part Three.

■ Lung 7 and Pericardium 6 strengthen the lungs and relax the chest.

AROMATHERAPY

For specific instructions on how to use aromatherapy, *see* PREPARING AROMATHERAPY TREATMENTS in Part Three.

■ A steam inhalation treatment made with basil, eucalyptus, pine, and/or tea tree oil can help to clear mucus and ease breathing.

■ Add a couple of drops of essential oils of eucalyptus, peppermint, and/or thyme to 1/4 cup of almond or sesame oil and blend. Rub this mixture over your back and chest to relax and increase circulation to the chest area.

Note: If you are using peppermint oil and also taking a homeopathic preparation, allow one hour between the two. Otherwise, the strong smell of the mint may interfere with the action of the homeopathic remedy.

GENERAL RECOMMENDATIONS

■ Avoid exposure to any kind of smoke, especially tobacco smoke.

■ Use a cool mist humidifier to moisten and soothe your respiratory tract and thin secretions so that they are easier to cough out. A drop or two of essential oil of thyme, eucalyptus, pine, or orange added to the water in the humidifier may also help to ease breathing. Be certain to clean the humidifier every few days to avoid the buildup of bacteria and fungi.

■ Applying a warm castor oil pack on the chest once or twice a week can be very useful in helping to eliminate mucus. Either warm castor oil and saturate several layers of clean white cloth with the oil, or saturate the cloth, place it on a clean plate, and warm it in a microwave oven for twenty to thirty seconds. The pack should be warm but not hot. Place it over your chest and leave it in place for fifteen to twenty minutes.

Leukemia

See under CANCER.

Liver Disease

See CIRRHOSIS; HEPATITIS.

Lockjaw

See TETANUS.

Lumbago

See under BACK PAIN AND STRAIN.

Lupus

Lupus erythematosus is a chronic inflammatory disorder of the connective tissue. It gets its name from the Latin word for "wolf," because some people who have it develop a butterfly-shaped rash over the cheeks and nose that was considered to give them a wolflike appearance (although this symptom actually appears in fewer than half of all people with the disease).

At least 90 percent of those who contract lupus are women, and it is most often diagnosed in young adulthood. It is more prevalent among people of African and/or Asian descent than among those of other ethnic

backgrounds. There are two types of lupus: discoid lupus erythematosus (DLE) and systemic lupus erythematosus (SLE).

DLE, the more common type of lupus, affects exposed areas of the skin, causing a rash that starts as one or more red, circular, thickened areas of the skin that later form scars. They may occur on the face, behind the ears, and/or on the scalp. If lesions lead to scarring on the scalp, there can be permanent hair loss in the affected areas.

SLE is a more serious form of the disease. It affects many systems of the body, especially the joints and the kidneys. Symptoms can include on-again, off-again low-grade fever, interspersed with periods of high fever, in addition to nausea, constipation and/or diarrhea, weight loss, general malaise, fatigue, skin rashes and lesions, and all-over muscle and joint pain similar to the aches and pains experienced by people with severe rheumatoid arthritis. There can also be neurological effects, including mental dysfunction, emotional instability, headaches, irritability, and depression. Recurrent urinary tract infections are common. More serious complications can include heart and lung problems, Raynaud's phenomenon, an enlarged spleen, and kidney damage. Like rheumatoid arthritis, SLE is characterized by alternating periods of remission and acute flare-ups. Because flare-ups are often triggered by exposure to sunlight, a worsening of symptoms is more likely to occur during spring and summer.

The underlying cause or causes of lupus are not clearly understood, but it is generally believed to be an autoimmune disease, in which the body—for reasons unknown—starts attacking its own cells. An enlarged spleen and lymph nodes are common. At least 10 percent of cases can be traced to a severe allergic reaction to certain drugs, including some vaccines, and there are some factors that appear to increase a person's risk of developing this disease. These include streptococcal infections, abnormal estrogen metabolism, pregnancy, and mental and physical stress.

The prognosis for people with lupus depends on the severity of the condition and whether any dangerous complications develop. Generally, the outlook is most promising if the disorder is diagnosed early and treatment is begun promptly. Mild cases of lupus respond very well to natural medicine, and even people with more serious illness can expect to achieve some relief of symptoms with natural approaches.

CONVENTIONAL MEDICINE

■ If you are diagnosed with lupus, it is wise to seek out and work closely with a rheumatologist or other physician who specializes, or at the very least has considerable experience, in the treatment of this condition.

■ Nonsteroidal anti-inflammatory drugs (NSAIDs) such as aspirin (Bayer, Ecotrin, and others) or ibuprofen (Advil,

Motrin, Nuprin, and others) may be recommended to reduce inflammation and control pain.

■ If skin rashes and joint pains are not adequately handled by NSAIDs, hydroxychloroquine (Plaquenil) may be prescribed. This is a drug originally used to combat malaria, but it can be helpful for people with lupus as well. This drug has the potential to cause considerable permanent damage to your vision, among other unwelcome effects, so you should be sure to work with a physician who is experienced in its use.

■ For acute lesions, topical steroid creams may be prescribed.

■ For serious cases, a regimen employing corticosteroids, such as prednisone (Deltasone), and possibly immunosuppressive drugs like cyclophosphamide (Cytoxan), may be needed to help ward off damage to the kidneys. Steroids modify the immune response, depress the adrenal glands, and have anti-inflammatory effects. They should be taken with food. If you must take either of these kinds of drugs, you must be monitored closely by your physician. Long-term use of steroids can lead to serious side effects, including glaucoma, cataracts, osteoporosis, skin changes, mental changes, ulcers, and an increased susceptibility to infection. Immunosuppressive drugs have even more serious toxic effects. Potential problems include kidney damage, liver damage, heart muscle damage, lung damage, nausea, vomiting, hair loss, and blood abnormalities.

DIETARY GUIDELINES

■ Follow a well-balanced, high-fiber diet plan that includes clean, lean, easily-digested high-protein foods, such as chicken and fish, and plenty of green vegetables.

■ Maximize your intake of raw and steamed vegetables. Some of the best choices include steamed broccoli, kale, arugula, artichokes, and beet and collard greens.

■ Drink eight 8-ounce glasses of pure water every day.

■ It is important to discover whether you have any allergies or sensitivities to foods that may be triggering flare-ups. For example, many people with lupus feel better when they avoid whole wheat and chocolate. See ELIMINATION DIET in Part Three for ways to track down foods that may be causing a problem.

■ Avoid alfalfa sprouts, which interfere with protein metabolism, as well as large amounts of raw cabbage, which depresses thyroid function. Proper thyroid function is very important for people with lupus. The thyroid is the body's "engine," encouraging the proper functioning of the endocrine system and processing of food. Also avoid eggplant, peppers, and other foods in the nightshade family, which can aggravate the symptoms of lupus.

NUTRITIONAL SUPPLEMENTS

■ Beta-carotene is converted by the body into vitamin A, which is required by the immune system and the adrenal glands for healthy functioning. If you are not getting a total of 15,000 international units of beta-carotene from other supplements, take a beta-carotene supplement to bring yourself up to that amount.

■ Many people with lupus have digestive problems that cause nutrients to be underutilized. Take a full-spectrum digestive-enzyme supplement providing 5,000 international units of lipase, 2,500 international units of amylase, and 300 international units of protease, plus 500 to 1,000 milligrams of pancreatin, immediately after each meal to enhance nutrient absorption.

Note: Long-term supplementation with pancreatin is not advised, as it can cause your pancreas to reduce its own production of this important enzyme. Overuse also has the potential to cause nausea or diarrhea. After two months on pancreatin, discontinue use and monitor your reaction. If you find that your problems recur, discuss pancreatin supplementation with your health-care provider.

■ People with lupus often have difficulty absorbing sufficient protein. Take a good amino-acid complex that supplies all the essential amino acids, plus additional cysteine, gamma-aminobutyric acid (GABA), and carnitine. Cysteine is a precursor of glutathione, one of the strongest antioxidants in the body. Some experts believe that free-radical damage is an integral part of the lupus syndrome. GABA is very useful for relaxing the nervous system and improving the transmission of nerve impulses. Many people with lupus have reported benefits from taking it. Carnitine is important for proper energy metabolism. Try the following program:

Month 1: Take a full free-form amino-acid complex daily, as directed on the product label. Also take 500 milligrams of L-cysteine twice daily.

Month 2: Continue taking the free-form amino-acid supplement. Also take 500 milligrams of N-acetylcysteine (NAC) daily.

Month 3: Take a free-form amino-acid complex plus 500 milligrams of GABA daily.

Month 4: Take a free-form amino-acid complex. Also take L-carnitine as follows: Start with 500 milligrams daily. After one week, increase the dosage to 500 milligrams twice a day.

■ Calcium is required for strong bones; magnesium protects the heart. Take a calcium and magnesium supplement that provides 800 milligrams of each mineral daily.

■ Essential fatty acids such as those found in black currant seed oil, borage oil, evening primrose oil, and flaxseed oil have an anti-inflammatory effect and are beneficial for the skin. Choose any of these oils and take 1 tablespoon (or 500 milligrams) daily for one month. After a month, add a second dose at a different time of day.

■ Glucosamine sulfate is very helpful for pain and cartilage repair. Try taking 500 milligrams three times daily.

■ Green-foods supplements contain important trace minerals missing in the ordinary diet. Select a formula that includes high amounts of carotene and take it as directed on the product label.

■ Acidophilus and bifidobacteria strengthen and stabilize the gastrointestinal system. Take a probiotic supplement as recommended on the product label. If you are allergic to milk, select a dairy-free product.

■ Proteolytic enzymes have notable anti-inflammatory action and are required for the digestion of protein. Take a proteolytic-enzyme supplement between meals, as directed on the product label.

■ Vitamin C has strong anti-inflammatory properties and helps strengthen collagen, an important constituent of connective tissue. Take 1,000 milligrams of vitamin C, in mineral ascorbate or esterified (Ester-C) form, three times daily.

■ Vitamin E promotes healing. It is also a strong antioxidant that helps prevent free-radical damage. Choose a product containing mixed tocopherols and start by taking 200 international units daily, then gradually increase the dosage until you are taking 400 international units once or twice daily.

Note: If you have high blood pressure, limit your intake of supplemental vitamin E to a total of 400 international units daily. If you are taking an anticoagulant (blood thinner), consult your physician before taking supplemental vitamin E.

■ Zinc is present in every cell in the body. It is integral to over 200 enzymes. For example, it participates in the formation of insulin, growth hormone, thyroid hormones, adrenal hormones, and sex hormones. Take 15 milligrams of zinc twice a day, with meals. If you take 30 or more milligrams of zinc on a daily basis for more than one or two months, you should also take 1 to 2 milligrams of copper each day to maintain a proper mineral balance.

■ Dehydroepiandrosterone (DHEA) is a hormone that, among other things, stimulates the adrenal glands. Adrenal function is often compromised in people with lupus. Discuss DHEA therapy with your physician. Age is a factor in deciding whether DHEA supplementation is suitable for you; levels of DHEA decline with age.

HERBAL TREATMENT

■ Aloe vera is very effective against abdominal pain, constipation, and pre-ulceration of the stomach. It helps soothe an irritated digestive tract. Select a food-grade product and take ⅛ cup twice a day.

■ If fatigue is your most prominent system, take an astragalus combination formula. Astragalus may be combined with a variety of herbs, such as Siberian ginseng, cordyceps, codonopsis, and others. Take it according to the directions on the product label.

■ Devil's claw is considered useful arthritic-type pain. Take 500 milligrams two or three times daily.

Note: Do not use cat's claw if you are pregnant or nursing, or if you are an organ transplant recipient. Use it with caution if you are taking an anticoagulant (blood thinner).

■ Pine-bark and grape-seed extracts are excellent natural anti-inflammatories. Take 50 milligrams of either twice daily.

■ Reishi or ganoderma mushroom enhances immune function. Research in laboratory animals suggest it may also improve parasympathetic nerve and heart function, and protect the central nervous system. Take a concentrate supplying the equivalent of 1,000 milligrams (1 gram) three times daily.

■ For energy enhancement and to overcome general malaise, take Siberian ginseng. Choose a standardized extract containing 0.5 percent eleutheroside E and take 100 milligrams twice daily, in morning and afternoon, as needed.

■ Turmeric is an excellent anti-inflammatory and effective against arthritic-type pain. Try taking 300 to 500 milligrams two or three times daily.

■ There are several very effective Chinese combination formulas that are recommended for lupus. See a doctor of Chinese medicine (OMD) or Chinese herbal practitioner for a prescription tailored to your symptoms.

■ Many people with lupus suffer from recurring urinary tract infections. Herbs that can be helpful for the urinary tract include cranberry, which has antibacterial properties; parsley root, which is a mild natural diuretic; and marshmallow root, which is soothing to both the bladder and the kidneys.

■ *Avoid* using echinacea. This herb stimulates the immune system, so anyone with an autoimmune disease, such as lupus, should not take it.

HOMEOPATHY

Lupus is a complicated problem. For substantial help, see a homeopathic physician for a constitutional remedy. The remedies that follow can be used to ease symptoms during acute flare-ups.

■ *Bryonia* is helpful for joints that hurt all the time, but feel worse with movement and better when resting. Take one dose of *Bryonia* 30x or 15c as needed.

■ *Natrum muriaticum* is good if you have mouth sores and

crave salty foods. Take one dose of *Natrum muriaticum* 30x or 15c as needed. If this remedy isn't sufficient, try *Mercurius solubilis*. This remedy is recommended for mouth sores accompanied by a sore throat. Take one dose of *Mercurius solubilis* 30x or 15c as needed.

■ If you have a rash on your cheeks, try *Psorinum* 30x or 15c or *Sulfur* 30x or 15c. Discuss the use of these remedies with a homeopathic physician before taking them.

■ *Rhus toxicodendron* is for joint pain that is worse upon awakening and better after moving around. Take one dose of *Rhus toxicodendron* 30x or 15c as needed.

BACH FLOWER REMEDIES

Select the remedy that most closely fits your emotional tendencies and concerns, and take it as needed, following the directions on the product label.

■ Holly (for anger) and/or Impatiens (for impatience and irritability) can be helpful if you have a skin rash that is very red and angry looking.

■ Hornbeam is the remedy for extreme fatigue and exhaustion.

■ Mimulus and/or Aspen is helpful if you are fearful, especially if you have problems with kidney function.

■ Mustard helps to relieve sadness and depression. You may be mourning a loss of some kind, perhaps the loss of well-being.

ACUPRESSURE

For the locations of acupressure points on the body, *see* ADMINISTERING AN ACUPRESSURE TREATMENT in Part Three.

■ All back Bladder points relax the nervous system.

■ Gallbladder 34 and 41 improve circulation and reduce pain in the joints.

■ Kidney 3 helps to strengthen the kidneys and bladder.

■ Pericardium 6 relaxes the body.

■ Spleen 4 and 10 strengthen and remove "heat" from the blood.

■ Stomach 36 improves digestion and the absorption of nutrients, helps to bring down fever, and strengthens overall well-being.

AROMATHERAPY

For specific instructions on how to use aromatherapy, *see* PREPARING AROMATHERAPY TREATMENTS in Part Three.

■ Soothing aromatherapy baths and massages can help to ease pain and inflammation. Choose up to three of the following essential oils to add to bath water or massage oil: basil, black pepper, elemi, myrrh, and pine.

GENERAL RECOMMENDATIONS

■ Schedule a daily rest period, whether for a nap, meditation, reading, or any other activity you find restorative.

■ Gentle daily exercise is important. Yoga, stretching exercises, and tai chi are good choices. (*See* STARTING AN EXERCISE PROGRAM in Part Three.)

■ As much as possible, avoid stress. Stress and aggravation can worsen symptoms. *See* RELAXATION TECHNIQUES in Part Three for ways you can deal with stress you cannot avoid.

■ Avoid contact with any environmental pollutants, including automobile exhaust, tobacco smoke, smoggy air, pesticides, herbicides, and household chemicals, even such harmless-seeming things as air fresheners and perfumes. Any of these substances can make symptoms worse.

■ Because sunlight worsens lupus—and may trigger a flare-up if you are in a period of remission—avoid exposure to the sun. Wear a hat and gloves. Never go out in the sun unless you are wearing clothing that covers your legs and arms. There is one line of sun protective clothing, called Solumbra, that is actually regulated as a medical device and has qualified for an SPF rating of over 30. The clothing comes in a wide variety of styles and sizes, and is widely accepted as good protection for the sun-sensitive. Solumbra is manufactured by Sun Precautions of Everett, Washington (see the Resources section at the end of the book).

■ Be extremely careful with over-the-counter sunscreens. People who have lupus often are allergic to common sun blocks. Ask your doctor to recommend a sun block suitable for hypersensitive skin.

■ Most physicians recommend that women with lupus not use oral contraceptives or hormone replacement therapy. Anything that manipulates your sex hormone levels can cause lupus to flare up, with unpredictable symptoms.

■ If you wear makeup, use only hypoallergenic products.

■ Use only unscented hypoallergenic shampoos. Avoid heavy fragrances.

■ Be sure your hairdresser or barber is very aware of scalp disorders. If you have lesions on your scalp, ignorance or carelessness on the part of a hairdresser or barber can make the problem worse.

Lyme and Other Tickborne Diseases

There are a number of diseases that can be transmitted by the bite of an infected tick. Lyme disease, probably the best known, is a potentially serious long-term illness caused by a spirochete (a slender, spiral-shaped bacterium) called *Borrelia burgdorferi*. This disease is spread by infected deer ticks, which are minute ticks that commonly feed on deer and mice. It was first identified as a distinct, separate illness in the area of Lyme, Connecticut (hence the name), but it is now found in most of the United States, and there have been cases in other countries as well. In some parts of the country, infected ticks may now readily be found in suburban back yards. Although the incidence of the disease in any given area seems to be related to the level of the deer population, other animals, including jackrabbits, lizards, and field mice, have been found to carry the infected ticks as well. Fortunately, the illness does not spread from one person to another.

A person becomes infected by being bitten by a tick that carries the bacteria. Because deer ticks are so tiny, however, it is quite possible to overlook their presence on the body, and the tick bites themselves are usually painless. The symptoms experienced vary from person to person, and they often mimic those of other ailments. As a result, a diagnosis of Lyme disease can easily be missed in the early stages.

The first sign noted in most people with Lyme disease is a characteristic "bull's-eye" marking at the site of the tick bite (usually, but not always, on the arm or leg). This is a round, raised reddish lesion that typically is paler, even white, in the center. In some cases, the bull's-eye rash gradually expands around the center; in others, a bumpy rash develops on the torso. These signs may come and go throughout the course of the disease. Often accompanying the development of the bull's-eye mark and/or rash are flulike symptoms, including fever, chills, headache, and overall achiness. Some people develop an enlarged spleen and lymph nodes, some complain of sore throat and severe headache, and some suffer from nausea and vomiting. The symptoms can occur singly or in any combination, and they can develop anywhere from three days to three weeks (or even more, in some cases) after the initial tick bite. The course of recovery is similarly variable. Some people get better after suffering the initial illness; others go on to develop long-term, even chronic, complications, including arthritis, neurological problems, and even enlargement of the heart and irregular heartbeat. The fatigue and achiness frequently last for weeks.

The critical factor in the treatment of Lyme disease is early diagnosis. Because early diagnosis is so important to the successful treatment of tickborne diseases, if you notice a bull's-eye-type lesion (a raised reddish bump that is paler in the center) or any other suspicious-looking bite or mark on your body, or if you develop flulike symptoms within a few days of spending time outdoors (particularly in a wooded area or an area with long grass or weeds), consult your doctor and explain the situation. There are several blood tests that can confirm whether or not you have been infected with *Borrelia burgdorferi* bacteria. The most sensitive is an enzyme-linked immunoadsorbent assay, or ELISA. If this test is inconclusive, a test called the Western blot may be recommended.

Rocky Mountain spotted fever is spread by different types of ticks, including the wood tick in the western United States and the dog tick in the eastern part of the country. The disease is also transmitted to other animals. Symptoms include fever, chills, headache, nausea, vomiting, muscle pains, and irritability. Later, cough, lethargy, seizures, and even coma may occur. A rash tends to occur soon after the fever starts, first around the wrists and ankles and then spreading to other parts of the body. If untreated it can progress to cause pneumonitis (inflammation of the lungs) and heart problems, and can be particularly dangerous in elderly people. In the acute stages of the illness, a biopsy of the skin lesions can confirm the diagnosis. Blood tests can diagnose the disease in its later stages.

Several more recently identified, and therefore less well known, tickborne diseases are human granulocytic ehrlichiosis (HGE), human monocytic ehrlichiosis (HME), and babesiosis. The symptoms of all three of these diseases are very similar to those of Lyme disease, including fever, chills, headache, muscle pain, and fatigue. However, with these more newly identified tickborne diseases, the symptoms are more severe and develop more quickly. In addition, the initial tick bites do not produce the bull's-eye-shaped rash that is characteristic of Lyme disease.

Like Lyme disease, HGE and babesiosis are spread by infected deer ticks, HME by lone-star ticks and dog ticks. Diagnosis is difficult because there are no immediately apparent signs and symptoms, and screening tests to identify the bacteria responsible for the disease are not always available. Further, if a tick carries more than one type of bacteria, a single tick bite can cause simultaneous infections, each requiring a separate blood test to pinpoint it.

CONVENTIONAL TREATMENT

■ Tickborne diseases generally are curable, but the key to the cure lies in prompt treatment. The major treatment is a course of oral antibiotics that can run from ten to twenty days in length, depending on the severity and/or stubbornness of symptoms. Tetracycline (also sold under the brand name Achromycin) is usually the antibiotic of choice for Lyme disease, although doxycycline (Doryx, Vibramycin, and others), cefuroxime (Zinacef), and amoxicillin (Amoxil, Augmentin, and others) may be prescribed as well. Erythromycin (ERYC, Ilotycin, Pediazole, and others) may be used but is thought to be somewhat less effective.

■ Though oral tetracycline or doxycycline is usually the

drug of choice, the administration of intravenous antibiotics, either in or out of the hospital, may be necessary in some cases.

■ In the case of Rocky Mountain spotted fever, intravenous treatment with the antibiotic chloramphenicol (Chloromycetin) may be required. This is an extremely powerful antibiotic, and it can cause life-threatening blood-cell changes, so it is used only when other drugs prove ineffective. Otherwise, doxycycline is usually preferred. Other possible side effects include liver toxicity, nausea, and vomiting.

■ A painkiller such as acetaminophen (Tylenol, Datril, and others), aspirin (Bayer, Ecotrin, and others), or ibuprofen (Advil, Motrin, Nuprin, and others) can help reduce fever and relieve achiness.

Note: In excessive amounts, acetaminophen can cause liver damage. Do not exceed the recommended dosage. Take aspirin or ibuprofen with food to prevent possible stomach upset.

DIETARY GUIDELINES

■ As when fighting any illness, take plenty of fluids and eat plenty of well-cooked whole grains and fresh vegetables.

■ To foster a more healing internal environment, reduce the amount of fat, sugar, refined carbohydrates, and dairy products in your diet.

NUTRITIONAL SUPPLEMENTS

■ Bromelain, a natural enzyme extracted from pineapple, acts as an anti-inflammatory. Take 500 to 1,000 milligrams two to three times daily, on an empty stomach.

■ A calcium and magnesium supplement may be helpful for relieving achiness. Take one dose of a formula supplying 500 milligrams of calcium and 250 milligrams of magnesium twice a day.

■ Chlorophyll is full of trace minerals that are helpful in the healing process. Take a chlorophyll or green-foods supplement as directed on the product label.

■ A person with a tickborne disease may have impaired digestion, resulting in stomach gas. Digestive enzymes can be of great help during the first month or two of treatment. Take a digestive-enzyme formula that includes bromelain and/or papain with each meal. Choose a formula *without* hydrochloric acid (HCl).

■ The B vitamins strengthen the body's overall nutritional status. Take a balanced vitamin-B complex supplement supplying 25 to 50 milligrams of each of the major B vitamins daily for two months.

■ Vitamin C is both antibacterial and anti-inflammatory; bioflavonoids stimulate the immune system and decrease inflammation, especially of the joints. Take 500 to 1,000 milligrams of each three times a day for two months.

■ Zinc promotes healing and stimulates the immune system. Take 15 to 20 milligrams of zinc, in tablet or lozenge form, twice a day for two weeks.

Note: Take zinc with food to prevent stomach upset. If you take over 30 milligrams of zinc on a daily basis for more than one or two months, you should also take 1 to 2 milligrams of copper each day to maintain a proper mineral balance.

HERBAL TREATMENT

■ Cat's claw enhances the immune response and has antibacterial properties. Take 500 milligrams of standardized extract three times a day until your condition improves.

Note: Do not use cat's claw if you are pregnant or nursing, or if you are an organ-transplant recipient. Use it with caution if you are taking an anticoagulant (blood thinner).

■ Garlic has antibacterial properties. Take the equivalent of 500 milligrams of fresh garlic twice a day for two months.

■ Goldenseal fights bacteria and tones the mucous membranes. Choose a standardized extract containing at least 5 percent total alkaloids and take 250 milligrams three times a day.

■ Oregano has antibacterial properties and helps to fight infection. Take 75 milligrams of standardized extract three times a day.

GENERAL RECOMMENDATIONS

■ Pay close attention to any suspicious-looking insect bites or other marks on your body, especially after you spend time outdoors. If you have any doubts, consult your physician.

■ If you have flulike symptoms, especially if they are severe, consult your physician to investigate the possibility of a tickborne infection. Often a diagnosis of a tickborne disease is missed or delayed because the symptoms are similar to those of other common diseases, but treatment is more likely to be successful if it is begun early. If your doctor doesn't suggest the possibility of a tickborne disease, don't hesitate to raise the subject.

PREVENTION

■ Anytime you will be walking or spending time in an area likely to have ticks, wear clothing that offers some protection. A long-sleeved shirt, long pants, a hat, and socks and shoes are recommended. It is a good idea to pull your socks up and over the bottoms of your pants legs, because ticks often climb up from the ground and will bite as soon as they find exposed skin. It may also be helpful

Tickborne Diseases by State

Your likelihood of contracting a tickborne disease depends to a certain extent on your geographical location. This is because the various ticks and microorganisms they carry thrive in different conditions. The following table lists individual tickborne illnesses and the states in which confirmed cases have been diagnosed. Be aware, however, that tickborne diseases can spread into new areas over time.

Disease	States in Which Cases Have Been Diagnosed
Babesiosis	California, Connecticut, Massachusetts, Minnesota, New York, Rhode Island
Human granulocytic ehrlichiosis (HGE)	California, Massachusetts, Minnesota, Rhode Island, Wisconsin
Human monocytic ehrlichiosis (HME)	Alabama, Arkansas, Delaware, Georgia, Illinois, Kentucky, Louisiana, Maryland, Mississippi, Missouri, New Jersey, North Carolina, Oklahoma, Pennsylvania, South Carolina, Tennessee, Texas, Virginia
Lyme disease	California, Connecticut, Delaware, Maryland, Massachusetts, Minnesota, New Jersey, New York, Pennsylvania, Rhode Island, Virginia, Wisconsin
Rocky Mountain spotted fever	All states *except* Alaska, Hawaii, Maine

to spray permethrin—a medication usually used for head lice—on your clothing before going outdoors. Permethrin is sold under the brand names Nix, Permanone, and Duranon. It is safe when used this way and is highly effective at repelling insects and ticks. Deet (diethyl toluamide) is generally an effective tick repellent as well, although it is potentially quite toxic. If enough of this chemical is absorbed through the skin, it can cause headaches and other problems. Read and follow package directions carefully, and be aware that some formulas containing deet may not be safe for children.

■ After walking, hiking, or otherwise spending time in a wooded or high-grass area, check your body, hair, and clothing thoroughly. Keep in mind that deer ticks are very tiny. Shower or bathe as soon as possible.

■ If you find a tick on your body, remove it by using tweezers. Grab the head of the tick, as close to the skin as possible, and firmly but gently pull it back and out of the skin. Try not to crush the tick, but save it in a small plastic bag or jar for identification. After removing the tick, wash your hands and the bite wound thoroughly with soap and water, and consult your physician.

Lymphedema

Edema is the swelling of tissues due to an accumulation of abnormally large amounts of fluid between the cells, usually in tissues under the skin. *Lymphedema* is a specific type of edema involving an accumulation of lymphatic fluid due to impairment of the movement of lymphatic fluid.

Most people think of circulation as involving blood only. But the body actually has a second circulatory system, the lymphatic system, which is part of an elaborate infection-fighting and cleansing system present throughout the body. Lymph is a clear, colorless fluid made up of protein, salts, glucose (sugar), urea, and white blood cells suspended in water. It begins as interstitial fluid, the fluid that constantly bathes virtually all of the body's cells. When it enters the lymphatic vessels, guiding channels that are similar to blood vessels but smaller and thinner, it becomes lymph. As it makes its way through these channels, the lymph flows through lymph nodes, also called lymph glands, which filter out toxins, harmful microorganisms, and waste materials. Eventually, the lymphatic vessels join up with the blood circulation, and the cleansed lymph drains into the blood. If anything interferes with the movement of lymph, this fluid can accumulate in the tissues, and lymphedema results.

Lymphedema can be present from birth, but it usually occurs as a result of infection or trauma to the lymphatic system. Cancer surgery in which lymph nodes are removed is a common cause. Radiation therapy also can lead to lymphedema, as can cancer itself. Once the blockage starts, valves within the channels become ineffective, which makes the situation worse. Fluids leak into the surrounding tissues, and swelling begins. This is not usually painful, but the swelling can be extreme—a limb or body part may expand to several times its normal size. In addition, it renders the skin and underlying tissues much more vulnerable to infection and inflammation than normal, and over time the skin can become hard and thickened.

The extent of damage to the lymphatic system can be determined by either of two methods: lymphangiography and radioactive isotope studies. Lymphangiography is a technique in which a dye is injected and its progress through the lymphatic system tracked by x-rays. Radioactive isotope studies are similar, but use a radioactive fluid that can be detected by a sophisticated camera designed to pick up the radioactivity and convert it into a picture.

CONVENTIONAL TREATMENT

■ Many doctors recommend elevating the affected body part above the level of the heart to improve the flow of lymph. This usually yields only temporary results, however, and does not address the underlying problem.

■ There are a variety of approaches to treating lymphedema. The best results appear to be achieved with a technique known variously as manual lymph drainage (MLD), complete decongestive physiotherapy (CDP), or complex lymphedema therapy (CLT). MLD is a specific massage technique that gently and gradually encourages the lymph to drain out of the swollen tissues. Technically, it is only part of CDP, which also involves skin cleansing, bandaging, a specific set of exercises, and the wearing of a compression garment, a tightly knit piece of elasticized cotton fabric, similar to the type of stockings that are worn for varicose veins. This type of treatment should be performed by a professional who has specific training in CDP.

■ Some doctors recommend the use of a pumping device to "milk" fluid out of the extremity. By itself, use of the pump does not seem to be as effective as comprehensive lymphedema therapy. Pumps have also been known to worsen the damage in some cases.

■ Diuretics are not generally effective in treating lymphedema, but they may be helpful in certain situations, such as if menstrual periods or seasonal effects temporarily make the situation worse.

■ Infections and cellulitis can be recurring problems for people with lymphedema. It is important to monitor the affected area for possible developing infections, and to treat any infections early and aggressively. Some doctors recommend ongoing treatment with low doses of antibiotics as a preventive.

■ In some cases, microsurgery to anastomose (join) lymphatic vessels to normal veins can help improve the situation.

■ Though it is not common, a person with lymphedema may develop lymphangiosarcoma, or cancer of the lymphatic vessels. In such cases, amputation may be necessary.

DIETARY GUIDELINES

■ Eat plenty of fresh vegetables and fruits to supply the nutrients needed for healthy skin and circulation.

■ Drink at least six 8-ounces of pure, clean water every day.

■ Avoid saturated fats and greasy fried foods, which make circulation more sluggish.

■ Avoid alcohol, caffeine, and refined sugar. All of these affect the body's fluid balance.

NUTRITIONAL SUPPLEMENTS

■ Bromelain, an enzyme derived from pineapple, is an effective anti-inflammatory. Take 400 milligrams three or four times daily, between meals.

■ Pine-bark and grape-seed extracts are natural anti-inflammatories. Take 100 milligrams of either three times daily while symptoms are acute.

■ Vitamin C affects several aspects of immune function, which is impaired in people with lymphatic disorders such as lymphedema. This vitamin enhances the functioning of white blood cells, increases antibody levels, increases the secretion of thymic hormone, and boosts the level of interferon in the body. Moreover, when the body is under stress, as it is with lymphedema, losses of vitamin C through excretion increase. To correct this problem, take 500 to 1,000 milligrams of vitamin C with 500 milligrams of mixed bioflavonoids four to six times daily, especially when symptoms are acute.

■ Vitamin E is a natural anti-inflammatory and antioxidant that protects cell membranes from damage by free radicals. Choose a product containing mixed tocopherols and start by taking 200 international units daily, then gradually increase the dosage until you are taking 400 international units in the morning and another 400 international units in the evening.

Note: If you have high blood pressure, limit your intake of supplemental vitamin E to a total of 400 international units daily. If you are taking an anticoagulant (blood thinner), consult your physician before taking vitamin E.

HERBAL TREATMENT

■ Herbal diuretics such as corn silk, shavegrass, and uva ursi, taken individually or in any combination, are sometimes helpful, especially if lymphedema is aggravated by ordinary fluid retention.

■ Echinacea has a long history of use for lymphatic congestion. It is best to use it together with bromelain and/or turmeric. Take 300 to 500 milligrams three times daily for one week. Take two weeks off, then use it again for one week, and so on.

■ Turmeric is a strong natural anti-inflammatory. Take 500 milligrams four times daily while symptoms are acute.

HOMEOPATHY

Apis mellifica is the remedy for swelling with redness and burning and/or stinging pain. Take one dose of *Apis mellifica* 12x or 6c three to four times daily for up to three days at a time.

Aqua marina is homeopathic sea water, taken miles from shore and at a great depth from the surface, then filtered and diluted. It is considered to be a great blood purifier and vitalizer. Take one dose of *Aqua marina* 30x or 15c three to four times daily for up to three days at a time.

Baryta carbonica is good for lymphedema originating from damage to the lymphatic vessels under the arm that is accompanied by numbness or burning pain in the limbs and/or a numb feeling that spreads from the knees to the groin. Take one dose of *Baryta carbonica* 12x or 6c three to four times daily for up to three days at a time.

BACH FLOWER REMEDIES

Select the remedy that most closely fits your disposition and emotional tendencies and concerns, and take it as needed, following the directions on the product label.

Chicory is good if you tend to be insecure and have your feelings hurt easily.

Mimulus helps to ease fearfulness, shyness, and timidity.

Choose Scleranthus if you are troubled by feelings of uncertainty and have difficulty making decisions.

ACUPRESSURE/MASSAGE

Massage is an essential part of comprehensive lymphedema therapy. However, unless it is done with the proper technique, known as manual lymph drainage (*see under* Conventional Treatment in this entry), exerting any pressure on a body part with lymphedema risks making the problem worse. You should therefore consult a professional who has specific training in treating lymphedema. If desired, he or she may be willing to instruct a friend or family member in techniques that can be used at home.

AROMATHERAPY

For specific instructions on how to use aromatherapy, *see* PREPARING AROMATHERAPY TREATMENTS in Part Three.

■ Grapefruit and rosemary oils are detoxifying. Use either or both as inhalants or diffuse them into the air.

GENERAL RECOMMENDATIONS

■ Take care to avoid anything that exposes the affected body part to the risk of cuts, scratches, scrapes, and other injuries. Even minor injuries pose a risk of infection.

■ Wear clothing that is loose and comfortable, and avoid anything that might be constricting. This can make the problem worse.

■ As much as possible, avoid exposing the affected area to heat, which can increase swelling. Avoid spending time in direct sunlight. In hot weather, try to stay in an air-conditioned environment as much as possible. Take showers and baths that are warm rather than hot. If lymphedema affects the hand or arm, use long oven mitts when working around a hot stove. Wear rubber gloves for cleaning chores involving hot water.

■ If you have lymphedema of the leg, avoid standing for long periods of time. If walking causes pain, stop.

■ If you have lymphedema of the arm, avoid lifting heavy objects.

■ Avoid exposing the affected area to potential irritants such as cleaning products and strong detergents. Use only gentle soap to wash your skin. If your skin is dry, use only mild, hypoallergenic lotion to moisturize it.

■ If the skin in the affected area shows any signs of infection, including redness or blotchiness, sensitivity to touch, a feeling of warmth, or pain or achiness, consult your physician immediately. Any infections should be treated very aggressively.

PREVENTION

■ If you have sustained any damage to your lymphatic system, whether through an accident or as a result of surgery, take care not to do anything that would place stress on the affected part of the body. If you have had lymph nodes removed from under your arm, for example, avoid picking up heavy objects with that arm, and do not do anything to compress the arm, whether wearing constricting clothing or having blood-pressure readings taken. If you are unsure about whether an accident or medical procedure may have affected your lymphatic system, ask your physician.

Lymphoma

See under CANCER.

Macular Degeneration

The macula is a small yellowish area approximately one-quarter inch in diameter in the center of the retina of the eye that is responsible for registering fine detail in the center of the field of vision (*see* illustration, page 306). In the condition known as macular degeneration, the macula begins to break down, resulting in a progressive loss of visual clarity that begins in the center of the visual field and gradually expands outward toward the periphery.

There are two types of macular degeneration: exudative (often referred to as "wet") and atrophic ("dry"). The wet type begins when blood vessels, for reasons unknown, begin to proliferate abnormally beneath the retina, and may invade retinal nerve tissue as well. These vessels leak fluid and may bleed, leading to scarring that destroys the macula. In the dry type of this disorder, macular tissue simply breaks down and wastes away, without any signs of fluid leakage, bleeding, or scarring.

Macular degeneration is associated with aging, and the underlying cause is not known. However, many experts believe this disorder is a result of free-radical damage, specifically from exposure to ultraviolet light rays, much as cataracts are. Some people may have an inherited tendency to develop this condition. Other known risk factors include diabetes, hardening of the arteries, and high blood pressure.

While macular degeneration is a leading cause of serious vision loss, it rarely leads to total blindness. Even in advanced cases, people usually retain some peripheral vision and the ability to distinguish colors.

CONVENTIONAL TREATMENT

■ A procedure known as *photocoagulation* may help some people with the wet type of macular degeneration. In this technique, a krypton laser is used to destroy the "runaway" blood vessels causing the leaking and bleeding and, therefore, the scarring of the macula. Unfortunately, this procedure is suitable only for certain people.

■ For the dry type of macular degeneration, unfortunately, medical science has yet to devise any type of treatment. Although this condition is considered irreversible, it can only help to take steps to fight free-radical damage with some of the natural treatments outlined in this section.

DIETARY GUIDELINES

■ Eat a diet that emphasizes fresh whole foods such as vegetables, whole grains, and fruits.

■ Increase the amount of fiber in your diet. Fiber assists the body in eliminating toxins; fruits and vegetables contain many valuable phytochemicals that act as antioxidants. Especially emphasize foods high in the carotenoids, beta-carotene, lycopene, and especially lutein. Some of the carotenoids are found in high concentrations in eye tissue, where they act as antioxidants. Some researchers believe that carotenoids act as filters, protecting eye tissue from blue light, a potentially destructive band of radiation in sunlight. Two carotenoids in particular, lutein and zeaxanthin, may be of particular value in preventing or slowing age-related macular degeneration. Among the foods highest in lutein are corn, kiwis, zucchini, spinach, yellow squash, red grapes, green peas, cucumbers, butternut squash, green bell peppers, and celery. Good sources of zeaxanthin are orange bell peppers, corn, orange juice, honeydew melon, mango, and oranges. Include plenty of these foods in your diet. The food richest of all in both of these carotenoids is egg yolk. If you have been shunning eggs because of their cholesterol content, you may want to reconsider.

■ Eat foods rich in vitamin C and the bioflavonoids. Vitamin C is an anti-inflammatory and is required for the formation of connective tissue. It also helps prevent hemorrhaging. The bioflavonoids boost the action of vitamin C and help strengthen capillaries. Both of these nutrients also fight free radicals. Citrus fruits, berries, and cherries are good sources.

■ Drink six to eight 8-ounce glasses of pure water daily.

■ Avoid saturated, hydrogenated, and partially hydrogenated fats, which lead to the generation of free radicals in the body. Also avoid caffeine, sugar, and alcohol.

NUTRITIONAL SUPPLEMENTS

■ Lutein, a carotenoid usually extracted from the marigold flower, has strong antioxidant properties and has been shown to be effective in maintaining and restoring ocular health. Take 5 milligrams three times daily.

■ N-acetylcysteine (NAC) is an antioxidant that chelates heavy metals so they can be excreted from the body. Take 500 milligrams twice daily.

■ Selenium is a potent antioxidant. Take 200 micrograms daily.

■ Shark cartilage may help people with the wet type of macular degeneration, particularly if the disorder is detected early. This supplement suppresses the formation of new blood vessels; if the vessels do not proliferate, they cannot leak and bleed onto the macula. Each day, take one 750-milligram capsule per 11 pounds of body weight (or 1 gram of powder per 15 pounds of body weight), divided into three equal doses.

■ Vitamin A and beta-carotene are effective free-radical fighters. These nutrients protect against oxidative damage caused by the absorption of light in the eye. Low levels of carotenoids and antioxidant vitamins in the body have been shown to increase the risk of age-related macular degeneration. Take 10,000 international units of vitamin A and 10,000 to 20,000 international units of beta-carotene daily.

Note: If you are pregnant, or intend to get pregnant, or if you have liver disease, consult your doctor before taking supplemental vitamin A. Pregnant women should not ingest a total of more than 25,000 international units of supplemental vitamin A *per week* from all sources.

■ Vitamin C and bioflavonoids provide antioxidant protection and strengthen tissue. Take 1,000 milligrams (1 gram) of vitamin C plus 500 milligrams of bioflavonoids three times daily.

■ Vitamin E strengthens connective tissue and assists in the healing of damaged membranes. Choose a product containing mixed tocopherols and start by taking 200 international units daily, then gradually increase until you are taking 400 to 800 international units of vitamin E daily.

Note: If you have high blood pressure, limit your intake of supplemental vitamin E to a total of 400 international units daily. If you are taking an anticoagulant (blood thinner), consult your physician before taking supplemental vitamin E.

■ Zinc is an important trace mineral that is needed for the formation of antioxidant enzymes in the body. A study of 151 people with macular degeneration published in 1995 showed that those who took 100 milligrams of zinc sulfate twice daily experienced significantly less visual loss over a two-year period than those who did not. Take 100 milligrams of zinc twice a day, with meals. If you take 30 or more milligrams of zinc daily, you should also take supplemental copper to maintain a proper mineral balance. Take 1 to 2 milligrams of copper daily.

HERBAL TREATMENT

■ Bilberry contains anthocyanidins, phytochemicals that have been shown to help protect against age-related (and diabetes-related) macular degeneration and cataracts. Select a standardized preparation containing 25 percent anthocyanidins (also called PCOs) and take 80 milligrams twice daily.

■ Ginkgo biloba may help inhibit macular degeneration. It has strong free-radical-scavenging activity. Select a formula containing at least 24 percent ginkgo heterosides (sometimes also called flavoglycosides) and take 40 to 60 milligrams two to three times daily.

HOMEOPATHY

■ See a homeopathic practitioner for a constitutional remedy. Constitutional treatment can help prevent further degeneration.

ACUPRESSURE

For the locations of acupressure points on the body, *see* ADMINISTERING AN ACUPRESSURE TREATMENT in Part Three.

■ Large Intestine 4 improves circulation to the head.

■ Liver 3 and 10 improve circulation. In Chinese medicine, the eyes are "fed" by good liver function, so by improving liver function, you improve eye health.

■ Spleen 6 and Stomach 36 strengthen immune function.

GENERAL RECOMMENDATIONS

■ If you smoke, quit, and avoid secondhand smoke. Studies of both men and women have shown that smoking cigarettes significantly increases the risk of developing macular degeneration, and the risk increases with every year a person smokes.

■ Get regular exercise. Exercise increases tissue oxygenation, which is critical for the health of the eyes.

■ Relaxation techniques of any type—whether meditation, biofeedback, breathing exercises, yoga, prayer, creative visualization, or anything else—help to revitalize the body and, ultimately, the eyes.

PREVENTION

■ Because there is increasing evidence that free-radical damage leads to macular degeneration, take measures to minimize the levels of free radicals your body must deal with. Eat a healthy low-fat, high-fiber diet that is rich in natural antioxidant nutrients. Several studies have shown that people who regularly eat large amounts of fruits and vegetables are less likely to develop macular degeneration than those who do not. You can also supplement your diet with antioxidants to boost your level of protection. Do not smoke, and avoid secondhand smoke. Also avoid exposure to other environmental pollutants and toxins, as well as excessive exposure to sunlight. Wear sunglasses guaranteed to protect against the sun's ultraviolet (UV) rays when you spend time outdoors on sunny days.

■ Take ginkgo biloba (*see under* Herbal Treatment in this entry).

Malabsorption/ Malnutrition

Malabsorption is a general term for the failure to properly convert food into usable nutrients. This can lead to nutritional deficiencies and even, ultimately, malnutrition, even if a person is eating a healthful diet.

Digestion begins in the mouth, with chewing and the mixing of foods with enzymes present in saliva. In the stomach, acid and pepsin continue the process. Further breakdown of foods occurs within the small intestine, where pancreatic enzymes and bile from the gallbladder, as well as enzymes secreted by the intestinal lining itself, get fats, proteins, and carbohydrates ready for absorption. Nutrients then cross through the mucosa, or intestinal wall, into the blood and lymph, which are responsible for delivering them to the cells.

Anything that interferes with any of these processes can result in malabsorption. If the pancreas is weakened by disease, such as pancreatitis, cystic fibrosis, or cancer, it may not produce sufficient enzymes for proper digestion. Or there may be an inadequate supply of bile as a result of obstruction (gallstones) or liver disease, or cancer in the lower small intestine may inhibit the reabsorption of bile salts. Any of these problems will result in inadequate conversion of fats, proteins, or carbohydrates into forms that can cross the intestinal wall into the bloodstream.

An insufficient supply of enzymes in the small intestine can impair absorption as well. Lactose intolerance is probably the most common problem of this type (see LACTOSE INTOLERANCE). Another possible cause is the removal of a portion of the intestine due to cancer, celiac disease, Crohn's disease, Whipple's disease (a rare bacterial infection of unknown origin), or lymphoma in the lower small intestine. Also, an overgrowth of yeast or bacteria can alter the intestinal environment in such a way that bile is broken down and rendered less effective, beneficial bacteria are crowded out, and the intestinal wall may be damaged. Enzyme deficiencies can also be congenital or result from other health problems, including AIDS and many other chronic illnesses, as well as from cancer chemotherapy.

Another condition that can lead to malabsorption is obstruction of the lymphatic system that prevents the fats and proteins normally carried by the lymph from being transported adequately. Cancer and its treatments, including surgery and radiation therapy, are the most common causes of this problem, though it can also be congenital. Enzyme deficiencies, whether congenital or the result of other health problems (chronic illness, AIDS, or chemotherapy, for example) and other causes can be involved here.

The signs and symptoms of malabsorption vary widely in both type and severity. They can result directly from the malabsorption itself, or from resulting nutritional deficiencies. Direct symptoms can include weight loss; glossitis (a slick, shiny tongue); a tendency to bruise easily; bloating; gas; pale, foul-smelling stools; diarrhea; and decreased reflexes. Nutritional deficiencies can be manifested as anemia (a result of iron, vitamin-B_{12}, or folic-acid

deficiency); calcium deficiency and resulting loss of bone mass (inadequate vitamin-D or fatty-acid absorption); difficulty seeing at night and in dim light (vitamin-A deficiency); numbness and tingling (vitamin-B_1 [thiamine] deficiency); dry skin and other skin problems (vitamin-B_2 [riboflavin], vitamin-B_3 [niacin], vitamin-B_6 [pyridoxine], biotin, vitamin-E, and/or fatty-acid deficiency); swelling (protein deficiency); bleeding problems (vitamin-K deficiency); cessation of menstrual periods (generalized deficiency); and many other problems.

Because there are so many factors involved in digestion and absorption, diagnosis of malabsorption can be a complicated process. Probably the most reliable indicator of malabsorption is a high level of fat in the stool. This is direct evidence that the body is not absorbing fats properly. Usually a three- or four-day stool collection is necessary for accurate assessment. Inspection of the stool can also show whether food particles are being excreted undigested and reveal the presence of parasites. A xylose absorption test may be done to assess absorption in the jejunum, the portion of the small intestine near the stomach. In this test, you are given a dose of xylose, a type of sugar, and urine or blood samples are then taken over a period of a number of hours. Blood tests may be done to determine the levels of individual nutrients. Another test that may be performed is the glycocholic acid breath test, in which you are given a dose of glycocholic acid tagged with radioactive carbon 14 and the amount of tagged carbon in subsequent exhalations is measured. If the tagged carbon exceeds a certain level, it is likely that you have an overgrowth of bacteria in your intestinal tract, which in turn may point to the existence of certain small-bowel disorders. X-ray testing and direct visualization may be used to find anatomical abnormalities that may be causing malabsorption. There are also specific tests for pancreatic function, cystic fibrosis, problems with stomach-acid secretion, and many other factors that can lead to problems with the absorption of nutrients. Biopsy of the small intestine, in which a sample of tissue is removed through a fiber-optic endoscope and studied under a microscope, is now fairly routine.

CONVENTIONAL TREATMENT

■ Treatment for malabsorption depends on the underlying cause. This can range from supplementation with missing enzymes to surgical correction of anatomical abnormalities, and can also include treatment of diseases such as cancer or cystic fibrosis.

DIETARY GUIDELINES

■ The appropriate diet depends on the cause of the problem. A varied and healthy diet based on lean proteins, fresh vegetables and fruits, whole grains, and legumes is best, but if malabsorption is related to digestive difficulty, you may need to modify your diet depending on what your body is able to digest. It may be advisable to consult a professional nutritionist who can devise the best diet for you.

NUTRITIONAL SUPPLEMENTS

■ Take a good multivitamin and mineral supplement daily. Choose a powder or capsule form, which is more easily assimilated.

■ Alpha-lipoic acid is an antioxidant and is helpful against fatigue. Take 50 milligrams three times daily.

■ Take a full-spectrum digestive enzyme-supplement with meals. Malabsorption is often linked to an inadequate supply of digestive enzymes.

■ If you have any symptoms of malabsorption, it is important to provide your intestinal tract with an ample supply of probiotics (beneficial bacteria). Take a probiotic supplement as recommended on the product label.

■ Fructooligosaccharides (FOS) supply a special form of carbohydrate that can be digested by friendly bacteria but not by yeast. This allows the good bacteria to grow rapidly, without the risk of encouraging the growth of yeast and other harmful microorganisms. Start by taking 1/4 teaspoon of FOS twice a day and work up to 1 teaspoon twice a day over a period of one to two weeks. (If you start taking too much too quickly, you may develop bowel gas.)

■ Glutamine is an amino acid that is both soothing to the gastrointestinal tract and helpful for mental "fuzziness." Take 3,000 milligrams three times daily.

■ To ensure an adequate supply of protein, take a whey-protein supplement as directed on the product label.

HERBAL TREATMENT

■ Cat's claw benefits the immune system, which can be weakened by nutritional deficiencies. Take 500 milligrams of standardized extract three times a day.

 Note: Do not use cat's claw if you are pregnant or nursing, or if you are an organ-transplant recipient. Use it with caution if you are taking an anticoagulant (blood thinner).

■ Chamomile, dandelion root, gentian root, and peppermint are all good for promoting proper digestion. Take any of these herbs in tea form with meals.

■ Olive leaf also benefits the immune system, and is helpful for fatigue. Take 250 milligrams of standardized extract three times a day.

■ Consider consulting a professional herbalist who can tailor an herbal prescription to meet your specific needs.

HOMEOPATHY

The best way to treat malabsorption problems homeo-

pathically is to see a homeopathic physician who can prescribe a constitutional remedy for you. For acute symptoms of digestive distress, try one of the remedies below.

■ *Carbo vegetablis* is for indigestion and pain in the stomach. Take one dose of *Carbo vegetabilis* 30x or 15c twenty minutes after eating—up to three or four times a day, as needed.

■ *Glycerinum* improves the absorption of nutrients. Take one dose of *Glycerinum* 12x three times a day for up to five days at a time.

■ *Lycopodium* is helpful for lower abdominal bloating that is usually worse between 4:00 and 8:00 PM. You may also have a craving for sweets. Take one dose of *Lycopodium* 30x or 15c three times daily for up to three days.

BACH FLOWER REMEDIES

Select the remedy that most closely fits your disposition and emotional tendencies and concerns, and take it as needed, following the directions on the product label.

■ Hornbeam helps to lift exhaustion.

■ Larch is good if you have low self-esteem and lack self-confidence.

■ Mustard helps to ease sadness and depression, possibly related to a loss of some kind.

ACUPRESSURE

For the locations of acupressure points on the body, *see* ADMINISTERING AN ACUPRESSURE TREATMENT in Part Three.

■ The back Bladder points, Spleen 6, and Stomach 36 enhance digestion.

AROMATHERAPY

For specific instructions on how to use aromatherapy, *see* PREPARING AROMATHERAPY TREATMENTS in Part Three.

■ A number of essential oils are known for stimulating the appetite and enhancing digestion, among them basil, black pepper, ginger, orange, and thyme. Use any or all of these oils as inhalants or diffuse them into the air shortly before meals.

GENERAL RECOMMENDATIONS

■ The proper treatment for problems with nutrient absorption depends on the underlying cause. *See* ALCOHOLISM; ANOREXIA NERVOSA; BULIMIA; CANCER; CANDIDA INFECTION; CELIAC DISEASE; CIRRHOSIS; COLITIS, ULCERATIVE; CROHN'S DISEASE; FOOD ALLERGIES; GALLBLADDER PROBLEMS; and/or PARASITES, INTESTINAL for suggestions of treatments for malabsorption related to any of those conditions.

■ Malabsorption can lead to a number of other health problems, among them anemia, easy bruising, recurring colds and other infections, depression, dry skin, dry eyes, recurring headaches, and even such serious problems as abnormal heart rhythms. See the appropriate entries for ways to deal with those problems.

Manic-Depressive Disorder

Manic-depressive disorder (also known as bipolar depression or bipolar mood disorder) is characterized by periods of depression alternating with periods of mania—a feeling of elation, invincibility, and tremendous energy. A person in a manic state may go for days without sleeping. Both the height of the highs and the depth of the lows can vary, as can the length of these cyclic mood changes. In relatively mild cases, this condition may not be recognized as a disorder, but merely considered a quirk of personality. In severe cases, however, a person may alternate between nearly catatonic depression and apparent psychosis, spending little or no time on an emotional level. In some people, the manic phase is manifested more as irritability, even hostility, than as elation. No matter how it is experienced, however, a person in a manic state is unlikely to believe anything is wrong with him or her, and in fact may have the sensation of functioning at his or her best.

Most people who develop manic-depressive disorder first suffer from ordinary (unipolar) depression, then at some point experience an episode of mania, which often comes on quite suddenly. The underlying cause of this disorder is not known, but it is likely linked to biochemical imbalances in the brain, and it can run in families. There are certain things that are known to be potential triggers of manic episodes, however, including a lack of sleep, hormonal changes, and reactions to certain drugs.

CONVENTIONAL TREATMENT

■ If you are suffering from symptoms of depression or mania, see your doctor. The first step in diagnosis is to rule out the possibility that a physical disorder is causing your symptoms. Your doctor will probably do blood tests to check your hormone levels, thyroid function, and other indicators of possible problems.

■ If symptoms persist and/or get worse, seek help from a mental-health professional with experience in treating manic-depressive disorder. The prognosis is good for most people with this problem. A knowledgeable mental-health professional will tailor your treatment to your individual situation.

■ Lithium has long been the standard treatment for manic-depressive disorder. It alters the manic-depressive cycles so that mood is more stable. Though lithium is a natural trace mineral, it must be prescribed by a physician. Because it can take some time for lithium to take effect, acute mania may require treatment with an antipsychotic drug such as haloperidol (Haldol), at least for a short time.

■ Bupropion (Wellbutrin) and paroxetine (Paxil) are widely considered to be the most effective antidepressants for people with manic-depressive disorder, as they appear to pose less of a risk of producing acute mania.

DIETARY GUIDELINES

■ Follow a healthy, well-balanced diet that provides a good balance of all important nutrients. Be sure to include plenty of green, yellow, and orange vegetables and fruits, as well as clean, lean protein foods such as chicken, fish, and tofu.

■ It is important to keep your blood-sugar levels in balance. Eat five or six small meals a day rather than three large ones, and eat healthy snacks whenever you feel hungry.

■ Avoid the artificial stimulation produced by alcohol and caffeine. While both of these substances are stimulating initially, the stimulation is ultimately followed by a depressed state.

NUTRITIONAL SUPPLEMENTS

■ Take a good multivitamin and mineral formula daily to make sure your body has all the basic nutrients it requires.

■ Calcium and magnesium are essential to the central nervous system. They work best when taken together. Take 500 to 600 milligrams of calcium and 250 to 300 milligrams of magnesium once or twice daily.

■ Chromium helps keep blood sugar levels in balance. Take 200 micrograms once or twice daily for up to two months.

■ The B vitamins are important for the proper functioning of the nervous system and can affect mood. Take a good B-complex formula supplying 25 to 100 milligrams of each of the major B vitamins once or twice daily.

■ The amino acid tryptophan can help with manic episodes. This supplement is available by prescription only. Speak with your physician about trying a course of 500 to 2,000 milligrams of L-tryptophan daily, taken on an empty stomach.

■ An alternative to tryptophan that is available over the counter is 5-hydroxytryptophan, or 5-HTP. Recommended doses of this supplement are in the range of 25 to 50 milligrams, taken at bedtime. However, the effects of 5-HTP are highly individual, and it may not be as nontoxic as its precursor, tryptophan. It can increase blood levels of sero-tonin instead of the desired brain levels, and the long-term effects of that are unknown.

HERBAL TREATMENT

■ Bupleurum and dong quai make up a Chinese herbal formula that helps reduce anxiety, irritabillity, and depression. Take a bupleurum and dong quai combination formula twice daily, as directed on the product label.

Kava kava eases mental anguish and anxiety, and can be useful in the manic phases of the disorder. Choose a product containing 30 percent kavalactones and take 200 to 300 milligrams daily.

Note: In excess amounts, this herb can cause drowsiness. Do not exceed the recommended dose. Do not use kava kava if you are pregnant or nursing, if you have Parkinson's disease, or if you are taking a prescription medication for depression or anxiety.

Oat straw is high in silica, which helps support and strengthen the central nervous system. Take 500 milligrams two to three times daily.

St. John's wort gently alters brain chemistry in such a way as to improve mood and ease depression. Start by taking one 300-milligram capsule of standardized extract containing 0.3 percent hypericin daily. At two-week intervals, you can add another 300-milligram capsule, taken at a different time of day, up to a total of four capsules a day or until you achieve the desired effect.

If sleeplessness is a problem, take 200 to 250 milligrams of standardized valerian extract containing 0.5 percent isovalerenic acids one-half hour before bedtime.

HOMEOPATHY

The best approach to treating manic-depressive disorder homeopathically is to consult a homeopathic physician who can prescribe a constitutional remedy.

BACH FLOWER REMEDIES

Select the remedy that most closely fits your emotional tendencies and concerns, and take it as needed, following the directions on the product label.

Rescue Remedy is the first choice to ease acute anxiety.

■ Choose Agrimony if you tend to maintain a smiling appearance while suffering inner anguish and despair.

Centaury is helpful for depression accompanied by feelings of intimidation.

■ Cherry Plum relieves feelings of fearfulness, whether of things real or imagined.

■ Mustard is the remedy for sadness and feelings of ineffectuality.

AROMATHERAPY

For specific instructions on how to use aromatherapy, *see* PREPARING AROMATHERAPY TREATMENTS in Part Three.

■ Many essential oils can affect mood. Geranium, jasmine, neroli, rose, and ylang ylang oils lift the spirits. Lavender oil helps to ease mood swings, restore emotional balance, and promote sound sleep. Elemi, frankincense, myrrh, and vetiver oils have calming and centering effects. Depending on your individual needs, use any or all of these oil as inhalants or in baths, diffuse them into the air, add them to massage oil, or use them in any other way you choose.

GENERAL RECOMMENDATIONS

■ Be aware that a person with this disorder truly may not realize he or she has a problem. If a friend or family member you trust expresses genuine concern about your moods and/or behavior, see your physician to rule out any underlying disorder that could be causing a problem. If no physical disorder is identified, consider seeking a professional evaluation by a qualified mental health care provider to determine whether you may have a disorder that requires treatment.

■ Exercise. Regular physicial activity eases depression, reduces nervous tension and feelings of anxiety, and is an aid to restful sleep. *See* STARTING AN EXERCISE PROGRAM in Part Three.

Measles

Measles is a highly contagious viral infection. It begins with fever, malaise, cough, runny nose, and, sometimes, red and/or itchy eyes that may be sensitive to light. These symptoms get worse over a period of a few days, and on approximately the fourth day, a rash appears. The rash is raised, splotchy, reddish-brown or purplish-red in color, and mildly itchy. It usually begins on the face and neck and spreads to the trunk, extremities, and feet, lasting about five to seven days. Red spots with a bluish-white center (known as Koplik's spots) appear on the inside of the mouth about twelve hours before the red rash first appears.

Once a person is infected with the measles virus, it can incubate for nine to fourteen days before signs of illness develop. A person with measles is considered contagious for at least seven days after the beginning of the illness.

Measles is most often contracted in childhood. However, it is possible to get it at any age, and if you **have** measles as an adult, you are likely to have more **severe** symptoms than a child would. Nevertheless, the disease usually is self-limiting and runs its course within ten days. The fever falls, making you feel more comfortable in general, and the rash fades to a brownish color that gradually disappears as the outer layer of skin is shed. Once this happens, you are no longer contagious.

While measles itself does not usually pose a serious danger, it can lead to complications afterward. Ear infections are a common complication. Pneumonia and encephalitis (an inflammation of the lining of the brain) are also possible. If your fever climbs to a very high level, if you have a seizure, or if you notice any changes in your level of consciousness or mental function, seek medical advice immediately. These may be symptoms of encephalitis.

Note that the treatment recommendations given in this section are intended for adults. To determine correct treatment regimens for children, consult your physician or *Smart Medicine for a Healthier Child* (Avery, 1994).

CONVENTIONAL TREATMENT

■ Treatment for measles is primarily aimed at alleviating symptoms while the virus runs its course. A painkiller such as acetaminophen (Tylenol, Datril, and others), aspirin (Bayer, Ecotrin, and others), or ibuprofen (Advil, Motrin, Nuprin, and others) may be recommended to reduce fever and achiness.

Note: In excessive amounts, acetaminophen can cause liver damage. If the recommended amount does not give the relief you want, do not increase the dosage, but try a different medication. Take aspirin or ibuprofen with food to prevent possible stomach upset.

■ Because measles is a viral illness, antibiotic therapy is ineffective and therefore not appropriate. If your doctor confirms that you have developed a secondary, bacterial infection, he or she may prescribe antibiotics to fight the secondary infection.

DIETARY GUIDELINES

■ Drink lots of fluids to prevent dehydration. Take pure water, herbal teas, soups, and diluted juices. During the recovery period, immune-boosting astragalus and vegetable soup is a good choice as well (*see* THERAPEUTIC RECIPES in Part Three).

■ As much as possible, eliminate fats from your diet. Fats are difficult to digest under normal circumstances, and are even harder to digest when the digestive system is weakened by infection. Undigested fats contribute to a toxic internal environment.

NUTRITIONAL SUPPLEMENTS

■ Vitamin A aids in healing mucous membranes. Take 10,000 international units of vitamin A twice daily for ten days.

Note: If you are pregnant, or intend to get pregnant, or if you have liver disease, consult your doctor before taking supplemental vitamin A. Pregnant women should not ingest a total of more than 25,000 international units of supplemental vitamin A *per week* from all sources.

■ Vitamin C and bioflavonoids help to stimulate the immune system. Three to four times a day, take 500 to 1,000 milligrams of vitamin C, in mineral ascorbate form, and an equal amount of bioflavonoids. Do this for one week. The following week, take the same dosage, but two to three times a day. During the third week, take the same dosage two or three times daily every other day. Then continue to take one-half dose once a week for three weeks.

■ Zinc stimulates the immune system and promotes healing. Take 25 milligrams twice a day for ten days. Take zinc with food to prevent stomach upset. If you take over 30 milligrams of zinc on a daily basis for more than one or two months, you should also take 1 to 2 milligrams of copper each day to maintain a proper mineral balance.

HERBAL TREATMENT

■ If you are feeling restless and uncomfortable, take a cup of chamomile tea as needed.

■ Echinacea and goldenseal help to clear infection, support the immune system, and soothe the skin and mucous membranes. Echinacea is also a powerful antiviral. Take one dose of an echinacea and goldenseal combination formula supplying 350 to 500 milligrams of echinacea and 150 to 300 milligrams of goldenseal every two hours until the fever breaks. Then take one dose three times a day for one week.

■ An herbal fever-reducing tea will help to bring down fever, decrease chills, and increase perspiration. Prepare a tea using equal parts of some or all of the following: chamomile flower, elder flower, lemon balm leaf, licorice root, and peppermint leaf (*see* PREPARING HERBAL TREATMENTS in Part Three). To improve the flavor, add a little honey. Take one cup four times a day for two or three days.

Note: If you have high blood pressure, omit the licorice. Also, if you are using peppermint in the tea and also taking a homeopathic preparation, allow one hour to elapse between the two treatments. Otherwise, the strong smell of the mint will decrease the effectiveness of the homeopathic remedy.

■ Ginger tea can be effective against a fever. It is most helpful if you tend to feel cold, especially in your hands and feet. Take a cup of tea four times a day for one day. If you find the taste too pungent, mix the tea with fruit juice. To decrease chills and increase perspiration, curl up under light covers after drinking the tea.

■ Take cool oatmeal baths to lessen the itching. Wrap a handful of oatmeal in a washcloth and let it soak in the bath water. For extra relief, gently rub the oatmeal-filled washcloth over your skin.

■ Shiitake, maitake, and cordyceps have immune-stimulating properties. You can add whole shiitake or maitake mushrooms to foods, such as soups, or you can take any of these in capsule form. Take 250 to 500 milligrams three times a day as long as signs of infection are present.

HOMEOPATHY

Choose the most appropriate symptom-specific remedy from the suggestions that follow and take one dose, as directed on the product label, every two hours, up to a total of four doses a day for up to two days.

Apis mellifica 30x or 9c is recommended if you have a swollen throat, difficulty breathing, and a cough that causes pain in your chest. You probably do not feel thirsty and are less comfortable in a warm room.

Choose *Arsenicum album* if you are restless but weak, feel worse after midnight, and want frequent small drinks. Your skin may be itchy, and you may have diarrhea as well.

Belladonna 30x or 9c is the remedy for a high fever accompanied by red eyes, a flushed face, a throbbing head, and difficulty swallowing.

Gelsemium is for a fever with droopy eyes and a croupy cough, a feeling of being chilled, and a runny nose. Your rash is likely to be very red and itchy, and you may have a headache.

Pulsatilla 30x or 9c is helpful if your eyes are teary, sticky, discharging, and very sensitive to light. Your rash is likely dark red and spotty, and you probably have thick yellow nasal mucus and a cough that is dry at night but looser during the day. You may have an upset stomach as well.

ACUPRESSURE

Four Gates can help you to relax.

GENERAL RECOMMENDATIONS

Make sure you get plenty of rest. Because measles often causes a heightened sensitivity to light, you will probably be more comfortable if you keep the lights dim.

Be alert for signs that a secondary infection may be developing. If symptoms seem to get worse, of if new symptoms develop, seek the advice of your health-care provider.

PREVENTION

■ A vaccine that protects against measles is available. It is usually given in the form of the MMR vaccine, which also contains vaccines against mumps and rubella (German measles), when a child is approximately fifteen months old. An additional dose is recommended either before a child enters school or when he or she is between the ages of eleven and thirteen.

■ A person who has recently been exposed to measles and may be incubating the disease should not be given the measles vaccine at that time. It may suppress the rash at the time, but it could leave you vulnerable to developing a more serious case of the illness later.

Melanoma

See under SKIN CANCER.

Memory Problems

Memory is the mental registration, storage, and recall of information, experiences, ideas, sensations, and thoughts. Mental registration, or encoding, depends on a clear perception of information at the time you are presented with it. Storage is the transfer of newly perceived material to one of the brain's memory cells. Though this complex process is not completely understood, it is known that brain chemicals called neurotransmitters play a key role, and that it results in the creation of new connections between brain cells. Retrieval is the process by which you can access the stored memory at will. Each phase of the memory process depends on the previous one—obviously, you cannot store a memory of something you have not perceived, and you cannot retrieve a memory that has not been properly stored. Anything that interferes with any aspect of this three-stage process can result in lost or impaired memories.

Probably the most common reason we fail to remember things is that we often do not register information well. If you are presented with a piece of information while your mind is wandering and you aren't really paying attention, recalling this information will be a lot more difficult than summoning a memory of an intensely pleasurable (or tragic) event that affected you deeply. Your recall can also fail you if you simply don't want to remember. Some experiences are so painful that your mind protects you by preventing you from summoning up the memory of them. This is why some people require hypnosis or extensive psychoanalysis to bring forth certain memories.

Many people find they have increasing difficulties with memory as they get older. In the past, memory loss in older adults was attributed to "senility," and it was believed to be an inevitable part of aging. Today, however, thanks to a better understanding of the brain and how it works, we know that this need not be so. It is possible to improve the ability to remember by giving the body what it needs to support brain function.

Brain cells communicate with one another by means of neurotransmitters, special chemicals that the cells produce from certain nutrients. It is true that the brain suffers some degree of degeneration during the normal aging process. As we age, the body not only produces fewer neurotransmitters, but the brain becomes less sensitive to their effects. Concentration becomes more difficult, learning suffers, memories are not well registered or stored, and recall becomes hazy. However, if you provide your brain with an increased supply of the nutrients required to produce neurotransmitters, you may be able not only to protect your brain from the effects of aging, but possibly even to reverse, at least partially, degeneration that has already occurred. Studies have shown that even young people can benefit from the right nutrients.

Other factors can contribute to age-related memory loss as well. For example, it is believed that free-radical damage over a period of many years plays a part, and having blood that is thick with cholesterol and triglycerides may impair circulation and result in an insufficient supply of oxygen and nutrients reaching the brain. Certain drugs, including some blood-pressure medications, antihistamines, antidepressants, antianxiety drugs, antipsychotic agents, hormones, painkillers, muscle relaxants, diet pills, alcohol, and recreational drugs can affect memory. It is well known that alcoholics and drug abusers often suffer from memory "blackouts"—periods of time for which they have no memory, despite having appeared conscious.

There are also a number of medical conditions that can have an adverse effect on memory. Among these are allergies, head injury, toxic-metal buildup, candidiasis, stress, thyroid disorders, and hypoglycemia. If you start having difficulties with memory, it is wise to consider the possibility that other conditions may be causing memory impairment.

CONVENTIONAL MEDICINE

■ Conventional approaches are primarily concerned with ruling out correctable causes of memory loss. Your doctor may recommend a variety of tests to rule out possible underlying conditions. Depending on your medical history, your doctor may want to rule out alcohol use, liver damage, infections such as meningitis or syphilis, thyroid disease, adrenal disease, low blood sugar, pituitary disease, electrolyte imbalances, nutritional deficiencies, head trauma, embolism, stroke, cancer, seizures, autoimmune diseases, AIDS, Parkinson's disease, multiple sclerosis, and/or Alzheimer's disease. He or she will also review any medications you are taking, as many different drugs have an effect on mental function. Changing your prescription or altering the dosage may help. Do not discontinue prescription medications or change dosages on your own, however. Always consult with your physician first.

DIETARY GUIDELINES

■ Eat a healthy, well-balanced high-fiber diet, with an emphasis on raw vegetables, whole grains, and the clean, lean protein supplied by fish and chicken. Fish has long been known as "brain food," and it turns out that there is something to this old belief. Fish contains choline, which the brain converts to acetylcholine, a neurotransmitter that plays an important role in memory, learning, and long-term planning.

■ Eat five or six small high-protein meals per day rather than three large ones. Avoid overeating.

■ To help flush toxins from your body, drink eight 8-ounce glasses of pure water daily.

■ Avoid processed foods, refined sugars, and alcohol.

NUTRITIONAL SUPPLEMENTS

■ To ensure an adequate supply of all major nutrients, take a good multivitamin and mineral complex daily.

■ Antioxidant nutrients fight the free radicals that cause cellular damage in every part of the body, including the brain. Take up to 10,000 international units of beta-carotene, 100 micrograms of selenium, and 1,000 milligrams of vitamin C daily.

■ Choline enhances the production of acetylcholine, an important neurotransmitter. Take 200 to 350 milligrams two or three times daily.

■ Dehydroepiandrosterone (DHEA) is a hormone that has been shown to enhance memory in some cases. Ask your doctor about DHEA therapy. Be aware, however, that some researchers caution that taking DHEA in supplement form can damage the body's ability to manufacture this hormone. In addition, taking too much DHEA can cause serious damage to the liver. Therefore, we advise that DHEA be taken only under the supervision of a physician experienced in its use. If you do decide to experiment with DHEA on your own, start by taking a small amount such as 5 milligrams daily for five days out of the week, then gradually increase to the manufacturer's recommended dose. If you experience any adverse effects, stop taking the supplement.

■ Huperzine-A, a compound isolated from club moss, inhibits the breakdown of the neurotransmitter acetylcholine and reduces the death of nerve cells caused by excess amounts of glutamine in the brain. Take 50 micrograms twice a day.

Note: Do not use this supplement if you are pregnant or have high blood pressure.

■ Lecithin improves brain function. It is a good source of choline and important B vitamins. Take 1,200 milligrams two or three times daily, with meals.

■ Low levels of phosphatidylserine, a type of lipid, in the brain are commonly associated with memory loss. This is an important brain nutrient and is essential for effective neurotransmission. Sufficient levels of vitamin B_{12}, folic acid, the essential fatty acids, and the amino-acid derivative s-adenosylmethionine (SAM or SAMe) are all essential for the production of phosphatidylserine. With age, one or more of these nutrients often becomes less available. To remedy possible deficiencies that may be contributing to memory loss, take 50 to 100 milligrams of phosphatidylserine three times daily; a B-complex formula that provides at least 500 micrograms of vitamin B_{12} and 800 micrograms of folic acid daily; a dose of black currant seed, borage, evening primrose, or flaxseed oil that supplies the equivalent of 250 milligrams of gamma-linolenic acid (GLA) twice daily; and 100 to 300 milligrams of s-adenosylmethionine two to three times daily. Try this program for two months.

■ The amino acid tyrosine stimulates thyroid function and helps improve mood. The brain uses tyrosine to make norepinephrine, a vital neurotransmitter that affects memory and learning capacity. Take 500 milligrams of L-tyrosine first thing in the morning for one to two months.

Note: If you are taking a monoamine oxidase (MAO) inhibitor drug, do not take supplemental tyrosine, as a sudden and dangerous rise in blood pressure may result.

HERBAL TREATMENT

■ Ginkgo biloba is an oxygenating herb that increases the blood supply to the brain. Choose a product containing at least 24 percent ginkgo heterosides (sometimes called flavoglycosides) and take 40 to 60 milligrams two or three times daily.

■ Gotu kola enhances choline production and can help improve mental function and concentration. In Ayurvedic medicine, this herb is considered to be a prime nerve tonic that promotes mental clarity and calmness. Choose a standardized extract containing 16 percent triterpenes and take 200 milligrams two to three times daily for up to six weeks. Gotu kola and ginkgo biloba are available in a combination formula that also contains choline and vitamin B_{12}. This powerful formula is a better choice than either of the two herbs alone.

■ Siberian ginseng enhances energy and improves mood. Choose a standardized extract containing 0.5 percent eleutheroside E and take 100 milligrams twice daily, in the morning and the afternoon.

HOMEOPATHY

■ A constitutional remedy is the best way to treat memory loss homeopathically. Consult a qualified a homeopathic practitioner who can formulate a remedy tailored to your particular needs.

BACH FLOWER REMEDIES

■ Impatiens can help if you tend to be tense, impatient, nervous, and easily irritated. Take one dose as needed, following the directions on the product label.

ACUPRESSURE

For the locations of acupressure points on the body, *see* ADMINISTERING AN ACUPRESSURE TREATMENT in Part Three.

■ Gallbladder 20 improves circulation to the head.

■ Kidney 1, 3, and 7 improve circulation in the kidney meridian. In traditional Chinese medicine, the brain is "fed" and strengthened by the kidneys. Improving kidney function thus ultimately improves brain function.

■ Large Intestine 4 has a beneficial effect on the head and face.

■ Spleen 6 and Stomach 36 together improve circulation and the utilization of nutrients.

AROMATHERAPY

For specific instructions on how to use aromatherapy, *see* PREPARING AROMATHERAPY TREATMENTS in Part Three.

■ Essential oils of basil, peppermint, and rosemary are reputed to enhance memory. Use any or all of them as inhalants or in baths, or diffuse them into the air in your home, particularly when you are engaged in learning activities.

GENERAL RECOMMENDATIONS

■ If following the recommendations in this entry do not help substantially within two months, consider the possibility that you may have an underlying condition that is contributing to your memory problems. See your healthcare provider for an evaluation.

■ Ask your physician about "smart drugs," such as hydergine and selegiline (Eldepryl, also known as deprenyl), which may be helpful for memory loss.

■ Exercise both your body and your mind. Regular physical exercise helps to increase the oxygen supply to the brain. But your mind needs "exercise" just as much as your body does. If all you ask of your mind is to follow the story line of the latest sitcom on television, your brain will become lazy. Read a newspaper regularly; join a book discussion group; do word puzzles; take an adult-education class and learn a new skill. If mobility is a problem, consider connecting with the outside world via computer.

PREVENTION

■ The most important thing you can do to prevent age-related memory impairment is to make sure your brain has the nutrients it needs to function normally. Follow the suggestions under Dietary Guidelines, above, and take appropriate dietary supplements.

Meniere's Disease

Meniere's disease is a disorder of the inner ear that causes intermittent episodes of vertigo (dizziness and loss of balance) that may be accompanied by nausea, vomiting, hearing loss, sound distortion, a feeling of pressure or fullness in the ear, and, possibly, a sensation of buzzing or ringing in the ear. Making sudden movements often adds to the vertigo, and you may become so dizzy that you require help to walk or remain standing. Attacks can last from a few minutes to a few hours. Some people have the condition for a matter of days or weeks, while others suffer recurrences throughout their lives. In most people, Meniere's disease affects only one ear, but it is possible to have it in both ears.

The cause of Meniere's disease is not known, but it is known that it often occurs after a middle-ear infection or a head injury. Upsets in the inner ear, including bleeding, fluid imbalances, or blood-vessel spasms, may also contribute to the problem. Acute attacks can be triggered by a variety of factors, including allergies, eyestrain, stress, and nutritional deficiencies. Many people with Meniere's disease have been found to have deficiencies of the B vitamins, especially vitamin B_3 (niacin). In addition, hypoglycemia (low blood sugar) is more common among people with this disorder than in the population as a whole. High blood-cholesterol levels and impaired circulation may also be contributing factors. It is interesting to note that the incidence of gallbladder disease in people with Meniere's disease is twice that in the general population. If you have symptoms of Meniere's disease, see your doctor to determine if you have any underlying conditions, such as gallbladder problems, hypoglycemia, or high cholesterol, that require treatment.

CONVENTIONAL MEDICINE

■ Since the underlying cause of this condition is not known, treatment focuses on easing symptoms. To help lessen the vertigo, your doctor may prescribe a type of drug classified as an anticholinergic. The way these drugs work is not understood, but they are thought to act on the vestibular area of the inner ear, the cerebral cortex itself, or an area called the *chemoreceptor trigger zone* (CTZ). Examples include atropine and scopolamine. These agents can cause side effects, most notably drowsiness and dry mouth.

■ Antihistamines, such as diphenhydramine (Benadryl), meclizine (Antivert), and hydroxyzine (Atarax, Vistaril) may be used. These drugs appear to act on the nerve pathway within the inner ear. They tend to be less effective than anticholinergics, but their effects last longer. Possible side effects include drowsiness and dry mouth.

■ If you suffer very severe attacks of vertigo, you may benefit from an antianxiety medication such as diazepam (Valium) or a sedative such as pentobarbital (Nembutal).

■ Some physicians believe that lowering fluid pressure in the inner ear can help to alleviate this disorder. Your doctor may recommend that you switch to a low-sodium diet and, possibly, take a diuretic.

■ If Meniere's disease becomes seriously disabling, surgery may be recommended. There are two types of procedures that may be used: vestibular neurectomy, in which the affected nerve is cut, and labyrinthectomy, in which the hearing and balance organ in the affected ear is removed. Labyrinthectomy is generally used only if hearing is poor; neurectomy may preserve hearing.

DIETARY GUIDELINES

■ Eat a well-balanced high-fiber diet with lean protein and plenty of fresh vegetables and fruits. Avoid foods that contain cholesterol or saturated fat. (*See* CHOLESTEROL, HIGH.)

■ Investigate the possibility that hypoglycemia may be contributing to symptoms. Follow a hypoglycemic diet (*see* HYPOGLYCEMIA) and see if your symptoms improve.

■ Eat five or six small, nutrient-dense meals daily instead of two or three large meals. This will help keep your blood sugar levels stable.

■ Beware of excess sodium. Consuming too much salt can cause your body to retain too much fluid, which can contribute to this disorder.

■ Avoid caffeine and alcohol, which are known to worsen symptoms.

NUTRITIONAL SUPPLEMENTS

■ Chromium helps to normalize blood-sugar levels, which are often low in people with Meniere's disease. Take 200 micrograms of chromium once or twice daily.

■ Coenzyme Q_{10} improves tissue oxygenation and aids circulation. Take 30 to 100 milligrams daily.

■ To improve your body's absorption and utilization of all nutrients, take a full-spectrum digestive-enzyme supplement providing 5,000 international units of lipase, 2,500 international units of amylase, and 300 international units of protease, plus 500 to 1,000 milligrams of pancreatin, with each meal.

Note: Long-term supplementation with pancreatin is not advised, as it can cause your pancreas to reduce its own production of this important enzyme. Overuse also has the potential to cause nausea or diarrhea. After two months on pancreatin, discontinue use and monitor your reaction. If you find that your problems recur, discuss pancreatin supplementation with your physician.

■ The essential fatty acids found in black currant seed oil, borage oil, evening primrose oil, and flaxseed oil help to normalize metabolism. Choose one of these oils and take 500 to 1,000 milligrams two to three times daily.

■ Magnesium deficiency has been implicated in some cases of Meniere's disease. Take 200 milligrams of magnesium citrate or magnesium aspartate twice daily.

■ A deficiency of manganese may be a factor in Meniere's disease. Take 5 milligrams daily for up to three months.

Note: Do not take manganese at the same time as calcium. Calcium can interfere with manganese absorption.

■ N-acetylcysteine (NAC) helps with the chelation of heavy metals, whose presence can contribute to this condition. Take 500 milligrams two or three times daily.

■ The B vitamins are very important. Take a good B-complex formula supplying 50 to 100 milligrams of each of the major B vitamins once or twice daily, plus an an additional 50 milligrams of vitamin B_6 (pyridoxine) twice a day, and enough additional vitamin B_3 (niacin) to bring your intake to a total of 200 milligrams daily from all sources. If you are bothered by the flush this nutrient can produce, take niacinamide instead.

Note: Do not take supplemental niacin if you have gout or liver dysfunction.

HERBAL TREATMENT

■ Chinese (Korean) and Siberian ginseng have normalizing properties and act as whole-body tonics. The ginsengs promote recovery from illness and ease stress, both physical and mental. Choose a standardized extract of Chinese ginseng containing 7 percent ginsenosides or a Siberian ginseng containing 0.5 percent eleutheroside E and take 100 milligrams twice daily for two to three weeks. Stop taking the preparation for two weeks, then repeat.

Note: Do not use Chinese ginseng if you have high blood pressure, heart disease, or hypoglycemia. If you are sensitive to the effects of caffeine and other stimulants, you may want to consult with a qualified herbalist before using ginseng.

■ Ginkgo biloba improves circulation and helps to treat symptoms of tinnitus, or ringing in the ears. Choose a product containing at least 24 percent ginkgo heterosides (sometimes called flavoglycosides) and take 40 milligrams three times daily.

■ Mullein oil, warmed and mixed with equal parts of homeopathic *Chenopodium anthelminthicum* in liquid form (see below) and applied as eardrops, often brings relief.

HOMEOPATHY

Choose an appropriate symptom-specific remedy from the list below and take one dose three times a day for up to five days. Wait one month, then repeat. If you notice even the slightest improvement at any time while you are taking the remedy, stop taking it.

■ *Chenopodium anthelminthicum* is good if your hearing changes from normal to weak and back again for no apparent reason. You find it easier to hear a high-pitched voice than one in a lower register.

■ *Chininum sulfuricum* is effective against vertigo, nausea, vomiting, and the typical ringing and buzzing in the ears.

■ Choose *Cocculus* is you are a fair-complexioned woman whose dizziness is worse when sitting or riding in a car, with a metallic taste in your mouth and nausea that may progress to vomiting. You probably have very strong emotions, may complain of pain in your lower back, and usually feel weak during your menstrual period.

■ If your hearing alternates between being normal and being weak and you find it easier to hear low-pitched sounds, take *Natrum salicylicum* 12x or 6c.

■ *Salicylicum acidum* is for a roaring noise in the ears, possibly accompanied by dizziness, digestive problems, and a lot of bowel gas. This remedy is commonly prescribed for Meniere's disease. Take one dose of *salicylicum acidum* 30x or 15c three to four times daily. If you experience no improvement after three days, discontinue it and select another remedy.

ACUPRESSURE

For the locations of acupressure points on the body, *see* **ADMINISTERING AN ACUPRESSURE TREATMENT** in Part Three.

■ Gallbladder 20, 34, and 41 increase circulation to the head.

■ Large Intestine 4 helps to relieve congestion and relax tension in the head.

GENERAL RECOMMENDATIONS

■ If you are overweight, slim down. Many experts believe that obesity is a contributing factor in Meniere's disease.

See OBESITY for recommendations that can help you lose the excess pounds.

■ Don't smoke. All ear disorders are more common in smokers than nonsmokers.

■ Never ignore a suspected ear infection. If you experience ear pain or a feeling of fullness that doesn't go away in several days, consult your physician to determine whether you have an ear infection that requires treatment.

■ Consider having a hair analysis done to check for the presence of heavy metals. The accumulation of heavy metals in the body has been linked to Meniere's disease.

PREVENTION

■ Exposure to loud sounds causes trauma to the ears, whether the sound comes from music you enjoy or a jackhammer that jangles your nerves. Avoid loud noises whenever possible, and protect your ears by using earplugs or other protective devices whenever you are in an environment with a high noise level.

Meningitis

Meningitis is an inflammation of the three meninges, which are thin membranes that cover the brain and spinal cord. It can be caused by any of a number of different infectious agents, including viruses, bacteria, and fungi; it can also have noninfectious causes, including brain tumor, stroke, and lead poisoning. If the same condition affects the spinal cord and brain as well as the meninges, it is called *encephalomyelitis*.

The classic symptoms of meningitis include rising fever, chills, achiness, vomiting, irritability, headache (often severe), and/or a stiff neck and back, often coming on during or just after another viral infection. Seizures and changes in consciousness, such as stupor or coma, are possible as the infection progresses. Some people develop a form of meningitis that develops more slowly, over several weeks, and that may not cause significant fever. This form of the illness most often affects people with depressed immune function, such as people who have certain forms of cancer and/or who are undergoing cancer treatment; those who must take immune-suppressing drugs following organ transplantation; and people with HIV disease.

Meningitis is a serious condition that can be life threatening in the acute phase and can also cause such long-term consequences as hearing or vision problems. However, if you are treated promptly and appropriately, there is good chance you will recover completely, even if you are very ill.

CONVENTIONAL TREATMENT

■ To determine whether you have meningitis, a physician will look for signs of infection and the presence of an infectious organism in your spinal fluid. This involves a spinal tap, a procedure in which the doctor inserts a needle into a space between two vertebrae and withdraws a small amount of fluid for inspection. The process can be difficult, as it requires you to curl up and lie very still. To lessen the pain, the doctor will use a numbing medicine on your skin before inserting the needle, but it still feels like pressure in the back. Your doctor will probably also take a sample of your blood to look for other signs of infection.

■ If your physician suspects meningitis, he or she will likely start antibiotic therapy immediately after the spinal-fluid and blood samples are taken. Doctors generally do not wait for the test results because the risk of failing to treat a possible bacterial infection immediately is too great. The antibiotic will be given intravenously, usually for a minimum of seven days. Ampicillin, penicillin, and chloramphenicol are commonly used for this purpose.

■ When the test results come back and the infecting organism is identified, your treatment may change. This may involve switching to a different type of antibiotic or, if the meningitis is determined to be viral in origin, discontinuing the antibiotic and substituting intravenous treatment with the antiviral drug acyclovir. If a fungal organism is found, your doctor will likely switch to an antifungal medication such as amphotericin B.

■ Rest and measures to restore your body's electrolyte balance, control fever, and relieve pain will be prescribed to ease discomfort and aid in recovery.

■ While adequate fluid intake is important, it may be restricted somewhat if there are signs of abnormal fluid levels in your brain.

NUTRITIONAL SUPPLEMENTS

The nutritional supplements listed below are aimed at supporting recovery from meningitis. They should not be considered a substitute for appropriate antibiotic therapy.

■ Acidophilus and bifidobacteria are very good for restoring bowel health after a regimen of potent antibiotics. Take them as recommended on the product labels for one month. If you are allergic to milk, select a dairy-free formula.

■ Green-foods products supply trace minerals and beta-carotene, and help to restore strength. Follow the directions on the product label.

■ Kidney glandular extract helps to strengthen kidney function, which is often compromised in meningitis. Take 300 milligrams two or three times daily for ten days to two weeks.

■ The B vitamins help to restore strength. Take a B-complex supplement supplying 25 milligrams of each of the major B vitamins three times daily.

■ Vitamin C and bioflavonoids help to stimulate the mmune system. Take 500 milligrams of each four times daily for two weeks, then reduce to 500 milligrams of each twice daily.

■ Zinc boosts immune function. Take 25 milligrams of zinc aspartate, chelate, citrate, or picolinate twice daily for two weeks. Take zinc with food to prevent stomach upset.

HERBAL TREATMENT

Herbal treatment for meningitis is aimed at supporting recovery from the illness. It should not be considered a substitute for appropriate antibiotic therapy.

■ Garlic has antibiotic properties that help to resolve infection. Take 500 milligrams (or one garlic clove) at least three times daily until the infection clears.

■ If you have a problem with water retention, a tea of dandelion root, nettle leaf, and/or parsley leaf can help. Make a tea using equal parts of these herbs (*see* PREPARING HERBAL REMEDIES in Part Three) and take one cup three times daily until the symptoms subside.

■ Once the infection is gone, you can use American ginseng and/or astragalus. Both of these herbs are excellent sources of trace minerals and micronutrients, and also support and strengthen the immune system. Take 500 milligrams of either or both three times a day for two weeks.

Note: These herbs should be used during recovery only. Do not take them if you have a fever or any other signs of acute infection. Do not use American ginseng if you have high blood pressure, heart disease, or hypoglycemia. If you are sensitive to the effects of caffeine and other stimulants, you may want to consult with a qualified herbalist before using ginseng.

HOMEOPATHY

Homeopathic treatment for meningitis is aimed at supporting recovery from the illness once the acute phase of the infection has passed. It should not be considered a subsitite for appropriate antibiotic therapy. Choose a symptom-specific remedy and take one dose, as directed on the product label, four times a day for up to two days.

■ *Belladonna* 30x or 9c is helpful if you have a fever, dilated pupils, and, perhaps, delirious behavior.

■ *Bryonia* 30x or 9c is good if you experience eye pain, constipation, and arthritis-like pain.

GENERAL RECOMMENDATIONS

■ During the acute phase of meningitis, resting in a quiet, dimly lit room will help ease the headache pain.

■ If you contract bacterial meningitis, be aware of the possibility that it can leave you with a subtle injury to the brain. Don't hesitate to talk to your doctor if you notice hearing loss, problems with balance or coordination, difficulties at work, or similar problems.

PREVENTION

■ There is a vaccine against *Hemophilus influenzae*, an organism that is often implicated in meningitis, that is now routinely given to children in a series of four immunizations, starting when they are two months of age.

Menopause

With the end of menstruation, the reproductive period of a woman's life comes to a close and menopause—also known as the "change of life"—occurs. Some women welcome it, others dread it, but it is a phase of life that comes to all women. For most, the menses stop naturally when they are between forty-five and sixty years of age with the decline of monthly hormonal cycles. However, menopause may occur earlier in life, often as a result of illness, the surgical removal of the uterus or ovaries (or both), eating disorders such as anorexia and bulimia, and intense, ongoing, and physically stressful activity.

During the five or so years before menopause—a period known as the *perimenopause*—the ovaries become increasingly insensitive to the hormonal signals that stimulate them to produce the sex hormones estrogen and progesterone. This process generally starts when a woman is between the ages of forty-two and fifty-five. As a result, although the average woman's ovaries still contain thousands of immature eggs at this point, these eggs fail to mature, making it impossible for the the ovaries to release a mature egg every month as they did during the woman's younger childbearing years. The menstrual cycles become irregular. Eventually, the ovaries become incapable of producing significant amounts of estrogen, and menstrual cycles cease altogether. At this point, menopause has arrived. Generally, doctors consider a woman menopausal if she has had no periods for twelve months and blood tests show high levels of follicle-stimulating hormone (FSH) and low levels of estrogen. The average woman in an industrialized Western nation can expect to spend approximately one-third of her lifetime in the menopausal and postmenopausal states.

It is worth emphasizing that menopause is *not* a disorder, but a natural part of life. However, it can cause a variety of symptoms and sensations that may range from mildly uncomfortable to inconvenient to downright maddening. Although some women breeze through the transition and scarcely notice it, most do experience some symptoms. The majority of women—estimates range from 50 to 80 percent—experience hot flashes. In these episodes, a woman has a sensation of being intolerably hot and unable to cool down. Her face (and sometimes other parts of her body) flushes and she may perspire profusely. Hot flashes usually last from two to three minutes, and tend to be at their most intense during the first two years of the perimenopause. Other common problems associated with menopause include fatigue, headaches, nervousness, irritability, insomnia, emotional stress, heart palpitations, aches and pains, and vaginal dryness. Some authorities list depression among the possible difficulties of menopause. However, there are as yet no studies that objectively support this belief. In fact, research indicates that women and men both are much more likely to experience depression in their twenties and thirties than later in life. Some women experience changes in their sexual needs and desires during menopause. For some, this translates into decreased desire (sometimes due to discomfort during intercourse caused by vaginal dryness), but many find they feel more sexually liberated and their libido increases.

Most if not all of the uncomfortable symptoms associated with menopause can be traced to the decline in estrogen production. While estrogen is vital for reproduction, that is not its only role in the body. It also has effects on the brain, cardiovascular system, skin, bones, and other vital tissue. Because of these effects, the decline in the body's supply of estrogen can have certain serious long-term effects, especially osteoporosis and cardiovascular disease. Estrogen causes the bones to hold on to the calcium and other minerals that give them their strength. Without sufficient estrogen, the bones start to lose their mineral mass and become weak and brittle. Estrogen also helps to keep the arteries pliable and relatively free of plaque. This is why, as a group, women in their childbearing years suffer less cardiovascular disease than men of the same age. It is also why, after menopause, women's rate of heart disease begins to climb until it is on a par with that of men. Less serious, but nevertheless distressing, long-term consequences of menopause include dry, aging skin and vaginal atrophy (wasting away of vaginal tissue). These problems occur because estrogen keeps skin and vaginal tissues plumped-up and pliable. Without estrogen, these tissues thin and become fragile.

When considering the use of any treatment, whether conventional or alternative, for menopausal symptoms, it is a good idea to focus on five basic points:

1. Digestion.

2. Energy level.

3. Mood.

4. Appetite.

5. Sleep.

If the treatment improves all of these, it is in all likelihood a good one for you. However, if a treatment relieves your hot flashes but leaves you depressed, tired, and unable to sleep, you would want to consider a different approach.

CONVENTIONAL TREATMENT

■ The most common conventional treatment for alleviating menopausal symptoms is hormone replacement therapy (HRT). Most programs for taking HRT are similar to those for taking oral contraceptives in that they follow a monthly cycle: On days 1 through 15, you take estrogen alone; on days 16 through 25, you take both estrogen and progesterone; and on days 26 through 30, you rest, taking no supplemental hormones at all. Then the regimen begins again. Hormones are most often taken in oral form, but skin patches that are applied once a week to provide a steady influx of hormones are also available. The most popular form of oral estrogen, Premarin, is derived from the urine of pregnant horses. However, with the advent, or rather return, of compounding pharmacists—pharmacists who actually mix prescribed ingredients instead of merely dispensing prepared pills and other products—more natural forms of HRT are now available. "Triple-estrogen" therapy using estrone, estriol, and estradiol (forms of estrogen identical to those found naturally in the human body) appears to yield excellent results for many women. Similarly, the most commonly used form of progesterone is the synthetic progestin (Provera), which is associated with such side effects as weight gain, bloating, irritability, depression, and headaches, as well as unhealthy changes in blood-fat levels. Natural progesterone, available from compounding pharmacies, is preferable.

In addition to relieving such acute symptoms as hot flashes, HRT can reduce women's risk of death from coronary artery disease and hip fractures due to osteoporosis. However, this treatment is not suitable for all women. Women with a history of liver disease, estrogen-dependent breast or endometrial cancer, or phlebitis or other blood-clotting problems are generally advised not to seek this type of treatment. You should be aware that there are natural alternatives to HRT that have been shown to be safe, nontoxic, and very effective in easing menopausal symptoms. Certain lifestyle changes also are known to be beneficial.

DIETARY GUIDELINES

■ Eat a diet that is high in fiber. Increase your consumption of fruits and vegetables. Prepare cooked foods simply. Steaming and baking are best.

Avoid refined sugars, red meat, chocolate, alcohol, and caffeine. These foods worsen menopausal symptoms and stress the body.

One of the best measures you can take is to increase your consumption of water. Consuming six to eight 8-ounce glasses of pure water can yield a mild reduction in many menopausal symptoms. Hot flashes can cause dehydration. In a kind of vicious cycle, the more dehydrated you become, the more difficulty you will have with hot flashes, headaches, fatigue, and dry skin.

Increase your consumption of foods rich in phytoestrogens (plant estrogens). Among the best sources of these compounds are soy foods. Phytoestrogens appear to function much like natural estrogens in many ways. For example, they have been found to increase cell growth in the vaginal walls and also to raise the body's level of high-density lipoproteins (HDL, the so-called "good cholesterol"). They may also help to decrease the risk of breast and endometrial cancer. The lower incidence of menopausal problems among Japanese women has been attributed to their greater consumption of soy products, including tofu, miso, aburage, koridofu, and, of course, soybeans themselves. Eating about 2 ounces of soy products each day may be enough to reduce menopausal symptoms and reduce the risk of cancer and heart disease. Other foods that contain phytoestrogens include apples, barley, beets, cabbage, fennel, flaxseeds, oats, olives and olive oil, papaya, pumpkin, adzuki and kidney beans, red clover, rice, sesame seeds, split peas, sunflower seeds, and yams.

If you suffer from hot flashes, increase your consumption of green vegetables and consider adding sea vegetables to your menu. The minerals in these foods replenish necessary electrolytes lost through perspiration.

If you suffer from depression, scrutinize your diet to make certain that your blood-sugar level remains as constant as possible. If you have a problem stabilizing your blood sugar, you may want to take supplemental chromium (see under Nutritional Supplements, below).

NUTRITIONAL SUPPLEMENTS

Take a good multivitamin and mineral supplement daily.

Bioflavonoids have been used successfully to reduce hot flashes, as well as to reduce heavy bleeding. They also help protect and strengthen capillary walls. Take 500 milligrams three times daily, with 500 milligrams of vitamin C, as long as you have symptoms.

■ Boron is a trace mineral that is required for strong bones and the full absorption of calcium. Take 1 to 2 milligrams daily.

■ Calcium helps to protect the bones from osteoporosis, which is common in postmenopausal women; magnesium is necessary for the absorption and utilization of calcium. Take 500 to 600 milligrams of calcium and 300 to 400 milligrams of magnesium twice daily. Avoid dolomite, as it is harder to absorb and may contain small amounts of lead.

■ Chromium helps to improve the efficient use of insulin and keep blood-sugar levels steady. Take 100 to 200 micrograms of chromium once or twice daily.

■ Black currant seed, borage, and evening primrose oil contain gamma-linolenic acid (GLA), one of the most powerful essential fatty acids. GLA is essential for the production of hormonelike chemicals called prostaglandins that are necessary for bone formation. Flaxseed oil contains two essential fatty acids, linoleic acid and linolenic acid, which are precursors for many enzymes and hormones. They promote bone formation, increase resistance to toxins and viruses and abnormal blood clotting, and are involved in the proper functoning of the cardiovascular system. Many women have found these oils helpful for reducing menopausal symptoms as well. Take 500 to 1,000 milligrams of black currant seed, borage, or evening primrose oil two to three times daily, plus 1 tablespoonful (or 500 to 1,000) milligrams of flaxseed oil twice daily.

■ Glucosamine and chondroitin promote joint repair, and help to relieve aches and pains in the muscles and joints. Take 500 milligrams of glucosamine sulfate or glucosamine hydrochloride (HCI) two or three times daily and 500 milligrams of chondroitin sulfate twice a day.

■ Genistein is a phytoestrogen derived from soybeans or red clover. Plant estrogens have much milder effects than human estrogens do. However, it has been observed that Japanese women, who eat a lot of soy foods, have relatively high levels of phytoestrogens in their blood, and also have fewer menopausal symptoms than their Western counterparts. If you find it difficult to increase your intake of soy foods, consider taking 250 milligrams of soy isoflavones three times a day.

■ The amino acid glutamine helps to improve mental clarity and lift depression. Take 500 to 1,000 milligrams of L-glutamine twice daily for up to three months.

■ If you feel you have tried everything and are still feeling overwhelmed by menopausal symptoms, consider trying hypothalamus protomorphogen. The hypothalamus is the "commander in chief" of the hormonal system. Many women have found great relief by taking 100 milligrams of hypothalamus protomorphogen one-half hour before breakfast and again one-half hour before lunch.

■ The combination of magnesium and malic acid helps to increase energy and combat fatigue. These nutrients are precursors to the Krebs cycle, a series of enzyme reactions that are a key part of the production of energy on the cellular level. Take 100 to 200 milligrams of magnesium and

200 to 300 milligrams of malic acid one-half to one hour before breakfast and again at bedtime.

■ Pantothenic acid is useful for relieving hot flashes. Take 250 milligrams twice daily for up to one week at a time, as needed to relieve symptoms. If you take any of the B vitamins individually, you should also take a B-complex supplement at a different time of day.

■ Royal jelly is rich in nutrients and hormonal factors that help optimize hormone balance in both sexes. Take 500 milligrams twice daily.

■ Selenium is an antioxidant trace mineral that protects the body from free-radical damage. Take 200 micrograms daily.

■ Soy isoflavones, phytochemicals derived from soybeans, may aid in maintaining hormonal balance. Take 250 milligrams three times a day.

■ The amino acid tryptophan helps to tame anxiety and relieve insomnia. The recommended dose is 500 milligrams of L-tryptophan, taken once daily at bedtime, for one month. This supplement is currently available only by prescription, however. You may want to discuss it with your doctor.

■ Vitamin A can reduce excessive bleeding and thus help to prevent anemia. If you experience exceptionally heavy bleeding as menopause approaches, take 25,000 international units of vitamin A twice daily for one week before the anticipated onset of your period.

Note: If you are pregnant, or intend to get pregnant, or if you have liver disease, consult your doctor before taking supplemental vitamin A. Pregnant women should not ingest a total of more than 25,000 international units of supplemental vitamin A *per week* from all sources.

■ Vitamin B_6 (pyridoxine) works with magnesium in a multitude of reactions that assist in the control of menopausal symptoms. Take 50 to 100 milligrams once or twice daily for up to three weeks (you should not take a separate B_6 supplement on a daily basis for more than three weeks without the guidance of a health-care professional). If you take any of the B vitamins individually, you should also take a B-complex supplement at a different time of day.

■ Vitamin B_{12} and folic acid help to improve energy levels. If fatigue and/or depression is a problem, take 250 to 500 micrograms of vitamin B_{12} and 800 micrograms of folic acid daily. You might also consider asking your doctor for vitamin-B_{12} injections to be given twice weekly for one month. If you take any of the B vitamins individually, you should also take a B-complex supplement at a different time of day.

■ Vitamin E helps to alleviate hot flashes and other menopausal symptoms. It is essential for healthy metabolism, and is also a primary antioxidant that protects against free-radical damage. Choose a product containing mixed tocopherols or d-alpha-tocopheryl succinate, and begin by taking 200 international units daily, then gradually increase the dosage until you are taking 400 to 800 international units daily.

Note: If you have high blood pressure, limit your intake of supplemental vitamin E to a total of 400 international units daily. If you are taking an anticoagulant (blood thinner), consult your physician before taking supplemental vitamin E.

HERBAL TREATMENT

■ Black cohosh acts to enhance the production of estrogen and helps to diminish hot flashes. It has been used as a remedy for menopausal difficulties for centuries. Choose an extract standardized to contain 2.5 percent triterpenes (calculated as 27-deoxyaceteine) per tablet, and take 20 to 40 milligrams twice a day.

■ The combination of bupleurum, white peony, and atractylodes root is a very old Chinese remedy that is helpful against many menopausal symptoms. Bupleurum has a harmonizing effect on the liver. White peony is a blood tonic used in Chinese medicine to regulate menstrual irregularities, and is also a relaxant, useful in allaying nervous conditions. Atractylodes root aids digestion and is a natural diuretic that rids the body of excess fluids. Take one dose of this remedy, as directed on the product label, three times daily, as needed.

■ Chamomile, passionflower, and valerian are botanical relaxants that can help if you are unable to sleep due to recurrent hot flashes and insomnia. You can take them in extract form or brewed into a strong tea. Take 300 to 500 milligrams of chamomile, 250 milligrams of standardized passionflower extract containing 0.7 percent flavonoids, or 200 milligrams of standardized valerian extract containing 0.5 percent isovalerenic acids one-half hour before bedtime. Or you can take a cup of chamomile, passionflower, and/or valerian tea, as needed.

■ Chaste tree berry (also known by its Latin name, *Vitex agnus-castus*) balances hormones by promoting the production of progesterone and reining in the production of estrogen. It is effective in helping to reduce excessive bleeding during the perimenopausal period, as well as in minimizing symptoms. During menopause and perimenopause, when both estrogen and progesterone levels drop, this herb combines well with dong quai to relieve menopausal symptoms. If you are still menstruating, take 200 milligrams two or three times daily for the two weeks before the anticipated onset of your period. If you are no longer having periods, take 400 milligrams daily.

■ Dong quai, sometimes referred to as "female ginseng,"

is a highly effective blood tonic and estrogen modulator. It helps to minimize menopausal symptoms such as hot flashes, nervousness, insomnia, and anxiety by providing an available form of phytoestrogen (plant estrogen). Take 200 milligrams of standardized extract daily. You should not take it if you are experiencing heavy menstrual bleeding, however.

■ Ginkgo biloba enhances circulation and mental clarity. Choose a standardized extract containing at least 24 percent ginkgo heterosides (sometimes called flavoglycosides) and take 40 milligrams three times daily.

■ Kava kava helps to relieve anxiety and promotes sound sleep. Choose a product containing 30 percent kavalactones and take 100 to 200 milligrams twice a day, in the morning and again at bedtime.

Note: In excess amounts, this herb can cause drowsiness. Do not exceed the recommended dose. Kava kava should not be used by women who are pregnant or nursing, or by people who have Parkinson's disease or are taking prescription medications for depression or anxiety.

■ Licorice is a harmonizing herb that appears to modulate estrogen much as dong quai does. Take 100 milligrams twice a day.

Note: Do not take licorice on a daily basis for more than five days at a time, as it can elevate blood pressure. Do not use it at all if you have high blood pressure.

■ Oat straw is high in silica, which aids the absorption and assimilation of calcium. This herb is also a well-known nerve tonic. Take 500 milligrams twice a day.

■ St. John's wort is a natural antidepressant. Choose a product containing 0.3 percent hypericin and take 300 milligrams one-half hour before breakfast and again one-half hour before lunch and dinner.

■ Siberian ginseng is an energizing herb that is useful for fatigue. Choose a standardized extract containing 0.5 percent eleutheroside E and take 100 milligrams twice daily, the first dose before breakfast and the second before lunch.

■ Skullcap is calming and strengthens the nervous system. Take 300 to 500 milligrams twice a day.

■ Valerian is a relaxant and an aid to sleep. If insomnia is a problem, take 200 milligrams of standardized extract containing 0.5 percent isovalerenic acids one-half hour before bedtime.

NUTRITIONAL/HERBAL COMBINATION TREATMENT

■ Try the following rotating program:

Week 1: Take one dose of a bupleurum and peony or bupleurum and dong quai combination formula three times daily. Also take a multivitamin and mineral supplement each day, plus 200 to 400 international units of vita-

min E and 50 to 100 additional milligrams of pantothenic acid three times daily.

Week 2: Take black cohosh extract (choose a product standardized to 2.5 percent triterpenes per tablet, and take 40 milligrams twice a day). Also take 500 to 1,000 milligrams of borage, evening primrose, or flaxseed oil twice daily. Continue taking the multivitamin and mineral and vitamin E supplements.

Week 3: Take 500 milligrams of chaste tree berry three times a day. Also take 500 milligrams of vitamin C and an equal amount of bioflavonoids three or four times daily. Continue taking the multivitamin and mineral supplement.

Week 4: Apply $1/4$ teaspoon of progesterone cream three times daily. Also take 2,500 milligrams of flaxseed oil twice a day. Continue taking the multivitamin and mineral supplement.

HOMEOPATHY

■ *Aurum muriaticum* is helpful if you are menopausal and find yourself in the throes of intense depression. Take one dose of *Aurum muriaticum* 30x or 15c three times daily for three days, as needed.

■ *Lachesis* is an excellent remedy for hot flashes, anxiety, and headaches. Take one dose of *Lachesis* 30x or 15c three times daily for three days, as needed.

■ *Natrum muriaticum* is for dry skin and dry mucous membranes. You probably have cravings for salt and salty foods. Take one dose of *Natrum muriaticum* 30x or 15c three times daily for three days, as needed.

■ Choose *Pulsatilla* if you find yourself becoming upset and crying easily. Take one dose of *Pulsatilla* 30x or 15c three times daily for three days, as needed.

■ *Sanguinaria* is the remedy for the woman who suffers periodic occipital headaches (headaches originating in the back of the head), usually weekly, that travel to over the eyes. The pain may be worse on the right side. You may also suffer from hot flashes and have hot hands and feet. Take one dose of *Sanguinaria* 30x or 15c three times daily for three days, as needed.

■ *Sepia* is useful if you are a dark-complected woman who enjoys exercise and are feeling irritable. Take one dose of *Sepia* 30x or 15c two to three times daily, as needed.

■ If your symptoms are not addressed by any of the above remedies, consult a homeopathic physician for a constitutional remedy.

BACH FLOWER REMEDIES

Select the remedy that most closely fits your emotional tendencies and concerns, and take it as needed, following the directions on the product label.

Aspen will ease fear of the unknown—fears you cannot (or cannot bear to) name.

- Centuary helps to overcome feelings of intimidation.
- Cerato combats timidity and a lack of self-confidence.
- Mimulus will help if you have fears that you can name.
- Sweet Chestnut is the remedy of choice to chase away feelings of anguish and torment.

White Chestnut is the remedy for obsessive thoughts that go around and around in your head.

ACUPRESSURE

For the locations of acupressure points on the body, see ADMINISTERING AN ACUPRESSURE TREATMENT in Part Three.

Bladder 60 increases circulation to the urinary tract and reproductive organs.

The combination of Gallbladder 21 and 41, Liver 3, Pericardium 6, and Spleen 6 aid in balancing hormones and relaxing the nervous system.

AROMATHERAPY

For specific instructions on how to use aromatherapy, see PREPARING AROMATHERAPY TREATMENTS in Part Three.

Essential oil of peppermint has cooling properties; geranium and lavender oils are centering, either calming or energizing, depending on your needs. Add several drops of any or all of these oils to a lukewarm bath to cool hot flashes—or, if that is not possible, simply add them to cool water in a spray bottle and give yourself a cooling spritz. You can also use these oils as inhalants, diffuse them into the air in your home, or add a few drops to massage oil and use them in conjunction with massage.

Geranium, jasmine, myrrh, neroli, and vetiver oils are good for counteracting the visible signs of aging. Make a skin oil using one or several of these oils, or add a few drops of them to your favorite skin-care products (no more than 10 drops per ounce of product).

GENERAL RECOMMENDATIONS

Exercise! Not only does exercise keep your muscles toned and lift the spirits, but it is an important part of a program for preventing osteoporosis and cardiovascular disease. Weight-bearing exercise increases bone density; regular aerobic exercise keeps your entire body functioning better. Running, walking briskly, or doing low-impact aerobic workouts for at least thirty minutes three times each week is all it takes to benefit. If you suffer from insomnia, do your exercising in the early part of the day.

- Learn strategies to deal with stress, whether it be taking a walk, meditating, doing breathing exercises, practicing yoga, learning biofeedback, or any other approach.

- To enhance all-over circulation, use a loofa or friction mitt in the shower or bath. Massage yourself briskly all over your body, then shower.

- For hot flashes, some combination of the following is often helpful:

  - Increased consumption of green vegetables and water.
  - Mild exercise to support circulation and relieve stress.
  - Stress-relieving strategies such as meditation, breathing exercises, and others.
  - A multivitamin and mineral supplement, plus supplemental pantothenic acid, vitamin E, and flaxseed or evening primrose oil.
  - An herb such as black cohosh, chaste tree berry, dong quai, or red clover.

- For fatigue, some combination of the following is often helpful:

  - A multivitamin and mineral supplement, plus supplemental magnesium and malic acid and royal jelly.
  - Siberian ginseng and/or ginkgo biloba.

- For anxiety and/or insomnia, some combination of the following is often helpful:

  - Regular exercise (done in the early part of the day only).
  - Stress-relieving strategies such as meditation, breathing exercises, and others.
  - A multivitamin and mineral supplement, plus supplemental L-tryptophan.
  - The herbs kava kava, oat straw, valerian, linden flower, passionflower, and/or lemon balm.

- For depression, some combination of the following is often helpful:

  - Regular exercise.
  - Dietary measures to keep blood-sugar levels even and, if necessary, supplemental chromium picolinate.
  - A multivitamin and mineral supplement, plus supplemental vitamin B_{12} (in injections, if possible) and L-glutamine.
  - St. John's wort.

- For aches and pains in the muscles and/or joints, some combination of the following is often helpful:

  - Mild exercise, including weight-bearing exercise.
  - A multivitamin and mineral supplement, plus supplemental glucosamine sulfate, chondroitin sulfate, and/or evening primrose or flaxseed oil. In addition, make certain that your calcium intake equals approximately 1,200 milligrams daily, and your magnesium intake 600 to 800 milligrams daily.

- If you are interested in exploring hormone replacement therapy, discuss with your doctor the possible use of natural hormone replacement using triple-estrogen, or "triest," and natural progesterone. These are available from compounding pharmacists. Excellent books on the subject are *The HRT Solution* by Marla Ahlgrimm and John M. Kells (Avery, 1999) and *Natural Hormone Replacement* by Jonathan V. Wright and John Morgenthaler (Smart Publications, 1997). Also consider reading *What Your Doctor May Not Tell You About Menopause* by John R. Lee (Warner Books, 1996).

■ If you are suffering from a depressed sex drive, you may want to speak with your gynecologist about the possibility of trying topical testosterone gel or cream.

PREVENTION

■ Menopause is a natural part of life, and therefore cannot be prevented. However, it can be a more pleasant experience than many people believe. Consider learning stress-management techniques or joining a support group. Remember, this is not an illness, but a transition. As such, it offers you a good opportunity to identify and explore changes you may need to make in your life and lifestyle.

Menstrual Problems

The menstrual cycle is a normal and predictable cycle that involves the shedding of the uterine lining once a month. The cycle repeats itself throughout a woman's reproductive years. A complete menstrual cycle can be anywhere from twenty-one to thirty-five days long, with a twenty-eight-day cycle being average. The menstrual period, which marks the beginning of the cycle, lasts from three to seven days. During the rest of the cycle, intricate physical and hormonal changes occur that prepare the body for the possibility of pregnancy.

During the first half of the cycle, the ovary prepares to release an egg. The body increases production of the hormone estrogen, and the pituitary gland releases follicle-stimulating hormone, causing an egg-bearing follicle in the ovary to develop. About halfway into the menstrual cycle, ovulation occurs and an egg is released from the follicle. This is followed by a rise in the hormone progesterone, which prepares the uterus for the implantation of a fertilized egg, and a drop in the level of estrogen. Progesterone influences the lining of the uterus to become rich in blood vessels and glandular tissue—a nourishing soft, spongy "nest." If the egg is not fertilized, however, the nest the body has prepared is not needed and, about a week after ovulation, the level of progesterone begins to drop. This drop culminates in menstruation, and the enriched spongy lining of the uterus leaves the body as menstrual blood. About one-quarter cup of blood is lost with the average menstrual period.

The most frequent problem experienced by women during menstruation is abdominal cramping. Medically, menstrual cramps are known as *dysmenorrhea,* which literally means "painful menstruation." Menstrual cramps usually occur just before the cycle starts or with the onset of menstruation. They can last anywhere from a few hours to a few days. Menstrual cramps feel like muscle contractions or sharp spasms in the lower abdomen. They may radiate to the back or down the thighs, and range from mildly achy to wrenchingly painful. In women with severe menstrual problems, cramping may be accompanied by nausea, vomiting, headache, nervousness, fatigue, diarrhea, fainting, bloating, breast tenderness, mood swings, backache, and/or dizziness.

Women who suffer from cramps seem to produce greater amounts of prostaglandins, which are hormones secreted by the uterine lining, than other women do. These hormones affect the smooth muscle of the uterus, causing an increase in uterine contractions. The contractions interfere with blood flow, reducing the amount of oxygen reaching the uterus and resulting in pain. A large increase in prostaglandins can also cause strong gastrointestinal contractions, which may be responsible for the diarrhea, nausea, and vomiting associated with severe menstrual cramps.

An estimated half of all women experience menstrual cramps at some point in their lives, and more than 10 percent of those who suffer from menstrual cramps have pain severe enough that it interferes with their usual daily routines. While irregular periods are common among young girls just entering puberty, cramps are not. Cramps usually begin with the onset of ovulatory cycles, which typically happens six months to two years after the first menstrual period. It is not known why some women suffer from cramps and others do not. However, we do know that physically active, athletic women are less likely to suffer from menstrual cramps, as are women who have had children. Anemia, fatigue, obesity, and diabetes are other factors that may predispose a woman to menstrual cramps. In some cases, the tendency to suffer from cramps seems to run in families.

If you are having menstrual cramps, you may not feel up to socializing or participating in your usual daily activities. Suffering through a day or two of menstrual cramps can be difficult, but can usually be managed using the remedies outlined in this entry. If you ever experience severe abdominal pain, however—as opposed to cramping or an achy feeling—you should consult a health-care provider for advice. This can be a sign of a more serious problem, such as an internal infection, ectopic pregnancy, endometriosis, pelvic adhesions, or cysts in the genitourinary tract. A professional diagnosis is essential, especially if you are fitted with an intrauterine device (IUD) or are taking birth control pills.

Other types of menstrual problems include persistently irregular menstrual cycles, a change in the normal pattern of cycles, or an unusual amount of blood loss. If you have any of these problems, consult your health-care provider. Irregular or changing cycles may indicate an endocrine problem. Prolonged or excessive bleeding can lead to anemia.

Menstrual irregularities are common in the first few years after menstruation begins and as menopause approaches (*see* MENOPAUSE). Other difficulties associated with the menstrual cycle fall under the general term *premenstrual syndrome,* or PMS (*see* PREMENSTRUAL SYNDROME).

In most cases, menstrual cramps are a short-term annoyance that can be treated successfully at home.

CONVENTIONAL TREATMENT

■ The drugs most often suggested for menstrual cramps are nonsteroidal anti-inflammatory drugs (NSAIDs), including ibuprofen (available in Advil, Motrin, Nuprin, and other products), naproxen (Aleve, Anaprox, Naprelan, Naprosyn), and mefenamic acid (Ponstel). Some are available over the counter; others require a prescription. These medications work by blocking the production of prostaglandins, thereby decreasing the intensity of uterine contractions. Because they typically take up to two hours to work, they should be taken as soon as cramping starts. These drugs are generally well tolerated, although they can cause gastrointestinal upset and bleeding in the stomach in some cases. These drugs are not recommended for people with ulcers, asthma, or liver or kidney disease. Take them with food to lessen possible stomach upset.

■ Oral contraceptives are sometimes recommended for the relief of menstrual cramps. They work by interfering with the hormonal process that leads to ovulation. As a result, the body does not build up or shed the lining of the uterus, so fewer cramp-inducing prostaglandins are released. A doctor may recommend oral contraceptives for a woman with menstrual cramps who cannot tolerate NSAIDs, or for a woman who wants birth control coupled with pain relief. Oral contraceptives are associated with many different side effects, some of them potentially dangerous. They should not be taken for menstrual cramps without serious consideration, especially if you smoke and/or are over thirty-five.

DIETARY GUIDELINES

■ Dietary treatment is directed toward making the lower abdomen a friendly and relaxed place prior to the onset of the menstrual period. Cramps are often exaggerated by a poor diet. Many women experience tremendous relief from cramps when they improve their diets. A good diet is so beneficial that it alone may completely resolve menstrual cramps. (*See* DIET AND NUTRITION in Part One.)

■ Avoid foods that cause gas. These include sugar, fats, and any other foods that make the lower abdomen uncomfortable, such as cucumbers, peppers, and the like. These foods, especially if eaten during the week before menstruation, will often exacerbate cramps. Fats in particular are difficult to digest and contribute to a toxic environment. Saturated fats promote the production of the types of prostaglandins that contribute to cramping.

■ Eat a diet high in fiber to promote regularity. Constipation can make menstrual cramps worse.

■ Eat plenty of lightly steamed green vegetables, which are rich sources of vitamins and minerals.

■ Avoid alcohol, caffeine, and refined sugar, all of which promote inflammation and can increase cramping.

NUTRITIONAL SUPPLEMENTS

■ Bioflavonoids protect and keep the capillaries healthy, and help to prevent excessive bleeding. With heavy bleeding, take 500 milligrams of mixed bioflavonoids and an equal amount of vitamin C four to six times daily.

■ Borage oil, evening primrose oil, and flaxseed oil supply gamma-linolenic acid (GLA), which helps to balance out the inflammatory prostaglandins by acting as a source of their anti-inflammatory counterparts. Take 500 to 1,000 milligrams of any of these oils twice a day for three months.

■ Fish oil is a very effective anti-inflammatory. Some experts have compared it to aspirin and accetaminophen in its effectiveness. Take 500 to 1,000 milligrams two or three times daily. If it causes digestive upset, reduce the dosage or discontinue the supplement.

■ Magnesium relaxes the uterine muscles and is a very helpful nutrient for menstrual cramps. Beginning one week before the expected onset of menstruation, take 100 milligrams of magnesium two to three times daily. The day before menstruation begins, take 100 milligrams three times daily, and on the first day of menstruation, take 100 milligrams four to five times daily. If the magnesium causes loose stool, reduce the dosage. Try it again, at a lower dose and in combination with calcium, during the next cycle.

■ If you are unable to tolerate taking magnesium orally, try taking an Epsom salts bath each day on the two days before the expected onset of menstruation and on the first day of your period.

■ Fish-oil supplements are rich in omega-3 essential fatty acids (EFAs), which help ease menstrual problems. An adequate intake of omega-3 EFAs is associated with fewer menstrual problems in general. Take 500 to 1,000 milligrams of fish oil twice daily.

■ Vitamin B$_6$ (pyridoxine) is often used as a supplement

in the treatment of menstrual cramps and other menstrual symptoms. Beginning five days before the anticipated onset of menstruation, take 50 milligrams twice daily, between meals. If you take any of the B vitamins individually, you should also take a B-complex supplement at a different time of day.

■ Vitamin C is a mild anti-inflammatory; bioflavonoids enhance the action of vitamin C. Five days before the expected onset of menstruation, start taking 250 milligrams of mineral ascorbate vitamin C and an equal amount of bioflavonoids three times a day, and continue until the cramping subsides.

■ Vitamin E, the B vitamins, and zinc can also be helpful against menstrual cramping, especially if you cannot resist the temptation to eat junk foods. Starting ten days before the anticipated onset of menstruation, take 100 international units of vitamin E twice a day (once in the morning and again at bedtime); plus a vitamin-B complex that contains 25 milligrams of each B vitamin and 5 to 10 milligrams of zinc twice daily. Take zinc with food to prevent stomach upset. Continue taking these supplements for as long as cramping lasts.

■ Menorrhagia, or excessive bleeding, can cause serious problems, including anemia, if too much blood loss occurs month after month. Bioflavonoids can reduce excessive menstrual discharge. They also act to protect and strengthen the capillaries. Take 500 milligrams twice daily, with an equal amount of vitamin C. By the second cycle after you start taking them, you should notice an improvement. If not, consult your doctor.

■ To reduce heavy bleeding and control menorrhagia, take 25,000 international units of vitamin A twice daily for one week before your period starts.

Note: If there is a chance you might be pregnant, or if you have liver disease, consult your doctor before taking supplemental vitamin A. Pregnant women should not ingest a total of more than 25,000 international units of supplemental vitamin A *per week* from all sources.

■ Women with a heavy menstrual flow are often deficient in vitamin B_{12}. If menorrhagia is a problem, take 250 micrograms of sublingual vitamin B_{12} once or twice daily for one week, then reduce to 1,000 micrograms once weekly. If you take any of the B vitamins individually, you should also take a B-complex supplement at a different time of day.

HERBAL TREATMENT

■ Butiao, a Chinese patent medicine, has been used for more than 1,000 years to treat menstrual cramps associated with excessive menstrual bleeding. For six months, take the equivalent of 500 milligrams three times daily during the two weeks before the anticipated onset of your period.

■ Chamomile is an herbal relaxant. Drink a cup of chamomile tea as needed.

■ Chaste tree berry (also known by its Latin name, *Vitex agnus-castus*) helps to regulate the hormonal cycle. Take 200 milligrams of standardized extract twice a day for the ten days preceeding the anticipated onset of your menstrual period.

■ Prepare a soothing herbal bath. Mix 1 quart of strong chamomile tea and 1 quart of ginger tea with warm to hot bath water, and enjoy a leisurely soak.

■ The Chinese herb dong quai helps to regulate the menstrual cycle by balancing female hormones. When taken for a few months, particularly if taken in combination with red raspberry leaf, it helps to alleviate cramping. Begin by taking 500 milligrams of dong quai or a dong quai and red raspberry leaf combination formula twice daily from day six through day twenty of the menstrual cycle (day one of the cycle is the first day of menstrual bleeding). Continue taking this dose twice daily for three weeks of each menstrual cycle. If your cycles are irregular, take the herbs for two to three weeks out of every month. Repeat this program for at least three menstrual cycles. Do not take this remedy during the menstrual period itself, however.

■ A hot ginger-tea compress placed on the lower abdomen helps to relax muscle cramping. Boil 6 ounces of fresh ginger root in 1 quart of water for fifteen to twenty minutes. Put a washcloth or hand towel in the hot ginger water and take it out when it is cool enough to handle. You can either place the saturated cloth directly on your abdomen or wrap it first with a dry cloth. Ginger is warming and increases circulation in the lower abdomen. This compress will feel like a deep-heating rub.

■ True cramp bark, a little-known botanical, is effective in treating menstrual cramps. Take a cup of true cramp bark tea twice daily for three days before the expected onset of your menstrual period, and three times daily during your period if you get cramps.

HOMEOPATHY

For long-term relief of menstrual cramps, it may be most helpful to consult a homeopathic physician for a constitutional remedy. Otherwise, try the most appropriate of the symptom-specific remedies below.

■ *Colocynthis* is especially effective against cramps that cause a sharp, stabbing pain and for those that feel better with mild pressure on the abdomen. Take one dose of *Colocynthis* 6x, 12x, or 6c every fifteen minutes for one hour. Then take one dose three times daily until the cramping subsides.

■ *Magnesia phosphorica* relieves menstrual cramps that feel better with heat on the lower abdomen. Start by taking one dose of *Magnesia phosphorica* 6x or 6c every fifteen minutes for one hour. Thereafter, take one dose three times daily until the cramping subsides.

■ You can alternate between *Colocynthis* and *Magnesia phosphorica* to relieve menstrual cramps. Take one dose of *Colocynthis* 6x, 12x, or 6c. Fifteen minutes later, take one dose of *Magnesia phosphorica* 6x or 6c. Repeat the cycle, alternating the remedies every fifteen minutes, for one hour or until the cramping is relieved. Resume the regimen if the cramps return.

■ Try *Pulsatilla* if you are a fair-haired, blue-eyed young woman with late and/or irregular periods and menstrual cramps. You are probably somewhat timid, perhaps frightened of men, and may tend to cry easily, especially during the premenstrual period. The day before the expected onset of your period, take one dose of *Pulsatilla* 30x or 9c three times daily. During your period, take one dose three times daily, as needed.

■ Choose *Sepia* if you are a brown-eyed, dark-haired woman. You are probably thin, enjoy exercising, and often experience low back pain with menstrual cramping. The day before the expected onset of your period, take one dose of *Sepia* 30x or 9c three times daily. During your period, take one dose three times daily, as needed.

■ *Viburnum* 30x or 9c is recommended if your period comes late, with diminished blood flow and pain in the abdomen that extends into your legs. Take one dose of *Viburnum* 30x or 9c three times daily for up to three days.

ACUPRESSURE/MASSAGE

For the locations of acupressure points on the body, *see* ADMINISTERING AN ACUPRESSURE TREATMENT in Part Three.

■ Bladder 20 to 28 relax the nerves of the uterus.

■ Gallbladder 34 helps to relax muscles.

■ Large Intestine 4 removes energy blocks in the large intestine, thus promoting a healthier lower abdomen. Massaging this point also relaxes the nervous system.

■ Liver 3, Spleen 6, and Stomach 36 is the most common acupressure point combination used for relief of menstrual cramps.

■ The points along either side of the spine relax the entire body.

■ Massaging the abdomen and lower back can be beneficial. Massage can be particularly helpful for relieving lower back pain.

AROMATHERAPY

For specific instructions on how to use aromatherapy, *see* PREPARING AROMATHERAPY TREATMENTS in Part Three.

■ Essential oils of clary sage, cypress, and lavender can help ease the pain of menstrual cramps. Use any or all of them to prepare a soothing bath or add them to massage oil and gently massage your abdomen with the oil.

■ If you experience heavy bleeding, try aromatherapy baths prepared with cypress, geranium, and/or rose oil.

GENERAL RECOMMENDATIONS

■ Get regular exercise. Swimming, biking, and walking are all very helpful.

■ Try using sanitary pads instead of tampons, at least during the first two days of your period. The presence of a tampon can sometimes cause cramping by itself. The use of tampons can also lead to a low-grade infection that exaggerates cramping. It may be helpful to try going without them for a couple of months to see if there is any change in symptoms.

■ Acupuncture has been shown to relieve menstrual cramps. Licensed acupuncturists have established practices in most larger cities. Ask your health-care provider to recommend one. If he or she is unable to provide a referral, an organization such as the American Association of Oriental Medicine or the National Commission for Acupuncture and Oriental Medicine may be able to help (see the Resources section at the end of the book).

■ Simple stretching will often relieve the abdominal cramps and lower back pain that can accompany menstruation. One helpful exercise is to put your hands on your hips and rotate your hips in a circle 15 times in one direction and then 15 times in the other direction. You can do up to a total of 120 circles. Start doing this exercise one week before menstruation begins and continue throughout your period. The idea is to keep energy moving in your pelvis and abdomen.

■ Yoga can be very helpful. *A Gem for Women* by Geeta S. Iyengar (Timeless Books, 1990) is a good resource book.

■ Investigate biofeedback, visualization, and other relaxation techniques. All can be very effective.

■ Welcome the menstrual cycle as a natural and important part of your body's functions. Tension and negative feelings can make cramping worse. This is a good time to learn about and get in touch with your body. *Understanding Your Body* by Felicia H. Stewart (Bantam, 1987) is a good, readable reference that thoroughly covers topics such as anatomy, physiology, the menstrual cycle, birth control, premenstrual syndrome, and menstrual discomfort.

PREVENTION

■ Follow a healthy diet, starting with the suggestions under Dietary Guidelines, above.

■ Get plenty of vigorous exercise. Women who are physically active are less likely to suffer from menstrual cramps.

■ Take dong quai and red raspberry leaf herbal combination as suggested under Herbal Treatment, above.

Migraine

See under HEADACHE.

Milroy's Disease

See LYMPHEDEMA.

Mitral Valve Prolapse

See under CARDIOVASCULAR DISEASE.

Mononucleosis

Infectious mononucleosis, commonly called "mono," is an acute infection of the throat and lymph nodes caused by the Epstein-Barr virus (EBV). Mono is often mistaken for a case of the flu. In childhood, the disease is mild and can pass unnoticed. However, when an adult contracts mononucleosis, the symptoms are usually more severe.

Because the virus is transmitted through infected saliva, mononucleosis is sometimes called "kissing disease." As a result, some people are initially amused when they come down with mono—until they discover that their activities must be severely restricted to ensure a full recovery. Actually, the virus may be spread through coughing or sneezing as well as kissing.

The condition gets its name from a characteristic increase in the number of mononuclear white blood cells. The symptoms of mononucleosis often resemble those of other infectious illnesses, but tend to be more persistent. They include a vague feeling of achiness and discomfort, a pronounced feeling of fatigue or weakness, headache, a tendency to feel chilled, moderate to high fever, sore throat, lymph nodes that become enlarged and remain that way for a week or more, and a bumpy red rash. A doctor's examination may reveal an enlarged spleen and

abnormal liver function. A person who has mononucleosis usually feels weak and very tired.

The infection generally lasts from two to four weeks, although the older a person is when it strikes, the more severe the symptoms and the longer the recovery time. It is not uncommon to feel more tired than usual for several months afterward. Potential complications of the disease include obstruction of the upper airway, difficulty swallowing, depression of the immune system, and liver disease. In exceptionally severe cases, the spleen may become very enlarged and then rupture (usually after a fall or similar trauma), making emergency surgery necessary.

Mononucleosis must be diagnosed by a blood test that detects an elevated concentration of antibodies to the Epstein-Barr virus, an elevated lymphocyte (white blood cell) count, or other characteristic abnormalities. If these tests confirm a diagnosis of mono, your liver function will probably be measured as well, and your doctor will do a physical examination to check for an enlarged spleen or liver, and to look for pus and inflammation in the back of your throat.

Note that the treatment recommendations in this section are intended for adults. To determine appropriate treatment approaches for a child or teenager, consult your physician or *Smart Medicine for a Healthier Child* (Avery, 1994).

CONVENTIONAL TREATMENT

There is no cure for mononucleosis. Treatment is aimed at relieving the symptoms and being alert for the development of complications while the virus runs its course.

■ To prevent serious damage to your liver and spleen, your health-care provider will prescribe bed rest, probably for one to four weeks. As long as your spleen is enlarged, you must avoid strenuous exercise, especially contact sports.

■ If you are uncomfortable or have a fever, aspirin (in Bayer, Ecotrin, and many other products) or ibuprofen (Advil, Motrin, Nuprin, and others) may be helpful. Acetaminophen (Tylenol, Datril, and others) is another possibility, but check with your doctor first. If your liver is inflamed, acetaminophen may add to your problems.

Note: In excessive amounts, acetaminophen can cause liver damage. Do not exceed the recommended dosage. Take aspirin or ibuprofen with food to prevent possible stomach upset.

■ Steroids such as dexamethasone (Decadron) are sometimes used, but only if you have such severe complications as an airway obstruction.

■ A strep throat often accompanies mononucleosis. If a throat culture reveals a strep infection, your doctor will prescribe an oral antibiotic. Although penicillin (sold under the brand names Bicillin, Pfizerpen, Wycillin, among others) is often the drug of choice for strep, it can cause an allergic rash in some people with mononucleosis and should be used cautiously. Erythromycin (ERYC, Ilotycin, and others) is a better choice.

DIETARY GUIDELINES

Drink plenty of pure water to flush toxins from your body. If swallowing is difficult, as it often is for people with mononucleosis, take frequent small sips of fluids to prevent dehydration.

Lemonade made with freshly squeezed lemon juice helps to dilute mucus and soothes the throat. Frozen fruit-juice popsicles also are soothing to an inflamed throat. Take pure fruit juices and fresh, whole fruits as well.

To support the healing process, eat healthy, nutrient-rich whole foods. Base your diet primarily on lean proteins, grains, fruits, and vegetables. Hot soups are a good source of nutrients, and are easier to take than whole foods.

Reduce your consumption of fats, especially saturated and hydrogenated fats. This virus affects the spleen and the liver. The liver has to work very hard to metabolize fats. Give your liver time to rest and heal.

■ Eliminate sugary foods, commercially prepared and additive-laden convenience foods, soft drinks, and all processed foods from your diet. All of these contribute to a toxic internal environment.

NUTRITIONAL SUPPLEMENTS

Green-foods supplements such as spirulina or chlorella have many vitamins and trace minerals that speed healing. Take a chlorophyll supplement as directed on the product label.

Lipoic acid improves energy metabolism by facilitating better conversion of carbohydrates to energy. This mechanism is often not working as it should in people who have mononucleosis. Take 500 to 100 milligrams two or three times daily.

■ Magnesium and malic acid act to improve energy levels, often quite remarkably. Take a combination formula supplying 100 milligrams of magnesium and 300 milligrams of malic acid three times daily, one-half to one hour before each meal.

Nicotinamide adenine dinucleotide hydrogen (NADH) is an important energizing coenzyme that stimulates the production of the neurotransmitters dopamine, noradrenaline, and serotonin, thereby helping to improve alertness, mental clarity, and concentration. Taking 10 milligrams one-half hour before breakfast often improves concentration, stamina, and energy.

■ The B vitamins increase energy. Once the fever has sub-

sided and the acute phase of the infection is resolved, take a B-complex supplement supplying 25 to 50 milligrams of each of the major B vitamins twice a day.

■ Vitamin C and bioflavonoids have antiviral and anti-inflammatory properties. Take 1,000 milligrams of mineral ascorbate vitamin C with an equal amount of bioflavonoids three to four times a day during the acute phase and twice a day thereafter, until the illness is completely resolved.

■ Vitamin E boosts the immune response and helps to protect the liver from inflammation. Choose a product containing mixed tocopherols and begin by taking 200 international units daily, then gradually increase the dosage until you are taking 400 international units twice a day. Maintain this dosage for one month.

Note: If you have high blood pressure, limit your intake of supplemental vitamin E to a total of 400 international units daily. If you are taking an anticoagulant (blood thinner), consult your physician before taking supplemental vitamin E.

■ Zinc helps to stimulate the immune system. Take 10 to 25 milligrams twice a day for one month. Take zinc with food to prevent stomach upset. If you take over 30 milligrams of zinc on a daily basis for more than one or two months, you should also take 1 to 2 milligrams of copper each day to maintain a proper mineral balance.

HERBAL TREATMENT

■ Yin Qiao is a Chinese herbal formula that is the first remedy to give in the initial stages of mononucleosis. It is helpful for relieving the initial feeling of achiness associated with mono. Take 2 or 3 tablets three times daily for the first three days.

■ Echinacea and goldenseal have antiviral and antibacterial properties. They help to boost the immune system and fight infection. Take one dose of an echinacea and goldenseal combination formula supplying 250 to 500 milligrams of echinacea and 150 to 300 milligrams of goldenseal three times daily for the first week. The second week, discontinue it, and then resume it for the third week.

■ Garlic has antiviral properties helpful in the treatment of mononucleosis. Take 500 milligrams twice a day for two to three weeks.

■ Marshmallow root and licorice root are soothing for a sore throat. Make a combination herbal tea and drink a cup two or three times a day for two days to relieve throat pain, or use it as a throat spray two or three times daily.

Note: Do not use licorice on a daily basis for more than five days at a time, as it can elevate blood pressure. Do not take it at all if you have high blood pressure.

■ Milk thistle contains silymarin, which helps to restore

and protect the liver. If you have liver inflammation and blood tests show elevated levels of liver enzymes, silymarin will help to resolve this. Choose an extract standardized to contain 80 percent flavonoids (silymarin) and take 200 to 300 milligrams twice a day for one month.

■ Olive leaf extract has powerful antiviral properties. Take 250 milligrams of standardized extract three times a day for two months.

☐ Shiitake mushrooms help the immune system fight off viruses. After the fever has subsided, take 250 to 500 milligrams three times daily for two weeks. Then take the same dosage twice daily for one month.

☐ Astragalus is a Chinese botanical that helps to strengthen the immune system and increase energy and is helpful in the recovery stage. You should not use this herb if you have a fever or any other signs of acute infection, however. After the fever subsides, take 500 milligrams of standardized extract in the morning and again in the afternoon for one month.

HOMEOPATHY

☐ If you have a persistent sore throat, take one dose of *Mercurius corrosivus* or *Mercurius solubilis* 12x or 6c three to four times daily for up to three days.

☐ For swollen lymph glands in the neck, take one dose of *Phytolacca* 12x or 6c four times daily for up to four days.

☐ If you have heavy, droopy eyes; feel weak and tired; and have aches and chills running up and down your back, take one dose of *Gelsemium* 9x or 30c three to four times a day for two days.

■ Consult a homeopathic physician for a constitutional remedy.

ACUPRESSURE

For the locations of acupressure points on the body, *see* ADMINISTERING AN ACUPRESSURE TREATMENT in Part Three.

☐ Gallbladder 20 and 21 help to bring down energy from the head and keep it circulating throughout the body to promote healing.

☐ Liver 3 helps to ease headache pain.

☐ Liver 4 helps to bring down a fever.

■ Stomach 36 energizes the digestive and immune systems, and helps to bring down fever.

■ Massaging down both sides of the spine helps to relax the nervous system.

BACH FLOWER REMEDIES

Select the remedy that most closely fits your emotional tendencies and concerns, and take it as needed, following the directions on the product label.

■ Holly helps to tone down feelings of anger at being sick.

■ Impatiens is good if you are feeling extremely impatient to be well.

■ Wild oat helps to counteract fatigue and difficulty reentering your daily routine.

AROMATHERAPY

For specific instructions on how to use aromatherapy, *see* PREPARING AROMATHERAPY TREATMENTS in Part Three.

■ A lukewarm bath prepared with elemi, myrrh, pine, and/or tea tree oil can help to ease a fever and achiness.

■ Peppermint oil helps to relieve headache pain. Add a few drops of peppermint oil to massage oil and gently massage the mixture into your temples. Be sure to keep the oil away from your eyes, and do not use it on broken skin. Or add peppermint oil to cool water and use it to make a compress. Apply the compress to your forehead (avoiding your eyes) or the back of your neck and leave it in place for at least ten minutes.

■ Essential oil of basil, elemi, geranium, lavender, patchouli, peppermint, pine, thyme, and vetiver are energizing and stimulating. If fatigue is a problem once the acute phase of the disease is over, add one or more of these essential oils to bath water or massage oil, use them as inhalants, or diffuse them into the air in your home.

GENERAL RECOMMENDATIONS

■ For a full recovery, unlimited rest is absolutely essential. Limit your physical activity in accordance with your doctor's orders. In the acute stage, you will probably be glad to rest. When you begin to feel restless, keep yourself busy with "effort-free" distractions such as movies, books, and magazines.

■ A bath prepared with 2 pounds each of Epsom salts and baking soda is very relaxing. Remain in the bath for ten to twenty minutes.

■ Remember that recovery is a gradual process. Returning to full activity too soon can prolong the time it takes for full healing.

■ Make sure you avoid strenuous exercise until your doctor certifies that recovery is complete. The spleen can become enlarged with mononucleosis, and an enlarged spleen can rupture easily, necessitating surgery.

■ Once you are able to be up and about, a modest twenty-minute walk every day will help to increase circulation and build strength.

■ *See* FEVER; HEADACHE; and/or SORE THROAT for additional suggestions regarding those symptoms. A mild form of hepatitis is also a possible complication (*see* HEPATITIS).

Motion Sickness

Whether you are traveling by car, boat, train, or plane, motion sickness can spoil a good time. Motion sickness is caused by excessive stimulation of the vestibular apparatus, located in the inner ear, which is responsible for maintaining a sense of balance and equilibrium.

Abnormal or irregular body motions or postures, as well as repeated acceleration and deceleration, such as occur in a moving car, on the deck of a boat, or in an airplane, disturb the delicate balance mechanisms in the inner ear. Because the eyes transmit messages to this seat of balance, visual cues also play a part. When the body is passively being transported while the landscape rushes by, the contradictory stimuli can confuse and disrupt the vestibular apparatus, resulting in symptoms of motion sickness.

Symptoms vary from person to person. Motion sickness usually starts with a general sense of discomfort and uneasiness. You may look noticeably pale, even a little green. You may feel dizzy and complain of a "sick headache." Motion sickness can escalate into vomiting and unremitting nausea.

Unfortunately, instant relief doesn't occur at journey's end. It can take several hours for the body to recover completely from motion sickness, even after the trip is over.

This condition is easier to prevent than it is to cure. If you are subject to motion sickness, keep in mind that whatever treatment you choose, it is best to begin using it before the trip begins.

CONVENTIONAL TREATMENT

■ Antihistamines like dimenhydrinate (Dramamine), meclizine (Antivert, Bonine), or diphenhydramine (Benadryl) are usually the first conventional medicines recommended for motion sickness, and they may be effective. You must take this type of product before symptoms arise, however; they are not as effective if you are already feeling sick. Common side effects include drowsiness and dry mouth, although these drugs can cause agitation in some people. You should not take them without first consulting with your physician if you have asthma, glaucoma, or an enlarged prostate. Avoid alcohol while taking these medications.

■ Antiemetics (drugs that stop vomiting) can be very effective for motion sickness, but can also cause more serious side effects. Promethazine (Phenergan) is one exam-

ple. In addition to drowsiness, these agents can cause blood abnormalities, liver damage, and, paradoxically, nausea. These drugs also are not suitable if you have glaucoma. Avoid alcohol while taking them.

■ A patch containing scopolamine (Transderm Scop) that can be placed behind one ear was very popular in the past, but the use of this belladonna derivative has decreased somewhat in recent years because of its side effects, which can include drowsiness and dry mouth, as well as confusion and disorientation, especially in older adults. This drug too should not be used by anyone with glaucoma, and you should avoid alcohol while using it. Also, when you apply or remove the patch, you must take care not to touch anywhere near your eyes without thoroughly washing your hands first, as a sudden and disconcerting (and, for glaucoma patients, dangerous) dilation of the pupils can occur.

DIETARY GUIDELINES

■ Use your judgment. Some people travel best on a full stomach, while others seem less bothered when traveling with an empty stomach.

■ Avoid fried or fatty foods before traveling. Greasy foods are more likely to cause an upset stomach.

HERBAL TREATMENT

■ Ginger is an effective treatment for nausea and motion sickness. Prepare and carry a Thermos of warm or room-temperature ginger tea and take it as needed. Or take a 500-milligram capsule every one to two hours until symptoms are eased.

HOMEOPATHY

Choose the most appropriate of the following symptom-specific homeopathic remedies and take one dose, as directed on the product label, one hour before traveling. Take a second dose upon entering the vehicle and another one hour into the trip.

■ *Cocculus* 12x or 6c will help if you feel nauseated and the mere smell of food makes you feel sick. You probably feel better under warm blankets.

■ If you feel better after eating, when resting quietly with your eyes closed, and when you know the trip will soon be over, take *Petroleum* 12x or 6c.

■ If you are pale, in a cold sweat, feel faint, and are nauseated and vomiting, take *Tabacum* 6x, 12x, or 5c.

ACUPRESSURE

For the locations of acupressure points on the body, *see* ADMINISTERING AN ACUPRESSURE TREATMENT in Part Three.

■ Four Gates will help you relax during a trip.

- Large Intestine 4 removes energy blocks in the large intestine, promoting a healthier lower abdomen.

- Liver 3 relaxes the nervous system and tones the digestive tract.

- Pericardium 6 helps relieve nausea.

AROMATHERAPY

For specific instructions on how to use aromatherapy, *see* PREPARING AROMATHERAPY TREATMENTS in Part Three.

- Essential oils of ginger and peppermint combat nausea. Carry either or a combination of both to use as an inhalant when you travel.

GENERAL RECOMMENDATIONS

- Plan ahead. When it comes to motion sickness, prevention is easier—and more likely to be successful—than treatment.

- Sometimes motion sickness can make you restless, and you may think that moving around will ease the discomfort. Don't. Movement actually makes motion sickness worse.

- Many people who suffer from motion sickness also experience severe pain in their ears when flying, particularly during ascent and descent. The pain is caused by air pressure changes that affect the inner ear as the air pressure in the cabin changes. Although ordinary ear plugs won't help, Ear Planes by Travel Smart are very effective. They act by maintaining an even air pressure within the ears. The same effect may be achieved by holding foam drinking cups very tightly over each ear. If you ask a flight attendant for two foam cups for your ears, she or he will understand. Some attendants will even wet paper towels with very hot water, wring them out well, and insert them in the bottom of the cups for you. The warmth is comforting, but this small addition is unnecessary.

PREVENTION

- Learn to hold your head very still while traveling. A strategically placed pillow will help.

- To avoid the confusion arising in the balance mechanism when the body is being passively transported and the eyes are viewing the landscape rushing by, focus on a fixed point on the far-distant horizon. The horizon is a constant and will appear to remain still.

- Having air blowing across your face can be very helpful in preventing and/or lessening motion sickness. Open a car window. Sit on the open deck of a boat. On an airplane, direct the air valve above your seat toward your face.

- Avoid anything involving reading while in a moving vehicle. This can often bring on an attack of motion sickness.

- You may be able to ward off an attack of motion sickness altogether by resting your head on the back of your seat, closing your eyes, and remaining very still.

Multiple Sclerosis

Multiple sclerosis (MS) is a disease of the central nervous system. Protective sheaths composed of a fatty substance called myelin cover nerve-cell fibers. In this disorder, myelin sheaths degenerate, leaving nerve fibers in the brain, the spinal cord, and the optic nerves vulnerable to damage and scarring. Areas of accumulated scarring are known as plaques. The nerve damage results in impairment and/or loss of function in the areas controlled by the affected nerves. Because nerve impulses sent from the brain via the spinal cord control the functioning of all parts of the body, damage to these nerves can affect any function or any organ. If the optic nerves are involved, vision can be impaired, and blindness is a possibility.

As many as 250,000 Americans are diagnosed with MS every year, usually in early adulthood. Approximately two-thirds of the people who currently have MS received their diagnoses when they were between the ages of twenty and forty, and more women than men are affected. Interestingly, this disorder is significantly more common among people who live in temperate climates than among those living in tropical areas of the world.

The severity and nature of symptoms a given individual experiences with MS depend on which nerves are affected. Neuromuscular symptoms of MS include muscle weakness, fatigue, slurred speech, clumsiness, unsteadiness, pins-and-needles sensations, numbness, tingling, feelings of constriction, dizziness, and memory loss. Your arms and legs may feel heavy and become weak. Stiffness and muscle spasms are common. If the nerve fibers controlling the bladder or bowels are involved, incontinence can be a problem, as can a loss of sexual desire and, for men, impotence. If the nerves in the brain are involved, symptoms can include blurred or double vision (or vision loss), and pain in the facial area. Mental changes, including wild mood swings ranging from euphoria to depression, are not uncommon. Digestive problems such as nausea, vomiting, and gastric reflux are a possibility also. Any of these symptoms can appear singly, but most people have two or more in combination.

As with symptoms, the course of this disease is extremely variable and impossible to predict. Most people have periods of remission punctuated by acute attacks, called exacerbations, but the duration of exacerbations, the length of time between them, and the degree to which normal functioning returns in the remission periods are all highly individual. An unfortunate minority become significantly disabled during the first year; others gradually develop increasing degrees of disability as attacks continue intermittently over the years; some have a series of flare-ups and suffer degrees of disability, but then never have another attack; still others have mild relapses followed by long periods when they remain symptom-free. A few experience a single attack and never have a second episode.

Although medical science has determined what is happening to the body in MS, why the myelin sheaths degenerate in the first place, and exactly what triggers this, have not yet been discovered. Currently, most researchers believe that the loss of myelin is caused by a virus or an autoimmune process, in which the body mistakenly reacts to some part of itself as foreign and attacks it. Some scientists believe that MS may result from a combination of a viral infection and autoimmunity complications—that infection with some as-yet-unidentified virus triggers the immune system, which then attacks myelin rather than destroying the virus. Heredity appears to play a role; relatives of people with MS are eight times more likely to contract it than other people are. Other theories that have been advanced include the possibility that chemical or heavy-metal poisoning may be involved—mercury poisoning has been shown to produce symptoms similar to MS in some people—and that food allergies, such as those experienced by people who cannot digest dairy products or wheat, may be a factor.

There is no single diagnostic test that can conclusively confirm MS. Diagnosis therefore is a process of elimination—excluding other conditions that can produce similar symptoms. A neurologist may do a spinal puncture and take fluid for laboratory analysis to check for characteristic abnormalities, and he or she may order a magnetic resonance imaging (MRI) scan to check for signs of the characteristic plaques.

Although there is no cure for MS, careful attention to diet, the right nutritional supplements, natural remedies, and the avoidance of stress are known to be helpful, particularly for those in the early stages of the disease. Also helpful is moderate, well-selected exercise.

CONVENTIONAL MEDICINE

■ Corticosteroids can sometimes shorten the length of time that an acute attack lasts, but they have no effect on how much you recover between episodes. A drug called interferon beta (Avonex, Betaseron) can reduce the frequency of episodes for some people. It is expensive, however, and not widely available. This drug is not recommended for anyone under the age of eighteen. Possible side effects include flulike symptoms, depression, palpitations, nausea, vomiting, blood-cell changes, shortness of breath, and burning on urination.

■ There is some question whether drugs that suppress the immune system might have a beneficial effect on long-term progression of the disease. Evidence of their benefit is incomplete, however, and they are still being studied in clinical trials. These agents, including cyclophosphamide (Cytoxan) and azathioprine (Imuran), have extremely serious side effects, including cancer, liver damage, kidney damage, and hair loss, so you should discuss the potential risks and benefits thoroughly with your physician before deciding to take one of these drugs.

■ Injections of glatiramer copolymer (Copaxone) may help prevent flare-ups and slow the progression of MS, though studies of this drug are still under way. It is not recommended for anyone under eighteen years of age. Possible side effects include infections, joint pains, chest pain, nausea, dilation of the blood vessels, and reactions immediately following the injections.

DIETARY GUIDELINES

■ Follow a healthy low-fat, high-fiber dietary plan. Especially avoid saturated fats, such as those in meat (especially red meat) and dairy products, as well as all hydrogenated and partially hydrogenated fats. Instead of butter, margarine, and salad dressings containing hydrogenated fats, use olive oil.

■ Eat as many fresh vegetables as you can, especially leafy greens such as spinach, kale, and broccoli. Also maximize your intake of fresh fruits.

■ Try avoiding foods containing gluten for several months and see if your condition improves. This protein, which is present in wheat, rye, oats, and barley, can irritate the intestinal lining and may interfere with the absorption of nutrients. For grains, stick to brown rice, corn, and other grains such as millet, amaranth, and quinoa. Substitute rice, soy, or potato flour for wheat flour in recipes. Also be aware that gluten can be a hidden ingredient in processed food products, showing up on the label as "hydrolyzed protein," "textured vegetable protein," "cereal fillers," "malt," and "modified food starch," among other things.

■ Avoid packaged and processed foods that contain synthetic colorings, flavorings, preservatives, and other additives. These chemicals add to the stress your body must deal with and drain the system.

■ Avoid alcohol and caffeine, which stress the body and can worsen MS symptoms.

■ A program developed by Roy Swank, M.D., Ph.D., which is based on strict adherence to a diet very low in fat (and particularly in saturated fat) combined with fish-oil supplementation, regular rest periods, and stress reduction, has been reported to be very successful in slowing the progress of the disease and preventing or minimizing exacerbations. For detailed information about this program, you can consult *The Multiple Sclerosis Diet Book* by Dr. Swank and Barbara Brewer Dugan, R.N. (Doubleday, 1987).

NUTRITIONAL SUPPLEMENTS

■ Take a high-potency multivitamin and mineral supplement daily.

■ To make sure of complete utilization of all important nutrients, take a full-spectrum digestive-enzyme supplement providing 5,000 international units of lipase, 2,500 international units of amylase, and 300 international units of protease, plus 500 to 1,000 milligrams of pancreatin, with each meal.

Note: Long-term supplementation with pancreatin is not advised, as it can cause your pancreas to reduce its own production of this important enzyme. Overuse also has the potential to cause nausea or diarrhea. After two months on pancreatin, discontinue use and monitor your reaction. If you find that your problems recur, discuss pancreatin supplementation with your health-care provider.

■ Acidophilus and bifidobacteria are friendly bacteria essential for digestive and intestinal health. Take a probiotic supplement as recommended on the product label. If you are allergic to milk, select a dairy-free formula.

■ Black currant seed oil, borage oil, evening primrose oil, fish oil, and flaxseed oil are all good sources of essential fatty acids (EFAs). EFAs act as natural anti-inflammatories, improve immune function, and are important for the integrity of the brain and spinal cord. Taking 500 to 1,000 milligrams of one or more of these oils twice daily may reduce the severity of flare-ups and lengthen the period of remission in some people with MS.

■ Green-foods supplements supply important trace minerals and beta-carotene, which are often lacking in the diet. Take a green-foods supplement daily as directed on the product label.

■ N-acetylcysteine (NAC) helps to chelate toxic heavy metals so that they can be excreted from the body. Take 500 milligrams two or three times a day.

■ Selenium is an important antioxidant. Take 200 micrograms daily.

■ Taking thymus glandular extract helps to strengthen the thymus and enhance the activity of T-cells, which are key components of the immune system. Take 500 milligrams three times a day for two months, then cut back to 250 milligrams a day.

■ The B vitamins are essential for healthy nerve function. Take a good B-complex formula daily, as directed on the label, and ask your doctor about injections of vitamin B_{12}, which is often deficient in people with MS. If your doctor does not favor injections, take 500 micrograms of

vitamin B_{12} daily in addition to the complete B-complex formula.

■ Vitamin C and bioflavonoids maintain healthy collagen, fight infection, and improve the functioning of the immune system. Take 500 milligrams of vitamin C with bioflavonoids twice daily.

■ Zinc fights free-radical damage and supports the immune system. Take 15 to 25 milligrams twice daily.

Note: Take zinc with food to prevent stomach upset. If you take over 30 milligrams of zinc on a daily basis for more than one or two months, you should also take 1 to 2 milligrams of copper each day to maintain a proper mineral balance.

HERBAL TREATMENT

■ American and Chinese (Korean) ginseng help to improve energy levels, as well as to improve digestion. You can use either or both. Begin by taking half the manufacturer's recommended dose and gradually increase the amount until you are taking it as directed on the product label.

Note: Do not use American or Chinese ginseng if you have high blood pressure, heart disease, or hypoglycemia.

■ Astragalus is valuable if you have a history of fatigue and breathing difficulties. This herb improves energy levels and helps strengthen the respiratory system. Take 500 milligrams in the morning and again in the afternoon for one month. There are also many herbal formulas available that combine astragalus with Siberian ginseng, cordyceps, codonopsis, and/or other herbs. Follow the dosage directions on the product label.

Note: Do not take astragalus if you have a fever or any other signs of acute infection.

■ Bupleurum and dong quai improve the digestion and absorption of food, and also help to relax the nervous system. Take 1,000 milligrams of a bupleurum and dong quai combination formula two or three times daily for two weeks out of every month (if you are a woman, take it for the two weeks prior to the anticipated onset of your menstrual period).

■ Ginkgo biloba enhances the flow of oxygen to the brain and helps protect brain cells from the harmful effects of free radicals. Select a standardized extract that supplies 24 percent ginkgo heterosides (sometimes also called flavoglycosides) and take 40 milligrams three times daily.

■ Olive leaf extract has antiviral and antifungal properties. This may help to reestablish healthy intestinal flora in individuals in whom it is compromised. The digestive tract may be a source of immune-triggering reactions than could heighten MS symptoms. Take 250 milligrams of standardized extract three times a day for two months. Cat's claw can also be used for this purpose. Take 500 milligrams of standardized extract three times a day for two months.

■ Siberian ginseng supports proper blood-sugar regulation, and is gentler on the system than the more active American and Chinese ginseng. It has been shown to have a balancing or regulating effect on the endocrine system, especially the thyroid and adrenal glands. Select a standardized extract containing 0.5 percent eleutheroside E and take 100 milligrams twice daily.

HOMEOPATHY

When dealing with a serious, chronic disorder such as MS, it is best to consult a homeopathic practitioner for a constitutional remedy. You may also find one or more of the following symptom-specific remedies helpful. If you feel considerably better with any of these remedies, you may wish to consult a homeopath who can prescribe a higher potency remedy.

■ *Argentum nitricum* is valuable for weakness, trembling, unsteadiness when walking, difficulty with voluntary motion, nervousness, indigestion, numbness and stiffness of the arms and legs, and twitching muscles. You may have a salty taste in your mouth, and, because your mind is sluggish, you often find yourself having difficulty connecting with what is going on around you. Take one dose of *Argentum nitricum* 30x or 15c three times daily for three or four days, as needed.

■ *Aurum muriaticum* 30x or 15c is helpful for irritability, severe nervousness and agitation, suicidal fantasies, and a pronounced sensitivity to cold. Take one dose of *Aurum muriaticum* 30x or 15c three times daily for three days, as needed.

■ *Plumbum metallicum* is for lightning-like pain in the extremities, atrophying muscles, difficulty with speech, and obstinate constipation. You likely feel worse at night and with movement, better with massage and pressure. Take one dose of *Plumbum metallicum* 200x or 30c twice daily for two days out of every ten, through a total of forty days.

BACH FLOWER REMEDIES

Select the remedy that most closely fits your emotional tendencies and concerns, and take it as needed, following the directions on the product label.

■ Beech is the remedy of choice if you are feeling cranky and impatient.

■ Chicory will tame a need for constant attention.

■ Gorse helps to lift feelings of deep despair that strike from time to time.

■ Holly can help if you are filled with anger that bursts outward in fits of temper.

■ Hornbeam eases feelings of deep exhaustion.

ACUPRESSURE

For the locations of acupressure points on the body, *see* ADMINISTERING AN ACUPRESSURE TREATMENT in Part Three.

■ All back Bladder points increase circulation and relax the nervous system.

■ Gallbladder 34 and 41 help to relax the muscles.

■ Liver 3 relaxes the nervous system and relieves muscle cramps and spasms.

■ Stomach 36 energizes the digestive and immune systems, gradually improves absorption of nutrients, and strengthens overall well-being.

GENERAL RECOMMENDATIONS

■ Many people with MS find great relief from acupressure and massage. Ask a loved one to consider learning these techniques and practicing them regularly. If that is not possible, ask your physician for a referral to a qualified acupuncturist, acupressurist, and/or massage therapist.

■ Avoid tobacco smoke, which is toxic and can make MS symptoms worse.

■ Do not permit yourself to get too fatigued. Adequate rest is important.

■ A program of moderate exercise, such as walking, swimming, or yoga, can help to maintain mobility and prevent further degeneration. Light stretching exercises also are acceptable, and may be helpful. Tiring calisthenics and other strenuous exercise should be avoided, however, especially during flare-ups.

■ As much as possible, avoid stress, whether physical or psychological. Exposure to toxins, pollution, and extremes of temperature (especially heat) can all make symptoms worse. Relaxation techniques may be helpful for dealing with psychological stresses that cannot be avoided (*see* RELAXATION TECHNIQUES in Part Three).

Mumps

Mumps is a viral infection that affects the salivary glands, most commonly the parotid glands, which are located near the ears (hence its medical name, *parotitis*). The illness begins with a fever, headache, loss of appetite, malaise, and muscle aches. Pain in the ear and under the jaw begins about twenty-four hours later. Over the next one to three days, the salivary glands swell and become very tender. The swelling typically lessens over a course of three to seven days.

The illness is spread by contact with infected saliva. Once a person is infected with the virus, it can incubate for two to three and a half weeks before signs of infection appear. A person is contagious from about six days before the onset of illness to nine days after the glands have become swollen.

Mumps is most common in children between the ages of five and fifteen, although a person can get it at any age, and, like measles and chickenpox, it tends to cause greater discomfort if contracted in adulthood. Nevertheless, it is usually self-limiting and runs its course without complications. One possible long-term complication that does exist occurs in men and boys. If the virus attacks the testicles, it can cause pain and swelling while the disease is active and, in some cases, infertility in the long run.

Note that the different treatments recommended in this section are intended for adults. To determine correct treatment regimens for children, consult your physician or *Smart Medicine for a Healthier Child* (Avery, 1994).

CONVENTIONAL TREATMENT

■ Treatment of mumps focuses on easing discomfort as the virus runs its course. Acetaminophen (Tylenol, Datril, and others), aspirin (Bayer, Ecotrin, and others), or ibuprofen (Advil, Motrin, Nuprin, and others) will bring down a fever and ease the headache, muscle aches, and malaise that accompany the disease.

Note: In excessive amounts, acetaminophen can cause liver damage. If the recommended amount does not give the relief you want, do not increase the dosage, but try a different medication. Take aspirin or ibuprofen with food to prevent possible stomach upset.

■ Because mumps is a viral illness, antibiotic therapy is ineffective and therefore not appropriate.

■ Applying warm or cool compresses to the site of the swollen glands may help relieve the pain and tenderness.

■ If mumps causes testicular pain, bed rest is important. It may help lessen the pain if you support the scrotum using cotton held in place by an adhesive-tape "bridge" between the thighs, and/or if you apply ice packs. If pain and swelling are extremely severe, your doctor may prescribe a corticosteroid to combat these symptoms.

DIETARY GUIDELINES

■ Because mumps causes pain when you chew or swallow, and because the parotid glands cannot work efficiently to moisten the food you are eating when you have this disease, eat a diet of soft, moist foods. Puréed foods are a good choice.

■ Avoid citrus fruits and other acidic foods. These stimulate the parotid glands to secrete saliva, which can be a painful process if you have mumps.

■ Keep yourself well hydrated. The increased metabolic rate that results from a fever causes the body to lose fluids

rapidly. Take plenty of spring water, herbal teas, soups, and diluted fruit juices. Once the acute phase of the infection has subsided, immune-boosting astragalus and vegetable soup is very good for supporting recovery (*see* THERAPEUTIC RECIPES in Part Three).

■ Eliminate fats from your diet as much as possible. Fats are difficult to digest under normal circumstances, and are even harder to digest when the digestive system is weakened by infection. Undigested fats contribute to a toxic internal environment.

NUTRITIONAL SUPPLEMENTS

■ Vitamin A helps to heal mucous membranes. Take 10,000 international units of fish-oil vitamin A twice a day for ten days.

Note: If you are pregnant, or intend to get pregnant, or if you have liver disease, consult your doctor before taking supplemental vitamin A. Pregnant women should not ingest a total of more than 25,000 international units of supplemental vitamin A *per week* from all sources.

■ Vitamin C and bioflavonoids help to stimulate the immune system. For one week, take 500 milligrams of mineral ascorbate vitamin C with an equal amount of bioflavonoids three or four times a day. (If you develop loose stools, cut back on the dosage.) The following week, take the same dosage, but two to three times a day. During the third week, take the same dosage once or twice a day. Then continue to take one-half dose daily for the fourth week, and three times a week for the next two weeks.

■ Zinc stimulates the immune system and promotes healing. Take 15 to 25 milligrams twice a day for one week to ten days. Take zinc with food to prevent stomach upset. If you take over 30 milligrams of zinc on a daily basis for more than one or two months, you should also take 1 to 2 milligrams of copper each day to maintain a proper mineral balance.

HERBAL TREATMENT

■ Liquid arnica extract, used as a rub, can help to relieve headache. Simply rub it into your temples or forehead. Be very careful to keep it away from your eyes, and do not use it on broken skin.

■ Castor-oil packs can be soothing to swollen glands. Heat castor oil to a soothing (but not too hot) temperature, soak clean cotton cloths in it, and apply these compresses as often as needed.

■ If you are feeling uncomfortable and restless, take a cup of chamomile tea three or four times a day, as needed.

■ Echinacea and goldenseal help to fight infection and boost the immune system. They also soothe mucous membranes. Take one dose of an echinacea and goldenseal combination formula supplying 250 to 500 milligrams of echinacea and 150 to 300 milligrams of goldenseal three times a day for up to one week, until the fever goes down and your salivary glands have returned to their normal size.

■ Shiitake mushrooms, available in capsule form, have immune-stimulating properties. Choose a product that is standardized and concentrated for 3 percent KS-2 poly-saccharides and take 250 to 500 milligrams three times a day for up to ten days.

HOMEOPATHY

Choose a symptom-specific remedy from the suggestions that follow, and take one dose four times a day until your symptoms improve. If the remedy produces no improvement within forty-eight hours, discontinue it and try another remedy.

■ Choose *Belladonna* 30x or 9c if your right gland is much more swollen than your left, you have a high fever and a flushed face, and you are easily chilled.

■ *Bryonia* 30x or 9c is good if your right gland is more swollen than the left, you are constipated, and your symptoms are worse with movement.

■ *Mercurius solubilis* 12x or 6c is for swollen glands and a sore throat. If you are a male, you may have testicular swelling as well.

■ *Phytolacca* 12x or 6c is for glands that are swollen and hard, with pain that goes into your ears. You tend not to want anything hot to drink.

■ *Rhus toxicodendron* 30x or 9c is the remedy to try if your left gland is much more swollen than your right, and you feel stiff and achy in the morning.

ACUPRESSURE

For the locations of acupressure points on the body, *see* ADMINISTERING AN ACUPRESSURE TREATMENT in Part Three.

■ Four Gates is relaxing.

■ Large Intestine 4 controls the head. This acupressure point can be helpful for relieving the headache that may accompany mumps.

AROMATHERAPY

For specific instructions on how to use aromatherapy, *see* PREPARING AROMATHERAPY TREATMENTS in Part Three.

■ Essential oil of peppermint can help to relieve headache. Add a few drops of peppermint oil to jojoba oil and gently rub the mixture into your temples. Be sure to keep the oil away from your eyes, and do not use it on broken skin. Or add peppermint oil to cold water and use it to make a com-

press. Apply the compress to your forehead (avoiding your eyes) or the back of your neck and leave it in place for at least ten minutes. Repeat as often as needed.

Note: If you are using peppermint oil as well as a homeopathic preparation, allow one hour between the two. Otherwise, the strong smell of the mint may interfere with the action of the homeopathic remedy.

GENERAL RECOMMENDATIONS

■ Be alert for signs that a secondary infection may be developing. If your symptoms seem to get worse, or if new symptoms develop, consult your health-care provider.

PREVENTION

■ A vaccine that protects against mumps, usually given in a combination vaccine that also protects against measles and rubella, is routinely recommended for children. The initial dose is given at the age of around fifteen months and a second dose either between the ages of four and six or a little later, between the ages of eleven and thirteen.

Muscle Sprain, Strain, and Pain

A sprain is an injury to the ligaments surrounding a joint. In the joints, tendons and ligaments are bands of fibrous tissue that connect, respectively, muscle to bone and bone to bone; the muscles power the joints' movement. All of these structures are important for stabilizing the joints and keeping them working properly. A sprain causes painful swelling around the joint, and the affected part cannot be moved without increasing the pain.

The most commonly sprained joint is the ankle, though other high-stress sites may be involved, such as knees and wrists. Over 20,000 ankle sprains occur each day in the United States. Ankle sprains are usually caused by the twisting of an ankle. About 85 percent are inversion sprains, in which the foot twists inward and the outside ligaments are stretched or torn. Eversion sprains occur when the foot twists outward, and affect the ligaments on the inner side of the ankle.

Ankle sprains are divided into three classes, depending on severity. In a first-degree sprain, there is stretching and minimal tearing, with mild pain and disability, tenderness, and swelling, but no bruising or loss of function. Recovery takes four to six weeks. With a second-degree sprain, you feel a tearing sensation, pop, or snap at the time of injury. The ankle swells and becomes tender, and bruising develops three to four days later. Walking may be difficult. It takes four to eight weeks for the injury to heal. In a third-degree sprain, the joint may slip out of place and then back in. There is usually massive swelling, severe tenderness, and instability, and you may be unable to walk at all. Recovery usually takes from six to twelve weeks.

Muscle strain occurs when muscle fibers are physically stressed—stretched too far or asked to bear too much weight—for too long. Overactivity, forcing the muscles to continue past exhaustion, or making sudden pulling or jerking motions that involve a group of muscles or their tendons can result in a strain. This type of injury is sometimes referred to as a "pulled muscle." Athletes often strain their muscles, but it can happen to anyone, especially if regular exercise is not part of your lifestyle. Strains most commonly occur during exercise, whether an intense weekend game of basketball, a jog around a city block, weight training, or an organized jazzercise class. The most common symptom of muscle strain is localized aches and pains that interfere with free movement, but there can also be swelling and inflammation. In addition, a strained muscle may spasm. Having a constricted muscle that fails to relax back into its normal configuration can be very painful.

Every movement you make involves your muscles. Your muscles are strongest when you are around the age of twenty-five, but you can keep them strong and healthy throughout life. It is well known that, without sufficient exercise, muscles shrink and become weaker. The old adage *use it or lose it* certainly applies here. However, if what you're doing hurts, you are probably injuring muscle tissue.

EMERGENCY/FIRST AID TREATMENT

■ If you suffer a severe sprain, try to get into a comfortable position and elevate the injured body part. Apply an ice pack or cold compress. Leave it in place for thirty minutes, or until it is removed by a health-care professional. With the ice pack or compress in place, have someone take you to see your doctor or to the emergency room of the nearest hospital, or call for emergency help.

■ A mild or moderate ankle sprain can usually be treated at home. Ice the injury as soon as possible. Cover your ankle with a wet towel and place a plastic bag full of ice over it. Ice it for ten to thirty minutes intermittently for forty-eight to seventy-two hours. Keep your foot elevated so that it is slightly higher than your hips, and stay off your feet. Between ice applications, compress the injury with an elastic bandage.

■ For muscle strain, use ice first. Applying ice for thirty minutes after the strain occurs temporarily decreases blood flow to the area, thereby reducing inflammation and swelling. Cold also eases pain. After twenty-four hours,

switch to applying heat. Heat increases blood flow, which helps loosen up stiff and sore muscles and joints. It also improves flexibility and makes movement easier.

CONVENTIONAL MEDICINE

■ If you suspect a sprain, begin emergency first-aid measures immediately.

■ Medical personnel will x-ray the joint to make sure no bones are broken. Once this has been ruled out, your physician will immobilize the joint with an elastic bandage, tape, a splint, or, possibly, a cast, depending on the severity of the injury.

■ To lessen the discomfort and decrease inflammation, your doctor will likely recommend a painkiller. An over-the-counter medication such as aspirin (Bayer, Ecotrin, and others), acetaminophen (Tylenol, Datril, and others) or ibuprofen (Advil, Motrin, Nuprin, and others) is likely to be recommended first. If pain is extremely severe, you may need a stronger prescription painkiller.

Note: In excessive amounts, acetaminophen can cause liver damage. If the recommended amount does not give the relief you want, do not increase the dosage, but try a different medication. Take aspirin or ibuprofen with food to prevent stomach upset.

■ A muscle relaxant such as diazepam (Valium), methocarbamol (Robaxin), or carisoprodol (Soma) may be prescribed as an adjunct to other therapy, to decrease discomfort. These drugs can cause considerable drowsiness, so they are generally reserved for injuries severe enough to require bed rest. Avoid all alcohol while taking these medications.

■ Pain and swelling can be controlled with injections of cortisone. However, this is not the preferred way of treating these injuries, as it also inhibits the functioning of the body's natural repair mechanisms and sometimes reduces blood flow to the affected area as well. This type of treatment is usually reserved for specific situations in which the sprain causes impingement on parts of the joint capsule that can develop into chronic inflammation as a result of friction.

■ If muscles, tendons, and/or ligaments are actually torn, they may need to be repaired surgically.

■ Strained muscles usually heal on their own in a matter of days to weeks, and the aches and pains subside as healing progresses. A painkiller may help to make this process more bearable.

DIETARY GUIDELINES

■ In order to build up your muscles and keep them in shape, you need sufficient clean, lean protein. Protein is necessary for tissue building and tissue repair. Include chicken, fish, whole grains, and legumes in your diet.

■ To flush toxins from your body, drink eight 8-ounce glasses of pure water every day.

NUTRITIONAL SUPPLEMENTS

■ To make sure your body has the full range of nutrients it needs for healing, take a good multivitamin and mineral formula daily.

■ Bromelain, an enzyme extracted from pineapple, helps to counteract inflammation, inhibit swelling, enhance healing, and reduce pain. It also assists the digestive process, helping to ensure absorption of other nutrients essential for healing. Take 250 to 500 milligrams three times daily, between meals, until the swelling goes away.

■ Calcium and magnesium help repair connective tissue. Take a calcium and magnesium combination formula supplying 500 to 1,000 milligrams of calcium and 250 to 500 milligrams of magnesium once or twice daily.

■ Pine-bark and grape-seed extracts are powerful anti-inflammatories. Take 50 to 100 milligrams of either three times daily for one week.

■ Vitamin C is required for tissue repair and fights inflammation. Select a formula that contains the bioflavonoids and take 1,000 milligrams four or five times daily for one week, then reduce to 500 to 1,000 milligrams two or three times daily until healing is complete.

■ Zinc helps the healing process. Take 25 milligrams twice daily for two weeks.

Note: Take zinc with food to prevent stomach upset. If you take over 30 milligrams of zinc on a daily basis for more than one or two months, you should also take 1 to 2 milligrams of copper each day to maintain a proper mineral balance.

HERBAL TREATMENT

■ A poultice of onion and comfrey is an old-time remedy that has anti-inflammatory action. It also stimulates the blood and gets it moving. Make a poultice with a combination of chopped onion and comfrey (*see* PREPARING HERBAL TREATMENTS in Part Three) and apply it to the affected area. Overwrap it with a clean white cloth and allow the poultice to remain in place for at least an hour.

Note: Do not use this treatment if the skin is broken.

■ Turmeric contains curcumin, a strong natural anti-inflammatory. Take 300 milligrams of standardized extract two or three times daily.

HOMEOPATHY

■ *Arnica* is useful for all sprains, strains, and pains that afflict the muscles. Take one dose of *Arnica* 30x, 200x, 15c, or 30c three to six times daily for the first forty-eight to seventy-two hours. *Arnica* ointment or gel can also be used topically. Apply it as directed on the product label. Do not use it topically if the skin is broken, however.

BACH FLOWER REMEDIES

Select the remedy that most closely fits your emotional tendencies and concerns, and take it as needed, following the directions on the product label.

■ Choose Holly if your injury is making you irritable and difficult to be around.

■ Impatiens is good if you are feeling impatient and cranky and are greatly annoyed that you are suffering.

ACUPRESSURE

For the locations of acupressure points on the body, *see* ADMINISTERING AN ACUPRESSURE TREATMENT in Part Three.

■ Gallbladder 34 helps to relax muscles.

■ Large Intestine 4 and Liver 3 act synergistically in relaxing muscles.

AROMATHERAPY

For specific instructions on how to use aromatherapy, *see* PREPARING AROMATHERAPY TREATMENTS in Part Three.

■ Essential oil of black pepper, eucalyptus, lavender, peppermint, and thyme are good for soothing painful muscles, reducing swelling and spasms, and enhancing blood circulation. Add any or all of these oils to a hot bath or massage oil, or blend a few drops in warm or cool water to make a comforting compress.

■ Inhaling lavender oil is particularly relaxing during the first forty-eight hours after an injury.

GENERAL RECOMMENDATIONS

■ If you are recovering from a sprain, follow your doctor's advice concerning rest, restrictions on activity, and other measures to promote healing.

■ If a strain is widespread and severe, resume your regular exercise routine and other activities slowly. Ease back gradually.

PREVENTION

■ Take time to warm up your muscles. You can minimize the risk of muscle strain by performing warm-up exercises before you engage in any strenuous physical activity, including heavy exercise.

■ Don't force your muscles to perform past their capacity. If you feel pain or your muscles begin trembling, ease up.

■ Cool down after exercising. During exercise, the muscles generate lactic acid. If lactic acid builds up in the muscles, which can occur if too little oxygen reaches the muscles during strenuous exercise, it can cause cramps and muscle spasms. To help your muscles release the lactic acid and receive the oxygen they need, cool down gradually with a less strenuous version of your exercise routine. Continue the cool-down period until your breathing is back in its normal rhythm. Taking methylsulfonylmethane (MSM) can also help by making it easier for lactic acid to pass out of muscle cells and be eliminated from the body. Take 500 milligrams three or four times daily, with meals.

Myasthenia Gravis

Myasthenia gravis (MG) is a disorder that causes progressive weakness of the voluntary muscles that tends to improve with rest and worsen with activity. This occurs because of interference with the action of acetylcholine, a neurotransmitter involved in the transfer of information concerning muscle activity. MG is believed to be an autoimmune disease in which the immune system produces antibodies that attack the body's acetylcholine receptors; if the receptors are damaged or blocked, acetylcholine cannot transmit its messages properly, and the body cannot act on the brain's commands.

Myasthenia gravis affects about 3 people in 10,000. Though most common among young women, it can occur in persons of any age and either sex. The underlying cause of autoimmune disorders such as myasthenia gravis is unknown. It can occur alone or in concert with other disorders, including rheumatoid arthritis, lupus, hyperthyroidism, or thymoma (a tumor of the thymus gland, most common in elderly men). The onset is usually slow, but it can come on rapidly in response to a trigger such as infection, pregnancy, or even a menstrual period.

The first signs and symptoms of MG often are drooping eyelids and/or double vision. Other possible symptoms include a drooping head, difficulty chewing or swallowing that may lead to choking or gagging, difficulty speaking, difficulty walking and lifting objects, and/or weakness in the upper or lower extremities. The severity of symptoms can fluctuate over the course of the day, and the weakness can become generalized or remain localized. Symptoms also may worsen with pregnancy or menstrual periods. There can be remissions, but the disease tends to be progressive. The greatest danger lies in the possibility of weakness of the muscles involved in breathing, which can be life-threatening.

Diagnosis involves the injection of a drug that stops the breakdown of acetylcholine for a short time. If muscle strength increases for several minutes, MG is likely. Since thymoma is not uncommon in people with MG, x-ray studies may be done to look for signs of such a tumor.

CONVENTIONAL TREATMENT

■ Treatment of myasthenia gravis is a difficult and intricate process. If you are diagnosed with MG, you would be wise to seek out a physician who specializes in, or at the very least has a great deal of experience with, this disorder.

■ The anticholinesterase drugs neostigmine (Prostigmin) and pyridostigmine (Mestinon) can be useful for decreasing symptoms in the short term. These drugs work by blocking the action of the enzyme cholinesterase, which breaks down acetylcholine. They cannot alter the progression of the disease, however. The use of these drugs must be carefully monitored and the dosage tailored to the individual. They should usually be taken thirty minutes before meals to maximize the ability to eat and swallow. Possible side effects include nausea, vomiting, increased salivation and bronchial secretions, sweating, and muscle cramps and weakness.

■ Surgical removal of the thymus gland may cause remission. This is not usually done immediately upon diagnosis, but is saved for when a person is older, or after a period of observation to see if he or she experiences spontaneous remission.

■ If the above treatments yield poor results, treatment with a steroid such as cortisone or prednisone (Deltasone) may be tried. Steroids are usually taken on alternate days, as they are better tolerated this way. These drugs depress the adrenal-gland function and the immune response, but this may be necessary for people with MG. Potential side effects include masking of infection, electrolyte abnormalities, blood-sugar problems, and an increased risk of developing peptic ulcers, glaucoma, cataracts, and osteoporosis. Another immune-system depressant, azathioprine (Imuran) may also be tried. This is a serious immunosuppressant with potentially severe side effects, including a drastic decrease in white blood cells, nausea, pancreatitis, liver toxicity, rash, hair loss, and others.

■ If you are unresponsive to other therapies, plasmapheresis may be used to remove harmful constituents in the plasma. This procedure is similar to dialysis. In this technique, blood plasma (the noncellular fluid part of the blood) containing the damaging antibodies is removed from the body and replaced with an equal amount of normal plasma, along with your own red blood cells. Plasmapheresis can result in remission in some cases. It may also be done to prepare you for thymus surgery.

■ Antibiotics of the class known as aminoglycosides are known to make the disease worse, so their use is to be *avoided* if at all possible. Drugs of this type include amikacin (Amikin), gentamicin (Garamycin), spectinomycin (Trobicin), and tobramycin (Nebcin).

DIETARY GUIDELINES

■ Eat a diet that is high in protein and fiber. Include plenty of high-potassium foods such as fresh fruits and vegetables, which help to preserve muscle strength.

■ Have three regular meals and two healthful snacks each day to keep your blood-sugar level in balance and your energy as high as possible.

■ Drink at least six 8-ounce glasses of pure water daily.

 Avoid salt, sugar, and concentrated saturated fats, which place stress on the body.

NUTRITIONAL SUPPLEMENTS

■ Take a good multivitamin and mineral supplement that includes the trace minerals daily.

 Colostrum strengthens immunity, improves energy, and increases the utilization of nutrients. Take 500 to 1,000 milligrams two or three times daily.

 To ensure proper digestion, take a full-spectrum digestive-enzyme supplement with each meal.

 Black currant seed oil, borage oil, evening primrose oil, and flaxseed oil contain essential fatty acids needed for the health of every cell in the body. Take 500 to 1,000 milligrams of any of these oils three times daily.

 The combination of magnesium and malic acid helps to generate energy at the cellular level. Take a supplement supplying 100 milligrams of magnesium and 250 to 500 milligrams of malic acid each morning, an hour before eating breakfast.

GENERAL RECOMMENDATIONS

 Plan activities, whether for work or recreation, to allow for scheduled rest periods. Don't allow yourself to overdo to the point of exhaustion.

 If double vision is a problem, you can use an eye patch to eliminate the extra image.

 Avoid exposure to toxins such as pesticides and cleaning chemicals. These not only stress the body, but can cause breathing problems.

■ Make baths and showers warm, not hot, and avoid saunas and hot tubs. The heat can be weakening.

 Get adequate regular sleep.

■ Get regular exercise, but take care to stay within the range of your fitness ability. Don't overdo.

■ Have regular dental checkups with a dentist familiar with your condition.

■ As much as possible, avoid stress, both physical and psychological. Avoid infections by practicing good hygiene, especially frequent hand-washing, and by calling ahead to make sure anyone you are planning to visit is healthy during cold and flu season. Try to avoid extremes of temperature as well. Learn and practice techniques to help you deal with stresses you cannot avoid, whether yogic breathing, meditation, yoga, or any other such discipline.

■ Consider joining a support group. There are MG support groups throughout the country, as well as online support resources.

Myocardial Infarction

See under CARDIOVASCULAR DISEASE.

Myxedema

See HYPOTHYROIDISM.

Nail Problems and Injuries

The finger- and toenails are hard platelike structures designed to protect the tips of the fingers and toes, areas that are full of nerve endings and more vulnerable than many other parts of the body to injury and pain. Fingernails are also useful for certain fine-motor tasks that would be impossible to perform with the fingertips alone. There are a variety of different problems that can affect the nails; there are also other health problems, including heart disease, respiratory problems, anemia, and nutritional deficiencies, that can cause telltale changes in the nails. This entry addresses poor nail growth, brittle nails, and nail injuries and infections.

 Anything that impairs the body's absorption and use of proteins for tissue repair can cause abnormal nail growth. Inadequate production of stomach acid or digestive enzymes, poor protein intake, nutritional deficiencies, acute or chronic illness, repetitive nail trauma (including excessive exposure to water, chemicals, even persistent biting), and allergies can all play a part. Usually this results in nails that grow very slowly, have horizontal or vertical ridges, and/or become brittle. Identifying and correcting these elements can make a visible difference in nail structure, sometimes within weeks.

 Nail problems can also be a result of an an underlying

physical disorder. There are many different health problems can affect the condition of the nails. For example:

- Blackish, splinterlike bits in the nails can be a sign of bacterial endocarditis, a serious infection of the heart.

- Easily broken nails can be a sign of deficiency of calcium, silica, and/or certain other trace minerals.

- Horizontal ridges can be an indicator of injury, infection, or illness.

- Pitted nails may be associated with psoriasis.

- Spoon-shaped nails are associated with iron deficiency.

- Vertical ridges may point to poor absorption of nutrients.

- Very pale colored nail beds may be a sign of anemia.

- White spots in the nails may signify a zinc deficiency.

If you develop any of these problems, you may wish to bring it to the attention of a health-care professional.

Injuries to the fingernails and toenails are common. Depending on the extent and type of injury, a bruise may form immediately. The area may appear red and swollen, or white and scraped. More seriously, a nail can be completely torn off. Any injury to tissue makes infection a possibility. Fungal infections are a particular problem, especially with the toenails. Fungal infection of the nail, or *onchomycosis*, is an infection caused by microscopic organisms that grow on the nail bed, beneath the nail. It causes the nail to become brittle, discolored, and deformed, with surrounding skin that is dry and peeling. If left untreated, fungal infection can actually destroy the entire nail. If a nail injury does not improve within twenty-four hours, or if the area begins to show increasing redness, warmth, swelling, or other signs of infection, call your physician.

Changes in the normal growth of a toenail can cause it to become ingrown. The big toe is the most likely to develop this problem. It can be a result of fungal infection, injury, inflammation, poor nail-cutting technique, or poorly fitting shoes. It can even follow a bout of anemia or other systemic illness. Whatever the cause, the edge of the nail digs into the surrounding soft tissue instead of staying above it, causing swelling, pain, inflammation, and sometimes infection and/or the formation of excess soft tissue around the irritated area.

CONVENTIONAL TREATMENT

■ Because anemia can cause nail distortions, your doctor may recommend a blood test to assess your body's iron stores.

■ If you have horizontal ridges in your nails, it may be wise to test your thyroid function, especially if you have other symptoms of an underactive thyroid as well. (*See* HYPOTHYROIDISM.)

■ If you injure a nail, hold it under running water to cleanse the area. If there is bleeding, use cold water. Unless you can readily see a foreign object protruding from under or around the nail, do not try to remove anything that might be under the skin. Poking and probing can result in infection later on.

■ Unless the nail is completely torn at the base, do not remove it. Even a badly broken nail can and should be taped in place to provide protection for the very tender nail bed underneath until the tissue has healed. Keep the area protected against further injury with a small splint or finger cup. If part of the nail bed is exposed, or if there is an open wound, apply an antibiotic ointment before bandaging. Keep the area bandaged until the injury heals. The nail will eventually fall off by itself, or else grow out again.

■ If the wound involves a puncture or is dirty, cleanse it with hydrogen peroxide, gently pat dry, and apply an antibiotic ointment such as bacitracin or Betadine before covering it.

■ For other nail problems, close examination is necessary to determine whether any inflammation, cosmetic allergy, fungal infection, or other treatable disorder is present.

■ For a fungal infection of the nail, your doctor may prescribe a liquid antifungal such as naftifine (Naftin) or ciclopirox (Loprox) for topical use. This kind of treatment takes diligence and time to be successful, especially for toenails. Infections in the nails can be resistant to treatment because it is difficult to deliver the medicinal agents to the site of infection.

■ Itraconazole (Sporanox), fluconazole (Diflucan), and terbinafine (Lamisil) are oral antifungal medications that are effective for fungal nail infections, though they also take time to work. They must be taken daily for three months or, if the problem is less severe, possibly one week of each month. The results are not seen on the old nail but only on the new emerging nail. You begin to see a small piece of clear nail emerging from the base of the nail after about a month. It takes about twelve months before a full toenail grows in. Possible side effects of these drugs include upset stomach, headache, liver stress, and sticker shock—these drugs are expensive. Older medications such as griseofulvin (Fulvicin, Grifulvin, Grisactin, Gris-PEG) and ketoconazole (Nizoral) are somewhat cheaper, but the side effects tend to be worse. Discuss your options with your doctor to determine which is best for your particular situation.

■ An ingrown toenail may require surgical removal of all or part of the nail. Nails nearly always regrow after this type of procedure. Careful treatment by shaving or notching the top of the nail and removing pressure on it can sometimes eliminate the need for more aggressive treatment. If infection develops, you may need a course of oral antibiotic treatment.

DIETARY GUIDELINES

■ For brittle or poorly growing nails, increase your intake of quality protein. If your cholesterol level is not too high, add up to two eggs a day to your diet. Eggs are a good source of sulfur-containing amino acids, which are excellent for supporting nail growth. Try to keep the yolk intact while cooking, as this keeps the cholesterol in a more benign form.

■ Avoid refined sugar and flour. This helps to keep blood-insulin levels under control, which in turn permits better absorption of proteins.

NUTRITIONAL SUPPLEMENTS

■ For brittle nails, try using a digestive-enzyme formula containing betaine hydrochloride for three months. Take 1 or 2 capsules immediately after each meal. If you develop indigestion, discontinue the supplement. If you notice that the addition of the enzymes makes a difference in the new nail forming, you may want to use a botanical enzyme combination to enhance digestion for three more months. Also take 10,000 international units of vitamin A daily for three to six months.

Note: If you are pregnant, or intend to get pregnant, or if you have liver disease, consult your doctor before taking supplemental vitamin A. Pregnant women should not ingest a total of more than 25,000 international units of supplemental vitamin A *per week* from all sources.

■ Methylsulfonylmethane (MSM) is a good source of sulfur, a trace mineral that is necessary for strong nails. Take 500 milligrams three or four times daily, with meals.

■ If you have white spots under your nails, try taking 50 milligrams of vitamin B_6 (pyridoxine) and 30 milligrams of zinc daily for three to six months. If you take any of the B vitamins individually, you should also take a B-complex supplement at a different time of day. Take zinc with food to prevent stomach upset. If you take over 30 milligrams of zinc on a daily basis for more than one or two months, you should also take 1 to 2 milligrams of copper each day to maintain a proper mineral balance.

HERBAL TREATMENT

■ If a nail injury becomes slightly infected, apply a green clay and goldenseal poultice to help draw out the infection (*see* PREPARING HERBAL TREATMENTS in Part Three). Apply the poultice for fifteen minutes twice a day until the infection is resolved. A nail injury can develop into a serious problem, so if you suspect infection and are experiencing pain, see a physician.

■ For any infection, take one dose of an echinacea and goldenseal combination formula supplying 350 to 500 milligrams of echinacea and 150 to 300 milligrams of goldenseal three to four times daily for four or five days.

HOMEOPATHY

■ *Antimonium tartaricum* is the remedy for thick and brittle nails. Three days out of each week for three weeks, take one dose of *Antimonium tartaricum* 12x or 6c three times daily.

■ *Silicea* is for thin and peeling nails with white spots. Your fingertips may be dry as well. Three days out of each week for three weeks, take one dose of *Silicea* 30x or 15c three times daily.

■ *Graphites* is the remedy for thick, brittle, cracked, and rough nails, possibly accompanied by an inflamed nail bed. Three days out of each week for three weeks, take one dose of *Graphites* 12x or 6c three times daily.

■ *Arnica* helps to alleviate acute pain. As soon as possible after an injury to a nail, administer one dose of *Arnica* 200x or 30c, as directed on the product label.

■ *Hypericum* helps to lessen the pain in an injured finger or toe. Take one dose of *Hypericum* 12x or 6c three times a day for two to three days after an injury.

■ *Ledum* helps to alleviate bruising. Take one dose of *Ledum* 12x or 6c three times daily for two to three days after a nail injury.

■ *Hepar sulfuris calcareum* helps to resolve a minor infection following a nail injury. Take one dose of *Hepar sulfuris calcareum* 12x or 6c three times daily for up to three days.

AROMATHERAPY

For specific instructions on how to use aromatherapy, *see* PREPARING AROMATHERAPY TREATMENTS in Part Three.

■ Tea tree oil, applied topically, is an effective treatment for fungal infection. In fact, a double-blind study comparing tea tree oil with clotrimazole, a prescription antifungal, found the two were equally effective. Twice a day, paint the affected area with undiluted tea tree oil. If the nail is dry, you can mix the tea tree oil with olive oil.

GENERAL RECOMMENDATIONS

■ Avoid exposing your nails to environmental stresses, such as chemicals, trauma, and even excessive immersion in water.

■ For brittle nails, there are topical nail oils available that can help, though it takes time. Plain olive oil is also beneficial.

PREVENTION

■ Don't use your nails as a prying tool.

■ Paying attention to nail hygiene and proper nutrition may help you avoid infection, ingrown toenails, and other nail problems.

Narcolepsy

Narcolepsy is a syndrome characterized by some combination of four specific symptoms that are, in effect, intensified versions of normal phenomena. These are:

1. Sleep attacks. These can come on quite suddenly and during any type of activity, and usually last only about fifteen minutes. You may feel wide awake afterward, but another attack can occur at any time.

2. Cataplexy. This is a disturbing and abrupt loss of muscle tone, manifested as momentary paralysis and/or profound muscular weakness. It can affect only certain muscles or the entire body. It usually seems to be triggered by strong emotions, such as intense laughter, fear, or anger, with an element of surprise. It does not involve losing consciousness. These episodes can look like seizures, but they are not.

3. Sleep paralysis. This is a phenomenon in which you are neither totally asleep nor totally awake (it usually occurs just as you are falling asleep or as you are awakening), and find that you cannot move any part of your body. Though temporary, this condition can be terrifying.

4. Hypnagogic phenomena. These are very vivid, believable auditory or visual hallucinations. They usually occur just before you fall asleep or during a sleep attack, and are followed immediately by rapid-eye-movement (REM) sleep, a normal phase that occurs during deep sleep.

A person with narcolepsy may experience any combination of these symptoms, though not all actually experience all four. Sleep paralysis and hypnagogic phenomena can also occur in people who do not have narcolepsy or any other sleep disorder.

Narcolepsy usually begins in adolescence or young adulthood. It often eases somewhat around age thirty. The cause is unknown.

CONVENTIONAL TREATMENT

■ The standard attempt to control narcolepsy consists of the use of stimulants such as dextroamphetamine (Adderall, Dexedrine) or methylphenidate (Ritalin). Side effects of these drugs can include increased heart rate and blood pressure, general overstimulation, and rashes. There is also significant potential for abuse.

■ Imipramine (Tofranil) is sometimes prescribed for cataplexy, though it is not effective for the other symptoms of narcolepsy. This is an antidepressant drug with potential side effects that include drowsiness, low blood pressure, insomnia, nausea, headache, jerky movements, jaundice, and bone-marrow depression.

DIETARY GUIDELINES

■ It is important not to eat too much at mealtimes. Many people with narcolepsy find that if they eat five small meals each day rather than three larger ones, they can handle their sleepiness better. Keeping blood-sugar levels relatively even throughout the day makes it easier to remain awake.

■ Focus on protein foods during the day. This promotes the production of norepinephrine, a hormone that is instrumental in stimulating pushing the sympathetic nervous system, which in turn promotes alertness. Eating excessive amounts of carbohydrates at any one time, in contrast, promotes sleepiness.

NUTRITIONAL SUPPLEMENTS

■ To ensure an adequate supply of all basic nutrients, take a multivitamin and mineral supplement daily.

■ Adrenal glandular extract supports the functioning of the adrenal glands. According to Chinese medicine, weak kidney and adrenal function is at the root of sleepiness during the day. Try taking 100 to 200 milligrams of adrenal extract twice a day, the first dose between breakfast and the second between lunch and dinner.

■ Nicotinamide adenine dinucleotide hydrogen (NADH) helps to promote energy production. Take 5 milligrams twice a day.

■ The B vitamins are essential for the proper functioning of the nervous system. Take a B-complex supplement supplying 25 milligrams of each of the major B vitamins twice a day, the first dose between breakfast and lunch and the second between lunch and dinner.

HERBAL TREATMENT

■ Siberian ginseng helps the body adapt to stress and increases energy levels. Choose a standardized extract containing 0.5 percent eleutheroside E and take 100 milligrams twice daily, in morning and afternoon.

Note: It is not necessary to use both Siberian ginseng and adrenal extract, at least initially. Choose one and take it for two weeks. If this proves insufficient, begin taking the other as well.

HOMEOPATHY

■ Nux moschata is helpful for extreme drowsiness and various mental and physical complaints that result in sleepiness. Take one dose of Nux moschata 12x or 6c three times daily, up to a total of ten doses.

ACUPRESSURE

For the locations of acupressure points on the body, *see* ADMINISTERING AN ACUPRESSURE TREATMENT in Part Three.

Stomach 36 helps to improve the utilization of nutrients from food. According to Chinese medicine, if food is utilized, transformed, and transported throughout the body successfully, you are less likely to experience narcoleptic episodes.

BACH FLOWER REMEDIES

Select the remedy that most closely fits your disposition and emotional tendencies and concerns, and take it as needed, following the directions on the product label.

Clematis counteracts apathy, a short attention span, and a tendency to daydream.

Olive helps to ease utter exhaustion.

Wild rose is helpful for a lack of vitality and feelings of tiredness and resignation.

AROMATHERAPY

For specific instructions on how to use aromatherapy, *see* PREPARING AROMATHERAPY TREATMENTS in Part Three.

Essential oil of lavender is strengthening to the nervous system. It also combines well with some of the more stimulating essential oils, such as rosemary and pine. You can use these oils as inhalants, in baths and/or massage, or diffuse them into the air in your home or workplace.

GENERAL RECOMMENDATIONS

Making basic lifestyle adjustments—regulating your sleep schedule, improving your diet, increasing the amount of exercise you get, and avoiding overstimulating situations—may help to reduce the effects of excessive daytime sleepiness and cataplexy. Go to bed and wake up at the same time each day. Take scheduled short naps once or twice daily as needed. Increase your activity level. Avoid repetitive and/or boring activities, however.

Ask your doctor to check your thyroid function. Subclinical hypothyroidism (thyroid function that is in the low normal range) may be a root cause of narcolepsy.

Nausea and Vomiting

Nausea is the queasy, uncomfortable feeling that you are about to vomit. It may be accompanied by abdominal pain, an inability to tolerate certain smells, a too-full feeling, and/or cramping. It often is followed by vomiting, in which contractions of the abdominal muscles force food and other ingested substances back up and out of the body through the mouth. Nausea is often felt in waves that peak right before a vomiting episode. After vomiting, you are likely to feel better, at least temporarily. Though distinctly unpleasant, vomiting actually has a positive value; it is a natural defense mechanism that helps to protect the body from harmful substances.

Nausea and vomiting can result from many causes, among them food poisoning, overeating, motion sickness, viral or bacterial infection, hepatitis, HIV disease, appendicitis, constipation, muscle strain, sleep deficit, fatigue, food allergies, a reaction to cancer treatments, or the accidental ingestion of drugs and poisons. Anxiety, worry, or great emotional shock can trigger nausea and vomiting as well.

A single episode of nausea or vomiting is likely to be a reaction to spoiled food or a sign of emotional upset. If nausea is severe or persists for more than a few hours, the most likely cause is either food poisoning or an intestinal infection. Food poisoning and infection can both be caused by a wide variety of organisms, including *Campylobacter, Escherichia coli* (*E. coli*), *Salmonella, Shigella,* or *Staphylococcus* bacteria, either by the bacteria themselves or by toxins they produce (*see* FOOD POISONING). Most often, nausea and vomiting related to a bacterial infection of the intestine are accompanied by diarrhea and fever. Food poisoning, which is usually caused by a toxin produced by bacteria rather than direct infection with the bacteria, is less likely to cause a fever. Viral infections can cause diarrhea in addition to vomiting.

Most episodes of nausea and vomiting can be eased with the remedies outlined in this section and run their course in a relatively short time. However, if you have persistent vomiting, blood in the vomit, abdominal pain so severe that it keeps you from your normal activities, persistent abdominal pain that lasts more than a few hours, or any other symptoms that are sufficiently abnormal to invite real concern, call your health-care provider for advice. A physical examination and laboratory tests may be required to diagnose the cause of persistent nausea and/or vomiting. If you experience nausea and vomiting with progressive pain and tenderness in your lower right abdomen, seek medical help immediately. This can sometimes be a sign of developing appendicitis (*see* APPENDICITIS).

CONVENTIONAL TREATMENT

■ Your doctor will perform an examination to determine whether the nausea and vomiting are caused by an infection or toxin, emotional distress, or an internal obstruction. He or she will look for signs of dehydration, fever, abdominal tenderness, or blood in the stools. If you have diarrhea, a stool culture may help to determine if the vomiting is related to a bacterial infection. Your doctor will recommend treatment based on the likely cause of your distress.

■ Antiemetics are drugs that are sometimes prescribed to ease nausea and stop vomiting. Trimethobenzamide (Tigan), prochlorperazine (Compazine), and promethazine (Phenergan) are among the ones most commonly used. They can be given in tablet or suppository form, or by injection. Because these drugs can have serious side effects, they should be used with caution. Never take more than the prescribed dose.

■ Emetrol is a safe, over-the-counter syrup that settles the stomach. It is useful for relief of nausea caused by infection, overeating, or emotional upset, and produces no side effects. Take it every few hours as directed on the product label.

■ Bismuth subsalicylate, more commonly known as Pepto-Bismol, absorbs toxins and provides a protective coating along the gastrointestinal tract. It is helpful for relief of nausea as well as of diarrhea. Take it as directed on the product label.

■ Unless your doctor specifically prescribes one, do not take any type of painkiller, whether prescription or over-the-counter, if you have an upset stomach. In relieving stomach pain whose cause has not been diagnosed, you may mask an underlying condition that could become worse without treatment.

DIETARY GUIDELINES

■ Guard against dehydration. Fluids are lost at an alarming rate when the body is coping with episodes of vomiting or diarrhea. Refer to the guidelines for fluid intake in DIET AND NUTRITION in Part One to learn how much fluid your body needs. Do not try to drink a whole glass of liquid at one time, however. Instead, take frequent small sips. Choose liquids that are relatively high in glucose and salts, such as soups and fruit juices. Avoid carbonated beverages, which stretch the stomach and may aggravate the condition.

■ Raw honey or barley malt extract can be used to settle an irritated stomach. Take 1 teaspoon of either every hour, as needed.

■ As long as you are vomiting, take only clear liquids to give your gastrointestinal tract time to heal and rest. Once the vomiting is under control, slowly progress to solid foods to give the digestive tract time to readjust itself.

■ If you don't feel like eating, don't force yourself. Your body often instinctively knows what's best. When your appetite improves, start with a bland, simple diet. Thin cooked oatmeal, dry toast, applesauce, and yogurt are good foods to begin with. Once you begin to feel better, you will start to feel hungry and will most likely want specific foods.

NUTRITIONAL SUPPLEMENTS

■ Probiotic acidophilus and bifidobacteria can help ease an upset stomach by restoring healthy flora to the intestines. Take a probiotic supplement as recommended on the product label for at least two to three weeks. If you are allergic to milk, select a dairy-free formula.

HERBAL TREATMENT

■ If you are feeling sick and restless, take a cup of soothing chamomile tea twice daily, between meals.

■ A 2,000-year-old Chinese herbal formula, available today as a product called Curing Pills, is effective for any stomach upset. Follow the dosage directions on the product label.

■ Ginger is helpful for nausea, vomiting, and stomachache. Take a cup of ginger tea as needed. If the tea tastes too strong, mix it with apple juice or make it with equal amounts of ginger and licorice root to sweeten the taste. Or choose a standardized extract containing 5 percent gingeoles and take 200 milligrams three times daily.

Note: Do not add licorice if you have high blood pressure.

■ Green tea has antibacterial properties and is helpful for nausea and vomiting related to food poisoning. Take a cup of strong green tea as needed.

■ Licorice root is very settling to the stomach. Take a cup of licorice root tea up to three times a day for one day.

Note: Do not take licorice on a daily basis for longer than five days at a time, as it can elevate blood pressure. Do not use it at all if you have high blood pressure.

■ Peppermint tea is an effective and safe digestive aid. It is especially helpful for nausea or vomiting that occurs after a heavy meal. Take a cup of tea twice daily, with or between meals.

■ For an upset stomach that is accompanied by gas, brew a stomach tea. Blend one part each anise seed, fennel, peppermint, and thyme, and take a cup of tea as needed. (*See* PREPARING HERBAL TREATMENTS in Part Three.)

■ Umeboshi plum paste is very settling to an upset stomach. (*See* THERAPEUTIC RECIPES in Part Three.) Take $^1/_4$ teaspoon every thirty to sixty minutes.

HOMEOPATHY

The following symptom-specific homeopathic remedies are useful for combating nausea. Please note that if you are also taking a tea containing peppermint, you should allow one hour between the tea and any homeopathic preparation. Otherwise, the strong smell of the mint may interfere with the action of the homeopathic remedy.

■ Take *Arsenicum album* if you have vomiting with diarrhea. Take one dose of *Arsenicum album* 30x or 9c every hour, up to a total of six doses.

■ *Carbo vegetabilis* is good if you have nausea accompanied by a specific pain in the center of your stomach, gas with burping, possibly heartburn, and a distended abdomen. Take one dose of *Carbo vegetabilis* 30x or 9c three times a day, up to a total of eight doses. There are also homeopathic combination remedies available containing both *Nux vomica* and *Carbo vegetabilis*.

Ignatia is effective for stress- or emotion-based nausea. You may feel a lump in your throat. Take one dose of *Ignatia* 30x or 9c three times a day for up to three days.

If you are experiencing incessant vomiting and heaving, homeopathic *Ipecac* can bring relief. It also helps to relieve unrelenting nausea. Take one dose of *Ipecac* 12x or 6c every hour, up to a total of three or four doses.

Caution: Do not confuse homeopathic *Ipecac* with conventional syrup of ipecac. That is an entirely different product, and it should never be used except at the direction of a doctor or Poison Control Center.

■ *Nux vomica* can help if you develop an upset stomach after overeating, after eating too many sweets, or after eating too much fried or fast food. You feel nauseated, may have a headache, and feel irritable. Take one dose of *Nux vomica* 30x or 9c three times a day, up to a total of six doses.

ACUPRESSURE

For the locations of acupressure points on the body, *see* ADMINISTERING AN ACUPRESSURE TREATMENT in Part Three.

Pericardium 6 helps to lessen nausea and vomiting.

Stomach 36 harmonizes and tones the digestive system.

AROMATHERAPY

For specific instructions on how to use aromatherapy, *see* PREPARING AROMATHERAPY TREATMENTS in Part Three.

Peppermint oil helps to relieve nausea; lavender is relaxing to the nervous system. Use either or both as an inhalant or diffuse them into the air in your home.

GENERAL RECOMMENDATIONS

To comfort and soothe stomach and/or abdominal muscles that are sore from vomiting, put a hot water bottle on your stomach. Don't fill the bottle so full that it becomes hard. Instead, fill it only about halfway, so that the bottle remains light enough to mold to your body.

■ Take Emetrol syrup, barley malt, or rice syrup. A teaspoon of honey every hour or two also can help settle the stomach.

See also CONSTIPATION or DIARRHEA if the nausea is accompanied by either of these symptoms.

■ *See also* APPENDICITIS; EMOTIONAL UPSET; FOOD ALLERGIES; FOOD POISONING; HEPATITIS; or MOTION SICKNESS, if you have reason to believe your nausea or vomiting may be related to any of these problems.

PREVENTION

■ Wash your hands regularly and thoroughly, especially before eating.

■ Guard against overeating. Practice portion control. Eat appropriate amounts of healthy whole foods, and limit sugar and fats.

Nephritis

See under KIDNEY DISEASE.

Nicotine Addiction

Few people would argue with the statement that smoking is bad for you. The image of concentrated particles of burning leaves sticking to moist, sensitive lung tissue is hardly compatible with a picture of optimal health. The link between smoking and diseases of the lungs, such as lung cancer and emphysema, is well known. Smoking has also been implicated in high blood pressure, heart disease, stroke, hardening of the arteries, osteoporosis, cervical cancer, and complications of pregnancy, and it can worsen heartburn.

So why do people smoke? Most people know about the risks, but people who smoke generally begin in their teens and early adulthood—sometimes even before that—when they perceive smoking as something "cool" or rebellious, or as something to do to fit in with a particular group of their peers. At this age, most people tend also to feel invincible and immortal, and genuinely believe that all of the well-known dangers of smoking somehow will not happen to them—or, at least, are something to worry about only in the distant future. Unfortunately, once you have smoked for any period of time, quitting can be very difficult. The primary reason for this is nicotine, the active ingredient in cigarette smoke. Most people who smoke will be the first to tell you that nicotine is addictive and that discontinuing its use causes cravings that can seem nearly unbearable.

As a drug, nicotine use enhances alertness, constricts the blood vessels, and allows muscles to relax. Once the body has become used to a steady supply of nicotine, there are physical symptoms if the nicotine is withdrawn. In addition to an intense craving for nicotine, these include nervousness, irritability, headache, difficulty concentrating, stomach cramps, tremors, disrupted sleep, and others. Quitting means getting past this period of withdrawal and beating the nicotine addiction. The good news is that, if you have made the decision to stop smoking, there is a lot you can do to lessen the cravings and handle the withdrawal symptoms.

CONVENTIONAL TREATMENT

■ Nicotine chewing gum (Nicorette) can be used to ease cravings during the withdrawal period. The idea, of course, is to taper off your use of the gum gradually as the ingrained habit of smoking diminishes. Problems may include damage to the teeth, dental work, or mouth tissue; nausea; an increased heart rate; and others.

■ Nicotine patches, sold under the brand names Habitrol and Nicoderm CQ, allow nicotine to be absorbed at a steady rate through the skin. As with nicotine gum, this is meant to lessen withdrawal symptoms. You apply a new patch each day and gradually, over a period of weeks, decrease the dosage until your body can function normally without nicotine. Possible side effects of this treatment can include nausea, fatigue, increased heart rate, joint pains, miscarriage, and skin irritation at the patch site.

■ A nicotine nasal spray (Nicotrol NS) works in a similar fashion to the patch. This should *not* be inhaled into the lungs.

■ The antidepressant bupropion (Zyban) helps some people to handle some of the symptoms of withdrawal. The combination of bupropion and nicotine patches appears to yield better results than either one alone. Bupropion can interact with a number of other drugs, so discuss your medication list carefully with your doctor. You should not take bupropion if you have seizures or an eating disorder such as anorexia or bulimia, as they increase the likelihood

---

Nicotine Addiction Self-Test

If you are a smoker, take the following quiz to help you determine how dependent you are on nicotine. Answer the eight questions below, and add up your score.

1. How soon after you wake up do you smoke your first cigarette?

    within 30 minutes = 1 point   after 30 minutes or more = 0 points   Points _____

2. Do you find it almost impossible to refrain from smoking in public places where it is forbidden, such as movie theaters, houses of worship, shopping malls, etc.?

    yes = 1 point   no = 0 points   Points _____

3. Which cigarette would you most hate to give up?

    the first in the morning = 1 point   any other = 0 points   Points _____

4. How many cigarettes do you smoke in the average day?

    26 or more = 2 points   16 to 25 = 1 point   15 or fewer = 0 points   Points _____

5. Do you smoke more frequently during the morning than during the rest of the day?

    yes = 1 point   no = 0 points   Points _____

6. Do you smoke if you are sick enough to stay in bed?

    yes = 1 point   no = 0 points   Points _____

7. What is the nicotine level of your usual brand of cigarettes?

    1.3 mg or more = 2 points   1.0 to 1.2 mg = 1 point   0.9 mg or less = 0 points   Points _____

8. Do you inhale?

    always = 2 points   sometimes = 1 point   never = 0 points   Points _____

If your total score is 6 or above, you are probably seriously addicted to nicotine and should seek the help of a health-care practitioner to guide you through the withdrawal process.   **TOTAL** _____

of seizures. In addition to the increased seizure risk, possible side effects include dry mouth, dizziness, constipation, insomnia, and allergic skin reactions.

■ Behavior modification programs such as biofeedback may be combined with any of the above medications. Ask your physician for a referral. If he or she is unable to supply one, an organization such as the Biofeedback Certification Institute of America may be able to help.

DIETARY GUIDELINES

To give your adrenal glands a chance to restore themselves, avoid caffeine and other stimulants.

Smoking causes the creation of harmful free radicals and depletes many nutrients, especially vitamin C. Include in your diet a wide variety of fresh fruits and vegetables to supply a full range of vitamins and minerals, as well as phytochemicals that have antioxidant properties.

Nicotine addiction can be worse if you are allergic to other plants in the nightshade family, of which tobacco is a member. These include potatoes (except for sweet potatoes), all types of peppers, eggplant, tomatoes, and paprika. As a test, eliminate nightshade vegetables from your diet for seven days to see if cravings lessen. You may also notice other symptoms you had not associated with food sensitivity abating. Afterward, reintroduce the foods one at a time to see if you experience any reactions. These can take many forms, from runny nose, sneezing, and itching to irritability to nausea and bloating to increased pulse rate. Any food that provokes a reaction should then be permanently banned from the menu.

Many naturopathic physicians feel all nightshade plants should be deleted from the diet to make the withdrawal from nicotine easier. After seven days, acute physical withdrawal should be past so, unless allergies are a problem, these foods can be returned to the diet.

Try chewing on raw sunflower seeds as a substitute for the nerve-calming effect of smoking a cigarette.

While cravings are acute, try dissolving a tablespoon of baking soda in 12 ounces of water and sipping the mixture slowly over the course of a twelve-hour day. This is an old naturopathic technique that works surprisingly well to reduce cravings, although why it works has never been determined.

NUTRITIONAL SUPPLEMENTS

■ To correct possible nutritional deficiencies, take a good multivitamin and mineral supplement daily. Be sure to choose a formula that contains the major antioxidant nutrients, including vitamins A, C, and E; bioflavonoids; and zinc.

Vitamin-B_3 (niacin) therapy can lessen cravings consid-erably while you are trying to quit. Relatively high doses are needed however, in the range of 250 to 500 milligrams three times a day, which can cause adverse reactions in some people. It is best to undertake this treatment under the supervision of a nutritionally oriented physician.

Note: Do not take supplemental niacin if you have gout or liver dysfunction.

■ Smoking depletes the body's supply of vitamin C. This vitamin can also help to both detoxify and relax someone withdrawing from nicotine. Take 1,000 milligrams of vitamin C three times daily. Choose a magnesium ascorbate formula if possible.

■ Vitamin E is an excellent antioxidant that protects against damage from the free radicals generated by smoking. If you are still smoking, take 400 international units of vitamin E daily. Choose the mixed-tocopherol or d-alpha-tocopherol form, not dl-alpha-tocopherol. Also take 100 micrograms of selenium daily to support the action of vitamin E.

Note: If you are taking an anticoagulant (blood thinner), consult your physician before taking supplemental vitamin E.

HERBAL TREATMENT

■ Bupleurum and dragon bone is an old Chinese herbal combination that has strong calmative powers and is very useful for people suffering from anxiety caused by withdrawal from nicotine. Twice a day, take one dose of a bupleurum and dragon bone combination remedy as directed on the product label. This formula is very strong, however, so if you have a troublesome and/or weak digestive system, you may wish to select a different remedy.

■ If you can tolerate the pungent taste, sucking on a clove can help reduce cravings.

■ Chewing on a small piece of fresh ginger root (about $1/8$ teaspoon) can help to both fight cravings and improve breath.

■ Pine-bark and grape-seed extracts have a powerful antioxidant effect. Take 50 milligrams of either two or three times daily.

■ Plantain (also known by its Latin name, *Plantago major*), taken as a tea, can help reduce cravings. Take a cup of plantain tea three times daily, as needed.

HOMEOPATHY

■ *Lobelia* reduces cravings for tobacco, especially if the cravings are made worse by cold and better by rapid walking. Take one dose of *Lobelia* 6x or 3c three to four times daily during the first seventy-two hours of withdrawal. After that, take one dose up to three times daily, as needed.

■ *Nicotiana tabacum* helps to reduce cravings accompanied by nausea and difficulty sleeping. This remedy is for symptoms that are better in the fresh air, and cravings and mood that tend to be worse in the evening. Take one dose of *Nicotiana tabacum* 6x, 12x, 3c, or 6c three to four times daily during the first seventy-two hours of withdrawal. After that, take one dose up to three times daily, as needed.

■ *Nux vomica* is helpful if you suffer from irritability, sullen mood, and/or headaches associated with smoking cessation. Symptoms tend to be worse in the morning and better after a nap. Take one dose of *Nux vomica* 12x, 30x, 6c, or 15c up to three times daily, as needed.

■ *Staphysagria* helps to reduce tobacco cravings. It seems to be more effective for female smokers, especially those who are very sensitive about what others say about them, prefer to be alone, have a tendency to develop styes and/or bladder infections, and/or desire stimulants. Take one dose of *Staphysagria* 30x or 15c three times daily for up to three days.

BACH FLOWER REMEDIES

Select the remedy that most closely fits your emotional tendencies and concerns, and take it as needed, following the directions on the product label.

■ Holly helps to reduce anger. It is beneficial if you find quitting has given rise to feelings of anger.

■ Impatiens helps to lessen anxiety.

■ Wild oat is good if you have difficulty sticking to the routine of smoking cessation.

ACUPRESSURE/MASSAGE

For the locations of acupressure points on the body, *see* ADMINISTERING AN ACUPRESSURE TREATMENT in Part Three.

■ Massaging along the Bladder meridian (the inner and outer Bladder points) helps to relax the entire body. Reducing tension is important, especially during the first seventy-two hours after your last cigarette.

■ Liver 3 relaxes the nervous system.

■ Large Intestine 4 and Liver 3 together help to relax the nervous system.

■ Massaging along the lung and pericardium meridians helps to relax the chest. Conception Vessel 17 also helps to relax the chest.

AROMATHERAPY

For specific instructions on how to use aromatherapy, *see* PREPARING AROMATHERAPY TREATMENTS in Part Three.

■ Essential oil of lavender promotes calmness and reduces stress reactions; orange oil is relaxing; and peppermint oil reduces nausea. Take a handkerchief and put 3 drops of lavender oil, 2 drops of orange oil, and 1 drop of peppermint oil on it. Keep this in your pocket. Throughout the day, whenever you feel you want a cigarette, take it out and inhale briefly. This is also effective for headaches associated with nicotine withdrawal, especially when combined with a quick walk.

GENERAL RECOMMENDATIONS

■ Exercise, even if you do not normally do so. Daily exercise is of tremendous benefit in helping to relieve stress

---

Cigars, Cigarettes, and Nicotine Addiction

It is widely accepted that the addictive quality of nicotine is responsible for the difficulty in quitting cigarette smoking. Yet cigars also contain nicotine, but seem not to cause the same degree of addiction. Could there be something in cigarettes other than tobacco that causes this problem?

Possibly, but the main reason for the greater addictiveness of cigarettes probably lies in the fact that cigarette smoke is inhaled deeply into the lungs, while cigar smoke is not. As a result, the cigarette smoker receives repeated potent jolts of nicotine (and other substances) that go directly from the lungs into his or her bloodstream. This greater exposure is more likely to lead to addiction, and in short order.

Does that mean cigar smoking is better for you— or at least less harmful—than smoking cigarettes? Some people certainly persist in believing so. And cigars have become quite trendy in recent years, having gained an image as a symbol of prosperity and success. If you are considering taking up cigar smoking, either because you think it might help you dodge the ills associated with cigarette smoking or because you think it's glamorous and sophisticated, consider that in 1996, over 58,000 new cases of oral cancer were diagnosed, and about 9,000 people died. Tobacco—whether in cigars, cigarettes, or "smokeless" forms—is a major risk factor for this disorder, which often necessitates remarkably disfiguring surgery. For more information about oral cancer, you can contact the American Association of Oral and Maxillofacial Surgeons at 800–467–5268. They will send you a free pamphlet on oral cancer as well as instructions for self-examination. They can also be contacted through their website, http://www.aaoms.org.

and enhance tissue oxygenation. It also can reduce cravings. Every time you have a craving, get up from your desk, chair, bed, or whatever, walk out the door, and run. Even if you run for only two minutes, you will find your craving reduced. Of course, you will first want to warn coworkers and household members that your are quitting smoking and may be acting strangely for several days.

■ Consider joining a stop-smoking group. It is often easier to go through a difficult experience like nicotine withdrawal if you have access to the support and practical advice of others who are going through the same thing.

■ It can be difficult to do, but try to have patience. When cravings strike, remind yourself that an individual craving has a limited lifespan and that, with time, they will cease, as long as you continue to abstain from smoking.

PREVENTION

■ Nicotine addiction is entirely preventable—all you have to do is *not* start smoking. Once you take that first cigarette, however, the only way to prevent nicotine addiction is not to take the next.

Night Blindness

Night blindness is a condition characterized by difficulty seeing well at night or in dim light, even though your vision is normal (with or without corrective lenses) in bright light or daylight.

Night blindness is usually brought on by a deficiency of vitamin A. The retina of the eye—the screen on which images form when light enters the eye—has literally millions of specialized nerve cells called rods and cones that respond to light. The rods are cylindrical-shaped cells on the surface of the retina. They contain a special chemical called visual purple, or rhodopsin, that is responsible for vision in low-light conditions. Rhodopsin is formed from protein and retinol, a form of vitamin A. It breaks down and is lost when struck by light, but it normally is replenished almost immediately—just closing your eyes momentarily is a natural reflex that stimulates the process. However, if you lack sufficient vitamin A, the production of rhodopsin suffers, leading to increased difficulty seeing in dim light. If the deficiency is severe enough, it may cause abnormally dry eyes and, possibly, the appearance of foamy white patches called *Bitot's spots* on the surface of the eye.

Though night blindness is often caused by a deficiency of vitamin A, it can be a sign of other problems, such as developing cataracts, glaucoma, or retinitis pigmentosa. Many people experience increasing difficulty with dark adaptation as they get older, but this is often actually a sign of chronic low-level deficiency of vitamin A rather than a normal part of the aging process. It can also be a result of stress or a reaction to medication, and may be accompanied by myopia (nearsightedness).

In diagnosing night blindness, your doctor will likely ask many questions, such as the following:

- When did you first notice the problem?
- Did it occur suddenly or gradually?
- Is it constant or occasional?
- Is your vision impaired even in a dimly lit room?
- Are you nearsighted?
- Do you have a fear of the dark?
- Are you under considerable stress?
- Does the use of corrective lenses improve your night vision?
- Have you had any changes in your daytime vision?
- Do you have photophobia (light sensitivity)?
- Do you have cataracts?
- What medicines are you currently taking?
- Do you use recreational drugs?
- Do you have a family history of diabetes?
- Do you eat a healthy diet?

If you prepare to answer these questions before your doctor visit, your physician will probably find it easier to make a correct diagnosis and appropriate recommendations.

CONVENTIONAL TREATMENT

■ Whenever you have a problem with your vision, consult an ophthalmologist. He or she will examine your eyes to determine your visual acuity, check for any signs of injury, and, most important, identify any underlying disease that may require treatment.

■ If vitamin-A deficiency is identified, your doctor will likely prescribe therapeutic doses of this vitamin. Follow your doctor's recommendations. Sometimes, though, deficiency can be severe enough to cause problems but not severe enough to show up on conventional tests. That can make this condition difficult to diagnose correctly.

DIETARY GUIDELINES

■ Eat plenty of clean, lean protein, such as that found in chicken and fish, as well as ample amounts of foods rich in beta-carotene, including fresh yellow and orange fruits and vegetables, to supply plenty of the basic ingredients your body needs to produce visual purple.

■ Avoid excess sugar and caffeine. These substances contribute to eye irritation and worsen the symptoms caused by many eye problems.

NUTRITIONAL SUPPLEMENTS

■ The essential fatty acids (EFAs), found in black currant seed oil, borage oil, evening primrose oil, and flaxseed oil, are required by every cell in the body. Take 500 to 1,000 milligrams of any of these oils twice daily.

■ Glutathione is a natural antioxidant normally present in high concentrations in healthy eye tissues. Glutathione levels are often lower than normal in the eyes of older individuals with compromised night vision. Take 100 milligrams of glutathione twice daily.

■ Without sufficient vitamin A, the eyes are more sensitive to variations in light intensity and more susceptible to infection, ulcerations, and even blindness. Even a slight deficiency can cause problems. Take 10,000 international units of vitamin A three times a day for two months. Then cut back to a maintenance dosage of 5,000 international units twice daily.

Note: If you are pregnant, or intend to get pregnant, or if you have liver disease, consult your doctor before taking supplemental vitamin A. Pregnant women should not ingest a total of more than 25,000 international units of supplemental vitamin A *per week* from all sources.

■ Beta-carotene is a precursor of vitamin A; the body converts it to vitamin A as needed. Taken as a supplement, it has many of the same properties as vitamin A, but it does not become toxic in large doses. Take 10,000 to 25,000 international units of beta-carotene twice daily.

■ Deficiencies of the B vitamins can contribute to light-related eye problems. While symptoms are acute, take a B-complex supplement supplying 50 milligrams of each of the major B vitamins twice daily. When symptoms improve, reduce the dosage to 25 milligrams twice daily.

■ Zinc supports the immune system and is beneficial for the eyes. A combination of vitamin A, the B vitamins, and zinc can sometimes alleviate night blindness if vitamin A alone is not successful. While symptoms are acute, take 25 to 50 milligrams daily. When symptoms improve, reduce the dosage to 15 to 20 milligrams daily.

Note: Take zinc with food to prevent stomach upset. If you take over 30 milligrams of zinc on a daily basis for more than one or two months, you should also take 1 to 2 milligrams of copper each day to maintain a proper mineral balance.

HERBAL TREATMENT

■ Bilberry provides important nutrients that nourish the eyes and enhance visual function. Taking bilberry extract can help the eyes make a quicker adjustment to changes in light levels and improve night vision. Extracts of this herb are believed able to provide protection against macular degeneration, cataracts, and glaucoma, and may slow the loss of sight in those with retinitis pigmentosa. Select a preparation containing 25 percent anthocyanosides and take 80 milligrams twice daily.

■ Eyebright is rich in vitamin A and vitamin C. It also contains moderate amounts of the B-complex vitamins, vitamin D, and traces of vitamin E. It helps maintain healthy eyes and good vision. Take 500 milligrams twice daily.

HOMEOPATHY

■ *Gelsemium* is good for tired or lazy eyes coupled with poor nighttime vision. Take one of *Gelsemium* 30x or 15c, as directed on the product label, three times daily for up to three days.

■ *Lycopodium* is good if you have poor night vision and also suffer from poor digestion. Take one dose of *Lycopodium* 30x or 15c three times daily for up to three days.

■ *Phosphorus* is for night blindness accompanied by exhaustion. You may feel so tired you "can't see straight." Take one dose of *Phosphorus* 30x or 15c three times daily for up to three days.

ACUPRESSURE

For the locations of acupressure points on the body, *see* ADMINISTERING AN ACUPRESSURE TREATMENT in Part Three.

■ Gallbladder 20 improves circulation to the head.

■ Large Intestine 4 has a beneficial effect on the head and face.

AROMATHERAPY

For specific instructions on how to use aromatherapy, *see* PREPARING AROMATHERAPY TREATMENTS in Part Three.

■ Essential oils of lavender and orange are calming, and may help if eye problems are associated with or made worse by stress. Use either or both as inhalants. There are also diffusers available that are designed to be used in cars that you may find useful.

GENERAL RECOMMENDATIONS

■ If you take the recommended amounts of vitamin A, the B-complex vitamins, and zinc for three months without seeing an improvement, see your ophthalmologist to rule out any serious eye problems, such as early-stage glaucoma or retinitis pigmentosa.

■ Avoid substances known to irritate the eyes, such as

smog and smoke. Whether it comes from cigars, pipes, cigarettes, or sweet-smelling wood burning in a fireplace, smoke is very hard on the eyes and can worsen symptoms.

■ As long as your night vision is compromised, avoid driving at night or performing any intricate or potentially dangerous tasks in low-light conditions. If you get up in the middle of the night, even for a few minutes, turn on a light so that you can see what you are doing.

PREVENTION

■ A deficiency of vitamin A, the "eye vitamin," is a major factor in the development of night-vision difficulties. As a preventive measure, take 5,000 international units of this important vitamin daily.

Nosebleed

There are a great many tiny blood vessels in the delicate lining of the nose. These small capillaries are easily broken. Any number of things can rupture some of these small vessels and cause a nosebleed.

An accident or assault that results in a blow to the nose can cause your nose to bleed. If you put something in your nose, bleeding can result form the trauma. Even just blowing your nose can start a nosebleed. Inflammation from a cold, an allergy, or dry winter air can cause the vessels to swell and rupture. You may even awaken with blood on your sheets or staining your nightclothes. When a nosebleed occurs from one of these causes, it seldom hurts. More uncomfortable causes include local infection, such as sinusitis, or systemic infections such as scarlet fever, malaria, or typhoid fever.

Blood can be swallowed during a nosebleed, especially one that occurs during the night. If enough blood is involved, you may vomit it up or pass a dark, tarry-looking stool after the nosebleed has stopped.

The blood coming from the nose during a nosebleed can be a continuous stream or a small trickle. It may look as if you are losing a lot of blood, but not much blood is actually lost during the typical nosebleed. Although a bloody nose, especially one that comes on suddenly and without warning, can be unnerving, nosebleeds can usually be managed easily at home. Like most wounds, ruptured capillaries inside the nose will heal completely in about ten days.

Certain medical conditions can increase the likelihood of nosebleeds, among them high blood pressure, aplastic anemia, hemophilia, leukemia, Hodgkin's disease, rheumatic fever, thrombocytopenia, and severe liver disease. The use of certain drugs, notably anticoagulants (blood thinners) and aspirin, may be involved as well. Other factors that increase the possibility of nosebleeds include the prolonged use of nose drops, exposure to irritating chemicals, vitamin-C deficiency, high altitude, and/or a dry climate.

EMERGENCY TREATMENT

See How to Stop a Nosebleed on page 446.

CONVENTIONAL TREATMENT

■ In the event of a severe nosebleed, your doctor may pack your nose with gauze and instruct you to leave the packing in for one or two days.

■ For an exceptionally serious nosebleed, your physician may recommend cauterizing the broken blood vessels within the nose. This involves applying an electrical current or silver-nitrate stick directly to the broken vessel to solidify the blood at the site.

■ In very rare cases of severe, recurrent nosebleeds, a surgical tie-off of one of the larger blood vessels that supplies the tiny capillaries in the lining of the nose may be recommended. Fortunately, this procedure is rarely necessary.

DIETARY GUIDELINES

■ Eat plenty of green leafy vegetables, both raw and cooked. These are good sources of vitamin K, which is necessary for proper blood clotting.

■ Eliminate refined sugars from your diet. Sugar makes the body more acidic, which slows healing.

NUTRITIONAL SUPPLEMENTS

■ Take a good multivitamin and mineral complex supplement daily for one month.

■ Green-foods supplements, available in health-food stores, supply an abundance of trace minerals as well as small amounts of bioavailable vitamin K. Take a green-foods supplement two to three times daily as directed on the product label.

■ Vitamin C and bioflavonoids help prevent capillary fragility. Take 500 to 1,000 milligrams of each four times daily for two days after a nosebleed. Then take 500 milligrams of each twice a day for at least one month.

■ Vitamin K helps the blood to clot more efficiently. If you suffer from recurring nosebleeds, take 25 micrograms once or twice daily for one month.

HERBAL TREATMENT

■ An aloe vera nasal douche can be very soothing. Take 1 teaspoon of aloe vera gel and instill some into each nostril with a dropper.

How to Stop a Nosebleed

■ If you develop a nosebleed, do the following:

1. Calmly sit down in an upright position, not back in the chair. This will help to keep blood from going down the back of your throat. Breathe through your mouth.

2. Tilt your head forward (*not* backward).

3. Place your thumb and forefinger on either side of the bridge of your nose and pinch the soft part of your nose firmly for ten minutes without releasing. Apply pressure firmly enough to slow bleeding, but not so strongly as to cause discomfort. Pressure decreases the blood flow through the affected area, slowing bleeding. You can also place a cold compress on the bridge of your nose. This has not been proven to be effective but seems to help constrict the local blood vessels.

4. After ten minutes, release the nostrils slowly and check to see if the bleeding has stopped. Avoid touching or blowing your nose. If the bleeding has *not* stopped, apply pressure for another ten-minute period.

5. If your nose is still bleeding steadily after twenty minutes of pressure, call your health-care provider.

■ Another way to stop a nosebleed is to wet a bit of cotton or plain sterile gauze with white vinegar and place it in your nose. Leave it in place for at least ten minutes. The acid of the vinegar will gently cauterize the inside of the nose and stop the bleeding.

HOMEOPATHY

■ *Ferrum phosphoricum* will help resolve a nosebleed and speed local healing of the injured tissue. Take one dose of *Ferrum phosphoricum* 6x, 12x, or 6c, as directed on the product label, every ten minutes for a total of three or four doses.

GENERAL RECOMMENDATIONS

■ Do not blow your nose for twelve hours after bleeding subsides.

■ For a minor nosebleed associated with dry air, such as results from having the heat on during the winter months, try *gently* applying a small amount of petroleum jelly (Vaseline) to the interior of your nostrils each night for a week or two. It may also help to use a humidifier in your bedroom at night.

PREVENTION

■ Never put any foreign object in your nose.

■ Do not smoke, and avoid secondhand smoke.

■ If you are prone to recurring small nosebleeds, take a cup of nettle-leaf several times a week as a preventive. Nettle contains vitamins A and C, which strengthen the mucous membranes, as well as many trace minerals, including an easily absorbed form of iron.

Note: Some people experience stomach upset as a result of taking nettle. If that happens, stop taking it.

■ Take Vitamin C and bioflavonoids.

■ To keep the lining of your nose moist and lessen the chance of small capillaries swelling and rupturing, humidify the air in your home, particularly during the dry winter months. Use a humidifier in your bedroom, making sure to fill it with purified distilled water only. Clean your humidifier once a week to keep bacteria from building up and to make certain that it is not spreading allergens.

■ Moisten the lining of your nose with a salt-water spray. Follow the procedure for NASAL SALINE FLUSH in Part Three to flush the nasal membranes twice daily (*do not* suction out mucus afterward). Over-the-counter saline (salt-water) nasal sprays, such as Ocean, Ayr, and Salinex, serve the same purpose. A small amount of an ointment such as Aquaphor, calendula, or aloe vera gel applied after a saline spray can help nasal membranes heal.

■ Avoid the use of decongestant nasal sprays. They constrict blood vessels and can lead to bleeding.

■ For some ways you can reduce the possibility that you will suffer an accident that leads to a nosebleed, *see* PERSONAL SAFETY in Part One.

Obesity

A person is considered obese if he or she weighs 20 percent more than the average for a person of the same sex, height, and body build. Obesity is considered a health problem, rather than merely a cosmetic concern, because it increases a person's risk of many serious disorders. For example, heart disease, high blood pressure, and stroke are twice as likely to strike obese people as those of normal weight. Obesity is also associated with low levels of high-density lipoproteins (HDL, the so-called "good cholesterol") and high levels of low-density lipoproteins (LDL, or "bad cholesterol," which builds up on arterial walls). Adult-onset diabetes is five times more common among obese individuals. Obese women show a progressive increase in risk of cancer of the breast, uterus, and cervix. Osteoarthritis is aggravated by obesity, because excess weight on the hips, knees, and back places a high degree of strain on these susceptible joints.

In the simplest terms, obesity results from an imbalance in energy exchange: Too much energy is taken in (food) without an equal amount of energy output (activity). The body takes these excess calories, turns them into fat, and stores them, which can lead to a weight problem. Though we know how this happens, people have been trying for years to determine the underlying causes—that is, why certain people become obese and others do not. Two main theories have emerged: the fat-cell theory and the theory that obesity is a hereditary condition.

The fat-cell theory postulates that if you have been programmed to overeat since childhood, or if you consume a high-fat and/or high-sugar diet, particularly during growth spurts, your body is stimulated to manufacture an excessive number of new fat cells. According to the fat-cell theory, every fat cell your body manufactures stays with you for life and, short of surgery, there is no way to rid yourself of even a single fat cell once your body has manufactured it. The heredity theory holds that some people are simply destined to be obese because overweight runs in families. Indeed, studies have shown that just 7 percent of children born to normal-weight parents grow up to be overweight, while if one or both parents has a weight problem, there is a 40- or 80-percent chance, respectively, that their child also will have a weight problem.

Both of these theories probably contain elements of the truth, but there is reason to doubt that either of them is entirely correct or accounts for all cases of obesity. Recent research shows that it may be possible to reduce the number of fat cells in the body, if there is a major weight loss. Other studies suggest that even obese people who had two obese parents can slim down to healthy proportions when they modify their diets and begin to exercise regularly. In other words, an inherited tendency to pack on the pounds does *not* mean that you have no choice but to become (or stay) overweight, just as the number of fat cells in your body is probably not a life sentence. In the final analysis, the experts say, eating and exercise habits are the greatest determinants of which individuals end up overweight.

People overeat for many reasons. Some simply love food. Many people subconsciously equate food with emotional comfort, and eat to cope with feelings of depression, failure, or low self-esteem. Some use food to reward themselves for minor accomplishments. Many people overeat simply out of habit. A particular problem these days is a dependence on convenience and junk foods, which supply lots of calories but very little nutrition. Heavy consumption of these foods creates an obese individual who—despite the excess weight—may also be malnourished, because he or she is missing the essential nutrients found in fresh, whole foods.

There are certain metabolic and endocrine imbalances, including hypothyroidism and hypopituitarism, that can cause abnormal weight gain. How the body uses insulin is another factor. If your body lacks the ability to clear insulin from the bloodstream quickly, you may feel hungry even when you have eaten enough. If you have a real reason to suspect that your excess weight is a result of something other than eating habits or lack of exercise, consult your physician.

CONVENTIONAL TREATMENT

■ In rare cases, an underlying medical condition may be causing weight gain. A doctor's examination and blood testing may be worthwhile to rule out endocrine or metabolic problems, such as hypothyroidism, adrenal disease (Cushing's syndrome), pituitary disorders, or genetic diseases.

■ There is mounting evidence that food allergies and intolerances may also contribute to weight gain for may people. Ask your physician about testing for these conditions. One excellent method of testing for food allergies is the ALCAT test, in which a sample of blood is drawn and sent to a laboratory that detects sensitivities by measuring changes in the blood in response to different test substances.

■ If there are no signs of underlying problems, your doctor will probably recommend dietary changes and regular exercise. Many will design a special diet and, in severe cases, supervised fasting. Some will mandate specific periods of exercise.

■ Behavior modification is a commonly used tool for weight problems. (*See* BEHAVIOR MODIFICATION FOR WEIGHT CONTROL in Part Three).

■ Medications to suppress appetite, whether prescription or over-the-counter drugs, are to be avoided. They do nothing to address the behavior patterns that led to obesity in the first place, and they can produce serious side effects. Amphetamines, once commonly prescribed for dieters, were notorious for causing hyperactivity, nervousness, dry mouth, insomnia, elevated blood pressure, and, ultimately, psychological dependence. More recently, use of the diet-drug combination of fenfluramine and phentermine (better known as "fen-phen,") was found to lead to serious heart damage in an alarming number of people who took it, and the U.S. Food and Drug Administration (FDA) banned its use. A newer diet drug, sibutramine (Meridia), has most of the side effects of its predecessors, and may have addictive properties.

■ Surgery is sometimes used as a last resort for severe obesity that responds to no other measures. The procedures used include gastric banding, in which a portion of the stomach is stapled closed, and gastric bypass, which also decreases the stomach's capacity. Weight loss immediately following surgery can be impressive. However, long-term success is only in the 50-percent range.

■ Liposuction is a surgical procedure in which fat cells are suctioned out from specific areas of the body by means of a tube called a cannula inserted through a small incision. Under ideal circumstances, liposuction is reputedly safe. However, cosmetic surgery is a very lucrative practice, and there have been problems with procedures performed by physicians with inadequate training and experience. If you are interested in liposuction, ask your physician to refer you to a qualified surgeon.

DIETARY GUIDELINES

■ Don't go on a crash diet, and don't skip meals. These tactics simply don't work. When you provide your body with too few calories (or no calories at all), it will automatically slow down its metabolic rate to conserve and use every nutrient. Instead, follow a diet regimen that provides 500 to 1,000 calories less than your energy requirements—a level that should yield a weight loss of no more than one or two pounds per week. This will cause your body to burn stored fat for energy, and should result in a safe and steady weight loss.

■ Eat nutrient-rich whole foods, which satisfy the appetite far better than processed or junk foods. A diet of whole foods keeps blood-sugar levels on an even keel, minimizing cravings and keeping energy levels high. Also, simple whole foods generally have fewer calories than manufactured food products, and the fiber they contain provides low-calorie, stomach-filling bulk, making it easier to eat less. Base your meals on fresh vegetables and fruits, lean protein foods (fish and skinless white-meat poultry), and whole grains. A simple technique that can help: Shop the perimeter of your supermarket. If you stay out of the middle of the store and do your shopping around the edges of your market, chances are you will be buying vegetables and fruits, dairy products (select the low-fat and nonfat varieties), and eggs, plus fish and poultry. Make an occasional foray into the aisles for bread, cereals, and whole grains, and you are well on your way to bringing home only wholesome whole foods.

■ If you must use prepared foods, check the labels carefully for the number of calories per serving, as well as fat (especially the percentage of calories that come from fat), sugar, and sodium content.

■ Eat a diet that is low in saturated fats, hydrogenated and partially hydrogenated fats, and cooked fats. Avoid creamed dishes, foods with creamy fillings, and rich gravies. Do not add cream or prepared salad dressings to foods. Instead of prepared salad dressings, use lemon juice or apple-cider vinegar and olive oil to dress your salads.

■ Your choice of cooking techniques is important. Eat vegetables either steamed or raw. Do not deep-fry your foods. Bake, broil, poach, or steam them instead. Deep-fried foods are both high in calories and more difficult to digest. Stir-frying, in which only a tablespoon or two of oil (preferably olive oil) is needed to cook an entire meal quickly, is acceptable. Using no-stick cookware can help reduce the amount of oil you need for cooking.

■ Eat slowly, and chew each bite thoroughly. Food that has been well chewed is more easily digested and is therefore more valuable as nourishment.

■ To help flush toxins from your system and fill a hungry stomach, drink at least eight 8-ounce glasses of pure water every day.

■ *Avoid* all foods with additives, preservatives, or sugar, as well as sodas, soft drinks, caffeine, chocolate, and all sweets. Sugar and caffeine cause a tremendous surge in blood sugar levels—followed by a great downward crash. When blood sugar levels are low, you may be tempted to eat undesirable foods. A simple rule of thumb: If you can't recognize (or pronounce) it, don't eat it.

■ Avoid eating heavy evening meals. Overeating at dinner and late-night snacking are primary factors in weight gain. The body burns very few calories while you are sleeping.

NUTRITIONAL SUPPLEMENTS

■ It is best to satisfy the body's vitamin and mineral needs with a healthy diet. However, if you experience a notable drop in your energy level, take a good multivitamin and mineral supplement that supplies at least the recommended daily allowance (FDA) of all the basic vitamins and minerals.

■ Carnitine helps transport fats in the bloodstream into the mitochondria (the "power plants" of the cells) for burning. It also helps to reduce cravings for sweets and fats. Though the body naturally produces carnitine, people who are overweight rarely make enough. Taking 500 milligrams two to three times daily, especially in conjunction with exercise, can be very rewarding.

■ Chromium, or glucose tolerance factor, helps to control blood-sugar levels and diminishes cravings for sugar. Take 200 micrograms of chromium once or twice daily for up to one month.

■ Conjugated linolenic acid (CLA) helps with fat metab-

Conquering Common Cravings

If you go into your local bookstore and look in the self-help category, you will find more books about weight loss than any other subject. That's because they sell. Unfortunately, many of these books contain a mixture of fact and fiction, and it is difficult to know what's true and what's not. Most diets that restrict your intake of calories will make you lose weight. However, if you feel deprived and hungry all the time, chances are you will not stay with a given diet very long. If you need different percentages of certain nutrients than a diet dictates in order to feel satisfied, the result can be food cravings that are very hard to ignore. Following are some strategies for dealing with common food cravings.

IF YOU CRAVE SWEETS

Cravings for sweets often reflect blood-sugar imbalances and a desire for a "quick-fix" stimulant.

• Astragalus provides a lift without artificially stimulating the body. Take 100 milligrams three times daily, at 9:00 AM, 11:00 AM, and 1:00 PM.
• Chromium controls blood-sugar metabolism and helps reduce body fat. Take 100 to 200 micrograms twice daily.
• *Garcinia cambogia* is an herbal remedy that reduces a craving for sweets. Take 500 milligrams twice daily.
• Taking one dose of homeopathic *Lycopodium* 30c can help tame cravings for sweets.

IF YOU CRAVE FATS

Cravings for fatty foods are often a sign that you are eating the wrong kinds of fats and/or not digesting fat properly.

• Flaxseed oil contains alpha-linoleic acid, which promotes the efficient use of carbohydrates and fats for energy. Take 500 to 1,000 milligrams twice daily.
• *Garcinia cambogia* is an herbal remedy that helps suppress appetite and rid the body of excess fat. Take 500 milligrams twice daily.

IF YOU CRAVE CHOCOLATE

Chocolate is a mild stimulant and mood elevator and it tastes good, but chocolate cravings may be related to nutritional deficiencies.

• Many "chocoholics" crave chocolate because they are low in chromium and magnesium. When these nutrients are provided, cravings often become manageable. Take 200 micrograms of chromium and 500 milligrams of magnesium daily.

• A Chinese herbal formula called *Bu Zhong Yi Qu Wan* raises chi, improves mood, and can radically diminish chocolate cravings. Take 3 pellets twice daily, in the morning and afternoon.

IF YOU CRAVE SALT

A single teaspoon of salt contains 2,360 milligrams of sodium (the main nutrient in salt), whereas the body requires only 250 to 350 milligrams daily. Moreover, sodium occurs naturally in all foods except for fruits. Salt cravings therefore most often are not a sign of nutritional deficiency, but of taste buds that have become accustomed to the overuse of salt.

• If your doctor has advised you to eliminate salt, or to tame a craving for salt, use kelp powder instead. Kelp is a naturally salty-tasting sea vegetable that is nevertheless low in sodium.
• Support adrenal function with adrenal glandular extract. Take 200 milligrams twice a day for two months. Or take 200 milligrams of standardized Siberian ginseng extract containing 0.5 percent eleutheroside E and take 200 milligrams once or twice daily for one month.
• Unless you must abandon salt immediately for medical reasons, you can reduce cravings by retraining your taste buds. Slowly cut back on your consumption of salt over a period of weeks.

Note: Sodium deficiency is very rare, but it can occur. If you become overheated and sweat excessively during strong physical exertion or due to extreme heat and then crave salt, your body may be alerting you to an imbalance in your electrolytes.

IF YOU'RE ALWAYS HUNGRY

Constant feelings of hunger are most often a sign that you are not ingesting the right foods—foods that satisfy your body and turn off your appestat.

• Increase your intake of fiber. A high-fiber diet that provides from 30 to 50 grams of fiber per day can ward off the hunger pangs that cause many people to overeat.
• Eat small, more frequent meals. Eating five or six small, well-balanced meals instead of three large ones can keep your stomach from growling "feed me" between meals.
• Fluctuating blood-sugar levels can trigger the appestat to emit hunger signals. Chromium helps to keep blood sugar in balance. Take 100 to 200 micrograms of chromium daily.
• *Garcinia cambogia* helps to control appetite. Take 250 milligrams twice daily.

olism, improving the ratio of lean to fat tissue. Take 1,000 to 2,000 milligrams (1 to 2 grams) three times a day, before meals.

■ Lecithin is a natural nutrient that helps the body metabolize fat. Take 1,200 milligrams twice daily, with meals.

■ The lipotropics, including choline, inositol, and methionine, help to control blood-sugar levels, improve liver function, and enhance fat and carbohydrate metabolism. They help the body use nutrients more efficiently, making it easier to eat less. Take a lipotropic combination supplement supplying 350 milligrams of choline, 100 milligrams of inositol, and 200 milligrams of methionine twice daily, with meals, as directed on the product label.

■ The amino acid phenylalanine stimulates the metabolism and helps suppress the appetite. Take 500 milligrams of DL-phenylalanine (DLPA) once or twice daily for three weeks.

■ Pyruvic acid helps the body to burn calories more effectively. Take a total of 5,000 to 6,000 milligrams (5 to 6 grams) daily.

■ Tyrosine, another amino acid, stimulates the thyroid and strengthens metabolic function. Take 500 milligrams of L-tyrosine each morning for three weeks.

Note: If you are taking a monoamine oxidase (MAO) inhibitor drug, do not take supplemental tyrosine, as a sudden and dangerous rise in blood pressure may result.

HERBAL TREATMENT

■ Alisma, astragalus, and atractylodes is a Chinese herbal combination that helps to encourage weight loss. Alisma is a diuretic; astragalus enhances energy; atractylodes helps the digestion of carbohydrates. These three herbs work best when taken together. Select a combination formula and take one dose, as directed on the product label, two to three times daily.

■ Dandelion helps lower cholesterol, improves liver function, and acts as a diuretic. Take 500 milligrams three times a day, with meals, for two months.

■ *Garcinia cambogia* helps reduce the appetite, inhibits the production and storagae of fat, and works to lower cholesterol. Select an extract of this herb that supplies 50 percent hydroxycitric acid (HCA) and take 500 to 750 milligrams three to four times daily.

■ Green tea enhances the ability of the body to burn fat. Choose a standardized extract containing 50 percent catechin and 90 percent total polyphenols and take 300 milligrams thirty minutes before breakfast and another thirty minutes before lunch.

■ Guggul is an herb that helps to lower cholesterol and that may stimulate thyroid function. Take 500 milligrams three times a day.

Note: Do not use this herb if you have a thyroid disorder.

■ Kelp and bladderwrack contain iodine, which helps to enhance thyroid function. Select either one and take 150 milligrams at breakfast and another 150 milligrams lunch for two months.

Note: If you are allergic to shellfish and/or sensitive to iodine, do not take these herbs.

■ Licorice root strengthens the adrenal glands, thus helping to sustain a regulated blood-sugar level and reduce cravings for sweets. Licorice tastes sweet. Take a cup of licorice daily, one week out of every month for up to three months. Licorice can also be added to other teas to sweeten them.

Note: Do not take licorice by itself on a daily basis for more than five days at a time, as it can elevate blood pressure. Do not take it at all if you have high blood pressure.

■ Cleansing and chlorophyll-rich parsley tea is a mild diuretic. Take one cup daily for one week when beginning a new dietary routine.

■ Plantain helps reduce the body's absorption of fats. Take a cup of plantain tea twice a day, three days per week, for two months.

■ Red clover aids in detoxifying a body burdened with excess pounds. Take 500 milligrams daily, one week out of every month, for up to three months.

■ Red raspberry leaf tea reduces appetite, increases energy, and acts as a diuretic—and it tastes good. Take a cup twice a day, one week out of each month, for up to three months. Do not take it before bed, though; it may be too energizing.

■ Siberian ginseng helps to stabilize blood sugar and reduce cravings for sweets. It is also a natural energizer. Choose a standardized extract containing 0.5 percent eleutheroside E and take 100 milligrams daily, two weeks out of every month, for up to three months.

■ Do *not* use herbal diet products that contain ephedra. This is a central nervous system stimulant, and should be avoided.

HOMEOPATHY

■ *Antimonium crudum* is good if you become peevish and irritable if anyone warns you not to overeat. You are also subject to belching and diarrhea, and may have a coated tongue. Take one dose of *Antimonium crudum* 30x or 7c each morning and another in late afternoon for up to five days.

■ *Argentum nitricum* reduces cravings for sweets. Take one dose of *Argentum nitricum* 30x or 9c twice daily for up to one week.

■ *Calcarea carbonica* can help if you have difficulty controlling your appetite and eat to calm your nerves. Take one dose of *Calcarea carbonica* 12x or 6c three times daily for up to one week when beginning a new dietary program.

■ *Coffea cruda* is good if you are excitable and nervous, and eat primarily to calm down. If *Calcarea carbonica* and/or *Ignatia* has not helped, try taking one dose of *Coffea cruda* 12x or 6c three times daily for up to three days.

■ *Graphites* 30x or 9c is the remedy for the perimenopausal woman fighting weight gain. You are probably pale and very sensitive to cold. Take one dose of *Graphites* 30x or 9c each morning and another in the afternoon for up to five days.

■ *Ignatia* is helpful if you are anxious and fearful, and feel you simply must eat when you are tense and nervous. Take one dose of *Ignatia* 30x or 9c each morning and again in the afternoon for up to five days.

■ *Staphysagria* is good if you tend to eat out of repressed anger. There may be oppressive, even abusive, relationships in your life that are contributing to the problem. Take one dose of *Staphysagria* 30x or 9c each morning and another in the late afternoon for up to five days.

ACUPRESSURE

For the locations of acupressure points on the body, *see* ADMINISTERING AN ACUPRESSURE TREATMENT in Part Three.

■ Four Gates relaxes the nervous system.

■ Neck and Shoulder Release will help to relax and calm you as you make the transition to a new dietary and exercise regime.

AROMATHERAPY

For specific instructions on how to use aromatherapy, *see* PREPARING AROMATHERAPY TREATMENTS in Part Three.

■ Essential oils of bergamot, fennel, and patchouli can help to regulate the appetite. Use any or all as inhalants or in baths or massage oil, or diffuse them into the air in your home.

GENERAL RECOMMENDATIONS

■ Avoid chewing gum. The calories in gum are few, but chewing increases the appetite by fooling the stomach into "thinking" that food is on the way. The stomach begins to prepare. It floods the area with digestive juices and churns and growls. Appetite increases. Because hunger signals have been activated, you are more likely to end up eating.

■ Keep in mind that no single diet that will work for everyone. In fact, a "diet" as such is rarely the answer at all, since the very idea of "going on a diet" implies that, at some point, you will go *off* the diet. Instead, work toward

creating a lifestyle that suits you and that will make you healthy and fit over the long run. Similarly, learn to respect the uniqueness of your body. There is no "right" body shape or size. Remember that losing weight is about being healthy, not about appearances. Only when you learn to truly love and care for yourself are you likely to succeed with a weight-loss regimen.

■ Physical activity increases the metabolic rate so that more calories are burned more efficiently. Remarkably, this higher rate of caloric burn continues even after the physical activity ceases. Basal metabolism, the rate at which the body burns calories while at rest, varies from person to person. There is no standard or norm. On the whole, though, naturally active people—the ones who never seem to sit still—use up more calories, and burn calories faster and more efficiently, than ones who prefer quiet activities. An active person will typically burn 10 percent more calories per hour than a sedentary person. Exercise also reduces appetite. The appetite-control center of the body is the hypothalamus, or "appestat," the portion of the brain that tells the body when it is hungry and when the stomach is full. The appestat's hunger signals are triggered by specific levels of certain substances in the blood, including glucose, serotonin, noradrenaline, adrenaline, and dopamine. Physical activity reduces the levels of the hunger-stimulating chemicals that cause the appestat to start the stomach growling for food, and increases the levels of the chemicals that signal to the appestat that the body is humming along at peak efficiency and doesn't require food. In fact, research indicates that exercise can inhibit hunger for as long as six hours after a high level of physical activity. If you are a sedentary person whose favorite activity is eating, commit yourself to at least a twenty-minute period of physical activity each day. Pleasant and fun forms of exercise to try include dancing, hiking, walking, yoga, swimming, bicycling, roller skating, and team sports. If you are self-conscious and prefer to exercise alone, you might want to investigate some of the video workout tapes on the market—there are plenty to choose from.

■ If your favorite way of rewarding yourself is with food, find calorie-free substitutes that give you pleasure. A vigorous massage is a wonderful way to pamper yourself, whether you are dieting or not. Use a natural vegetable-fiber (loofah) mitt or brush. In addition to keeping you in touch with your body, a dry-brush massage before showering enhances circulation, stimulates a sluggish nervous system, and hastens detoxification of the system, as well as getting rid of dead skin cells and making the skin shine.

■ Don't neglect your emotional side. Sharing thoughts, accomplishments, and frustrations with a friend or family member can help you keep yourself on track. If you need an extra boost, look into joining a support group or seeing a professional counselor. Also, pay attention to how your feelings and food habits relate to each other. For example, many people eat to calm or comfort themselves when they are nervous, worried, and/or depressed. Once you realize what it is that is driving you to overeat, you can work on finding other strategies for dealing with these feelings.

■ Explore biofeedback, meditation, and visualization exercises. All of these techniques can help you stay with your new program. For example, spend a certain period of time each day visualizing yourself having a slimmer, fitter body, and feeling stronger and healthier.

■ Americans spend over six billion dollars every year on fraudulent weight-loss programs and products. Always remember that the miraculous claims for many food products and/or services are designed to sell the product or service, not to transform an overweight individual into a slim one. A simple rule of thumb is: If it sounds too good to be true, it probably is.

PREVENTION

■ When it comes to obesity, prevention is easier than cure. A healthy lifestyle that includes a healthy diet, regular exercise, self-discipline, and supportive family and friends can help prevent weight problems. But these same measures can also help you lose those excess pounds, and it is never too late to begin.

Obsessive-Compulsive Disorder

Obsessive-compulsive disorder (OCD) is a psychological syndrome characterized by constantly recurring thoughts (obsessions) and actions that are performed repetitively (compulsions). Whether the thoughts and/or actions are considered "acceptable" is unimportant; the mere frequency of them makes them abnormal. A person with OCD is likely to recognize the absurdity of his or her routine, and may even hate it, but violating it causes severe anxiety that can be reduced only by returning to the obsessive thought or compulsive action.

People with OCD tend to be highly ordered and intelligent, and may have an underlying fear of losing control. Major depression is associated with the disorder, and affects an estimated two thirds of people with OCD at some point in their lives. At times of high stress, more serious psychological problems can occur, such as paranoia or delusions. OCD may also be associated with involuntary movements such as tics or tremors, and fine motor coor-

dination may be altered. For many people, symptoms seem to go away on their own from time to time, but then return. This disorder is often diagnosed in childhood or adolescence, although it can develop in adulthood as well.

CONVENTIONAL TREATMENT

■ Drugs known as selective serotonin reuptake inhibitors (SSRIs), which increase the levels of the neurotransmitter serotonin in the brain, are helpful for some people. These include fluoxetine (Prozac), fluvoxamine (Luvox), paroxetine (Paxil), and sertraline (Zoloft), which are commonly prescribed for depression. It may be necessary to take a higher dosage for OCD than for depression. Possible side effects include headache, loss of appetite, anxiety, sleepiness, tremor, nausea, weakness, diarrhea, rash, and blood-sugar changes.

■ Clomipramine (Anafranil), a tricyclic antidepressant, may also be tried. This drug too can cause side effects, including seizures, dizziness, loss of sex drive, nervousness, nausea, weight gain, and blood-cell changes.

■ If antidepressant therapy is not effective, buspirone (BuSpar) may be added. This is an antianxiety drug. Unlike some antianxiety agents, it is not a tranquilizer, and does not seem to cause depression or dependence or impair motor skills. It can, however, cause side effects of dizziness, nausea, nervousness, disturbed dreams, nasal congestion, and ringing in the ears. You have to take it for up to three weeks before experiencing a beneficial effect.

■ Drug therapy is often combined with behavioral therapy. While traditional psychotherapy has not been found to be very effective for OCD, a technique called exposure therapy appears to be useful for many people. This involves intentional exposure, in a clinical setting, to things that have caused anxiety and triggered obsessive-compulsive behavior in the past while preventing yourself from engaging in that behavior. The anxiety and undesirable behavior eventually start to diminish, and the effects can last for quite a long time.

■ In the most extreme cases, surgery may be recommended. This can involve cutting an area of the brain called the cingulum, which is involved in pain and other functions. This is obviously an extreme measure, and is reserved for situations in which the disorder is seriously disabling and does not respond to any other treatments.

DIETARY GUIDELINES

■ Maintaining a stable blood-sugar level is very important. Avoid refined sugar (and anything that contains it) and stimulants such as caffeine, which cause rapid fluctuations in blood sugar.

■ Consider the possibility that food allergies may be aggravating symptoms. Use an Elimination Diet to uncover possible sensitivities (*see* ELIMINATION DIET in Part Three).

NUTRITIONAL SUPPLEMENTS

■ Calcium and magnesium help to strengthen the nervous system. Take 600 milligrams of calcium and 300 milligrams of magnesium twice a day.

■ Gamma-aminobutyric acid (GABA) is an amino acid that acts as a calming neurotransmitter in the brain. Taking 500 milligrams one hour before bedtime improves sleep and helps to restore the nervous system.

■ Taurine is another amino acid that assists in improving brain function and reducing anxiety. Take 500 milligrams two or three times daily, between or before meals.

■ The B vitamins are essential for a properly functioning nervous system. Take a B-complex supplement containing 50 to 100 of each of the major B vitamins three times daily.

HERBAL TREATMENT

■ Bupleurum and dong quai is a Chinese herbal combination that restores the blood, strengthens the spleen, and helps to regulate the liver. In Chinese medicine, obsessive-compulsive disorder is due to liver stagnation and a weak spleen. Take 300 to 500 milligrams three times daily.

■ Oat straw is high in silica and aids in the utilization of calcium. Take 500 milligrams twice a day.

■ St. John's wort has shown some usefulness in mild cases of obsessive-compulsive disorder. Select a standardized extract containing 0.3 percent hypericin and take 300 milligrams two or three times daily.

HOMEOPATHY

■ The best approach to treating this disorder homeopathically is to consult a homeopathic physician who can prescribe a constitutional remedy designed specifically for you.

BACH FLOWER REMEDIES

■ White Chestnut is helpful if you are troubled by obsessive thinking and repetitive thoughts that seem to go around and around in your head long after they should have been forgotten. Use it as directed on the product label.

ACUPRESSURE

For the locations of acupressure points on the body, *see* ADMINISTERING AN ACUPRESSURE TREATMENT in Part Three.

■ The combination of Liver 3, Pericardium 6, Spleen 6, and Stomach 36 helps to relax and strengthen the nervous system.

AROMATHERAPY

For specific instructions on how to use aromatherapy, *see* PREPARING AROMATHERAPY TREATMENTS in Part Three.

■ Aromatherapy baths made with essential oil of chamomile can help you to relax.

■ Lavender, orange, and rose oils are simultaneously uplifting, calming, and centering. Use any or all of these oils as inhalants, diffuse them into the air, or use them in baths or massage oil.

GENERAL RECOMMENDATIONS

■ If you are under a doctor's care for obsessive-compulsive disorder, do not make changes in your treatment regimen without consulting him or her. If you decide to discontinue medication or stop seeing your doctor because you seem to be doing much better, you may suffer a relapse of symptoms. Successful treatment of this condition almost always requires the involvement of a professional.

PREVENTION

■ The cause or causes of OCD are not known, so preventing it may not be possible. It is wise, however, to be aware of its characteristic signs and symptoms so that you can recognize them if they arise, and can seek treatment promptly.

Osteoarthritis

See under ARTHRITIS.

Osteoporosis

Osteoporosis is a condition in which the bones become porous and brittle and, as a result, more likely to break, bend, or become compressed, leading to pain and disability. Although it can occur in men and even in children, it is most common in postmenopausal women.

Doctors distinguish between two major types of osteoporosis, depending on which part or part of the bones are affected. Bones consist of two layers: the cortical bone, formed primarily from calcium and other minerals, and cancellous bone, formed of bone cells and interlacing fibers of collagen, a type of protein. The cortical bone (the outer shell) is hard and dense, but the inside collagen layer is soft and spongy. Type I osteoporosis is characterized by a loss of cancellous bone mass; type II by a loss of both cancellous and cortical bone mass.

Bone is complex living tissue. Our bones provide structural support for muscles, protect vital organs, and store calcium. The most important years for building bone mass are from preadolescence to about age thirty.

The body is in a constant state of bone repair, laying down new bone while reabsorbing the old. Normally, a steady level of bone mass is maintained. An overall loss of bone mass can be due to the body breaking down too much bone tissue or failing to form enough bone tissue—or both. Some loss of bone is a normal part of the aging process for both sexes; it begins at around age thirty and by the age of seventy, bone density has diminished by about one-third in the average adult. However, it is a particular problem for women after menopause. When the ovaries stop producing estrogen, which helps maintain bone mass, osteoporosis becomes a real threat. Other factors in osteoporosis are deficiencies of calcium and vitamin D (which enhances the absorption of calcium) and lack of sufficient physical activity. If you do not provide your body with enough calcium for its needs, it will "steal" calcium from your bones. Exercise, particularly weight-bearing exercise such as walking, stimulates the body to build up the bones and keep them strong.

Osteoporosis can also be caused by certain hormonal disorders and prolonged treatment with corticosteroid drugs. Although medical science cannot explain why, this condition is more common in people with chronic obstructive lung disorders such as bronchitis and emphysema. Smoking and alcohol consumption are additional risk factors, as are early menopause (whether natural or surgically induced) and a history of eating disorders such as anorexia and bulimia. Body build also plays a part—the more fine-boned you are to start with, the greater the chance that loss of bone mass will be a problem—as does ethnicity. Women of Caucasian and Asian descent are far more likely to develop osteoporosis than women of African ancestry are, though no ethnic group is immune.

Some people with osteoporosis experience an achiness in their bones, but most have no symptoms, at least in the early stages. The first sign is often a broken bone caused by a fall that would not cause injury to a normal adult. Although broken hips are often held up as a typical injury from undiagnosed osteoporosis, fractures of the wrist and thigh are more common. Spontaneous compression fractures of one or more vertebrae can lead to a progressive loss of height and/or pain due to a pinched spinal nerve.

CONVENTIONAL TREATMENT

■ Conventional treatment often begins with a bone mineral density test. This is a quick, painless low-dose radiological exam that shows the extent of bone loss. A newer ultrasound test may also be used for this purpose.

■ Hormone replacement therapy (HRT) is often recommended for postmenopausal women who have, or are considered at risk for, osteoporosis. HRT does slow bone loss, and in some cases can increase bone density. Unfortunately, HRT is not without side effects (*see* MENOPAUSE for a discussion of hormone replacement therapy).

■ Alendronate (Fosamax) and etidronate (Didronel) are drugs classified as bisphosphonates. They force the body to stop reabsorbing existing bone, thus helping to increase relative bone density. Possible side effects include nausea and diarrhea. Though it is generally the more effective of the two, alendronate must be taken exactly according to the instructions or ulceration of the esophagus may result.

■ Calcitonin (Miacalcin, Calcimar) is a synthetic version of a hormone secreted by the thyroid gland that inhibits the reabsorption of bone tissue. Its ability to markedly affect bone density appears to be pretty limited, however. Possible side effects include nausea, vomiting, rashes, and flushing sensations.

■ The drug raloxifene (Evista) is a newer agent approved for the prevention of osteoporosis. Raloxifene is one of a new class of drugs known as selective estrogen receptor modulators, or SERMs, which have estrogenlike efects in some parts of the body but not others. SERMS have been shown to prevent bone loss in the spine, hip, and even in the body as a whole. They may also benefit the heart. Possible side effects include hot flashes and the formation of blood clots in the veins.

■ According to report published in the September 1998 issue of the *Journal of the American Medical Association*, estrogen-deficient women may be able to prevent bone loss by taking supplements of human parathyroid hormone. You may wish to discuss this finding with your health-care provider.

DIETARY GUIDELINES

■ A diet high in calcium helps to protect against bone loss. Milk and dairy products, including yogurt, are dependable sources of natural calcium. If you do not eat dairy products, include in your diet plenty of sea vegetables, such as kelp and dulse; green leafy vegetables such as collards, kale, parsley, and watercress; tofu; and broccoli. (See the table on page 455 for the calcium content of selected foods.)

■ Avoid salt. A high salt intake not only contributes to high blood pressure, but increases the likelihood of osteoporosis.

■ Monitor your caffeine consumption carefully (or better yet, avoid caffeine entirely). It has been shown that women who drink more than two cups of regular coffee or caffeinated sodas per day suffer a loss of bone density that can lead to bone fractures later in life.

Calcium Content of Selected Foods

Food (quantity)	Calcium Content
Yogurt, plain nonfat (8 oz)	450 mg
Sardines, with bones (3 oz)	370 mg
Orange juice, calcium-fortified (8 fl oz)	300 mg
Yogurt, fruit-flavored (8 oz)	300 mg
Milk (8 fl oz)	300 mg
Swiss cheese (1 oz)	270 mg
Salmon, with bones (3 oz)	225 mg
Cheddar cheese (1 oz)	205 mg
Turnip greens, cooked (1 cup)	200 mg
Ice cream/ice milk (8 oz)	175 mg
Cottage cheese (8 oz)	150 mg
Tofu (2 oz)	115 mg
Kale, cooked (1 cup)	95 mg
Broccoli, cooked (1 cup)	90 mg
Bread (1 slice)	20–40 mg

■ If you consume alcohol, do so in moderation only. An occasional glass of wine is fine, but heavy alcohol use is associated with a higher risk of osteoporosis.

■ Avoid carbonated beverages and other foods that contain phosphoric acid, which has a detrimental effect on the bones.

NUTRITIONAL SUPPLEMENTS

■ Calcium is a vital raw material for building healthy bones; boron, magnesium, and vitamin D_3 are necessary for its effective absorption and assimilation. Take 250 milligrams each of calcium citrate, calcium carbonate, calcium aspartate, and calcium chelate daily, for a total of 1,000 milligrams of calcium (1,500 milligrams for postmenopausal women not taking hormone replacement therapy). By taking calcium in its many forms, you will assure the effective utilization of this vital mineral. Also take 1 or 2 milligrams of boron citrate daily; 200 milligrams each of magnesium oxide, magnesium citrate, and magnesium chelate daily, for a total of 600 milligrams of magnesium; and 400 international units of vitamin D_3 daily.

■ Research suggests that soy isoflavones can help to maintain bone density. They are also good for reducing menopausal discomforts, the risk of certain types of cancer, and, possibly, cardiovascular risk. Take 1,000 milligrams once or twice daily. Ipriflavone, a synthetic supplement based on soy isoflavones, has been reported to show promising results in stopping bone loss as well. The recommended dose is 200 milligrams three times a day.

■ A natural trace mineral combination is an excellent adjunct to your calcium supplement. More and more research is showing that trace minerals such as boron, vanadium, and manganese are crucial for the proper use of calcium in the body.

HERBAL TREATMENT

■ Horsetail and oat straw are high in silica, which is needed for strong bones and also assists in the assimilation of calcium. Take 500 milligrams of either twice daily.

■ Nettle is a good source of important trace minerals. Take 500 milligrams twice daily. It is best to rotate between this herb and horsetail or oat straw on a weekly basis.

BACH FLOWER REMEDIES

■ Hornbeam is good if you feel so exhausted that you miss out on enjoyable activities.

ACUPRESSURE/MASSAGE

For the locations of acupressure points on the body, *see* ADMINISTERING AN ACUPRESSURE TREATMENT in Part Three.

■ Massaging the Bladder meridian, as well as the feet and hands, increases circulation.

■ If certain areas are especially painful, local massage can prove beneficial.

GENERAL RECOMMENDATIONS

■ Exercise! Regular weight-bearing exercise can stop, or at least slow, bone loss in postmenopausal women. A half-hour of jogging, aerobics, or brisk walking daily is sufficient. In one study, a group of previously inactive postmenopausal women were able to increase their bone density by 5.2 percent in nine months by engaging in fifty to sixty minutes of weight-bearing exercise three times each week. At the end of twenty-two months, their bone density was up by 6.1 percent. In contrast, a similar group of women who did not exercise *lost* an average of 1.1 percent of bone density.

■ Research on the use of natural progesterone cream has found that it can be very successful in helping postmenopausal women to regain some bone density. Discuss the possibility of using natural progesterone with your health-care provider.

PREVENTION

■ Ideally, prevention of osteoporosis should begin early in life—before the age of thirty, when you achieve your maximum bone mass. But it is never too late to start. Make sure your diet includes sufficient amounts of calcium, vitamin D_3, and the trace minerals mentioned in this section, as well as sufficient (but not excessive) amounts of lean protein. If foods containing these vitally important nutrients are not often featured on your menu, take quality supplements regularly.

■ To prevent osteoporosis, women should make sure to get adequate amounts of calcium, magnesium, and vitamin D throughout life, not just after menopause. The recommended daily intake of calcium and vitamin D for adult women is as follows:

Age	Calcium	Magnesium	Vitamin D
25–35	800 mg	400 mg	200 IU
35–50	1,000 mg	500 mg	200 IU
50–65	1,500 mg	750 mg	400 IU
66+	1,500 mg (1,200 mg if on HRT)	750 mg (600 mg if on HRT)	400–800 IU

It is best to take calcium before or at the begining of meals, plus a dose at bedtime. If you are prone to constipation, you may wish to increase the amount of magnesium somewhat. For vitamin D, spending ten to fifteen minutes in direct sunlight twice a week should be adequate for a forty-year-old. After the age of sixty-five, this increases to approximately one-half to one hour two or three times a week.

■ Adopt a program of regular exercise and stick to it. Exercise keeps bones strong.

■ Don't smoke. Smoking is an proven risk factor associated with a whole host of diseases, including osteoporosis.

Overweight

See OBESITY.

Paget's Disease of Bone

Also called *osteitis deformans*, this chronic disease afflicts up to 3 percent of people over the age of forty. Somewhat more men than women are affected. The cause is unknown, though an as-yet-unidentified virus is suspected.

Though we often think of bones as static, inanimate structures, they are actually in the process of remodeling themselves all the time. Old bone cells are destroyed and new bone cells grow to take their place. In people with Paget's disease, turnover in localized areas of bone becomes somewhat hyperactive, and the new bone tends to be larger but softer than the normal bone it replaces. Any part of the body may be affected, but the most common sites are the long bones, pelvis, skull, and vertebrae. The skull may enlarge, and load-bearing bones may weaken and become bowed as the disease progresses.

Many people with Paget's disease have no symptoms, especially in the early stages, but some experience a deep, aching pain that comes on gradually, along with fatigue, and stiffness and deformity may develop over time. If the skull is affected, you may experience headaches and some degree of hearing loss, and your skull may increase in size. Sometimes this disorder is mistaken for bone tumors or multiple myeloma (cancer of the blood-forming tissues), but Paget's disease is not cancerous. While the defective bone can fracture more easily than normal, fractures usually heal well. Most cases of Paget's disease are mild and allow for a long life. Occasionally, however, the kidneys can be adversely affected, or bone cancer may develop. In rare cases, the pain can be severe, and there may be marked deformities and even heart failure.

Diagnosis of Paget's disease is based on x-ray studies that show the typical lesions of overgrowth, changes in bone density, and alterations in bone shape. A blood test may be performed to determine whether levels of alkaline phosphatase, an enzyme involved in bone remodeling, are elevated. In many cases, the disorder is found by accident during either a routine physical exam or testing for other conditions.

CONVENTIONAL TREATMENT

■ If there are no symptoms, no treatment is required.

■ Pain may be treated with nonsteroidal anti-inflammatory drugs (NSAIDs) such as aspirin (Bayer, Ecotrin, and others), ibuprofen (Advil, Motrin, Nuprin, and others), ketoprofen (Orudis, Oruvail), or naproxen (Aleve, Anaprox, Naprelan, Naprosyn). These drugs can cause gastric distress, peptic ulcers, and other adverse effects, especially with long-term use. Take them with food to prevent stomach upset.

■ Braces or other orthotic devices may be recommended if the disease leads to alterations in gait.

■ If a hip or the spine is severely affected, orthopedic surgery may be needed.

■ Calcitonin (Calcimar, Miacalcin) is a hormone that reduces the activity of osteoclasts, cells that break down bone for remodeling and repair, and may slow the progression of the disease. Side effects may include nausea and flushing. In addition, this drug may become less effective over time.

■ Drugs classified as bisphosphonates, including alendronate (Fosamax) and etidronate (Didronel), also inhibit the breakdown of bone by osteoclasts. Alendronate has become more popular than etidronate in recent years, as etidronate can adversely affect both bone remineralization and bone pain over time. Alendronate can cause nausea, vomiting, abdominal pain, headache, esophageal ulcers, and other effects.

■ In severe cases, gallium nitrate (Ganite) may help. This

drug inhibits the removal of calcium from bone. However, it is potentially dangerous to the kidneys, so it is reserved for serious disease that responds to little else.

DIETARY GUIDELINES

■ Eat fresh pineapple frequently. Fresh pineapple is high in bromelain, a natural anti-inflammatory.

■ Avoid vegetables in the nightshade family, such as eggplant, tomatoes, and potatoes, which can promote inflammation.

■ Avoid carbonated beverages. Carbonated drinks are high in phosphates, which force the body to excrete calcium.

NUTRITIONAL SUPPLEMENTS

■ Calcium, magnesium, boron, manganese, zinc, and phosphorus are all essential for bone formation; vitamin D aids in the assimilation of calcium. Take 500 milligrams of calcium and 300 milligrams of magnesium three times daily; 400 international units of vitamin D daily; 1 milligram of boron and 15 milligrams of zinc twice daily; and 2 milligrams of manganese daily. Assess your diet to see whether you are getting 1,200 milligrams of phosphorus daily. If not, take a supplement that will raise your intake to that level.

■ Gamma-linoleic acid (GLA) has anti-inflammatory properties. Take 250 milligrams twice a day.

■ Glucosamine and chondroitin are beneficial for the joints and connective tissue. Take 500 milligrams of glucosamine sulfate and 350 milligrams of chondroitin sulfate three times daily. If you weigh more than 200 pounds, take the same amount four times daily.

■ Green-foods supplements, available in health-food stores, are high in trace minerals essential to the laying down of bone. Take a green-foods supplement twice a day, as directed on the product label.

HERBAL TREATMENT

■ Horsetail is high in silica, which is important for the proper formation of bone and connective tissue. Take 500 milligrams twice a day for three months.

■ Passionflower calms the nervous system; white willow bark is an anti-inflammatory. To help reduce pain, take 250 milligrams of standardized passionflower extract containing 0.7 percent flavonoids, plus 350 milligrams of white willow bark, three times daily, as needed.

Note: Do not use white willow bark if you are allergic to aspirin or are taking an anticoagulant (blood thinner).

HOMEOPATHY

■ *Floricum acidum* is good for pain and inflammation in finger joints and for pain in shins and buttocks. It is especially suitable for individuals over age sixty-five. Take one dose of *Floricum acidum* 30x or 15c three times daily for three days. Do this once each month for four to six months.

■ *Silicea* relieves pain in spine, hips, legs, and feet. Your extremities are probably cold, yet your feet may be sweaty. Take one dose of *Silicea* 6x or 3c three times daily for three days. Do this once each month for four to six months.

BACH FLOWER REMEDIES

■ Hornbeam helps to ease exhaustion. Take it as needed, following the directions on the product label.

ACUPRESSURE

■ Kidney 3 and Kidney 7 help to improve the condition of the bones. Chinese medicine teaches that the kidneys are responsible for keeping bones healthy.

■ Stomach 36 and Spleen 6 improve the utilization of nutrients necessary for bone formation.

GENERAL RECOMMENDATIONS

■ Work with your health-care practitioner to develop an exercise program that is right for you, and follow it faithfully.

■ If pain and/or debility as a result of Paget's disease force you to spend prolonged periods in bed, make certain you change position at least every hour. (*See* BEDSORES.)

PREVENTION

■ If possible, avoid taking prescription tranquilizers. Individuals over sixty-five who use tranquilizers regularly have been shown to suffer 70 percent more hip fractures than other people their age. It is believed that repeated use of prescription tranquilizers may diminish bone strength.

■ Avoid carbonated beverages.

Pain

Pain is nature's alarm system, a signal that something is hurt and needs to be attended to. Pain in the form of a headache can signal muscle tension. Other types of pain can alert you to a strained muscle, a broken bone, an infection, or an inflamed appendix. Pain is a response that helps protect the body from harm. For example, it is the lightning-fast transmission of a pain signal that causes you to snatch your hand away from a fire or hot stove. Even before the brain signals "danger" or the hurt fully registers consciously, the body knows what action to take. Similarly, if you have broken a bone, the pain will convince you to avoid moving it, which could worsen the injury.

Pain can also be a signal that something has gone wrong internally. It is a basic symptom of inflammation, and can be an important clue to many disorders. There are a variety of sensations that may be described as painful, including throbbing, stabbing, and aching. Pain may be localized at the site of an injury, or "referred" to another part of the body. It may be acute and resolve after a short time, or chronic, lasting for six months or more, and it can be anywhere from mild to severe in intensity.

Both the physical and emotional aspects of pain need to be addressed and respected. The physical component of pain is relatively straightforward; it is the result of information being transmitted from the site of injury or illness to the brain. At the same time, however, another impulse runs through the central nervous system to another part of the brain, the limbic system. This system transmits the perception of pain and generates an emotional reaction to it. For example, when you stub a toe, you feel the immediate pain of the injury. But you also have an emotional reaction that may cause you to feel angry, afraid, sick to your stomach, or even sad. Because both physical and emotional aspects are involved when you are in pain, recognizing and dealing with your emotional response may be as important as anything else you can do.

The suggestions offered here are intended to help you deal with mild to moderate pain that may be related to an injury, acute illness, or recovery from surgery or a broken bone. If you experience pain that gets progressively worse, does not improve with ordinary pain-control measures, interferes with your normal activity level, and/or starts in a small area and involves an increasingly larger area, or if the pain is severe and unremitting, consult your doctor. Chronic pain (pain that lasts longer than three months) should be addressed by a health-care professional. An estimated 10 to 30 percent of all Americans suffer chronic pain severe enough to interfere with their ability to function.

CONVENTIONAL TREATMENT

■ Acetaminophen (available in Tylenol, Datril, and many other over-the-counter medications) is generally thought to be the safest conventional painkiller for mild to moderate pain, as long as you take only the recommended dose. In excessive amounts, however, it can cause serious liver damage. If the recommended amount does not give the relief you want, do not increase the dosage, but try a different medication.

■ Aspirin, the old home standby for treating pain, also can be effective for mild to moderate pain. It can cause stomach irritation, however, so it is probably best taken with food. You should not take aspirin during the last three months of pregnancy unless directed to do so by a physician, as it can complicate labor and delivery, and may cause harm to the developing child.

■ Ibuprofen (Advil, Motrin, Nuprin, and others) is a nonsteroidal anti-inflammatory drug (NSAID) that some doctors consider to be the most effective medication for many common types of pain, including muscle pain and headaches. Like all medications, it can have side effects for some people, among them gastrointestinal irritation and/or ulceration and kidney damage, especially with long-term use. Take ibuprofen with food to prevent possible stomach upset.

■ Codeine is a prescription narcotic that is effective for moderate to severe pain that is not relieved by less potent medications. Narcotics like codeine work by binding with opiate receptors in the central nervous system to alter the perception of pain. In other words, the pain still exists, but the narcotic tricks the body into not recognizing it. Possible side effects of codeine include sedation, slowed breathing, low blood pressure, stomach upset, and constipation. If your doctor prescribes codeine, increase your intake of fluids and fiber to avoid constipation. (*See* CONSTIPATION.)

■ An acetaminophen and codeine combination can be very effective and is sometimes prescribed for pain control. Acetaminophen works at the site of the illness or injury, lessening pain and inflammation, while codeine works in the central nervous system and blocks the perception of pain. Needless to say, this combination can also have the side effects of both acetaminophen and codeine.

■ Pain-management centers evaluate chronic pain and design individualized treatments for sufferers. Often, they use a variety of treatments, including such drug-free therapies as biofeedback, meditation, acupuncture, and exercise. If the recommendations in this entry do not provide sufficient relief from pain, consider scheduling an appointment at a pain-management center that embraces all protocols, both medical and alternative therapies.

■ Extremely severe pain, such as can occur with cancer and certain end-of-life situations, is usually handled within medical facilities, with such therapies as high doses of narcotics and even, in some cases, surgical intervention to sever nerves if excruciating pain cannot be resolved otherwise.

DIETARY GUIDELINES

■ Avoid foods containing saturated, hydrogenated, and partially hydrogenated fats. In the body, these fats are transformed into a type of hormonelike compound called a prostaglandin that promotes inflammation and pain. This means eliminating from your diet butter, red meat, shellfish, margarine and shortenings (or anything that contains them), tropical oils such as coconut and palm oil, and *all* fried foods. Moderate amounts of baked, broiled, or poached fish and white-meat poultry, as well as low- or nonfat dairy products such as yogurt, are acceptable.

■ Include fresh pineapple in your diet. Fresh pineapple is high in bromelain, which has anti-inflammatory properties.

■ Soups made with plenty of garlic, onions, and green leafy vegetables, plus burdock root, ginger root, and turmeric root, are natural pain relievers with anti-inflammatory and diuretic properties.

NUTRITIONAL SUPPLEMENTS

■ Bromelain is a natural enzyme that reduces inflammation. Take 300 to 500 milligrams three times daily, between meals.

■ Calcium and magnesium can be effective for pain associated with muscle spasms. Take 500 milligrams of each three times daily. These minerals are best taken with vitamin C to improve bioavailability.

■ Flaxseed oil contains essential fatty acids that have an anti-inflammatory effect. Take 1 tablespoonful (or 500 to 1,000 milligrams in capsule form) twice a day.

■ Glucosamine sulfate is a safe and effective natural alternative to aspirin and other nonsteroidal anti-inflammatory drugs (NSAIDs). It is especially helpful for arthritis-type pain. Take 500 milligrams three times daily. If you weigh over 200 pounds, take the same dose four times daily.

■ Pain, particularly low back pain, sometimes responds to high doses of vitamin C. Take 1,000 milligrams of vitamin C and an equal amount of bioflavonoids three times daily.

HERBAL TREATMENT

■ Brew a pain-relief tea as follows: Simmer 1 tablespoon of white willow bark in 1 quart of water for fifteen minutes. Add 1 tablespoon of chamomile, 1 tablespoon of skullcap, 1 tablespoon of valerian root, and ¹/₂ tablespoon of licorice root. Simmer for another ten minutes; then strain and cool. To help relieve generalized pain, take 1 cup every hour for four consecutive hours. White willow bark is an anti-inflammatory similar to aspirin; chamomile is an effective relaxant; skullcap and valerian have sedative and antispasmodic properties; licorice is an anti-inflammatory and enhances the action of the other herbs, in addition to sweetening the tea.

Note: Do not use licorice on a daily basis for more than five days at a time, as it can elevate blood pressure. Do not use it at all if you have high blood pressure. Do not use white willow bark if you are allergic to aspirin.

■ Capsaicin, a compound derived from cayenne pepper (capsicum) and available in cream or gel form, is especially good for pain associated with rheumatoid arthritis or shingles. Apply it as directed on the product label.

■ Curcumin, the compound in turmeric that gives Indian curry its color, has distinct anti-inflammatory abilities. Take 500 milligrams three times daily.

■ Kava kava is a relaxing herb that helps to ease pain. Choose a standardized extract containing 30 percent kava lactones and take 250 milligrams three times a day.

■ Pine-bark and grape-seed extracts have anti-inflammatory properties. Take 50 to 100 milligrams of either two or three times daily.

HOMEOPATHY

■ *Arnica* is very helpful for pain related to overexertion, injury, or bruising. Take one dose of *Arnica* 30x or 9c, as directed on the product label, every hour for three to four hours or until the pain subsides.

■ *Hypericum* benefits an injury to fingers or toes, pain after surgery, or injury to a nerve. Take one dose of *Hypericum* 12x or 6c three times daily for up to two days.

■ *Ledum* is good for a puncture wound that results in bruising. Take one dose of *Ledum* 12x or 6c three times daily for two days.

ACUPRESSURE

For the locations of acupressure points on the body, *see* ADMINISTERING AN ACUPRESSURE TREATMENT in Part Three.

■ Four Gates helps to calm and relax the body.

■ Neck and Shoulder Release helps to release pain centered in the head, neck, and shoulder area, and will help you relax.

GENERAL RECOMMENDATIONS

■ Try to relax. Stress, tension, and worry make pain worse. As much as possible, keep stressors such as noise, drafts, uncomfortable temperatures, glaring (or too-dim) lighting, and emotions such as anger, anxiety, and fear to a minimum. A quiet room, soothing music, a warm bath, or a gentle massage can be helpful. Slow, deep breathing is also recommended. Relaxation exercises and visualization techniques are very helpful. (*See* RELAXATION TECHNIQUES in Part Three.)

■ Explore the possibility of acupuncture, biofeedback, and/or hypnotherapy. Certain types of pain can be managed very effectively with these approaches. Ask your health-care provider for a referral to a qualified practitioner, or see the Resources section at the end of the book for professional organizations you can consult for assistance.

■ Practice distraction. Any kind of pleasant distraction—whether an engrossing book or movie, an addictive computer game, or a conversation with a good friend—can help take your attention away from the discomfort.

Pancreatitis

Pancreatitis is a term for inflammation of the pancreas, an elongated organ approximately four to six inches in length located in the upper abdomen, surrounded by the stomach and small intestine. The pancreas has two vital functions: It produces digestive enzymes that are released into the small intestine, and it produces two hormones, insulin and glucagon, that are released into the bloodstream to regulate blood-sugar levels.

Enzymes are delivered from the pancreas to the intestines by means of the same duct used to transport bile from the gallbladder. Pancreatitis can result if there is a gallstone blocking this passage. It can also be a result of damage to the pancreas from alcohol consumption. In either case, digestive enzymes become trapped in the pancreas and can actually begin to digest the tissues there, causing inflammation. Some enzymes may ooze out and find their way into the bloodstream and/or the abdominal cavity. Symptoms of pancreatitis include upper abdominal pain and tenderness, back pain, nausea, vomiting, fever, and distention of the abdomen. Blood tests may show elevated levels of pancreatic enzymes, and the red blood cell count may be affected as well. Pancreatitis may be complicated by liver problems, with jaundice, as well as kidney failure. If the damage is severe enough, the pancreas can become infected, a potentially life-threatening situation, and pockets of fluid may form.

Another scenario that can lead to the development of pancreatitis is exposure to certain chemicals, such as petrochemicals, diesel fuel, gasoline, acetone, and trichloroethylene, a solvent. This type of exposure is most often linked to the work environment, although there have been instances in which children who played in a diesel fuel shed or rode their bicycles long distances to school on busy roads where they were exposed to automobile exhaust ultimately contracted pancreatitis. This is particularly a problem in developing countries, where an estimated one person in twenty suffers from pancreatic disease, though it can happen anywhere.

Pancreatitis can be either acute or chronic, and the problem can recur, especially in people who are alcoholics or are prone to developing gallstones. About 10 percent of cases of acute pancreatitis eventually become chronic, which involves scarring and permanently decreased pancreatic function. Because the pancreas produces substances necessary for digestion and blood-sugar regulation, both digestive difficulties and diabetes are often the result, and both may be severe.

CONVENTIONAL TREATMENT

■ Mild pancreatitis can often be treated successfully with

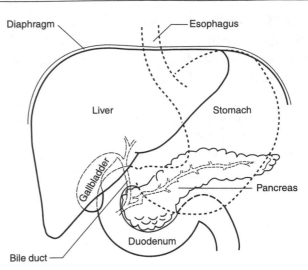

The Upper Digestive Tract

bed rest, no food or liquid taken by mouth (eating or drinking will stimulate the pancreas to release more digestive enzymes), and, possibly, suctioning out of the contents of the stomach if there is pain or intestinal obstruction. It can take anywhere from several days to several weeks to recover.

■ For pain, meperidine (Demerol) may be prescribed. This is a narcotic that is effective for moderate to severe pain. Possible side effects include dizziness, nausea, vomiting, dry mouth, low blood pressure, and urinary retention. Meperidine is also potentially habit-forming.

■ For more severe cases, the administration of intravenous fluids may be necessary, along with plasma and/or serum protein and, possibly, supplemental calcium.

■ If infection develops, aggressive treatment with antibiotics is necessary.

■ More severe cases usually require treatment in a hospital intensive-care unit because there are many biochemical abnormalities that can occur, and very quickly, and that can lead to difficulty breathing, electrolyte imbalances, infection, kidney failure, and other serious problems.

■ If there is ulceration, a gallstone blocking the outflow tract, or a fluid-filled cyst, surgery may be used to correct the problem. Some problems can be corrected using an endoscope, a fiber-optic scope inserted through the mouth into the upper intestinal tract.

■ If you have chronic pancreatitis, you may need to take lipase (fat-digesting enzymes) orally with meals. Flare-ups are treated as attacks of acute pancreatitis would be.

DIETARY GUIDELINES

■ Whether pancreatitis is acute or chronic, adhere to a low-fat diet and avoid all alcohol. Your doctor should give you specific dietary instructions.

■ Simplify your diet. Avoid all fried foods, saturated and hydrogenated fats, and refined sugars.

■ Include in your diet plenty of yellow and orange vegetables and dark leafy greens, which are high in antioxidants such as the carotenes, vitamin C, and bioflavonoids.

NUTRITIONAL SUPPLEMENTS

■ To assure a supply of all basic nutrients, take a multivitamin and mineral supplement supplying 50 milligrams of each of the major B vitamins twice a day. For the first ten days, take an additional 250 milligrams of pantothenic acid twice a day as well.

Chromium helps to keep blood-sugar levels in balance and enhance the efficiency of insulin, which is important if insulin production is compromised as a result of pancreatitis. Take 200 micrograms of chromium twice a day for two weeks, then reduce to 100 micrograms twice a day for six weeks.

Lecithin aids in the digestion of fats. Take 1,200 milligrams with the largest meal of the day.

■ Lipoic acid, vitamin E, and selenium are all valuable antioxidants. Take 100 milligrams of lipoic acid twice a day for two months. Also take 400 international units of vitamin E and 100 micrograms of selenium daily, at bedtime.

Note: If you are taking an anticoagulant (blood thinner), consult your physician before taking vitamin E.

Methionine is important for the metabolism of fats. Take 500 milligrams twice a day, with meals, for up to three months.

N-acetylcysteine (NAC) is a strong antioxidant that helps to protect the liver. Take 500 milligrams twice daily for two months.

Pancreatic enzymes are important for digestion. Choose 10X strength non-enteric-coated enzyme tablets or capsules, and take 500 milligrams immediately before each meal. Make sure the label states that the tablet or capsule contains amylase (an enzyme that breaks down starch molecules into smaller, more easily digested sugars), lipase (an enzyme that assists in the digestion of fats), and proteases (enzymes that break down proteins).

Vitamin C is an anti-inflammatory that aids healing. Take 500 milligrams three times daily. Choose a powder or capsule form, which is more easily digested.

HERBAL TREATMENT

■ Cat's claw acts as an anti-inflammatory and immune stimulant. Take 500 milligrams of standardized extract three times a day.

Dandelion root assists in the production of bile, thereby improving the digestion of fats. Take a cup of dandelion-root tea twice a day, with meals, for six weeks.

■ Goldenseal and the Chinese patent medicine Huang Lian Su contain berberine alkaloids, which have antibiotic effects, stimulate the secretion of bile, and are helpful in the treatment of gallstones (*see* GALLBLADDER PROBLEMS). Take 500 milligrams of goldenseal or two tablets of Huang Lian Su three times daily for three days to one week. If you take either of these herbs for more than three days, be sure to take a probiotic supplement, such as bifidobacteria, to renew the bowel flora and improve your utilization of nutrients.

■ Licorice has long been used for its anti-inflammatory properties. It has the effect of stimulating the production of two natural steroids, cortisone and aldosterone. Licorice also stimulates the production of bile by the liver and can relieve indigestion and even ulceration. This herb can be particularly helpful for people with chronic pancreatitis. Choose deglycyrrhizinated licorice (DGL) and take 300 milligrams three times daily.

Note: Ordinary licorice can elevate blood pressure, and should not be taken on a daily basis for more than five days in a row. DGL should not have this effect, however.

HOMEOPATHY

■ *Arsenicum album* relieves nausea and vomiting after eating or drinking that makes you unable to bear the sight and smell of food. You may have heartburn, crave coffee and acidic foods, and get indigestion from vinegar, ice water, and tobacco. Take one dose of *Arsenicum album* 30x or 15c three times daily for up to three days.

■ *Phosphorus* is good for pain and inflammation in the stomach and/or pancreatic area. You experience sour burping after eating and fatigue after bowel movements, and may feel fearful and oversensitive. Take one dose of *Phosphorus* 30x or 15c three times daily for up to three days.

BACH FLOWER REMEDIES

Select the remedy that most closely fits your disposition and emotional tendencies and concerns, and take it as needed, following the directions on the product label.

■ Mimulus eases fear and apprehension.

■ Red Chestnut helps to tame feelings of worry.

AROMATHERAPY

For specific instructions on how to use aromatherapy, *see* PREPARING AROMATHERAPY TREATMENTS in Part Three.

■ Inhaling a combination of lavender and orange oil is relaxing and mildly rehabilitating to the digestion.

ACUPRESSURE

For the locations of acupressure points on the body, *see* ADMINISTERING AN ACUPRESSURE TREATMENT in Part Three.

■ Stomach 36 and Spleen 6 work to restore digestion.

PREVENTION

■ If you drink alcoholic beverages, do so in moderation only. Chronic alcohol consumption is the leading cause of pancreatitis in North America.

■ If you are prone to gallstones, *see* GALLBLADDER PROBLEMS for suggestions that may help to prevent them.

Parasitic Disease

See CHLAMYDIA; PARASITES, INTESTINAL; SCABIES; TRICHOMONIASIS. *Also see* Hookworms; Toxoplasmosis; and/or Pets and Your Health under HOME AND PERSONAL SAFETY in Part One.

Parasites, Intestinal

Parasites have become increasingly prominent as a cause of disease in recent years. This is particularly true of parasites that inhabit the gastrointestinal (GI) tract. Apparently, years of poor eating habits, overuse of medication, and, possibly, increased exposure to these organisms have combined to create an unsettling rise in the number of people suffering symptoms of parasitic invasion. Many Americans think of parasitic infections as something that occurs only in other, less developed parts of the world. While that may be true for certain individual parasitic diseases (malaria is one example), in fact some experts estimate that as many as 85 percent of all North Americans have at least one kind of parasite—many, obviously, without knowing it.

There is an amazing assortment of parasites that can infest various parts of the human body. This entry concerns intestinal parasites, those organisms that invade the digestive tract, particularly protozoa (including giardia, cryptosporidia, and entamoebas) and different types of worms (flatworms [tapeworms], flukes, hookworms, pinworms, and roundworms). Protozoa are simple single-celled organisms. Worms are elongated round or flat, flexible multicellular organisms that can be as small as several millimeters or as long as thirty feet, depending on the species. Regardless of size or type, all parasitic organisms survive by feeding on the cells and tissues of the infected host, and all types of parasitic infestation are more common among children, people who live in institutional settings, and those with immune-system dysfunction.

The range of symptoms that have been traced to intestinal parasites can be mind-boggling. They include indigestion, constipation, gas, bloating, nausea, diarrhea, fatigue, depression, skin rashes, headaches, insomnia, anemia, joint pains, and a vague overall feeling of being unwell, to name a few. There have even been cases in which people with all the symptoms of other disorders—among them allergies, asthma, irritable bowel syndrome, attention deficit hyperactivity disorder (ADHD), heart disease, and cancer—were found really to be suffering from the presence of parasites.

Giardiasis, or infestation with the protozoan *Giardia lamblia,* is one of the more common parasitic disorders that afflicts human beings. It can be transmitted through contaminated food or water as well as by direct or indirect contact with body fluids of an infected person. Symptoms, which are usually relatively mild, can include general abdominal discomfort, burping, flatulence, and foul-smelling diarrhea. If the infestation is severe, it can lead to problems with the absorption of nutrients.

Cryptosporidia are tiny (only a few thousandths of a millimeter in diameter) protozoal organisms that are spread primarily through contaminated water and food, though they can also be spread from person to person. In a previously healthy person, they cause explosive watery diarrhea and abdominal cramping. Symptoms come on quickly and also resolve quickly, usually about a week later. For people with depressed immune function, such as cancer patients and people who are HIV-positive, cryptosporidia pose a particular problem. In such individuals, the diarrhea is usually more severe and the condition can become chronic and even life-threatening. Further, while most municipal water supplies are tested to make sure they contain no more than "acceptable" levels of these parasites—levels deemed not likely to make a healthy person sick—levels lower than that may very well cause illness in a person with low immune function. Numerous cases of cryptosporidiosis are believed to have been caused by drinking supposedly safe tap water. There have also been incidents in recent years in which cryptosporidia in ground water have proliferated beyond the so-called acceptable point, causing entire communities to be advised to either boil their tap water before using it or, preferably, to use bottled water instead.

Infection with entamoebas is a more chronic problem, even in previously healthy people. While in some these organisms cause no specific symptoms, others experience periodic flare-ups of gas, abdominal pain, cramping, and diarrhea, often alternating with constipation—symptoms that can be confused with those of ulcerative colitis or irritable bowel syndrome. Some people notice blood or mucus in the stools, and the abdomen may be tender to the touch. In severe cases, a fever may be present. Without treatment, symptoms can recur for life and lead to nutritional deficiencies such as anemia.

Infestation with any of the various forms of worms most often starts with accidental ingestion of worm eggs, embryos, or cysts (structures containing larvae sealed within a protective shell or envelope), usually a result of contaminated or improperly prepared food. Hookworms, however, are contracted when worm larvae from contaminated soil penetrate the skin. Whatever the port of entry, the organisms eventually migrate to the intestines and attach themselves to the intestinal wall, where they begin to feed. They may or may not cause such symptoms as abdominal pain, nausea, vomiting, or diarrhea. If the infestation is severe enough, weight loss and malnutrition may occur. In particularly severe or long-standing cases, the worms can grow to such a size that they cause blockage of the digestive tract.

Pinworms, a comparatively common type of worm infestation that is seen mainly in children, also cause severe anal itching as the female worms migrate to the anus at night to lay their eggs. The egg deposit is itchy and irritating to the delicate tissues in the area. This makes it likely the affected person will scratch, and if some of the eggs end up on the hands, he or she may spread the infection to others or reinfect him- or herself.

Getting an accurate diagnosis of intestinal parasites is made complicated by the fact that the symptoms are so variable and mimic those of other diseases. Then, too, many doctors simply do not think of the possibility of parasites as a cause of health problems unless other possibilities have been exhausted. We believe that testing to rule out the presence of parasites is always wise, especially if you are dealing with a problem that is chronic or difficult to treat. There are laboratories that have specific tests for tracking down parasitic infections. (See the Resources section at the end of the book.) Some laboratories appear to get more accurate results than others, so it is best to use a facility that has an established reputation.

CONVENTIONAL TREATMENT

■ Giardiasis may be treated with the antibiotic metronidazole (Flagyl, Metric, Protostat), furazolidone (Furoxone), or quinacrine (Atabrine). The success of these treatments varies. All of these drugs can cause side effects. Quinacrine can cause nausea, vomiting, and dizziness. In rare cases, it can cause psychotic reactions. Furazolidone can cause high or low (sometimes considerably so) blood pressure, blood-sugar problems, nausea, vomiting, headache, rash, fever, and joint pains.

■ There is no reliable treatment for cryptosporidiosis. Fortunately, it usually goes away by itself. If dehydration becomes severe, intravenous fluids may be necessary. In persons with depressed immune function, various antibiotics may be tried, but none is clearly effective in all cases.

■ Amoebic infection is usually treated with metronida-

zole. Sometimes, an additional drug—iodoquinol (Yodoxin) or paromomycin (Humatin)—may be added. Metronidazole interacts badly with many other drugs. If you must take it, you should avoid all alcohol, as it can have an effect similar to that of disulfiram (Antabuse), a drug used to treat alcoholism that causes intense nausea, vomiting, headaches, and other symptoms if a person taking it consumes even the smallest quantity of alcohol. Side effects of metronidazole can include seizures, nerve damage, nausea, vomiting, constipation, headache, and urinary discomfort.

■ Roundworm infections are usually treated with the anthelmintic (anti-worm) drug pyrantel pamoate (Antiminth) or mebendazole (Vermox). Pyrantel pamoate is often effective in just one dose and is generally well tolerated, causing only mild side effects of nausea, diarrhea and headache, if any. Mebendazole (Vermox) is usually prescribed for a three-day course. This drug can cause abdominal pain and diarrhea, and should not be used during pregnancy.

■ Threadworms require a longer course of treatment than other types of roundworms do, at least five days in many cases. Thiabendazole (Mintezol), the best-known treatment, often causes side effects including nausea, vomiting, dizziness, headache, weakness, and other side effects in a large proportion of patients. More recently, the drug ivermectin (Stromectol) has been used successfully, and with far fewer side effects.

■ Tapeworm infestations are usually treated with one of two drugs, niclosamide (Niclocide) and praziquantel (Biltricide). Both are generally well tolerated and have few side effects. Usually a single dose is all that is required.

■ With any type of parasitic infestation, it is wise to have a follow-up examination at the interval recommended by your doctor to be sure the treatment has been effective.

DIETARY GUIDELINES

■ Use crushed garlic liberally. The allicin it contains is known to have activity against several invading organisms.

■ When you get the urge to snack, choose raw pumpkin seeds, which can be helpful in fighting parasitic and worm infestation.

NUTRITIONAL SUPPLEMENTS

■ Glutamine is an amino acid that helps to repair the cells of the intestinal tract. Take 1,000 to 2,000 milligrams of L-glutamine three times daily for two months.

■ All of the treatments for parasitic organisms have a tendency to disturb the normal intestinal flora, which can lead to an overgrowth of yeast. To restore the friendly bacteria, take a probiotic supplement for two months, as recommended on the product label, before breakfast and at bedtime.

■ Vitamin C can be an excellent intestinal cleanser. Start by taking 2,000 to 4,000 milligrams (2 to 4 grams) of vitamin-C powder or capsules (ascorbic acid). Each hour thereafter, take more vitamin C, increasing the dose gradually until you develop gas, then diarrhea. Then decrease the dose to the greatest amount that does *not* cause these symptoms, and continue taking it three or four times a day for a day or two. Make sure to drink plenty of quality water throughout this process. If you develop any stomach distress, you may need to switch to an ascorbate form of vitamin C, such as calcium, magnesium, or potassium ascorbate (or mixed ascorbates).

HERBAL TREATMENT

■ Black walnut extract has a long history of use for intestinal worms. Take 15 to 25 drops three times daily for ten days to two weeks.

■ Ginger root can help relieve nausea associated with some parasitic infections, such as roundworm. Drink a cup of ginger tea up to three times daily, as needed. If you dislike the tea, you can take 100 milligrams of an extract containing 5 percent gingerols three times daily for several days.

■ Goldenseal contains berberine, an alkaloid that has strong antimicrobial properties. It prevents microorganisms from adhering to the walls of host cells. Choose an extract standardized to contain 8 to 10 percent total alkaloids (including berberine, hydrastine, and canadine) and take 500 milligrams three times daily for three days. This is exceptionally effective for diarrhea associated with intestinal parasites, as it reduces inflammation of the mucous membranes of the digestive tract.

■ Grapefruit-seed (or citrus-seed) extract is a powerful treatment for many sorts of intestinal parasites. Read the product instructions carefully, as most brands must be diluted considerably before use—usually, a few drops in 8 ounces of water is enough.

■ Oregano extract has both antifungal and antiparasitic properties. Take 50 to 100 milligrams of standardized extract three times a day.

HOMEOPATHY

■ *Cina* helps to relieve symptoms associated with pinworms, including hunger pangs soon after eating, vomiting, diarrhea, and an intense craving for sweets. Take one dose of *Cina* 12x or 6c three times daily for up to three days, as needed to control symptoms.

■ *Cinchona officinalis* helps to alleviate abdominal gas, acid reflux, bloating, and general debility associated with parasitic infection. Take one dose of *Cinchona officinalis* 30x or 9c three times daily for up to three days.

■ *Teucrium* is helpful for restlessness in bed, very dry skin, and anal itching, especially in the evening, associated with parasites. Take one dose of *Teucrium* 12x or 6c three times daily for up to three days, as needed to relieve symptoms.

PREVENTION

■ Do not eat raw seafood. As good as it may taste, eating sushi is like playing Russian roulette when it comes to parasites. Raw oysters also are a risky venture.

■ When using any type of food processor, especially if raw meat is involved, clean the device thoroughly before using it for a different food-processing task.

■ Be careful about pets. Never let an animal lick you on the mouth. Many parasites are carried in animals' digestive tracts—and you know where your pet's tongue has been. Do your best to keep your pet free of fleas, which can carry the larvae of different types of worms. Don't sleep with your pet, and be compulsive about cleaning up after it. If you just wipe up an "accident," there's no telling what you may have left on the carpet.

■ You can use grapefruit-seed extract once or twice a year as a preventive against intestinal parasites. When you travel to locations where parasites may be a problem, take grapefruit-seed extract with you and add a drop to your drinking water three times a day.

Parkinson's Disease

Parkinson's disease, sometimes called palsy or paralysis agitans, is caused by damage to certain nerve-cell clusters in the brain. The degeneration of nerve cells in the basal ganglia—islands of gray matter located in the lobes of the cerebrum, the large, wrinkled section that caps the entire brain—causes a deficiency of the neurotransmitter dopamine within this part of the brain. Normally, dopamine works together with another neurotransmitter, acetylcholine. Together, these two brain chemicals act to transmit messages between the nerve cells that control the functioning of muscles throughout the body. Acetylcholine sends messages that induce the muscles to contract, while dopamine moderates these signals to manageable levels. In people with Parkinson's disease, however, there is an imbalance between dopamine and acetylcholine—specifically, there is too much acetylcholine and too little dopamine. As a result, nerves that control muscle contraction send inappropriate signals, causing involuntary tremors and muscle rigidity. Parkinson's disease can also result if the receptors to which dopamine must bind to exert its effects become blocked.

Parkinson's disease usually comes on slowly. Early symptoms include a slight tremor, usually of one hand, arm, or leg. The trembling is worse when the affected body part is at rest, but may be hardly noticeable when that part is in motion. As the disease progresses, both sides of the body become affected. Stiffness, muscle weakness and rigidity, shaking of the head, and trembling increase. A "pill-rolling" movement of the fingers—in which the thumb and first finger rub together as if rolling a pill or tiny ball bearing between them—is typical of the disease. Over time, the posture becomes stooped, and the affected individual moves with a stiff, shuffling walk, though he or she may break into tiny uncontrollable running steps at times. Cramplike pains in the arms, legs, and spine are common. Constipation is very often a problem as well. In the later stages, a person with Parkinson's disease may drool and have an unblinking, fixed expression and oily skin. Eventually, everyday activities become difficult or impossible to manage without help, and speech becomes impaired. If untreated, the disease progresses over ten to fifteen years to severe weakness and incapacity. Despite these difficulties, the ability to think and reason are unaffected in most cases.

This disorder is more common in men than women. It most often affects persons over sixty years of age, although it can occur in younger people as well. When it does, it is usually as a result of encephalitis (brain inflammation) or poisoning by carbon monoxide, heavy metals, or drugs. The incidence of Parkinson's disease is rising. In the mid-1970s, among people over the age of sixty, one person in 1,000 was diagnosed with Parkinson's disease. By the mid-1980s, that figure had increased to one in every 200 people, and today, an estimated one person in every 100 over the age of sixty is affected. While no one knows what causes the nerve cells to degenerate, these statistics would seem to support a recent theory suggesting that increased exposure to environmental toxins may be a factor in this disease. Proponents of this theory believe that brain cells may be destroyed by the cumulative effects of toxins absorbed over the years. Malnutrition and incomplete utilization of nutrients have also been suggested as contributing factors to this disease.

CONVENTIONAL MEDICINE

■ If you suffer from Parkinson's disease, it is wise to seek out and work closely with a neurologist or other physician who specializes, or at the very least has considerable experience, in the treatment of this condition.

■ The primary treatment for Parkinson's disease is aimed at correcting the imbalance between dopamine and acetylcholine in the brain. Levodopa (often called L-dopa; also sold under the brand name Larodopa), which the body converts into dopamine, has proven to be the most effective drug treatment. Because much of this substance is taken up by other parts of the body before it reaches the brain, high doses are required to achieve the desired effect. Because some amino acids prevent this drug from reaching the brain, L-dopa should not be taken with food. Possible side effects include nausea, vomiting, low blood pressure, and irregular heartbeat. And unfortunately, the beneficial effects of levodopa diminish with prolonged use, while there is an increase in longer term side effects, including dyskinesias (abnormal movements) and confusion. After about two years, it no longer works well and another drug, such as bromocriptine (Parlodel) or a combination of levodopa and carbidopa (Atamet, Sinemet), is usually substituted. These substitute drugs are not as effective as the initial levodopa therapy. When residual amounts of levodopa in the system are diminished, usually after about a month, your doctor may advise you to resume taking it once again. At this point, the side effects may take awhile to return, though the progression of the disease is not stopped. The variability of drug treatment stems from a well-known phenomenon called the *on-off effect*, in which Parkinsonian symptoms can suddenly get worse and then improve again. This may be helped by taking lower doses of medication at more frequent intervals.

■ The most common secondary drugs used against Parkinson's disease include levodopa plus carbidopa, bromocriptine, amantadine (Symadine, Symmetrel), and pergolide (Permax). Carbidopa prevents levodopa from being broken down before it reaches the brain; amantadine enhances the release of dopamine; and bromocriptine stimulates dopamine receptors. All of these drugs can have serious side effects, including uncontrollable movements, mood or mental changes, irregular heartbeat, difficulty urinating, and nausea accompanied by vomiting. Both carbidopa and amantadine are ineffective alone, and must be used in conjunction with levodopa. The dosages of all of these drugs must be carefully regulated, and your condition closely monitored.

■ The most interesting advances in the treatment of this disease are two relatively new surgical procedures, thalamotomy and pallidotomy. Thalamotomy corrects severe tremors, while pallidotomy reduces rigidity and small tremors. Both procedures require only local anesthetic. A neurosurgeon creates a very small opening in the skull and uses a probe to send electrical impulses into the areas of the brain that are causing the symptoms, "disconnecting" pathways that transmit their disordered messages to the muscles. A reported 90 percent of people undergoing thalamotomy find their tremors disappear, while 80 percent of those having pallidotomy have less rigidity and find their small tremors relieved. The effects of both procedures are immediate, and most patients are ready to go home within twenty-four hours. These procedures appear to be relatively safe, even for older adults.

DIETARY GUIDELINES

Eat a well-balanced, high-fiber diet. Maximize your intake of fresh green vegetables.

As much as possible, buy organic fruits, vegetables, and grains to minimize your exposure to pesticide residues.

Limit your intake of high-protein foods to no more than six ounces per day, taken mostly at dinner.

Vitamin B_6 (pyridoxine), found in bananas, beef, fish, liver, oatmeal, peanuts, potatoes, and whole grains, interferes with the action of L-dopa. If you are taking L-dopa, take these foods only in moderation, if at all.

Avoid all alcohol, caffeine, and sugar. All these substances create an acidic internal environment and are overstimulating to a stressed nervous system.

Drink at least six to eight 8-ounce glasses of pure water daily to help flush toxins from your body.

NUTRITIONAL SUPPLEMENTS

To prevent or correct possible nutritional deficiencies, take a high-potency multivitamin and mineral supplement daily. Choose a form that is easily digested, such as a soft gel-cap.

Acidophilus and bifidobacteria are friendly bacteria that ensure a healthy gastrointestinal tract. Probiotics are especially helpful for preventing constipation, which is often a problem for people with Parkinson's disease. Take a probiotic supplement as recommended on the product label. If you are allergic to milk, select a dairy-free formula.

Alpha-lipoic acid is an antioxidant that also helps to "recharge" other antioxidants in the body. Take 50 to 100 milligrams three times a day.

Calcium and magnesium are imperative for maintaining a healthy nervous system. Take a multimineral supplement that supplies 500 milligrams of calcium and 250 milligrams of magnesium, as well as trace minerals, twice daily.

■ Coenzyme Q_{10} is an oxygenating antioxidant that helps prevent free-radical damage. Take 30 milligrams two or three times daily.

■ People with Parkinson's disease often do not utilize nutrients effectively. To insure complete digestion and assimilation of the nutrients in the food you eat, take a digestive-enzyme supplement with each meal.

■ Evening primrose oil and flaxseed oil contain valuable essential fatty acids (EFAs), which are often deficient in people with Parkinson's disease. Take 1 tablespoonful (or 500 to 1,000 milligrams) of either or both twice daily.

■ Gamma-aminobutyric acid (GABA) is an amino acid that acts as a neurotransmitter. It helps both to strengthen and relax the nervous system. Take 500 milligrams up to three times daily for up to three months in a row.

■ Green-foods supplements supply chlorophyll and important trace minerals. Take a green-foods supplement as directed on the product label.

■ Marine alginate concentrate and N-acetylcysteine may help in the process of chelating (binding to) heavy metals in the body so that they can be excreted. If you or your health-care provider suspects heavy metal toxicity, take 500 milligrams of marine alginate concentrate three times a day and 500 milligrams of N-acetylcysteine twice daily.

■ Nicotinamide adenine dinucleotide hydrogren (NADH) is an enzyme that helps to improve neurotransmitter function. Take 5 to 10 milligrams twice daily.

■ Phosphatidylserine is a type of lipid important for normal brain function and the effective transmission of nerve impulses. Low levels of phosphatidylserine are associated with Parkinson's disease. Take 50 milligrams of phosphatidylserine three times daily.

■ Pine-bark and grape-seed extracts fight free-radical damage and have anti-inflammatory properties. Many people consider Parkinson's disease to be a consequence of degeneration of nerve cells due to free-radical damage. Take 25 to 50 milligrams of either three times daily.

■ The B vitamins are very important for brain and nerve function. Take a B-complex supplement so that you are getting 25 milligrams of each of the major B vitamins three times a day from all sources. In addition, take 50 milligrams of vitamin B_6 (pyridoxine) and pantothenic acid three times daily, between meals, plus 100 milligrams of niacinamide twice daily (morning and evening).

Note: If you are taking L-dopa, talk to your physician before taking any supplemental B vitamins, and do not take additional vitamin B_6, as this vitamin interferes with the action of L-dopa.

■ Vitamin C and the bioflavonoids are powerful antioxidants that fight free radicals. Take 1,000 milligrams of vitamin C with bioflavonoids three times daily for one month. Then gradually increase your intake to the highest level you can tolerate.

■ Vitamin E is a powerful antioxidant that prevents free-radical damage. Choose a product containing mixed tocopherols and start by taking 200 international units daily, then gradually increase the dosage until you are taking 400 international units in the morning and another 400 international units in the evening.

Note: If you have high blood pressure, limit your intake of supplemental vitamin E to a total of 400 international units daily. If you are taking an anticoagulant (blood thinner), consult your physician before taking supplemental vitamin E.

■ Selenium is an antioxidant that works with vitamin E. It also helps to increase circulation and tissue oxygenation, thereby limiting damage to nerve cells. Take 200 micrograms of selenium daily.

HERBAL TREATMENT

■ Ginkgo biloba scavenges free radicals and boosts circulation to the brain. Select a product containing at least 24 percent ginkgo heterosides (sometimes called flavoglycosides) and start by taking 40 milligrams three times daily. If you feel fine at that dosage, you can gradually increase to as much as 80 milligrams three times daily.

HOMEOPATHY

■ *Agaricus* is for limbs that are stiff but tremble and twitch. You likely feel itchy, and your back, especially your spine, is probably very sensitive. Take one dose of *Agaricus* 30x or 15c, as directed on the product label, three times daily for up to three days, as needed to relieve symptoms.

■ Choose *Gelsemium* if you have considerable trembling and eyelids so droopy that you may appear to be asleep. You stagger when walking and feel weak and fatigued much of the time. Take *Gelsemium* 30x or 15c three times daily for up to three days, as needed to relieve symptoms.

■ *Hyoscyamus* is for the person who exhibits inappropriate behavior at inopportune times. You have a lot of twitching, are restless, and tend to be jealous and very suspicious. Take one dose of *Hyoscyamus* 30x or 15c three times daily for up to three days, as needed to relieve symptoms.

■ *Mercurius corrosivus* is for trembling hands and excessive salivation. You tend to be very sensitive to heat and cold, and have difficulty concentrating. Take one dose of *Mercurius corrosivus* 30x or 15c three times daily for up to three days, as needed to relieve symptoms.

■ *Rhus toxicodendron* is good for mild tremors and stiffness that feels better with movement, worse with dampness. Take one dose of *Rhus toxicodendron* 30x or 15c three times daily for up to three days, as needed to relieve symptoms.

BACH FLOWER REMEDIES

Select the remedy that most closely fits your emotional tendencies and concerns, and take it as needed, following the directions on the product label.

■ Beech is the remedy for impatience and intolerance of your affliction. You have a tendency to be a perfectionist and like an orderly life.

■ Holly will prove helpful if you are angry, prone to fits of temper, and feel jealous and insecure underneath.

■ Impatiens will ease nervous tension, feelings of impatience, irritability, and a tendency to fidget.

■ White Chestnut helps to counteract a tendency to obsess on problems without letup.

ACUPRESSURE

For the locations of acupressure points on the body, *see* ADMINISTERING AN ACUPRESSURE TREATMENT in Part Three.

■ Four Gates relaxes the muscles.

■ Stomach 36 improves the absorption of nutrients and strengthens overall well-being.

GENERAL RECOMMENDATIONS

■ Exercise. Moderate daily exercise helps to maintain muscle tone and function. Stretching exercises, deep breathing, yoga, and tai chi are all excellent. *See* STARTING AN EXERCISE PROGRAM in Part Three.

■ Physical therapy, including active and passive range-of-motion exercises, can be immensely valuable. If you cannot exercise on your own, you may need a therapist to perform the movements for you.

PREVENTION

■ Because the root cause of Parkinson's disease has not been determined, there is no known way to prevent it. However, maintaining a healthy lifestyle that includes eating a wholesome diet and drinking only pure water, getting regular exercise, and avoiding toxins and pollutants as much as possible, plus taking antioxidant supplements to prevent free-radical damage, are probably prudent precautions.

Pelvic Inflammatory Disease

Pelvic inflammatory disease (PID) is an infection of the internal female reproductive organs. It can be either acute or chronic. It occurs when infectious organisms, usually bacteria or chlamydia, enter the uterus and spread to infect the fallopian tubes, ovaries, and surrounding tissues. Although PID itself is not sexually transmitted, it is most often a complication of a sexually transmitted disease such as chlamydia or gonorrhea. A pelvic infection of this type can also develop after miscarriage or induced abortion. PID is most common among sexually active young women and women who have been fitted with intrauterine devices (IUDs) for contraception. It seldom occurs in women who have passed menopause.

Symptoms include a heavy, rank-smelling vaginal discharge; fever; pain and tenderness in the lower abdomen; backache; and abnormal bleeding. Menstrual periods may arrive early and the bleeding is often heavy. In both the acute and chronic forms of the disease, sexual intercourse may be painful.

Diagnosis involves a pelvic examination, during which your doctor will take a swab of material from inside your vagina. Laboratory analysis can identify the infectious agent, which in turn will guide your doctor in prescribing appropriate treatment. In addition, your physician may wish to view your interior organs with a laparoscope to see the extent of inflammation and other signs of infection.

PID should always be treated promptly. If the ovaries or fallopian tubes become infected, it can cause scarring that may lead to infertility.

CONVENTIONAL MEDICINE

■ Antibiotics are the mainstay of therapy for PID. If the infection is severe, they may have to be administered intravenously at a hospital. Because there are many drug-resistant infectious agents out there today, most doctors use a combination of two or more different antibiotics to treat this infection.

■ If abscesses are found within the internal reproductive organs, surgery may be required to remove them.

■ If an acute pelvic infection causes severe pain, your doctor may prescribe narcotics to relieve the pain and bed rest during treatment.

■ If you have blocked fallopian tubes or an abscess as a result of the infection, you may need surgery to open the tubes or drain the abscess.

■ If you are sexually active, your partner or partners should be examined and, if necessary, treated as well. They may need treatment even if they are not having any symptoms at all.

DIETARY GUIDELINES

■ To flush toxins from your body, drink eight 8-ounce glasses of pure water daily.

■ Eat many and varied fresh vegetables to assure a full complement of phytonutrients. Eat them either raw or steamed. If you steam them, save the resulting broth to use in soups or gravies, or for cooking rice and other grains that absorb water.

NUTRITIONAL SUPPLEMENTS

■ PID places considerable stress on the body. Take a good multivitamin and mineral complex daily, with meals, to ensure you have all the basic micronutrients you need.

■ Digestive enzymes help to ensure complete digestion of foods and enhance the assimilation of nutrients, providing more nutrients to help rebuild damaged tissues. Take a full-spectrum digestive-enzyme supplement providing 5,000 international units of lipase, 2,500 international units of amylase, and 300 international units of protease, plus 500 to 1,000 milligrams of pancreatin, with each meal.

Note: Long-term supplementation with pancreatin is not advised, as it can cause your pancreas to reduce its own production of this important enzyme. Overuse also has the potential to cause nausea or diarrhea. After two months on pancreatin, discontinue use and monitor your reaction. If you find that digestive problems recur, discuss pancreatin supplementation with your health-care provider.

■ Vitamin C helps the body fight infection and acts as an anti-inflammatory. Take 1,000 milligrams (1 gram) of vitamin C three times daily.

HERBAL TREATMENT

■ Butiao is a Chinese herbal remedy that is very effective in reducing excessive bleeding and menstrual pain. Take 3 tablets twice a day for three months.

■ Carthamus and persica is a Chinese herbal combination that improves digestion and helps relax the lower abdominal cavity. Although it is not a specific treatment for PID, many women with a history of this condition have found it useful in speeding recovery. Take two capsules two or three times daily.

■ Applying warm castor-oil packs can help to reduce inflammation. Prepare a warm castor-oil pack by saturating several layers of clean white cloth with the oil. You can either warm the oil before preparing the pack or prepare the pack, place it on a clean plate, and warm it in a microwave oven for twenty to thirty seconds. Make sure the pack is warm, not hot. Place the warm pack on your lower abdomen and leave it in place for fifteen to twenty minutes. Do this once a day for five to seven days.

■ Echinacea and goldenseal are natural antibiotics that are especially useful if you have lingering symptoms of infection after antibiotic therapy. Take one dose of an echinacea and goldenseal combination formula supplying 200 to 350 milligrams of echinacea and 100 to 300 milligrams of goldenseal two or three times daily for one week.

■ If your symptoms are aggravated by poor digestion, take a cup of ginger-root tea two or three times daily. It is especially helpful for people with a history of poor lower bowel function and a fondness for raw foods and juices.

■ Grapefruit-seed extract has antibacterial, anviral, and antifungal activity. Take 1,000 milligrams two or three times a day.

■ Nettle and yellow dock are herbs that are very high in minerals. They are traditionally used to revitalize the blood. Native Americans used these two herbs for women recovering from PID. Take 500 milligrams of nettle and 250 to 500 milligrams of yellow dock twice daily for one week.

HOMEOPATHY

PID is a complicated and potentially serious problem that should not be self-diagnosed or self-treated. We strongly advise that you see a homeopathic practitioner for a constitutional remedy. The following remedies may serve to help alleviate some of the acute symptoms in the meantime.

■ *Apis mellifica* may help relieve a burning pain that is worse on the right side, possibly accompanied by a swollen abdomen. Take one dose of *Apis mellifica* 30x or 15c three times a day for up to three days.

■ *Arsenicum album* can help if you are restless and anxious, and are experiencing diarrhea. Take one dose of *Arsenicum album* 30x or 15c three times a day for up to three days.

■ *Belladonna* is for fever and abdominal pain that is worse with movement. You are likely feeling restless and have a bright red, hot face. Take one dose of *Belladonna* 30x or 15c three times a day for up to three days.

■ *Colocynthis* may prove helpful if you have abdominal cramping that feels better if you curl your legs up to your chest. Take one dose of *Colocynthis* 12x or 6c three times a day for up to three days.

■ *Magnesia phosphorica* can ease abdominal cramping that feels better with applications of warmth. Take one dose of *Magnesia phosphorica* 12x or 6c three times a day for up to three days.

■ *Mercurius vivus* 12x or 6c can help if you have a strong body odor and alternate between feeling hot and cold. You may have a sore throat as well. Take one dose of *Mercurius vivus* 12x or 6c three times a day for up to three days.

BACH FLOWER REMEDIES

Select the remedy that most closely fits your emotional tendencies and concerns, and take it as needed, following the directions on the product label.

■ Elm is good if you feel simply incapable of doing things that need to be accomplished.

■ Choose Gentian if you are feeling discouraged and need praise and encouragement to succeed.

■ Holly helps to tame feelings of anger and insecurity that burst out in fits of bad temper.

■ Hornbeam helps relieve the kind of fatigue that is so strong it keeps you from participating fully and effectively in your normal daily activities.

■ Larch helps to overcome a lack of confidence that makes you want to stay in the background.

ACUPRESSURE

For the locations of acupressure points on the body, *see* ADMINISTERING AN ACUPRESSURE TREATMENT in Part Three.

■ Bladder 23, 25, 27, and 28 increase circulation to the genitourinary tract.

■ Four Gates calms the nervous system.

■ Gallbladder 41 is a "hormonal" point that helps to regulate the hormonal system.

■ Spleen 6 reduces uterine cramping.

■ Stomach 36 strengthens overall well-being.

GENERAL RECOMMENDATIONS

■ Follow your doctor's instructions regarding bed rest and activity restrictions. Adequate rest is very important in recovering from this disease.

■ Anytime you must take antibiotics, it is a good idea to try to keep high levels of beneficial bacteria present in the vagina. Moisten a tampon and sprinkle it with a powdered probiotic culture, then insert it and leave it in place overnight.

■ Avoid sexual intercourse until your treatment is over and the infection has cleared.

PREVENTION

■ The only sure way to avoid contracting a sexually transmitted disease is to abstain from sex entirely or to have a monogamous relationship with a healthy partner. If you have multiple sexual partners, or if you have sexual contact with anyone whose health status or background is not known to you, practice safer sex. Use a latex (not animal-skin) condom *every time*. For added protection, use a spermicide in addition to the condom.

■ If you have any suspicion you may have contracted a sexually transmitted disease or other type of genital infection, consult a health-care professional promptly for evaluation and treatment. Possible signs include itching and burning sensations in the genital area, pain on urination, and/or unusual vaginal discharge. Proper and timely treatment can prevent complications such as PID from developing.

Peptic Ulcer

A peptic ulcer is an area of erosion in the mucous membranes of the stomach or duodenum, the upper portion of the intestines, directly below the stomach. Ulcers are in part caused—and can be greatly worsened—by the corrosive action of gastric (stomach) juices. Gastric juices consist of hydrochloric acid and pepsin, an enzyme that helps break down food. To protect the mucous membranes lining the walls of the stomach and duodenum from contact with digestive acids, cells in the lining of the digestive tract secrete mucus. However, if either too much acid or too little mucus is produced, or if the stomach is subjected to substances that irritate the protective lining—including alcohol, tobacco, and certain drugs, especially nonsteroidal anti-inflammatory drugs (NSAIDs)—a peptic ulcer may develop.

Acid is not the only factor in peptic ulcers, however. It is now known that *Helicobacter pylori* (*H. pylori*), a type of bacteria commonly found in the lining of the stomach, is a primary cause of ulcers. Although these bacteria don't always cause problems, studies have shown that between 90 and 100 percent of those suffering from duodenal ulcers, and 70 to 75 percent of people with gastric ulcers, are under attack by *H. pylori*. Many experts now believe that *H. pylori* may be a factor in other stomach disorders, including gastritis, esophagitis, acid indigestion, and stomach cancer.

The primary symptom of a peptic ulcer is a burning or gnawing pain that usually occurs shortly before a meal, an hour or so after eating, or during the night. The pain is usually felt in the stomach or abdomen, but may also be experienced as discomfort in the back or chest. If the pain is severe enough, it can cause you to waken from a sound sleep. Some people feel nauseated and lose their appetite; others find they eat more than ever. The pain is usually relieved by eating or taking antacids. Some people find the pain is relieved by vomiting. Many find their pain follows a more or less predictable pattern, and that periods of stress make the problem worse.

Ulcers can occur anywhere in the digestive tract, but they are most common in the lower half of the stomach and upper part of the duodenum. About one in every ten Americans develops a peptic ulcer at some time in his or her life. Ulcers are roughly twice as common in men as in women.

CONVENTIONAL MEDICINE

■ The first treatment your doctor is likely to recommend is an over-the-counter antacid drug to neutralize excess acidity. Tums, Rolaids, and Maalox are well-known examples of this type of product. Read the label carefully before buying an antacid. Some antacids are aluminum-based. A calcium- or magnesium-based product is a better choice. Also, you should be aware that while antacids may provide temporary relief, there can be a rebound effect when you stop taking them that results in an increased production of stomach acids and more irritation.

■ If symptoms persist, your doctor may prescribe medication to reduce the production of stomach acid and/or a drug designed to form a protective covering over the ulcer. Histamine-blockers are drugs that reduce acid production by blocking receptors on acid-producing cells. Examples include cimetidine (Tagamet), famotidine (Pepcid), nizatidine (Axid), and ranitidine (Zantac). Lower dose over-the-counter versions of these drugs are available as well. Possible side effects of these medications include dizziness, diarrhea, headache, and liver damage. The long-term use of histamine-blockers may also be associated with an increased risk of stomach cancer.

■ A newer type of medication, known as a proton-pump inhibitor, stops far more production of acid than the histamine blockers do. This class of drugs includes omeprazole (Prilosec) and lansoprazole (Prevacid). Possible side effects include nausea, diarrhea, headaches, and abdominal pain. If you must take any drug designed to reduce the production of stomach acid, it is worth remembering that your body produces acid for a reason—it is necessary for proper digestion and absorption of nutrients—so these drugs should be used for the shortest time possible.

■ Sucralfate (Carafate), bismuth subsalicylate (Pepto-Bismol), and misoprostol (Cytotec) may be used to assist the mucus defenses in the intestinal tract. Though the actual protective mechanism is not well understood, it appears that an increased coating effect of the stomach lining is involved. You should not take misoprostol if you are pregnant, as it can cause miscarriage.

■ If an ulcer proves resistant to treatment, chances are that *H. pylori* is involved. Until the *H. pylori* bacteria are eliminated, ulcers will continue to recur. *H. pylori* infection is diagnosed by a blood test for antibodies that show the presence of the bacteria, and is treated with antibiotics.

■ *Avoid* taking any medications that contain aspirin, ibuprofen, or other nonsteroidal anti-inflammatory drugs (NSAIDs). These drugs are very irritating to the stomach lining and increase acidity.

DIETARY GUIDELINES

■ Although a bland diet was once prescribed as an "ulcer cure," that thinking is changing. A diet that is low in saturated and hydrogenated fats and high in fiber has been shown to be much more effective. If your symptoms are severe, or if you have been on a bland diet for some time, increase the amount of fiber in your diet gradually.

■ In order to create a successful diet—that is, one you can stick with—it is important to consider your personal dietary preferences, as well as the stage your ulcer is in. Steamed green vegetables are very beneficial, as are any vegetables high in vitamin K, including alfalfa and all leafy greens. People with digestive-tract problems are often deficient in this vitamin, which promotes healing and helps prevent bleeding.

■ Eat frequent small meals to avoid triggering excessive production of digestive acids, and to ensure these acids have something other than your stomach lining to go to work on.

■ Drink cabbage juice. In one controlled study, ulcers in subjects who drank a quart of raw cabbage juice daily (in divided doses) were found to have healed within ten days. The cabbage should be juiced and the juice taken immediately after preparation.

■ If you have a bleeding ulcer, eat organic baby food and sip barley water. Barley water is an age-old remedy that soothes the entire digestive tract. (*See* THERAPEUTIC RECIPES in Part Three.)

■ Drink plenty of pure water. Water dilutes excess stomach acid and helps flush it away. If you are feeling excessively acidic, drink 8 to 16 ounces of water at once. This will dilute stomach acid quickly and help minimize damage and pain.

■ Avoid milk. Although milk was once recommended for people with ulcers because it neutralizes stomach acids, milk also stimulates the production of gastric juices. The end result is increased irritation of the ulcerated lining.

■ Avoid coffee, alcohol, citrus juices, and sugar, as well as hot and spicy foods. These substances are irritating to the stomach lining and also cause additional secretion of digestive acids.

NUTRITIONAL SUPPLEMENTS

■ The amino acid glutamine helps to soothe stomach irritation. Take 1,000 milligrams of L-glutamine three times daily for two weeks, then decrease to 1,000 milligrams twice daily for two weeks. Then take 500 milligrams daily for two months.

■ Take a probiotic supplement containing acidophilus or bifidobacteria. Probiotics are especially important if you must take antibiotics, as antibiotics destroy the good bacteria along with the bad. Probiotic bacteria also help to crowd out the harmful *H. pylori* bacteria. Take a probiotic supplement as recommended on the product label. If you are allergic to milk, select a dairy-free formula.

■ Vitamin A is healing for mucous membranes. Take 5,000 international units two to four times daily for six weeks; then decrease the dosage to 5,000 units twice a day for one month. Then take a maintenance dosage of 5,000 international units daily. For better assimilation, select an emulsified form of vitamin A.

Note: If you are pregnant, or intend to get pregnant, or if you have liver disease, consult your doctor before taking supplemental vitamin A. Pregnant women should not ingest a total of more than 25,000 international units of supplemental vitamin A *per week* from all sources.

■ Vitamin E helps heal the stomach lining. Choose a product containing mixed tocopherols and take 200 to 600 international units twice daily.

Note: If you have high blood pressure, limit your intake of supplemental vitamin E to a total of 400 international units daily. If you are taking an anticoagulant (blood thinner), consult your physician before taking supplemental vitamin E.

HERBAL TREATMENT

■ Aloe vera has been used for many years to bring quick relief of excess stomach acidity. Select a food-grade product and take $1/4$ cup two or three times daily.

■ Chamomile is an antispasmodic and eases abdominal gas. It has a mild anti-inflammatory effect on the lining of the digestive tract and also has antimicrobial properties. Drink a cup of chamomile tea with meals.

■ If you cannot tolerate the taste or odor of fresh cabbage juice, you'll be glad to know there is an alternative. Fare You is a Chinese patent medicine prepared from dried cabbage juice that has been used successfully for centuries to resolve stomach acidity and ulceration. Take two tablets twice daily.

■ Goldenseal has antibiotic properties, which makes it valuable in resolving a variety of infections. If your doctor has told you that *H. pylori* infection is the cause of your peptic ulcer, choose a standarized extract containing 8 to 10 percent total alkaloids and take 300 to 500 milligrams three times daily for five days.

■ Licorice soothes and helps heal mucous membranes by stimulating production of the mucus that protects the digestive tract. Select chewable deglycyrrhizinated licorice (DGL) tablets and take 500 to 750 milligrams three times daily.

Note: Do not substitute ordinary licorice root for DGL. Ordinary licorice root contains glycyrrhizinic acid, which can elevate blood pressure, so it should not be taken on an ongoing basis and should not be used at all by persons with high blood pressure. With the glycyrrhizinic acid removed, DGL does not affect blood pressure.

■ Marshmallow root and slippery elm are very soothing to the lining of the stomach. Take 500 milligrams of either or both three times daily for ten days to two weeks.

Turmeric is a natural anti-inflammatory and helps to speed the healing process. Take 500 milligrams two to three times daily.

HOMEOPATHY

The most helpful approach to treating a peptic ulcer homeopathically is to consult a qualified homeopathic practitioner who can prescribe a constitutional remedy suited to your individual needs.

Carbo vegetabilis may be helpful for acute discomfort. This remedy is very useful for easing the sensation of excess stomach acidity. Take a dose of *Carbo vegetabilis* 30x or 15c as needed to relieve symptoms.

BACH FLOWER REMEDIES

Select the remedy that most closely fits your emotional tendencies and concerns, and take it as needed, following the directions on the product label.

Holly helps to tame anger that stems from underlying feelings of insecurity and jealousy, and bursts out in fits of temper.

Impatiens calms the impatience and hyperactivity typical of the tension-filled type-A personality.

Larch is helpful if you lack self confidence and hate being the center of attention. For example, you probably find giving a presentation or facing a job interview to be an agonizing ordeal.

White Chestnut counteracts a tendency to obsess on ideas or events long after they should have been forgotten.

ACUPRESSURE

For the locations of acupressure points on the body, *see* ADMINISTERING AN ACUPRESSURE TREATMENT in Part Three.

Pericardium 6 relaxes the upper digestive tract.

Spleen 6 increases yin.

Stomach 36 tones the digestive system and strengthens overall well-being.

AROMATHERAPY

For specific instructions on how to use aromatherapy, *see* PREPARING AROMATHERAPY TREATMENTS in Part Three.

■ Essential oils of lavender and orange are good for neutralizing stress, which can aggravate ulcers. Use any or all of these oils as inhalants, diffuse them into the air, use them to prepare a relaxing bath, or add a few drops to massage oil.

GENERAL RECOMMENDATIONS

Do not smoke, and avoid secondhand smoke. Tobacco smoke irritates the stomach lining and increases stomach acidity.

■ As much as possible, avoid stress, and learn ways to manage the stress you cannot avoid. Biofeedback, yoga, and meditation are techniques that many people have found helpful.

■ If you have been battling an ulcer for a long time without success, ask your doctor about testing (and, if necessary, treating) you for *H. pylori* bacteria.

PREVENTION

■ Regular supplementation with probiotic bacteria is the most effective way of protecting your body against the development of ulcers caused by *H. pylori* bacteria. Acidophilus and bifidobacteria can destroy many dangerous organisms before they can create problems.

■ Avoid stress as much as possible. Although it is now known that stress itself does not cause ulcers, stress does cause the body to increase production of the stomach acids that irritate an ulcer.

Periodontal Disease

The term *periodontal disease* refers to any disease of the periodontium, the tissues that surround and support the teeth, including the jawbone. These conditions are extremely common. An estimated 75 percent—or more—of Americans over the age of thirty-five have some degree of periodontal disease.

There are two primary categories of periodontal disease: gingivitis and periodontitis. Gingivitis is characterized by red, inflamed gums that are swollen, sore, and tender, and that tend to bleed, especially when you brush your teeth. It usually begins as a bacterial infection that thrives between the gums and teeth. Plaque, that sticky film of mucus and bacteria that adheres to the teeth, particularly along the gum line, is generally the source of the infection. Inflammation of the gums can also occur due to certain drugs, the hormonal changes of pregnancy, or leukemia. Poorly fitting dental appliances and misaligned teeth can be contributing factors. If gingivitis is left untreated, the gums can recede and the teeth can loosen.

In periodontitis (also sometimes called *pyorrhea*), the infection spreads to and erodes the underlying bone. If enough of the supporting bone is lost, tooth loss can follow. In fact, periodontitis is the leading cause of tooth loss among American adults. In addition, pockets of bacteria in the mouth can lead to a chronic low-grade bodywide infection that contributes to conditions as serious as heart disease and diabetes. One anti-aging study tracking 1,231 men determined that those who developed periodontal disease had a significantly higher chance of dying from heart disease than men whose gums remained healthy.

It is worth noting that although gingivitis almost always precedes periodontitis, periodontitis is *not* an inevitable consequence of gingivitis. Swollen and tender gums are a sign that you should pay more attention to your teeth and their support structure.

CONVENTIONAL MEDICINE

■ Meticulous oral hygiene, including daily brushing and flossing and regular dental visits for cleaning and scaling to remove plaque, is the most important element of treatment. An antimicrobial mouthwash may help as well. Listerine, an old standby that is available over the counter, contains a natural antibacterial called thymol (a derivative of the thyme plant), which can help to fight gingivitis. Another alternative is a prescription mouthwash containing the antimicrobial agent chlorhexidine (Peridex). Chlorhexidine is a drug with strong anti-plaque and anti-inflammatory properties. Your dentist can prescribe it if he or she believes it appropriate for you.

■ If poorly fitting dental appliances or restorations are contributing to the problem, they may have to be replaced or repaired.

■ If less aggressive techniques fail, surgical removal of swollen tissue may be required. This type of treatment is also used for inflammation of the gums due to certain drugs or leukemia.

■ In serious cases of periodontitis, loose teeth may need to be removed or splinted into place.

DIETARY GUIDELINES

■ Diet (and cleanliness) are important factors in sustaining good oral health. Avoid refined sugars and any foods that contain them, particularly foods with a sticky texture. Bacteria thrive on sugar, and it is particularly difficult to remove all residue from foods that adhere to the tooth surface. Simply avoiding the simple sugars that lead to tooth decay is a good place to start.

■ To maintain strong teeth and healthy gums, eat a diet that emphasizes high-fiber foods such as whole grains and fresh (preferably raw) vegetables. Chew your foods thoroughly before swallowing.

NUTRITIONAL SUPPLEMENTS

■ The antioxidants—beta-carotene, vitamins C and E, selenium, and zinc—all enhance oral health. Take an antioxidant formula that supplies at least 10,000 international units of beta-carotene, 500 milligrams of vitamin C, 200 international units of vitamin E, and 20 milligrams of zinc twice daily.

Note: If you are taking an anticoagulant (blood thinner), consult your physician before taking vitamin E.

■ Coenzyme Q_{10} increases the supply of oxygen to the tissues and can help heal a receding gumline. You should take 60 milligrams two or three times daily for a minimum of one month to see its beneficial effects. If you have serious periodontal problems, you may need more. Fortunately, side effects are minimal to nonexistent.

■ Folic acid fights plaque and can reduce gum inflammation, swelling, and bleeding. You can take it internally, chew the whole tablet, or dissolve a tablet or capsule in water to make a mouthwash. Take 400 micrograms twice daily.

HERBAL TREATMENT

■ Aloe vera is beneficial and soothing to the gums and tissues of the mouth. Use it as a mouthwash or take $1/8$ cup twice a day for one month. Be sure to select a food-grade product for this purpose.

■ Echinacea has antimicrobial properties that fight infection. Take 250 milligrams of standarized extract or one cup of tea three times daily for one week.

■ Hawthorn has a "tightening" effect on the gums when used over a period of time. Choose an extract standardized to 1.8 percent vitexin rhamnosides and take 100 to 200 milligrams twice daily. You can also add 2 tablespoons of liquid extract to 8 ounces of water to make a mouthwash.

HOMEOPATHY

■ *Carbo vegetubilis* is for gums that are receding and bleed when brushed. You may also have sluggish digestion and become nauseated easily. Take one dose of *Carbo vegetabilis* 30x or 15c, as directed on the product label, three times daily for up to three days, as needed.

■ *Mercurius solubilis* is helpful if you have bad breath and loose teeth with decay on the crowns. You feel thirsty, but your mouth is moist. Take one dose of *Mercurius solubilis* 12x or 6c three times daily for up to three days, as needed.

■ Choose *Pyrogenium* 12x or 6c if you have a red, dry tongue; foul breath; and a constant bad taste in your mouth. Take one dose of *Pyrogenium* 12x or 6c three times daily for up to three days, as needed.

ACUPRESSURE

For the locations of acupressure points on the body, *see* ADMINISTERING AN ACUPRESSURE TREATMENT in Part Three.

■ Gallbladder 20 improves circulation to the head.

■ Kidney 7 strengthens the kidneys. In Chinese medicine, the kidneys "rule" the bones and teeth.

■ Large Intestine 4 relieves face and tooth pain and helps to clear infection.

■ Spleen 6 strengthens yin.

■ Stomach 36 strengthens yang.

AROMATHERAPY

For specific instructions on how to use aromatherapy, *see* PREPARING AROMATHERAPY TREATMENTS in Part Three.

■ Essential oils of myrrh, tea tree, and thyme can be useful for fighting gum infections. Add 10 or 12 drops of any or all of these oils to 1 tablespoon of a carrier oil, such as plain canola or olive oil, and gently massage the mixture into your gums after brushing. Pay particular attention to the areas where the teeth meet the gums. Or you can add the same amount of oil to 8 ounces of distilled water to make an infection-fighting mouthwash.

GENERAL RECOMMENDATIONS

■ Brush your teeth carefully after eating, and floss thoroughly between your teeth at least once every day. As you do so, remember that your goal is to prevent plaque buildup by removing this bacteria from between your gums and teeth. If you are unsure of the best brushing and/or flossing technique, or if just you want to verify that you are doing it correctly, ask your dentist or dental hygienist to demonstrate. After brushing and flossing, rinse your mouth with your favorite mouthwash or with any of the mouthwashes suggested in this section.

■ Buy a new toothbrush twice each month until the infection is under control. Bacteria can cling to your toothbrush, causing you to reinfect yourself. Between brushings, you can disinfect your toothbrush by immersing it in hydrogen peroxide or a citrus-seed-extract solution (remember to rinse it thoroughly before using it again).

■ Use a rotary electric toothbrush instead of the standard hand-powered variety. These mechanical instruments can remove up to 95 percent of plaque, compared with 48 percent for hand-brushing.

■ A Water Pik—a hand-held device that shoots a jet of water to thoroughly rinse your teeth, especially between the teeth and at the gum line—is beneficial for thorough cleaning and good oral health.

■ Twice a day, make a paste by mixing a equal amounts of hydrogen peroxide and baking soda. Peroxide kills bacteria; baking soda is cleansing and deodorizing. If you wish, you can add powdered or liquid zinc, folic acid, hawthorn extract, and/or echinacea, as well as aloe vera juice—experiment to find the mixture that suits you best. Apply the paste to your gums, both inside and out. Then use a rubber-tipped gum stimulator between your teeth: Place the rubber point between two teeth and rotate in a circular motion for about ten seconds, then move on to the next space and repeat. When you have worked on all areas of your gums, rinse your mouth thoroughly. This procedure should take no more than ten or fifteen minutes each time, and the benefits can be enormous.

PREVENTION

■ Follow the suggestions under Dietary Guidelines in this entry, and chew thoroughly to stimulate your gums.

■ Practice good oral hygiene as detailed in this entry.

Pernicious Anemia

See under ANEMIA.

Perspiration, Excessive

Perspiration is one of the body's natural mechanisms for maintaining a proper internal temperature. This is why people sweat more in warm weather and when the metabolic rate increases, whether in response to physical exertion or nervousness. Some people, however, perspire more heavily than circumstances would seem to call for. Medically, this is known as *hyperhidrosis*.

Excessive perspiration can be a result of overactive sweat glands. It may be limited to certain areas—the palms of the hands, the soles of the feet, the armpits, the groin, or under the breasts—or it can affect the entire body. The cause of the localized type of hyperhidrosis is unknown, though there may be a psychological component. It is not considered a serious problem, but it can be an embarrassing one. Generalized hyperhidrosis can have a variety of causes, including fever and overactive thyroid or adrenal glands. Anyone with this problem should therefore have a thorough medical examination to look for an underlying cause.

Occasionally, bacteria and yeast in the skin act on decaying cellular debris and sweat in the skin, causing a foul odor. This condition is known to doctors as *bromhidrosis*, and it too can cause embarrassment.

CONVENTIONAL TREATMENT

■ Treatment for generalized hyperhidrosis depends on the underlying cause, though this is sometimes difficult to track down.

■ For a localized perspiration problem, your doctor may recommend treating the affected area with an aluminum chloride solution. This is generally applied at night and washed off in the morning. Bear in mind that aluminum may be absorbed through the skin, and this element has no known benefit to the human body. Though no connection has been proved conclusively, high levels of aluminum have also been linked to Alzheimer's disease.

■ If anxiety is a factor, your doctor may prescribe an anti-anxiety drug.

■ In severe cases, the sweat glands in the armpit may be surgically removed.

■ Bromhidrosis can often be treated successfully with a combination of careful hygiene, the application of topical antibacterial agents, and, possibly, shaving of underarm hair.

DIETARY GUIDELINES

■ Simplify your diet. Reduce your consumption of foods of animal origin, and emphasize fresh vegetables and fruits instead.

■ Include fresh pineapple and papaya in your diet. These fruits contain natural enzymes that aid in digestion. In Chinese medicine, body odor is linked to incomplete digestion.

NUTRITIONAL SUPPLEMENTS

■ Body odor is often correlated with low zinc levels. Take 15 milligrams of zinc two or three times daily. Take zinc with food to prevent stomach upset. If you take over 30 milligrams of zinc on a daily basis for more than one or two months, you should also take 1 to 2 milligrams of copper each day to maintain a proper mineral balance.

HERBAL TREATMENT

■ The combination of barberry, nettle, and yellow dock, taken as a tea, has traditionally been used to diminish sweating and perspiration odor. Take a cup of tea three times daily.

■ Taking grapefruit-seed extract can sometimes reduce perspiration odor. Take 3 drops three times daily.

HOMEOPATHY

■ See a homeopathic physician who can prescribe a constitutional remedy designed specifically for you.

■ *Sulfur* is good if you are sweaty, with hot, sweaty hands, and perspiration odor that smells like garlic. Take one dose of *Sulfur* 30x or 15c three times daily for up to four days.

BACH FLOWER REMEDIES

■ Holly is good for feelings of insecurity and jealousy that come out in displays of anger and bad temper. Use it as directed on the product label.

ACUPRESSURE

For the locations of acupressure points on the body, *see* ADMINISTERING AN ACUPRESSURE TREATMENT in Part Three.

■ The combination of Liver 3 and Spleen 10 relaxes the nervous system and detoxifies the blood.

AROMATHERAPY

For specific instructions on how to use aromatherapy, *see* PREPARING AROMATHERAPY TREATMENTS in Part Three.

■ Essential oils of cypress, geranium, grapefruit, and lavender are all known for their detoxifying properties. Take a daily bath prepared with one to three of these oils.

GENERAL RECOMMENDATIONS

■ Careful attention to hygiene is important, but be kind to your skin. Avoid scented and harsh detergent-based skin-care products. Thorough washing with ordinary soap is just as effective at removing dirt and bacteria, and poses less risk of irritation or drying.

■ Avoid using oily or heavy body lotions, which make it hard for the skin to "breathe" and can increase perspiration. If you use a body lotion, choose a water-based, hypoallergenic product.

■ Wear clothing, including underwear, made from lightweight woven fabrics that breathe, such as cotton. Avoid synthetics. In cooler weather, dress in several lighter layers rather than a single heavy one. That way, you can remove a layer if you find yourself becoming warm as a result of activity or an overly heated indoor environment.

PREVENTION

■ Since perspiration is part of the body's natural temperature-control mechanism, it is neither possible nor desirable to prevent it completely. Excessive and/or unusually odorous perspiration, however, can often be controlled with the measures outlined in this entry.

Phlebitis

Properly called *thrombophlebitis*, this is a partial or total blockage of a vein by a blood clot. The vein then becomes inflamed. Often, phlebitis is superficial, affecting veins close to the skin. It can be a result of trauma or an intravenous catheter that is left in for too long. It can also occur spontaneously after childbirth. Paradoxically, superficial phlebitis, the less serious form of the condition, usually causes more symptoms, including pain, swelling, redness, and warmth in the affected area.

About one in five cases of phlebitis involve clots in deeper veins. This is a more serious condition, and usually affects veins in the leg or pelvis. There may be dull aching pain and, possibly, swelling, though some people have no symptoms at all. Deep-vein phlebitis, also known as deep venous thrombosis, is most likely to occur following a period of prolonged inactivity or after surgery. Cancer, the use of oral contraceptives, prominent varicose veins, and a history of congestive heart failure increase the risk.

Deep-vein phlebitis can lead to embolism, in which bits of the clot break off and move through the bloodstream to other parts of the body, such as the lung or brain, where they can have extremely serious consequences. Another potential complication is venous insufficiency (inadequate drainage of blood through the veins), which can cause a worsening of varicose veins, edema (swelling of tissues due to the accumulation of fluid), and, possibly, the formation of skin ulcers in the parts of the leg below the site of the clot.

Diagnosis of phlebitis usually involves a Doppler ultrasound screen, a painless procedure in which a microphone-like probe is passed over the area in which a clot is suspected. Success with this technique requires a certain amount of training and experience on the part of the practitioner, however. Another type of testing that may be done is plethysmography, a noninvasive test that is done to look for differences in pressure within major veins. The most accurate test is contrast venography, in which a dye is injected into the vein system and its progress (or lack thereof) is tracked by means of x-ray studies.

CONVENTIONAL TREATMENT

■ For superficial phlebitis, bed rest, heat, and elevation of the limb may be all that is needed. To relieve pain, your doctor may recommend a nonsteroidal anti-inflammatory drug (NSAIDs) such as ibuprofen (Advil, Motrin, Nuprin, and others) or naproxen (Aleve, Anaprox, Naprelan, Naprosyn). Take these drugs with food to prevent possible stomach upset.

■ Deep venous thrombosis is treated in the hospital. Anticoagulation (blood-thinning) therapy is begun, at first with intravenous administration of heparin and later an oral anticoagulant such as warfarin (Coumadin), or low doses of aspirin to keep the blood from clotting. These therapies do not dissolve the current clot, but are used to stop future clot formation.

■ Thrombolysis, or clot-dissolving therapy, may be used. The drugs streptokinase (Streptase) and urokinase (Abbokinase), administered intravenously, can often dissolve some or all of the clot in twenty-four to forty-eight

hours. Before this treatment is used, however, the diagnosis must be certain. If you have a broken blood vessel, an aneurysm, or similar problem, these drugs can cause internal bleeding.

DIETARY GUIDELINES

■ Avoid all saturated and hydrogenated fats, which contribute to impaired circulation. This means cutting out dairy products (except for small amounts of the low-fat varieties), red meat, eggs, margarine, shortening, tropical oils such as coconut and palm oil, and all fried foods. For protein, choose fish, white-meat poultry, whole grains, and legumes.

■ Include beets in your diet. Grated raw beets are an old naturopathic remedy for healing and strengthening veins.

NUTRITIONAL SUPPLEMENTS

■ Carnitine improves the digestion of fats and protects the blood vessels against fat deposition. Take 500 milligrams of acetyl-L-carnitine two to three times daily.

■ Flaxseed oil contains essential fatty acids that act as natural anti-inflammatories. Take 1 teaspoon (or 500 to 1,000 milligrams) twice a day.

■ Pine-bark and grape-seed extracts have anti-inflammatory properties and thus help to alleviate discomfort. Take 50 to 75 milligrams of either two to three times daily.

■ Vitamin C and bioflavonoids strengthen the blood vessels and act as anti-inflammatories. They are especially effective if combined with butcher's broom (*see under Herbal Treatment in this entry*), Take 500 milligrams of vitamin C three to four times daily and 200 milligrams of mixed bioflavonoids three times a day.

■ Vitamin E is a natural anticoagulant (blood thinner) that reduces platelet aggregation, an early phase in the formation of blood clots. Choose a formula containing mixed tocopherols and begin by taking 200 international units, then gradually increase the dosage until you are taking 400 international units in the morning and another 400 international units at bedtime.

HERBAL TREATMENT

■ Butcher's broom is a natural anti-inflammatory that has been used for centuries to treat circulatory disorders. The saponins in butcher's broom, ruscogenin and neo-ruscogenin, are known to constrict the veins and decreases the permeability of the capillaries. Take 300 to 500 milligrams three times a day.

■ For pain, applying plasters prepared with cayenne, ginger, and/or mustard can be helpful. Mix cayenne, ginger, and/or mustard powder with enough warm water to achieve a pastelike consistency. Spread the paste on a thin cotton cloth, such as cheesecloth, and apply the cloth to the affected area. Do not apply the paste directly to your skin. Leave the plaster in place for up to fifteen minutes, then remove and rinse the skin. Do this every other day for two weeks.

■ Hawthorn has been used since the seventeenth century to treat heart disease and inflamed veins. It dilates the blood vessels and increases peripheral circulation. Choose a standardized extract containing 1.8 percent vitexin-2 rhamnosides and take 100 to 200 milligrams up to three times a day.

HOMEOPATHY

■ *Aesculus hippocastanum* is good for aching and soreness in the limbs, possibly accompanied by numbness in the fingertips, swelling in the hands and feet, and aching in the lower back and between the shoulder blades. Symptoms tend to worsen with walking. Take one dose of *Aesculus hippocastanum* 6x or 3c three times daily for up to three days. Wait for ten days, then repeat.

■ *Hamamelis virginiana* is helpful for phlebitis and venous congestion accompanied by a bruised, sore feeling in the affected area, tired legs, and very sore muscles and joints. Take one dose of *Hamamelis virginiana* 6x or 3c three times daily for up to three days. Wait ten days, then repeat.

BACH FLOWER REMEDIES

Select the remedy that most closely fits your disposition and emotional tendencies and concerns, and take it as needed, following the directions on the product label.

■ Holly eases feelings of anger that and fits of bad temper that may stem from underlying feelings of insecurity.

■ Hornbeam helps to lift fatigue.

ACUPRESSURE

For the locations of acupressure points on the body, *see* ADMINISTERING AN ACUPRESSURE TREATMENT in Part Three.

■ The combination of Liver 3, Spleen 6 and 10, and Stomach 36 improves circulation.

AROMATHERAPY

For specific instructions on how to use aromatherapy, *see* PREPARING AROMATHERAPY TREATMENTS in Part Three.

■ Essential oil of rosemary helps to increase circulation. Blend a few drops in warm water to make comforting compresses. Apply the compresses for fifteen minutes at a time while sitting with your legs elevated. Repeat as often as needed.

GENERAL RECOMMENDATIONS

■ Get regular exercise. Moderate activity such as swim-ming and walking helps to maintain good blood circulation.

■ One can purchase support hose made specfically for compromised veins.

■ If you smoke, stop now. Smoking impairs circulation.

■ If you take oral contraceptives, switch to another method of birth control. Oral contraceptives are associat-ed with an increased risk of phlebitis.

PREVENTION

■ If you must endure a prolonged period of inactivity, such as during illness, following surgery, or during a long airplane flight, stretch your legs and flex your ankles fre-quently.

■ If you have had a bout with deep-vein phlebitis, wear-ing elastic stockings that maintain support against weak vessel walls, along with elevation of the leg and mild exer-cise, can help prevent recurrences.

Photophobia

Photophobia is a condition characterized by an abnormal sensitivity or intolerance to light, especially bright light. Actually, it is normal for sudden exposure to bright light to cause momentary discomfort. This is why, if you come out of a dark movie theater into a bright sunlit day, you instinctively blink and reach up to shade your eyes. Most people's eyes then adapt to the light within a few mo-ments, however. For a person with photophobia, the dis-comfort caused by light, especially bright light, does not go away. It can cause actual pain as well as an inability to see clearly because of a constant glare before one's eyes.

In most cases, photophobia is not considered a serious disorder, though it can be annoying and inconvenient. It is more common in people with light-colored eyes, presum-ably because the light-colored iris admits more light into the eye. However, photophobia can be a symptom of cer-tain eye disorders, such as abrasion or ulceration of the cornea, uveitis, developing retinitis pigmentosa, and some forms of glaucoma. Some people develop photophobia in conjunction with migraines or measles, and it can also be a consequence of certain types of brain injury. An aversion to bright light is also a well-known morning-after conse-quence of overindulgence in alcohol.

CONVENTIONAL TREATMENT

■ If your eyes seem to be abnormally sensitive to bright light, especially if this is a sudden occurrence, consult an ophthalmologist for a thorough eye examination to detect any underlying disorders that may be causing this symptom. Treatment, if any, will depend on the results of the examination.

DIETARY GUIDELINES

Maximize your consumption of fresh fruits and vegetables. These healthy foods contain antioxidant phytochemicals that protect all the cells of the body, including those of the eyes, from free-radical damage.

Eat clean, lean protein, such as that found in chicken and fish. The retinal pigment necessary for adaptation to changing light conditions is composed of protein and vitamin A. Both protein and vitamin A are needed to maintain healthy eyes.

Limit your intake of sugar and caffeine. These substances contribute to eye irritation and worsen many eye problems.

NUTRITIONAL SUPPLEMENTS

Beta-carotene is a strong antioxidant and a precursor of vitamin A (see below). Take 10,000 to 15,000 international units daily.

Lutein, a carotenoid usually extracted from the marigold, has been shown to have a remarkable impact on ocular health. Take 5 milligrams three times daily.

Vitamin A protects against free-radical damage and is especially important to the eyes. Without sufficient vitamin A, the eyes are more sensitive to variations in light intensity. Take 5,000 international units of vitamin A three times a day for two months. Then reduce to a maintenance dosage of 5,000 international units daily.

Note: If you are pregnant, or intend to get pregnant, or if you have liver disease, consult your doctor before taking supplemental vitamin A. Pregnant women should not ingest a total of more than 25,000 international units of supplemental vitamin A *per week* from all sources.

Deficiencies of the B vitamins can contribute to an abnormal sensitivity to light. Vitamin B_2 (riboflavin), in particular, has been shown to reduce the incidence of floaters and "halos" around lights or objects. While symptoms are acute, take a vitamin-B complex that supplies 50 milligrams of each of the major B vitamins daily. When symptoms improve, reduce the dosage to 25 milligrams twice daily.

HERBAL TREATMENT

■ Bilberry extract can help the eyes make a quicker adjustment to changes in light levels. Select a preparation containing 25 percent anthocyanidins (also called PCOs) and take 80 milligrams twice daily.

■ Used as an eyewash, eyebright helps prevent excessive tearing and eases eyes that are overly sensitive to light.

Bring 3 ounces of sterile saline solution to a boil, and pour it over 1 tablespoon of dried cut herb (or one eyebright teabag). Allow it to steep for fifteen minutes, then strain out the herb. When the liquid has cooled to a comfortable temperature, use it as an eyewash. Or prepare a compress by moistening a sterile cloth in the warm infusion. Place the compress over your closed eyes, pressing down gently to achieve contact with the affected area. Relax for at least ten minutes. Then moisten a fresh sterile cloth in the eyewash tea and wipe away any crusts or scales. Throw away (or sterilize) each cloth after one use.

HOMEOPATHY

■ *Nux vomica* is for light sensitivity associated with the consumption of too much rich food and alcohol—especially when the aftereffects of the night before result in a hangover. Take one dose of *Nux vomica* 30x or 15c three times daily for up to three days.

■ *Phosphorus* is for light sensitivity accompanied by nervousness and fatigue. Take one dose of *Phosphorus* 30x or 15c three times daily for up to three days.

GENERAL RECOMMENDATIONS

■ Have a thorough eye examination to be sure you have no developing health problems that are contributing to your light sensitivity.

■ Invest in a good pair of sunglasses that blocks out both UVA and UVB rays, and keep them with you at all times so that you can put them on whenever you need to. A hat with a wide brim in front may also be helpful. If you find certain types of interior lighting, such as fluorescent lights, to be annoying, don't be shy about wearing your dark glasses indoors, if need be.

■ Avoid anything that can irritate your eyes, such as smog and smoke. Whether it comes from cigars, pipes, cigarettes, or sweet-smelling wood burning in a fireplace, smoke is very hard on the eyes and worsens symptoms.

PREVENTION

■ A deficiency of vitamin A, the "eye vitamin," is a factor in the development of many eye problems. Taking a maintenance dose of 5,000 international units of this important vitamin daily can be helpful. Consult your doctor first, however, if you are pregnant, intend to get pregnant, or have liver disease.

Pinkeye

See CONJUNCTIVITIS.

Pinworms

See under PARASITES, INTESTINAL.

Pleurisy

Pleurisy is inflammation of the pleura, a thin membrane that covers the lungs and lines the chest. Pleurisy can have a variety of causes, including pneumonia; pulmonary embolism (a blood clot lodged in the lung); an amoebic, viral, or bacterial infection in the pleural space (though not in the lung itself); the presence of tumor cells or toxins; lupus; rheumatoid arthritis; uremia (the presence of high levels of ammonia in the blood); and trauma such as from a broken rib. The chief symptom is chest pain, which can be severe, and that is usually worse with breathing and coughing.

CONVENTIONAL TREATMENT

■ The appropriate treatment depends on the underlying cause. Once the root problem is found and addressed, pleurisy usually gets better on its own and the pain is relieved.

■ While the pain persists, painkillers, including acetaminophen (in Tylenol, Datril, and many other products) and nonsteroidal anti-inflammatory drugs (NSAIDs) such as ibuprofen (Advil, Motrin, Nuprin, and others), ketoprofen (Orudis, Oruvail), and many others, are usually recommended. For severe pain, codeine may be used, but most doctors try to avoid it because it also suppresses coughing, which increases the likelihood of developing pneumonia.

■ It may be helpful to wrap the entire chest with elastic bandages so that chest movement is minimal during breathing. This encourages abdominal breathing.

■ If pneumonia is not already present, bronchial drainage may be recommended as a preventive. Coughing is encouraged. Having someone hold a pillow firmly against the chest can help minimize the pain the coughing causes.

DIETARY GUIDELINES

■ Simplify your diet. Base your meals on clean, lean protein, fresh vegetables and fruits, and whole grains.

■ Avoid dairy products and fried and greasy foods. These foods promote the formation of mucus.

■ Be sure to get plenty of fluids. Soups and fresh vegetable fruit juices are good choices.

■ Include fresh pineapple in your diet. Pineapple contains bromelain, an enzyme that is a natural anti-inflammatory.

NUTRITIONAL SUPPLEMENTS

■ Pine-bark and grape-seed extracts are natural anti-inflammatories. Take 100 milligrams of either three times daily for ten days.

■ Vitamin A and beta-carotene are useful in speeding the healing of mucous membranes. Beta-carotene has also been shown to enhance thymus function and increase the effectiveness of interferon, a natural immune system chemical that protects against viral infections. Take 25,000 international units of vitamin A twice daily for five days, then cut back to 25,000 international units daily for two weeks. During the same period, take 15,000 international units of mixed bioflavonoids twice daily.

■ Vitamin C is a mild anti-inflammatory and helps to resolve infection. Take 500 to 1,000 milligrams four or five times daily until you are better.

HERBAL TREATMENT

■ Comfrey root tea compresses can be applied to the chest to ease inflammation. Place 2 tablespoons of comfrey root in 6 ounces of water and simmer for twenty minutes. Soak a piece of cheesecloth or other thin cotton fabric in the resulting tea. Allow it to cool to a comfortable temperature, wring excess from the tea, and apply the compress to your chest for fifteen minutes.

Note: Comfrey is recommended for external use only. It contains substances that can cause liver damage if taken internally.

■ Cordyceps is a tonic herb that increases the oxygen supply to body systems, enhances immunity, and acts as an antioxidant. Take 1,000 milligrams of standardized extract twice a day.

■ A tea of corn silk and sage is excellent for helping to expel excess water from the system. Place 1 tablespoon (or tea bag) of each in 8 ounces of water and simmer for ten minutes. Strain and drink. Take a cup of tea up to three times daily.

HOMEOPATHY

■ *Bryonia* is good for tearing pain that is worse with motion and better with rest. Breathing is difficult, and you are likely to be thirsty and feel irritable. Take one dose of *Bryonia* 12x or 6c three times daily for up to three days.

■ *Cantharis* is helpful for breathlessness, burning pain, mild fever, and a dry cough. Take one dose of *Cantharis* 12x or 6c three times daily for up to three days.

■ Choose *Hepar sulfuris calcareum* if healing is slow and there is fluid in the lungs. Take one dose of *Hepar sulfuris calcareum* 30x or 15c three times daily for up to three days.

BACH FLOWER REMEDIES

Select the remedy that most closely fits your disposition and emotional tendencies and concerns, and take it as needed, following the directions on the product label.

■ Gentian is good if you are feeling discouraged and need a great deal of encouragement.

■ Mustard helps to lift sorrow and depression, possibly related to a loss of some kind.

■ Olive gently helps to overcome deep exhaustion.

■ Sweet Chestnut eases feelings of anguish, torment, and alienation.

ACUPRESSURE

For the locations of acupressure points on the body, *see* ADMINISTERING AN ACUPRESSURE TREATMENT in Part Three.

■ The combination of Liver 3, Lung 7, Pericardium 6, Spleen 6, and Stomach 36 helps to alleviate discomfort and pain in the chest.

AROMATHERAPY

For specific instructions on how to use aromatherapy, *see* PREPARING AROMATHERAPY TREATMENTS in Part Three.

■ Essential oils of bergamot, calendula, and chamomile have anti-inflammatory properties. They can be added to massage oil and used in gentle massage of the chest or back. You can also add them to a steam inhalation treatment to encourage healing.

■ Inhaling lavender oil during an attack helps to calm and fight infection.

GENERAL RECOMMENDATIONS

■ Before the advent of antibiotics, pleurisy was a life-threatening illness, especially for children. If you suspect you may have pleurisy and you do not feel better within twenty-four hours, consult your physician.

PMS

See PREMENSTRUAL SYNDROME.

Pneumonia

Pneumonia is an acute inflammation and infection of the lung tissue that can result in the tiny air sacs becoming filled with fluid, mucus, and pus. It can be caused by a number of different infectious agents, including viruses, bacteria, chlamydia, mycoplasma, and fungi.

Viral pneumonia often begins as an upper respiratory infection, such as the flu. The illness may progress suddenly or gradually, and may be accompanied by either a low-grade fever, cough, and mild fatigue, or by a high fever, severe cough, and lethargy. The cough is usually not productive until the later stages of the illness. There may also be some stomach upset. It is important to treat viral pneumonia, because if left untreated, it creates fertile ground for the development of a secondary bacterial infection in the lungs.

Bacterial pneumonia usually comes on more suddenly, often as a complication of other illnesses. Pneumococci and staphylococci are the types of bacteria most often involved. A person with bacterial pneumonia usually feels and appears very sick, with a high fever, lethargy, difficulty breathing, a cough, and possibly pain in the chest, particularly upon breathing. He or she is likely to be pale and sweating; in severe cases, the fingernails may turn bluish in color. Bacterial pneumonia is a dangerous illness, more dangerous than either viral or mycoplasmal pneumonia. Fortunately, it is much less likely than viral or mycoplasmal pneumonia to be transmitted from one person to another.

Chlamydial and mycoplasmal pneumonia have many features in common. The initial symptoms include sore throat, dry cough, and an all-over achy and sick feeling. Coughing gradually increases and becomes productive, and there may be blood in the sputum. Both of these types of pneumonia are most common in persons under the age of thirty-five, and most people recover without complications, although chlamydial pneumonia can sometimes be stubborn and persistent, and require longer treatment.

A full recovery from pneumonia, no matter what the cause, may take several weeks, and a cough can sometimes hang on for up to two months, even after the infection is gone.

CONVENTIONAL TREATMENT

■ If your doctor suspects pneumonia, he or she is likely to want to look at a chest x-ray (to determine which part of the lungs is involved), as well as a blood test and/or a sputum sample (to determine what type of infectious agent is responsible). This determination is essential for proper treatment.

■ If you are having difficulty breathing, an ear or finger oximetry test may be used. This is a quick and painless way to find out how much oxygen is in the blood, using a clip-on device with a photoelectric cell that measures oxygen saturation in the blood.

■ If you are diagnosed with viral pneumonia, treatment

will be aimed at promoting comfort and preventing bacterial pneumonia from developing. To lower fever and ease discomfort, your doctor may recommend acetaminophen (Tylenol, Datril, or the equivalent) or a nonsteroidal anti-inflammatory drug (NSAID) such as ibuprofen (Advil, Motrin, Nuprin, and others) or ketoprofen (Orudis, Oruvail), as well as plenty of bed rest. Chest physiotherapy to promote the drainage of mucus from the lungs may also be indicated.

Note: In excessive amounts, acetaminophen can cause liver damage. Do not exceed the recommended dosage.

■ If bacterial pneumonia is diagnosed, you have a serious infection that requires aggressive treatment with either intravenous or oral antibiotics. Oxygen therapy may be called for, as well as chest physiotherapy to promote the drainage of mucus from the lungs.

■ For mycoplasmal pneumonia, your doctor may or may not prescribe an antibiotic, most likely tetracycline (also sold under the brand name Achromycin) or erythromycin (ERYC, Ilotycin, and others). This treatment may reduce, to some extent, the length of time you have such symptoms as fever, cough, and general discomfort. However, it does not actually kill the mycoplasma responsible for the infection, and although the recovery period may be a little longer, it is possible that you may recover just as well without the antibiotics.

■ Like mycoplasmal pneumonia, chlamydial pneumonia is treated with either tetracycline or erythromycin. However, in persons who have heart failure or some other underlying disease, this type of pneumonia may become quite severe, even life-threatening, even with treatment.

■ Use cough suppressants with great care if you have pneumonia. It is important to be able to cough out the mucus that is in the lungs in order to recover, and any medication that interferes with this may slow recovery. However, if a persistent hacking cough keeps you from resting, a mild suppressant, such as benzonatate (Tessalon perles) may be a reasonable compromise.

DIETARY GUIDELINES

■ Be sure to get plenty of fluids. This will help prevent dehydration and will thin secretions so that they are easier to cough out. Try sipping lemon water sweetened with a bit of maple syrup. Try to take lots of soups and juices.

■ Avoid dairy products. These can increase the production of mucus. Also avoid foods that contain fats, refined sugar, refined carbohydrates, and caffeine.

■ Eat small, frequent meals featuring nutrient-dense foods such as whole grains, fruits, vegetables, and lean proteins. Hot soups are a good choice, because they are soothing and may be easier to take than solid foods.

NUTRITIONAL SUPPLEMENTS

■ Beta-carotene helps to protect, soothe, and repair mucous membrane tissue. It is also a precursor of vitamin A, which is essential for the health of the respiratory-passage linings. Take 15,000 international units up to three times daily for two weeks. Also take 10,000 international units of vitamin A daily for two weeks.

■ Vitamin C is an anti-inflammatory and helps to stimulate the immune system. Choose a mineral ascorbate form of vitamin C with bioflavonoids and 500 to 1,000 milligrams, plus an equal amount of bioflavonoids, three to four times a day for two weeks.

■ During the recovery phase, take a vitamin-B complex supplement supplying 25 milligrams of each of the major B vitamins three times daily for two weeks.

■ Also during the recovery phase, take 15 to 25 milligrams of zinc twice a day for two weeks. Take zinc with food to prevent stomach upset.

HERBAL TREATMENT

■ Astragalus enhances immunity and increases the amount of oxygen available to the body. Take 500 milligrams of standardized extract three times a day.

■ Cordyceps is a tonic herb that increases the oxygen supply to body systems, enhances immunity, and acts as an antioxidant. Take 1,000 milligrams of standardized extract twice a day.

■ Depending on the type and severity of the pneumonia, you can use a variety of herbs either along with conventional treatment or during the recuperation phase, once the conventional treatment regimen is completed. You can use these herbs on an alternating basis, taking one herb for the first two weeks, another for the second two weeks, and so on. Or you can make a tea that combines several or all of them. Use one, several, or all of the following, as appropriate.

- Ginger tea helps to break up mucus and enhance circulation. Take a cup of ginger tea three times a day for two weeks. Applying warm ginger compresses to the chest several times a day may also help to ease breathing.

- Isatis is a Chinese herb with antiviral properties. It can be useful if the pneumonia is viral or mycoplasmal. However, you may find it difficult to tolerate if you have a sensitive stomach. Take 300 milligrams three times daily, with food, for one week.

- Marshmallow root is soothing to the lungs. Take 300 to 500 milligrams three times a day for two weeks.

- Osha root helps to strengthen the lungs and decrease inflammation. Take 500 milligrams three times a day for two weeks.

■ Cordyceps helps to strengthen the immune system and lungs. Take 1,000 milligrams three times a day for three weeks.

■ Goldenseal fights bacteria and tones the mucous membranes. It has traditionally been used for upper respiratory disorders. Choose an extract standardized to at least 5 percent total alkaloids and take 250 milligrams three times a day.

Make a combination herbal tea by simmering 1 teaspoon each of licorice, osha root, slippery elm, and marshmallow root, plus $1/4$ teaspoon of wild cherry bark, in a quart of water. Simmer the mixture for fifteen minutes. If desired, sweeten with honey. Drink a cup of this tea three times a day for three days.

Note: If you are pregnant, omit the wild cherry bark. If you have high blood pressure, omit the licorice.

Astragalus helps the body to regenerate bronchial cells after a viral insult. Once the acute phase of the illness has passed, take 500 milligrams of standardized extract four times a day for three weeks.

HOMEOPATHY

If you have viral, mycoplasmal, or chlamydial pneumonia, choose the most suitable symptom-specific remedy from the list below and take one dose, as directed on the product label, four times a day for up to two days. If you have bacterial pneumonia, you may do the same once you are past the acute stage and are recovering from the illness. Be aware, however, that for acute bacterial pneumonia, homeopathic remedies should not be considered a substitute for appropriate antibiotic therapy.

Use *Arsenicum album* 30x or 9c if you are coughing with a wheeze, and feel anxious and restless.

If you developed pneumonia following exposure to cold wind or an episode involving great fear, and you are running a temperature, try *Belladonna* 30x or 9c.

Bryonia 30x or 9c is recommended if your chest hurts every time you move, you feel pain on inhaling, and are constipated.

Choose *Hepar sulfuris calcareum* 12x or 6c if you have a hacking cough and want hot drinks.

■ If you have a cough with ropy or stringy phlegm, take *Kali bichromicum* 12x or 6c.

■ *Nux vomica* 30x or 9c is for a dry cough accompanied by irritability, stomach upset, nausea, and, possibly, vomiting.

■ If you have a tickle in your throat, some vomiting, and a craving for cold drinks, try *Phosphorus* 30x or 9c.

■ *Pulsatilla* 30x or 9c is good if you are feeling fearful and weepy and want company. You may also be coughing up yellow and/or green phlegm.

■ *Spongia tosta* 30x or 9c is for a barking cough that feels better after you drink warm liquids.

ACUPRESSURE

For the locations of acupressure points on the body, *see* ADMINISTERING AN ACUPRESSURE TREATMENT in Part Three.

■ Four Gates is calming and relaxing.

■ Lung 7 helps to clear upper respiratory infections.

■ Pericardium 6 helps to relax the chest.

■ Stomach 36 supports and improves circulation and digestion.

AROMATHERAPY

For specific instructions on how to use aromatherapy, *see* PREPARING AROMATHERAPY TREATMENTS in Part Three.

■ Add a couple of drops of essential oils of eucalyptus, peppermint, and/or thyme to $1/4$ cup of almond or sesame oil and blend. Rub this mixture over your back and chest to relax and increase circulation to the chest area.

Note: If you are using peppermint oil and also taking a homeopathic preparation, allow one hour between the two. Otherwise, the strong smell of the mint may interfere with the action of the homeopathic remedy.

GENERAL RECOMMENDATIONS

■ Make sure to get plenty of rest. Rest is essential for the recovery process.

■ A cool mist humidifier will help to soothe your respiratory tract and thin secretions so that they are easier to cough out. A drop or two of essential oil of thyme, eucalyptus, pine, or orange added to the water in the humidifier may also help to ease breathing. Be certain to clean the humidifier every few days to avoid the buildup of bacteria and fungi.

■ Be cautious about contact with others. The microorganisms that cause the pneumonia may remain with you for several weeks. To avoid spreading the illness, avoid close contact with uninfected friends and family members as much as possible.

■ For further suggestions on relieving the symptoms of pneumonia, *see* COUGH and FEVER.

PREVENTION

■ Whenever you come down with a viral illness, especially an upper respiratory infection, be sure to treat it promptly. Keep physicial exertion to a minimum until recovery is complete. Be alert for any signs that pneumonia may be developing.

Poison Ivy, Poison Oak, and Poison Sumac

The rash associated with a case of poison ivy, oak, or sumac is an allergic reaction to a resin contained in the leaves, stems, and roots of these poisonous plants. Because these plants are most abundant during springtime, most cases occur at that time of the year.

The rash and treatment of these three conditions are similar. This entry focuses mainly on poison ivy, the most common of the three, but what is true for poison ivy is true also for poison oak and poison sumac.

You can get poison ivy from the plant itself or by touching anything that has come in contact with the plant and has some of the resinous oil on it. For example, if you pick up a rake that has been resting in a bed of poison ivy, the characteristic rash may develop. If clothing or the part of the body that touched the plant is not carefully washed, the oil can be spread to other parts of the body, or even be transmitted to another person. Another, and potentially quite serious, form of exposure can occur through the inhalation of smoke from burning leaves if there are parts of the poison ivy plant among them.

A poison ivy rash can appear anywhere from a few hours to a few days after contact with the resin. The rash first appears as red, very itchy pimples that may develop into small fluid-filled blisters. If the contact occurred with the edge of a leaf, the eruption may form in a straight line. The rash can last from one to four weeks, and is usually at its worst four to seven days after exposure. The severity of the condition depends on the amount of contact with the resinous oil, as well as how sensitive you are to the plant. Not everyone is allergic to poison ivy. The resin may not bother some people at all, while others develop a serious and extensive rash.

Most cases of poison can be treated successfully at home. However, if you experience pain or swelling on your face or genitals and are uncomfortable because of this, or if the rash is very extensive, medical care may be warranted. And as with all skin rashes and wounds, it is possible for the area to become infected. If you notice signs of local infection, such as increased redness, swelling, or warmth or tenderness at the site, seek the advice of your heatlh-care provider.

EMERGENCY TREATMENT

■ If there is any sign that you are developing difficulty breathing as a result of an allergic reaction to poison ivy, oak, or sumac, have someone take you at once to the emergency room of the nearest hospital, or call for emergency assistance.

CONVENTIONAL TREATMENT

■ Calamine lotion is an old standby that temporarily eases the itching of poison ivy. However, if used for more than one week, calamine lotion can harden and dry the skin, causing more problems.

■ Rhulicream and Rhuligel are over-the-counter preparations that may be more effective than calamine at relieving the itching of poison ivy. Follow the application directions on the product label.

■ Diphenhydramine (in Allerdryl, Benadryl, and many other over-the-counter products) and chlorpheniramine (Chlor-Trimeton and others) are antihistamines that can help with the itching and swelling of poison ivy. Possible side effects include drowsiness and dry mouth. The drowsiness may actually be a benefit, however, if the intense itching makes it difficult to sleep.

■ In severe cases, a physician may prescribe an oral or topical steroid such as prednisone to lessen itching and especially to decrease inflammation. Steroids are strong and work quickly. Because of potential side effects, however, they are not suitable for long-term use and are generally reserved for very serious cases. Also, steroids must be tapered off gradually. If they are stopped too soon or too abruptly, the rash may get worse as a result of a rebound effect.

■ If the rash is inflamed, red, and oozing, Burow's solution may help. This over-the-counter product is both astringent and antiseptic, but it is mild on the skin. You can dilute it even further than the label directions indicate if it seems to irritate your skin.

NUTRITIONAL SUPPLEMENTS

■ Calcium helps to dry up the rash. Take 2,000 to 5,000 grams (2 to 5 grams) of calcium lactate three or four times daily.

■ Vitamin C helps to reduce the inflammatory response. Take 500 to 1,000 milligrams three to four times daily.

HERBAL TREATMENT

■ Apply soothing aloe vera gel to the rash three or four times a day.

■ To relieve itching and help the skin heal more quickly, apply calendula gel or liquid extract to the rash several times a day, as needed.

■ Applying cold cucumber slices to the affected area can help dry out an oozing rash.

■ To relieve both itching and inflammation, apply jewelweed juice. Use the fresh plant. Simply slit the stem and put the juice on the rash. Jewelweed will also help keep the rash from spreading. Jewelweed is a native perennial wildflower that is sometimes also referred to as impatiens.

Recognizing Poison Ivy, Oak, and Sumac

The best way to prevent a bout with poison ivy, poison oak, or poison sumac is to know how to recognize these plants and avoid them.

Poison ivy (*Rhus radicans*), by far the most common of the three, is usually thought of as a vine, but it can also grow straight up, like a shrub, to a height of anywhere between two and seven feet. It grows equally happily in woods, partly wooded areas and thickets, and suburban backyards, and can be found virtually anywhere in the United States and southern Canada. Its leaves are often shiny bright green, but not always; the edges can be smooth or jagged. In the fall, the leaves can turn a brilliant bronze-red, and drooping clusters of white berries appear. The distinctive feature of poison ivy, and the thing to look for, is that its leaves always occur in groups of three, with the end leaflet pointed and on a slightly longer stalk than the side pair (see illustration). If you see any plant whose leaves match this description, stay away from it. Touching any part of the poison ivy plant is dangerous.

Poison oak (*Rhus toxicodendron*) is similar to poison ivy in most respects. The only important differences to note are that this plant always grows in shrub form, and that the leaves, while still occurring in trios, are shaped more like oak leaves (see illustration).

Poison sumac (*Rhus vernix*) is less common than either poison ivy or poison oak, which is a good thing, because it is much more toxic. Touching any part of the plant can result in a severe rash and allergic reaction. The poison sumac plant, which is found primarily in swampy, partly wooded areas in the eastern half of the United States and Canada, takes the form of a shrub or small tree with leaves consisting of seven to thirteen (but always an odd number) pointed leaflets. The edges of the leaflets are smooth, not jagged (see illustration). From late summer to early spring, the plant puts out berries that are whitish in color and occur in clusters.

If you come into contact with any of these plants, you should immediately take measures to wash off the resin with either soap and water or jewelweed juice (*see* General Recommendations, below).

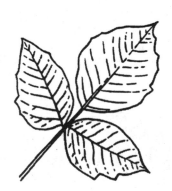

Poison Ivy

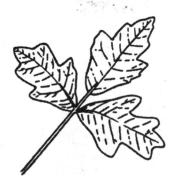

Poison Oak

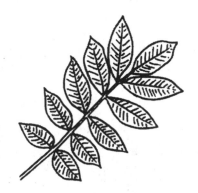

Poison Sumac

However, it should not be confused with the cultivated annual called impatiens that is commonly sold in nurseries and garden centers. That is an entirely different plant, and it has no usefulness in treating poison ivy. Jewelweed should be available at herb shops and through qualified herbalists. If you wish, you can use alternate applications of jewelweed juice and herbal or homeopathic calendula liquid or gel three times daily until the itching and discomfort are relieved.

HOMEOPATHY

■ In keeping with the basic principle of homeopathy—"like cures like"—*Rhus toxicodendron*, which is homeopathic poison ivy, will help relieve itching quickly. Take one dose of *Rhus toxicodendron* 12x or 6c three to four times daily until symptoms lessen.

ACUPRESSURE

For the locations of acupressure points on the body, *see* ADMINISTERING AN ACUPRESSURE TREATMENT in Part Three.

■ Four Gates promotes relaxation.

■ Spleen 10 helps detoxify the blood.

GENERAL RECOMMENDATIONS

■ If you know you have been exposed to poison ivy, thoroughly wash the area of contact with soap and water as soon as possible. Because unexposed areas of skin may come in contact with the oil as clothing is stripped off, a thorough shower is probably the best way to make sure all of the resin is washed off. If no washing facilities are available, do what you can to cleanse the area that made contact with the plant. Change your clothes as soon as possible, taking care to avoid contact with contaminated areas. Washing or rinsing with jewelweed juice may also be helpful. The resinous oil of poison ivy penetrates the skin in about ten minutes. After ten minutes, it cannot be washed off.

■ Applying cold compresses for fifteen to thirty minutes every few hours is useful for soothing and decreasing the swelling. If you wish, you can dissolve sea salt in the water before making the compress. Use 1 tablespoon of sea salt per pint of water.

■ Prepare an old folk remedy by making a solution of 2 tablespoons of sea salt and $\frac{1}{2}$ cup of buttermilk. Apply it to the affected area to reduce itching and promote healing.

■ Wash any clothing that has come in contact with the oil in a strong detergent with chlorine bleach added.

PREVENTION

■ When you will be in an area where poison ivy may be flourishing, wear shoes, socks, long pants, and a long-sleeved shirt to reduce the possibility of contact with the oil.

■ Learn how to identify poison ivy, oak, and sumac (see Recognizing Poison Ivy, Oak, and Sumac on page 484), and then avoid these plants.

Polycystic Ovary Syndrome

See under INFERTILITY.

Premenstrual Syndrome

Premenstrual syndrome (better known by the acronym PMS) is a condition in which various troublesome physical and emotional symptoms arise during the week or two before menstruation begins. Some women have symptoms for two weeks or more; others for a matter of only a few hours. Most fall somewhere between these two extremes. Women with PMS report a wide range of symptoms, both physical and emotional. On the physical side are breast pain and/or tenderness, fatigue, fluid retention (bloating),

swelling of fingers and ankles, headache, backache, abdominal pain, increased appetite, sugar cravings, acne, and weight gain. Emotional symptoms can include irritability, tension, mood swings, depression, and altered sex drive. All of these problems can be traced to the hormonal changes that occur within a woman's body during the seven to fourteen days prior to the onset of menstruation. Symptoms can occur singly or in any combination.

Experts estimate that over 90 percent of women experience some degree of PMS at some point in their lives. For most, PMS symptoms are a temporary annoyance. For an unlucky minority, however, symptoms are severe enough to disrupt their work and social relationships.

PMS can be divided into four types, depending on the predominant symptoms, as follows:

- *PMS-A (anxiety).* Symptoms include anxiety, irritability, mood swings, and nervous tension. Women with this type of PMS typically have an imbalance in the levels of the sex hormones estrogen and progesterone circulating in their bodies—specifically, too much estrogen and too little progesterone.

- *PMS-C (cravings).* During the week or two weeks before the onset of menstruation, some women experience an increase in appetite, especially for sugar and sweets. Other symptoms of this type of PMS include fatigue, a lack of energy, a feeling of faintness and/or dizziness, and, sometimes, heart palpitations. These problems can be attributed to low levels of hormonelike compounds called prostaglandins and changes in the way the body metabolizes carbohydrates, resulting in an increased tolerance for simple sugars.

- *PMS-D (depression).* Symptoms include depression, occasional crying fits, forgetfulness, and mild mental confusion, as well as episodes of insomnia. The hormonal factors responsible include low levels of estrogen and high levels of progesterone, plus elevated levels of adrenal hormones.

- *PMS-H (hyperhydration).* Hyperhydration, or fluid retention, manifests itself in swelling of the fingers and ankles, abdominal bloating, breast pain and/or tenderness, and weight gain that can total three pounds or more. The cause is an excess of aldosterone, an adrenal hormone that regulates the body's electrolyte and water balance.

The appropriate treatment for PMS depends on the precise nature of the symptoms you are experiencing. It is not necessary, however, to limit your treatments to those for one type of PMS or another. Many women have symptoms that place them in more than one subgroup.

CONVENTIONAL TREATMENT

■ Some conventional doctors focus on psychosocial

issues such as family stress, a type-A personality with a strong drive to achieve, or clinical depression as a cause of PMS. They advocate the use of reassurance, counseling, and self-help groups to help women gain insight into and learn to cope with these factors. This approach may or may not be beneficial for any individual woman.

■ Antianxiety drugs such as diazepam (Valium), once widely prescribed for women who complained of premenstrual symptoms, are falling more and more into disuse, primarily because they have the potential to cause dependency.

■ Many women have found relief from symptoms with the short-term use of an antidepressant such as fluoxetine (Prozac) or paroxetine (Paxil). While these drugs do not cause dependency as tranquilizers do, they nevertheless can have side effects, including anxiety, dizziness, tremors, and fatigue, among others.

■ Natural hormone therapy has been receiving increased prominence in the treatment of PMS. Many doctors report that natural progesterone (as opposed to the synthetic version of this hormone, progestin [Provera]), can successfully treat many PMS symptoms. Effective dosages of 50 to 400 milligrams daily (administered orally, vaginally, or topically), have been reported, with few to no side effects. However, there have not yet been any double-blind drug-comparison studies to verify this, most likely because natural hormones are not patentable, so they hold no promise of profit for pharmaceutical companies. Nevertheless, you may wish to discuss these findings with your doctor.

DIETARY GUIDELINES

■ Follow a healthy high-fiber diet plan. To keep your blood-sugar level on an even keel, eat meals at regular intervals through the day. Eat a lot of vegetables, especially leafy greens. They are full of trace minerals essential for the absorption of calcium. Calcium and magnesium are vital for proper nervous-system function. Green leafy vegetables are also good sources of bioavailable potassium and have a diuretic effect, which is useful if you suffer from water retention. However, you should avoid vegetables of the genus *Brassica*, such as cabbage, cauliflower, and Brussels sprouts, especially in their raw form. Raw brassicas depress thyroid function.

■ Increase your consumption of protein, but emphasize vegetable sources of protein such as legumes and soy foods. Fish is a good protein source also. The clean proteins from vegetables and fish help the body to excrete excess estrogen, which in turn helps keep estrogen and progesterone levels in balance.

■ Limit your consumption of refined carbohydrates, including sugar, honey, maple syrup, corn sweeteners, white-flour products, dried fruit, and fruit juice.

■ Reduce your consumption of dairy products. Consumption of large amounts of dairy foods may be associated with PMS symptoms of irritability, anxiety, and mood swings.

■ Keep to a minimum your intake of animal fats and the hydrogenated and partially-hydrogenated processed fats present in margarine, many salad oils, and shortenings. Better yet, avoid them entirely. The body uses the saturated fatty acids from animal fats and the trans fatty acids in hydrogenated fats to produce types of prostaglandins that promote inflammation and pain, and can impair circulation.

■ Eliminate meat, especially red meat, from your diet. Eating meat promotes the absorption of estrogens from the intestines, which in turn can lead to the type of imbalance in estrogen and progesterone levels that so often occurs in women with PMS.

■ Reduce your consumption of salt, especially if fluid retention is a problem.

■ Avoid all foods containing caffeine, including coffee, tea, chocolate, and caffeinated sodas. Caffeine causes fluctuations in blood sugar levels, contributing to cravings and adding to PMS stress.

■ Avoid alcohol and tobacco. Alcohol dehydrates the body, and dehydration can lead to increased premenstrual symptoms. Alcohol consumption also leads to hypoglycemia. Swings in blood sugar aggravate many premenstrual problems.

■ If you experience heavy menstrual bleeding, try taking the juice of one-half to one lemon in a glass of warm water half an hour to an hour before breakfast. Do this for two weeks before the anticipated onset of your menstrual period.

NUTRITIONAL SUPPLEMENTS

■ Many PMS-related symptoms are caused by deficiencies of the nutrients the body requires for hormonal regulation. If you are not already taking a high-quality multivitamin and mineral supplement, start now. Sometimes this alone can improve symptoms.

■ Acidophilus bacteria normalize the bowel flora and help decrease the reabsorption of estrogens from the intestines, thereby assisting in normalizing the estrogen-progesterone balance. Acidophilus also helps to relieve constipation, a premenstrual problem for many women. Take it as recommended on the product label. If you are allergic to milk, select a dairy-free product.

■ Black currant seed oil, borage oil, and evening primrose oil contain gamma-linolenic acid (GLA), which has anti-inflammatory, pain-reducing, and skin- and energy-enhancing properties. Many women have found that taking supplemental GLA helps to ease symptoms. Take 1,000 milligrams of borage, black currant seed, or evening primrose oil, and/or an equal amount of flaxseed oil, twice daily.

■ One recent study found that calcium supplementation can help to minimize premenstrual symptoms. Take 800 to 1,200 milligrams of calcium daily, in divided doses.

■ Many women with PMS have lower than normal levels of magnesium. Magnesium deficiency can increase the level of aldosterone in the body, which in turn promotes fluid retention. A lack of magnesium can also lead to heart palpitations, nervous tension, and a reduced ability to handle stress. Take 400 to 800 milligrams of magnesium aspartate or magnesium citrate daily.

■ Soy isoflavones provide phytoestrogens that help to balance hormone levels. Take 500 milligrams twice daily.

■ The B vitamins are essential to the health of the nervous system. Vitamin B_6 (pyridoxine) also acts as a coenzyme in many hormonal functions. Take a vitamin-B complex supplement supplying 25 milligrams of each of the major B vitamins two or three times daily, plus an additional 50 to 100 milligrams of vitamin B_6.

■ Vitamin C is a natural anti-inflammatory and helps to rid the body of excess estrogen. Take 500 milligrams of vitamin C with bioflavonoids two or three times daily.

■ Vitamin E protects against the adverse effects of saturated and trans fats, and can help reduce nervous tension, fatigue, breast tenderness, depression, headache, and even insomnia. Take 200 to 400 international units of vitamin E daily.

Note: If you are taking an anticoagulant (blood thinner), consult your physician before taking supplemental vitamin E.

■ Zinc deficiency is common in women with PMS. This mineral is particularly helpful in controlling acne associated with the premenstrual period. Take 15 milligrams of zinc picolinate once or twice daily.

Note: Take zinc with food to prevent stomach upset. If you take over 30 milligrams of zinc on a daily basis for more than one or two months, you should also take 1 to 2 milligrams of copper each day to maintain a proper mineral balance.

■ If you have PMS-A, in addition to the appropriate supplements above, take 500 milligrams of mixed bioflavonoids, twice daily. Bioflavonoids act as natural anti-inflammatories.

■ If you have PMS-C, add to your regimen 100 micrograms of chromium three times daily, plus 500 milligrams of evening primrose oil twice daily. Chromium helps normalize blood sugar levels, an important factor in controlling food cravings and mood swings. Evening primrose oil helps to regulate hormone synthesis and the body's

response to pain, inflammation, and swelling; direct hormones to their target cells; and regulate the transmission of nerve impulses. Also consider taking 250 to 500 milligrams of bromelain three times daily, between meals, for one week prior to the anticipated onset of menstruation. An enzyme extracted from pineapple, bromelain helps smooth muscles relax and aids in balancing prostaglandins.

■ If you have PMS-D, take 500 to 1,000 milligrams of tyrosine each morning starting one week before the anticipated onset of menstruation and continuing through the end of the menstrual period. If extreme moodiness and deep depression are particular problems during the two weeks prior to your menstrual period, take 500 milligrams of DL-phenylalanine (DLPA) three times a day. This nutrient is not effective for mild mood swings, but is helpful for persistent melancholia and severe depression.

Note: If you are taking a monoamine oxidase (MAO) inhibitor drug, do not take supplemental tyrosine, as a sudden and dangerous rise in blood pressure may result.

HERBAL TREATMENT

■ Black haw contains four compounds that relax the uterus and relieves muscle spasms, and can help relieve abdominal pain associated with PMS. Make a tea by simmering 1/2 ounce of herb in 1 cup of water for ten minutes, then strain and drink. Take a cup of tea three times daily.

■ Bupleurum and dong quai and bupleurum and peony are two Chinese herbal combinations that help to regulate the menstrual cycle and reduce bloating and irritability. Bupleurum and dong quai is generally recommended for women between the ages of fifteen and thirty-eight, bupleurum and peony for women aged thirty-eight and over. Take 1/2 to 1 teaspoon (or 1,000 milligrams) three times daily for two weeks before the anticipated onset of your menstrual period.

■ In one German study of over 1,500 women, chaste tree berry (*Vitex agnus-castus*) provided relief of PMS symptoms for 90 percent of participants after one month. Take 200 milligrams of standardized extract three times daily for the two weeks before the anticipated onset of your period.

■ False unicorn root has been used for hundreds of years to help balance female hormones. It is known as a uterine tonic and is helpful for menstrual cramps. The usual dosage is 1/4 to 1/2 teaspoon of herb taken two to three times daily, with meals, for one week before menstruation. This herb is very strong, however, and we recommend using it only under the supervision of a health-care professional. Excessive use can cause itching, rash, and stomach upset. It should not be used during pregnancy.

■ Kava kava contains two pain-relieving chemicals and is

effective as a relaxant for menstrual cramps and premenstrual anxiety. Choose a product containing 30 percent kavalactones and take 200 milligrams once or twice a day as needed to relieve symptoms.

Note: In excess amounts, this herb can cause drowsiness. Do not exceed the recommended dose. Do not use kava kava if you are pregnant or nursing, if you have Parkinson's disease, or if you are taking a prescription medication for depression or anxiety.

■ Milk thistle stimulates and protects the liver, which in turn promotes the proper regulation of the body's hormonal balance. Choose an extract standardized to contain 80 percent flavonoids (silymarin) and take 150 to 300 milligrams twice daily for two to three months.

■ Red raspberry leaf helps to ease menstrual cramps by relaxing the uterus. It is believed to be high in oligomeric proanthocyanidins (OPCs), flavonoids that act as natural anti-inflammatories. Take a cup of red raspberry leaf tea, or 500 milligrams in capsule form, two to three times daily, as needed.

HOMEOPATHY

■ *Lachesis* is good if you are very talkative and tend to lash out verbally during the premenstrual period. Your breasts are painful, and you feel considerably worse when you first awaken. Take one dose of *Lachesis* 30x or 15c, as directed on the product label, three times daily during the week prior to the expected onset of menstruation.

■ *Lycopodium* is the remedy for depression and irritability before a period, accompanied by flatulence. You are probably frugal, crave sweets, and love chocolate. Take one dose of *Lycopodium* 30x or 15c three times a day during the week prior to the expected onset of menstruation.

■ *Natrum muriaticum* is for the sadness, melancholy, and irritability accompanied by edema. Your ankles and breasts are likely to be swollen. Take one dose of *Natrum muriaticum* 30x or 15c three times a day during the week prior to the expected onset of menstruation.

■ *Pulsatilla* is good if you have irregular periods and a tendency to cry easily. You have painful breasts and find greasy foods distasteful. Take one dose of *Pulsatilla* 30x or 15c three times daily during the week prior to the expected onset of menstruation.

■ Choose *Sepia* if your premenstrual symptoms include feeling irritable, emotionally dull, and sexually apathetic. You crave salty, sweet, and vinegary foods, and feel better with exercise. Take one dose of *Sepia* 30x or 15c three times a day during the week prior to the expected onset of menstruation.

BACH FLOWER REMEDIES

Select the remedy that most closely fits your emotional tendencies and concerns, and take it as needed, following the directions on the product label.

■ Heather is the remedy for the kind of self-absorption that leads you always to bring the conversation back to your own personal cares and concerns.

■ Holly helps to tame anger that bursts out in fits of bad temper.

■ Impatiens is for hyperactivity, impatience, and irritability.

■ Olive stimulates gently to relieve a sense of being exhausted to the very core.

■ Rock Water can ease feelings of panic.

■ Vervain is for the tense and driven woman who is a perfectionist and may have trouble sleeping.

■ White Chestnut helps to counteract a tendency to obsess on subjects and events long after they should have been resolved and forgotten.

ACUPRESSURE

For the locations of acupressure points on the body, *see* ADMINISTERING AN ACUPRESSURE TREATMENT in Part Three.

■ Liver 3 relaxes the nervous system.

■ Pericardium 6 is useful for anxiety associated with PMS.

■ Spleen 6 reduces uterine cramping.

■ Stomach 36 helps to strengthen the body in times of stress.

GENERAL RECOMMENDATIONS

■ Exercise. Women who get regular moderate exercise throughout the menstrual cycle are less likely to suffer from PMS systems than those who do not. Many women report that a program of regular exercise eases PMS to a great degree. Walking briskly for thirty to forty-five minutes five days a week has been shown to make a real difference.

■ If mood swings, fatigue, and cravings are particularly troublesome, *see* HYPOGLYCEMIA for additional suggestions. Low blood sugar can be a factor in many of the symptoms of PMS.

Presbyopia

Presbyopia is a type of farsightedness that comes with age. It is an extremely common condition characterized by the gradual and progressive loss of normal visual accommodation, the ability of the eyes to change focus to see things that are either close or far away. As you grow older, the lens of the eye grows harder, and the ability to focus on close work declines. At around age forty-five, it is common to notice that reading small print at a normal distance has become difficult. As a result, you may find yourself holding books and newspapers at arm's length.

CONVENTIONAL TREATMENT

■ There is no treatment as such for presbyopia, but corrective lenses can help you see clearly despite it. You may need to have your prescription changed four or five times over a period of about twenty years after you first get reading glasses (or bifocals, which combine lenses for distance vision with lenses for close focus). By the time you are sixty-five or so, your eyes may lose their ability to focus entirely. If this occurs, you will have to depend on corrective lenses for visual accommodation.

DIETARY GUIDELINES

■ Maximize your intake of fresh fruits and vegetables. These healthy foods contain antioxidant phytochemicals that protect all the cells of the body, including those of the eyes, from free-radical damage.

■ Limit sugar and caffeine. These substances contribute to eye irritation and worsen the symptoms caused by many eye problems.

NUTRITIONAL SUPPLEMENTS

■ Beta-carotene is a strong antioxidant that prevents free-radical damage. It is related to vitamin A and has many of the same properties, but it does not become toxic in large doses. Take 10,000 to 25,000 international units of beta-carotene daily.

■ The essential fatty acids (EFAs), found in black currant seed oil, borage oil, evening primrose oil, and flaxseed oil, are required by every cell in the body. They help counteract the hardening effects of cholesterol on cell membranes. Take 500 to 1,000 milligrams of black currant seed, borage, or evening primrose oil, and/or an equal amount of flaxseed oil, two or three times daily.

■ Lutein, a carotenoid usually extracted from the marigold plant, is very useful in maintaining and restoring ocular health. Take 5 milligrams two or three times daily.

■ Selenium is an excellent antioxidant that helps prevent free-radical damage throughout the body, including the eyes. Take 100 micrograms daily.

■ Vitamin A protects against free-radical damage and is especially important to the eyes. Even a slight deficiency can contribute to eye problems. Take 5,000 international units of vitamin A twice daily.

Note: If you are pregnant, or intend to get pregnant, or if you have liver disease, consult your doctor before tak-

ing supplemental vitamin A. Pregnant women should not ingest a total of more than 25,000 international units of supplemental vitamin A *per week* from all sources.

■ Vitamin C helps to strengthen capillaries and maintains collagen, an important protein in connective tissue. Select a vitamin-C formula that includes bioflavonoids and take 500 to 1,000 milligrams three times daily.

HERBAL TREATMENT

■ Bilberry provides important nutrients that nourish the eyes and enhance visual function. Phytochemicals called anthocyanidins in this herb also help prevent damage to the structures of the eyes. Select a preparation containing 25 percent anthocyanidins (also called PCOs) and take 80 milligrams two or three times daily.

■ Eyebright is rich in vitamin A and vitamin C, and helps maintain healthy eyes and good vision. Take 200 milligrams two or three times daily.

■ Ginkgo biloba protects cellular membranes, improves circulation, and promotes cellular health by enhancing the use of oxygen and glucose by the cells. Select a preparation of ginkgo leaf extract containing at least 24 percent ginkgo heterosides (sometimes called flavoglycosides) and take 40 milligrams three times daily.

HOMEOPATHY

■ See a homeopathic practitioner for a constitutional remedy. Although homeopathic remedies cannot restore visual accommodation, a constitutional remedy can help make your eyes more comfortable.

GENERAL RECOMMENDATIONS

■ Most people need reading glasses as they grow older. Once you have had a thorough eye exam to rule out any serious conditions that may be affecting your ability to focus clearly, you can either have your prescription filled by an optician or purchase an inexpensive pair of glasses in your local drugstore or supermarket. Use the chart that accompanies the display to be sure you select the correct power. Be aware, however, if the vision in one eye differs from that in the other, these glasses will not help. You need prescription glasses to meet the specifications for each individual eye.

■ Eye exercises can sometimes help to halt the progression of presbyopia. These are done by focusing your eyes on a fingertip or pencil point held in front of your face at a distance of eight to twelve inches. Then you transfer your focus to a point at least eight feet away (the farther, the better). Repeat this about ten times in a row, all the while concentrating on actually focusing at the two distances. This is harder than you might think. You should perform three sets of ten repetitions several times each day. After a while the task gets easier, and you can perform more repetitions and sets.

Prostate Disorders

The prostate is a chestnut-shaped male reproductive gland that sits beneath the bladder, surrounding the urethra, which serves as a passageway for both urine and semen. The function of the prostate is to add secretions of fluid to the semen during ejaculation. Prostatic fluid is clear and slightly acidic. It contains calcium, sodium, potassium, and zinc.

There are a number of disorders that commonly affect the prostate. This entry addresses prostate enlargement, prostatitis, and prostate cancer.

When a man is around forty years of age, the prostate often begins a kind of growth spurt. The exact mechanism by which this happens is not completely understood, but it is believed to be related to shifts in hormone levels—at this time, a man's testosterone levels begin to decline and there is an increase in the level of a breakdown product of testosterone called dihydrotestosterone. High levels of the pituitary hormone prolactin may be involved as well, and levels of other hormones may rise or fall, too. The result is that the body overproduces prostate cells, which ultimately leads to an enlarged prostate, medically known as *benign prostatic hyperplasia* or *benign prostatic hypertrophy* (BPH).

At least 50 percent of men over the age of forty-five have some prostate enlargement, and the incidence increases with age. In the beginning stages, this condition often causes no symptoms. As it progresses, however, an enlarged prostate squeezes the urethra, partially obstructing the flow of urine and causing symptoms such as difficulty starting urination, a reduction in the force of the urine stream, dribbling after urination, frequent urination of small amounts, and an inability to completely empty the bladder. Even if a man has no noticeable symptoms, if his bladder is not emptied completely when he urinates, the leftover urine stagnates in the bladder and can set the stage for a bladder infection. *Prostatitis*—infection of the prostate gland itself—also becomes a possibility. In this disorder, the prostate becomes tender and inflamed. In addition to having difficulty urinating, a man with prostatitis may suffer fever, chills, back pain, pain in the area between the genitals and the anus, pain on urination, blood in the urine, and even bodily aches and pains.

Prostate cancer is the most common type of cancer in men. Like other prostate disorders, it primarily affects men in middle to later adulthood—it is rare before age fifty, and more than 80 percent of all cases are diagnosed in men over sixty-five. Many prostate cancers are very slow growing, and the condition often causes no symptoms, at least in the early stages. Later, symptoms of urinary blockage and, possibly, blood in the urine may appear. It is also possible for prostate cancer to spread to other parts of the body. Men who eat high-fat diets, are over sixty-five, are of African ancestry, and/or have close family members who have (or have had) prostate cancer have a higher than average risk of developing this disease. However, prostate cancer is extremely common among the male population as a whole, whether they have known risk factors or not.

CONVENTIONAL TREATMENT

■ Finasteride (Proscar) is the current prescription of choice for BPH. It inhibits the action of 5-alpha reductase, the enzyme that breaks down testosterone into dihydrotestosterone, and shrinks enlarged prostate tissue. Improvement in symptoms is often slow, however; it can take three to twelve months of therapy before it has optimal results. Once you start taking it, you must take it for life to maintain its effects.

■ Alpha-blockers are drugs that relax the smooth muscles of the prostate and bladder, making it easier to urinate. They can also be used in the treatment of high blood pressure. Examples include terazosin (Hytrin), doxazosin (Cardura), and prazosin (Minipress). Relief can be expected within two to four weeks.

■ If BPH causes severe constriction of the urethra, it may be impossible to urinate at all. In such cases, surgery may be necessary to restore function. There are a number of procedures that may be used:

• *Transurethral resection of the prostate* (TURP) involves the insertion of a loop of wire into the urethra through a tube. This allows the doctor to visualize the area and also to introduce fluids. The loop is then used to "shave" away excess prostatic tissue, which is flushed out the urethral/penile opening. TURP can cause complications, including urinary incontinence, retrograde ejaculation (in which ejaculate flows backwards, into the bladder), and impotence. In addition, 20 percent of men who undergo the procedure ultimately need another resection.

• An alternative procedure that may be suitable for some men is *transurethral incision of the prostate* (TUIP). This technique aims to relieve pressure on the urethra by making pressure-relieving cuts in the prostate instead of removing prostate tissue. TUIP appears to cause fewer ejaculatory problems than TURP does.

• *Transurethral needle ablation* (TUNA) also involves inserting a tube via the penile opening and threading it up to the prostatic portion of the urethra. At this point, multiple needle punctures of the urethra are performed, with heat applied through the needle to destroy portions of the prostatic tissue. Because of the heat involved in this procedure, you may require spinal or even general anesthesia before undergoing it.

- *Transurethral microwave thermotherapy* (TUMT) is similar to TUNA but may be less traumatic; a flexible catheter is used and the urethra itself is not punctured. Rather, microwave heat energy, alternated with cooling, is used to shrink the prostatic tissue.

■ Both diagnosis and treatment of prostatitis may involve prostate massage, in which pressure is applied directly to the gland to force the fluid out. When this procedure is done as part of diagnosis, the prostatic fluid is cultured to determine the nature of the infectious organism, if any, that is causing the problem.

■ Acute bacterial prostatitis is treated with antibiotics. If it comes on suddenly, causing fever and severe illness, you will probably first be treated in the hospital with intravenous antibiotics. Once the particular organism causing the infection has been identified, you will likely be switched to an appropriate oral antibiotic and continue treatment at home. If you cannot urinate at all due to prostatitis, your bladder may have to be drained by means of a tube inserted through the skin just above the pubic bone (a standard urinary catheter, which is inserted through the penile opening, is not suitable for men with acute prostatitis).

■ Chronic prostatitis is difficult to cure. Long-term antibiotic treatment is often used as "suppressive therapy" to help control recurrent urinary tract infections. If you must use such treatment, bear in mind that antibiotics kill the body's beneficial bacteria also, so you should take probiotic supplements during and after such a medication program (*see under* Nutritional Supplements, below).

■ Nonbacterial prostatitis is a common syndrome, though its cause is unknown. A short course of treatment with a broad-spectrum antibiotic such as erythromycin (ERYC, Ilotycin, and others) is often tried. A nonsteroidal anti-inflammatory drug (NSAID) such as ibuprofen (Advil, Motrin, Nuprin, and others) or ketoprofen (Orudis, Oruvail), along with sitz baths, may be recommended to help relieve symptoms.

■ If you are diagnosed with prostate cancer that your oncologist judges to be slow growing, he or she may recommend watchful waiting rather than immediate intervention with surgery or radiation treatment. There are also medications that may slow the progress of the disease. These drugs work by interfering with the production of hormones, principally testosterone, that promote the growth of prostate tumors.

■ If your doctor judges that aggressive intervention is needed and the cancer has not spread beyond the prostate, he or she may recommend radiation therapy. This can be done either by directing an external beam of radiation to the area or by implanting tiny particles of radioactive isotopes ("seeds") in the prostate tissue. Such implantation techniques are becoming more common.

■ Your doctor may advise prostatectomy (surgical removal of the prostate) as a treatment for prostate cancer (or for a very serious case of prostate enlargement). About 400,000 of these operations are performed in the United States each year, at an estimated cost of $4 billion. However, a recent American study determined that older men who had their prostates removed lived less than a year longer, on average, than those whose cancers were monitored by watchful waiting. If your doctor recommends prostatectomy, ask for a thorough explanation of why he or she feels this is the appropriate treatment for you.

DIETARY GUIDELINES

■ Enjoy tomatoes often. Eating at least four servings of tomato-based foods per week is associated with better prostate health.

■ Eat pumpkin seeds. They are high in zinc, which the prostate requires, and are an excellent snack food. Enjoy them raw, not toasted and salted.

■ Eliminate meat and other sources of saturated fats from your diet. Fats, especially saturated animal fats, are associated with all prostate disorders.

■ Avoid alcohol and caffeine, both of which are associated with urinary problems.

NUTRITIONAL SUPPLEMENTS

■ To promote overall good health and prevent nutritional deficiencies, take a good multivitamin and mineral complex that provides 100 percent of the recommended daily allowances (RDAs) of all the major vitamins and minerals.

■ Lycopene is a carotenoid, a type of phytochemical, that protects and nourishes prostate tissue. Take 3 milligrams twice a day.

■ Magnesium promotes a healthy prostate and aids the urinary tract. Take 200 to 600 milligrams of magnesium oxide, aspartate, or citrate daily.

■ Selenium is an important antioxidant nutrient that works with vitamin E. Take 200 micrograms of natural selenium daily.

■ Vitamin E is a powerful antioxidant that fights free radicals and supports the immune system. Choose a product containing mixed tocopherols and start by taking 200 international units daily. Then gradually increase the dosage until you are taking 400 international units twice daily.

Note: If you have high blood pressure, limit your

intake of supplemental vitamin E to a total of 400 international units daily. If you are taking an anticoagulant (blood thinner), consult your physician before taking supplemental vitamin E.

■ Vitamin B_6 (pyridoxine) promotes the absorption of zinc and can also help suppress the secretion of excessive amounts of prolactin. Take 50 to 100 milligrams of vitamin B_6 daily, between meals. If you take any of the B vitamins individually, you should also take a B-complex supplement at a different time of day

■ Zinc can be effective in reducing the size of the prostate and easing the symptoms of BPH. It works in two ways. First, it suppresses the activity of the enzyme 5-alpha reductase, an element in the trigger mechanism that causes the production of too many additional prostate cells. Second, it reduces the levels of prolactin. Recent studies have also shown a significant correlation between low levels of zinc in the prostate tissue and the occurrence of prostate cancer. Choose zinc picolinate or zinc oxide and take 15 to 60 milligrams daily. Take zinc with food to prevent stomach upset, and do not exceed the recommended dosage. Copper increases the beneficial effects of zinc and also promotes prostate health. If you take extra zinc on an ongoing basis, it is important to take a small amount of copper as well because these two minerals compete for absorption in the small intestine. Take 4 milligrams of copper daily.

HERBAL TREATMENT

■ Saw palmetto is the premier herbal remedy for prostate problems. A natural 5-alpha reductase inhibitor, it reduces the amount of testosterone that is transformed into dihydrotestosterone, thus helping to fight prostate enlargement. In one study, saw palmetto decreased nighttime urination by 45 percent, increased urinary flow rate over 50 percent, and reduced the retention of urine in the bladder by 42 percent. Choose an extract standardized to contain 85 to 95 percent essential fatty acids and plant sterols and take 150 to 250 milligrams twice daily.

■ Cat's claw enhances the immune response and has antibacterial properties that make it helpful for prostatitis. Take 500 milligrams of standardized extract three times a day until the infection clears.

Note: Do not use cat's claw if you are pregnant or nursing, or if you are an organ-transplant recipient. Use it with caution if you are taking an anticoagulant (blood thinner).

■ Goldenseal fights bacteria and tones the mucous membranes, and is also beneficial for prostatitis. Take 250 milligrams of standardized extract three times a day.

■ Nettle root has been used for over 200 years in Europe for prostatitis and BPH. Take 100 to 300 milligrams of nettle root extract two or three times daily.

■ Oregano has antibacterial properties and helps to fight infection. For prostatitis, take 75 milligrams of standardized extract three times a day.

■ Pygeum has notable anti-inflammatory properties and is helpful for enlargement and/or inflammation of the prostate. Take 100 milligrams twice a day.

HOMEOPATHY

■ *Causticum* 12x or 6c can ease a frequent desire to pass urine combined with difficulty in doing so. You may eject a small spurt of urine involuntarily when coughing, sneezing, or laughing. Take one dose of *Causticum* 12x or 6c three times daily for three days.

■ *Chimaphila umbelatta* is for a constant urge to pass urine, despite the fact that urination is difficult to start and urine is passed in small amounts. You may find passing urine is easier if you urinate with your legs wide apart. Take one dose of *Chimaphila umbelatta* 12x or 6c three times daily for up to three days.

■ *Clematis erecta* is good if the urine flows in a thin stream, as if the urethra is obstructed. You may feel the need to urinate frequently and experience dribbling after urination. Take one dose of *Clematis erecta* 12x or 6c three times daily for three days.

■ *Sabal serrulata* is helpful for frequent nighttime urination. Take one dose of *Sabal serrulata* 12x or 6c in the morning and another dose in the late afternoon for up to ten days.

BACH FLOWER REMEDIES

■ Mimulus should help if you have fears about your condition and worry about what the future may bring.

ACUPRESSURE

For the locations of acupressure points on the body, *see* ADMINISTERING AN ACUPRESSURE TREATMENT in Part Three.

■ The Bladder points in the lower back enhance circulation to the genitourinary tract.

■ Kidney 3 helps to strengthen the genitourinary tract.

■ Spleen 6 and Stomach 36 strengthen the body in times of stress.

AROMATHERAPY

For specific instructions on how to use aromatherapy, *see* PREPARING AROMATHERAPY TREATMENTS in Part Three.

■ An aromatherapy sitz bath prepared with essential oil of lavender, rosemary, and/or sandalwood can be soothing, while at the same time increasing circulation to the area and promoting healing. Some people recommend alternating hot and cold sitz baths for greatest effect.

GENERAL RECOMMENDATIONS

■ As much as possible, avoid stress, both physical and mental. Stress is a factor in the hormonal shifts that lead to enlargement of the prostate.

PREVENTION

■ Eat a low-fat diet and take red meat and other sources of saturated fat off the menu. A low-fat diet reduces your risk of developing prostate disorders, especially prostate cancer. Men who eat meat, especially red meat, have a nearly 80 percent greater risk of developing prostate cancer than men who eat a low-fat diet.

■ Enjoy tomatoes and tomato-based foods often. The phytochemicals found in tomatoes reduce the risk of developing prostate cancer dramatically.

■ Take zinc daily. When you feel like snacking, make a habit of munching on pumpkin seeds, which are high in zinc.

■ For prostate cancer, early detection is often the best protection. If it is caught and treated early—before it spreads into other areas of the body—the prognosis is excellent. The National Cancer Institute recommends that all men over the age of forty have a rectal exam once a year, which should include manual examination by a doctor and an ultrasound scan to detect growths that are too small to feel. In addition, men over fifty should have a yearly blood test for prostate-specific antigen (PSA). The levels of this compound in the blood rise in the presence of enlarged prostate or prostate cancer. Having a suspicious PSA test does not mean you have cancer, but it does mean that more detailed examination is warranted to rule out the possibility.

Psittacosis

See Pets and Your Health *under* HOME AND PERSONAL SAFETY in Part One.

Psoriasis

Psoriasis is a common skin disorder characterized by thick patches of reddened skin covered by silvery scales. The name comes from the Greek *psora*, which means "to itch." In this condition, the body produces new skin cells about ten times faster than normal, but the rate at which old skin cells on the surface are shed remains the same. Because they cannot reach the surface, underlying live skin cells accumulate and form thickened patches. The silvery scales appearing on the surface of the skin are old dead and dying cells that have not been shed.

The cause of psoriasis has so far eluded medical scientists, but theories and intriguing bits of evidence abound. For example, because psoriasis is rarely found in areas of the world where a low-fat diet is the norm, some researchers believe it may be related to a high-fat diet. Others say the problem is not so much the amount of fat in the diet, but the type of fat—that a diet deficient in the omega-3 and omega-6 essential fatty acids is to blame. Still other theories say that a buildup of toxins in the intestines fosters the development of psoriasis, or that a bodywide candida infection may be involved. People with impaired immune systems often have severe psoriasis. There appears to be a genetic component as well, as the disorder seems to run in families.

Psoriasis most often first appears in people between the ages of fifteen and twenty-five. This disorder affects an estimated 2 percent of the population. It generally follows a pattern of acute flare-ups and periods of healing, though it never disappears entirely. Flare-ups can be triggered by many different things, including stress, infections, illness, sunburn, and alcohol abuse. Certain drugs, such as nonsteroidal anti-inflammatories (NSAIDs), lithium, chloroquine (Aralen, an antimalaria drug), and beta-blockers can bring on an attack in susceptible individuals. The duration and spacing of both the flare-ups and the remissions vary, as does the extent of the disease. A given individual may have one or two isolated lesions, or scaly patches virtually all over his or her body—or anything in between. Any area of the body may be affected, but the most common sites are the scalp, elbows, knees, back, and buttocks. Some people develop an arthritic condition, *psoriatic arthritis*, in conjunction with psoriasis. The symptoms are similar to those of rheumatoid arthritis. *Pustular psoriasis* is a form of the condition that causes the formation of blister-like lesions, often just on the palms of the hands and the soles of the feet, but sometimes affecting a broader area.

Psoriasis can be managed effectively in most cases, but it is not considered to be conventionally curable. Though it is not a dangerous disorder, it can be unsightly and distressing.

CONVENTIONAL MEDICINE

■ The standard medical treatment for acute flare-ups of psoriasis is topical steroids, usually in high-strength formulas, such as clobetasol (Cormax, Temovate) or halobetasol (Ultravate). This treatment cannot be used in skin-fold areas or for extensive outbreaks, however. In some cases, such a high-strength formula is required that steroids can be used only intermittently, to avoid causing atrophy (wasting away) of skin tissue.

■ Complete occlusion of the site (blocking it off from air and water) by means of a plastic dressing for over a week may sometimes help, if repeated for several weeks. This may be used in conjunction with milder steroid creams, but may be effective alone in some cases.

■ A coal-tar product such as Fototar or Zetar may be helpful. These are sometimes used together with controlled ultraviolet-light treatment. There are also coal-tar shampoos that can be used for psoriasis affecting the scalp. Unfortunately, coal tar can stain clothing, irritate skin, and make skin sensitive to sunlight.

■ Anthralin (the active ingredients in the products Drithocreme and Dritho-Scalp) is a chemical that inhibits cell division, thereby slowing the growth of psoriatic lesions. It is applied topically and is appropriate only for chronic disease; if used for acute cases, it can cause irritation. It can also stain skin and clothing.

■ Calcipotriene (Dovonex) is a synthetic derivative of vitamin D_3 that has shown promising results in the treatment of psoriatic plaques. Unfortunately, it does not work in all cases, and can make some outbreaks of psoriasis worse. It can also irritate skin, particularly on the face, and prolonged use can lead to abnormally high levels of calcium in the blood.

■ Widespread disease is often treated with ultraviolet light. PUVA is a type of therapy that combines the use of ultraviolet light and psoralens, plant derivatives that can cause a skin reaction sometimes helpful in chronic disease. PUVA must be used repeatedly, and repeated exposure to ultraviolet rays can cause premature aging of the skin and even skin cancer in some individuals.

■ Etretinate (Tegison) is a synthetic relative of vitamin A. Taken orally, it can be very helpful for some cases of severe psoriasis. However, it also has potentially serious side effects, including liver damage. It should not be taken by women who are (or have even a chance of becoming) pregnant, as it can cause major birth defects.

■ For the most severe, bodywide cases of psoriasis that respond to no other treatment, a doctor may prescribe a kind of drug normally used for cancer chemotherapy or an immune-suppressing drug designed to prevent rejection after organ transplantation. Examples include methotrexate (Rheumatrex) and cyclosporine (Neoral, Sandimmune). These can be dramatically successful for some people, but they are extremely powerful drugs that can have other very serious, even life-threatening, effects, including liver damage, kidney damage, and bone-marrow suppression, in addition to the more mundane nausea, vomiting, and diarrhea. If you decide to try this approach, it is vital to work with a physician who is experienced in using these drugs to treat psoriasis and who can monitor all of their effects closely.

DIETARY GUIDELINES

■ Eat a well-balanced high-fiber diet that emphasizes clean, lean protein foods, whole grains, and fresh (preferably raw) fruits and vegetables.

■ Enjoy fish often. Fish oils contain essential fatty acids that reduce the inflammatory response.

■ Avoid dairy products and red meat. These foods contain arachidonic acid, which promotes inflammation and can cause psoriatic patches to become even more inflamed and swollen.

■ Avoid alcohol, caffeine, and refined sugar.

NUTRITIONAL SUPPLEMENTS

■ Take a multivitamin and mineral supplement that provides trace minerals daily.

■ Digestive enzymes enhance the utilization of the nutrients in your food. Take a full-spectrum digestive-enzyme supplement providing 5,000 international units of lipase, 2,500 international units of amylase, and 300 international units of protease, plus 350 milligrams of pancreatin, two to three times daily, with meals.

Note: Long-term supplementation with pancreatin is not advised, as it can cause your pancreas to reduce its own production of this important enzyme. Overuse also has the potential to cause nausea or diarrhea. After two months on pancreatin, discontinue use and monitor your reaction. If you find that your problems recur, discuss pancreatin supplementation with your health-care provider.

■ A deficiency of fumaric acid, a compound found naturally in some plants, may contribute to psoriasis. In healthy people, fumaric acid forms in the skin on exposure to sunlight. People with psoriasis, however, must spend a much longer time in sunlight to produce it. European researchers have been experimenting with fumaric acid ester supplements, with good results. Fumaric acid is not a quick-fix, however. It can take up to three months before yielding results, and it can produce some uncomfortable side effects. Its use should be monitored by a physician. If you are interested in trying this supplement, seek your doctor's advice.

■ Glutathione is an amino-acid compound that slows the runaway growth of underlying skin cells. Take 500 milligrams twice a day, between meals.

■ An adequate intake of omega-3 and omega-6 essential fatty acids can improve psoriasis in many cases. Unfortunately, many people do not get enough of these nutrients from the foods they eat. Fish oils are rich in the omega-3 acids; black currant seed oil, borage oil, evening primrose oil, and flaxseed oil are good sources of omega-6 essential fatty acids. Shark liver oil also contains compounds called alkylglycerols, or AKGs, which stimulate the immune system. Take 1,000 to 2,000 milligrams (1 to 2 grams) of fish oil and 500 milligrams of black currant seed, borage, evening primrose, or flaxseed oil three times daily.

Note: If you have diabetes, consult your doctor before taking supplemental fish oil. People with diabetes sometimes have difficulty digesting fish oil due to compromised gallbladder function.

■ Probiotic bacteria help to keep the intestines functioning efficiently and also keep candida under control. Strengthening the absorption and transport of nutrients is often very helpful for people with psoriasis. Take a probiotic supplement as recommended on the product label. For best results, take both acidophilus and bifidobacteria, on an alternating basis. If you are allergic to milk, choose a dairy-free formula.

■ The B vitamins help in the healing and repair of skin cells. Take a good B-complex formula supplying 25 milligrams of each of the major B vitamins twice daily.

■ Vitamins A and E are antioxidants that are beneficial for the skin. Take 10,000 international units of vitamin A and 15,000 international units of its precursor, beta-carotene, twice daily for one month. Then cut back to one dose of each daily. Also take 200 international units of vitamin E each day, in mixed-tocopherol form, and then gradually increase the dosage until you are taking 200 international units three times daily.

Note: If you are pregnant, or intend to get pregnant, or if you have liver disease, consult your doctor before taking supplemental vitamin A. If you have high blood pressure, limit your intake of supplemental vitamin E to a total of 400 international units daily, and if you are taking an anticoagulant (blood thinner), consult your physician before taking supplemental vitamin E.

■ Vitamin C is important for the formation of collagen and healthy skin. Take 500 milligrams of vitamin C with an equal amount of mixed bioflavonoids two or three times daily.

HERBAL TREATMENT

■ *Coleus forskohlii* is an Ayurvedic herb that can slow down the high rate of cell division that characterizes psoriasis. Using the whole herb yields the greatest benefits. Make an infusion (tea) from the the dried root (*see* PREPARING HERBAL TREATMENTS in Part Three) and take three to five cups daily. Or take 250 milligrams of 1-percent extract two or three times daily.

■ Gotu kola reduces inflammation and speeds wound healing. It has been used for centuries in Indian medicine for all kinds of skin conditions, including psoriasis. Choose a standardized extract containing 16 percent triterpenes and take 200 milligrams two to three times daily for one month.

■ Milk thistle contains silymarin, which acts to correct the abnormal cell replication involved in psoriasis. It also contains several anti-inflammatory compounds and enhances the liver's ability to filter toxins from the blood. Choose an extract standardized to contain 80 percent flavonoids (silymarin) and take 200 to 300 milligrams three times a day. If you develop loose stools, increase the amount of fiber in your diet or take a natural fiber supplement.

HOMEOPATHY

The best approach to treating psoriasis homeopathically is to see a qualified homeopath who can prescribe a constitutional remedy. Constitutional remedies can be tremendously effective in clearing psoriasis. The remedies that follow can provide short-term symptomatic relief. Choose an appropriate remedy and take one dose, as directed on the product label, three or four times daily for up to four days. If you fail to note an improvement in that time, discontinue the remedy and select another. Better yet, see a homeopathic physician.

■ *Arsenicum album* 30x or 15c is for red, hot burning skin accompanied by tiredness and anxiety.

■ *Graphites* 12x or 6c is for psoriasis with honey-colored pus that is likely worse behind the ears.

■ *Kali arsenicosum* 12x or 6c may prove valuable if you are suffering from intense itching that is worse with heat. You probably also tend to be nervous and may be anemic.

BACH FLOWER REMEDIES

Select the remedy that most closely fits your emotional tendencies and concerns, and take it as needed, following the directions on the product label.

■ Chicory helps to overcome feelings of insecurity and fears of being rejected that may manifest themselves in what appears to be selfishness.

■ Impatiens calms nervousness, tension, and impatience.

■ Red Chestnut counteracts a tendency to worry excessively.

■ Sweet Chestnut can ease anguish and feelings of alienation.

ACUPRESSURE

For the locations of acupressure points on the body, *see* ADMINISTERING AN ACUPRESSURE TREATMENT in Part Three.

■ Four Gates relaxes the nervous system. Psoriasis is linked to a sensitive nervous system.

■ Spleen 6 and 10 cleanse and strengthen the blood.

■ Stomach 36 improves digestion.

■ Triple Warmer 5 regulates hormonal function.

AROMATHERAPY

For specific instructions on using aromatherapy, *see* PREPARING AROMATHERAPY TREATMENTS in Part Three.

■ Many essential oils have the ability to promote healing and reduce inflammation and irritation of the skin. Among them are calendula, chamomile, lavender, and rose. Add one or more of these oils (you may wish to experiment to determine which oil or oils work best for you) to a soothing aromatherapy bath. For smaller areas, you can use compresses rather than a bath if it is more convenient. After the bath, apply a skin oil made by blending a total of 12 drops of essential oil into 1 ounce of jojoba oil to the affected areas to treat them and help lock in moisture.

Note: Do not expose the skin to water for very long periods, as this may dry it out even further, and always apply a moisturizer or skin oil after bathing. Be careful not to use too much essential oil in these treatments, and never apply pure essential oil directly to your skin. Always dilute it in water or oil first. If irritation results, reduce the amount of essential oil you are using or discontinue use of the suspect oil.

GENERAL RECOMMENDATIONS

■ Apply fish-oil salve or a light vegetable oil such as olive oil to the scales twice a day. This helps to relieve itching and softens the scales, making them easier to eliminate. After the scales have been softened sufficiently, scrub gently with a terry-cloth washcloth to remove them.

■ Expose the affected areas to direct sunlight for fifteen to thirty minutes each day to reduce scaling and inflammation. Be careful not to overdo it, however, or it may trigger a worse flare-up.

■ Get regular exercise. Exercise increases the supply of oxygen to all the body's tissues, including the skin, which ultimately helps to reduce inflammation.

■ When you exercise or engage in any other activity that causes sweating, it is important to wear loose clothing made of a natural, breathable fiber such as cotton.

■ As much as possible, avoid stress, which can provoke and worsen flare-ups.

■ Install a filter to remove chlorine from bath and shower water. Most municipal water supplies contain chlorine, which further dehydrates the skin and can contribute to skin problems.

Psychological Problems

See ANXIETY DISORDERS; DEPRESSION; MANIC-DEPRESSIVE DISORDER; OBSESSIVE-COMPULSIVE DISORDER; STRESS.

Purpura

See under BRUISING; VASCULITIS.

Pyorrhea

See under PERIODONTAL DISEASE.

Radiation Sickness

Radiation sickness is the result of exposure to radiation, whether accidental, as in the case of a nuclear power plant accident, or intentional, as in the case of radiation therapy for cancer. Radiation can damage, deform, and kill cells. It has the greatest effect on cells that have a high rate of turnover. This is why it is useful in cancer therapy, but it also poses significant danger to the bone marrow and mucous membranes, among other types of tissue. Exposure to radiation results in insufficient replacement of cells in these tissues. The specific symptoms this can manifest itself in vary, depending on the dosage of radiation received, the area of the body affected, and the individual's reaction, but they can include headache, nausea, vomiting, diarrhea, fatigue, shortness of breath, oral thrush, dry mouth, loss of the sense of taste, difficulty swallowing, gum disease, musculoskeletal pain, hair loss, dry cough, skin darkening, bleeding under the skin, anemia, loss of sex drive, impotence, and sterility.

CONVENTIONAL TREATMENT

■ In the case of accidental exposure to radiation, contaminated clothing and other materials should be removed at once, and extremely thorough washing begun to remove as much of the contamination as possible. If there are any breaks in the skin, these must be scrubbed vigorously, and some tissue may have to be removed until the area is clean. Blood transfusions and intravenous fluids may be necessary to support the body until it begins to recover somewhat. Antibiotic therapy is instituted as a prevention against infection, and oral medication may be administered to protect the thyroid. In some cases, a bone marrow transplant may ultimately be necessary, though it is often difficult to find a suitable donor.

■ In some cases, chelation therapy may be helpful for removing radioactive substances from the body.

■ Doses of radiation received in the course of treatment for cancer are calibrated so as not to be life-threatening. However, they still often cause extreme nausea, hair loss, and other symptoms of radiation sickness. In such cases, nausea is treated with drugs called antiemetics, which help to alleviate nausea and prevent vomiting. Examples include prochlorperazine (Compazine) and trimethobenzamide (Tigan). Fluids and electrolytes should be monitored and replaced, if necessary. Hair growth usually returns to normal once the treatment is over.

DIETARY GUIDELINES

■ Eat a balanced diet with an emphasis on antioxidant-, vitamin-, and mineral-rich foods such as fresh green, yellow, orange, and red vegetables and fruits.

■ Drink at least eight 8-ounce glasses of water daily to keep yourself well hydrated and flush toxins from your body.

NUTRITIONAL SUPPLEMENTS

■ Take a good multivitamin and mineral supplement daily to build up your nutritional status.

■ Exposure to radiation bombards the body with free radicals; antioxidants defuse free radicals and limit the damage they can cause. Take the following antioxidant nutrients: 25,000 international units of a carotene complex twice daily; 25,000 international units of vitamin A twice a day for two weeks; 500 milligrams of vitamin C with an equal amount of bioflavonoids three to four times daily; 400 international units of vitamin E twice daily, in morning and evening; 200 micrograms of selenium twice a day; and 15 milligrams of zinc twice a day. In addition, take 25 milligrams of pine-bark or grape-seed extract three times daily.

Note: If you are pregnant, or intend to get pregnant, or if you have liver disease, consult your doctor before taking supplemental vitamin A. When you start taking vitamin E, begin with 400 milligrams in the morning and gradually, over a period of two weeks, increase to the recommended amount. If you have high blood pressure, limit your intake of supplemental vitamin E to a total of 400 international units daily, and if you are taking an anticoagulant (blood thinner), consult your physician before taking supplemental vitamin E. Take zinc with food to prevent stomach upset. If you take 30 milligrams or more on a daily basis for more than one or two months, you should also take 1 to 2 milligrams of copper each day to maintain a proper mineral balance.

■ Lipoic acid protects the liver. It helps to improve liver function and, ultimately, to increase energy levels during and following radiation therapy. Take 100 milligrams three times daily.

■ Malic acid with magnesium, taken at least half an hour before breakfast in the morning, is most useful for enhancing energy and minimizing musculoskeletal pain. Take a combination that supplies 350 to 600 milligrams of malic acid and 100 milligrams of magnesium up to three times a day.

■ Marine alginate concentrate binds with heavy metals and helps to detoxify the body after occupational or accidental radiation exposure. Take 500 milligrams three times a day.

■ Taking thymus glandular extract helps to strengthen the immune system after exposure to radiation. Take 250 to 500 milligrams three times a day for two months, then cut back to 250 milligrams a day.

HERBAL TREATMENT

■ Ashwaganda helps to protect against the adverse effects of radiation and also may enhance the effectiveness of radiation treatment. Take 450 to 900 milligrams of standardized extract daily.

■ Astragalus has been reported to protect white blood cells during radiation treatment. Take 500 milligrams of standardized extract four times a day.

■ Ginger root tea helps to reduce nausea. Take a cup three times daily, as needed.

■ Green tea has known radioprotective effects. Choose a decaffeinated standardized extract containing at least 50 percent catechins and take 250 milligrams two to four times daily.

■ Milk thistle protects the liver when the body is attacked by radiation. Choose an extract standardized to contain 80 percent flavonoids (silymarin) and take 200 to 300 milligrams twice daily during radiation therapy and for two to three months afterwards.

■ Siberian ginseng increases energy and helps the body adapt to stress. Choose a standardized extract containing 0.5 percent eleutheroside E and take 100 milligrams once in the morning and again before lunch.

HOMEOPATHY

■ *Nux vomica* is very effective in minimizing nausea. Take one dose of *Nux vomica* 30x or 15c, as directed on the product label, three times daily for up to three days, as needed.

BACH FLOWERS

■ Hornbeam is helpful for fatigue. Take it as needed, following the directions on the product label.

ACUPRESSURE

For the locations of acupressure points on the body, *see*

ADMINISTERING AN ACUPRESSURE TREATMENT in Part Three.

■ Pericardium 6 helps to lessen nausea and vomiting.

AROMATHERAPY

■ Essential oils of lavender and rosemary, used in a bath, gently relax and mildly detoxify the body. Add 3 drops of each to a tubful of warm water and enjoy a relaxing soak.

GENERAL RECOMMENDATIONS

■ A warm bath made with 3 pounds of Epsom salts and 3 pounds of baking soda is an old naturopathic prescription for detoxifying the body and reducing acidity. Soak in the tub for 20 minutes. This is a relatively strong bath. Be careful when leaving the tub—some people find they get sleepy while in the bath.

■ If you know you will be exposed to radiation, such as from radiotherapy for cancer, begin at once to adhere to a healthy diet and take the supplements recommended above.

Rash

See SKIN RASH.

Raynaud's Phenomenon

Raynaud's phenomenon is a circulatory condition in which the small arteries that supply the fingers and toes, and sometimes the ears and nose, contract on exposure to cold. This interrupts the normal flow of blood and causes the affected area to suddenly become extremely pale, then to take on a bluish tinge. Then, as the arteries relax and the blood comes rushing back, the skin turns quite red. Feelings of tingling, numbness, burning, and pain may accompany the attack. The fingers, usually on both hands, are most often affected.

This condition affects more women than men, and younger women are more prone to have this problem than older women. Like carpal tunnel syndrome, Raynaud's phenomenon sometimes occurs in pianists, computer operators, and others whose fingers are continually in use. Because of repeated trauma to their hands and fingers, people who use vibrating machinery such as jackhammers and chain saws also have an increased risk of developing the condition. Smoking increases the risk because the nicotine in tobacco smoke constricts the blood vessels.

Sometimes Raynaud's phenomenon is associated with an underlying health problem such as rheumatoid arthritis, hardening of the arteries, lupus, hypothyroidism, scleroderma, or injury to the blood vessels. Certain drugs, including ergotamine (used for treating migraine) and beta-blockers (used for treating cardiovascular problems), can cause similar symptoms. In many cases, however, Raynaud's phenomenon occurs without any identifiable underlying cause. In such cases, it is called Raynaud's disease.

Both Raynaud's phenomenon and Raynaud's disease can have serious complications. In the advanced stages, the condition can be very painful and may interfere with the sense of touch. In rare cases, the walls of the arteries may thicken so severely that blood flow to the affected extremities may be permanently reduced. If this happens, ulcers can develop and gangrene may even set in, resulting in the death of tissue at the tips of the digits.

CONVENTIONAL TREATMENT

■ Appropriate treatment for Raynaud's phenomenon depends on the cause. If the underlying condition is treated successfully, the circulatory problems that cause the unpleasant symptoms may be resolved. The use of skin lotions, local applications of warmth, and, above all, stopping smoking are also likely to be recommended (*see* General Recommendations in this entry).

■ Vasodilators (drugs that cause blood vessels to relax and dilate) may be helpful for some people. The calcium-channel blocker nifedipine (Adalat, Procardia) is often prescribed for this purpose. Possible side effects include headaches, swelling, dizziness, nausea, cramping, and heart palpitations.

■ An operation to cut the nerves controlling the degree of constriction of blood vessels in the upper or lower extremities may offer relief for some people with Raynaud's disease. Unfortunately, the relief may not last. This procedure is not as effective in later stages of the disease.

DIETARY GUIDELINES

■ Eat a diet that is high in fiber and low in saturated, hydrogenated, and partially hydrogenated fats. Plan meals to include foods containing phytochemicals that lower cholesterol and thin the blood, such as onions, garlic, grapes, eggplant, red cabbage, and broccoli.

■ Avoid coffee, tea (except herbal teas), caffeinated sodas, and anything else that contains caffeine. Caffeine constricts blood vessels. The tiny ones that bring blood to the extremities are the most affected.

■ Although a hot toddy may seem like a good idea if your hands and face feel cold, avoid alcohol. The warming effect is an illusion. Alcohol actually lowers body temperature.

NUTRITIONAL SUPPLEMENTS

■ Take a multivitamin and mineral supplement each day. Choose a formula that contains trace minerals.

■ Fish oils contain omega-3 essential fatty acids that decrease inflammation and may improve circulation. Take 1,000 milligrams twice a day.

■ Grape-seed extract is an antioxidant and also improves circulation. Choose a standardized extract containing 90 percent proanthocyanidins (PCOs) and take 500 milligrams twice a day.

■ Green-foods supplements are full of important trace minerals that are essential to the health of the nervous system. Take a green-foods supplement as recommended on the product label.

■ The B vitamins are important for the proper transmission of nerve impulses and also enhance circulation. Three times a day, take a B-complex supplement that supplies 50 milligrams of each of the major B vitamins.

■ Vitamin B_3 (niacin or nicotinic acid) causes the blood vessels to dilate, allowing blood flow to increase for short periods of time. If you take a high enough dose, this form of vitamin B_3 causes a flushing sensation for about twenty minutes, starting about fifteen minutes after you take it. Niacinamide (nicotinamide), another form of vitamin B_3, does not cause flushing, but also does not dilate the blood vessels. Start with a dose of 200 milligrams daily. If this dose causes flushing, stay at that level; if not, increase the dose until you do experience the flush, and then stay with that dose. After several days you may cease to feel much effect at all. At this point, discontinue the supplement completely for two or three days, then resume taking the same dose that caused the flush originally. Do not use a timed-release form of niacin, as these can irritate the liver. If you take any of the B vitamins individually, you should also take a B-complex supplement at a different time of day.

Note: Do not take supplemental niacin if you have gout or liver dysfunction.

■ Vitamin E is a mild anticoagulant (blood thinner) and enhances circulation. Choose a product containing mixed tocopherols and take 200 international units twice daily for three weeks, then increase the dosage to 400 units twice daily.

Note: If you have high blood pressure, limit your intake of supplemental vitamin E to a total of 400 international units daily from all sources. If you are taking an anticoagulant, consult your physician before taking supplemental vitamin E.

HERBAL TREATMENT

■ Ginkgo biloba extract acts as a vasodilator to increase circulation through the small arteries of the body, such as occurs in Raynaud's disease. Select a standardized extract of this herb that contains at least 24 percent ginkgo heterosides (sometimes called flavoglycosides), and take 40 to 60 milligrams, three times daily.

■ Hawthorn improves peripheral circulation. Take 250 milligrams of standardized extract containing 1.8 percent vitexin-2 rhamnosides three times a day.

■ Siberian ginseng helps the body adapt to stress, regulates circulation and hormonal function, and helps to strengthen the nervous system. Choose an extract standardized to contain 0.5 percent eleutheroside E and take 100 milligrams twice daily, the first dose before breakfast and the second before lunch.

HOMEOPATHY

The best approach to treating Raynaud's disease homeopathically is with a constitutional remedy prescribed by a qualified homeopathic physician. The following remedies can be used as needed to provide relief of symptoms.

■ *Arsenicum album* is for burning pain in the extremities that is accompanied by feelings of anxiety and restlessness, and that is worse with cold. Take one dose of *Arsenicum album* 30x or 15c three to four times daily for three days. If there is no improvement after three days, stop taking it and try another remedy.

■ *Cactus* is for swollen, icy-cold hands and feet and restless legs that are worse at 11:00 AM and 11:00 PM. You may also be prone to getting a headache if you miss a meal. Take one dose of *Cactus* 3x three to four times daily for three days. If there is no improvement after three days, stop taking it and try another remedy.

■ *Crotalus horridus* is for hands that tremble and are generally swollen, accompanied by numbness in the extremities. Symptoms worsen with dampness. You probably have a history of poor nutrition as well. Take one dose of *Crotalus horridus* 12x or 6c three to four times daily for three days. If there is no improvement after three days, stop taking it and try another remedy.

■ If damp weather aggravates symptoms, choose *Dulcamara*. Take one dose of *Dulcamara* 12x or 6c three times a day for three days. If there is no improvement in three days, stop taking it and try another remedy.

■ *Lachesis* is good if your skin is bluish and you feel considerably worse upon awakening. Take one dose of *Lachesis* 30x or 15c three to four times daily for three days. If there is no improvement after three days, stop taking it and try another remedy.

■ *Secale* 12x or 6c is for very cold extremities that are bluish, accompanied by pain and, possibly, numbness in your fingertips. You may also be a smoker, or have smoked at one time. Take one dose of *Secale* 12x or 6c three to four times daily for three days. If there is no improvement after three days, stop taking it and try another remedy.

BACH FLOWER REMEDIES

Select the remedy that most closely fits your emotional tendencies and concerns, and take it as needed, following the directions on the product label.

Holly helps to tame insecurity and jealousy that burst out in fits of bad temper.

■ Hornbeam helps to alleviate exhaustion so deep that it makes you miss out on pleasurable activities.

Impatiens calms nervousness, hyperactivity, impatience, and irritability.

Willow is the remedy to select if you are feeling resentful and nothing seems to please you.

ACUPRESSURE

For the locations of acupressure points on the body, *see* ADMINISTERING AN ACUPRESSURE TREATMENT in Part Three.

Gallbladder 21 improves circulation.

■ Gallbladder 41 improves hormonal function.

■ Large Intestine 10 detoxifies the large intestine.

Lung 7 improves tissue oxygenation.

Pericardium 6 improves circulation in the upper body. This point is especially important if, despite all of the admonitions from your doctor and others, you are a smoker.

Spleen 6 strengthens the blood.

Stomach 36 improves the utilization of nutrients.

Triple Warmer 5 improves hormonal function.

GENERAL RECOMMENDATIONS

If you smoke, quit. Avoid secondhand smoke. The nicotine in tobacco smoke causes the blood vessels to constrict, which can seriously worsen Raynaud's.

Try to avoid the cold as much as possible. If you must spend time in a cold environment, take measures to keep your hands and feet warm. Wear two (or more, if necessary) pairs of socks and insulated shoes, and make sure each succeeding layer fits easily over the one before it (trapping air between the layers is vital for maintaining warmth). Wear mittens, not gloves. Gloves expose each finger to the cold, while mittens trap body heat. Again, if need be, wear multiple layers on your hands. If you are particularly affected, it may be a good idea to wear mittens even when you are shopping for frozen foods.

Do circulation-enhancing exercises during exposure to cold. Twirl your arms in a wide circle, back behind your body, then forward, at a fast rate. The combination of centrifugal force and gravity conspire to increase the flow of blood into the fingers. Stop when your fingers feel warm.

■ Transcutaneous electrical nerve stimulation (TENS) is a type of therapy in which a small battery-device administers electrical impulses to certain points on the body. This increases circulation, and has been found to be very effective for some people with Raynaud's. You may wish to discuss this with your doctor.

PREVENTION

■ There is no known way to prevent Raynaud's disease, but it may be possible to condition your hands so that the small blood vessels do not constrict as much in response to cold. Experiments with 150 people in Alaska involved the following procedure: First, the subjects soaked their hands in warm water for three to five minutes. Next, they were placed in a room with a temperature hovering around the freezing mark. There they again immersed their hands in warm water, this time for ten minutes. Although the low temperature would normally cause the arteries to constrict, the warmth of the water kept the blood flowing freely. This conditioning exercise was repeated three to six times every other day, for a total of fifty-four treatments. When the study was completed, the subjects' hands registered an average of seven degrees warmer on exposure to cold, even without immersion in warm water.

Restless Legs Syndrome

Restless legs syndrome (RLS) is a neurological condition characterized by sensations in the extremities that range from the mildly uncomfortable to the nearly unbearable. As the name implies, it primarily involves the legs, but the arms may also be affected. Symptoms of RLS can be difficult to describe precisely, but have been characterized as twitching, tugging, tingling, itching, pulling, and burning—even feeling as if worms are crawling inside one's legs. The symptoms occur most often in the evening and at night, especially if you are quite tired, but can also occur at other times, especially if you are lying down or attempting to sit still. Because the sensations are usually relieved by movement, sitting, resting, and sleeping can be difficult—sometimes completely impossible. People with RLS often find it necessary to move or stretch the affected limbs in order to find some measure of relief.

Restless legs syndrome is usually diagnosed in people between the ages of fifty and sixty, but in most cases it begins much earlier; many people who receive the diagnosis say their symptoms have been with them for many, many years. In fact, some report having been scolded as children because they wouldn't sit still, due to the same type of discomfort diagnosed as RLS later in life. It is likely that many people who have RLS do not realize that their symptoms actually have a name.

RLS can be divided into three basic categories: primary, secondary, and transient. Primary (also referred to as *idiopathic*) RLS is unrelated to any other underlying health problem. This form of the condition tends to run in families, and symptoms often intensify with age. If RLS is due to another health problem, it is considered secondary. There are a number of chronic disorders, including diabetes, alcoholism, rheumatoid arthritis, Parkinson's disease, kidney failure, and peripheral neuropathy (damage to the nerves in the hands and feet), that can cause RLS. The transient form of the condition is most often a result of pregnancy or anemia. With transient RLS, symptoms usually disappear after the baby is born or the anemia is corrected.

The cause of RLS is not understood, but it is believed to be related to a problem in the nervous system that originates in either the brain or the spinal cord. It may also be linked to a combination of mineral deficiency and some type of inflammatory process. There are no laboratory tests for RLS, so diagnosis must be made by a process of elimination. If other possible medical conditions are ruled out, and you have a history of RLS-type symptoms that get worse when you are at rest coupled with an irresistable urge to move around to get relief, you will likely be diagnosed with RLS.

Although RLS seldom disappears entirely, the vast majority of people who have it can be helped. A combination of drug therapies and natural treatments appears to be the most successful approach to managing this condition.

CONVENTIONAL TREATMENT

■ Drugs that boost the level of dopamine, a chemical that regulates the transmission of messages in the central nervous system, show promise against RLS. These drugs are also used to treat Parkinson's disease. Examples include levodopa plus carbidopa (Atamet, Sinemet), pergolide (Permax), and bromocriptine (Parlodel).

■ Benzodiazepines such as clonazepam (Klonopin) are tranquilizers that depress the central nervous system. Taken before bedtime, they do not eliminate symptoms, but they do dull the sensations, making it easier to sleep. Possible "morning-after" side effects, especially for older adults, include daytime drowsiness or confusion.

■ Anticonvulsants (drugs used to prevent seizures) can decrease the unpleasant sensations and inhibit the urge to move. Gabapentin (Neurontin), which is considered to be the most effective among the anticonvulsant drugs, is effective for some (but, unfortunately, not all) people with RLS, especially those who have daytime symptoms.

■ Narcotics such as codeine, propoxyphene (Darvon), oxycodone (often combined with a painkiller such as acet-

aminophen, aspirin, or ibuprofen, and sold under different brand names, including Percocet, Percodan, and Tylox), pentazocine (in Talacen and Talwin), and methadone are painkillers that work by blocking the body's perception of pain. They may be effective at relieving the discomfort of RLS, but they are powerful drugs with equally powerful side effects. They can also be addictive, so they are reserved for people whose symptoms are exceptionally severe.

■ Injections of magnesium sulfate can be helpful, especially if you have found taking magnesium orally to be beneficial (*see under* Nutritional Supplements, below), although you may have to seek out a nutritionally oriented physician in order to try it. Taking this mineral by injection improves its absorption and avoids the possibility of diarrhea, which can be a problem if you take high doses by mouth. This treatment is remarkably safe.

■ Because any medication that is used nightly over a long period of time will tend to lose some of its effectiveness, treatment with low doses of two or more different drugs may be more successful than taking standard doses of a single agent.

DIETARY GUIDELINES

■ Eat a well-balanced, high-fiber diet with an emphasis on green vegetables, which have high levels of folates. Low levels of folic acid are associated with RLS.

■ Avoid refined sugar, coffee, tea (except herbal teas), anything containing chocolate, and caffeinated sodas. Many people find that their symptoms are worse after consuming these substances. People with diabetes appear to be particularly susceptible to this effect. In some cases, simply avoiding caffeine is all that's needed to bring relief.

NUTRITIONAL SUPPLEMENTS

■ Take a multivitamin and mineral supplement twice daily to ensure a supply of all necessary nutrients. Vitamin B_{12} and folic acid in particular are important for the proper transmission of nerve impulses.

■ Black currant seed oil, borage oil, evening primrose oil, flaxseed oil, and fish oils contain essential fatty acids (EFAs) that can help normalize the transmission of nerve impulses. Take 500 to 1,000 milligrams of black currant seed, borage, or evening primrose oil, and/or an equal amount of flaxseed or fish oil, twice daily.

■ Calcium and magnesium strengthen muscle function and are essential to the central nervous system. Take 300 to 500 milligrams of calcium and 200 to 300 milligrams of magnesium citrate or malate three times daily.

■ Folic acid deficiency has been linked to RLS. Take 400

micrograms twice daily, with 250 micrograms of vitamin B_{12}. If you take any of the B vitamins individually, you should also take a B-complex supplement at a different time of day.

■ Iron deficiency can contribute to restless legs syndrome. Consult your physician for testing to determine whether you have this problem. If so, take an iron supplement as recommended by your doctor.

Note: Too much iron can be toxic. Do not take supplemental iron unless a deficiency has been diagnosed by your health-care provider, and do not take the supplement in higher amounts or for a longer period of time than he or she prescribes.

HERBAL TREATMENT

■ Kava kava is relaxing and promotes sound sleep. Choose a product containing 30 percent kava lactones and take 200 to 250 milligrams three times a day.

Note: This herb can cause drowsiness. Do not exceed the recommended dose. Do not use kava kava if you are pregnant or nursing, if you have Parkinson's disease, or if you are taking a prescription medication for depression or anxiety.

■ A combination of passionflower and valerian can help alleviate many symptoms of RLS. Passionflower, which has a long history of use for nerve-related disorders, is a nutritive tonic for the nervous system. Choose an extract standardized to contain 0.7 percent flavonoids and take 250 milligrams two or three times daily. Valerian helps relieve pain, cramps, and spasms, and also promotes healthy sleep. Select a standardized extract containing at least 0.5 percent isovalerenic acids and take 150 to 250 milligrams in the morning and again in the evening.

■ Pine-bark and grape-seed extracts are powerful anti-inflammatories with antioxidant properties. Take 50 milligrams of either two or three times daily.

HOMEOPATHY

■ *Cuprum metallicum* is the remedy for intense jerking and twitching, cramping in the calves and soles of the feet, and cold hands. Take one dose of *Cuprum metallicum* 12x or 6c three or four times daily for three days. If there is no improvement after three days, stop taking it and try another remedy.

■ *Phosphorus* should prove helpful if you suffer from weakness and trembling that is worse with physical or mental exertion, and worse yet with changes in the weather. Take one dose of *Phosphorus* 30x or 15c three or four times daily for three days. If there is no improvement after three days, stop taking it and try another remedy.

■ Choose *Tarentula hispana* if your legs are weak and trembling and your sleep is restless due to their twitching;

you tend to experience rapid changes in mood, and often feel discontented and irritable; and your legs feel better if you rub them. Take one dose of *Tarentula hispana* 12x or 6c three or four times daily for three days. If there is no improvement after three days, stop taking it and try another remedy.

■ If the above remedies are not helpful, see a homeopathic physician for a constitutional remedy.

BACH FLOWER REMEDIES

Select the remedy that most closely fits your emotional tendencies and concerns, and take it as needed, following the directions on the product label.

■ Agrimony is for the kind of person who smiles outwardly but suffers in silence inside.

■ Holly tames anger and a tendency to display bad temper.

■ Oak is helpful if you have a typical type-A personality and feel relentlessly driven to excel.

ACUPRESSURE

For the locations of acupressure points on the body, *see* ADMINISTERING AN ACUPRESSURE TREATMENT in Part Three.

■ Gallbladder 30 and 34 relax muscles and tendons.

■ Liver 3 relieves muscle cramps and spasms.

■ Spleen 6 reduces cramping.

■ Stomach 36 enhances the utilization of nutrients.

GENERAL RECOMMENDATIONS

■ Get regular exercise. Some people with RLS report this has been helpful in moderating symptoms.

■ When circumstances require a period of enforced sitting, practice distraction. At work, concentrate fully on the task at hand. At home, try a challenging video game or an absorbing novel with an intricate plot. A good book may help when you are traveling as well.

■ Many people who suffer from restless legs syndrome also have fibromyalgia, a disorder that causes aching and pain in muscles and joints throughout the body (*see* FIBROMYALGIA).

Retinal Disorders

The retina is a concave membrane situated over the inner surface of the back and sides of the eye. Packed with nerve fibers that respond chemically to various wavelengths and intensities of light, the retina is the "screen" on which images form when light enters the eye. Light waves striking the cells of the retina create a complex flow of impulses that are carried by the optic nerve to the brain, which transforms the images into vision. Because the retina has such a central role in the visual process, any disorder that compromises its functioning can threaten the sense of sight. This entry addresses three of the more common retinal disorders: detached retina, retinitis pigmentosa, and retinopathy.

Retinal detachment is a situation in which the light-sensitive inner surface of the retina separates from the outer layers. It is usually preceded by a hole or tear in the retina. This allows some of the vitreous fluid (the jellylike material that fills the back of the eyeball and maintains its round shape) to collect between the membrane and the underlying layer. A retina may detach after trauma such as a blow to the head or surgery, but it most often happens spontaneously, as a result of gradual degeneration of the tissues of the eye. It is more common in people with myopia (nearsightedness) and those who have undergone cataract surgery. The incidence increases with age.

A detached (or detaching) retina causes no pain. The first sign that a retina is becoming detached may be a shower of bright flashes of light glimpsed at the edge of the field of vision. This may be accompanied by the sudden appearance of cobweblike floaters—specks that appear to float across the field of vision. Some people never experience such early warnings, however. In some cases, the only indication that something is wrong is the characteristic loss of vision that makes it appear as if a black curtain is being pulled across part of the field of vision. If you develop signs that may indicate a detaching retina, consult an ophthalmologist *immediately*. This is considered an ophthalmic emergency.

Retinitis pigmentosa (RP) is a disorder characterized by the progressive degeneration of the retina. The first sign, which often develops in late childhood or in adolescence, is usually difficulty seeing at night or in dim light. Gradually, visual difficulty occurs in daylight also, as a ring-shaped blind spot develops in the field of vision and slowly extends to destroy an increasing area of the field, beginning with the peripheral vision. While the loss of vision is progressive and irreversible, it is generally slow. Complete loss of sight may not occur until the age of thirty or later—much later in some cases. The cause of RP is not known, but it does run in families.

Retinopathy is a general term for diseases of the retina. One of the most common of these disorders is diabetic retinopathy. Diabetic retinopathy can occur in two ways. First, the blood vessels in the retina can become more porous and leak, which decreases and/or blocks blood flow within the retina. Second, if diabetes-induced circulatory problems cause a reduction in the blood supply to the eyes, the body may attempt to restore circulation by releasing substances that stimulate the growth of new blood vessels. New vessels then begin to grow into and over various structures in the interior of the eye, including the retina, causing damage to the nerve tissues there. Further, these vessels tend to rupture easily, resulting in bleeding and scarring inside the eye.

Retinopathy can also be a result of other circulatory disorders, such as hypertension (high blood pressure) and arteriosclerosis (hardening of the arteries). Like diabetic retinopathy, these types of retinopathy can cause hemorrhages and scarring within the eye that damage retinal tissue. It is also possible for the tiny blood vessels within the eye to become blocked, starving the retina of oxygen and nutrients—much as heart tissue is starved during a heart attack—which can cause the death of tiny areas of retinal tissue and, consequently, blind spots in the field of vision.

In the early stages, retinopathy often causes no symptoms. Not until the damage is advanced and you start to lose vision are you likely to notice that something is wrong. However, changes in the eye characteristic of retinopathy can be detected by an opthalmologist during a thorough eye examination before vision is affected. This is why, if you have diabetes, you should have your eyes checked regularly by an ophthalmologist. Diabetic retinopathy cannot be cured, but if it is caught early, it can be treated and, in many cases, managed successfully. You should also work with your health-care provider to keep your blood-sugar level well controlled. People with insulin-dependent diabetes who effectively control their blood-sugar levels may be able to slow the progress of diabetic retinopathy dramatically.

CONVENTIONAL TREATMENT

■ If a hole or tear in the retina is detected early, it can be sealed by cryotherapy (freezing) or laser surgery. These procedures can usually be performed under local anesthetic.

■ If detachment has begun, any accumulating fluid may be drained away, allowing the retina to resume its normal position while the tear is being repaired. This procedure also is usually done under local anesthetic.

■ In severe cases of retinal detachment, the hole in the retina can be sealed and a technique called *scleral buckling* used to fold the wall of the eye inward so that the retina is brought back into its normal position. This operation may be done under local or general anesthetic.

■ There is no conventional treatment that can halt the loss of vision caused by retinitis pigmentosa. Your doctor may, however, recommend various types of therapies and assistive devices to help you learn to carry on your normal activities despite declining vision.

■ Leaking blood vessels due to diabetic retinopathy can be sealed and the progress of runaway blood vessels stopped by laser surgery. If blood has entered the vitreous fluid, this jellylike substance can actually be removed from the eye and replaced with a satisfactory substitute.

DIETARY GUIDELINES

■ Maximize your intake of fresh fruits and vegetables. These healthy foods contain antioxidant phytochemicals that protect all the cells of the body, including those of the eyes.

Eat clean, lean protein food such as chicken and fish. Both protein and vitamin A are necessary for maintaining healthy eyes.

Limit sugar and caffeine. These substances contribute to and worsen the symptoms caused by many eye problems.

NUTRITIONAL SUPPLEMENTS

Take a good multivitamin and mineral supplement once or twice daily.

Chromium helps to stabilize blood sugar. If you are battling diabetic retinopathy, take 200 micrograms twice daily for three months, then reduce the dosage to 100 micrograms daily. GTF chromium is probably the best absorbed form of this mineral; however, it can be expensive if taken on an ongoing basis. Fortunately, studies suggest that chromium chloride, a cheaper form, should be adequately effective.

■ Coenzyme Q_{10} is an antioxidant that fights free-radical damage and is a blood oxygenator. This is another nutrient that can help in cases of retinopathy. Take 50 milligrams of coenzyme Q_{10} twice daily for up to three months, then reduce the dosage to 30 milligrams daily.

The essential fatty acids (EFAs) found in black currant seed oil, borage oil, evening primrose oil, and flaxseed oil, are required by every cell in the body. Choose one of the above oils and take 1 tablespoon (or 500 to 1,000 milligrams) three times daily.

Lutein, a carotenoid usually extracted from the marigold plant, has been shown to improve ocular health. Take 5 milligrams two or three times daily.

Selenium is an excellent antioxidant that helps prevent free-radical damage throughout the body, including the eyes. Take 100 micrograms once daily.

■ Vanadium, in the form of vanadyl sulfate, aids in blood-sugar regulation, a factor in diabetic retinopathy. Take 250 micrograms three times a day.

■ Vitamin A protects against free-radical damage and is especially important to the eyes. Without sufficient vitamin A, the eyes are more susceptible to infection, ulcerations, and even blindness. Further, taking therapeutic doses of vitamin A may slow the loss of vision due to retinitis pigmentosa by about 20 percent per year. Take 5,000 international units two or three times daily, and be sure to eat plenty of green and yellow vegetables. Beta-carotene also is a strong antioxidant that prevents free-radical damage. It is a precursor of vitamin A and has many of the same properties, but it does not become toxic in large doses. Take 5,000 international units of beta-carotene two or three times daily.

Note: If you are pregnant, or intend to get pregnant, or if you have liver disease, consult your doctor before taking supplemental vitamin A. Pregnant women should not ingest a total of more than 25,000 international units of supplemental vitamin A *per week* from all sources.

■ The B vitamins are required for intracellular metabolism in the tissues of the eyes. Combined with vitamins C and E, the B-complex vitamins are especially beneficial to the eyes. Twice a day, take a B-complex supplement that supplies 25 milligrams of each of the major B vitamins.

■ Vitamin C helps to lower the pressure within the eye, strengthen capillaries, maintain connective tissue, and prevent hemorrhaging, and is notable for speeding healing. Select a vitamin-C formula that includes bioflavonoids, especially rutin, and take 500 to 1,000 milligrams three times daily.

■ A deficiency of vitamin E is believed to be a factor in some cases of detached retina. Choose a product containing mixed tocopherols and take 200 international units twice daily.

Note: If you are taking an anticoagulant (blood thinner), consult your physician before taking supplemental vitamin E.

■ Zinc supports the immune system and aids in the healing process. A deficiency of zinc may contribute to retinal detachment. Take 25 to 50 milligrams of zinc daily.

Note: Take zinc with food to prevent stomach upset. If you take over 30 milligrams of zinc on a daily basis for more than one or two months, you should also take 1 to 2 milligrams of copper each day to maintain a proper mineral balance.

HERBAL TREATMENT

■ Bilberry provides important nutrients that nourish the eyes and enhance visual function. Phytochemicals called anthocyanidins in this herb also help prevent damage to the structures of the eyes. Bilberry extract may also help to slow the loss of sight caused by retinitis pigmentosa. Select a preparation containing 25 percent anthocyanidins (also called PCOs) and take 80 milligrams three times daily, or follow the directions on the product label.

■ Ginkgo biloba extract contains flavonoids with an affinity for organs that are rich in connective tissue, including the eyes. Ginkgo protects cellular membranes and has notable antioxidant properties. It also enhances the use of oxygen and glucose by the cells, and works to normalize circulation in areas that are affected by small blood clots. Laboratory studies suggest that it may help protect against diabetic retinopathy. Select standardized ginkgo leaf extract that contains at least 24 percent ginkgo heterosides (sometimes called flavoglycosides) and take 60 milligrams three times daily for one month, then cut back to 40 milligrams three times daily.

■ Gotu kola contains compounds called triterpenes that have a remarkable ability to speed the healing of wounds. It exerts a balancing and strengthening effect on connective tissue. Because of these effects, the extract is believed to be valuable both before and after treatment for detached retina. Choose a standardized extract containing 16 percent triterpenes and take 100 to 200 milligrams two or three times a day.

HOMEOPATHY

■ *Arnica* can help to relieve pain and speed healing after surgery. After undergoing any procedure to repair a torn or detached retina, take one dose of *Arnica* 30x or 15c four times daily for two days.

■ If retinal detachment was accompanied by seepage of fluid into the space behind the retina, *Apis mellifica* can encourage any remaining fluid to drain away. After surgery to drain the fluid, take one dose of *Apis mellifica* 30x or 15c every thirty minutes, up to a total of four doses.

■ If you are diagnosed with retinitis pigmentosa, consult a homeopathic physician who can formulate a constitutional remedy for you. It may be possible to reduce the rate of retinal degeneration.

GENERAL RECOMMENDATIONS

■ If you are over thirty-five, schedule an eye examination annually (or follow the schedule recommended by your eye doctor). Many eye problems are age related. When it comes to the eyes, early detection and, if necessary, treatment of developing problems can save your sight.

■ Avoid substances known to irritate the eyes, such as smog and smoke. Whether it comes from cigars, pipes, cigarettes, or sweet-smelling wood burning in a fireplace, smoke is very hard on the eyes and worsens symptoms.

PREVENTION

■ It may be possible to prevent retinal detachment if you can catch a developing problem early enough. Be aware of the characteristic signals of a detaching retina (see page 503). If you develop any of these signs, consult an ophthalmologist immediately.

■ Since it is possible for a retina to tear or detach following a blow to the head, take measures to protect yourself from head injury. When traveling by car, always wear your seat belt; in a plane, keep your seat belt loosely fastened at all times except when you must leave your seat. Wear goggles when using power tools (including lawnmowers), and always wear protective headgear for such activities as biking and roller-blading.

Rheumatism

See ARTHRITIS; BACK PAIN AND STRAIN; FIBROMYALGIA.

Rheumatoid Arthritis

See under ARTHRITIS.

Ringworm

Ringworm is not actually a worm, but a fungal infection that thrives on the outer layers of the scalp, skin, and nails. This is the same fungus (tinea) that causes "jock itch" and athlete's foot. Ringworm is highly contagious. Like athlete's foot, it spreads from one person to another via contaminated gymnasium floors and shower stalls at health clubs, public swimming pools, and other communal facilities. Contact with an affected animal will also spread the infection.

This condition typically appears as a slightly scaly lesion on the skin. It starts out as a small round, itchy red spot. The infection heals from the inside of the circle to the outer rim, giving rise to the typical ringlike look. It often spreads from one area of the body to another.

Ringworm is not a serious infection, but it can be persistent. To confirm a diagnosis, your doctor may gently scratch off some scaly particles from a lesion and examine them under a microscope. The fungus also tends to have a characteristic glow under ultraviolet light. With prompt treatment, ringworm generally clears up in a few weeks. If the fungus is not treated correctly, however, it can lead to a chronic rash or hair loss.

A related problem, *tinea versicolor*, shows up as a blotchy white discoloration of the skin. The darker the skin tone of the infected person, the more obvious the discoloration is. In a very light skinned person, it may not be visible at all unless he or she gets a suntan (the affected areas will remain white) or unless it is looked at under ultraviolet light. Other than the characteristic skin discoloration, tinea versicolor produces few, if any, symptoms, but it is extremely persistent and difficult to get rid of completely. Normal color cannot return to the affected area unless the fungus is completely eradicated and the skin is exposed to the sun.

CONVENTIONAL TREATMENT

■ Topical antifungals, available in cream and lotion form, usually bring about an improvement in ringworm within seven days. To decrease the chance of a recurrence, however, it is best to continue applying the medication for a full course of treatment of up to three weeks. Over-the-counter antifungals include miconazole (in Micatin and Monistat-Derm), clotrimazole (Lotrimin, Mycelex), and undecylenic acid (Cruex, Desenex).

■ If thorough treatment with a topical antifungal medication does not resolve the problem, it may be necessary to use an oral medication such as griseofulvin (Fulvicin, Grifulvin, Grisactin, Gris-PEG). This drug can have significant side effects, however, including allergic reactions, gastrointestinal upset, and liver toxicity, so it should be reserved for severe, resistant cases.

■ If the ringworm is on your scalp, use a shampoo that contains selenium sulfide (such as Selsun Blue) for at least one week.

■ It is possible for a secondary infection to develop alongside a case of ringworm. If you are treating a ringworm infection and you notice that the area is getting increasingly red, warm, tender, or swollen, or if you develop a fever or swollen glands, consult your doctor for advice about further treatment.

■ Treatment for tinea versicolor is similar to that for ringworm. In addition, the overnight application of a selenium sulfide shampoo, such as Selsun Blue, for three or four days, is often recommended.

DIETARY GUIDELINES

■ Eat plenty of vegetables. Vegetables are high in important vitamins and trace minerals. Green and yellow vegetables are especially recommended. The beta-carotene they contain is an important nutrient for all conditions involving the skin.

NUTRITIONAL SUPPLEMENTS

■ Methylsulfonylmethane (MSM) is a good source of sulfur, a trace mineral that helps to fight parasites and fungi. It can be applied directly to the affected area in cream or spray form. Follow the directions on the product label.

HERBAL TREATMENT

■ Balsam of Peru is useful for many skin conditions. Apply it to the affected area two or three times a day for

two to three weeks. You can apply it either full strength or diluted with olive, almond, or sesame oil.

■ Calendula ointment can be used to moisten the affected area if the skin is dry.

■ Cat's claw enhances the immune response and has antifungal properties. Take 500 milligrams of standardized extract three times a day until the infection clears.

Note: Do not use cat's claw if you are pregnant or nursing, or if you are an organ-transplant recipient. Use it with caution if you are taking an anticoagulant (blood thinner).

■ Ginger contains some twenty-three antifungal compounds, of which caprylic acid is perhaps the most potent. Simmer 1 to 2 ounces of fresh ginger root in 6 to 8 ounces of water for fifteen to twenty minutes, and drink the resulting tea. You can also apply it directly to the lesions. Do this three times daily.

■ Olive leaf extract acts as an immune-system fortifier and has antifungal properties. Take 250 milligrams of standardized extract three times a day for one month while you are treating the infection topically.

■ Turmeric has noted anti-inflammatory properties. Take 300 milligrams of standardized extract three times daily.

HOMEOPATHY

■ Take one dose of *Sulfur* 30x or 9c three times a day for three days.

AROMATHERAPY

For specific instructions on how to use aromatherapy, *see* PREPARING AROMATHERAPY TREATMENTS in Part Three.

■ Tea tree oil is one of the strongest known natural antifungals, and is very effective against ringworm. Mix 8 to 10 drops of tea tree oil and 4 drops of grapefruit-seed extract in 2 tablespoons of spring or distilled water and apply the mixture to the affected area three times daily until the rash goes away.

Note: If you are using tea tree oil and also taking a homeopathic preparation, allow one hour between the two. Otherwise, the pungent odor of the tea tree oil may cancel out the action of the homeopathic remedy.

GENERAL RECOMMENDATIONS

■ Keep your skin clean, cool, and dry. Fungi thrive in warm, moist environments. Loose cotton clothing is best, as it allows air to circulate next to the skin.

■ To decrease the possibility of reinfection and to prevent the spread of ringworm to other members of the household, wash your clothing after each wearing. Do not share clothing, combs, hats, socks, pillows, or sheets with anyone else.

PREVENTION

■ Practice good hygiene, especially careful hand-washing.

■ Avoid contact with affected animals. The signs and symptoms of ringworm in animals are the same as in humans. If you notice the telltale ring or patches of hair loss on the household dog, cat, ferret, or other furry pet, take the animal to a veterinarian for examination and treatment.

Rocky Mountain Spotted Fever

See under LYME AND OTHER TICKBORNE DISEASES.

Rosacea

Rosacea is an inflammatory skin disorder that primarily affects the skin in the central portion of the face. On the surface, it often resembles acne, with redness, swelling, bumps, and pimples. However, it can also cause the small blood vessels beneath the skin to dilate and become visible as reddish blotches known as *telangiectasias*. If left untreated, it can lead to permanent thickening and redness of the skin tissue, especially of the nose, a condition called *rhinophyma*. And unlike acne, it does not cause the development of blackheads or whiteheads, those oily plugs that block the pores.

The cause of this condition is not known, but it is known that it is more common in lighter skinned people than in those with darker complexions. It is also more common in women than in men. Although rosacea may occur in children as young as ten years old, most people who get it are between thirty and fifty.

CONVENTIONAL TREATMENT

■ Medical treatment for rosacea usually begins with antibiotic gel or lotion applied directly to the affected area. Topical metronidazole (MetroGel) is usually tried first. If this is not effective, or if you are unable to tolerate it, topical clindamycin (Cleocin T) may be substituted. Response to either of these drugs normally takes five to eight weeks.

■ Occasionally, a 1-percent hydrocortisone cream may be used early in treatment to relieve inflammation. Stronger steroid preparations are *not* used, as these can make the problem worse.

■ If local treatment is not successful, your doctor may

also prescribe an oral antibiotic such as tetracycline (also sold under the brand name Achromycin). Tetracycline is not suitable, however, for women who are or who may become pregnant, as it can cause discoloration in the teeth of the developing fetus. It can also cause a rare but very dangerous form of diarrhea or colitis, so if you must take this drug, you should be alert for any signs that you may be developing abdominal distress.

■ If rosacea resists all types of antibiotic treatment, your doctor may recommend trying isotretinoin (Accutane), a synthetic compound that resembles vitamin A. This drug can have a wide range of potentially serious side effects, including arthritis, elevation of blood fats, liver toxicity, nosebleeds, cracking at the corners of the mouth, and extreme dryness of the eyes. It also causes severe birth defects if taken during pregnancy. As a result, doctors tend to avoid prescribing it for any woman of childbearing age. If they do, they are likely to require that such women use more than one form of birth control and take pregnancy tests monthly.

■ Telangiectasias may be treated with laser surgery.

■ If long-term, severe rosacea results in rhinophyma, plastic surgery may be recommended to improve appearance.

■ Be aware that certain drugs may cause rosacea flare-ups. For example, vasodilators, which are used in the treatment of cardiovascular disease, can cause "vasodilator rosacea." Discuss this possibility with your doctor.

■ *Avoid* using topical steroid creams on an ongoing basis. This can aggravate rosacea.

DIETARY GUIDELINES

■ Eat a well-balanced diet that emphasizes raw and lightly cooked vegetables. Green leafy vegetables in particular are good because they contain lots of fiber and valuable trace minerals.

■ Drink at least eight 8-ounce glasses of pure water every day.

■ Eat your food warm, but not steaming hot, and reduce the heat of hot beverages. Exposure to heat, especially drinking a very hot cup of tea or coffee, may aggravate your skin.

■ Keep your intake of animal fats and hydrogenated oils to an absolute minimum. That means avoiding dairy products, margarine, vegetable shortening, red meat, and all fried foods. These fats are used to produce a type of prostaglandin (a hormonelike body chemical) that promotes inflammation.

■ Be aware of how your body reacts to alcoholic beverages. Alcoholic beverages often induce flare-ups. Obviously, if alcohol aggravates your condition, you should limit or avoid alcohol.

■ Avoid hot, spicy foods such as white and black pepper, red pepper, and chilies.

■ Avoid junk foods, fast foods, refined sugars, and anything containing additives such as artificial flavorings, colorings, or preservatives. All of these contribute to an unhealthy internal environment, which may show up in the skin.

■ Investigate the possibility of hidden food sensitivities and allergies, which can cause increased inflammation. (*See* ELIMINATION DIET in Part Three.) Then avoid any foods that seem to cause a problem.

NUTRITIONAL SUPPLEMENTS

■ Take a good-quality multivitamin and mineral supplement daily.

■ If you must take antibiotics, be sure to take a supplement containing acidophilus and bifidobacteria to restore the normal friendly bacteria in the intestines. Take a probiotic supplement as recommended on the product label. Be sure to take this supplement at least one hour before or after taking antibiotics, as antibiotics kill off both good and bad bacteria.

■ Beta-carotene and vitamin A are healing to the skin. While vitamin A can be toxic in large doses, beta-carotene—which the body uses to produce vitamin A as needed— appears to be extremely safe. Take 25,000 international units of beta-carotene and 10,000 international units of vitamin A, twice daily, five days a week, for one month.

Note: If you are pregnant, or intend to get pregnent, or if you have liver disease, consult your doctor before taking supplemental vitamin A. Pregnant women should not ingest a total of more than 25,000 international units of supplemental vitamin A *per week* from all sources.

■ Flaxseed oil and fish oils contain essential fatty acids that are helpful for reducing inflammation. Take 1 teaspoon (or 500 to 1,000 milligrams) of either two or three times daily.

■ The B vitamins are essential for the synthesis of hormones and a healthy nervous system. Vitamin B_2 (riboflavin) is also essential for healthy skin, hair, and nails. Take a B-complex supplement supplying 50 to 75 milligrams of each of the major B vitamins two or three times daily.

■ Vitamin C promotes healing and helps strengthen connective tissue; bioflavonoids strengthen the blood vessels and act as a natural anti-inflammatory. Take 500 milligrams of each three times a day, between meals, for one month. After that, take 500 milligrams of each twice daily for one month. Then reduce the dosage to 500 milligrams of each once a day.

■ Zinc has a healing effect on skin cells. Take 25 milligrams of zinc twice daily (at the beginning of a meal) for two weeks. Then reduce the dosage to 25 milligrams daily.

Note: Take zinc with food to prevent stomach upset. If you take over 30 milligrams of zinc on a daily basis for more than one or two months, you should also take 1 to 2 milligrams of copper each day to maintain a proper mineral balance.

HERBAL TREATMENT

■ Cat's claw helps to reestablish a healthy intestinal environment so that food sensitivities may be reduced. It also acts as an anti-inflammatory. Take 500 milligrams of standardized extract three times a day.

Note: Do not use cat's claw if you are pregnant or nursing, or if you are an organ-transplant recipient. Use it with caution if you are taking an anticoagulant (blood thinner).

■ Chaste tree berry (also known by its Latin name, *Vitex agnus-castus*) aids in hormonal regulation. Take 200 milligrams of standardized extract two or three times daily for two weeks out of each month. If you are a woman of childbearing age, take it during the two weeks before the anticipated onset of your menstrual period.

■ Gotu kola promotes healing of the skin. Choose a standardized extract containing 16 percent triterpenes and take 100 milligrams two to three times daily for up to six weeks at a time.

■ Grape-seed extract aids in collagen formation and is an anti-inflammatory. Take 50 milligrams three times daily.

■ Jigucao is a Chinese herbal patent medicine that is very useful in the treatment of rosacea. Take 500 milligrams two or three times daily.

ACUPRESSURE

For the locations of acupressure points on the body, *see* ADMINISTERING AN ACUPRESSURE TREATMENT in Part Three.

■ Large Intestine 4 has a beneficial effect on the head and face.

HOMEOPATHY

■ *Arsenicum album* is for a dry, burning, face with scaly and flaky skin, possibly accompanied by feelings of restlessness. Take one dose of *Arsenicum album* 30x or 15c three times daily for up to three days.

■ Choose *Nux vomica* if symptoms are made worse by drinking coffee, tea, or alcoholic beverages.

■ *Rhus toxicodendron* is helpful for skin that is swollen and puffy, with itchy, painful red spots. Cold or wet weather makes symptoms worse. Take one dose of *Rhus toxicodendron* 12x or 6c three times a day for up to three days.

■ *Sanguinaria* is good for itching and burning skin that is aggravated by heat, especially for women whose menstrual periods are scanty. Take one dose of *Sanguinaria* 12x or 6c three times daily for up to three days.

■ *Sulfur* is for inflamed skin that becomes worse after exposure to heat or a hot bath. Take one dose of *Sulfur* 30x or 15c three times daily for up to three days.

■ There are also many homeopathic combination skin remedies that may be helpful for acute symptoms. Take as directed on the product label.

AROMATHERAPY

For specific instructions on how to use aromatherapy, *see* PREPARING AROMATHERAPY TREATMENTS in Part Three.

■ Calming oils such as chamomile and lavender can help to reduce stress, which often exacerbates this condition. Use either or both in soothing aromatherapy baths.

GENERAL RECOMMENDATIONS

■ Always protect your face from the sun. Wear a sunscreen with a sun protection factor (SPF) of 15 or higher year-round. You may have to use a product formulated for children to avoid irritation. Wear a broad-brimmed hat when outdoors, and minimize midday (10:00 AM to 2:00 PM) exposure to the sun, especially in the summer.

■ As much as possible, stay in a cool, air-conditioned environment on hot, humid days. Sip cool drinks and try not to exert yourself. Spray cool water on your face from time to time.

■ Beware of the cold—cover your cheeks and nose with a soft scarf when going out in cold weather. When participating in outdoor activities, you may want to wear a ski mask made of soft, hypoallergenic material.

■ Keep your skin clean, but treat it gently to avoid irritating it further. Using a mild soap or cleanser and cool to lukewarm (not hot) water, wash your face no more than twice a day. Castile and hypoallergenic soaps, or ones made with calendula or chamomile, are best.

■ Avoid touching, picking at, or scratching the affected area. This will only irritate the skin and make matters worse.

■ Use a moisturizer daily. This will protect against the drying effects of the wind and cold in the winter and dehydration during the summer months.

■ Avoid using facial products, such as witch hazel and isopropyl alcohol, that can sting, burn, or cause facial redness. Use only fragrance-free, hypoallergenic skin-care products.

■ If you feel you must wear makeup, use only water-based preparations made with gentle, natural ingredients. Harsh chemicals can worsen inflammation.

■ Men should shave with an electric razor rather than a blade. Avoid shaving lotions that burn or sting.

■ Take warm, not hot, showers, and avoid exposing your face to steamy heat, whether from relaxing in a hot bath, tending to hot pots cooking on the stove, or anything else. Avoid hot tubs, steam rooms, and saunas.

■ Get regular exercise, but avoid heavy exertion or high-intensity workouts that cause overheating and bring on flushing. Try low-intensity exercise routines (which often can be just as effective) and consider exercising for shorter periods. For example, you might work out for fifteen to twenty minutes three times a day rather than forty-five minutes to an hour all at once. If you exercise indoors, make sure the exercise room is well ventilated.

■ Consider yoga. Stretch out and relax your muscles.

■ When under stress, try deep breathing. Inhale to a slow count of ten, then exhale to a slow count of ten.

■ Use visualization techniques. Sit in a quiet place, close your eyes, and visualize a peaceful image. Hold this image for several minutes.

■ Consider consulting a physician who utilizes hyperbaric oxygen therapy. Many people with rosacea have found this treatment very beneficial.

Salmonella

See under FOOD POISONING.

Scabies

Scabies is a skin rash caused by a tiny crablike mite. The mites burrow into and lay eggs in soft areas of the skin, such as the buttocks, genitals, wrists, armpits, and between the toes and fingers.

The rash is characterized by small red lumps that may become dry and scaly. It can be very itchy, especially at night. You may also notice tiny, thin light-gray or pink lines on your skin. These are the burrowing tunnels.

Scabies is highly contagious and spreads through skin-to-skin contact or through contact with infested clothing, sheets, or towels. It can also be caught from infested animals. If you develop scabies, all close contacts and members of your household should be checked for this infestation.

Scabies can usually be treated successfully at home. If the inflammation persists after one week of treatment, if it becomes worse, or if new bumps develop, call your health-care provider for advice.

CONVENTIONAL TREATMENT

■ The diagnosis of scabies is made by examination of the distribution and characteristic appearance of the rash. Sometimes the mites can be scraped off and seen under a microscope.

Permethrin lotion (sold as Nix or Elimite) kills the mites by attacking their nervous systems. It is safer and more effective than the better known lindane, or gamma benzene hexachloride (found in Kwell), which is chemically related to DDT and can cause headaches and nervous-system damage. Another alternative is crotamiton cream (Eurax), which is safer than gamma benzene hexachloride and also has anti-itch properties.

An over-the-counter spray called RID is useful for treating infested clothes and bedding.

A topical steroid, such as cortisone, or an oral antihistamine, such as diphenhydramine (in Allerdryl, Benadryl, and many other over-the-counter products) or hydroxyzine (Atarax, Vistaril), may be suggested to help lessen the itching while the antiparasitic medication is taking effect. You should be aware that an antihistamine will also likely have the effect of making you sleepy.

An antibiotic is not necessary unless a bacterial secondary infection results from scratching and breaking the skin.

DIETARY GUIDELINES

To decrease your vulnerability to infestation and boost your immune system, make sure you eat foods that contain plenty of zinc. Foods that are high in zinc include egg yolks, fish, milk, blackstrap molasses, sesame seeds, pumpkinseeds, soybeans, sunflower seeds, turkey, wheat bran, wheat germ, whole-grain products, and yeast.

HERBAL TREATMENT

Balsam of Peru has antiparasitic properties and is useful against scabies. It can be applied either full strength or diluted with olive, almond, or sesame oil.

Calendula and goldenseal ointments are commercially available. The calendula is healing and soothing to the skin; the goldenseal helps to heal infection. Apply the mixture to the affected area three times a day.

■ Comfrey root makes an excellent topical salve. Apply this three times a day.

HOMEOPATHY

■ *Antimonium crudum* is good for a dry skin rash with pimples or vesicles. The itching is often worse at night.

Take one dose of *Antimonium crudum* 12x or 6c, as directed on the product label, three times a day for up to three days.

■ *Arsenicum album* is for a dry, rough, scaly rash. The itching may be accompanied by a burning sensation and restlessness, and the rash feels worse when you are exposed to cold. Take one dose of *Arsenicum album* 12x or 6c three times a day for up to three days.

■ *Sulfur* is for red, dry, hot-looking skin patches accompanied by sweating and a feeling of warmth. You typically throw off the covers when you sleep and want your skin exposed to the air. Take one dose of *Sulfur* 30x or 9c twice a day (at 11:00 AM and 3:00 PM) for up to three days.

AROMATHERAPY

■ Essential oil of tea tree is a strong disinfectant. Paint the affected area with tea tree oil twice a day.

GENERAL RECOMMENDATIONS

■ Thoroughly wash all bedding, towels, and clothing in very hot water. Spray them with RID according to the directions on the package.

■ Take cool oatmeal baths to help lessen the itching.

PREVENTION

■ Do not share clothes, bedding, or towels.

■ Avoid handling strange animals.

Sciatica

Sciatica is a form of low back pain characterized by discomfort that radiates down the buttock, often reaching as far down as below the knee, usually on only one side. The pain follows the pathway of the sciatic nerve, the longest nerve in the body, which connects the spinal cord with the leg and foot. Sciatica can be caused by herniation, or rupture, of one of the intervertebral disks. These are pads composed of a firm outer layer surrounding softer material. They sit between individual vertebrae in the spine. When a disk herniates, the outer layer ruptures and the interior of the disk bulges out of it, which in turn can irritate nerves at the site of the bulge. Sciatica can also be caused by arthritis of the vertebral joints; inflammation at the spot where the bones of the pelvis join together, known as sacroiliitis; scarring of the spinal canal in the area through which the nerves pass; and even external pressure on the lower back or buttock, a condition sometimes referred to as "wallet sciatica."

CONVENTIONAL TREATMENT

The primary goal of treatment is to relieve the pain. The appropriate type of painkiller depends on the pain's severity. Nonsteroidal anti-inflammatory drugs (NSAIDs) such as ibuprofen (Advil, Motrin, Nuprin, and others) and naproxen (Aleve, Anaprox, Naprelan, Naprosyn) are usually tried first, and are the cornerstone of pain treatment. Potential side effects of the NSAIDs are primarily gastrointestinal, and include nausea, vomiting, bleeding, and even ulcers. These drugs should be taken with food to minimize stomach upset.

■ If NSAIDs do not provide sufficient pain relief, stronger pain medication may be prescribed. Among these are hydrocodone and codeine, both of which are sold under different brand names, often combined with acetaminophen, aspirin, or ibuprofen. These are powerful narcotics, and can cause dizziness, drowsiness, nausea, vomiting, constipation, and other side effects. They also have the potential to be addictive.

If ordinary pain medications fail, a muscle relaxant such as diazepam (Valium) or carisoprodol (Soma) may be tried, though their effectiveness has not been conclusively proved. Side effects of these medications can include dizziness and drowsiness, and these drugs too can be habit-forming.

■ Recent research indicates that long periods of rest, even with controlled back exercises, seem to offer little benefit. Doctors now consider it preferable to carry on with your normal activities as much as possible.

Physical therapy can be very helpful.

If sciatica is due to a ruptured disk or other anatomical abnormality, surgery may be recommended.

DIETARY GUIDELINES

Eat a diet that is high in fiber, and that includes plenty of fresh vegetables and fruits, to ensure regular and healthy bowel movements. Poor bowel habits can make the pain of sciatica worse.

■ Avoid eating large meals.

NUTRITIONAL SUPPLEMENTS

Take a high-potency multivitamin and mineral supplement to ensure a full supply of all the nutrients needed to support healthy nerves.

■ Bromelain, an enzyme derived from pineapple, has a notable anti-inflammatory action. Take 300 to 500 milligrams three times daily, between meals.

Calcium and magnesium are useful for relaxing back muscles that have an impact on the sciatic nerve. Take 500 to 600 milligrams of each twice daily.

■ Lysine is an amino acid that inhibits viruses. Some experts believe that sciatic pain is associated with viral activity. Take 500 milligrams of L-lysine two or three times daily for two weeks during acute flare-ups.

HERBAL TREATMENT

■ Turmeric is a strong natural anti-inflammatory. Take 500 milligrams four times daily while symptoms are acute.

HOMEOPATHY

■ *Ammonium muriaticum* is helpful for pain that is significantly worse when sitting but improves when you are lying down or walking. You feel pain when you straighten the affected leg, the hamstring is contracted, and you may feel somewhat melancholy. Take one dose of *Ammonium muriaticum* 12x or 6c four times daily, up to a total of ten doses.

■ *Arsenicum album* is good for sciatica in older adults and in people with some degree of debility. The pain, which is burning and may be accompanied by trembling, twitching, and spasms, is typically worse in cold weather and at night, but better with moderate, gentle exercise. Take one dose of *Arsenicum album* 30x or 15c three times daily, up to a total of ten doses.

■ *Colocynthis* is for pain that shoots down the leg to the foot and that feels better with strong pressure and/or warmth. The muscles are contracted and in spasm, the joints are stiff, and there may be cramplike pain in the hip. Take one dose of *Colocynthis* 12x or 6c four times daily, up to a total of ten doses.

■ *Gnaphalium dioicum* is helpful for pain and cramps in the leg that are worse with movement and better with rest and while sitting down. The pain is accompanied by numbness. Take one dose of *Gnaphalium dioicum* 12x or 6c four times daily, up to a total of ten doses.

■ *Rhus toxicodendron* is for pain that is alleviated by heat and movement and worse with cold or damp and while sitting or in a stationary position. Take one dose of *Rhus toxicodendron* 30x or 15c four times daily, up to a total of ten doses.

■ There are also many combination sciatica remedies available that are effective for acute symptoms.

■ If you suffer from chronic sciatica, consult a homeopathic physician who can prescribe a constitutional remedy tailored specifically to your needs and symptoms.

ACUPRESSURE

For the locations of acupressure points on the body, *see* ADMINISTERING AN ACUPRESSURE TREATMENT in Part Three.

■ The combination of Gallbladder 20 and 30, Liver 3,

Spleen 6, and Stomach 36 is helpful for relaxing the nervous system and improving circulation.

AROMATHERAPY

For specific instructions on how to use aromatherapy, *see* PREPARING AROMATHERAPY TREATMENTS in Part Three.

■ Essential oils of ginger, lavender, marjoram, and rosemary help to stimulate circulation. Use one or more (up to a total of three) in massage oil or in baths.

GENERAL RECOMMENDATIONS

■ Wear comfortable shoes. Especially avoid wearing high heels

■ Swimming is excellent exercise for people with sciatica. Water physical therapy is even better. The water gives you buoyancy and allows you to exercise without placing stress on the spine.

PREVENTION

■ Do not sit in one position for too long at a time. Your muscles tighten when you assume a stationary position, such as sitting at a desk.

■ Stretch! Yoga and yoga-like stretching are very effective in preventing sciatic pain from returning.

■ Do exercises to strengthen your abdominal muscles. If your abdominal muscles are strong, your lower back is stronger and healthier. Sit-ups are a great preventive.

Scleroderma

Also called progressive systemic sclerosis, this is a disease that attacks the skin and connective tissue, and can also affect internal organs. The skin typically becomes thickened, stiffened, and taut, and often darkens. This may happen across wide areas of the body, or to the fingers and hands only. Eventually, the joints can contract and "freeze" in position as a result. The esophagus and the rest of the digestive tract are often affected as well, resulting in difficulty swallowing and poor motility of the entire gastrointestinal tract, which in turn can lead to an overgrowth of bacteria in the intestines and problems with nutrient absorption. Heartburn is also a common problem. Scarring and thickening can also affect the lungs and liver, potentially leading to shortness of breath and cirrhosis of the liver, and there can be abnormal changes in the kidneys and cardiovascular system that can result in high blood pressure, abnormal heart rhythm, heart failure, and pulmonary hypertension, a dangerous complication. Arthritis, fever, and swelling in areas of the skin are com-

mon. Most people with scleroderma also suffer from Raynaud's phenomenon, in which cold temperatures or emotional upset can cause a sharp drop in circulation to the fingers and toes, and sometimes the nose and ears (*see* RAYNAUD'S PHENOMENON).

The cause or causes of scleroderma are unknown, and the severity of symptoms and progression of the disease are both extremely variable. The condition is more common in women than in men. The most significant known factor in predicting the severity of the illness is whether you have full-system disease or only those facets of it that make up what is known as the CREST syndrome: *c*alcinosis cutis (deposits of calcium in the skin); *R*aynaud's phenomenon; *e*sophageal involvement; *s*clerodactyly (hardness and shrinking of the skin of the fingers); and *t*elangiectasias (the appearance of red spots in the skin due to the dilation of small groups of blood vessels). The consequences are usually less severe for people with the CREST syndrome than for those with full-system disease, which in the worst cases can become life-threatening in a matter of a few years as a result of scarring damage to vital internal organs. The prognosis tends to be poorer for elderly people, for men, and for people of African ancestry.

CONVENTIONAL TREATMENT

■ There is no known cure for scleroderma, and no specific treatment for the disease as a whole. Treatment focuses on relieving symptoms and providing supportive care as individual problems arise.

■ If you have great difficulty swallowing and suffer from acid reflux, your doctor will likely recommend switching to a diet of puréed foods, elevating the head of your bed, and avoiding late-night meals to minimize scarring as a result of acid in the esophagus. Antacids and acid-blocking agents such as cimetidine (Tagamet) and famotidine (Pepcid) are also used, though newer acid-blockers of the type known as proton-pump inhibitors appear to block acid in the stomach more completely. Examples include omeprazole (Prilosec) and lansoprazole (Prevacid). Unfortunately, these drugs can have side effects, including diarrhea, nausea, and abdominal pain.

■ If bacterial overgrowth develops in the intestinal tract, it may be treated with the antibiotic tetracycline (also sold under the brand name Achromycin). Potential side effects of this medication include nausea, dizziness, blood changes, rashes, and the possibility of secondary infection by organisms that are resistant to it.

■ High blood pressure is usually treated with angiotensin converting enzyme (ACE) inhibitors such as captopril (Capoten) and enalapril (Vasotec). Potential side effects of these drugs include a persistent dry cough, rash, disturbances in the sense of taste, and fatigue. (*See* HIGH BLOOD PRESSURE.)

■ Occasionally, the drug penicillamine (Cuprimine, De-pen) or cyclophosphamide (Cytoxan) may be suggested. Penicillamine is a drug sometimes used for rheumatoid arthritis; cyclophosphamide is an agent used in cancer chemotherapy. There is some evidence that these drugs may help to slow the skin changes and organ damage associated with scleroderma, though there is some controversy as to their effectiveness. Both are extremely powerful and highly toxic, and have a wide range of potentially serious side effects.

DIETARY GUIDELINES

■ Eat a diet that consists of fresh vegetables, fruits, lean protein foods, whole grains, and nuts, seeds, and legumes (if you are able to digest them).

■ Include in your diet cold-water fish such as salmon for their content of essential fatty acids.

■ Avoid any foods you have a sensitivity or allergy to. Use an elimination diet to investigate the possibility of hidden food allergies and sensitivities (see ELIMINATION DIET in Part Three).

■ Drink six to eight 8-ounce glasses of pure water daily to flush toxins from your system.

■ Avoid meat (especially red meat), dairy products, tofu, alcohol, caffeine, refined sugars, spicy foods, fried foods, sauces and gravies, and excessive amounts of salt, all of which place added stress on the body.

NUTRITIONAL SUPPLEMENTS

■ Take a good multivitamin and mineral complex daily. Choose a powder or capsule form, which is more easily absorbed.

■ DHEA is a hormone that has been found to useful for lupus, and that may also be helpful for other autoimmune diseases. You may want to try taking 5 milligrams in the morning for six out of the seven days of the week. The long-term effects of swallowing this hormone (rather than using only the amount your body makes) are not well established, however, so if you are interested in using it, we recommend that you consult a physician experienced in its use. DHEA is not recommended for people under forty.

■ To ensure proper digestion, take a full-spectrum digestive-enzyme supplement providing 5,000 international units of lipase, 2,500 international units of amylase, 300 international units of protease with each meal.

■ Evening primrose and flaxseed oils contain essential fatty acids that are vital for the health of the skin and connective tissue, and that also have anti-inflammatory effects. Take 1 tablespoon (or 500 to 1,000 milligrams) once or twice daily.

■ Fish oils contain essential fatty acids that aid in controlling the inflammatory response. Take 1,000 milligrams twice a day.

■ Probiotic supplements such as acidophilus or bifidobacteria promote intestinal health. Take a probiotic supplement twice a day, as directed on the product label.

■ Vitamin C is a mild ant-inflammatory and is needed for the production of collagen, a key protein in skin and connective tissue. Take 500 to 1,000 milligrams three times daily.

■ Vitamin E also is an antioxidant and aids in tissue healing. Choose a product containing mixed tocopherols and start by taking 200 international units daily, then gradually increase the dosage until you are taking 400 international units in the morning and another 400 international units in the evening.

Note: If you have high blood pressure, limit your intake of supplemental vitamin E to 400 international units daily. If you are taking an anticoagulant (blood thinner), consult your physician before taking vitamin E.

HERBAL TREATMENT

■ Cat's claw is an anti-inflammatory that is particularly useful if "leaky gut syndrome" is part of the picture. Take 500 to 1,000 milligrams three times a day.

Note: Do not use cat's claw if you are pregnant or nursing, or if you are an organ-transplant recipient. Use it with caution if you are taking an anticoagulant (blood thinner).

■ Gotu kola has been found to have some efficacy in the treatment of scleroderma. It appears to decrease skin hardening and improve joint pain. Choose a standardized extract containing 16 percent triterpenes and take 200 milligrams two to three times daily.

■ Pine-bark and grape-seed extract improve circulation and decrease inflammation. Take 50 milligrams of either two or three times daily.

HOMEOPATHY

The best approach to treating a chronic disorder such as scleroderma homeopathically is to consult a homeopathic physician who can prescribe a constitutional remedy. For relief of acute symptoms, try one of the symptom-specific remedies below.

■ *Graphites* is good for dry skin that is itchy and stinging, with red spots. Take one dose of *Graphites* 12x or 6c four times daily, up to a total of ten doses.

■ *Secale cornutum* is helpful for skin that is flaccid, rough, and dry. You may have sensations as if insects were crawling on your skin. Take one dose of *Secale cornutum* 12x or 6c four times daily, up to a total of ten doses.

■ *Calcarea fluorica* is for skin that is harsh and dry. Take one dose of *Calcarea fluorica* 6x four times daily, up to a total of ten doses.

AROMATHERAPY

For specific instructions on how to use aromatherapy, *see* PREPARING AROMATHERAPY TREATMENTS in Part Three.

■ Essential oil of orange is rejuvenating to the nervous system. Use it as an inhalant, add a few drops to massage oil and use it in conjunction with massage, or make soothing aromatherapy baths with it.

Seasonal Affective Disorder (SAD)

See under DEPRESSION.

Seborrhea

Seborrhea, or seborrheic dermatitis, is a skin disorder characterized by dry or greasy scaly patches that may be somewhat red or yellowish and may or may not be itchy. It most commonly occurs on the scalp and face (including the eyelids), as well as on the chest and back and within skin folds. In infants, it can occur on the scalp, and is known as cradle cap. This disorder has a tendency to recur intermittently for life, with outbreaks lasting from weeks to years. Symptoms tend to be worse in people infected with HIV. Scratching can cause the problem to spread, but it can also spread without scratching. Dry climates often make things worse. The cause is unknown, but in some cases nutritional deficiencies may be involved, particularly deficiencies of zinc, selenium, and/or essential fatty acids. Seborrhea also seems to have a hereditary component.

CONVENTIONAL TREATMENT

■ For seborrhea on the scalp, shampoos containing zinc pyrithione (such as DHS Zinc), selenium sulfide (Selsun Blue), tar (DHS Tar), or ketoconazole (Nizoral shampoo) can be tried to see which is most effective. Ketoconazole is an antifungal agent, and the fact that it can help suggests that a fungus may be involved, but this is not fully established.

■ Seborrheic patches on the face are usually treated with mild steroid creams or ointments containing 1 percent hydrocortisone. Stronger steroids should be avoided be-

cause they can cause thinning of the skin and/or a form of rosacea (*see* ROSACEA). Topical ketoconazole (Nizoral) may be helpful as well. If you use a steroid ointment, keep it away from your eyes to avoid possible complications.

■ For other areas of the body, low-potency steroid creams or lotions, along with ketoconazole lotion, are the mainstay of treatment.

■ If you are HIV-positive and suffer from seborrhea, it may respond to the use of both clotrimazole cream (Lotrimin) and mild steroid creams. People with HIV seem to respond to clotrimazole better than to other antifungals.

DIETARY GUIDELINES

■ Consider adding sea vegetables—such as granulated kelp as a seasoning, dulse and hijiki in salads, and kombu cooked with beans or other vegetables—to your diet. Sea vegetables contain good amounts of iodine and trace minerals, which are important for skin health.

■ Make sure your diet supplies sufficient clean, lean protein, which is vital for the healing and repair of the skin. If it doesn't, or if you are not sure, consider taking a free-form amino-acid supplement (*see under* Nutritional Supplements, below).

■ Avoid fried foods, refined sugars, and chocolate. All of these can contribute to skin problems.

■ Investigate the possibility that food allergies or sensitivities may be contributing to the problem. (*See* ELIMINATION DIET in Part Three.)

NUTRITIONAL SUPPLEMENTS

■ Coenzyme Q_{10} improves the transport of oxygen to skin cells. Take 60 milligrams of coenzyme Q_{10} twice daily for one month, then reduce the dosage to 30 milligrams once or twice daily.

■ Seborrhea is sometimes associated with poor digestion, which aggravates the condition. Try taking supplemental digestive enzymes for six to eight weeks to aid in the breakdown of food, and see if your condition improves. Take a full-spectrum digestive-enzyme supplement providing 5,000 international units of lipase, 2,500 international units of amylase, and 300 international units of protease, plus 500 to 1,000 milligrams of pancreatin, with the two largest meals of the day.

Note: Long-term supplementation with pancreatin is not advised, as it can cause your pancreas to reduce its own production of this important enzyme. Overuse also has the potential to cause nausea or diarrhea. After two months on pancreatin, discontinue use and monitor your reaction. If you find that your problems recur, discuss pancreatin supplementation with your health-care provider.

■ To assure a good supply of all basic nutrients, take a

multivitamin and mineral complex supplying at least 50 milligrams of each of the major B vitamins twice daily. This is particularly important if your physician has prescribed antibiotic therapy. In addition, consider taking a probiotic supplement twice daily to replace the good bacteria destroyed by antibiotic treatment.

■ Take supplemental probiotics such as acidophilus and/or bifidus to restore beneficial intestinal flora. Take them as recommended on the product labels. If you are allergic to milk, select dairy-free formulas.

■ Vitamin-A deficiency can lead to seborrhea. Take 25,000 international units of mycellized vitamin A twice a day for two weeks, then reduce to 25,000 international units once daily.

Note: If you are pregnant, or intend to get pregnant, or if you have liver disease, consult your doctor before taking supplemental vitamin A. A pregnant woman should not ingest a total of more than 25,000 international units of supplemental vitamin A *per week* from all sources.

■ Vitamin E helps to speed skin-tissue healing. Start by taking 200 international units daily and gradually increase the dosage until you are taking 400 international units once or twice daily.

Note: If you have high blood pressure, limit your intake of supplemental vitamin E to a total of 400 international units daily. If you are taking an anticoagulant (blood thinner), consult your physician before taking vitamin E.

■ Selenium is an antioxidant that works with vitamin E. Take 100 micrograms daily for two months.

HERBAL TREATMENT

■ Massaging burdock-root oil, available in health-food stores, into the scalp has long been used by herbalists in the treatment of seborrhea. This can be mixed with an equal amount of calendula oil for its soothing properties.

HOMEOPATHY

■ *Mezereum* is good if the skin is intensely itchy, with thick, leathery crusts. Take one dose of *Mezereum* 12x or 6c three times daily for three to five days.

■ *Psorinum* is the remedy for intolerable itching with oily skin due to overactive sebaceous glands. You may be extremely sensitive to cold and feel hopeless about the possibility of recovery. Take one dose of *Psorinum* 200x or 200c once weekly for three weeks.

■ *Sulfur* is helpful for dry, scaly, itchy, burning skin that is made worse by scratching. You may also complain of being forgetful and feeling irritable. Take one dose of *Sulfur* 30x or 15c three times daily, up to a total of twelve doses. If your condition shows improvement but relapses at a later date, consider repeating this regimen after one month.

BACH FLOWER REMEDIES

Select the remedy that most closely fits your disposition and emotional tendencies and concerns, and take it as needed, following the directions on the product label.

■ Crabapple helps to tone down difficulty tolerating disorder or untidiness.

■ Gorse helps to lift feelings of despair.

AROMATHERAPY

■ Essential oil of rosemary soothes itching and inflammation, promotes healing, and helps to normalize oil secretion. It is particularly useful for nourishing the scalp and hair. You can add it to jojoba oil and apply it to the skin or scalp, and/or add it to shampoo or conditioner and apply it that way. Use up to 5 drops of rosemary oil per ounce of shampoo or conditioner.

GENERAL RECOMMENDATIONS

■ Don't pick at or scratch your skin. This only makes seborrhea worse, and also creates a risk of infection.

■ Keep your skin clean, but avoid irritating soaps and harsh scrubbing. Castile and hypoallergenic soaps, or ones made with calendula or chamomile, are best.

Seizure

A seizure is an episode caused by chaotic firing of neurons (brain cells), resulting in a sudden and temporary change in brain function. Seizures vary in severity, from a slight change in consciousness, tingling or numbness in the limbs, and apparent clumsiness, to severe, rigid, and spastic muscle jerking and loss of consciousness. Twitching, weakness, a feeling of warmth, confusion, staring, garbled speech, vomiting, or a shrill cry may be part of a seizure.

If a seizure involves intense, uncontrolled spasmodic contractions of the muscles, it may be referred to as a *convulsion*. It is worth noting that while a convulsion is a type of seizure, not all seizures involve convulsions. Although the process usually lasts only a few minutes, seeing someone undergo a convulsive seizure is a frightening experience. He or she loses consciousness, and his or her entire body may twitch or shake. The eyes may roll back and the teeth may clench. Breathing may be labored and heavy. The individual may froth at the mouth, and may lose control of his or her bladder or bowels. After a seizure has run its course, the individual will sleep. Upon awakening, he or she will likely feel fatigued, disoriented, and dazed.

Seizures can have a variety of causes, including high fever, a head injury, poisoning, shock, epilepsy, brain infection, an allergic reaction, or withdrawal from drugs or alcohol. It may be an isolated occurrence or the result of a chronic disorder. Epilepsy is a chronic seizure disorder that affects approximately $\frac{1}{2}$ to 1 percent of the population. It is usually diagnosed in childhood or adolescence. Most people with epilepsy have the same type of seizure with each episode, although it is possible to experience more than one type over the course of the illness. Epilepsy can develop in the aftermath of head injury, but in most cases no underlying cause is ever found. A given individual is likely, however, to identify the specific factors that can trigger a seizure in him or her. Common seizure triggers include fever, illness, lack of sleep, low blood sugar, certain drugs, flashing or pulsating lights, and/or loud noises. Some people experience a characteristic series of symptoms that may include abdominal pain, nausea, dizziness, shakiness, fear, or changes in vision or hearing right before the onset of a seizure. This type of syndrome is called an *aura*.

An unusual type of seizure disorder is characterized by recurring seizures triggered by various types of music. This condition, called *musicogenic epilepsy*, was first identified in 1937. Rock-and-roll music and particular rhythms, for instance, are documented seizure triggers for certain individuals. One very interesting case involved a minister who had a seizure whenever he played a particular hymn.

Most seizures resolve themselves on their own. However, anyone who has a seizure should be examined by a doctor. An initial evaluation may include a thorough medical history, including a description of the seizure episode; a neurological examination; and certain blood and urine tests. Other tests that may be used include an electroencephalogram (EEG) to look for signs of abnormal activity in the brain; a magnetic resonance imaging (MRI) scan of the brain to evaluate any signs of possible neurological damage; and a spinal tap to examine the cerebrospinal fluid (the fluid that surrounds the brain and spinal cord) for signs of infection or other problems. The recommended course of treatment, if any, will depend on the cause of the seizure.

EMERGENCY TREATMENT

If you witness someone having a seizure, do the following:

■ If this is the person's first seizure, or if the individual is unknown to you, call a doctor or emergency medical personnel immediately.

■ Stay with the person. Talk reassuringly to him or her.

■ Watch closely for changes in breathing and color. Be sure the person's airway stays open.

■ Clear the area around the person to prevent injury. Move back tables, chairs, or anything else he or she could knock into. Do not try to hold the person down. Restrain-

ing someone who is having a seizure can cause additional injury.

■ Do not try to force anything into the person's mouth or hold down his or her tongue. You might cause choking or be bitten. To prevent the possibility of the individual choking on vomit, keep his or her head turned toward the side or roll the person onto his or her side.

■ Try placing a pillow, blanket, or other soft object under the person's head. If possible, loosen clothing to prevent injury and ease discomfort.

■ If the seizure lasts longer than ten minutes, or if the person seems to be having difficulty breathing, or if he or she is turning blue or injuring him- or herself, call for emergency help.

CONVENTIONAL TREATMENT

■ If seizures are chronic, as in epilepsy, or if recurrences are deemed likely, an anticonvulsant (seizure-preventing) medication will probably be prescribed. The most commonly used anticonvulsant medications include phenobarbital, phenytoin (Dilantin), primidone (Mysoline), carbamazepine (Tegretol), divalproex sodium (Depakote), valproic acid (Depakene), ethosuximide (Zarontin), and clonazepam (Klonopin). Which medication is prescribed will be determined by the particular symptoms you experience while having a seizure, possible drug interactions, and other factors. Generally, you begin by taking a relatively low dose of seizure medication. The dosage is then gradually increased until the seizures are under control. Anticonvulsant medications can have significant side effects, including drowsiness, irritability, nausea, suppressed immune function, and liver damage. Phenytoin can cause an overgrowth of gum tissue. If you must take this drug, careful tooth-brushing and regular visits to the dentist are especially important.

If you must take anticonvulsant medication, be certain you understand exactly how and when to take it. Ask questions of your doctor until you feel confident in your knowledge, and follow your doctor's instructions exactly. With all of these drugs, it is critical that blood levels of the drugs and specific blood tests be monitored, and follow-up appointments kept, so that the best seizure control can be maintained with the fewest side effects.

■ In extremely rare cases, surgery may be recommended. This is reserved for cases in which medication has not helped and a specialized test such as an MRI scan shows a lesion or tumor in the brain that may be causing the seizures.

DIETARY GUIDELINES

■ If you experience recurring seizures, investigate the possibility that food allergies or sensitivities may be involved. Keep a diet diary and use an elimination diet if you suspect certain foods may be implicated (*see* ELIMINATION DIET in Part Three).

■ Avoid foods containing the artificial sweetener aspartame (NutraSweet), an ingredient in a growing number of processed food products. Some people who are sensitive to the amino acid phenylalanine may react to aspartame with seizure activity.

NUTRITIONAL SUPPLEMENTS

Nutritional treatment for seizures is directed at supporting recovery once the seizure has run its course and emergency medical care, if appropriate, has been administered. It is not meant to be a substitute for appropriate medical treatment.

To ensure you are getting an adequate supply of all the major nutrients, take a good multivitamin and mineral supplement daily.

Borage oil is a good source of omega-6 fatty acids, which support nervous-system tissues. Take 1,000 milligrams twice a day.

■ Calcium and magnesium help to relax the nervous system. Take 500 milligrams of calcium and 250 milligrams of magnesium twice a day for one month. Then take the same dose once daily for six months.

■ Chromium helps to regulate blood-sugar levels. Take 200 micrograms two or three times daily.

■ Dimethylglycine (DMG), sometimes called pangamic acid or vitamin B_{15} (although technically it is not a vitamin), has been reported to reduce the frequency of seizures in people with chronic seizure disorders. Take 25 milligrams three times daily.

Fish oils are rich sources of omega-3 essential fatty acids, which act as mediators of the inflammatory response and nutrients for nerve tissue. Take 1,000 milligrams twice a day.

Manganese and zinc are trace minerals that are often deficient in people with epilepsy. Take 10 milligrams of manganese and 15 milligrams of zinc twice daily for six months.

■ S-adenosylmethionine (SAM or SAM-e) is an amino-acid derivative that has been reported to have promising results in improving mental clarity. Try taking it as follows:

Week 1: Take 400 milligrams three times a day.

Week 2: Take 400 milligrams twice a day.

Week 3: Reduce to a maintenance dosage or 200 milligrams twice a day.

■ The amino acid taurine has been shown in some studies to help anticonvulsant medications work more effec-

tively, so that a lower dose of the drug may successfully control seizures. The usual dose of taurine is 500 milligrams twice daily. Because epilepsy is a serious condition and these are complex interactions, however, and because it is not advisable to take a single amino acid for more than three months at a time, we recommend consulting your physician if you wish to try using this supplement.

■ The B vitamins help to strengthen the nerves and are vital for the healthy functioning of the nervous system. Take a B-complex supplement supplying 50 milligrams of each of the major B vitamins daily for six months.

HERBAL TREATMENT

Herbal treatments for seizures are directed at supporting recovery once the seizure has run its course and emergency medical care, if needed, has been administered. They are not meant to be a substitute for appropriate medical treatment.

■ Bitter melon is an herb that helps regulate blood sugar. It can be helpful if blood-sugar fluctuations act as a seizure trigger. Take 200 milligrams of standardized extract three times a day.

■ Chamomile, licorice, passionflower, skullcap, and valerian root are all herbs that help to relax the nervous system. Take 300 to 500 milligrams of chamomile; 500 milligrams of licorice; 250 milligrams of standardized passionflower extract containing 0.7 percent flavonoids; 300 to 500 milligrams of skullcap; and/or 200 to 300 milligrams of standardized valerian extract containing 0.5 percent isovalerenic acids twice a day for one week following a seizure.

Note: Do not use licorice on a daily basis for more than five days at a time, as it can elevate blood pressure. Do not use it at all if you have high blood pressure.

■ Bupleurum and dong quai is a Chinese herbal combination that helps to regulate the nervous system; taurine can enhance the effectiveness of seizure medications; and oat straw strengthens the nervous system. Use them as part of a twelve-week herbal regimen to support recovery from a seizure.

Weeks 1–2: Take one dose of a bupleurum and dong quai formula, as directed on the product label, twice a day.

Weeks 3–4: Take 500 milligrams of oat straw twice daily.

Weeks 5–7: Take 500 milligrams of taurine twice a day.

Weeks 9–12: Take one dose of a bupleurum and dong quai formula twice a day.

■ Ginkgo biloba increases circulation to the brain. Choose a product containing at least 24 percent gingko hererosides (sometimes called flavoglycosides) and take 40 to 60 milligrams three times daily.

■ Kava kava helps to relax the nervous system. Consider taking 250 milligrams of standardized extract containing 30 percent kavalactones two or three times a day for ten days after a seizure.

Note: In excess amounts, this herb can cause drowsiness. Do not exceed the recommended dose. Do not use kava kava if you are pregnant or nursing, if you have Parkinson's disease, or if you are taking a prescription medication for depression or anxiety.

■ If you are on medication to prevent seizures, take milk thistle for liver protection. Choose an extract standardized to contain 80 percent flavonoids (silymarin) and take 150 milligrams two to three times daily for two to three months. Take a month off, then repeat.

HOMEOPATHY

Homeopathic treatment for seizures is directed at supporting recovery once the seizure has run its course and emergency medical care, if needed, has been administered. It is not meant to be a substitute for appropriate medical treatment.

■ Take one dose of *Aconite* 200x following a seizure to ease fright and shock.

■ Ten minutes after taking the *Aconite*, take one dose of *Hyoscyamus* 6c. Continue taking one dose every ten minutes thereafter, up to a total of ten doses.

■ Working with a qualified homeopathic practitioner who can prescribe a constitutional remedy designed specifically for you can be very beneficial in strengthening overall health.

GENERAL RECOMMENDATIONS

■ In addition to following the course of treatment recommended by your doctor, be aware of those things that seem to have set off seizures in the past and avoid them, much as you would identify and avoid substances that cause allergic reactions.

■ If you have a history of seizures, it is wise to obtain a Medic Alert bracelet or necklace and wear it at all times so that others will be alerted to your condition, if necessary (see the Resources section at the back of the book for more information).

PREVENTION

■ Some cases of seizure disorder are the result of trauma to the head. Take measures to protect yourself against head injuries. When in a car, whether as passenger or driver, always wear your seat belt. In airplanes, keep your seat belt loosely fastened at all times except when you must leave your seat. Wear protective headgear for such activities as bicycle (or horseback) riding, roller-blading, football, and hockey.

Sexually Transmitted Disease

See CHLAMYDIA; GONORRHEA; HERPES; HIV DISEASE; SYPHILIS; TRICHOMONIASIS. *Also see under* CANDIDA INFECTION; EPIDIDYMITIS; VAGINITIS; WARTS.

Shingles

Chickenpox is caused by herpes zoster, a virus in the herpes family. Once you have chickenpox, the virus never leaves your body. Instead, it takes up residence on nerve roots somewhere in your body and becomes dormant. Later—often many years later—if you experience some type of physical or emotional stress that lowers your immune response sufficiently, the virus can become active again and flare up in an attack of shingles (or zoster). The trigger can be something obvious, such as cancer, HIV infection, or treatment with immunosuppressant drugs, but often no specific trigger can be identified. Shingles can occur at any age, but most people who develop it are in middle age or beyond.

Shingles begins with extreme pain and/or itching, usually on one side of the body at face or trunk level. It usually affects a specific, defined area—the area of skin served by the infected nerves. This entire area is likely to be excruciatingly sensitive to touch. Two or so days after the pain starts, an eruption of characteristic small reddish blisters appears. The blisters resemble tiny cold sores, and some people develop one or two; others develop many. The blisters usually last from two to three weeks before they dry, crust over, and heal.

An attack of shingles in the pelvic area can affect bladder or bowel function. If the outbreak occurs near the eyes, vision may be affected. Pain, numbing, scarring, and even paralysis can persist for up to a year after the lesions heal, a phenomenon known as *postherpetic neuralgia*. Attacks in the facial region can give rise to viral encephalitis. This is more likely to occur in elderly or immunocompromised persons. For such individuals, widespread dissemination of the virus can be life-threatening.

CONVENTIONAL TREATMENT

■ There is no cure for shingles, though antiviral agents such as acyclovir (Zovirax), famciclovir (Famvir), and valacyclovir (Valtrex) may shorten healing time and lessen pain somewhat if started early in the course of the disease.

These are most often reserved for elderly people and those with compromised immune systems, for whom shingles poses a greater danger. Potential side effects of these drugs include nausea, vomiting, abdominal pain, headache, and dizziness. For immunocompromised individuals, if oral antiviral therapy is not adequate, it may be necessary to administer the drugs intravenously. For cases that prove resistant to acyclovir, another antiviral, foscarnet (Foscavir), may be necessary. This drug causes some degree of kidney damage in nearly all those given it, and can also cause seizures, anemia, and other problems, so its potential benefits must be weighed against these adverse effects.

■ Calamine lotion can be applied to the area to help lessen the discomfort.

■ A painkiller such as acetaminophen (in Tylenol, Datril, and many other products), aspirin (Bayer, Ecotrin, and others), ibuprofen (Advil, Motrin, Nuprin, and others), or naproxen (Aleve, Anaprox, Naprelan, Naprosyn) may be recommended.

Note: In excessive amounts, acetaminophen can cause liver damage. If the recommended amount does not give the relief you want, do not increase the dosage, but try a different medication. Take aspirin, ibuprofen, or naproxen with food to prevent possible stomach upset.

■ If ordinary painkillers do not provide sufficient relief, codeine may be prescribed. This drug is sold under different brand names, often combined with acetaminophen, aspirin, or ibuprofen. It is a powerful narcotic that can cause drowsiness, dizziness, constipation, and other unpleasant side effects, and can also be addictive.

■ For severe pain, injected nerve blocks may be necessary.

■ If the area surrounding the eyes is affected, you should consult with an ophthalmologist. This is a serious, potentially sight-threatening problem.

■ Antidepressants such as amitriptyline (Elavil), fluphenazine (Prolixin), and others have been suggested as possible treatments for postherpetic neuralgia, but their effectiveness is controversial and potential side effects are numerous. These include alterations in sex drive, drowsiness, confusion, stroke, headache, heart-rhythm changes, and jerking movements.

DIETARY GUIDELINES

■ Avoid foods that are high in the amino acid arginine, including chocolate, peanuts, walnuts, and wheat. Too-high levels of arginine tend to diminish those of another amino acid, lysine, which inhibits viruses such as herpes zoster.

NUTRITIONAL SUPPLEMENTS

■ Alpha-lipoic acid is a powerful antioxidant and protector of nerve tissue. Take 100 milligrams twice a day.

■ Coenzyme Q_{10} fights free-radical damage to the nerves. Take 60 milligrams twice a day.

■ Fish oils contain essential fatty acids that are natural inhibitors of the inflammatory response. Take 1,000 milligrams twice a day.

■ Lysine is an amino acid that helps to strengthen adrenal function and fight herpes viruses. Take 500 milligrams three times daily.

■ The B-complex vitamins strengthen nerve function. Take a good B-complex supplement that supplies 50 milligrams of each of the major B vitamins three times daily.

■ Vitamin B_{12} in particular is vital for nerve health and repair. If possible, consult a nutritionally oriented physician and request a course of injections with vitamin B_{12} (preferably in the form of hydroxocobalamin) given on a daily basis for up to a week. This treatment is inexpensive, harmless, and may shorten the duration of the discomfort.

■ Vitamin C is a mild anti-inflammatory and boosts the immune response. Start by taking 1,000 milligrams of magnesium or calcium ascorbate powder every half hour, until you develop loose stools. Then cut back to the highest dosage your digestive system can tolerate.

■ Zinc enhances immune function. Take 25 milligrams of zinc twice a day until the condition resolves. Take zinc with food to avoid possible stomach upset. If you take 30 or more milligrams of zinc on a daily basis for more than one or two months, you should also take 1 to 2 milligrams of copper each day to maintain a proper mineral balance.

HERBAL TREATMENT

■ Capsaicin, an extract of cayenne (capsicum), can be helpful for postherpetic neuralgia. Choose a topical cream or ointment containing 0.025 percent capsaicin and apply it as directed on the product label.

■ Cat's claw has antiviral and anti-inflammatory properties. Take 1,000 milligrams three times a day for two weeks, then reduce to 500 milligrams three times a day until all pain and inflammation are gone.

Note: Do not use cat's claw if you are pregnant or nursing, or if you are an organ-transplant recipient. Use it with caution if you are taking an anticoagulant (blood thinner).

■ Oat straw calms and tones the nervous system. Take 500 milligrams three times daily.

■ Reishi mushroom stimulates the immune system. Take 500 milligrams three times daily.

■ St. John's wort has antiviral properties. Choose a product containing 0.3-percent hypericin and take 300 milligrams three times daily.

■ Turmeric helps to reduce the inflammatory response.

Take 300 milligrams of standardized extract three times a day.

HOMEOPATHY

■ *Mezereum* is helpful for severe pain and itching, burning skin that forms brown scabs. Take one dose of *Mezereum* 12x or 6c four times daily for up to three days, as needed.

■ *Rhus toxicodendron* is good for skin that is red and swollen, with pain and intense itching. The pain tends to be worse at night, better with warmth and movement. Take one dose of *Rhus toxicodendron* 30x or 15c four times daily for up to three days, as needed.

AROMATHERAPY

For specific instructions on how to use aromatherapy, *see* PREPARING AROMATHERAPY TREATMENTS in Part Three.

■ Essential oils of eucalyptus, geranium, and lemon help to alleviate inflammation. Add a few drops of one or more of these oils to olive oil and apply it to the affected area. Or add them to a tubful of water and enjoy a soothing aromatherapy bath.

GENERAL RECOMMENDATIONS

■ If an attack of shingles does not follow a localized pattern, but is generalized over your entire body, and you have no known immune dysfunction, consult your physician. This may indicate a problem such as a hidden malignancy or HIV infection.

PREVENTION

■ Since shingles is a long-term consequence of chickenpox, and nearly every adult today has had chickenpox at some time in his or her life, it may not be possible to prevent shingles.

■ If you are over sixty-five or have a compromised immune system, and you come into contact with someone who has shingles, take one dose of *Variolinum* 30c every twelve hours, for a total of three doses.

Shock

Although many people use the word to describe an emotional reaction, in medical terms, *shock* is a physical state in which circulation is so severely compromised that blood cannot reach the body's tissues and organs. Without the essential nutrients and oxygen carried by the blood, the body becomes less and less able to perform its vital functions. This creates an emergency situation that re-

quires immediate medical attention. If untreated, shock leads to complete circulatory collapse and death.

Shock can be caused by a variety of problems, including major blood loss, drug overdose, severe dehydration, serious infection, disturbances in heart rhythm, sudden and extreme dilation of the blood vessels, major emotional trauma (such as after a serious accident), or, in a person with diabetes, a sudden and dangerous rise in the amount of insulin in the body. Anaphylaxis, a dangerous type of allergic reaction, can also cause shock (*see* ANAPHYLACTIC SHOCK).

Signs and symptoms of shock include nausea, vomiting, weakness, cold and clammy skin, pale white or grayish skin color, dizziness, a cold sweat, increased breathing and heart rate, and restless or frightened behavior.

EMERGENCY TREATMENT

If you witness someone exhibiting signs of shock, do the following:

■ Call for emergency medical help immediately.

■ While waiting for emergency personnel to arrive, wrap the person in a warm blanket or extra clothes. Put a blanket between the person and the ground to help keep his or her body protected from the cool earth. If no blanket or extra clothing is available, use leaves, newspaper, or anything else on hand that can act as insulation.

■ Keep the person on his or her back and raise his or her feet about a foot off the ground, so that they are higher than the heart. If the individual has an injured arm or leg, raise it above heart level as well. These measures decrease the workload of a heart that is already under stress.

■ If the person is not breathing, turn to CARDIOPULMONARY RESUSCITATION (CPR) on page 593. Start CPR at once.

■ If the person is bleeding, turn to BLEEDING, SEVERE on page 138. Take action immediately to stop the bleeding.

■ If the person is unknown to you, look for a Medic Alert necklace or bracelet that might explain his or her condition. For example, a person with diabetes might have a bracelet relating this information, which would guide medical personnel in their treatment.

■ If the person vomits or begins bleeding from the mouth, turn him or her onto his or her side so that the fluid can drain without obstructing breathing.

CONVENTIONAL TREATMENT

■ If shock is related to a large blood loss, intravenous fluids will be given to increase blood volume. Cardiopulmonary resuscitation (CPR), blood transfusion, and/or a ventilator for breathing assistance may be required in severe situations. Depending on reactions and response during treatment, and on which organ systems become affected, treatment may also include pain-control measures, the administration of oxygen, placement of a urinary catheter to monitor urine production (this is often decreased in shock), heart-rhythm monitoring, administration of fluids, and a variety of drug treatments.

NUTRITIONAL SUPPLEMENTS

Nutritional supplementation is aimed at supporting recovery once the acute phase of the crisis is over and you are home from the hospital. If you suspect shock, seek emergency treatment.

■ Adrenal glandular extract supports the adrenal glands, which are instrumental in helping the body cope with stress. Take 200 milligrams twice daily for four weeks.

■ The B vitamins also support adrenal function. Take a B-complex supplement that supplies 50 milligrams of each of the major B vitamins daily for four weeks.

■ Vitamin C supports the immune system and adrenal function. Take 1,000 milligrams three times a day for four weeks.

HERBAL TREATMENT

Herbal treatment for shock is directed at supporting recovery once the acute phase of the crisis is over and you are home from the hospital. If you suspect shock, seek emergency treatment.

■ Astragalus helps to restore immune function after an episode of shock. It strengthens the body's overall ability to cope with physiologic or psychologic stress. Take 250 milligrams three times daily for two weeks.

■ Nettle and yellow dock help build healthy blood cells. After the crisis is over, take 250 to 500 milligrams of each twice daily for one week.

Note: Some people experience stomach upset as a result of taking nettle. If this happens, stop taking it.

■ American ginseng helps to restore energy. Try taking 500 milligrams (or 2 droppersful of liquid extract) twice daily for two days after the nettle and/or yellow dock.

Note: Do not use American ginseng if you have high blood pressure, heart disease, or hypoglycemia. If you are sensitive to the effects of caffeine and other stimulants, you may want to consult with a qualified professional before using ginseng.

HOMEOPATHY

Homeopathic treatment for shock is directed at supporting recovery once the acute phase of the crisis is over and you are home from the hospital. If you suspect shock, seek emergency treatment.

■ *Aconite* helps you to recover from shock, great fear, and anxiety. As soon as the crisis is over and you are well

enough to take something by mouth, take one dose of *Aconite* 200x or 200c.

■ *Ferrum phosphoricum* assists in recovery from a major blood loss. Take one dose of *Ferrum phosphoricum* 6x, as directed on the product label, three times daily for five days.

BACH FLOWER REMEDIES

■ Following any injury or crisis, Rescue Remedy helps to calm and stabilize. Once your doctor says you are well enough to take something by mouth, have someone mix a few drops of Rescue Remedy in a glass of water and sip from the mixture throughout the day. Or place one or two drops under your tongue directly from the bottle.

GENERAL RECOMMENDATIONS

■ The authors strongly recommend that everyone who possibly can take a good first-aid course that includes instruction in cardiopulmonary resuscitation (CPR). We hope that you will never be called upon to use these skills, but CPR is a technique that can literally make the difference between life and death, and it should be learned before the need arises.

■ Keep smelling salts on hand. These can be used to distinguish an episode of fainting from true shock. If an emergency arises when smelling salts are unavailable, try using a bottle of perfume or essential oil instead. Open the bottle and wave it under the person's nose. (*See* FAINTING.)

■ If you are prone to severe allergic reactions, ask your doctor to prescribe a home emergency kit containing epinephrine, such as the Ana-Kit or EpiPen, and learn how to administer it correctly. Having a supply of epinephrine on hand may someday save your life.

Sickle Cell Disease

See under ANEMIA.

Sinusitis

Sinusitis is an inflammation or infection that occurs in the sinuses. The sinuses are four sets of open spaces within the bones of the skull. They come in matched pairs. The *sphenoid sinuses* are centered in the skull, nestled just behind the bridge of the nose. The *ethmoid sinuses* are way back in the upper nose. The *frontal sinuses* are located in the forehead, just above the eyebrow. The *maxillary sinuses* are located under each eye, on either side of the nose. Sinusitis most often occurs in the frontal and/or maxillary sinuses.

The sinuses are lined with mucous membranes similar to the lining of the nasal passages. Their function is to warm, moisten, and filter incoming air on its way to the trachea and lungs. The trouble starts when the membranes lining the nasal passages swell and block the ducts that lead to the sinuses, preventing them from draining freely. Congestion results. The swelling, blockage, and congestion then predispose the sinuses to bacterial infection.

If your sinuses are blocked, congested, irritated, and inflamed, secondary symptoms may include headache, earache, toothache, and/or facial pain and pressure, with marked tenderness over the forehead and cheekbones. You may develop a high fever, lose your ability to smell, and have bad breath. Swelling and puffiness around the eyes, as well as drainage from the eyes, can be danger signals that a more serious condition is developing. If left untreated, sinusitis can lead to meningitis or pneumonia. Chronic sinusitis, even if mild, can also be an underlying factor in asthma. If it is, often the asthma will not improve until the sinusitis is treated.

Many cases of sinusitis occur after the onset of a cold. Hay fever and food allergies, especially a sensitivity to milk and dairy products, are common sources of allergic sinusitis. Exposure to environmental pollutants, including cigarette smoke, can also predispose a person to allergic sinusitis, as can nasal polyps.

The most reliable way to diagnose sinusitis is by a magnetic resonance imaging (MRI) or ultrasound scan, though computerized tomography (CT) scans can be adequate. X-rays are sometimes useful, but can be misleading. A physical examination and diagnostic tests may reveal other indicators of sinus infection, including teeth that are tender when tapped, tenderness in the maxillary area, puffy lower eyelids, thick green-yellow nasal discharge, and an elevated white blood cell count. A doctor may also use transillumination (transmission of light through the tissue) to examine the sinuses, and perform a culture of the nasal discharge to determine whether an infection is present.

CONVENTIONAL TREATMENT

■ For a bacterial infection, your doctor will prescribe an antibiotic. Most commonly used are amoxicillin (Omnipen, Polycillin) and sulfamethoxazole plus trimethoprim (Bactrim, Septra). For an acute infection, the medication is usually prescribed for ten to fourteen days, though two weeks or more may be needed to help prevent recurrences. A host of newer antibiotics have become available in recent years that are much more expensive—but not necessarily more effective—than the old standbys. Their

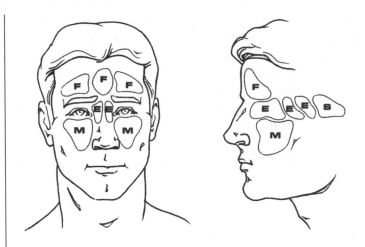

Location of the Sinuses
There are four sets of sinuses: the sphenoid (indicated by the letter S), the ethmoid (E), the frontal (F), and the maxillary (M).

primary usefulness is in treating people who are allergic to penicillin or sulfa drugs.

■ Decongestants may be suggested to help drain the sinuses. Topical decongestants such as Afrin and Neo-Synephrine are probably more effective than the oral variety, but decongestant nasal sprays or drops should not be used for longer than three days in a row. Their initial effect is an opening of nasal passages, but after several days the body can become dependent on them. Then, when use is discontinued, the nasal ducts may swell up and fail to respond as they normally would.

■ Over-the-counter painkillers such as aspirin (Bayer, Ecotrin, and others), acetaminophen (Tylenol, Datril, and others), ibuprofen (Advil, Motrin, Nuprin, and others), and others can be used to ease discomfort and to bring down a fever.

Note: In excessive amounts, acetaminophen can cause liver damage. Do not exceed the recommended dosage. Take aspirin or ibuprofen with food to prevent stomach upset.

■ A severe case of sinusitis that does not respond to antibiotics may have to be treated by a surgical procedure to open the sinuses and allow them to drain adequately.

■ Avoid using antihistamines if you have a sinus infection. These dry the mucous membranes and may thicken secretions so much that they will not drain, which can lead to them becoming impacted.

DIETARY RECOMMENDATIONS

■ To thin mucus, promote drainage, and relieve congestion, drink plenty of pure water and hot herbal teas.

■ Eat chicken soup made with lots of vetetables. Medical

science has confirmed what your mother always knew: Hot chicken soup contains substances that promote healing and sinus drainage.

■ No matter what the cause of sinusitis, eliminate milk and dairy products from your diet until you recover. Dairy products can increase the production of mucus and cause it to thicken, making drainage even more difficult.

■ To identify food sensitivities or allergies that may be fostering a chronic sinus condition, try a rotation or elimination diet (*see* ELIMINATION DIET or ROTATION DIET in Part Three). Start by targeting dairy products and wheat, two of the most common offenders. It is also possible to use a blood test to detect food allergies.

■ Make a drink of hot lemonade to help cut mucus and improve blood flow. Mix the juice of two freshly squeezed lemons with an equal amount of water, and sweeten the drink with a bit of maple syrup. Drink this three times a day. If you can tolerate it, add $1/8$ teaspoon of cayenne pepper.

NUTRITIONAL SUPPLEMENTS

■ Bromelain, an enzyme derived from pineapple, is a natural anti-inflammatory. Take 500 milligrams three times daily, between meals.

■ Beta-carotene helps to heal mucous membranes. Take 10,000 international units twice a day for four or five days.

■ Vitamin C and bioflavonoids help reduce inflammation and fight infection. Take 500 to 1,000 milligrams of each three to four times a day for four or five days.

■ Zinc boosts the immune system and aids tissue healing. Lozenges are a particularly good form. Take 15 to 25 milligrams two or three times a day for up to one week. Take zinc with food to prevent stomach upset.

■ If you have chronic sinusitis and suspect that food intolerances may be a contributing factor, try the following:

- Take a probiotic supplement such as acidophilus or bifidobacteria, as directed on the product label, twice a day for three months. Then cut back to a dose every other day.

- Take 1,000 milligrams of L-glutamine three times a day. This amino acid soothes and promotes repair of the cells of the intestinal tract.

- Take 250 milligrams of thymus glandular extract three times a day to strengthen your immune system.

HERBAL TREATMENT

■ Cat's claw enhances the immune response and has antibacterial properties. Take 500 milligrams of standardized extract three times a day until the infection is resolved.

Note: Do not use cat's claw if you are pregnant or nursing, or if you are an organ-transplant recipient. Use it with caution if you are taking an anticoagulant (blood thinner).

■ Echinacea and goldenseal stimulate the immune system, help in clearing infection, and soothe mucous membranes. They work very well when combined with bromelain (see under Nutritional Supplements, above). Take one dose of an echinacea and goldenseal combination formula supplying 250 to 500 milligrams of echinacea and 150 to 300 milligrams of goldenseal every two hours while symptoms (including fever and sinus pain) are acute, up to a total of six doses. After the acute phase is resolved, take one dose three times a day for up to ten days.

■ Make an herbal tea combining 1 tablespoon of fenugreek, 1 tablespoon of rose hips, 1 tablespoon of thyme, and $1/2$ tablespoon of licorice brewed in 8 ounces of water. (*See* PREPARING HERBAL TREATMENTS in Part Three.) Fenugreek and thyme help to relieve nasal and sinus congestion; rose hips contain vitamin C; and licorice sweetens the tea. Take a cup twice a day during the acute phase of the infection.

Note: Do not use licorice on a daily basis for more than five days at a time, as it can elevate blood pressure. Do not use it at all if you have high blood pressure.

■ Garlic has antibacterial properties and helps to clear infection. Select an odorless capsule variety and take 500 milligrams four times a day for up to ten days.

■ A warm, moist compress of water and ginger root placed over the sinuses helps to drain the area and relieve congestion. Grate a large ginger root into a pot containing 1 pint of water and simmer for fifteen minutes. Use the resulting tea to make a hot compress.

■ Grapefruit-seed extract is antibacterial, antiviral, and antifungal. Take 100 milligrams two or three times a day. You can also put 2 drops of liquid extract in an ounce of distilled water and instill a few drops in each nostril several times a day.

■ Menthol lozenges help to clear respiratory passages. Menthol is a purified and refined extract of peppermint. Lozenges made without sugar are preferable. Take one lozenge every two hours, as needed, up to a total of four lozenges a day.

Note: If you are using menthol lozenges and also taking a homeopathic preparation, allow one hour between the two. Otherwise, the strong smell of the mint may interfere with the action of the homeopathic remedy.

■ Oregano has antibacterial properties and helps to fight infection. Take 75 milligrams of standardized extract three times a day.

■ Pueraria (also known as kudzu) is a botanical used in Japan to help resolve nasal congestion. It is usually found as part of combination formulas designed for this purpose. Take it as directed on the product label.

Shiitake mushrooms have an immune-stimulating effect. Take 500 to 800 milligrams three times daily for one week after the acute infection is over. Then take the same dose twice a day for two months. Make sure you do not have an allergy or sensitivity to mushrooms before using any type of mushroom in supplement form.

HOMEOPATHY

Hepar sulfuris calcareum is helpful for sinus infection with a yellow or yellow-green nasal discharge. Take one dose of *Hepar sulfuris calcareum* 12x or 6c, as directed on the product label, four times a day for up to two days.

Kali bichromicum is good for a sinus infection with white, ropy mucus. Take one dose of *Kali bichromicum* 12x or 6c four times a day for up to two days.

Mercurius solubilis is for a stuffed nose that isn't getting better, possibly accompanied by bad breath. Take one dose of *Mercurius solubilis* 12x or 6c four times a day for up to two days.

Homeopathic combination sinus formulas are available that may offer relief. Follow the dosage directions on the product label.

ACUPRESSURE

For the locations of acupressure points on the body, *see* ADMINISTERING AN ACUPRESSURE TREATMENT in Part Three.

Large Intestine 4 clears the head and sinuses.

Large Intestine 20 clears the sinuses.

AROMATHERAPY

For specific instructions on how to use aromatherapy, *see* PREPARING AROMATHERAPY TREATMENTS in Part Three.

Alkalol is an over-the-counter "mucus solvent" made from salt water and a combination of aromatic oils. It is very soothing to the sinus membranes and helps clear out infection. Dilute it with an equal amount of water and gently flush your sinuses with the mixture three or four times daily. It is possible to obtain a special tip for a Water Pik from an ear, nose, and throat specialist that makes nasal irrigation much easier.

Give yourself a vapor inhalation treatment by adding 4 or 5 drops of essential oil of eucalyptus and/or rosemary to a sinkful or large pot of water (*see* PREPARING AROMATHERAPY TREATMENTS in Part Three).

GENERAL RECOMMENDATIONS

■ Use nasal saline flushes to cleanse the sinuses and thin mucus. (*See* NASAL SALINE FLUSH in Part Three.) You can do this four to six times a day, as needed.

Use the proper technique when blowing your nose. *Do*

not hold one nostril closed and blow with force. This can send mucus back up into the sinus cavities. A gentle blow with both nostrils open is more effective.

■ The use of a cool mist vaporizer may be helpful. To prevent the buildup of bacteria, keep the equipment scrupulously clean. During an acute infection, a humidifier can help to thin and drain secretions.

PREVENTION

■ Eliminate all known and suspected allergens from your environment.

■ Avoid exposure to cigarette smoke and wood smoke. Studies have shown that people who live in households where one or more members smoke and those who live in extremely well insulated homes with wood stoves have more upper respiratory infections than average.

Sjögren's Syndrome

Sjögren's syndrome is a disorder characterized by the dysfunction of certain glands, including the salivary glands, lacrimal (tear) glands, and pancreas. It is believed to be an autoimmune disorder, in which the immune system mistakenly attacks the body's own tissues. About 90 percent of people who have it are women, and the average age at diagnosis is about fifty.

The primary symptoms are dry mouth and dry eyes, symptoms sometimes referred to as *sicca components*. These problems in turn can lead to further symptoms, such as mouth ulcers, difficulty swallowing, tooth decay, and corneal damage. The salivary glands are often enlarged. Sjögren's syndrome can also cause dry skin, hair loss, and dryness of other mucous membranes throughout the body, such as those in the nose, throat, bronchial tubes, lungs, and vagina. In some cases, it attacks internal organs as well, affecting the liver, pancreas, kidneys, and even the heart.

Other autoimmune diseases, including rheumatoid arthritis and systemic lupus erythematosus, can be associated with this disorder. People with Sjögren's syndrome also have a higher than normal risk of developing lymphoma, cancer of the lymphatic system. In most cases, however, while it is chronic and can be uncomfortable, Sjögren's syndrome does not pose a serious danger.

CONVENTIONAL TREATMENT

■ There is no known cure for Sjögren's syndrome, so treatment is aimed at handling individual symptoms as they occur.

■ Artificial tears should be used regularly. It is wise to

consult an ophthalmologist who can monitor and help to manage the effects of this disorder on the eyes.

■ The mouth should be moistened regularly. The teeth may loosen and fall out if drying is severe. Also, mouth ulcers are less frequent if you pay careful attention to oral hygiene and lubrication.

■ If inflamed salivary glands cause discomfort, an over-the-counter painkiller such as acetaminophen (in Tylenol, Datril, and many other products), aspirin (Bayer, Ecotrin, and others), ibuprofen (Advil, Motrin, Nuprin, and others), or ketoprofen (Orudis) may be recommended.

    Note: In excessive amounts, acetaminophen can cause liver damage. Do not exceed the recommended dosage. Take aspirin, ibuprofen, or ketoprofen with food to prevent possible stomach upset.

■ Problems such as pancreatitis, pleurisy, kidney disease, heart problems, rheumatoid arthritis, and lupus are handled with the standard treatments for those conditions. (*See* ARTHRITIS; CARDIOVASCULAR DISEASE; KIDNEY DISEASE; LUPUS; PANCREATITIS; and/or PLEURISY.)

■ Any drugs that have drying effects, such as antihistamines and decongestants, should be *avoided.* If you are unsure about possible side effects of any medication, whether prescription or over-the-counter, ask your physician or pharmacist.

DIETARY GUIDELINES

■ A diet of soft foods is likely to be easier to eat. Consider consulting a professional dietitian who can work with you to develop a soft diet that supplies all the nutrition you need.

■ Avoid coffee, alcohol, and spicy food, all of which tend to dehydrate the body.

■ Drink at least eight 8-ounce glasses of water every day. Keep a glass of water near you at all times and take frequent sips.

NUTRITIONAL SUPPLEMENTS

■ Evening primrose oil is a source of essential fatty acids and sterols necessary for the health of the skin and mucous membranes. Take 1,000 milligrams three times daily.

HERBAL TREATMENT

■ Marshmallow root and slippery elm are soothing to inflamed tissues and mucous membranes. Take either or both in tea form. Drink a cup of tea two or three times daily.

■ Reishi mushroom improves immune function and helps the body deal with stress. Take 500 milligrams three times daily.

HOMEOPATHY

■ *Alumina* is helpful for dry mucous membranes accompanied by a general lack of vitality and energy. Symptoms tend to be worse upon arising in the morning. Take one dose of *Alumina* 200x or 200c twice a day for three days. Wait two weeks, then repeat.

BACH FLOWER REMEDIES

Select the remedy that most closely fits your disposition and emotional tendencies and concerns, and take it as needed, following the directions on the product label.

■ Hornbeam helps to ease feelings of deep exhaustion.

■ Choose Sweet Chestnut if you are feeling melancholy and alienated.

GENERAL RECOMMENDATIONS

■ Keep regular appointments with both a dentist and an eye doctor at the intervals they recommend. It is a good idea to seek out health-care professionals who have experience in treating patients with this condition.

■ Use a humidifier to keep the air in your home and/or work environment from becoming too dry, especially during the winter months. This can make symptoms worse. Clean the equipment frequently so that bacteria do not collect and spread through it into the air.

Skin Cancer

The skin is the body's largest organ, so it is perhaps not surprising that more people are diagnosed with skin cancer than with any other type of cancer. Like all types of cancer, skin cancer is characterized by the uncontrolled growth of cells. There are different forms of skin cancer. The most common types are basal cell carcinoma, squamous cell carcinoma, and melanoma. All of these originate in the outer layer of the skin, the epidermis, and all are often a result of overexposure to the sun's ultraviolet rays. Not surprisingly, they are most common among people with light-colored skin, who have less natural protection against the sun's rays, as well as among people who spend a great deal of time outdoors, whether for work or recreation.

    The three major forms of skin cancer are distinguished from one another based on the specific types of cells they originate in. Basal cells are located just under the outermost surface of the skin. Basal cell carcinomas account for approximately three-quarters of all skin cancers. They may appear as firm and shiny, ulcerated and scabbing, or hard and scarlike patches of skin. They often alternate between bleeding and seeming to heal—only to open and bleed again later. Basal cell carcinoma is very closely linked to sun exposure. It tends to grow slowly, and does not usually spread to other parts of the body in the way that other cancers can, although it can grow into adjacent tissues in some cases.

Squamous cells are found in the middle of the epidermis. Squamous cell carcinoma is the most common type of skin cancer after basal cell. Though also strongly linked to sun exposure, these cancers are sometimes found in areas of the body not normally exposed to the sun, such as the tongue and the inside of the mouth. They usually begin as small scaly, reddish bumps that gradually grow larger and may turn warty in appearance. As a squamous cell cancer progresses, the bump erodes and an ulcer forms in the middle. At this point, the cancer is also usually growing downward and invading deeper layers of tissue. This type of cancer does not usually spread to other parts of the body, but it can, and because much of the cancer is often under the surface of the skin, it can be more extensive than it appears. It is therefore considered a more serious condition than basal cell carcinoma.

Melanoma is the least common of the major skin cancers, but it is the most feared, and with good reason: While only 5 percent of skin cancers are melanomas, fully 75 percent of skin-cancer-related deaths are attributable to this type of cancer. The melanocytes, the cells in which melanoma originates, are the skin's pigment-producing cells. They are located near the bottom of the epidermis, in the area where the epidermis meets the dermis, or deeper skin layer. This is where such structures as hair follicles and sweat glands are located. These tumors can grow rapidly and invade surrounding tissue. Tumor cells can also break off and spread through the bloodstream to other parts of the body, creating new tumors there. Generally, the thicker the growth, the more likely this is to happen.

Though overexposure to the sun doubtless plays a part in their formation, melanomas can be found on both sun-exposed and non-sun-exposed parts of the body. There are different subtypes of melanoma. Most have, at least initially, a flat, molelike appearance, though they have little bumps within them as well. The color can be black, brown, reddish, bluish, or even pearly white. Often, a single lesion will combine several colors. A significant percentage of melanomas originate in preexisting moles, although it should be emphasized that the vast majority of moles do not become cancerous.

Another type of skin cancer is Kaposi's sarcoma. Though much less common than the cancers discussed above, its incidence has been rising sharply since the early 1980s. Prior to that time, it was a rare syndrome seen primarily in older men of Mediterranean ancestry. Today, however, it is known as one of the opportunistic illnesses associated with AIDS. It appears as slightly raised spots that may be pink, red, bluish, or even purple in color, and can affect the skin anywhere on the body. It can also affect the mucous membranes.

CONVENTIONAL TREATMENT

■ Basal cell carcinoma is treated by removing the affected tissue. There are different techniques that may be used to do this, depending on the location and size of the cancer, as well as other factors. The goal is to completely remove the tumor while removing as little normal tissue as possible.

■ Squamous cell carcinoma also is treated by removing the tumor, though in some cases, local injection of small amounts of a chemotherapeutic agent such as methotrexate or fluorouracil may be an effective substitute.

■ As with the other major types of skin cancer, treatment of melanoma requires surgical removal of the cancerous tissue. However, more surrounding skin is taken than with other skin masses, and lymph nodes in the area may be removed to check for any signs that the cancer may have spread to other parts of the body, though the effect of doing so on the ultimate outcome is still controversial.

■ Treatment for Kaposi's sarcoma depends on the extent of the disease. If it is limited to the skin, watchful waiting may be the first approach, as this disease can progress very slowly. If more aggressive treatment is warranted, local cryotherapy (freezing), injections of chemotherapeutic agents, laser treatment, or radiotherapy may be used to shrink the lesions and slow the progression of the disease.

DIETARY GUIDELINES

■ Eat a healthy high-fiber diet with lots of fresh fruits and vegetables, which contain valuable vitamins, minerals, and, perhaps most important, phytonutrients that may benefit the skin and have anticancer properties.

■ Avoid sugar and saturated, hydrogenated, and partially hydrogenated fats and oils. These substances foster a toxic internal environment.

NUTRITIONAL SUPPLEMENTS

■ To ensure an adequate supply of all major nutrients, take a good high-potency multivitamin and mineral supplement daily.

■ Alpha-lipoic acid is an antioxidant that neutralizes several of the most damaging free radicals and also reactivates other antioxidants. Also, unlike many other antioxidants, it is both both lipid- and water-soluble, which means that it can go virtually anywhere in the body. Take 150 milligrams three times a day.

■ Antioxidants help protect against potentially cancer-causing free radicals. Take a good antioxidant combination formula that supplies 200 micrograms of selenium daily.

■ Beta 1, 3 glucan, a compound derived from the cell walls of yeast, is an important immune-system supporter. Take 24 to 40 milligrams two or three times daily.

Coenzyme Q_{10} is an antioxidant. Preliminary studies suggest it may have some success in fighting cancer. Take 60 to 100 milligrams three times a day.

Flaxseed and fish oils contain essential fatty acids needed for healthy skin. Take 1 tablespoon daily, or 500 to 1,000 milligrams in supplement form two or three times daily.

N-acetylcysteine (NAC) stimulates detoxification in the liver. Take 500 milligrams twice a day.

Pine-bark and grapeseed extracts are good antioxidants. Take 50 milligrams of either three times a day.

Spleen glandular extract supports the activity of B-cells, which are important elements of the immune system. Take 200 to 300 milligrams three times a day.

Thymus glandular extract can help to boost immunity. Take 500 milligrams in the morning and again in the afternoon.

■ Vitamin C is an antioxidant and promotes healing because it boosts the immune system and is essential for the production of collagen, a key component of the skin. Take 500 milligrams of vitamin C with bioflavonoids three times daily.

Vitamin E also is a valuable antioxidant. Choose a product containing mixed tocopherols and start by taking 200 international units daily, then gradually increase the dosage until you are taking 400 international units twice daily, in morning and evening.

Note: If you have high blood pressure, limit your intake of supplemental vitamin E to a total of 400 international units daily. If you are taking an anticoagulant (blood thinner), consult your physician before taking supplemental vitamin E.

HERBAL TREATMENT

Cat's claw has a positive impact on the immune system. Preliminary hopes that it can kill cancerous cells without damaging normal ones are currently being researched as well. Take 1,000 milligrams three times a day.

Note: Do not use cat's claw if you are pregnant or nursing, or if you are an organ-transplant recipient. Use it with caution if you are taking an anticoagulant (blood thinner).

■ Maitake, reishi, and shiitake mushrooms offer immune support. Take 250 to 500 milligrams of standardized extract three times a day.

Milk thistle supports the liver and aids in detoxifying the body. Choose an extract standardized to contain 80 percent flavonoids (silymarin) and take 150 milligrams three times a day for two to three months.

■ Red clover has been known historically as a blood cleanser. In order for tumors to grow, they need a blood supply, so they send out chemical messages that induce the body to grow new blood vessels into and around them. This process is known as *angiogenesis*. Red clover contains genistein, a compound that has been found to have an antiangiogenic effect. Take 500 milligrams four times daily for three months. You can also apply a liquid extract to the affected area twice a day.

HOMEOPATHY

■ *Aceticum acidum* is helpful for a lesion that is dry, red, and hot, though the rest of the skin is pale. You may be irritable and have a tendency to develop nervous headaches with bulging blood vessels in your temples. Take one dose of *Aceticum acidum* 6x or 3c three times daily for up to three days. Do this monthly for four months.

■ *Gallium aparine* can help modify cancerous lesions and ulcers. The skin lesions may be associated with chronic urinary problems and/or edema. Take one dose of *Gallium aparine* 6x or 3c three times daily for up to three days. Do this monthly for four months.

■ If the cancer has caused ulceration, take *Hydrastis* to help dry up the site. Take one dose of *Hydrastis* 6x or 3c three times daily for up to three days. Do this monthly for four months.

ACUPRESSURE

■ All back Bladder points relax the nervous system to enhance and speed healing.

■ Spleen 10 takes the "heat" out of the blood.

AROMATHERAPY

For specific instructions on how to use aromatherapy, *see* PREPARING AROMATHERAPY TREATMENTS in Part Three.

■ *Avoid* using bergamot oil if you will be spending time outdoors. This essential oil can increase the skin's sensitivity to the sun.

GENERAL RECOMMENDATIONS

■ Above all else, be careful about sun exposure. Avoid spending time outdoors in the middle of the day. Regardless of the day or season, always use a sunscreen on all uncovered areas of skin. Choose a product that protects against both UVA and UVB rays and has an SPF of 10 or higher, and reapply it several times throughout the day. When you are outside, wear a broad-brimmed hat to shield your face and cover up as much as possible. Loose, light-colored clothing made of tightly woven fabric is best.

Be aware, however, that the sun's rays can reach you even through clothing, so if you must be outdoors for a long period, apply sunscreen before getting dressed.

■ If you have been treated for skin cancer, be alert for recurrences so that they can be treated promptly, if necessary.

PREVENTION

■ It's never too late to start protecting yourself against harm from the sun's rays. Use a good sunscreen regularly. Don't let that give you a false sense of security about sun exposure, though. You should still limit the amount of time you spend outdoors during daylight, particularly in the middle of the day. Similarly, don't count on a suntan or a naturally dark skin tone to protect you. While light-colored skins burn more easily and are more prone to developing skin cancer, all kinds of skin are subject to sun damage. Moreover, sun damage is cumulative, so while you may not see its effects immediately, they may show up at some later date in the form of skin cancer.

Skin Rash

The skin is the largest organ of the body. If bears made "human-skin" rugs, the skin of the average adult would cover about twenty-two square feet of the bear's lair, and the "rug" would weigh between eight and ten pounds. Your skin provides you with a waterproof covering, protects the interior of your body by moderating temperature extremes, and guards against invasion by harmful bacteria. Your skin grows faster than any other organ, and it keeps renewing itself for life. The skin is so important that the loss of more than one third of it from burns can be fatal.

Rash is a general term that describes an eruption of the skin. A rash can be flat, raised, or blistered. It may be pink, red, purple, or brown in color. It may be made of separate, distinct spots or consist of a diffuse reddened area. It can be moist and "weepy" or dry and scaly. Some rashes start on one part of the body and spread to other parts; others appear in one area only. There may be no sensation with it, or it may be itchy or burning.

Many different things can cause a rash to develop. A rash can be a result of infection or allergies, whether a bacterial infection such as impetigo, a viral infection such as chickenpox or herpes, a fungal infection such as ringworm or yeast, or an airborne or contact allergy to foods, mold, a plant, or a drug. *Contact dermatitis* is the medical term for a contact allergy that results in skin rash. Common allergens involved in contact dermatitis include cosmetics, detergents, certain plants and metals, and household chemicals.

Rashes can also be due to physical and environmental agents. Sun poisoning (not the same thing as sunburn) can cause a localized rash consisting of tiny white itchy bumps. Exposure to wind, especially cold wind, can cause the reddened skin condition known as windburn. Friction, caused either by two parts of the body rubbing against each other or a part of the body rubbing against some external item, can provoke a skin rash as well. Skin disorders such as psoriasis and eczema are responsible for many rashes.

The more you know about the rash, the better able you will be to treat it. Look at it closely and observe what it looks like. Take note of where it appears on the body, whether it spreads or not, and any other symptoms you have, even if they seem unrelated. Also take into account where you were and what you were doing in the day or days before the rash appeared, as well as environmental factors such as the temperature or exposure to possible allergens. All of these clues can be important for the correct diagnosis of a rash.

If you feel unsure about the cause of a skin rash, consult your health-care provider for advice. If you develop a rash accompanied by a high fever, weakness, and lethargy, seek medical attention immediately.

CONVENTIONAL TREATMENT

■ Your doctor should first take a complete history. Depending on what he or she determines to be the cause of the rash, your doctor may prescribe simple comfort measures, antibiotic cream, an antifungal agent, and/or antihistamine lotion.

■ If no definitive cause can be found, your doctor may prescribe a cortisone or hydrocortisone ointment, or an oral steroid such as prednisone (Deltasone) or dexamethasone (Decadron). These can be amazingly effective for many kinds of skin rashes. However, you should bear in mind that whether they are applied topically or taken by mouth, these drugs should be be taken only for short periods of time and must be tapered off gradually rather than stopped abruptly. They suppress the functioning of the adrenal glands, depress immune function, and, if used locally, can cause thinning and aging of the skin.

GENERAL RECOMMENDATIONS

■ Appropriate treatment, if any, depends on the cause of the rash. For example, a rash resulting from a viral infection usually doesn't need any specific treatment except for comfort measures, while a rash caused by a bacterial infection may need to be treated with antibiotic cream and herbs with immune-stimulating properties. For specific recommendations, refer to the relevant entries in this book. *See* ACNE; ALLERGIES; ATHLETE'S FOOT; BITES AND STINGS, INSECT AND SPIDER; CANDIDA INFECTION; CHICKEN-POX; DERMATITIS; ECZEMA; FOOD ALLERGIES; HERPES;

Common Skin Rashes

In order to know how to treat a rash, it is best to know the cause. The following table lists some of the conditions that most commonly cause rashes, together with a description of characteristic features. It is not meant to be a list of all possible causes of skin rash, however. Consult your health-care provider for a definitive diagnosis of your rash.

Cause of Rash	Description
Acne	Inflammation and pimples, possibly with whiteheads and/or blackheads, usually on the face but possibly also on the chest and back. In severe cases, pus-filled cysts and bumps can accompany the pimples.
Allergy (food or drug)	Pink or red flat and raised lesions. The skin may appear swollen, and it may be itchy. Usually goes away once the offending food or drug is identified and avoided, but in rare cases a drug allergy can lead to a prolonged skin disease called Stevens-Johnson syndrome.
Athlete's foot	Clusters of tiny blisters and scaly sores that appear on the feet, especially between the toes. Itchy and burning. Goes away with treatment, but can be persistent; a complete cure can take up to a month in some cases.
Candida infection	Inflamed, splotchy red patches that may itch and/or be tender to the touch, most often in such areas as the underarms, groin, beneath the breasts, and other places with skin-to-skin contact. Gets better with treatment, but can be persistent.
Chickenpox	Appears first as a flat, reddish rash, then turns into batches of tiny pimples and blisters that crust over as they heal. Usually preceded by a day or two of typical viral symptoms—fever, headache, fatigue, and general malaise. In most cases the rash begins on the trunk and spreads to the extremities. Usually there are comparatively few lesions on the neck and head. Very itchy.
Contact dermatitis	Redness, itching, swelling, often followed by blisters of varying size at the site of contact with the agent responsible.
Eczema	A raised red rash that may be dry and scaly or composed of weepy, fluid-filled lesions. Itching can be severe. Usually an allergic reaction that improves once the allergen is identified and avoided.
Heat rash	Small, raised red lesions with tiny blisters at the center. Appears suddenly, usually in hot weather, and resolves quickly. May be itchy and stinging.
Herpes	Small blisters and ulcers, either around the mouth or in the genital area, that may be preceded by an itching or burning sensation. Itchy and painful. An outbreak usually lasts four to ten days, but outbreaks can be a recurring problem.
Lupus	Discoid lupus erythematosus (DLE): Starts as one or more red, circular, thickened areas of the skin that later form scars, most often on the face, behind the ears, and/or on the scalp. If lesions lead to scarring on the scalp, there can be permanent hair loss in the affected areas. Systemic lupus erythematosus (SLE): a red butterfly-shaped rash over the cheeks and nose. There can also be reddening on the palms and fingers; flat or raised red lesions on the face, neck, upper chest, and/or elbows; and circular markings similar to those of DLE.
Lyme disease	A round, raised reddish lesion that is usually paler or whitish in the center occurs at the site of the tick bite that transmits this disease. May or may not be accompanied by flulike symptoms, including headache, fever, and general malaise. The rash may come and go throughout the illness.

Cause of Rash	Description
Measles	A splotchy purplish-red rash of irregularly shaped raised and flat lesions. Begins as small spots that coalesce into larger patches. Usually preceded by several days of viral symptoms, including fever, cough, and general malaise, as well as conjunctivitis. In most cases, the rash begins on the face and spreads to the trunk and extremities. Lasts four to seven days, then fades away as the virus runs its course.
Poison ivy, oak, or sumac	Small fluid-filled lesions, with redness and swelling, weeping and crusting. Can appear several hours or several days after contact with the plant. Itching and burning can be severe. Lasts from two to four weeks, then gradually heals.
Psoriasis	Patches of reddened skin covered by thick, scaly clumps, most often on the scalp, elbows, knees, back, and buttocks, though any part of the body can be affected. Cannot be cured, but can usually be managed with treatment.
Ringworm	Small, flat lesions that grow to be approximately $\frac{1}{4}$-inch circular lesions. The skin may appear scaly; there may be fluid-filled blisters. Itchy. Usually appears on the face, arms, and/or trunk. Goes away with treatment.
Rosacea	Areas of redness and swelling, possibly with bumps and pimples, principally in the center of the face. Dilated blood vessels beneath the skin may appear as reddish blotches. Cannot be cured, but can usually be managed with treatment.
Scabies	Small red lumps that may become dry and scaly. You may also see thin light-gray or pinkish lines under the skin. Often very itchy. Most commonly occurs on the buttocks, genitals, wrists, armpits, and between the fingers and toes. Resolves with treatment.
Seborrhea	Dry scaling over underlying redness, usually on the scalp or face or in skin folds.
Shingles	Tiny vesicles that erupt following two days or so of pain and itching at the site, usually on one side of the face or trunk.
Warts	Common warts: Raised, sharply outlined rough bumps, often brown or gray in color. Most often found on the hands, feet, face, and/or neck. Genital warts: Clusters of small rubbery, usually pinkish-colored, cauliflower-shaped growths in the genital area. Plane warts: Small, flat lumps, often found in clusters. Plantar warts: Painful hard round areas in and on the soles of the feet and bottoms of the toes.

LUPUS; LYME DISEASE; MEASLES; POISON IVY, OAK, AND SUMAC; PSORIASIS; RINGWORM; ROSACEA; SCABIES; SEBORRHEA; SHINGLES; and/or WARTS, as appropriate.

■ Regardless of the cause, if the rash is itchy and/or inflamed, cool compresses can often provide quick relief. Soak a clean cloth in cool water, wring it out, and apply it to the affected area for ten minutes. Repeat as often as necessary.

PREVENTION

■ Some types of skin rashes may not be preventable. However, it can only help to avoid contact with any substances to which you know you are sensitive. Also avoid having your skin come in contact with harsh and potentially irritating substances such as detergents, cleansers, and household chemicals.

Sleep Apnea

See under SNORING.

Sleep Problems

See INSOMNIA; NARCOLEPSY; RESTLESS LEGS SYNDROME; SNORING.

Smoking

See under NICOTINE ADDICTION.

Snakebite

See BITES, SNAKE.

Snoring

Snoring is that annoying buzzing, rattling, snorting, and wheezing noise that some people make during sleep. These harsh sounds are caused by the vibration of the uvula, the small, conical piece of flesh that projects downward from the soft palate in the middle of the mouth. Each inhalation and exhalation of breath causes the uvula to vibrate.

An estimated 40 million Americans snore. Almost twice as many men as women snore, but women are not immune. Most people who snore sleep with their mouths open, usually because their throats or nasal passages are partially obstructed. Possible causes of snoring include nasal congestion, enlarged tonsils or adenoids, nasal polyps, a deviated septum, or loose dentures. Obesity increases the likelihood of snoring by a factor of three. Although people who sleep on their sides sometimes snore, you are much more likely to snore if you sleep on your back. Sleeping on your back causes your jaw to drop open and your tongue to fall backward, setting up even more vibration of the uvula and also partially closing the windpipe.

CONVENTIONAL MEDICINE

■ Your doctor is first likely to recommend commonsense lifestyle measures such as those outlined under General Recommendations, below.

■ For severe snoring due to obstruction, treatment may involve surgery to remove tonsils and adenoids, or excision of excess tissue at the back of the throat. In extreme conditions, tracheostomy (surgery to create an opening into the windpipe that allows air to flow directly into the lungs during sleep) may be necessary.

■ *Avoid* taking antihistamines, tranquilizers, or any other type of medication that depresses the central nervous system.

DIETARY GUIDELINES

■ Avoid eating within two hours of bedtime.

■ Minimize your consumption of salt and salty foods, especially before bedtime. If sodium levels are high, potassium levels are relatively low. Low levels of potassium are associated with snoring.

■ Avoid alcohol. If you do drink, limit it to at least two hours away from bedtime. Alcohol causes a snorer to sleep more heavily and snore more loudly.

NUTRITIONAL SUPPLEMENTS

■ Take a good multivitamin and mineral supplement daily. Choose a product that supplies at least the recommended daily allowance (RDA) of all major vitamins and minerals.

■ Calcium and magnesium are essential to the central nervous system and have calming properties. Take 500 milligrams of calcium and 250 to 500 milligrams of magnesium twice daily.

■ Some cases of snoring are associated with poor digestion. Take a full-spectrum digestive-enzyme supplement providing 5,000 international units of lipase, 2,500 international units of amylase, and 300 international units of protease, plus 500 to 1,000 milligrams of pancreatin, immediately before each meal to improve digestion.

Note: Long-term supplementation with pancreatin is not advised, as it can cause your pancreas to reduce its own production of this important enzyme. Overuse also has the potential to cause nausea or diarrhea. After two months on pancreatin, discontinue use and monitor your reaction. If you find that your problems recur, discuss pancreatin supplementation with your health-care provider.

■ Green-foods supplements provide minerals, such as potassium, that are often lacking in a normal diet. Take a green-foods supplement as directed on the product label.

HERBAL TREATMENT

■ The best approach to treating snoring with herbs is to consult a knowledgeable herbalist who can formulate a remedy for your particular symptoms.

HOMEOPATHY

■ There are several effective anti-snoring homeopathic formulas available. If these do not give you satisfactory results, you may wish to see a homeopathic practitioner for a constitutional remedy.

GENERAL RECOMMENDATIONS

■ If you are overweight, try to slim down. Obesity contributes to snoring.

Sleep Apnea

Sleep apnea is a potentially dangerous condition in which breathing stops for periods lasting some ten seconds to two minutes during sleep. It is often considered to be related to snoring because most people with obstructive sleep apnea, the most common form of the condition, are overweight men between the ages of thirty and fifty who are heavy snorers. Apnea is not limited to this group of people, however; it has also been implicated in sudden infant death syndrome (SIDS).

When breathing stops, the oxygen content of the blood falls, prompting the brain to take steps to reinitiate breathing. Breathing usually starts again with a snort and a quick intake of breath. Though this gasping for air often causes momentary waking, the person is unlikely to remember it. This sequence of events can happen again and again throughout the night. An affected individual may have as many as 200 episodes during a single night, yet—because it happens during sleep—not be aware of the problem. He or she is likely, however, to be aware of fatigue and drowsiness the following day, results of insufficient good-quality sleep the night before.

Obstructive sleep apnea can be caused by overrelaxation of the muscles controlling the soft palate and uvula. As the muscles sag, the airway becomes obstructed, breathing becomes labored, and snoring escalates. It can also be a result of enlarged tonsils and/or adenoids. Although it is rare, some people with this condition have larger than usual tongues and smaller than normal airway openings.

In *central sleep apnea,* a less common form of the condition, the airway is open and clear but the diaphragm and chest muscles fail to work properly. A person with central sleep apnea may or may not snore. The cause of central sleep apnea is not completely understood, but experts believe it is related to a disturbance in the brain's automatic regulation of breathing.

Most people who suffer from sleep apnea have a combination of obstructive and central sleep apnea, in which a short episode of central apnea usually precedes a longer period of obstructive apnea. In those with mixed apnea, snoring is common.

Although not everyone with apnea feels drowsy during the daylight hours, excessive sleepiness during the day is a primary symptom. Drowsiness may be so extreme that it makes working difficult and driving hazardous. In fact, people with sleep apnea are significantly more likely to be involved in automobile accidents than other people, probably due to the exhaustion it creates. Problems with concentration and memory are not uncommon. Sleep apnea contributes to the risk of high blood pressure, cardiovascular problems, and stroke.

If you suffer from extreme drowsiness and fatigue for which you can find no explanation, you may be suffering from sleep apnea and should seek a doctor's evaluation, diagnosis, and, if appropriate, treatment. Some of the treatments for sleep apnea include the use of a device that continuously pumps air into the airway to keep it open during sleep; surgery to remove obstructions and/or enlarge the airway; and respiratory stimulants. If you are overweight, your doctor will recommend that you lose the excess pounds, since obesity often contributes to the problem. In addition, people who suffer from sleep apnea should not take sleeping pills of any kind, and should avoid alcoholic beverages, antihistamines, and anything else that causes drowsiness.

■ Sleep on your side, not your back. Sometimes this alone is enough to fix the problem.

■ Try adding an extra pillow. Elevating your head can sometimes relieve snoring.

■ There are devices available that adhere to the bridge of the nose and hold the sides of the nasal passages open wider than normal to increase air flow. These can be worth a try.

■ Hundreds of gadgets have been invented over the years to prevent snoring. One cure for snoring that dates back to the American Revolution, and possibly before, is to sew a pocket onto the back of your nightclothes and then to place a ball in the pocket. When you roll over onto your back and end up in the prime snoring position, the ball should cause enough discomfort to prompt you to choose another position. The "ball in the pocket" remains a popular home remedy. There are also many other anti-snoring devices on the market today, including aids that hold the lower jaw forward, adhesive patches that open nasal air passages, and even some that supposedly can condition snorers to stop by causing unpleasant sensations when they snore. A little experimentation may reveal what works for you.

Sore Throat

The medical terms for sore throat are *pharyngitis* (inflammation of the throat), *laryngitis* (inflammation of the larynx, or voice box), and *tonsillitis* (inflammation of the tonsils). The throat, or pharynx, is a tubelike passageway that separates into the breathing and digestive tracts. It is made of smooth muscle and lined with a mucous membrane. The throat facilitates speech by changing shape to allow the formation of vowel sounds. It also contains openings for the eustachian tubes, which drain secretions from the middle ear; the nasal space, or posterior nares; and the larynx, esophagus, and tonsils.

A sore throat can feel vaguely scratchy, sharply hot and painful, or anything in between. Pain and swelling may make swallowing difficult, and spots may be visible on the tonsils. If the tonsils are infected, the pain may be felt more in the ears than in the throat, and swallowing can be extremely painful. If the larynx becomes inflamed, you are likely to lose your voice temporarily.

Most sore throats are caused by viruses or bacteria. Other possible causes include overuse of the voice and local irritation such as that from exposure to cigarette smoke, environmental pollutants, dust, or dry winter air. A sore throat can also be caused by an abscess in the back of the throat or on the tonsils.

Sore throats occur most often in late winter and early spring. The majority of sore throats are minor viral illnesses that can be treated easily at home. However, about one-third of sore throats are diagnosed as "strep" throat, an infection caused by *Streptococcus* bacteria. The strep bacteria is highly contagious and persistent. The distinguishing signs and symptoms of strep infection, as opposed to a viral infection, are not always consistent, so definitive diagnosis must be based on a throat culture. But there are some general features that can help you make an initial evaluation (*see* Strep Infection Versus Viral Infection on page 534). If left untreated, a strep infection can lead to a number of complications. The most serious of these is rheumatic fever, an inflammatory disease that can cause heart damage. If you are recovering from a sore throat and develop a fever, joint pain and/or achiness, a rash, or muscle spasms, call your doctor. These can be signs of rheumatic fever. If you have a history of rheumatic fever, you should consult your physician immediately if you develop a sore throat of any kind.

CONVENTIONAL TREATMENT

■ A throat culture provides the only conclusive diagnosis of *Streptococcus* infection. Using a swab, the physician gently removes mucus from the back of the throat for examination. In a modern laboratory, a culture can be done very quickly, and the results can be in your doctor's hands within twenty-four hours. There are also newer tests that can be performed in a doctor's office and that can give results in as little as fifteen minutes.

■ If the diagnosis is strep, your doctor will prescribe an antibiotic. Penicillin (Bicillin, Pentids, Pfizerpen, Wycillin, and others) is usually the antibiotic of choice. Your physician may give you a course of penicillin in pill form, to be taken over a ten-day period, or he or she may opt for a one-dose injection of penicillin. If you are allergic to penicillin, erythromycin (ERYC, Ilotycin, and others) is the preferred alternative. If your doctor prescribes pills, it is important that you take the entire ten-day course to ensure complete eradication of the bacteria. Don't stop taking the pills after a few days, even if you feel much better.

■ If a strep throat is ruled out, the sore throat is most likely caused by a viral infection. If this is the case, antibiotics are ineffective and therefore not appropriate. Medical science has not yet discovered medications that fight most viral infections effectively. Fortunately, though viral infections can be quite uncomfortable, most are self-limiting. Treatment for a viral infection is aimed at helping you stay as comfortable as possible while it runs its course.

■ A pain reliever, such as acetaminophen (found in Tylenol, Tempra, and other medications), aspirin (Bayer, Ecotrin, and others), or ibuprofen (Advil, Motrin, Nuprin, and others) can help to control fever and ease the pain of a sore throat, as well as any other accompanying aches and pains.

Note: In excessive amounts, acetaminophen can cause liver damage. Do not exceed the recommended dosage. Take aspirin or ibuprofen with food to prevent possible stomach upset. Do not take aspirin during the last three months of pregnancy unless directed to do so by a physician.

■ Chloraseptic, available in lozenge and spray form, is an oral anesthetic and antiseptic that can help relieve the pain of a sore throat. Follow the directions on the product label. Use it sparingly, however. This product contains phenol, which can slow healing.

DIETARY GUIDELINES

■ Enjoy ice-cold frozen-fruit-juice popsicles. These can be effective temporary anesthetics for a sore throat.

■ Take plenty of fluids. Warm miso soup and chicken soup are excellent choices.

■ Eat lots of whole grains, fresh vegetables, and fruits. Cut out sugar, refined carbohydrates, and dairy products.

NUTRITIONAL SUPPLEMENTS

■ Vitamin C is both antibacterial and anti-inflammatory.

Strep Infection Versus Viral Infection

Although not all viral or strep infections cause identical symptoms, there are some general tendencies to look for when you have a sore throat. Review the following symptoms to see which match your condition. If you suspect a strep infection, contact your doctor. Only a throat culture can accurately confirm a diagnosis of strep.

Sign	Strep Infection	Viral Infection
Onset	Comes on suddenly. One minute, you feel fine; the next, tired, listless, and uncomfortable.	Comes on gradually, escalating from a mild scratchiness to a full-fledged sore throat.
Symptoms	A very painful sore throat, often accompanied by headache, stomach pain, vomiting, and/or tender or very firm lymph nodes. You may have much difficulty swallowing, and you will look and feel very sick.	A sore, thick, or scratchy-feeling throat that may be accompanied by cough, headache, a runny nose, hoarseness, enlarged lymph nodes, some difficulty swallowing, and/or conjunctivitis.
Fever	A temperature that escalates to 102°F (or even higher) is possible.	Mild to moderate fever, if any.
Tonsils	Most likely red and swollen, with white splotches.	May or may not be swollen; may or may not have a white coating.

Dissolve 1 teaspoon (1,000 milligrams) of buffered vitamin-C powder in 8 ounces of water and sip this throughout the day. Do this for the first forty-eight hours of a sore throat.

■ Bioflavonoids help to ease inflammation in the throat and fight infection. Take 500 milligrams of mixed bioflavonoids three or four times a day for the first three to four days.

■ Sugar-free herbal-based lozenges fortified with vitamin C or zinc, a mineral that speeds healing, are very helpful. Lozenges increase saliva production and help soothe a dry, irritated throat. Take one lozenge every hour, as needed, up to a total equivalent to 50 or 60 milligrams of zinc daily, for up to one week. Avoid lozenges made with unnecessary chemicals and sugar.

HERBAL TREATMENT

■ Echinacea and goldenseal stimulate the immune system and are important for helping to clear any kind of infection. Take one dose of an echinacea and goldenseal combination formula supplying 350 to 500 milligrams of echinacea and 250 to 500 milligrams of goldenseal every two hours during the acute phase. Then cut back to one dose three times a day for up to one week.

■ Elderberry extract works well against viruses. Choose an extract standardized to contain 5 percent total flavonoids and take 500 milligrams twice daily. Or take 1/2 to 1 teaspoonful of liquid extract every four to six hours.

■ Garlic is antibacterial and supports the immune system. Many people find the odorless capsule forms are easier to take. Take the capsules whole or open them and dissolve the liquid in hot water or soup. Take 500 milligrams at least three times daily until you recover.

■ Grapefruit-seed extract can be taken internally or used as a gargle. A highly concentrated form, such as Citricidal, Nutrabiotic, or Paramicrocidin, is preferred. Place 5 to 10 drops in a glass of water for a gargle (for extra benefit, add 3 drops of tea tree oil as well). Or drink 3 to 5 drops of extract in 6 ounces of water. Do this three or four times daily for up to three days. Or use a gargle made by dissolving 1/4 teaspoon of salt in 4 ounces of water and adding a small pinch each of cayenne pepper, lemon juice, and honey.

■ Olive leaf extract is an excellent antibacterial and antiviral agent. Take 250 milligrams of standardized extract four times a day, starting at the first sign of a sore throat.

■ Drink an herbal sore-throat tea containing some or (preferably) all of the following: slippery elm bark, hyssop, licorice root, and sage. Hyssop and sage detoxify the blood; licorice and slippery elm soothe irritated mucous membranes and ease a sore throat. Take a cup of the tea three times daily for a couple of days or until you feel better. You can also cool the tea and use it as a gargle.

Note: Do not use licorice on a daily basis for more than five days at a time, as it can elevate blood pressure. Do not use it at all if you have high blood pressure.

■ Yarrow may be helpful because it promotes sweating and helps to lower fever. Take 500 milligrams three times a day, as needed, for the first one or two days.

HOMEOPATHY

■ *Apis mellifica* is good for a sore throat that comes on suddenly and is accompanied by swollen, red tonsils. Your tongue may be red as well. You have little thirst, although your mucous membranes are dry, and there is no coating on your throat. Take one dose of *Apis mellifica* 30x or 9c every one or two hours, up to a total of four doses, as long as symptoms last.

■ *Belladonna* also is for a sore throat that comes on suddenly, with extremely red tonsils, throat, and uvula; a fever; and, possibly, dilated pupils. Take one dose of *Belladonna* 30x or 9c every one to two hours, up to three doses in six hours.

■ *Hepar sulfuris calcareum* is for a sore throat accompanied by a cough that brings up thick white or yellow plugs of mucus, and a throat coated with mucus. You feel better with a hot washcloth on your throat. Take one dose of *Hepar sulfuris calcareum* 30x or 9c three times a day for two days.

■ *Lachesis* will benefit a sore throat that is localized on the left, or one that moves from left to right, with a dark-red throat and tonsils. You are understandably in a very bad mood; you are in a lot of pain and don't want to be touched. Take one dose of *Lachesis* 30x or 9c three times a day for up to two days.

■ *Lycopodium* will help a sore throat that is localized on the right side, or that moves from the right to the left side. You probably feel worse during late afternoon and early evening, between the hours of 4:00 and 8:00 PM. Take one dose of *Lycopodium* 30x or 9c three times a day for up to two days.

■ If the sore throat is accompanied by hoarseness and worsens in the evening, take one dose of *Phosphorus* 30x or 9c three times a day for up to two days.

■ *Phytolacca* is for a very dark, red throat and much pain with swallowing, accompanied by swollen glands and pain that radiates to the ears. Take one dose of *Phytolacca* 12x or 6c four times a day for up to two days.

■ If you have a mild to moderate fever along with a sore throat, take one dose of *Ferrum phosphoricum* 6x three times daily until the fever is resolved, in addition to one of the other symptom-specific remedies recommended above.

ACUPRESSURE

For the locations of acupressure points on the body, *see* ADMINISTERING AN ACUPRESSURE TREATMENT in Part Three.

■ Large Intestine 4 helps to clear infection.

■ Lung 7 moistens a dry and irritated throat.

GENERAL RECOMMENDATIONS

■ Get plenty of rest. A rested body generally heals more quickly than an active one.

■ Use a cool mist vaporizer to humidify the air. Humidified air soothes irritated respiratory membranes and helps relieve coughing and hoarseness.

■ *See also* COMMON COLD; COUGH; or FEVER if your sore throat is accompanied by these symptoms.

PREVENTION

■ Protect yourself from environmental pollutants and respiratory irritants, such as cigarette smoke and wood smoke.

■ If recurrent strep infections are a problem, consider checking out your pets. Cats have been known to harbor *Streptococcus* bacteria.

■ As soon as you recover from a strep infection, replace your toothbrush to avoid reinfecting yourself.

Spider Bite

See under BITES AND STINGS, INSECT AND SPIDER.

Spider Veins

See under VARICOSE VEINS.

Sprains

See under MUSCLE SPRAIN, STRAIN, AND PAIN.

Stomach, Upset

See INDIGESTION; NAUSEA AND VOMITING.

Stress

Stress is anything that disturbs your mental, emotional,

social, economic, and/or physical equilibrium. It causes your body to boost production of the hormones cortisol and adrenaline, which speed up your heart rate, raise your blood pressure, and increase your metabolic rate, among other things. Theses changes are part of what is called the "fight-or-flight" response. Presumably, in prehistoric times, this built-in protective mechanism provided the sudden rush of energy required to grab a spear and meet a challenger from the next cave (fight), or the extra burst of speed needed to run away from an enraged woolly mammoth (flight). Once the stressful event was resolved, our ancient ancestor's adrenaline was used up and his or her body slowly returned to normal.

Most of the stress we face today is mental and psychological, not physical. One psychiatric handbook gives a list of forty-three stress-producing events that commonly occur during a lifetime. Death of a spouse tops the list, followed by divorce or separation. Other stressful events include pressure at work, trouble with the boss, losing a job, a new marriage, the birth of a baby, too many bills and not enough money, a problem with your health or the health of a loved one, too much pressure at home, a change in financial status, retiring, and major holidays. Note that not all of these are bad experiences. The birth of a baby, for instance, is usually a joyful event, but because it represents a major change in one's life, it is nevertheless a source of stress.

Even though our stresses are not usually physical, stress still triggers the physical fight-or-flight response meant to prepare you to face challenges and improve your performance under pressure. Stress hormones circulate in your system, keeping you in a heightened state of readiness, and creating still more feelings of stress. Worse yet, when these hormones reach a certain level, instead of helping you cope, they actually have the opposite effect, reducing your ability to handle a tough situation. It stress persists for too long a time, it can literally wear your body out.

It has long been recognized that persons who suffer from high levels of stress are more likely to develop heart disease than those who lead calmer lives. One recent study found that accountants and tax professionals had a greater incidence of artery-clogging blood clots during tax season, which is a period of extreme stress for these individuals, than at other times of the year. This too is related to the body's stress response. When stress threatens, the composition of the blood actually changes slightly to make it clot more easily—presumably in preparation for dealing with physical danger. Even though the danger faced by the accountants amounted to piles of paperwork and a looming deadline, their bodies still responded by readying them for battle. What this means is that, due to the tremendous changes in the lives of humans over the past ten thousand years or so, a mechanism that once helped us survive is now a liability.

The stresses of modern life can cause a variety of direct symptoms. The most common include high blood pressure, sexual dysfunction, heart problems, fatigue, backaches, headaches, moodiness, irritability, sleep disturbances, gastrointestinal distress, and skin conditions. In addition, stress can contribute to many other illnesses, including cardiovascular disease, cancer, irritable bowel syndrome, glandular problems, and infectious diseases. Stress also taxes the endocrine system, so that many people, especially women, experience depressed thyroid function, even hypothyroidism, as a result. And, of course, stress is a major factor in virtually all psychological disorders.

There is no way to eliminate all the stress in your life, but there are ways to defuse tension and handle stress more effectively. This entry focuses on the natural nutrients, remedies, and strategies that can help.

CONVENTIONAL TREATMENT

■ If stress manifests itself as anxiety or depression, your doctor may recommend a short-term course of medica-

Adaptogens

Adaptogen is a term used for herbal remedies that strengthen or improve the body's overall ability to cope with the effects of stress. They do this by supporting and strengthening various organs, making the body more resilient in recovering from the stress response. Numerous herbs have long traditions of use for this purpose. Some of the best known include the following:

- Ashwaganda.
- Astragalus.
- Corcyceps.
- Chinese (Korean) ginseng.
- Dong quai.
- Schizandra.
- Siberian ginseng.

Adaptogens are valuable whether the stresses you face are emotional, biochemical, or environmental in origin. Used properly, and at the right time, they can reduce the toll that stress takes on your body.

tion. An antianxiety agent such as lorazepam (Ativan) or diazepam (Valium), or an antidepressant such as amitriptyline (Elavil), may help you get through a single very stressful episode. Both types of medications have a multitude of potential side effects, however, including drowsiness, agitation, and weakness. Lorazepam and diazepam can also cause blood abnormalities; amitriptyline has also been known to cause nausea, hair loss, and changes in sex drive, as well as more serious problems such as stroke and coma. Also, if your doctor prescribes medication, it is important not to use it as a substitute for dealing with the stressful event, or the stress will never really be resolved. If you have difficulty doing this on your own, working with a qualified therapist or counselor may be helpful.

■ Handling long-term, repeated stress requires strengthening the body and mind to deal with it. This is best accomplished through diet, lifestyle modification, and other natural techniques, as outlined in the rest of this entry.

■ If you are under stress and start noticing such symptoms as fatigue, abnormal intolerance to cold, hair loss, and dry skin, hair, and nails, consult your physician. You may have developed a thyroid problem.

DIETARY GUIDELINES

■ Because stress, especially chronic stress, depletes nutrients, a healthy diet is especially important when you are under pressure. Eat a well-balanced diet that emphasizes clean, lean protein; fresh vegetables and fruits; and whole grains. Eating five small meals and one or two healthy snacks spaced out throughout the day is usually better than having three large meals.

■ Avoid processed foods and food products that contain chemical additives, refined sugar and/or flour, red meat, and all fried foods. These substances put additional stress on the body. Do not allow yourself to use stress or a busy schedule as an excuse for unhealthy eating habits.

■ Avoid caffeine and alcohol. Caffeine affects the central nervous system and adds to stress. Alcohol may seem to relax you and temporarily relieve stress, but this effect is an illusion. In reality, it depresses the nervous system and may actually increase stress.

■ Avoid eating under stressful conditions. A relaxed eating atmosphere is very important for sufficient blood flow and digestive function throughout the gastrointestinal tract.

NUTRITIONAL SUPPLEMENTS

■ Take a good multivitamin and supplement daily to ensure that you get at least the recommended daily allowance (RDA) of all the major vitamins and minerals. Stress, especially long-term stress, depletes nutrients and can lead to multiple deficiencies.

■ Stress is usually associated with compromised adrenal function. Taking small amounts of adrenal glandular extract for a short time tends to give these important glands a jump-start. This supplement is especially important if stress is accompanied by fatigue. Take 150 to 200 milligrams twice a day for three weeks.

■ Calcium and magnesium are required by the central nervous system, and they are depleted by stress. Twice daily, take a good calcium and magnesium formula that provides 1,000 milligrams of calcium and 500 milligrams of magnesium.

■ Gastrointestinal problems often associated with stress, such as stomach ulcers, diarrhea, and inflammatory bowel disorders, often benefit from the amino acid glutamine. Take 1,000 to 2,000 milligrams of L-glutamine two to three times daily for up to three months.

■ Stress often results in depleted friendly bacteria in the intestines, which in turn compromises digestion. To replenish it, take a probiotic supplement such as acidophilus or bifidobacteria as recommended on the product label. If you are allergic to milk, be sure to select a dairy-free formula.

■ The B vitamins are vitally important for a properly functioning nervous system. Take a good B-complex formula that supplies 25 to 50 milligrams of each of the major B vitamins daily, or talk to your doctor about weekly injections. You can often get results faster by receiving intramuscular injections than by taking vitamins orally. In addition to the full B complex, take 250 milligrams of stress-fighting pantothenic acid twice daily plus 500 micrograms of vitamin B_{12} twice a day for up to one month. Better yet, talk to your doctor about weekly injections of these vitamins as well.

■ Vitamin C and bioflavonoids support the adrenal glands, which are overburdened during periods of long-term stress. Take 1,000 to 3,000 milligrams (3 to 10 grams) of vitamin C with bioflavonoids daily.

■ Vitamin E is a powerful antioxidant that supports immune function, which can be depressed by stress. Choose a formula containing mixed tocopherols, and start by taking 200 international units daily. Then gradually increase the dosage until you are taking 400 international units of vitamin E twice daily.

Note: If you have high blood pressure, limit your intake of supplemental vitamin E to a total of 400 international units daily. If you are taking an anticoagulant (blood thinner), consult your physician before taking supplemental vitamin E.

■ Zinc supports the immune system and helps defuse free radicals, which proliferate during periods of stress. Take up to 100 milligrams of zinc daily from all sources.

Note: Take zinc with food to prevent stomach upset,

and do not exceed the recommended dosage. If you take over 30 milligrams of zinc on a daily basis for more than one or two months, you should also take 1 to 2 milligrams of copper each day to maintain a proper mineral balance.

HERBAL TREATMENT

■ Astragalus supports the immune system and helps the body cope with stress. Take 250 milligrams three times a day.

■ Chinese (Korean) ginseng helps the body adapt to stress, alleviates fatigue, and improves mood. Select a standardized extract containing 7 percent ginsenosides and take 100 milligrams twice daily for two to three weeks. Stop taking the preparation for two weeks, then repeat.

Note: Do not use Chinese ginseng if you have high blood pressure, heart disease, or hypoglycemia. If you are sensitive to the effects of caffeine and other stimulants, you may want to consult with a qualified health-care professional before using ginseng.

■ Kava kava is a calming herb that helps alleviate mental anxiety. Choose a standardized extract containing 30 percent kavalactones and take 200 milligrams twice a day, in morning and evening.

Note: In excess amounts, this herb can cause drowsiness. Do not exceed the recommended dose. Do not use kava kava if you are pregnant or nursing, if you have Parkinson's disease, or if you are taking a prescription medication for depression or anxiety.

■ St. John's wort has valuable calming and antidepressant properties. Choose a standardized extract containing 0.3 percent hypericin and take 200 to 300 milligrams two or three times daily.

■ Siberian ginseng has the remarkable ability to reduce the fight-or-flight response to stress. It also helps prevent stress-induced damage to the thymus gland. Choose a standardized extract containing 0.5 percent eleutheroside E and take 100 milligrams half an hour before breakfast. Take this herb in a cyclical fashion: four weeks on, one week off.

■ Valerian can relieve insomnia, a common symptom of stress. If you have trouble sleeping, choose a standardized extract containing at least 0.5 percent valerenic acids and take 250 to 500 milligrams one-half hour before bedtime.

HOMEOPATHY

■ *Coffea cruda* can help relieve stress accompanied by obsessive thoughts. Take one dose of *Coffea cruda* 12x or 6c, as directed on the product label, one-half hour before bedtime for three to five consecutive nights. If you find your symptoms improve before then, stop taking the remedy.

BACH FLOWER REMEDIES

■ Select the remedy that most closely fits your emotional tendencies and concerns, and take it as needed, following the directions on the product label.

■ Rescue Remedy helps relieve any crisis-caused stress, as well as feelings of panic and anxiety.

■ Beech is good if you tend to be a perfectionist who is impatient with others, and you experience stress when there is an upset in your schedule.

■ Holly helps to tame anger that bursts out in fits of temper.

■ White Chestnut helps to counteract stress due to obsessing incessantly on upsetting events long after they should have been forgotten.

ACUPRESSURE

For the locations of acupressure points on the body, *see* ADMINISTERING AN ACUPRESSURE TREATMENT in Part Three.

■ The back Bladder points relax the nervous system.

■ Gallbladder 20 and 21 help to relax the mind.

■ Liver 3 helps to quiet the nervous system.

■ Pericardium 6 helps relax the mind and alleviate nervousness.

■ Stomach 36 strengthens overall well-being.

AROMATHERAPY

For specific instructions on how to use aromatherapy, *see* PREPARING AROMATHERAPY TREATMENTS in Part Three.

■ There are many essential oils that help to calm and counteract stress. Bergamot, elemi, frankincense, geranium, jasmine, lavender, myrrh, neroli, patchouli, sandalwood, vetiver, and ylang ylang are all good for this purpose. They can be used singly or in combinations of up to three different oils—you may want to experiment a bit to find the mixture you like best. There are also many ways you can use essential oils to reduce stress. Add a few drops to a hot bath or massage oil, inhale directly from the bottle, or diffuse them into the air.

GENERAL RECOMMENDATIONS

■ Don't take home-related problems to work, and don't take work-related problems home. Each environment has its own set of problems. Try to keep each in its place.

■ You may not be able to fight (though some people find punching a pillow or other soft object helpful), but you can take flight: Exercise. Exercise is a powerful stress-buster. Physical activity helps dissipate the stress-induced chemicals affecting your body. Regular exercise is best for keeping yourself on an even keel over the long term, but a brisk walk, several trips up and down stairs, or even some jumping jacks in your office or your living room can prove helpful.

■ Relaxation techniques are very helpful against both acute and chronic stress. Select a soothing phrase and repeat it silently to yourself whenever you feel stressed. Try this the next time you're late and stuck in traffic, when the boss is on the rampage, when there's too much to do and not enough time, or even after you read a newspaper article that makes you furious. Simply repeating a preselected phrase or word over and over again boosts the relaxation response. Slow, even deep breathing also initiates the relaxation response and helps slow a racing heart. You must concentrate on your breathing, though. Don't just breathe automatically; make a conscious effort. Think, "In comes the good air" on the inhale, and "out goes the bad air" on the exhale. For more information about inducing relaxation, *see* RELAXATION TECHNIQUES in Part Three.

■ Change your thinking. A technique called cognitive restructuring requires you to interrupt your thought process whenever you find yourself focusing on a subject that causes you to feel stressed. As soon as the banned thoughts cross your mind, deliberately and immediately begin thinking about something pleasant, even if it's just something as simple as deciding what type of luscious ripe fruit you are going to pick up at the farmer's market to have for dessert.

Stroke

A stroke occurs when the blood supply to the brain is interrupted, depriving the brain of the oxygen it needs to function. If oxygen deprivation continues for more than a few minutes, areas of brain tissue die, causing permanent damage. About 80 percent of all strokes are caused by atherosclerosis, which results in a gradual buildup of fatty plaques on artery walls. The plaques narrow the arteries and can block them; alternatively, a blood clot can become lodged in the narrowed portion of a blood vessel, causing blockage. A stroke can also result if a blood vessel serving the brain ruptures, interrupting the normal flow of blood.

The risk of suffering a stroke is increased by certain factors. The two most important risk factors are atherosclerosis and high blood pressure, which weakens the walls of the arteries. Hyperlipidemia (a higher than normal level of fatty substances in the blood) increases the risk. Diabetes and smoking also increase the likelihood of stroke because they increase the risk of high blood pressure and atherosclerosis. Other serious problems that add to the risk of stroke include an irregular heartbeat and/or

a damaged heart valve. These situations can cause disruptions in the flow of blood in the heart's chambers that lead to the formation of clots or even bacterial growths that can break off and travel through the arteries, and ultimately block the flow of blood to the brain. A recent heart attack also increases the risk. Women who take oral contraceptives are at higher risk of stroke than those who practice different methods of birth control.

The lasting consequences of a stroke, if any, depend on whether the brain suffers permanent damage and, if it does, exactly which area of the brain is affected. If your brain is deprived of oxygen only briefly, you may experience a temporary loss of speech, visual problems, confusion, weakness, and/or tremors, but then return to normal once the flow of blood to the brain is restored. This type of episode is termed a *transient ischemic attack,* or TIA. Sometimes TIAs are a sign of further trouble to come, but not always; some people have them repeatedly without appearing to suffer any serious consequences. A full-blown stroke that causes brain damage may happen within minutes or seconds, or may develop slowly over a period of hours or even a day or two. In either case, you may be left with impairment in bodily sensations, movement, vision, and/or speech. In one way, the slowly developing type of stroke can be the more dangerous of the two, because you may not recognize it as an emergency right away, and delaying treatment can affect the outcome.

Symptoms of stroke usually include one or more of the following: a sudden, intense headache; numbness, dizziness, weakness, and/or paralysis of the face, arm, or leg, often affecting only one side of the body; blurred vision or loss of vision in one or both eyes; difficulty swallowing; difficulty speaking or slurred speech; sudden confusion and/or difficulty understanding simple statements; and dizziness, unsteadiness, and loss of balance and coordination, possibly leading to a fall. It is possible for a person having a stroke to lose consciousness altogether.

Roughly one-third of people who suffer strokes do not survive the attack. Another third are left with some degree of disability, and the remaining third recover completely. Quick treatment is the key to survival and recovery.

EMERGENCY TREATMENT

■ To be effective, treatment must be initiated within three hours of the onset of the stroke. After that period, the window of opportunity closes and permanent damage is likely. If you develop one or more of the symptoms of stroke outlined in the introduction above, have someone take you immediately to the emergency room of the nearest hospital or call for emergency medical assistance and stress the urgency of the situation.

■ Appropriate emergency treatment depends on whether a stroke is due to a blood clot or bleeding from a ruptured blood vessel. A computerized tomography (CT) scan is likely to be the first measure taken, as it can usually differentiate between the two.

■ If the stroke is determined to be due to a clot, medical personnel may administer intravenous clot-dissolving medication such as tissue plasminogen activator (TPA) or streptokinase. The idea is that, if used properly within the first three hours after a stroke occurs, these drugs may relieve the blockage in time to help you avoid some damage to the brain. This promising treatment has been used for some time for heart attacks, but is still relatively new in the treatment of stroke. For a slowly evolving stroke, the blood thinner heparin may be administered to try to lessen the magnitude of the completed stroke. The calcium channel blocker nimodipine (Nimotop) may also be used, as there is some evidence that it can lessen the amount of brain damage caused by a stroke. Other agents that are still considered experimental, but that may be in regular use soon, include drugs called N-methyl-D-aspartate (NMDA) receptor blockers, which may make nerve cells less sensitive to oxygen deprivation.

■ If an abnormality in blood vessel formation is found, such as an aneurysm (weakness in a spot in the wall of an artery) or a congenital malformation, immediate neurosurgery may be done to place a clip at the site and stop further bleeding.

■ If needed, treatment to reduce blood pressure, supply oxygen, and deal with other problems will be administered.

CONVENTIONAL TREATMENT

■ Once the acute crisis has been handled and your condition has stabilized, conventional treatment focuses on recovery and the prevention of recurrences. Physical and/or speech therapy should be begun as early as possible. Depending on the area of the brain that is affected, it may be possible to "reroute" the transmission of nerve impulses and improve functioning. Physical therapy is designed to improve muscle memory, stimulate limb movement, and build overall strength. Speech therapy is designed to help you remember words and recall how to pronounce them. To do this, it may be necessary to start by relearning basic letter recognition and phonics (letter sounds).

■ If the stroke was due to a blood clot, your doctor may recommend that you take a blood thinner such as warfarin (Coumadin) on an ongoing basis.

■ If blockage is found in a major artery that serves the brain, your doctor may recommend surgery to remove it.

■ It is not uncommon for disturbances in mood, such as depression and/or anxiety, to occur after a stroke. These can be due to the stroke's physical effects on the brain, to the psychological impact of having had such an attack and, perhaps, facing some degree of disability, or to all of the above. If such problems persist after your physical condition has become stable, your doctor may suggest antidepressant or antianxiety medication to treat them.

■ After a stroke, treatment of any chronic disorders you have that may have been contributing factors, such as high blood pressure or diabetes, should be evaluated and modified, if necessary, to keep them well controlled.

DIETARY GUIDELINES

■ Eat a well-balanced diet with an emphasis on fresh vegetables and fruits; lean, clean protein foods; and whole grains. This is important for the health of the blood vessels as well as for ensuring an abundant supply of important vitamins, minerals, and phytochemicals (antioxidant compounds in plants) that fight free-radical damage and help increase the oxygenation of tissues, including those of the brain.

■ Enjoy carrots often. In a study of 87,000 nurses conducted by Brigham and Women's Hospital and Harvard University, subjects who ate five or more servings of carrots every week had a 68-percent lower risk of suffering a stroke compared with those who ate no more than one serving a month.

■ Make sure your diet includes the blue and purple fruits and vegetables, such as Concord grapes, eggplant, and red cabbage. These foods contain pigments called anthocyanidins. The anthocyanidins in wine grapes are believed to explain why having a glass of red wine with dinner can help lower the risk of stroke (and heart attack).

■ Avoid saturated and hydrogenated fats. This means cutting out dairy products (except for small amounts of the low-fat varieties), red meat, eggs, margarine, shortening, tropical oils such as coconut and palm oil, and all fried foods. Saturated and hydrogenated fats raise cholesterol levels, especially that of LDL (the so-called "bad cholesterol") and promote the buildup of fatty plaques in the arteries. Fish and moderate amounts of skinned white-meat poultry are acceptable; other good sources of protein are whole grains and legumes.

NUTRITIONAL SUPPLEMENTS

Nutritional supplements are intended to support recovery from a stroke, rather than to treat an acute episode. If you suspect you may be having a stroke, seek emergency medical treatment immediately.

■ Coenzyme Q_{10} is noted for increasing the flow of oxygenated blood to the brain. Take 30 to 60 milligrams three times daily.

■ The essential fatty acids found in black currant seed,

borage, evening primrose, fish, and flaxseed oils have important antioxidant and anti-inflammatory properties. Choose one of these oils and take 500 to 1,000 milligrams two or three times daily. If you are taking an anticoagulant (blood thinner), be sure to have your clotting time checked regularly.

■ Green-foods supplements are filled with trace minerals that both improve and speed healing. Take a green-foods supplement as directed on the product label.

■ Lecithin helps improve the digestion of fats. Take 1,200 milligrams two or three times daily, with meals.

■ Vitamin C and the bioflavonoids, especially rutin, strengthen weak blood-vessel walls and help to initiate healing of the arterial system. Take 500 to 1,000 milligrams of vitamin C and an equal amount of mixed bioflavonoids three times daily. If you wish, you can gradually increase your intake to the highest level you can tolerate (the highest dosage that does not result in loose stools).

■ Vitamin E protects the cells from free-radical damage and is necessary for nerve health. Start by taking 100 international units daily. After two weeks, gradually increase the dosage until you are taking 200 international units in the morning and another 200 international units in the evening.

Note: If you are taking an anticoagulant (blood thinner), consult your physician before taking supplemental vitamin E.

HERBAL TREATMENT

Herbal treatments are intended to support recovery from a stroke, rather than to treat an acute episode. If you suspect you may be having a stroke, seek emergency medical treatment immediately.

■ Astragalus acts to improve tissue oxygenation. Take 250 milligrams of standardized extract four times a day.

■ Cayenne improves circulation and heart function without raising blood pressure. It also enhances the power of other herbs taken at the same time. Take 100 milligrams twice daily, with meals.

■ Garlic helps lower high blood pressure and also helps thin the blood. Take 500 milligrams three times daily.

■ Ginkgo biloba is used both to prevent and treat stroke. It helps to prevent blood clots from developing and increases blood flow to the brain. This herb has also been shown to inhibit free-radical formation. Select a product containing at least 24 percent ginkgo heterosides (sometimes called flavoglycosides) and take 40 to 80 milligrams three times daily.

■ Green tea may act as one of the most potent free-radical scavengers to protect against the peroxidation of lipids, a contributing factor in atherosclerosis. Choose a decaffeinated standardized extract containing at least 50 percent catechins and 90 percent total polyphenols, and take 300 to 500 milligrams daily.

■ With regular use, hawthorn has been reported to prevent or slow the progression of arteriosclerosis. Choose a standardized extract containing 1.8 percent vitexin-2 rhamnosides and take 100 to 200 milligrams two or three times a day.

■ Kava kava helps to protect the brain against oxygen deprivation. Choose a standardized extract containing 30 percent kavalactones and take 250 milligrams twice a day.

Note: In excess amounts, this herb can cause drowsiness. Do not exceed the recommended dose. Do not use kava kava if you are pregnant or nursing, if you have Parkinson's disease, or if you are taking a prescription medication for depression or anxiety.

■ Pine-bark and grape-seed extract are high in proanthocyanidins (also known as OPCs) that increase the structural strength of weakened blood vessels. Take 25 to 50 milligrams of either two or three times daily.

HOMEOPATHY

Homeopathic treatments are intended to support recovery from a stroke, rather than to treat an acute episode. If you suspect you may be having a stroke, seek emergency medical treatment immediately. The best approach to treating the aftermath of stroke homeopathically is to consult a qualified homeopathic practitioner who can prescribe a constitutional remedy. The remedies that follow can be helpful as well.

■ *Aconite* can help alleviate the panic, fright, and shock that accompany a stroke; *Arnica* helps to initiate bodywide healing. As soon as your doctor signals that you can take something by mouth, take one dose of *Aconite* 200x or 30c. Follow this with one dose of *Arnica* 30x or 15c three to four times daily for three to five days.

■ *Aurum muriaticum* is good if your predominant symptom is depression. Take one dose of *Aurum muriaticum* 30x or 15c three times daily for up to three days, as needed. If you notice an improvement before that time, stop taking the remedy.

■ *Baryta carbonica* is helpful for both physical and mental weakness and fatigue following a stroke. Take one dose of *Baryta carbonica* 30x or 15c three times daily for up to three days, as needed. If you notice an improvement before that time, stop taking the remedy.

■ *Gelsemium* can help if you have numbness and trembling, and have lost the ability to speak. Take one dose of *Gelsemium* 30x or 15c three times daily for up to three days, as needed. If you notice an improvement before that time, stop taking the remedy.

If none of the symptom-specific remedies listed here bring about any improvement after two or three days, discontinue the remedy and consult a health-care practitioner experienced in homeopathy.

BACH FLOWER REMEDIES

Select the remedy that most closely fits your emotional tendencies and concerns, and take it as needed, following the directions on the product label. Note that Bach remedies are intended to support recovery from a stroke, rather than to treat an acute episode. If you suspect you may be having a stroke, seek emergency medical treatment immediately.

Rescue Remedy is the first remedy to apply in any crisis situation. Take it as soon as it is safe for you to take something by mouth. This remedy is helpful also for family members and friends, who are understandably anxious and upset.

Agrimony can help if you are suffering inside but are determined to appear cheerful to others.

Beech is valuable if you find yourself impatient and intolerant over upsets in schedule.

Holly helps to defuse anger that is rooted in feelings of insecurity but that is expressed in fits of bad temper.

Mimulus helps to ease fears of things you can clearly identify. You may be somewhat timid and shy.

Mustard can help to lift feelings of sadness, sorrow, and depression.

ACUPRESSURE

Acupressure is intended to support recovery from a stroke, rather than treating an acute episode. If you suspect you may be having a stroke, seek emergency medical treatment immediately. For the locations of acupressure points on the body, *see* ADMINISTERING AN ACUPRESSURE TREATMENT in Part Three.

All of the back Bladder points stimulate circulation.

Gallbladder 20 improves circulation to the head.

Large Intestine 4 relaxes tension in the head.

Liver 3 relaxes the nervous system.

The Ting points are the points at the tips of the fingers and toes. They can be very helpful in aiding recovery following a stroke.

GENERAL RECOMMENDATIONS

■ If you require physical, occupational, and/or speech therapy, be as cooperative with your therapist as you can. Keep in mind that recovery from stroke is a gradual process. It can be frustrating at times, but do your best not

to feel discouraged. Perseverence is often the key to long-term success.

■ Consider consulting a professional acupuncturist who can use electrical stimulation to work the Ting points. This treatment can be dramatically effective in reversing some of the effects of stroke.

PREVENTION

■ If you have high blood pressure and/or diabetes, work with your health-care provider to keep these conditions under control. Take any medication exactly as prescribed, and keep regular follow-up appointments as recommended by your physician. If you think you are having side effects due to medication, advise your physician promptly. You may need an adjustment in dosage or even a different prescription. *Do not* stop or reduce the dosage of prescription medication on your own, however. Always consult with your physician first.

■ Keep your weight down and get regular exercise. If you are an overweight couch potato, the nicest thing you can do for yourself (and your loved ones) is to adopt a healthy weight-loss plan and stick to it. (*See* OBESITY.)

■ As much as possible, avoid stress, and learn how to deal with the stress you cannot avoid. Any method that helps promote the relaxation response can help reduce your chances of suffering a stroke. Meditation and yoga are both good choices. (*See* RELAXATION TECHNIQUES in Part Three.)

■ Don't smoke. Smoking constricts the blood vessels, increasing the likelihood of high blood pressure and, consequently, stroke. Actually, it is an unnecessary risk factor in almost any health problem you can name. (*See* NICOTINE ADDICTION for suggestions that can help you quit and regain your health.)

Stye

A stye is an infection on the edge of the eyelid that occurs in an oil-secreting gland located near the root of an eyelash. Styes are usually bacterial in origin and are primarily caused by *Staphylococcus* bacteria. An emerging stye appears as a red, swollen, tender area on the rim of an eyelid. As pus forms, the red area may develop into a fluid-filled blister with a small but visible yellowish spot in the center, and the eye may water. When the blister opens and drains, healing can begin. A stye should improve within two or three days.

It is possible for a stye to form in a gland located deeper under the skin. This may be referred to as an internal stye, and it usually causes greater pain. Due to its location, it is less likely to open and drain on its own than an ordinary stye, so it may need a doctor's treatment.

A *chalazion* is a condition that starts out very much like a stye, with pain, redness, and swelling in the eyelid. However, these symptoms soon clear up and in their place a small round lump appears and begins to grow. There may also be a reddish or grayish spot on the underside of the eyelid. A chalazion is not the result of infection, but of blockage of one of the oil-secreting glands that causes the gland to become hard and enlarged.

CONVENTIONAL TREATMENT

■ Applying hot moist compresses for ten minutes three or four times per day can help bring the infection to a head (see the suggestions under Herbal Treatment, below, for ways of enhancing the effectiveness of this treatment).

■ If the stye is persistent or the infection worsens, an ophthalmic-formula antibiotic, such as erythromycin (Ilotycin), tobramycin (Tobrex), sodium sulamyd, or Polysporin, may be prescribed.

■ In rare cases, a stye may have to be opened with a needle to facilitate drainage. This procedure must be performed by a physician.

■ Chalazions usually clear up on their own, though they may take up to six weeks to do so. Using hot compresses as described above may speed the process. If a chalazion is not better after six weeks, your doctor will likely recommend removing it. This involves a minor, in-office surgical procedure.

NUTRITIONAL SUPPLEMENTS

■ Vitamin C is an important supplement whenever any type of infection is present. When the body is fighting an infection, its vitamin-C requirements may climb to as much as five or six times higher than normal because white blood cells use up its vitamin-C stores. Take 500 to 1,000 milligrams three times a day until the infection clears.

HERBAL TREATMENT

■ Cat's claw enhances the immune response and has antibacterial properties. Take 500 milligrams of standardized extract three times a day until the infection clears.

Note: Do not use cat's claw if you are pregnant or nursing, or if you are an organ-transplant recipient. Use it with caution if you are taking an anticoagulant (blood thinner).

■ Echinacea has antiviral and antibacterial properties; goldenseal is antibacterial and helps soothe mucous membranes. Take one dose of an echinacea and goldenseal combination formula supplying 500 milligrams of echinacea and 350 milligrams of goldenseal four times daily for five days.

■ Goldenseal fights bacteria and tones the mucous membranes. Take 250 milligrams of standardized extract three times a day.

■ Oregano has antibacterial properties and helps to fight infection. Take 75 milligrams of standardized extract three times a day.

■ Make hot herbal compresses by simmering 1 teaspoon of a selected herb or herbal extract (see below) in 1 pint of water for ten minutes. Cool the infusion to a tolerable temperature, soak a clean cloth or piece of sterile cotton in it, and wring the cloth or cotton out so that it isn't dripping. Apply the warm, wet compress to the stye for ten minutes four to six times a day. The following herbs may be used:

- Eyebright helps relieve redness and swelling, and helps to clear infection.
- Goldenseal is antibacterial and is a good source of berberine, a potent natural antibiotic.
- Oregon grape root also is a source of berberine.

Wash your hands both before and after the treatment. If you use a cotton ball, throw it away after removing the compress; if you use cloth, wash the compress in detergent and hot water (with chlorine bleach added if possible), separately from all other laundry, before using it again. Always be very cautious when using warm liquids around your eyes. The skin of the eyelid is thin and tender and can burn easily.

HOMEOPATHY

As soon as you notice a stye developing, take one dose of *Aconite* 30x or 9c. Then choose one of the following symptom-specific remedies.

■ *Apis mellifica* is for an eyelid that is red and swollen. Take one dose of *Apis mellifica* 30x or 9c three times daily for up to two days.

■ *Hepar sulfuris calcareum* will help the stye to drain when it is about to burst. Take one dose of *Hepar sulfuris calcareum* 12x or 6c three times daily for up to two days.

■ *Myristica* is useful for a stye that is taking a very long time to open. Take one dose of *Myristica* 12x or 6c three times daily for up to two days.

■ *Staphysagria* helps to relieve the pain of stye. Take one dose of *Staphysagria* 12x or 6c four times daily, as needed.

GENERAL RECOMMENDATIONS

■ Do not squeeze or try to puncture the blister. This only worsens the infection.

■ If a stye begins to spread, or shows no improvement after three days, consult your health-care provider.

■ If what appeared to be a stye gave way to a slowly growing round lump in the eyelid, and the bump does not go away on its own in six weeks, consult your health-care provider.

Sunburn

Sunburn is caused by exposure to radiation from the sun. It is usually a first-degree burn. In other words, it involves the epidermis, the outer (superficial) layer of the skin. Sunburned skin is hot, red, and painful. If the skin blisters and swelling develops, a second-degree burn has occurred, and the dermis, the underlying layer of skin, has been affected (*see* BURNS).

The radiation that causes sunburn comes down to the earth in the form of ultraviolet (UV) rays. There are two types of UV radiation: ultraviolet-A (UVA), which is present year round, and ultraviolet-B (UVB), which is present primarily in the summer months. While it was once believed that only UVB radiation presented the danger of damage from the sun, it is now known that UVA radiation is harmful also. As a result, experts recommend taking precautions against sun exposure no matter what the season.

Without the protection of sunscreen, clothing, or a hat, the skin can burn quickly. The sun's rays are further intensified when they are reflected by water or sand, or by suntan oils and lotions that do not contain sunscreen. Reflected radiation is real. Even if you are wearing a T-shirt and sitting under a beach umbrella, you can burn.

The long-term hazards of sun exposure have long been well known. More recent evidence suggests that skin cancer may be even more closely related to sunburn—even a single bad case—than to total long-term sun exposure. And just because you don't seem to be getting burned while you are outside, you cannot assume that you are being unaffected by the sun's rays. A sunburn can develop and deepen even after you are home and in bed. The pain of sunburn is most intense between six and forty-eight hours after exposure to the sun. Skin that is lightly pinked when you go to bed may turn red, burning, and painful by the next morning. A severe sunburn can cause nausea, chills, and fever, as well as intense stinging. If you develop such symptoms along with a sunburn, or if the skin becomes blistered and/or swollen, you should consult your health-care provider for advice.

CONVENTIONAL TREATMENT

■ A painkiller such as acetaminophen (in Tylenol, Datril, and many other over-the-counter products), aspirin (Bayer, Ecotrin, and others), or ibuprofen (Advil, Motrin, Nuprin, and others) can decrease the severity of pain if taken soon after exposure, but before a full-blown burn develops.

Note: In excessive amounts, acetaminophen can cause liver damage. Do not exceed the recommended dosage. Take aspirin with food to prevent possible stomach upset. Do not take aspirin during the last three months of pregnancy unless directed to do so by a physician.

■ Cool showers, baths, and compresses are very soothing, and may keep the burn from getting worse, especially if used soon after sun exposure.

■ If you suffer from itching as a sunburn heals, an antihistamine such as hydroxyzine (Atarax, Vistaril), diphenhydramine (Benadryl), or chlorpheniramine (Chlor-Trimeton) may help. Possible side effects include drowsiness and dry mouth, although the drowsiness can help you sleep if you are feeling uncomfortable.

■ Anesthetic sprays that contain benzocaine sometimes help, especially if sunburn pain is severe. These medications can cause an allergic skin reaction and eczema in some people, however, and should not be used routinely.

■ For an extremely severe sunburn, your doctor may prescribe a cortisone-like drug such as prednisone, either to be taken orally or to be used in a topical spray. Although this can be dramatically effective when used early on, there are potentially serious side effects, so it should be reserved for the worst cases.

DIETARY GUIDELINES

■ Dehydration often accompanies excessive exposure to the sun. Make sure you get sufficient fluids after spending time in the sun.

NUTRITIONAL SUPPLEMENTS

■ Beta-carotene helps to heal the skin and protect against burns. Take 25,000 international units of beta-carotene twice a day for three days after a sunburn. On the fourth day, cut back to 10,000 international units twice daily and maintain that dosage for two weeks. Then cut back again, to 2,500 to 5,000 international units.

■ Selenium is an antioxidant and free-radical scavenger. Be sure to get 200 micrograms of this importat mineral daily.

■ Vitamin C and bioflavonoids are essential for the production of collagen, a protein that is a major component of skin tissue, and aids healing. Take 500 to 1,000 milligrams of mineral ascorbate vitamin C and an equal amount of bioflavonoids three to four times a day for two weeks following a sunburn.

■ Zinc boosts the immune system and aids in healing. Take 15 to 30 milligrams of zinc once or twice a day for up to two weeks after a sunburn. Take zinc with food to prevent stomach upset.

HERBAL TREATMENT

■ Aloe vera has been used for centuries to soothe and cool burns. To soothe and cool a sunburn quickly, gently rub 100-percent aloe vera gel over the burned area. Apply it as often as needed.

■ To take the heat out of the skin and help promote healing, soak a clean white cloth in cool comfrey-root tea and apply the compress to the affected area. Comfrey is high in allantoin, a compound that helps to promote healing.

■ Infection-fighting gotu kola is effective against sunburn. Take a cup of gotu kola tea once or twice a day, or take 200 milligrams of standardized gotu kola extract containing 16 percent triterpenes twice daily.

■ Nettle is soothing, and relieves stinging and burning. Apply nettle lotion or ointment directly to the burned area as needed.

HOMEOPATHY

■ *Urtica urens,* homeopathic stinging nettle, will quickly reduce the stinging and burning pain of sunburn. Take one dose of *Urtica urens* 12x or 6c, as directed on the product label, every fifteen minutes. After the first four doses, cut back to one dose every hour, up to a total of three more doses.

■ If you develop a slight fever after the pain has been relieved, *Ferrum phosphoricum* will help. Take one dose of *Ferrum phosphoricum* 12x or 6c every hour, up to a total of four doses.

AROMATHERAPY

For specific instructions on how to use aromatherapy, *see* PREPARING AROMATHERAPY TREATMENTS in Part Three.

■ Essential oil of lavender is particularly healing for sunburned skin. Add lavender oil to cool-to-lukewarm bath water and enjoy a leisurely soak, or make cool compresses with lavender oil. You can also add 10 to 20 drops of lavender oil to an ounce of bland, lightweight oil (jojoba oil is best, as it is nongreasy and well absorbed by the skin) and gently apply the mixture to the affected area.

GENERAL RECOMMENDATIONS

■ If you have been overexposed to the sun, a soak in a cool bath, followed by the application of aloe vera gel, will help to take the heat out of the burn, lessen the pain, and moisturize parched skin.

■ For an extra-soothing soak, treat the bath water with $\frac{1}{2}$ cup of oatmeal or with Aveeno, a commercial product that is an oatmeal derivative. Wrap the oatmeal in a washcloth and let it soak in the tub. You can also *gently* rub the oatmeal-filled washcloth over your skin.

■ To soothe the worst areas of the burn, apply cool compresses where needed. For added benefit, add lavender oil to the water you use to make the compresses.

PREVENTION

■ Always apply a sunscreen when you will be spending time in the sun. Make sure you select a formula that screens out both UVA and UVB rays, and that has an SPF of 10 or higher. Apply it generously to *all* exposed areas of skin before going out in the sun, and reapply the sunscreen every three to four hours throughout the day.

■ Wear loose, light-colored clothing made of tightly woven fabric, and also wear sunglasses and a hat, preferably one with a broad brim. Like sunscreen, sunglasses should screen out both UVA and UVB rays to provide effective protection.

■ Limit outdoor activities during the middle of the day (between 10:00 AM and 2:00 PM), when the sun is at its highest and strongest point.

■ Divide your outdoor time between sunlight and shade. Spend no more than a total of three or four hours on any day in the sun.

■ Don't be fooled by cloudy or hazy days. Approximately 80 percent of the sun's rays pass through clouds. Take the same precautions on hazy days as you would on bright, sunny days.

■ Be aware of the dangers of sunbathing, and especially tanning salons. Tanning salons sometimes advertise that their machines are "safe" because they emit only UVA rays. This is simply not true. Exposure to UVA radiation can cause skin cancer just as well as UVB radiation can. Both should be avoided. As one dermatologist put it, a suntan is really just a sign of skin damage.

Sunstroke

See HEAT EXHAUSTION.

Surgery, Recovering From

There may be a time in your life when surgery is a necessary intervention. After any surgery, no matter how minor, a certain amount of time is required for the body to heal itself. You can support and speed that process by implementing a healthy regimen both before and after the surgery, and by following your doctor's suggestions.

CONVENTIONAL TREATMENT

■ Your surgeon or primary-care physician may give you specific instructions for diet, activity level, or special exercises, as well as any precautions you should take to guard against complications after surgery. Take these recommendations seriously, especially those regarding your activity level.

■ After a surgical procedure, even a minor one, you may suffer pain. The pain may be mild and easily managed with an analgesic such as acetaminophen (Tylenol, Tempra, or the equivalent) or ibuprofen (Advil, Nuprin, and others). If the surgery was extensive, however, the pain associated with the healing process may be severe and require stronger, perhaps prescription, medication. Talk frankly with your doctor about any pain you are experiencing. If not relieved, pain is a source of stress, and stress can slow down the healing process. If you require powerful medication for pain, such as a narcotic, keep in mind that it is rare for anyone to become addicted to pain medications if they are used to treat a short-term problem. Also, be aware that taking a painkiller *before* surgery may reduce the amount of pain you feel afterward. A study done at the University of Pennsylvania School of Medicine found that up to 81 percent of subjects given pain medication before surgery felt no pain nine and a half weeks after the procedure, whereas only 44 percent of those not given an analgesic prior to surgery were pain-free at that point. You may wish to discuss these findings with your doctor and ask him or her to administer pain medication before your operation, rather than waiting and treating pain afterwards.

DIETARY GUIDELINES

■ Depending on the type of surgery, your physician may prescribe a specific diet for you. Follow your doctor's instructions.

■ Even after your doctor gives full permission for you to eat, you may have little or no appetite. Once you do start to feel hungry, begin with clear liquids such as broth, fruit juices, and herbal teas. Applesauce and toast also make good "starter" foods.

■ Eat whole foods that are full of the many vitamins and minerals your body needs to heal itself and regain energy. To allow your gastrointestinal tract to readjust to food, begin with foods that are easier to digest, such as bananas, applesauce, and puréed foods, and work up to a normal diet gradually. As you recover, eating a healthy whole-foods diet can help you feel better than you did before the operation.

■ Unless your doctor restricts fluids, get plenty of liquids to ensure that you stay well hydrated. Water, nourishing broths, apple juice, and herbal teas are good choices. Even if you aren't thirsty, try to make yourself sip water or juice through a straw.

■ If you are a regular coffee drinker, you should be aware that withdrawal from caffeine can cause headaches after surgery. An estimated 25 percent of coffee drinkers complain of headaches after surgery, even if they drink as little as one cup of coffee a day. If possible, it is a good idea to taper off your coffee drinking before surgery to prevent this. If this is not possible, you may wish to ask your physician to administer an amount of caffeine equivalent to that in a cup of coffee soon after surgery, or to drink a cup as soon as possible once you are able to take fluids by mouth.

NUTRITIONAL SUPPLEMENTS

■ If you need surgery, you can help your body prepare for and recover from it with a simple program of nutritional supplements and natural remedies. Begin the following program anytime up to two weeks before the day of surgery, and maintain it for one month afterward:

- Beta-carotene, a precursor of vitamin A, soothes injured mucous membranes and helps heal tissue. Take 10,000 international units twice a day.
- Vitamin C and bioflavonoids help with tissue repair and in decreasing inflammation. Take 500 to 1,000 milligrams of each two to three times a day.
- Zinc hastens wound and tissue healing. Take 25 milligrams two to three times a day for two weeks. Take zinc with food to prevent stomach upset. If you take over 30 milligrams of zinc on a daily basis for more than one or two months, you should also take 1 to 2 milligrams of copper each day to maintain a proper mineral balance.

■ If you have had gastrointestinal surgery, take an acidophilus or bifidobacteria supplement for one month following the operation, as recommended on the product label. If you are allergic to milk, be sure to select a dairy-free formula.

■ Vitamin E is an antioxidant nutrient and is a mild but effective anti-inflammatory. Choose a formula containing mixed tocopherols and start by taking 200 international units daily, then gradually increase the dosage to 400 international units twice a day. Maintain that dosage for up to one month following surgery.

Note: If you have high blood pressure, limit your intake of supplemental vitamin E to a total of 400 international units daily. If you are taking an anticoagulant (blood thinner), consult your physician before taking supplemental vitamin E.

HERBAL TREATMENT

■ The following fifteen-day plan can help the body recover from surgery:

Days 1–4: Take one dose of an echinacea and goldenseal combination formula supplying 500 milligrams of echinacea and 350 milligrams of goldenseal two to three times daily. Echinacea and goldenseal help to detoxify the blood after anesthesia and can help prevent infection of the surgical wound. These herbs also support the immune system.

Days 5–7: Take 500 milligrams of astragalus three times daily. Astragalus contains a rich concentration of trace minerals and micronutrients. It also strengthens the immune system and supports healing.

Note: Do not take astragalus if you have a fever or other signs of acute infection.

Days 8–15: Take 500 milligrams of American ginseng three times daily. American ginseng is an excellent source of trace minerals and micronutrients, and supports and strengthens the body's internal defenses.

Note: Do not take American ginseng if you have high blood pressure, heart disease, or hypoglycemia. If you are sensitive to the effects of caffeine and other stimulants, you may want to consult with a qualified herbalist before using ginseng.

■ Gotu kola is a general tonic that also speeds wound healing. Take a cup of gotu kola tea once or twice daily, or take 200 milligrams of standardized gotu kola extract containing 16 percent triterpenes two or three times daily for three to four weeks after surgery.

■ Grape-seed extract stimulates the synthesis of collagen, a key protein in skin and connective tissue, which aids in proper scar formation. Starting one week after surgery, take 50 milligrams three times a day until healing is complete.

HOMEOPATHY

■ If you received general anesthesia, use the following regimen:

- To begin detoxifying the blood after general anesthesia, take one dose of *Nux vomica* 30x or 200x as soon as possible after you awaken. This homeopathic will also help to reduce the nausea associated with anesthetics. If you are still feeling nauseated three hours after the first dose, take one more dose.
- *Phosphorus* helps to detoxify a liver that is overloaded as a result of general anesthesia. The liver is the organ responsible for clearing anesthetic chemicals from the body. One to two hours after the second dose of *Nux vomica*, take one dose of *Phosphorus* 30x or 200x.

■ The following regimen will support and hasten the healing process following surgery:

Days 1–2: Take one dose of *Arnica* 30x or 9c three to four times daily to help decrease inflammation following surgery and speed the healing process.

Day 3: To further hasten healing of tissues injured by surgery, take one dose of *Ledum* 12x or 6c three to four times during the day.

Days 4–5: For nerve pain following surgery, take one dose of *Hypericum* 12x or 6c three to four times daily.

■ If your abdomen is bloated and you are feeling weak following surgery, take one dose of *China* 30x or 9c three times a day for up to two days.

■ *Thuja* can help inhibit the formation of keloids, which are raised pinkish overgrowths of scar tissue at the site of a wound. Young women and people of African ancestry are more likely than other people to form keloid tissue. If you fall into either of these groups, or if you have a known tendency to develop keloids, take one dose of *Thuja* 200x or 30c once a week for six to eight weeks following surgery. Once the incision wound is completely closed, homeopathic 1-percent *Graphites* cream can also help. After your physician gives you the okay, apply it as directed on the product label.

BACH FLOWER REMEDIES

■ As soon as possible following the procedure (as soon as your doctor says it is safe to take something by mouth), take one dose of Bach Flower Rescue Remedy. One hour later, take one dose of homeopathic *Arnica* 30x, 200x, 9c, or 15c.

GENERAL RECOMMENDATIONS

■ If you are scheduled for surgery, ask if you can donate your own blood in advance to be used in a transfusion, if one is needed. While the risk of any problem developing due to being transfused with donated blood is very small, if you donate your own blood prior to surgery, it is a risk you will not have to face.

■ To ensure a full and strong recovery after surgery, adequate rest is essential. Limit visitors and minimize distractions. A calm and familiar environment is best. A cozy, dimly lighted room, thick blankets, and soft music are conducive to rest and relaxation. If you are feeling restless and uncomfortable, listening to books on tape can be a good way to engage your attention and take your mind off your discomfort.

■ A surgical wound, like any wound, can become infected. Watch for signs and symptoms of a local infection. If the area becomes red, warm, swollen, or tender, or if you develop a fever, call your surgeon or physician.

Syphilis

Syphilis is a sexually transmitted disease caused by the bacteria *Treponema pallidum*. During sexual contact, the bacteria are transferred to the moist mucous membranes of the vagina, the urethra, the mouth, or the anus, where they burrow in and enter the body.

Syphilis progresses in three stages. In the first stage, called *primary syphilis,* a small red, painless, pus-forming bump appears at the site where contact with the infection occurred. This most often takes place between ten and ninety days after exposure. A sore on the penis is usually visible, but if a sore forms in the vagina or cervix, it is not likely to be noticed. The sore then turns into a painless, bloodless ulcer called a chancre (pronounced shanker), which releases a fluid that is swarming with the *Treponema pallidum* bacteria. Because the chancre is painless, it may not be noticed, but it is highly infectious. The chancre usually heals by itself within one to five weeks.

The second stage, or *secondary syphilis,* usually develops about two months after the chancre heals. At this stage, the bacteria have traveled throughout the body, where they cause symptoms that can include loss of appetite, nausea, fever, headache, hair loss, bone and joint pain, a rash that does not itch, and flat grayish-white patches of skin that appear in the mouth, throat, and/or anus. Pimples may occur in the moist areas of the skin. These symptoms usually continue for two to six weeks, and then they too disappear. During this period, the infected individual is highly contagious.

Third-stage, or *tertiary syphilis,* can take as long as many years to resurface, and can flare up without warning. This stage can last anywhere from two years to a lifetime. Soft, rubbery tumors, called gummas, may develop anywhere on the surface of the body, including the eyes, liver, lungs, stomach, and/or sexual organs. Gummas fester and then heal by scarring over, resulting in noticeable saucerlike depressions. Except for the soft tumors, third-stage syphilis may be painless and unremarkable. However, as time goes on, there may be a deep "burrowing" pain as the bacteria begin a process of damaging or destroying various parts of the body, including the nervous system and the heart. This can give rise to mental or physical disorders and premature death. Oddly enough, by the time it reaches the third stage, syphilis is no longer contagious except by blood-to-blood contact.

Congenital syphilis, caused by infection of the fetus in the womb, can result in the birth of a child with serious physical abnormalities and disabilities, including blindness. In some cases, an infant with congenital syphilis may appear normal at birth, but symptoms usually appear within several weeks. He or she may develop bloody "sniffles" and skin sores on the palms, soles of the feet, and genitalia. Visual and/or hearing problems are common. Such a child may develop progeria, a condition in which aging takes place at a greatly accelerated rate.

Syphilis is diagnosed by a blood test. Early treatment is the key to recovery. If you develop a sore in your mouth or in the genital area that you cannot identify, see a physician without delay.

CONVENTIONAL MEDICINE

■ Penicillin is still the treatment of choice for syphilis, though far higher doses are used today than in the past. If you are sensitive to penicillin, tetracycline or doxycycline may be used instead. Primary syphilis is easily cured with antibiotic injections. Secondary syphilis requires additional injections and is usually cured as well, although some cases are resistant to treatment. In tertiary syphilis, the goal of antibiotic treatment is to prevent additional damage to the body; existing damage to the heart and/or nervous system may not be reversible.

■ Sexual activity is strictly off-limits until blood tests reveal you have been cured.

■ If you are being treated for syphilis, anyone you had sexual contact with since contracting the infection must be notified and, if necessary, treated.

■ Your doctor is likely to recommend testing for HIV, the virus that causes AIDS, as well. These two diseases often occur together.

DIETARY GUIDELINES

■ Eat a high-fiber diet of whole foods that contain no chemicals that add stress to the body. Maximize your intake of fresh vegetables and fruits. Include in your diet clean, lean protein foods such as chicken and fish.

■ Add sea vegetables to your diet. Besides improving thyroid function, the high iodine content of sea vegetables enhances circulation and helps detoxify the blood.

■ Avoid refined sugar, alcohol, and caffeine. These substances increase the acidity of the body, which adds to inflammation and worsens symptoms.

NUTRITIONAL SUPPLEMENTS

■ Take a good multivitamin and mineral supplement daily to correct or prevent deficiencies of basic nutrients.

■ Green-foods supplements such as chlorella and spirulina supply cleansing chlorophyll and trace minerals that may be missing in the diet. Take a green-foods supplement as directed on the product label.

■ Take supplemental probiotics (acidophilus and/or bifidobacteria). This is important any time you must take antibiotics. Antibiotics kill the friendly bacteria your body needs right along with the dangerous organisms. Take a probiotic supplement as recommended on the product label. If you are allergic to milk, select a dairy-free formula.

■ Proteolytic enzymes reduce inflammation and aid in the repair of damaged tissue. Take proteolytic enzymes with each main meal of the day, and also twice a day between meals.

■ Vitamin A helps heal mucous membranes and is necessary for the repair of injured tissue. Take 25,000 international units twice a day for three weeks.

Note: If you are pregnant, or intend to get pregnant, or if you have liver disease, consult your doctor before taking supplemental vitamin A. Pregnant women should not ingest a total of more than 25,000 international units of supplemental vitamin A *per week* from all sources.

■ Vitamin C and bioflavonoids have anti-inflammatory action and stimulate healing. They also fight free-radical damage. For three weeks, take 1,000 milligrams of a vitamin-C formula that contains rutin and other bioflavonoids four to five times daily.

■ Vitamin E improves circulation, stimulates healing, and is required for tissue repair. It also has antioxidant properties and scavenges free radicals. Choose a product containing mixed tocopherols and start by taking 200 international units daily, then gradually increase the dosage until you are taking 400 international units once or twice daily.

Note: If you have high blood pressure, limit your intake of supplemental vitamin E to a total of 400 international units daily. If you are taking an anticoagulant (blood thinner), consult your physician before taking supplemental vitamin E.

HERBAL TREATMENT

■ Cat's claw supports the immune system and has reported effects against bacteria as well as viruses. Take 500 milligrams of standardized extract three times a day for one week, then increase to 1,000 milligrams three times a day for two weeks.

Note: Do not use cat's claw if you are pregnant or nursing, or if you are an organ-transplant recipient. Use it with caution if you are taking an anticoagulant (blood thinner).

■ Echinacea and goldenseal make a powerful combination that supports the immune system and offers antibacterial, antifungal, and antiviral action. They are also useful if there are any lingering symptoms of infection after antibiotic therapy. Take one dose of an echinacea and goldenseal combination formula supplying 500 milligrams of echinacea and 350 milligrams of goldenseal three times daily for one week.

■ Grapefruit-seed extract has antiviral, antifungal, and antibacterial properties. Take 100 milligrams three times a day.

■ Oregano has antibacterial properties and helps to fight infection. Take 75 milligrams of standardized extract three times a day.

■ Uva ursi, or bearberry, is a diuretic and urinary tract antiseptic with antiviral and antibacterial action. It contains allantoin, a substance that soothes and helps to repair

inflamed tissue. Take 300 to 500 milligrams two or three times daily for three to four days.

HOMEOPATHY

Syphilis is best treated constitutionally. See a homeopathic physician for a constitutional remedy. The following remedies can provide symptomatic relief during the acute phase of the infection.

■ *Cantharis* is the remedy for burning and stinging of the genitals and intense pain on urination. Take one dose of *Cantharis* 12x or 6c three times a day, as needed, for up to three days.

■ *Rhus toxicodendron* is for itching and burning of the genitals that feels worse with cold and damp. Take one dose of *Rhus toxicodendron* 12x or 6c three times a day, as needed, for up to three days.

■ *Sempervivum tectorum* is the remedy to choose if the whole genital area is very tender and very painful, especially at night. Take one dose of *Sempervivum tectorum* 12x or 6c three times a day, as needed, for up to three days.

■ If the preceding remedies do not match your symptoms or fail to bring relief, try *Sulfur*. Indications for this remedy include urethral burning and frequent urination, with mucus and pus in the urine. In women, there is much itching and burning in the vaginal area; in men, there is spasmodic pain in the penis. Take one dose of *Sulfur* 30x or 15c three times a day, as needed, for up to three days.

BACH FLOWER REMEDIES

Select the remedy that most closely fits your emotional tendencies and concerns, and take it as needed, following the directions on the product label.

■ Holly helps to tame anger and fits of bad temper that may reflect underlying feelings of jealousy and insecurity.

■ Hornbeam helps to lift exhaustion so extreme that it makes you miss out on interesting activities.

■ Impatiens calms hyperactivity, impatience, and tension.

■ White Chestnut helps to counteract a tendency to obsess on ideas or events long after the subject should have been forgotten.

ACUPRESSURE

For the locations of acupressure points on the body, *see* ADMINISTERING AN ACUPRESSURE TREATMENT in Part Three.

■ Conception Vessel 4 and 12 improve circulation in the genitourinary area.

■ Kidney 3 and 7 increase circulation in the genitourinary tract.

- Liver 3 relaxes the nervous system.
- The combination of Spleen 6 and Stomach 36 improves immune function.

GENERAL RECOMMENDATIONS

- Take the entire course of antibiotics. Even if your symptoms seem to disappear, do not fail to take your medication on schedule. Only the weaker bacteria succumb early; the stronger and more powerful organisms may survive to create future problems. Always take all your prescribed antibiotics.

- Be sure to see your doctor at the appointed time for a follow-up visit to make sure your treatment is working.

PREVENTION

- Abstinence (or a monogamous relationship with a partner who is known to be healthy) is the only way to avoid contracting a sexually transmitted disease. Using a latex (not animal-skin) condom is your next best choice. Be aware, however, that the use of a condom is not an absolute guarantee of protection against STDs.

Temporomandibular Joint Syndrome

The temporomandibular joint is one of two joints that connect the lower jawbone to the skull. It is a combined hinge and gliding joint. If the jaw joints and the muscles and ligaments that control and support them do not work together smoothly, temporomandibular joint, or TMJ, syndrome is the result. Symptoms can include headaches (often mistaken for sinusitis), chronic neck pain, toothaches, a dull pain in the affected area of your face, soreness of the jaw muscles, and severe pain in or around your ears. Dizziness, hearing problems, and ringing in the ears are not uncommon. Some people have trouble opening their mouths widely; their jaws sometimes lock in certain positions, and yawning and/or chewing may cause popping and even sudden pain.

TMJ syndrome can be caused by a malocclusion (misalignment) of the jaw or teeth. If your teeth are out of alignment, your muscles must make adjustments in how they work to compensate. Over a long period of time, this can cause the joints to become misaligned. However, the most common cause of TMJ syndrome is believed to be frequent clenching of the jaw muscles and bruxism (tooth-grinding). These behaviors are often associated with stress, although there is some question as to whether the stress itself causes them or whether an underlying maloc-clusion causes a person to respond to stress in this way. For some people, clenching the teeth together seems to be merely a habit. Hypoglycemia (low blood sugar) can be a contributor; people tend to clench their jaws and grind their teeth more when their blood sugar is low. Regardless of the cause, clenching, grinding, or gritting the teeth, or even chewing or crunching hard foods, can exert tremendous pressure in the area. Over time, the cartilage that cushions the joint can wear down, causing additional stress. If this happens, the bones rub against each other, instead of sliding past one another.

Other factors that have been implicated in TMJ syndrome include bad posture; habitually cradling a telephone between the ear and the shoulder; poor dental work and/or badly fitted bridgework or dentures; and displacement of the joint as a result of an injury to the jaw, head, or neck, such as a whiplash. In rare cases, arthritis causes TMJ syndrome. If so, symptoms are typically worse in the morning, but ease as the day goes on.

If you have any of the symptoms described above and have been wondering if you might have TMJ syndrome, try the following test: Put your little fingers into your ears and press forward. Then, with your fingers in place, open and close your mouth. If you hear a clicking or popping noise and feel your jawbone pushing against your fingers, you probably have TMJ syndrome. A definitive diagnosis can be made by x-ray. Arthrography, a technique that involves injecting a dye into the joint for examination with a fluoroscope, can show any misalignment. However, many people who suffer from symptoms of TMJ syndrome are not found to have any obvious structural abnormalities.

CONVENTIONAL MEDICINE

- Consult a qualified dentist or oral surgeon to determine whether any structural problems, including misaligned teeth, are present. For some fortunate individuals, curing TMJ syndrome is as simple as fixing one or two teeth that are too high or too low.

- If the condition causes significant pain, your doctor will likely recommend painkillers to make you more comfortable. For mild to moderate pain, acetaminophen (Tylenol, Datril, and others), aspirin (Bayer, Ecotrin, and others), or ibuprofen (Advil, Motrin, Nuprin, and others) is usually sufficient.

Note: In excessive amounts, acetaminophen can cause liver damage. If the recommended amount does not give the relief you want, do not increase the dosage, but try a different medication. Take aspirin or ibuprofen with food to prevent possible stomach upset. Do not take aspirin during the last three months of pregnancy unless directed to do so by a physician.

- If over-the-counter painkillers do not provide sufficient

relief, it may be necessary to resort to prescription medications.

■ Switching to a soft diet (*see under* Dietary Guidelines, in this entry) and applying moist heat several times a day, along with gentle massage over the temples, the back of the jaw, and the upper neck, may help in the short term.

■ If the problem is a result of severe malocclusion, surgical correction may be considered. An oral surgeon can cut the lower jaw and realign it to meet the upper with a proper fit. Obviously, this type of treatment is suitable only for certain severe circumstances.

DIETARY GUIDELINES

■ Eat a soft diet consisting of steamed vegetables, fresh fruits, nutritious homemade soups, and well-cooked whole grains and cereals. Select foods that don't require hard chewing. Include plenty of lean, clean protein in the form of baked or poached fish and chicken. Poaching may be best, because the liquid keeps the food moist and therefore easier to chew.

■ Avoid chewy foods, such as red meat and bagels.

■ Avoid anything containing caffeine, including coffee, green and black tea, chocolate, and caffeinated soft drinks, as well as sugar and alcohol, in the six to eight hours before bedtime. All of these substances increase the likelihood of bruxism and worsen TMJ syndrome.

NUTRITIONAL SUPPLEMENTS

■ Take a good multivitamin and mineral supplement daily.

■ Bruxism is often associated with weak adrenal-gland function. Take 100 to 200 milligrams of adrenal glandular extract at breakfast and again at lunch.

■ Calcium and magnesium help relax the nervous system and can decrease bruxism. Take 400 to 500 milligrams of calcium and 200 to 300 milligrams of magnesium two to three times daily. Take the last dose just before bedtime.

■ The B vitamins support and strengthen the nervous system. Two to three times daily, take a B-complex formula that supplies 25 to 50 milligrams of each of the major B vitamins.

■ Niacinamide, a form of vitamin B_3, helps to strengthen the relaxation response. Take 100 milligrams of niacinamide at bedtime, along with your last dose of calcium and magnesium.

■ Pantothenic acid strengthens adrenal function, which is often compromised in people with TMJ syndrome. In addition to the B complex and niacinamide, take 100 milligrams of pantothenic acid twice daily, between meals, for one month. Stop for one month, then repeat. Follow this cycle for a total of six months.

HERBAL TREATMENT

■ Bupleurum and dong quai is an ancient Chinese remedy that helps to relax the nervous system. Take 500 milligrams of a bupleurum and dong quai combination formula two or three times daily for two weeks out of every month. If you are a woman, take it for the two weeks prior to the anticipated onset of your menstrual period.

■ Kava kava is the choice for TMJ syndrome associated with anxiety. Choose a stardardized extract containing 30 percent kavalactones and take 100 to 250 milligrams in the morning and another 100 to 250 milligrams at bedtime.

　Note: In excess amounts, this herb can cause drowsiness. Do not exceed the recommended dose. Do not use kava kava if you are pregnant or nursing, if you have Parkinson's disease, or if you are taking a prescription medication for depression or anxiety.

■ Oat straw is high in silica. If taken over a long period of time, this herb can help strengthen the entire central nervous system. Take 500 milligrams twice a day.

■ St. John's wort is an herbal calmative that is especially helpful for TMJ syndrome accompanied by depression. Choose a standardized extract containing 0.3 percent hypericin and take 200 to 300 milligrams three times daily.

■ Valerian, passionflower, and skullcap help to strengthen and relax the nervous system, and are known for their ability to promote restful sleep. Choose an herbal formula that combines valerian with either of the other two herbs and take a dose supplying 350 to 500 milligrams of valerian plus 200 to 300 milligrams of the other herb twice daily. Take the second dose before bedtime.

　Note: Do not use both these herbs and kava kava at the same time.

HOMEOPATHY

■ *Arnica* is very effective for the symptomatic relief of pain. Take one dose of *Arnica* 12x or 6c three times daily for up to three days. If you experience improvement before that, stop taking the remedy. You can also use *Arnica* gel topically on the affected area. Follow the directions on the product label.

■ *Arsenicum album* is for anxiety and tooth-grinding that takes place mostly between 12:00 midnight and 3:00 AM. You may tend to be quite particular, even fussy, about many things in your life. Take one dose of *Arsenicum album* 30x or 15c three times daily for up to three days. If you experience improvement before that, stop taking the remedy.

■ *Cina* is for TMJ syndrome accompanied by pinworms. Take one dose of *Cina* 30x or 15c three times daily for up to three days. If you experience improvement before that, stop taking the remedy.

■ *Ignatia* is good if you feel tension in your jaw, especially when you are sad, such as after hearing bad news. Take one dose of *Ignatia* 12x or 6c three times daily for up to three days. If you experience improvement before that, stop taking the remedy.

Phytolacca helps to counteract a tendency to clench your teeth at any time of the day or night. You may be quite unaware of this habit. Take one dose of *Phytolacca* 12x or 6c three times daily for up to three days. If you experience improvement before that, stop taking the remedy.

■ *Ruta graveolens* is helpful for sharp pain and achiness caused by overuse or trauma. Take one dose of *Ruta graveolens* 12x or 6c three times daily for up to three days. If you experience improvement before that, stop taking the remedy.

Spigelia anthelmia is good for nerve pain in the cheek and temple. Take one dose of *Spigelia anthelmia* 12x or 6c three times daily for up to three days. If you experience improvement before that, stop taking the remedy.

BACH FLOWER REMEDIES

Select the remedy that most closely fits your emotional tendencies and concerns, and take it as needed, following the directions on the product label.

Holly tames anger that may be due to underlying feelings of insecurity and that is expressed in outbursts of bad temper.

Impatiens calms impatience, nervousness, and irritability.

Vervain helps to counteract perfectionistic tendencies and tension related to a drive to excel, as well as difficulty sleeping normally.

ACUPRESSURE

For the locations of acupressure points on the body, *see* ADMINISTERING AN ACUPRESSURE TREATMENT in Part Three.

Large Intestine 4 relaxes tension in the head, relieves face and tooth pain, and calms a stressed nervous system.

Liver 3 relaxes the nervous system, relieves muscle cramps and spasms, and helps to ease headache pain.

The temporomandibular joint lies along the Stomach meridian; Stomach 36 is a strategic point that helps to move energy along this meridian.

GENERAL RECOMMENDATIONS

If your work keeps you in a sitting position, watch your posture. Keep your back straight, don't lean on your desk, and don't hold a telephone between your jaw and your ear. Pay attention to how you hold your jaw. The correct way is to keep your lips together and your teeth apart. This keeps the jaw relaxed and in the proper position.

■ Don't chew gum, and don't chew your food on only one side of your mouth. Both of these habits can contribute to TMJ syndrome.

■ Try using a mouth guard. You can find inexpensive mouth guards in most sporting-goods stores. Immerse the guard in hot water until it becomes pliable, then put it in your mouth and bite down on it. Sleep with it for a few nights and see if your symptoms are less troublesome. If it helps, talk with your dentist about fitting one to your mouth.

■ Many people who have TMJ syndrome habitually sleep on their sides. Instead, try to train yourself to sleep on your back to give your neck, back, and shoulder muscles a rest.

■ If you can find a chiropractor who is skilled in this area, give chiropractic a try. This is one area in which a competent chiropractor may be able to take you right off the surgeon's schedule.

■ Stress-management techniques have proven effective for many people with TMJ syndrome. (*See* STRESS; *also see* RELAXATION TECHNIQUES in Part Three.)

PREVENTION

■ It may not be possible to prevent TMJ syndrome, since it can be due to an anatomical anomaly. However, adopting the habits outlined under General Recommendations in this entry may help.

Tendinitis

Tendinitis is the inflammation of a tendon. Tendons are cords of fibrous tissue that connect muscles to bones. They are extremely strong and flexible, but they cannot stretch. Tendons are composed principally of bundles of collagen, a protein that is a key constituent of all the connective tissues of the body.

Tendinitis can occur anywhere a tendon joins muscle to bone. The tendons most likely to become inflamed include the Achilles tendon, located at the back of the ankle, and tendons in the knee, elbow, and rotator cuff, which stabilizes the shoulder. The inflammation is usually caused by overexertion in sports or other physical activity, and can be acute or become a chronic problem from long-term overuse. If you place too much stress on a tendon, it can become inflamed and swell, causing pain, soreness, tenderness, and impaired motion of the muscle attached to the affected tendon. *Tennis elbow,* one type of tendinitis, is caused by straining the tendon on the outside of the elbow; *golfer's elbow* is caused by straining the tendon on the inside of the elbow. *Painful arc syndrome* results from injury to the tendons of the rotator cuff, causing pain in the shoulder when you raise your arm above a certain point. Similar problems include repetitive-stress-induced tendinitis of the forearms and/or wrists, which plagues many people who work at computer keyboards and in light assembly jobs. In chronic tendinitis, calcium deposits can occur within tendinous tissue, causing increased pain and decreased range of motion.

CONVENTIONAL MEDICINE

■ The RICE (*rest, ice, compression, elevation*) technique can help either an acute or a chronic problem.

- *Rest.* If something you're doing hurts, stop and rest the affected area as soon as possible. "No pain, no gain" is bad advice.
- *Ice.* Cold can help hold down swelling and inflammation. Do not apply ice directly to the skin, however. Cover the area with a towel first. Ice the area for twenty minutes, then remove the ice for twenty minutes. Repeat this over a period of a few hours or as needed.
- *Compression.* Wrap the area in an elastic bandage or strips of cloth, firmly enough to provide support and limit swelling, but not so tightly that you interfere with circulation. Compress the area for thirty minutes, then remove the compression for fifteen minutes to allow full circulation. Repeat this process over a period of a few hours or as needed.
- *Elevation.* To ensure drainage of fluids from the injured area, elevate the affected part to a level above your heart. Rest and relax for thirty minutes.

You can do these steps simultaneously or individually as the injury heals.

■ If the pain does not diminish within seven days, see your doctor. You may have ruptured a tendon, a condition that requires medical attention.

■ For pain relief, your doctor will likely recommend a nonsteroidal anti-inflammatory drug (NSAID) such as ibuprofen (Advil, Motrin, Nuprin, and others), naproxen (Aleve, Anaprox, Naprelan, Naprosyn), or fenoprofen (Nalfon). Some of these are available over the counter, others by prescription only. All have the potential to cause such undesirable side effects as nausea, heartburn, bleeding in the gastrointestinal tract, ulcers, kidney damage, and liver damage.

■ If the pain is severe, your doctor may recommend an injection of cortisone, probably mixed with a long-lasting anesthetic. This can be dramatically effective for relieving pain, but it should not be done repeatedly, as injected corticosteroids can cause local wasting and decrease the body's immune response.

■ If calcification has set up in the soft tissue, physical therapy is important to regain full mobility.

DIETARY GUIDELINES

■ Eat lean, clean protein foods such as chicken, fish, and tofu.

■ Maximize your intake of fresh vegetables, especially dark-green vegetables, and fruits.

■ Avoid refined sugar and anything containing caffeine. Sugar and caffeine contribute to an acidic internal environment, which slows healing.

■ Avoid saturated, hydrogenated, and partially hydrogenated fats, which promote inflammation and pain. That means avoiding red meat, dairy products, margarine, vegetable shortening, and foods containing them.

NUTRITIONAL SUPPLEMENTS

■ Beta-carotene and vitamin A help reduce inflammation and are necessary for tissue repair. Take 5,000 international units of each twice daily for one month.

Note: If you are pregnant, or intend to get pregnant, or if you have liver disease, consult your doctor before taking supplemental vitamin A. Pregnant women should not ingest a total of more than 25,000 international units of supplemental vitamin A *per week* from all sources.

■ Bromelain is a natural anti-inflammatory. Take 400 milligrams three times daily, between meals, while symptoms last.

■ Flaxseed and fish oils are rich in omega-3 essential fatty acids that help to moderate the inflammatory response. Take 1,000 milligrams of either twice daily.

■ Manganese is a trace element that is essential for rebuilding connective tissue. Take 3 to 5 milligrams twice a day while the problem persists.

■ Pine-bark and grape-seed extracts act as antioxidants and anti-inflammatories. Take 50 milligrams of either, two or three times daily while symptoms last.

■ Vitamin C is important in the production of collagen and helps speed repair of tissue; bioflavonoids strengthen connective tissue. Take 1,000 milligrams of vitamin C with bioflavonoids three times daily for two weeks. Then take 500 milligrams three times daily for three weeks.

■ Vitamin E is an active anti-inflammatory. Choose a product containing mixed tocopherols and start by taking 200 international units, then gradually increase to 400 international units daily.

Note: If you have high blood pressure, limit your intake of supplemental vitamin E to a total of 400 international units daily. If you are taking an anticoagulant (blood thinner), consult your physician before taking supplemental vitamin E.

■ Zinc supports the immune system and works with vitamin A to ease inflammation. Take 15 milligrams of zinc daily, preferably at the same time as you take vitamin A and beta-carotene. Take zinc with food to prevent stomach upset.

HERBAL TREATMENT

■ Boswellia is an herb that has noted anti-inflammatory effects. Take 200 milligrams of standardized extract three times a day.

■ Horsetail is rich in silica, which increases circulation and strengthens tendons, ligaments, and bones. Research shows this herb can hasten healing. Take 500 milligrams two or three times daily.

■ Turmeric also is known for its anti-inflammatory properties. Take 300 milligrams of standardized extract three times a day.

HOMEOPATHY

■ *Arnica* is the first remedy to reach for to reduce acute pain and swelling. Take one dose of *Arnica* 30x or 15c four times daily for the first forty-eight hours after an injury.

■ *Rhus toxicodendron* is for pain that feels better with modest movement and better still with continued movement, but worse after a long rest and in damp weather. Take one dose of *Rhus toxicodendron* 30x or 15c three or four times daily, as needed. If you notice no improvement after three or four days, discontinue it and select another remedy.

■ *Ruta graveolens* is helpful if you experience a sensation of painful tearing and feel bruised. Take one dose of *Ruta graveolens* 12x or 6c three or four times daily, as needed. If you notice no improvement after three or four days, discontinue it and select another remedy.

BACH FLOWER REMEDIES

■ Rescue Remedy can help relieve stress and feelings of anxiety that arise due to injury.

ACUPRESSURE

For the locations of acupressure points on the body, *see* ADMINISTERING AN ACUPRESSURE TREATMENT in Part Three. If points near the site of an injury are too sensitive to touch, you can work only the corresponding point on the opposite side of the body.

■ Gallbladder 30 nourishes tendons in the lower half of the body.

■ Gallbladder 34 nourishes the tendons.

■ Liver 3 nourishes the muscles and tendons.

■ Spleen 6 and Stomach 36 together improve the transformation and absorption of nutrients. Spleen 6 also improves circulation in the lower limbs.

■ Large Intestine 10 improves circulation in the arm.

GENERAL RECOMMENDATIONS

■ Rest the affected area and give it time to heal, especially in the beginning. If you continue to stress an inflamed tendon, you will make the injury worse.

■ After the initial pain and inflammation have eased—which can take a week or longer—ease back into exercising. *Gentle* and *gradual* are the operative words here. Gradually begin to exercise the affected area with gentle movements. If you keep the area immobilized for too long, healing will be delayed. On the other hand, if you force yourself to move too soon or too vigorously, healing will take even longer. Moderation is the key.

■ To keep the area limber, apply warmth for thirty minutes after mild exercise. Use warm, moist cloths or a heating pad set on the lowest setting.

■ Be patient. A strained and overused tendon can be slow to heal. The pain generally disappears with time, but soreness and pain can persist a lot longer than you might think. An injured tendon may take as long as two to three months to heal properly.

PREVENTION

■ Warm up before exercising or playing sports. This allows the tendons and muscles to become more flexible, which makes strains less likely.

■ Be careful when engaging in any activity that involves using the same joint repeatedly. If it hurts, stop.

■ Consider using the RICE technique (*see under* Conventional Treatment in this entry) after any particularly stressful physical activity. It's been reported that this is a good way to avoid ending up on the injured list.

■ If your job or favorite activity causes you to be subject to recurring bouts of tendinitis, it might be helpful to consult a coach or occupational therapist who can help you modify your movements in order to avoid stressing the vulnerable area.

Tetanus

Tetanus, also known as lockjaw, is a consequence of infection by *Clostridium tetani*, an organism found in soil, manure, and everyday dirt. It enters the body through open wounds, particularly puncture-type wounds, and releases a toxin that travels to the central nervous system, causing severe muscle stiffness and spasms. Once the organism enters the body, the incubation period can be from one to twelve days, or even longer in some cases. Tetanus is not transmitted from one person to another.

The wound through which the organism enters the

body often heals before other symptoms appear. The illness begins with muscle stiffness in the neck and jaw, and progresses over the next twenty-four hours into painful muscle rigidity and spasms. Normal muscle function can be so impaired that breathing may stop during the first three to four days. This can be a life-threatening situation that requires hospitalization and close medical attention.

If you suffer a puncture wound, you should see a doctor promptly. You may need to have your tetanus immunization updated and the wound properly cleaned and debrided. If you develop any symptoms of tetanus, even if you don't remember any injury that could have exposed you to a risk of the disease, call your doctor right away. Tetanus requires professional medical treatment.

CONVENTIONAL TREATMENT

■ If you develop tetanus, you will probably have to be hospitalized for treatment. This is a complex process that involves the administration of medications including antitoxin, antibiotics, painkillers, and drugs that relax muscles and decrease spasms; measures aimed at supporting nutrition and elimination and preventing the development of secondary infections such as pneumonia; and continuous monitoring of bodily functions. Other treatments may be added as the need arises.

■ Having the disease does not give you a lifelong immunity to it. Once you recover, your physician will recommend a full course of immunization to protect you against future illness.

DIETARY GUIDELINES

■ Do not consume any refined sugars or anything containing caffeine while you are recovering. Both of these substances make the body more acidic, which slows healing.

NUTRITIONAL SUPPLEMENTS

The nutritional supplements listed below are aimed at supporting recovery from a puncture wound. They are not intended as substitutes for appropriate tetanus immunization or professional wound treatment.

■ Mineral ascorbate vitamin C and bioflavonoids help heal skin tissue and prevent infection after an injury. Take 500 to 1,000 milligrams of each three times a day for one week following a puncture wound. Then take the same dosage twice a day for two weeks.

■ Vitamin E and beta-carotene help to promote healing and support the immune system. Start by taking 200 international units of vitamin E daily, and gradually increase the dosage until you are taking 400 international units once or twice daily. Also take 5,000 international units of beta-carotene twice a day. Continue this regimen until the wound heals.

Note: If you have high blood pressure, limit your intake of supplemental vitamin E to a total of 400 international units daily. If you are taking an anticoagulant (blood thinner), consult your physician before taking supplemental vitamin E.

■ Zinc helps to boost the immune system. Take 15 to 25 milligrams twice a day for up to ten days following a puncture wound. Take zinc with food to prevent stomach upset.

HERBAL TREATMENT

The herbal treatments outlined below are aimed at supporting recovery from a puncture wound. They are not intended as substitutes for appropriate tetanus immunization or professional wound treatment.

■ Apply calendula ointment or collagen gel as neded.

■ Echinacea and goldenseal boost the immune system. Take one dose of an echinacea and goldenseal combination formula supplying 500 milligrams of echinacea and 350 milligrams of goldenseal three to four times daily for three days.

■ Garlic has antibacterial properties. Choose an odorless capsule form and take 500 milligrams three times daily. Or eat a clove of fresh garlic three or more times daily.

■ Make an herbal poultice. Add 1 tablespoon of any or all of the following to 1 cup of water: goldenseal, marshmallow root, Oregon grape root, and plantain. Bring the water to a boil and simmer for twenty minutes. Cool the infusion to a comfortably warm temperature. Soak a washcloth in the mixture and apply it to the affected area for twenty to thirty minutes. Do this three times a day for two to three days.

HOMEOPATHY

■ *Ledum* is a homeopathic remedy specifically for puncture wounds. Take one dose of *Ledum* 12x or 6c every thirty minutes, up to a total of three doses. Then take one dose four times a day for up to two days. Note that this homeopathic remedy is aimed at supporting recovery from a puncture wound. It is not intended as a substitute for appropriate tetanus immunization or professional wound treatment.

BACH FLOWER REMEDIES

■ If you suffer a puncture wound, take a dose of Rescue Remedy as soon as possible. This wonderful natural remedy helps to calm and ease any anxiety or fright you may experience as a result of an injury.

PREVENTION

■ The tetanus toxoid vaccine, which prevents tetanus, is

usually administered at intervals throughout childhood. Thereafter, a booster may be given every ten years or after an injury that results in an open wound.

■ Any injury that breaks the skin, especially a puncture, should immediately be washed with plenty of water to which a small amount of hydrogen peroxide or povidone-iodine solution (Betadine) has been added.

Thalassemia

See under ANEMIA.

Thrombophlebitis

See PHLEBITIS.

Thrush

Thrush is a fungal infection of the mouth. It is caused by the yeastlike fungus *Candida albicans*, which can also cause vaginal yeast infections and systemic candidiasis. Thrush is most often seen in babies and in individuals with compromised immune systems, such as people with HIV disease or certain types of cancer, people undergoing cancer chemotherapy, and organ-transplant recipients who must take antirejection drugs.

Thrush appears as white, flaky, cheesy-looking patches covering all or part of the tongue and gums, the insides of the cheeks, and, sometimes, the lips. These patches do not scrape off easily. When they are picked or scraped off, they leave a red, inflamed area that may bleed. The pain of thrush may interfere with eating.

CONVENTIONAL TREATMENT

■ The most commonly prescribed medication for thrush is a liquid antifungal, such as nystatin (in the medications Mycostatin and Nilstat), taken four times daily until the infection clears.

■ To ease the pain of the infection, a pain reliever such as acetaminophen (Tylenol, Datril, and others), aspirin (Bayer, Ecotrin, and others), or ibuprofen (Advil, Motrin, Nuprin, and others) may be useful.

■ Gentian violet in a 1-percent solution can help clear a thrush infection. This is a purple dye that is swabbed on the affected area. Be careful when applying it—it stains.

DIETARY GUIDELINES

■ Reduce the amount of sugar in your diet. Better yet, eliminate it entirely. Fungi thrive on sugar and proliferate in its presence.

■ Reducing or eliminating fats also can be helpful, with one notable exception: A diet that includes uncooked cold-pressed olive oil may inhibit the growth of yeast.

NUTRITIONAL SUPPLEMENTS

■ Acidophilus and bifidobacteria are friendly bacteria that help clear the body of fungi. Take a probiotic supplement as recommended on the product label. You can also use probiotics as a mouthwash. Mix $1/8$ teaspoon of acidophilus and/or bifidobacteria in $1/2$ cup of water and rinse your mouth well with it two or three times daily. For thrush in hard-to-reach places, you can use an eyedropper to apply the solution.

■ The antioxidant nutrients beta-carotene, vitamin C, bioflavonoids, vitamin E, selenium, and zinc can help to control yeast. Take a good antioxidant formula that supplies 15,000 international units of beta-carotene, 3,000 milligrams of vitamin C, 1,500 milligrams of bioflavonoids, 400 international units of vitamin E, 200 micrograms of selenium, and 30 to 50 milligrams of zinc daily.

■ Caprylic acid, a short-chain fatty acid, helps to kill yeast. Take 200 milligrams three times a day, immediately before meals, for three to four weeks.

HERBAL TREATMENT

■ Aloe vera gel has been shown to have antifungal properties. Try dipping your finger in aloe vera gel and applying it topically to the thrush two or three times a day. Use a food-grade product for this purpose.

■ Cat's claw enhances the immune response and has antifungal properties. Take 500 milligrams of standardized extract three times a day until your condition improves.

Note: Do not use cat's claw if you are pregnant or nursing, or if you are an organ-transplant recipient. Use it with caution if you are taking an anticoagulant (blood thinner).

■ Garlic fights fungal infection. Take 500 milligrams three to four times daily for two to three weeks.

■ Ginger also has fungus-fighting capabilities. Drink a cup of ginger tea with meals.

■ Grapefruit-seed extract is helpful for reducing the amount of yeast in the body. Take 100 to 200 milligrams in capsule form, or 10 drops of liquid in $1/4$ cup of water, two or three times a day for three weeks.

HOMEOPATHY

■ *Arsenicum album* is good for thrush accompanied by

restlessness and/or fatigue. Take one dose of *Arsenicum album* 30x or 9c three times a day for up to three days.

■ *Sulfur* is for thrush with a general feeling of being overheated. Take one dose of *Sulfur* 30x or 9c three times a day for up to two days.

GENERAL RECOMMENDATIONS

■ Do not try to scrape or pick off patches of thrush. You will only leave behind a painful, inflamed, and, possibly, raw and bleeding area.

■ Discuss with your physician the possibility of an underlying condition that may be depressing your immune function.

PREVENTION

■ Antibiotics alter the normal flora of the mouth and body, and can lead to an overgrowth of candida. Any time you must take antibiotics, eat yogurt regularly or supplement your diet with acidophilus and/or bifidobacteria to maintain the friendly bacteria that help control candida within the body.

■ If you have a tendency to develop thrush, keep your consumption of refined sugars to an absolute minimum. Drinking ginger tea with meals may also help.

Thyroid Disorders

See HYPERTHYROIDISM; HYPOTHYROIDISM.

Tinnitus

The term *tinnitus* comes from the Latin *tinnit*, which means "tinkling." In this condition, the acoustic nerve transmits impulses to the brain as the result of stimuli that originate inside the head or within the ear itself, rather than coming from perceptible sounds, causing you to hear sounds that no one else can hear. In some people, the ability to hear normally is not affected, but in others, tinnitus may precede or accompany hearing loss.

Tinnitus can involve just one ear, but it is more common to have it in both. At the onset, the noises may come and go and be nothing more than an occasional annoyance that is scarcely noticed. As time goes on, however, the sounds usually become constant. These sounds range from the characteristic tinkling through a whole gamut of other noises that have been described as ringing, buzzing, roaring, chirping, or hissing, or likened to the sound of rushing water, splashing water, grasshoppers, crickets, wood being sawed, an engine running, and the ringing of bells or the telephone.

Though tinnitus is quite common, its causes are not well understood. It is sometimes linked to *presbycuscis*, or the gradual loss of hearing due to the aging process. Some people develop tinnitus as a result of an unusual toxic reaction to certain drugs and other substances, especially salicylates. Aspirin, which is primarily salicylate, and foods containing salicylates are the most common offenders. These include apples, cucumbers, grapes, tomatoes, and many others. Besides aspirin, other drugs that can cause this disorder include atropine, an antispasmodic; ergot derivatives, which are used to treat migraine; quinidine, a heart medication; and chloroquine and quinine, which are used to treat malaria. Caffeine and nicotine are also known to cause tinnitus in some people.

Tinnitus can occur by itself, or it can be a symptom of virtually any ear disorder, including Meniere's disease, labyrinthitis, and middle-ear infection. It can also be a result of exposure to loud noises or blockage of the ear canal with a buildup of earwax. People with high blood pressure, a dysfunctional thyroid gland, or hypoglycemia may occasionally suffer from tinnitus as well. Some people develop tinnitus as a result of an injury to the brain, such as can occur in a fall or car accident. It is also possible, although extremely unusual, to have tinnitus due to a tumor that affects the nerves inside the ear.

CONVENTIONAL MEDICINE

■ The first step in medical treatment of tinnitus is determining whether an underlying disorder is causing the problem. Appropriate treatment will then depend on the nature of any condition identified. If you are taking any medications, including aspirin, on an ongoing basis, you should discuss this with your physician as well. Sometimes a change of dosage or medication is enough to eliminate the characteristic ear sounds associated with this condition. *Do not* discontinue or reduce the dosage of prescription medication on your own, however. Always consult with your physician first.

■ If an examination fails to reveal the source of the condition, your doctor may recommend one or more of the measures outlined elsewhere in this entry. Some doctors recommend trying a course of an antidepressant such as nortriptyline (Aventyl, Pamelor) or desipramine (Norpramin), taken at bedtime. Since there is no specific treatment for tinnitus, doctors have tried many different drugs to see if they would help, and antidepressants have surfaced as the agents with the most positive effect. Possible side effects of these drugs include dry mouth, nausea, rash, fatigue, headache, low or high blood pressure, blood-sugar problems, and liver damage.

DIETARY GUIDELINES

■ Follow a diet low in mucus-forming foods. That means holding to a minimum your intake of dairy products and other sources of saturated fats of animal origin, such as eggs and red meat.

■ Avoid all foods containing salicylates—including almonds, apples, apricots, cherries, cucumbers, grapes, nectarines, oranges, peaches, pickles, plums, prunes, raisins, tomatoes, many kinds of wine, and all berries—for one month and monitor your reaction. If your symptoms lessen, chances are that salicylates are the offenders, and you should eliminate them from your menu.

■ Avoid anything that contains caffeine, including coffee, green and black tea, caffeinated sodas, and chocolate. Caffeine has been known to cause tinnitus in some people.

■ Avoid alcoholic beverages. Alcohol can make tinnitus worse.

NUTRITIONAL SUPPLEMENTS

■ Vitamin C and bioflavonoids have been successfully used against labyrinthitis, an inflammation of the fluid-filled canals of the inner ear that is known to contribute to tinnitus. Take 500 milligrams of each three or four times daily for one month.

■ Calcium and magnesium are important for the proper transmission of nerve impulses and soothe irritated nerve endings. Take 800 to 1,200 milligrams of calcium and 400 to 800 milligrams of magnesium daily.

■ Cysteine, an amino acid, helps drain excess fluid from the ear. It also protects the liver, which is associated with ear problems in Chinese medicine. N-acetylcysteine is the preferred form of this nutrient. Take 500 milligrams two to three times daily.

■ Kelp contains iodine, which stimulates and supports the thyroid gland. Tinnitus is sometimes associated with depressed thyroid function. Take 150 milligrams of kelp twice daily for one month and see if your symptoms improve. If they do, gradually cut back on the amount to the lowest dose that maintains the effect. You should also consult your physician to determine whether you have a problem with thyroid function.

■ People with ear disorders often have deficiencies of trace minerals. Take a trace-mineral complex that includes 5 milligrams of manganese and 100 milligrams of potassium daily.

■ Some people with tinnitus report they have benefited from vitamin-A therapy. Take 25,000 international units of vitamin A daily for one month and monitor your reaction. If symptoms improve, continue taking vitamin A, but reduce the dose to 10,000 international units a day.

Note: If you are pregnant, or intend to get pregnant, or if you have liver disease, consult your doctor before taking supplemental vitamin A. Pregnant women should not ingest a total of more than 25,000 international units of supplemental vitamin A *per week* from all sources.

■ Deficiencies of the B vitamins are common among people with tinnitus. Twice a day, take a B-complex formula supplying 25 to 50 milligrams of each of the major B vitamins.

HERBAL TREATMENT

■ Ginkgo biloba can be valuable in the treatment of tinnitus. This herb has been shown to increase oxygen supply and promote the proper transmission of nerve impulses. Select a standardized extract containing 24 percent ginkgo heterosides (sometimes called flavoglycosides) and take 40 to 60 milligrams three times daily.

HOMEOPATHY

■ *Carboneum sulfuratum* is good if your hearing is impaired and you hear buzzing and singing noises like those of a harp. Take one dose of *Carboneum sulfuratum* 12x or 6c three to four times daily. If you experience no improvement after three days, discontinue it and select another remedy.

■ *Chininum salicylicum* 30x or 15c is helpful for noises in the ears with a subnormal body temperature and fatigue. Take one dose of *Chininum salicylicum* 30x or 15c three to four times daily. If you experience no improvement after three days, discontinue it and select another remedy.

■ *Chininum sulfuricum* is for violent ringing and buzzing in the ears, possibly accompanied by itchy skin, pain in the head and neck, a lower than normal body temperature, and/or great sensitivity in the spine. Take one dose of *Chininum sulfuricum* 30x or 15c three to four times daily. If you experience no improvement after three days, discontinue it and select another remedy.

■ *Kali iodatum* is for tinnitus of long standing, possibly accompanied by irritability and a congested head. You probably feel better in the open air. Take one dose of *Kali iodatum* 12x or 6c three to four times daily. If you experience no improvement after three days, discontinue it and select another remedy.

■ Salicylic acid is for a roaring noise in the ears, possibly accompanied by dizziness, digestive problems, and a lot of bowel gas. This remedy is commonly prescribed for Meniere's disease as well. Take one dose of salicylic acid 30x or 15c three to four times daily. If you experience no improvement after three days, discontinue it and select another remedy.

BACH FLOWER REMEDIES

Select the remedy that most closely fits your emotional tendencies and concerns, and take it as needed, following the directions on the product label.

- Beech helps to tame a tendency to be impatient and intolerant. It is particularly good if you are the type of person who hates having his or her schedule upset.

- Impatiens eases nervousness, tension, and irritability.

ACUPRESSURE

For the locations of acupressure points on the body, *see* ADMINISTERING AN ACUPRESSURE TREATMENT in Part Three.

- Gallbladder 20 improves circulation to the root of the ear and helps to relieve head congestion.

- Kidney 3 and 7 strengthen circulation to the ears.

- Spleen 6 and Stomach 36 support and improve circulation, and strengthen overall well-being.

- Triple Warmer 5 is connected to the inner ear.

GENERAL RECOMMENDATIONS

- If you smoke, quit. Nicotine is known to cause tinnitus in some people.

- Playing a radio or white-noise machine is often helpful because it helps to mask the annoying sounds of tinnitus. There are even devices called tinnitus maskers, designed to be worn like external hearing aids, that are made specifically for this purpose. This type of tactic can be particularly helpful at bedtime if tinnitus keeps you awake.

- Consider trying biofeedback. Some people with tinnitus have found biofeedback techniques helpful, either in learning to ignore the sound or actually altering the perception of sound.

PREVENTION

- Protect your ears from loud noises, whether from power machinery, loud music, or anything else. Exposure to high-decibel sound is known to cause tinnitus. If you are going to be in an environment with a high noise level, wear earplugs. Damage to the ears caused by loud noise cannot be remedied—it must be prevented from the outset.

Toenail, Ingrown

See under NAIL PROBLEMS AND INJURIES.

Tonsillitis

See under SORE THROAT.

TMJ Syndrome

See TEMPOROMANDIBULAR JOINT SYNDROME.

Tooth, Broken or Knocked Out

We often look at the structures of the mouth in a rather mechanical way—there are baby teeth, permanent teeth, cavities, and at some point, perhaps, braces, dentures, and other dental appliances. However, fully one-third of the motor and sensory areas of the human brain are devoted to the mouth and oral structures. Disturbances here can therefore have far-reaching implications. Consequently, dental problems deserve serious attention.

A car accident or a fall that causes the mouth to collide with a hard surface can result in a tooth being fractured or knocked out. Even biting into something harder than expected can chip or fracture a tooth. If you suffer a tooth injury, you should see a dentist, even if you seem to be fine afterwards. Complications, such as an infection or abscess under the gum, can develop and must be treated promptly. In addition, any tooth that has suffered trauma will have to be watched closely afterward by your dentist. Orthodontia and/or cosmetic dentistry may be necessary to treat the situation.

If you suffer an injury that knocks out or damages a tooth, take action at once. The speed of response is important.

EMERGENCY TREATMENT

- If you suffer an injury to the mouth, wipe away any blood with a cool, clean, wet cloth and look at your teeth. If they are all present and properly aligned, check the frenum (the tissue that connects the lip to the gums) for lacerations.

- If a tooth has been knocked out and you find it within minutes, rinse it briefly to remove debris, but do not scrub it. Use one of the following to rinse the tooth:

• Save•A•Tooth solution, a nutrient-based solution designed specifically for this purpose (*see under* Prevention in this entry).

• Saline solution (commercial eyewash).

• 8 ounces of water with $^1/_2$ teaspoon of table salt dissolved in it.

• Your own saliva.

Immediately after rinsing the tooth, replace it in the

tooth socket, checking its position with respect to adjacent teeth. Then call your dentist to explain the situation and arrange an emergency visit. If at all possible, it is better not to take the tooth to the dentist for reimplantation, but to replace it yourself and then seek your dentist's treatment. This will save precious time and prevent clotting from taking place in the socket. Also, immediately after an injury, the shock will cause your face to feel somewhat numb. If the tooth is reimplanted after the numbness has passed, this process can be needlessly difficult and painful.

■ If all of your teeth are present but one appears to have been displaced deeper into the socket than normal, clasp the bone and palate above the tooth firmly between your thumb and finger. Firmly but gently squeeze/massage with a downward motion to encourage the tooth to return to a normal position. Call your dentist to explain the situation and arrange an emergency visit.

■ If you suffer a deep tooth fracture, if possible, rinse the broken part quickly and hold it in place until it can be treated. If the injury is bleeding, place clean plastic wrap over the bleeding area and secure it by biting steadily on a piece of folded gauze. This will seal off and protect the injured area until you can get to your dentist's office. If possible, save the broken piece of tooth; it may be possible for your dentist to reattach it. Call your dentist to arrange an emergency visit.

CONVENTIONAL TREATMENT

■ Rely on your dentist to treat the injury and advise you on any measures you need to take to promote recovery.

■ Appropriate treatment for a tooth fracture depends on the severity of the fracture. A chip or very shallow fracture may require only cosmetic treatment—the fracture smoothed out to eliminate rough or sharp edges. In time, the newly exposed area of tooth will calcify and become less sensitive, as long as it is kept clean, brushed with a mineralizing toothpaste, and kept from contact with decalcifying foods such as carbonated sodas (see TOOTH DECAY).

■ If the fracture is somewhat deeper, your dentist may recommend restoring it with filling material or by means of bonding techniques.

■ If a fracture is particularly severe, root-canal therapy may be advised. A root canal is a procedure in which the nerve is removed and replaced with a sterile material such as a heavy wax or paste. The tooth is then capped. Root canals are a source of controversy in dentistry, as they expose the immune system to mixtures of different metals and other foreign substances, some of which may have toxic or immune-compromising effects. Before agreeing to root-canal therapy, it is a good idea to discuss with your dentist all of the available treatment options and the pros and cons of each for your individual situation. Unfortu-

nately, if a tooth is injured badly enough, there may be no alternative to extraction.

DIETARY RECOMMENDATIONS

■ Be sure to get plenty of lean protein, plus healthy concentrations of calcium, phosphorus, and vitamin D. Calcium-rich foods include all the familiar dairy products, plus green leafy vegetables, broccoli, cabbage, and Brussels sprouts. Figs, kelp, oats, prunes, sesame seeds, and tofu contain calcium as well. Phosphorus can be obtained from bananas, whole-grain breads and cereals, nuts, eggs, fish, and poultry. Vitamin D is present in fortified dairy products, eggs, and saltwater fish. The body also produces this vitamin as a result of exposure to the sun.

■ Eliminate carbonated soft drinks and sugary foods from the menu. The phosphoric acid most sodas contain can cause the depletion of calcium from tooth enamel, making teeth weaker and slowing recovery. The dangers of sugar are well known.

NUTRITIONAL SUPPLEMENTS

■ Take a good-quality multimineral supplement that is in amino acid chelate form. It should contain 1,000 milligrams of calcium (preferably in malate, hydroxyapatite, or citrate form) and 600 milligrams of magnesium per daily dose.

HOMEOPATHY

■ Immediately after an injury, take one dose of *Aconite* 200x to alleviate some of the initial shock.

■ Take one dose of *Calcarea carbonica* or *Calcarea fluorica* 6x three times a day for five days to aid the healing process.

BACH FLOWER REMEDIES

■ Taken as soon as possible after any type of injury or accident, Rescue Remedy helps to ease stress and anxiety. Add a few drops to a glass of water and sip it gradually, or place one or two drops of the undiluted remedy under your tongue.

PREVENTION

■ Practice proper oral hygiene and visit your dentist regularly to be sure your teeth are healthy and in good condition (see PERIODONTAL DISEASE; TOOTH DECAY). A decaying tooth is much more likely to chip or fracture than a healthy tooth.

■ It may not be possible to prevent all injuries that can damage the teeth, but certain commonsense measures can help. When in a car, always wear your seat belt, whether you are a passenger or the driver. Wear appropriate headgear for activities like roller-blading or riding a bicycle or motorcycle, and a helmet plus mouth guard for contact sports such as football or hockey. Don't use your teeth as a cutting tool—for cutting off thread or fishing line, for example, or opening cellophane packaging.

■ As a precaution, keep Save•A•Tooth solution on hand. It is available in many drugstores and can also be ordered from the manufacturer, Biological Rescue Products (see the Resources section at the end of the book). While it cannot prevent a tooth from being knocked out or fractured, this nutrient-based product can keep a lost or broken tooth alive for hours (without protection, a knocked-out tooth will often die in about fifteen minutes). This reduces the risk of permanent tooth loss and years of expensive dental procedures and exposure to metal bridgework.

Tooth Decay

Tooth decay—known to doctors and dentists as *dental caries*—is a process by which the tooth enamel (the outer covering of the tooth) and the dentin (the body of the tooth) gradually disintegrate. Tooth decay does not happen all at once. It takes months for the bacterial plaque on the surface of the teeth to dissolve its way through the outer enamel and into the dentin. After that happens, the bacteria can travel through structures called dentinal tubules toward the pulp, where it can lead to deep infection, the formation of abscesses, and possible tooth loss.

Tooth decay is a two-faceted disease. It requires, first, that a concentration of certain bacteria be left for long periods of time on the surface of the teeth. The bacteria most often involved are a strain of *Streptococcus* bacteria known as *Streptococcus mutans*, which for unknown reasons seem to be more prevalent in some people's mouths than others. Second, it requires that an individual's teeth be susceptible to decay. This can be caused by a number of factors, including poor-quality tooth enamel, mineral imbalances in the blood, and/or acidic, mineral-deficient saliva. Certain foods are implicated in the decay process as well. At the top of the list of culprits are fermentable carbohydrates—refined starches and sugars, including fruits. Also, while a certain level of phosphorus is necessary for healthy teeth, an excessive amount of this mineral can be a problem because it may cause the depletion of calcium from tooth enamel. A person who consumes large quantities of meat, milk, and, above all, carbonated beverages is probably getting more phosphorus than is good for his or her teeth. Finally, acidic foods, including carbonated beverages and certain types of fruit, such as citrus fruits and pineapple, as well as chewable vitamin C tablets also cause the loss of calcium from tooth enamel when held in the mouth. You'll notice that sweetened carbonated bev-

erages—a favorite of many people, unfortunately—are actually a triple threat to healthy teeth.

On the other hand, there are foods that can help fight and prevent tooth decay. Mineral-rich vegetables, nuts, and whole grains enhance the buffering (neutralizing) action of the saliva, and promote recalcification of the teeth. They also preserve teeth from the inside by helping to maintain proper balances of calcium, magnesium, and phosphorus. And tannin, which is found in black teas, grapes, and certain herbs, fights the bacteria that are involved in the decay process.

In the early stages of tooth decay, there are likely to be no symptoms. In fact, until a developing cavity is pretty far advanced, you will probably not be aware of it. Then the tooth may become sensitive to heat and cold, and you may feel discomfort after eating sugary foods. Since symptoms develop only after significant decay has occurred, you have to have periodic dental examinations to prevent your teeth from developing a serious decay problem. A dentist can detect early signs of decay either visually or by probing (the spot on the surface of tooth where decay is beginning will feel softer than it should). At this stage, the problem is simpler and relatively painless to treat. Your dentist should then also be able to help you identify and change the decay-promoting elements in your oral environment so that you can reduce the chances of other cavities developing in the future.

CONVENTIONAL TREATMENT

■ When decay is found, treatment involves two steps: removal of the decay and restoration (filling) of the cleaned spot to seal out further decay and reconstruct the surface of the tooth.

Decay removal has traditionally been done by drilling, though some dentists today use lasers for this purpose. Because laser treatment doesn't cause the pressure and vibration of a drill, this is reportedly the first truly painless method of removing decay. Another advantage is that the laser can make a smaller hole than a drill, so a smaller filling is required.

Many different materials can be used to fill teeth. Most commonly used in the United States are amalgams, which are silver-colored mixtures of metals that contain copper, tin, and zinc, among others, plus approximately 50 percent mercury. Because of the potential toxicity of these metals, especially mercury, there is growing concern about the safety of amalgam as a dental material. Some European countries, in fact, have made the transition to mercury-free dental fillings. As a result, a number of effective nonmetallic and less potentially toxic filling materials called *composites* have been developed. Unfortunately, these are more expensive than amalgam fillings, and in order to use them, a dentist must spend a certain amount of time learning to handle them properly, something not all dentists are willing or able to do. If you need a filling, ask your dentist about the materials he or she uses. If you are concerned about metal fillings, you may wish to seek a dentist who shares your concern.

■ If the decay has reached the pulp of a tooth, the tooth may be removed or a procedure called pulpotomy may be recommended. In a pulpotomy, enough of the infected pulp is removed to avoid inflammation and the formation of an abscess, thus saving the tooth, which is then restored with a crown. Most of the crowns used for this purpose are made of stainless steel or nickel-chromium. Both of these metals contain nickel, which can cause a variety of sensitivity or allergic reactions either in the mouth or, more commonly, on the skin elsewhere on the body. If avoiding these materials is important to you, discuss this with your dentist.

■ It is possible for teeth, particularly molars, to develop deep decay that is not detectable by regular visual examination or even probing, but that can be seen with the use of an x-ray or special transilluminating lights or lasers. These can often be treated by careful removal of the decay followed by the placement of a sedative dressing. As long as the pulp is still vital, this procedure will usually preserve the tooth and allow it to heal. If the decay is very deep into the pulp, a dentist may try a pulpotomy (see above), or may recommend root-canal treatment or extraction of the tooth. Root-canal therapy involves removal of the nerve underlying the tooth. The resulting empty space is filled with a heavy wax or paste. Root canals expose the body to different mixtures of metals and other substances that may cause toxicity or immune-system reactions in some people. There is some research that suggests root canals may be better tolerated if they are performed before a tooth becomes seriously degenerated. Before agreeing to root-canal therapy, discuss with your dentist all of the available treatment options and the pros and cons of each.

■ Your dentist may recommend that a local anesthetic be injected into your gums to numb your mouth during a dental procedure. The injection of anesthetic itself is a source of anxiety for some people. Most small cavities should be able to be treated with minimal discomfort using modern cleaning and filling techniques, so it is probably better to bypass anesthesia in favor of less invasive measures, including distraction and the use of guided imagery. Certain procedures, however, such as pulpotomy or root canal, or the filling of deep and/or extensive decayed areas, may simply be too painful if performed without anesthesia. In some cases, general anesthesia may be recommended. This is a subject you should discuss in advance with your dentist. What you decide will depend on the type of treatment needed as well as your feelings about and past experiences with dental treatment.

DIETARY GUIDELINES

■ Eliminate sodas and sugary foods from the menu, and keep your consumption of refined carbohydrates to a minimum. These foods promote tooth decay. Be especially wary of sticky foods that linger in the mouth. They are much more likely to cause problems than nonsticky foods.

■ Make sure you eat plenty of vegetables and whole grains.

NUTRITIONAL SUPPLEMENTS

■ After you undergo any kind of dental procedure, take 400 milligrams of bromelain three times a day, between meals, to reduce inflammation.

HOMEOPATHY

■ If you require dental work and are feeling nervous and apprehensive, take one dose of *Ignatia* 200x or 200c before going to the dentist.

■ After you undergo a dental procedure, take one dose of *Arnica* 30x, 200x, 15c, or 30c to help lessen residual pain and heal any traumatized tissue.

■ *Nux vomica* is helpful if you have lingering effects from dental anesthesia. Take one dose of *Nux vomica* 30x or 15c twice a day for one or two days.

BACH FLOWER REMEDIES

■ If you are fearful or apprehensive about dental treatment, take one dose of Rescue Remedy immediately before and after a visit to the dentist.

ACUPRESSURE

For the locations of acupressure points on the body, *see* ADMINISTERING AN ACUPRESSURE TREATMENT in Part Three.

■ If you are suffering from pain as a result of a cavity, massage Large Intestine 4. This acupressure point relieves face and tooth pain and calms a stressed nervous system.

■ Four Gates will help you relax if you are anxious or uncomfortable.

AROMATHERAPY

For specific instructions on how to use aromatherapy, *see* PREPARING AROMATHERAPY TREATMENTS in Part Three.

■ Clove oil is a time-honored remedy for toothaches. If you are suffering from pain as a result of tooth decay, place a drop of clove oil directly on the crown of the affected tooth and dab another drop on the gum around the tooth to anesthetize the area until you can see your dentist. Tea tree oil can also be rubbed or dabbed on with cotton for pain relief.

GENERAL RECOMMENDATIONS

■ Discuss your dentist's treatment plan thoroughly in advance, especially if you need more than one procedure performed. Many dentists routinely treat the worst cavity first, for example, but there is no reason that this has to be done, and it can be easier on your nerves if the procedure done first is the one that is least likely to be unpleasant.

PREVENTION

■ When it comes to tooth decay, prevention is of paramount importance, as there is currently no way to remineralize a cavity. Avoid frequent snacking and the consumption of refined sugars and carbohydrates and sticky foods. If you take vitamin-C supplements, avoid the chewable types, which can erode tooth enamel and promote decay. And make sure to practice good oral hygiene. Brush your teeth well, preferably after each meal (ask your dentist or dental hygienist for a demonstration of proper brushing technique). Exercise care in your choice of toothpaste. Avoid toothpastes that contain sugar or artificial sweeteners. Also avoid toothpastes with strong flavors, which can numb the tongue and create a deceptive feeling of cleanliness that wears off a short time later, when you are away from the brush. One recommended product is Merfluan. This is a baking-soda-based tooth powder with myrrh, natural oils, sea salt, calcium, and magnesium. Brush your tongue as well as your teeth, and floss daily. Again, ask your dentist or dental hygienist to demonstrate the proper technique.

■ Some dentists recommend fluoride treatments for the prevention of cavities. Fluoride is a mineral found in nature that, in small concentrations, stabilizes the structure of the tooth material and helps teeth to resist decay. In too-large concentrations, however, fluoride can cause the teeth to develop abnormal color and form, and the enamel to become softer, though still decay-resistant. You and your dentist are a team that must weigh the benefits and risks of fluoride treatment, as well as other alternatives.

■ Another technique recommended by some dentists to protect against tooth decay involves the use of sealants. These are resins or other similar materials that are applied to form a hard, invisible covering over the teeth, especially the grooves and pits that occur naturally on the tops of the molars. These pits and grooves are the areas in which decay is most likely to begin, because they are easily missed during brushing and therefore tend to collect cavity-causing bacteria. Sealants prevent bacteria from getting to the teeth and causing cavities. If applied properly, sealants should be undetectable and should last for at least two years.

■ Most municipal water supplies in this country today contain added fluoride, intended to prevent tooth decay. Studies of the efficacy of this approach have yielded conflicting results, however. Fluoride also carries with it considerable potential for toxicity, which can show up as white mottling of the teeth and deposits in the bones that allow fractures to occur more easily. Most other countries of the world have declined to fluoridate their water for this reason. It is best not to count on fluoridated water as a preventive against cavities, but to take other measures, especially eating a healthy diet and praticing meticulous oral hygiene, to promote strong and healthy teeth.

Tooth-Grinding

See under TEMPOROMANDIBULAR JOINT SYNDROME.

Toxoplasmosis

See under PETS AND YOUR HEALTH in Part One.

Trichomoniasis

Trichomoniasis is an infection caused by the protozoan *Trichomonas vaginalis*. The principal site of infection is the vagina; in fact, trichomoniasis is the second most prevalent type of vaginal infection in the United States. Although trichomoniasis is most often sexually transmitted, it can also be contracted from an infected washcloth or towel, or transmitted from mother to baby during childbirth.

T. vaginalis may be present in the vagina for some time without causing obvious symptoms. When symptoms arise, they are similar to those of a yeast infection, including vaginal discharge and painful inflammation and itching of the vagina and vulva. However, while the discharge caused by a yeast infection is relatively odor-free, trichomoniasis produces a profuse, greenish-yellow, frothy discharge with a foul odor. Sexual intercourse is often painful, and there may be a burning sensation on urination.

Men also are subject to trichomoniasis, but most have no symptoms of the infection. If symptoms do occur, there may be some urethral discomfort, often diagnosed as *nonspecific urethritis,* and the head of the penis may become inflamed.

A firm diagnosis of trichomoniasis is made by laboratory testing of a sample of the discharge or of swabs taken from the urethra. Since the condition rarely causes a discharge in men, diagnosis of the infection in males is difficult.

CONVENTIONAL TREATMENT

■ The antibiotic metronidazole (Flagyl, Metric, Protostat) is generally effective in treating trichomoniasis. Even if your sexual partner has no symptoms, he or she should be treated at the same time so that you do not end up passing the infection back and forth to each other.

■ As an adjunct to antibiotic treatment, you can use a douche made by adding 2 tablespoons of povidone-iodine concentrate (Betadine) to 1 quart of water. Povidone-iodine, available at most pharmacies, is an antibacterial agent that can fight certain vaginal infections, including trichomoniasis. Douche once a day for one week.

DIETARY GUIDELINES

■ Low to low-normal thyroid function has been associated with increased susceptibility to a wide variety of infections. Iodine strengthens thyroid function. Maximize your intake of kelp and other sea vegetables, such as dulse, hijiki, and kombu, which are high in iodine. (*See* HYPOTHYROIDISM for additional information.)

NUTRITIONAL SUPPLEMENTS

■ To restore the friendly bacteria that keep the vaginal flora in balance, take a probiotic supplement containing acidophilus and bifidobacteria, as directed on the product label. This is especially important if you must take antibiotics. You can also apply the probiotics directly to the affected area. Moisten a tampon and sprinkle it with a powdered probiotic culture, then insert it and leave it in place overnight. If you are using a daily douche as part of your treatment, do this right after using the douche.

HERBAL TREATMENT

■ There are several vaginal boluses that may be helpful, including 3-percent peroxide solution, oil of garlic, grapefruit-seed extract, goldenseal, vitamin A, vitamin C, aloe vera, acidophilus, bifidobacteria, and others. Vaginal boluses are small waxy, tamponlike suppositories designed to deliver various herbs and nutrients directly to the site of the infection. They can be found in various combinations at specialty health-food stores, or you can ask your pharmacist to order one for you. Usually one to three are used daily, depending on the severity of the problem. Follow the instructions on the product label.

■ Nettle and yellow dock are high in trace minerals and help revitalize the blood. They are especially valuable following any type of antibiotic therapy. Take a nettle and yellow dock combination formula supplying 300 to 500 milligrams of each herb per dose, and take it three times daily for up to two weeks.

■ St. John's wort is very useful if you feel depressed following a course of antibiotics and/or if your immune system appears to be vulnerable—for example, if you suffer an outbreak of herpes. Choose a product containing 0.3 percent hypericin and take 300 milligrams two or three times daily for six to eight weeks.

HOMEOPATHY

■ *Alumina* is good if you have an itchy light-yellow discharge that is exaggerated before and after menstruation, and if you feel better with a cold-water wash. Take one dose of *Alumina* 30x or 15c three times a day, as needed, for up to three days.

■ *Mercurius corrosivus* is the remedy for a burning discharge with a strong odor. You feel cold yet sweaty, and may have a sore throat. These secondary symptoms may cause you to think you have the flu. Take one dose of *Mercurius corrosivus* 12x or 6c three times a day, as needed, for up to three days.

■ *Sepia* is for a burning yellow discharge accompanied by irritability, fatigue, and, possibly, swelling of the lower abdomen. Take one dose of *Sepia* 30x or 15c three times a day, as needed, for up to three days.

■ *Sulfur* should help if you have a yellowish discharge that causes a burning sensation, possibly accompanied by abdominal cramping with discomfort centered around the navel. You usually feel worse immediately before menstruation. Take one dose of *Sulfur* 30x or 15c three times a day, as needed, for up to three days.

BACH FLOWER REMEDIES

Select the remedy that most closely fits your emotional tendencies and concerns, and take it as needed, following the directions on the product label.

■ Hornbeam eases the kind of exhaustion that causes you to miss out on normal daily activities.

■ Mimulus is for shyness, timidity, and many specific fears.

■ Sweet Chestnut is the remedy for alienation and a feeling of being very much alone in your suffering.

■ White Chestnut helps to counteract a tendency to obsess on things long after they should have been forgotten.

ACUPRESSURE

For the locations of acupressure points on the body, *see* ADMINISTERING AN ACUPRESSURE TREATMENT in Part Three.

■ Liver 3 detoxifies the blood.

■ Spleen 3 and 10 also detoxify the blood.

■ Spleen 6 and Stomach 36 together strengthen immune function.

AROMATHERAPY

For specific instructions on how to use aromatherapy, *see* PREPARING AROMATHERAPY TREATMENTS in Part Three.

■ Use tea tree oil sitz baths to fight infection. Add a dozen or so drops of tea tree oil to a shallow bath, and soak in the bath for fifteen minutes. Do this several times daily.

GENERAL RECOMMENDATIONS

■ At the first sign of symptoms, see your doctor. Although trichomoniasis is not considered a serious infection, its symptoms, especially in the early stages, are similar to those of other sexually transmitted diseases that are serious. Early diagnosis and early treatment are your best protection.

■ Refrain from sexual intercourse until your symptoms are gone.

■ Do not wear tight jeans, nylon underwear, or pantyhose. Warmth and moisture create a favorable environment for all types of infections. Wear looser fitting cotton underwear that permits air circulation. If you must wear pantyhose, cut a vertical slit in the crotch area to ensure air circulation. Most pantyhose are constructed with an inset crotch panel that is seamed on all four sides. Slitting this panel will not cause the stockings to run, and it should not change the fit of the garment.

PREVENTION

■ The only way to avoid contracting a sexually transmitted disease is to abstain from sex entirely or practice monogamy with an uninfected partner. If you have sex with more than one partner, or change partners often, use a latex condom *every time,* and ask your physician about having periodic physical examinations to insure your continuing good health.

Tuberculosis

Tuberculosis (TB) is a chronic bacterial infection, almost always of the lungs, caused by *Mycobacterium tuberculosis.* Although the incidence of tuberculosis in this country has decreased significantly over the last century, outbreaks still occur, primarily in large metropolitan areas such as New York, Boston, and Los Angeles. The AIDS epidemic is also implicated in recent outbreaks, because people with impaired immune systems are more likely to contract (and therefore to spread) the disease.

Tuberculosis is transmitted when an infected person coughs or sneezes and microscopic droplets containing the infecting organism dry in the air and are inhaled by others. Crowded living conditions are therefore conducive to the spread of the disease.

Tuberculosis generally affects the lungs, but it can spread to the joints and to other parts of the body, creating serious illness. Symptoms include fatigue, a chronic cough, bloody sputum, lack of appetite, weight loss, headache, and fever. A tuberculin skin test, chest x-ray, and a culture of sputum are used to confirm the diagnosis.

CONVENTIONAL TREATMENT

■ If you have active tuberculosis, your doctor will prescribe treatment with several different antibiotics simultaneously, to be taken over a long period of time (usually six to nine months). To achieve a cure, you must take the drugs exactly as prescribed and for the full course of treatment. Antibiotics kill off the most susceptible bacteria first. This may be enough to make you start to feel better, but the least susceptible—or most resistant—bacteria still remain. If you then stop taking the antibiotics, the most resistant bacteria are allowed to survive and reproduce. This is what gives rise to so-called drug-resistant strains of bacteria, which cause infection that is difficult, even potentially impossible, to treat. Recent years have seen an increase in drug-resistant strains of tuberculosis bacteria. Therefore, a combination of drugs is now used routinely to treat all cases of the disease. Increasing numbers of bacteria now resist being killed by one drug or another, so only with a combination can you kill all of them.

All of the drugs used to treat tuberculosis can have serious side effects. Isoniazid can cause liver toxicity, so your liver function must be monitored periodically for as long as you take it. Rifampin (Rifadin) can cause drowsiness and may turn bodily fluids such as urine and sweat a red-orange color. Pyrazinamide can cause liver damage, gout, joint pain, nausea and vomiting. Ethambutol (Myambutol) can result in visual problems, nausea, vomiting, itching, and joint pain. Streptomycin often causes nausea, vomiting, vertigo, rashes, unusual facial sensations, fever, and hives.

■ While the disease is active, your doctor will recommend isolation so that you do not spread the disease to others. Once your sputum and gastric secretions are clear of the bacteria, you are no longer considered contagious, so isolation is no longer necessary.

■ If you have tested positive for tuberculosis but have no symptoms, your doctor will likely prescribe a twelve- to eighteen-month course of isoniazid to prevent the illness from developing. It is also generally recommended that all household members of a person diagnosed with tuberculosis take isoniazid for twelve months.

■ Vaccination with BCG (a weakened form of the tuberculosis bacteria) is sometimes suggested to increase the resistance of a child who is living with an adult who has the disease. This vaccine is used routinely in some parts of the world where the incidence of tuberculosis is high, but is rarely used in the United States. A person who is given a BCG vaccine can later have a false positive result to a TB skin test.

DIETARY GUIDELINES

Drink as much fluid as possible. Herbal teas, chicken soup, and vegetable soups help to support the body during recovery.

■ Avoid concentrated animal fats and greasy or fried foods.

NUTRITIONAL SUPPLEMENTS

The nutritional supplements listed below are intended to support recovery from tuberculosis. They should not be considered a substitute for appropriate antibiotic therapy.

Take a good multivitamin and mineral complex daily.

Beta-carotene helps to heal mucous membranes. Take 10,000 international units daily while the disease is active.

■ Coenzyme Q_{10} increases tissue oxygenation. Start by taking 50 milligrams a day, between meals. After ten days, increase to 50 milligrams twice daily, between meals.

Colloidal silver is considered to have antibacterial properties. Take it as directed on the product label. Do not take this supplement for more than two weeks at a time.

Green-foods supplements such as chlorella and spirulina supply trace minerals that are imperative for healing tissue and restoring energy. Take a green-foods supplement as directed on the product label.

N-acetylcysteine helps to protect the liver against the damaging effects of the antibiotics used for tuberculosis. Take 500 to 600 milligrams daily for three months.

Because it depletes vitamin B_6 (pyridoxine), isoniazid can cause nerve damage. Taking supplemental vitamin B_6 can help prevent this. Take 50 to 100 milligrams daily (one hour away from food) throughout the course of treatment with this medication. If you take any of the B vitamins individually, you should also take a B-complex supplement at a different time of day.

■ Vitamin C and bioflavonoids decrease inflammation and build the immune system. During the first month, take 500 milligrams of mineral ascorbate vitamin C and an equal amount of bioflavonoids three to four times a day. During the second month, take the same amount, but twice a day. During the third and fourth months, take one dose daily.

■ Zinc helps to build up the immune system. Take 25 milligrams twice a day for three months. Take zinc with food to prevent stomach upset. If you take 30 or more milligrams of zinc on a daily basis for more than one month,

you should also take 1 to 2 milligrams of copper each day to maintain a proper mineral balance.

HERBAL TREATMENT

Herbal treatment for tuberculosis is aimed at supporting recovery from the illness. It should not be considered a substitute for appropriate antibiotic therapy. For best results, do not use a single herb continuously, but set up a rotating schedule using the herbs listed here, so that you take one herb a week for six months.

■ American and Siberan ginseng are both excellent sources of trace minerals and micronutrients, and also help to strengthen the immune system. Twice a day, take 300 to 500 milligrams of American ginseng or 100 milligrams of standardized Siberian ginseng extract containing 0.5 percent eleutheroside E, or a combination of the two. Take the first dose one-half hour before breakfast and the second one-half hour before lunch. Continue taking it for up to three months.

Note: Do not use these herbs until fever and other signs of acute infection are no longer present. Do not use American ginseng if you have high blood pressure, heart disease, or hypoglycemia. If you are sensitive to the effects of caffeine and other stimulants, you may want to consult with a qualified herbalist before using ginseng.

■ Ashwaganda, an herb sometimes referred to as "Indian ginseng," has been used for centuries to treat the symptoms of tuberculosis. Take 500 milligrams twice a day.

■ Astragalus has a rich concentration of trace minerals and micronutrients, and helps to strengthen the immune system. Take 300 to 500 milligrams twice a day, one-half hour before breakfast and again one-half hour before lunch, for up to three months.

Note: Do not take astragalus until fever and other signs of acute infection are no longer present.

■ Cat's claw enhances the immune response and has antibacterial properties. Take 500 milligrams of standardized extract three times a day.

Note: Do not use cat's claw if you are pregnant or nursing, or if you are an organ-transplant recipient. Use it with caution if you are taking an anticoagulant (blood thinner).

■ Cordyceps is a tonic herb that increases the oxygen supply to body systems, enhances immunity, and acts as an antioxidant. Take 1,000 milligrams of standardized extract twice a day.

■ Goldenseal fights bacteria and tones the mucous membranes. Take 250 milligrams of standardized extract three times a day.

■ Licorice soothes the throat and respiratory tract, has antibacterial properties, and tastes sweet. For a cough, licorice works best when taken warm. Take a cup of licorice tea three times daily.

Note: Do not use licorice on a daily basis for more than five days at a time, as it can elevate blood pressure. Do not use it at all if you have high blood pressure.

■ Marshmallow root lessens lung inflammation and coats and soothes an irritated throat. Make a tea and take a cup twice daily. You can also make a tea that combines marshmallow root with licorice.

■ Milk thistle helps to protect the liver. Choose an extract standardized to contain 80 percent flavonoids (silymarin) and take 200 to 300 milligrams twice daily for three months.

■ Oregano has antibacterial properties and helps to fight infection. Take 75 milligrams of standardized extract three times a day.

■ Osha root has a long history of use to strengthen the lungs and entire pulmonary system. Take 500 milligrams three times a day.

■ Reishi mushroom helps the body adapt to stress, including the stress of serious illness. Taking 500 milligrams three times daily should help to improve vitality.

HOMEOPATHY

■ When dealing with tuberculosis, it is most valuable to visit a homeopath who can prescribe a constitutional remedy. A constitutional remedy can help strengthen your overall vitality as you recover. Be aware, however, that homeopathic treatment for tuberculosis should not be considered a substitute for appropriate antibiotic therapy.

GENERAL RECOMMENDATIONS

■ Rest is an important part of treatment and healing from tuberculosis. Get as much rest as possible.

■ It is important to prevent the spread of this highly contagious disease from one person to another. As long as you are contagious, keep away from others and sleep alone. Wash your sheets, pillowcases, and towels separately from other laundry and in hot water with chlorine bleach added. Your dishes should be disposed of or sterilized. Used tissues should be disposed of carefully.

■ Routine screenings are an important tool used by public health departments to track, and thereby limit, cases of tuberculosis. Ask your doctor how frequently he or she would recommend you have yourself tested.

■ *See also* COUGH; FEVER.

Ulcer

See BEDSORES; CANKER SORES; PEPTIC ULCER.

Ulcerative Colitis

See COLITIS, ULCERATIVE.

Underweight

Some people consistently weigh less than they would like to (and less than most other people of the same age and height); others experience unwanted weight loss. The chief concern in evaluating this type of situation is finding the underlying cause. It may be that you are perfectly healthy, but simply thinner than most people. However, it is also possible that you may not be eating enough to supply your body with the calories and nutrients it needs. Or you may have a food allergy, or a problem with nutrient metabolism or absorption, that makes it impossible for your body to get the nutrition it needs, even from a healthy and sufficient diet. Underweight can also be one sign of intestinal parasites; certain chronic illnesses, such as cystic fibrosis, celiac disease, heart disease, and problems with thyroid function; or emotional issues, such as stress, depression, anxiety, or an eating disorder. A person who is undernourished—whether as a result of insufficient intake or inadequate absorption of nutrients—may feel tired and weak. If you are chronically deficient in various nutrients, you may feel dizzy and have a difficult time concentrating.

Of greater concern than chronically low weight is an unexplained, unwanted weight loss. This can be a result of any of the illnesses mentioned above. It can also signal the development of a potentially serious health problem, such as cancer. People undergoing cancer treatment often lose significant amounts of weight. This is generally a byproduct of the nausea and deep fatigue the treatments cause, which can make eating seem distasteful and a tremendous chore at the same time. People with HIV disease frequently experience weight loss as well. For some, it is a consequence of having chronic nausea, diarrhea, and/or painful mouth sores. Some develop a progressive, ultimately drastic loss of weight known as *wasting syndrome* (*see* HIV DISEASE).

CONVENTIONAL TREATMENT

■ The first step in treating underweight is to discover the underlying cause, if any. This is a job for your doctor. He or she will probably take a complete medical history, discuss your dietary routine, and order blood tests to determine your nutritional status and check your thyroid function, glucose levels, and other key markers to either rule out or identify any metabolic disorders. A stool analysis is sometimes used to check for absorption problems or parasites. Depending on the results of these tests, additional testing or treatment may be recommended to correct the problem.

■ If you suffer a very severe weight loss, you may need to be hospitalized in order to receive nutrition and close medical care and attention.

DIETARY GUIDELINES

■ Do not eat lots of sweets or fatty foods in an attempt to gain weight. Even if you are truly underweight, you require a well-balanced, healthy diet consisting of three meals a day plus two or more healthy snacks—but be sure to time your snacks so that they don't interfere with your appetite at mealtimes.

■ Be sure to get adequate amounts of quality protein. If you don't, your body may start breaking down muscle tissue to obtain the protein it needs. Include in your diet ample amounts of poultry, fish, whole grains, legumes, and soy foods.

■ Eliminate coffee, tea (except for caffeine-free herbal types), chocolate, and anything that contains caffeine from your diet.

■ Try taking smaller initial portions at meals. Facing a large amount of food can actually cause you to lose your appetite. You can always have more if you are still hungry after finishing the first serving.

■ Consider consulting a nutritionist who can help you plan meals that take into account your individual needs and tastes. This can be especially valuable if you are battling a disease, such as AIDS or cancer, that causes eating to be an ordeal for certain specific reasons. For instance, if you find swallowing difficult, a nutritionist can devise a nutritionally complete, high-calorie diet of soft, nonirritating foods that are easier to eat. A nutritionist may also be able to counsel or advise you concerning emotional and practical issues that may be affecting your weight.

NUTRITIONAL SUPPLEMENTS

■ To correct any possible nutritional deficiencies, take a good multivitamin and mineral supplement daily.

■ Acidophilus and bifidobacteria often help improve nutrient absorption. Take a probiotic supplement as recommended on the product label. If you are allergic to milk, be sure to select a dairy-free formula.

■ Digestive enzymes help to improve nutrient absorption, which is often poor in people who are underweight. Try taking one dose of a full-spectrum digestive-enzyme supplement that contains betaine hydrochloride with each meal for at least one month, and see if your health or

weight improves. If it does, continue to take digestive enzymes for a second month, then begin cutting back slowly.

■ Glutamine is an amino acid that helps to fuel intestinal cells so that they maintain their integrity. Take 1,000 milligrams three times daily.

■ Whey protein is a high-quality source of proteins that are easily absorbed and may help improve immune function in the digestive tract. Try supplementing your diet with a whey-protein drink containing 25 grams of protein per serving. Take one or two drinks per day.

HERBAL TREATMENT

■ Gentian root has been used by Europeans for centuries to stimulate the appetite and improve digestion. Take 500 milligrams three times daily, with meals.

■ Goldenseal stimulates digestive function and many people find it increases appetite. Try taking a cup of goldenseal tea before meals for a week.

ACUPRESSURE

For the locations of acupressure points on the body, *see* ADMINISTERING AN ACUPRESSURE TREATMENT in Part Three.

■ Massaging the Bladder meridian (adjacent to the spine) and then Stomach 36 gradually improves the absorption of nutrients.

AROMATHERAPY

For specific instructions on how to use aromatherapy, *see* PREPARING AROMATHERAPY TREATMENTS in Part Three.

■ A number of essential oils are known for stimulating the appetite. Most of these are oils distilled from various parts of plants also used for food and as spices, such as basil, black pepper, ginger, orange, and thyme. Use any or all of these oils as inhalants or diffuse them into the air shortly before meals.

GENERAL RECOMMENDATIONS

■ Eat in a relaxed setting and enjoy your meals as much as possible. Try not to feel as if you are forcing yourself to eat. This will only cause additional stress and make eating all the more distasteful.

■ Consider weight training to build and maintain muscle mass. In addition to enhancing appearance, strength training increases cardiovascular fitness. It may also help to improve appetite.

■ For suggestions on dealing with weight loss related to eating disorders, *see* ANOREXIA NERVOSA and/or BULIMIA.

■ If you find eating difficult due to nausea, *see* NAUSEA AND VOMITING for additional suggestions.

Urethritis

See under TRICHOMONIASIS; URINARY TRACT INFECTION.

Urinary Tract Infection

A urinary tract infection is a bacterial infection of the urethra, ureters, kidneys, or bladder. An infection of the bladder, called *cystitis,* is the most common type of urinary tract infection. *Urethritis,* or infection of the urethra, is also very common, and may occur either on its own or in combination with cystitis.

If you have a urinary tract infection (UTI), you may experience a burning pain upon urination, and your urine may be foul-smelling, dark, and/or bloody. It is common to feel the urge to urinate frequently, but void only a small amount each time. Additional symptoms can include abdominal pain and backache. Occasionally, a person with a urinary tract infection may experience fever, vomiting, diarrhea, lethargy, and/or irritability.

Because of the structure of the female urinary tract, UTIs are much more common among women than men. The urethra is the small tube that drains urine from the bladder and out of the body. In the female body, the urethra lies close to the rectum and vagina. Bacteria from the lower intestine or vagina thus can easily migrate to and travel up the urethra into the bladder. In fact, this happens quite frequently, but it does not usually result in infection. First, urination washes the bacteria out of the body. Second, the lining of the bladder resists the invasion of bacteria, and urine itself is bacteriostatic, meaning that it inhibits bacterial growth. If these natural defense mechanisms are not successful, however, infection of the bladder can result. In more serious situations, bacteria continue to migrate from the bladder, up through the ureters, and into the kidneys, causing inflammation or infection of kidney tissue.

Factors that can increase the likelihood of a UTI include constipation, malnutrition, and sexual intercourse, especially for women who use the diaphragm for birth control. Even the chemicals in bubble baths and the scents and dyes in some toilet tissue can cause local irritation that leads to an infection. Recurrent UTIs can be a sign of a structural problem in the urinary tract system that causes reflux to occur. That is, the urine moves back up through the urethra to the bladder, and sometimes into the kidneys, instead of moving out of the body. Continuous reflux creates a perfect environment for bacterial growth.

In males, the symptoms of local irritation caused by scratching, masturbating, or an injury to the area can often mimic those of a UTI. If a man develops these symptoms as a result of a true UTI, it is important to have a complete medical investigation, including ultrasound and x-rays. UTIs are uncommon enough in men that a search for an underlying problem is indicated. In women, urinary tract infections are relatively common, and most often do not signal a serious problem. However, if a woman experiences two or three episodes within a matter of months, she should be evaluated closely for a possible anatomical abnormality or other underlying problem.

Regardless of your gender, if you develop a UTI, it is important to have it treated thoroughly, so that it does not spread to the kidneys. To determine whether or not an infection is present, and which specific bacteria are involved, your doctor will recommend both a urinalysis and urine culture. You may be tested again after treatment to be certain that the treatment was successful.

CONVENTIONAL TREATMENT

■ UTIs are usually treated with antibiotics. Nitrofurantoin (Furadantin, Macrobid, Macrodantin), sulfamethoxazole (Gantanol), sulfamethoxazole plus trimethoprim (Bactrim, Septra), and amoxicillin (Amoxil, Augmentin, and others) are commonly prescribed. Most antibiotics are excreted through the urinary tract, so they make their way to the site of the infection and wash over it on their way out of the body, killing the organism responsible for the infection. Treatment of "simple" cystitis usually is uncomplicated and consists of a short (one- to three-day) course of antibiotics. A persistent infection may need a longer course of treatment, up to ten days in some cases. Antibiotics can have a variety of side effects, including allergic reactions, diarrhea, upset stomach, and intestinal or vaginal yeast infections.

■ Phenazopyridine (Pyridium, Prodium), a urinary tract analgesic, is sometimes prescribed to anesthetize the urethra. This eases the uncomfortable feeling of urgency that can accompany a urinary tract infection, and makes it less painful to urinate. It also turns the urine a reddish-orange color. It may be prescribed to alleviate discomfort during the two- or three-day period before antibiotic therapy has an effect on symptoms.

■ An infection of the kidney itself (pyelonephritis) requires more aggressive treatment with intravenous antibiotics, plus possible hospitalization, extensive radiological examination, and/or catheterization. Ultrasound and x-rays of the kidney area may be ordered. These tests allow a doctor to see the anatomy of the kidneys and the rest of the urinary tract, and may help him or her to identify any anatomical abnormalities. (*See also* KIDNEY DISEASE.) Intravenous pyelography (or IVP, a procedure in which dye is injected intravenously, then observed via x-ray as it passes through the system), voiding cystourethrography (VCUG), renal ultrasound, and renal scanning are further x-ray studies used to evaluate the structure and functioning of the urinary system. IVP is usually recommended for any man who develops a UTI. For women, x-rays are usually considered necessary if there are recurrent infections, suspicion of anatomic abnormalities, or kidney disease.

DIETARY GUIDELINES

■ To help flush out your system, drink as much pure water as you can—a minimum of eight 8-ounce glasses a day. This is one of the most comforting things you can do for a urinary tract infection. It dilutes the urine, making it easier on the urinary tract and resulting in much less pain as the urine leaves the body.

■ Cranberries and blueberries both contain a compound that prevents bacteria from sticking to the bladder wall. They also have diuretic and antibiotic properties. Take at least three 8-ounce glasses of pure unsweetened cranberry or blueberry juice daily.

■ Make and eat a clear soup with parsley, celery, carrots, and/or watercress. This is high in minerals, particularly potassium, and is both diuretic and nutritive to the urinary tract.

■ Avoid citrus fruits and acidic foods, which can be irritating to the urinary tract.

■ Avoid alcoholic beverages and all refined sugar. Bacteria thrive on sugar.

NUTRITIONAL SUPPLEMENTS

■ Antibiotics kill both friendly and infectious bacteria. During antibiotic therapy and for two weeks afterward, take a probiotic agent such as acidophilus or bifidobacteria (or a mixture) to maintain and restore beneficial flora in the digestive and urinary tracts. Probiotics are available in either capsule or powder form. Do not take probiotics at the same time as antibiotics; allow at least two hours between the two. If you are allergic to milk, be sure to select a dairy-free formula.

■ Vitamin A supports the health of mucous membranes and epithelial tissues. Take 25,000 international units daily until the infection clears.

Note: If you are pregnant, or intend to get pregnant, or if you have liver disease, consult your doctor before taking supplemental vitamin A. Pregnant women should not ingest a total of more than 25,000 international units of supplemental vitamin A *per week* from all sources.

■ Vitamin C is an important nutrient whenever you are fighting an infection of any type. Take 1,000 milligrams of vitamin C in calcium ascorbate form three to four times daily.

HERBAL TREATMENT

■ Cat's claw enhances the immune response and has antibacterial properties. Take 500 milligrams of standardized extract three times a day until the infection clears.

Note: Do not use cat's claw if you are pregnant or nursing, or if you are an organ-transplant recipient. Use it with caution if you are taking an anticoagulant (blood thinner).

■ If you cannot tolerate drinking cranberry juice (see under Dietary Guidelines in this entry), take cranberry extract. Take 500 milligrams two or three times daily until the infection clears.

■ Grapefruit-seed extract is an excellent antibacterial. Take 100 to 200 milligrams three times a day for ten days.

■ Goldenseal may reduce the ability of invading bacteria to adhere to the lining of the urethra. Choose a goldenseal extract standardized to contain at least 5 percent total alkaloids and take 250 milligrams four times a day.

■ Oregano has antibacterial properties and helps to fight infection. Take 75 milligrams of standardized extract three times a day.

■ Uva ursi has been used for decades by Native Americans for urinary disorders. It has antiseptic and astringent properties that can be very effective for treating mild UTIs and for preventing recurrences. Take 100 milligrams of standardized extract two or three times daily for three to four days. Because uva ursi can be irritating to the urinary tract, it is best to combine it with a soothing herb, such as corn silk.

■ Pipsissewa, although harder to find, is less potentially irritating than uva ursi and is just as effective. Take 500 milligrams three to four times a day for three to four days.

HOMEOPATHY

■ *Cantharis* is the premier homeopathic remedy for urinary tract infection. It helps to relieve the burning pain experienced before, during, and after urination. Take one dose of *Cantharis* 12x or 6c, as directed on the product label, three to four times a day for two to three days.

■ *Apis mellifica* is helpful for burning and a feeling of soreness on urination. Take one dose of *Apis mellifica* 12x or 6c three to four times a day for up to three days.

■ *Berberis vulgaris* is good if you have a burning sensation between urination. Take one dose of *Berberis vulgaris* 4x three to four times a day for up to three days.

■ *Pulsatilla* aids stitching, burning pain during and after urination. Take one dose of *Pulsatilla* 6x three to four times a day for up to three days.

■ *Staphysagria* is helpful for cystitis that developed following sexual relations. Take one dose of *Staphysagria* 12x or 6c three to four times a day for up to three days.

ACUPRESSURE

For the locations of acupressure points on the body, *see* ADMINISTERING AN ACUPRESSURE TREATMENT in Part Three.

■ Bladder 28 helps to regulate the bladder.

■ Kidney 3 helps to strengthen the kidneys and bladder.

■ Stomach 36 is useful if a UTI is related to a disturbance in the digestive tract.

AROMATHERAPY

For specific instructions on how to use aromatherapy, *see* PREPARING AROMATHERAPY TREATMENTS in Part Three.

■ Sitz baths made with essential oil of bergamot, tea tree, and/or thyme can be helpful for fighting infection. Use them several times daily.

GENERAL RECOMMENDATIONS

■ If urination is very painful, sitting in a tub of warm water can help to relax the muscles and dilute the urine so that it is easier and less uncomfortable to urinate.

PREVENTION

■ To prevent bacteria from migrating through the urethra, women should always wipe from front to back after defecating. Buy and use only unscented white toilet tissue, and avoid potential irritants such as bubble baths.

■ If you seem to be prone to urinary tract infections, include acidophilus-rich foods such as sweet acidophilus milk and yogurt in your diet. Be sure to select brands containing active cultures. You can also take an acidophilus or bifidus supplement to help prevent recurrences.

■ A woman should empty her bladder before and within fifteen minutes after sexual intercourse. She should also drink an 8-ounce glass of pure water both before and after sex.

■ If you use a diaphragm for contraception, consider switching to a different method. Women who use diaphragms are more likely to suffer UTIs than those who do not.

Uveitis

Uveitis is a general term for inflammation affecting the uvea, the middle layer of the eye. The uvea consists of three distinct structures: the iris, the ciliary body, and the choroid. The iris is the colored part in the front of the eye; the choroid is a thin layer of blood vessels covering the back and sides of the eye; and the ciliary body is a ring-shaped structure between the two that joins the iris with the retina, the inner layer of the eye. The ciliary body has two main functions: its muscles serve to focus the lens, and it also produces the aqueous humor, a nourishing liquid that bathes the front of the eye. Uveitis may affect all or any of these three parts of the eye.

The primary symptom of uveitis affecting the choroid, known as posterior (rear) uveitis, is a vague feeling of fading or hazy vision. Some people see black spots that seem to float before their eyes. *Iritis*, also known as anterior (front) uveitis, is a type of uveitis that affects the iris, although the term is sometimes used for inflammation that includes the ciliary body as well. Iritis can cause redness, pain, blurred vision, an intolerance to light, and, sometimes, headaches.

Uveitis is often linked to an autoimmune disorder such as rheumatoid arthritis, but it can also be the result of infection. More often than not, there is no obvious cause. Uveitis can be a precursor of other eye problems, including glaucoma and detached retina. If you suspect you may have uveitis, consult an ophthalmologist for a thorough eye examination.

CONVENTIONAL TREATMENT

■ If you are diagnosed with uveitis, your doctor will likely prescribe a corticosteroid. Depending on the specific location of the inflammation, the drug may be applied topically, injected, or taken by mouth. However you take them, if you must use steroids for an eye problem, you need to be monitored by a medical professional. These drugs are generally quite effective, but there are potential negative effects. If you have a herpes infection of the eye, the use of steroids can be disastrous. Steroid use is also associated with an increased risk of glaucoma.

■ In some cases, steroids are not able to suppress the inflammation and a stronger inhibitor of the immune system such as azathioprine (Imuran) or cyclosporine (Neoral, Sandimmune), which are used to prevent rejection in organ-transplant recipients, may be necessary. Potential side effects include an increased susceptibility to infection, low blood counts, and others. Fortunately, however, when these drugs are used to treat a condition such as uveitis, they are normally not used for a long enough period to cause the more serious problems.

■ If an infection is found to be the root of the problem, your doctor will prescribe an appropriate antibiotic.

DIETARY GUIDELINES

■ Maximize your intake of fresh fruits and vegetables. These healthy foods contain antioxidant phytochemicals that protect all the cells of the body, including those of the eyes.

■ Avoid sugar and caffeine. These substances contribute

to eye irritation and worsen the symptoms caused by many eye problems.

NUTRITIONAL SUPPLEMENTS

■ Take a good multivitamin and mineral supplement daily.

■ Beta-carotene is a strong antioxidant that prevents free-radical damage. It is related to vitamin A and has many of the same properties, but it does not become toxic in large doses. Take 10,000 to 25,000 international units of beta-caroteneor mixed carotenoids daily.

■ The essential fatty acids (EFAs), found in black currant seed oil, borage oil, evening primrose oil, and flaxseed oil, are required by every cell in the body. They have been shown to reduce pain, inflammation, and swelling. EFAs also help counteract the hardening effects of cholesterol on cell membranes. Choose one of the above oils and take 500 to 1,000 milligrams two to three times daily.

■ Selenium is an excellent antioxidant that helps prevent free-radical damage throughout the body, including the eyes. While symptoms are acute, take 100 micrograms twice daily. When symptoms improve, reduce the dosage to 100 micrograms once daily.

■ Vitamin A protects against free-radical damage and is especially important to the eyes. Without sufficient vitamin A, the eyes are more susceptible to infection and other problems. Take 10,000 international units of vitamin A three times a day for two months. Then reduce to a maintenance dosage of 5,000 to 10,000 international units daily.

Note: If you are pregnant, or intend to get pregnant, or if you have liver disease, consult your doctor before taking supplemental vitamin A. Pregnant women should not ingest a total of more than 25,000 international units of supplemental vitamin A *per week* from all sources.

■ The B vitamins are required for intracellular metabolism in the tissues of the eyes. Combined with vitamins C and E, the B-complex vitamins are especially beneficial to the eyes. While symptoms are acute, take a B-complex supplement supplying 50 milligrams of each of the major B vitamins twice daily.

■ Vitamin C helps to prevent and clear up infections. It also helps to strengthen capillaries, maintain collagen, and prevent tissue hemorrhaging, and is notable for speeding healing. Select a vitamin-C formula that includes bioflavonoids, especially rutin; these nutrients work best together. While symptoms are acute, take 1,000 to 3,000 milligrams of a vitamin-C complex three times daily. When symptoms improve, reduce the dosage to 500 to 1,000 milligrams three times daily.

■ Vitamin E is an antioxidant and is essential in cellular respiration. It has been shown to improve eyesight in clinical studies. Start by taking 200 international units daily, then gradually increase to 400 international units twice daily. When symptoms improve, reduce the dosage to 200 international units twice daily.

Note: If you have high blood pressure, limit your intake of supplemental vitamin E to a total of 400 international units daily. If you are taking an anticoagulant (blood thinner), consult your physician before taking supplemental vitamin E.

■ Zinc supports the immune system and aids in the healing process. While symptoms are acute, take 25 to 50 milligrams of zinc daily. When symptoms improve, reduce the dosage to 15 to 20 milligrams daily. Take zinc with food to prevent stomach upset. If you take over 30 milligrams of zinc on a daily basis for more than one or two months, you should also take 1 to 2 milligrams of copper each day to maintain a proper mineral balance.

HERBAL TREATMENT

■ Bilberry provides important nutrients that nourish the eyes and enhance visual function. Phytochemicals called anthocyanidins in this herb also help prevent damage to the structures of the eyes. Select a preparation containing 25 percent anthocyanidins (also called PCOs) and take 80 milligrams three times daily.

■ Eyebright is rich in vitamin A and vitamin C. It also contains moderate amounts of the B-complex vitamins, vitamin D, and traces of vitamin E. Eyebright has been used for centuries both as an eyewash and in tea form as a tonic for the eyes. Taken internally, it helps maintain healthy eyes and good vision. Take 300 to 500 milligrams three times daily.

■ Ginkgo biloba extract contains flavonoids with an affinity for organs that are rich in connective tissue, including the eyes. It also protects cellular membranes, has notable antioxidant properties, and enhances the use of oxygen and glucose by the cells. Select a ginkgo leaf extract containing at least 24 percent ginkgo heterosides (sometimes called flavoglycosides) and take 40 milligrams three times daily.

HOMEOPATHY

■ *Mercurius corrosivus* is for an inflamed iris accompanied by a profuse and burning discharge and headache. The eyelid may also be inflamed. Take one dose of *Mercurius corrosivus* 12x or 6c four times daily, as needed, up to a total of ten doses.

■ *Rhus toxicodendron* can relieve swelling and inflammation that occurs after eye surgery or after exposure to cold and damp. Take one dose of *Rhus toxicodendron* 12x or 6c four times daily, as needed, up to a total of ten doses.

ACUPRESSURE

For the locations of acupressure points on the body, *see* ADMINISTERING AN ACUPRESSURE TREATMENT in Part Three.

■ Gallbladder 20 and Large Intestine 4 improve circulation to the head.

■ Liver 3 nourishes the eyes.

■ Spleen 6 and Stomach 36 together improve immune function.

GENERAL RECOMMENDATIONS

■ Avoid substances known to irritate the eyes, such as smog and smoke. Whether it comes from cigars, pipes, cigarettes, or a sweet-smelling wood fire, smoke is very hard on the eyes and worsens symptoms.

PREVENTION

■ A deficiency of vitamin A, the "eye vitamin," is a factor in the development of many eye problems. As a preventive, take 5,000 international units of this important vitamin daily.

■ Using contaminated eye makeup can lead to infection. For example, every time a mascara wand is used and replaced in the tube, it picks up more and more bacteria, some of which is later transferred to the eyelashes. If you use makeup, minimize your risk of bacterial infection by replacing your cosmetics—especially mascara, eyeliner, and other forms of eye makeup—at least every three months.

Vaginitis

Almost all women have vaginitis at some point in their lives. Essentially, this is an infection that causes inflammation of the vaginal lining. Although vaginitis can result from such factors as local trauma or irritation, the condition most commonly occurs when an infectious microorganism invades the vaginal environment and irritates or inflames the sensitive vaginal walls. Itching, tenderness, burning, pain with urination, and pain with sexual intercourse are the most common symptoms of vaginitis. There may also be a vaginal discharge.

Many of the organisms that can cause vaginitis are present in the vagina normally, but the vagina is able to maintain the delicate healthy balance required to prevent infection. Vaginal secretions are basically acidic, which inhibits the growth of most organisms. However, the balance can become disrupted, allowing an overgrowth of the normal flora or allowing an organism from outside the body to invade and start an infection. Antibiotics are one of the greatest culprits when it comes to changes in the vaginal environment. Other things that change the flora and increase the likelihood of infection include stress, the

use of birth-control pills or steroids, diabetes, pregnancy, tight clothing, pantyhose, warm weather, and a decrease in overall immune function.

The infectious agents that cause more cases of vaginitis than any other are monilia (a type of yeast), *Gardnerella vaginalis* (bacteria), and *Trichomonas vaginalis* (protozoa). The yeast organism most commonly involved, *Candida albicans*, normally lives in the vaginas of up to 20 percent of all women without creating symptoms, but under certain circumstances can proliferate and result in infection. Yeast vaginitis often causes intense itching and burning accompanied by a white discharge that resembles cottage cheese.

Some types of vaginitis are sexually transmitted. Vaginitis can also be a symptom of a more serious infection such as chlamydia or gonorrhea.

If untreated, any type of vaginal infection can travel up the genital tract to cause pelvic inflammatory disease or an infection of the fallopian tubes. Recurring vaginitis, especially recurring yeast infections, can be a sign of an underlying immune deficiency or other serious health problem, such as diabetes. If you suffer from recurring yeast infections, consult your physician to check for an underlying health problem. Depending on your history and other symptoms, your doctor may order a blood-sugar test, a blood test for HIV antibodies, and/or other diagnostic work.

Because there are different kinds of vaginitis, it is important to get a precise diagnosis. A physician or nurse practitioner will take a sample of discharge from the vagina or cervix and look at it under a microscope to determine what is causing the problem.

CONVENTIONAL TREATMENT

■ The appropriate treatment depends on the type of organism that is causing the infection. For a yeast infection, antifungal creams or vaginal suppositories (Femstat, Monistat, and Gyne-Lotrimin, among others) are generally recommended. Some of these products are available by prescription, others over the counter. Both the creams and suppositories can be inserted with an applicator. A suppository is warmed and melted by the body so that it can be dispersed throughout the vagina. Antifungal creams also are dispersed throughout the vagina. All of these products tend to be messy and can leak; wearing a mini-pad may be helpful. If you are menstruating, it is best not to wear a tampon while using these medications, as the tampon may absorb the medication.

■ For vaginitis caused by bacteria or protozoa, your physician will likely prescribe an antibiotic such as metronidazole (Flagyl, Metric, Protostat).

■ Some physicians recommend douching with a povidone-iodine solution (Betadine) to wash out the vagina.

Mix the solution according to the directions on the product label. Be aware that this is a strong chemical mixture, and it can adversely affect the vaginal environment by killing the normal flora that should be present. Following it with a probiotic retention douche should help to correct this problem. Povidone-iodine should not be used as a retention douche, and it should not be used during pregnancy.

■ Depending on the type of vaginitis you have, it may be necessary for your sexual partner or partners to be examined and treated as well.

DIETARY GUIDELINES

■ Eat a nutrient-dense diet of lean proteins, fresh vegetables, and whole grains.

■ Eliminate all refined foods, alcohol, sugars, dairy products, and simple carbohydrates from your diet. Yeast and bacteria thrive on sugar.

■ If you experience recurrent yeast infections, use an elimination or rotation diet to identify foods you may be allergic or sensitive to (*see* ELIMINATION DIET and/or ROTATION DIET in Part Three).

NUTRITIONAL SUPPLEMENTS

■ Acidophilus and bifidobacteria help to add friendly flora to the vaginal area and restore the healthy balance of organisms in the vagina. Take a probiotic supplement as recommended on the product label. You can also make a retention douche by mixing 1 teaspoon of acidophilus powder with 1 ounce of water or milk. (*See* ADMINISTERING A DOUCHE in Part Three.) Use this once daily for three days.

■ Vitamin A and beta-carotene help to soothe and heal mucous membranes. Take 10,000 international units of beta-carotene and 10,000 international units of vitamin A twice a day for two weeks.

Note: If you are pregnant, or intend to get pregnant, or if you have liver disease, consult your doctor before taking supplemental vitamin A. Pregnant women should not ingest a total of more than 25,000 international units of supplemental vitamin A *per week* from all sources.

■ Vitamin C and the bioflavonoids have anti-infective and anti-inflammatory properties. Take 1,000 milligrams of each three or four times daily for three days.

HERBAL TREATMENT

■ Cat's claw enhances the immune response and has antibacterial and antifungal properties. Take 500 milligrams of standardized extract three times a day until the infection clears.

Note: Do not use cat's claw if you are pregnant or nursing, or if you are an organ-transplant recipient. Use it with caution if you are taking an anticoagulant (blood thinner).

■ An herbal douche is one of the most helpful treatments for a yeast infection. Try one of the following mixtures:

• Mix 40 drops each of liquid extract of echinacea, goldenseal, and calendula and 2 tablespoons of aloe vera gel in 16 ounces (1 pint) of water. Echinacea and goldenseal are antibacterial; calendula helps to soothe and heal inflammation; aloe vera is soothing to the tissues. Any of these herbs can be used separately, but they seem to work best as a combination.

• Add 20 drops of an echinacea and goldenseal combination extract, 6 drops of tea tree oil, and 1 tablespoon of liquid calendula extract to 16 ounces (1 pint) of water. Again, you can use one or all of these ingredients.

• Add 1 capful of grapefruit-seed extract and 6 drops of tea tree oil to 16 ounces of water. Douche with this mixture twice a day for five days, then once a day for five days.

• Add 4 tablespoons of white or apple-cider vinegar to 8 ounces (1 cup) of water. This can be used as either a standard or a retention douche.

■ Garlic has antibacterial and antifungal properties. Take 500 milligrams of aged garlic extract three times a day for a week to ten days.

■ Olive leaf has known antifungal effects. Take 250 milligrams of standardized extract four times a day for one week.

HOMEOPATHY

■ *Cantharis* helps to relieve the burning and sense of urgency (needing to go to the bathroom frequently and quickly) that often accompanies a vaginal infection. Take one dose of *Cantharis* 12x or 6c three times a day for two to three days.

■ If *Cantharis* is not helpful, or if you suffer from recurrent vaginitis, try *Sulfur*. This remedy will help if the vagina is red, feels hot, and is itchy. It will also help clear up the odor of the vaginal discharge. Take one dose of *Sulfur* 30x or 9c twice a day for up to five days.

■ If you are experiencing burning and itching, with a milky discharge, try *Calcarea carbonica*. Take one dose of *Calcarea carbonica* 12x or 6c three times a day for three days.

■ If the discharge is yellow and has an acrid odor, take one dose of *Kreosotum* 12x or 6c three times a day for three days.

■ If you are suffering from a burning sensation and the discharge is creamy, with an acrid odor, take one dose of *Pulsatilla* 12x or 6c three times a day for three days.

ACUPRESSURE

For the locations of acupressure points on the body, *see* ADMINISTERING AN ACUPRESSURE TREATMENT in Part Three.

Bladder 23 and 60 and Kidney 3 all increase circulation to the urinary tract and reproductive organs.

Spleen 10 detoxifies the blood.

AROMATHERAPY

For specific instructions on how to use aromatherapy, *see* PREPARING AROMATHERAPY TREATMENTS in Part Three.

Essential oil of tea tree has notable antimicrobial properties. Add a dozen or so drops to a sitz bath. To soothe irritation, add an equal amount of lavender oil to the bath. Or use tea tree oil suppositories as directed on the product label.

GENERAL RECOMMENDATIONS

Wear 100-percent cotton clothing and underwear that breathes. Loose-fitting clothing is best. Wash your underwear in hot water with chlorine bleach added, if possible, to kill the microorganisms that cause vaginitis. If you must wear pantyhose, make sure the crotch is made of cotton—or cut a slit lengthwise across the crotch. This is especially important in warm weather.

Try taking sitz baths to soothe the burning and itching. For added benefit, add liquid calendula and goldenseal extract or tea tree and lavender oils.

Use yogurt as a retention douche to get friendly bacteria directly into the vagina. This can be quite soothing to inflamed tissue, and is especially effective for yeast infections. Be sure to buy plain, unflavored nonfat yogurt that contains live cultures. Apply about 1 tablespoon at night.

An alternative to douching is to prepare a bath with $1\frac{1}{2}$ cups of salt and $1\frac{1}{2}$ cups of apple-cider vinegar added. Soak in the bath for fifteen to twenty minutes once or twice a day for two or three days.

PREVENTION

Since many of the organisms that cause vaginitis are normally present in the vagina, it may not be possible to prevent all infections. However, there are things you can do to help make the vaginal environment less conducive to the overgrowth of these organisms. Wear cotton clothing and underwear, and avoid tight-fitting clothing. If for any reason you must take antibiotics, also take an acidophilus or bifidobacteria supplement to help maintain a healthy balance in the flora of the vagina.

Varicose Veins

A varicose vein is a vein that has become swollen, twisted, and distorted. The most common site for varicose veins is on the inside of the leg and on the back of the calf. Varicose veins are considered unsightly, and they can also cause symptoms ranging from a feeling of heaviness in the legs to deep aching to severe pain accompanied by swollen ankles and feet. Shoes that fit in the morning may be too tight by afternoon. The distended vein may be sore to the touch, and itching of the skin in the affected area is common. Symptoms tend to become progressively worse as the day wears on, and worse yet with prolonged standing; elevating the legs most often eases symptoms. It is interesting to note that the appearance of the veins does not necessarily correspond to the severity of symptoms. Some people with many and very obvious varicose veins experience no discomfort, while some with only the slightest appearance of the condition complain of severe pain.

In order to understand how varicose veins form, it is necessary to know something about the design and function of the veins. Blood is pumped from the heart to the various parts of the body by means of the arteries, delivers oxygen and nutrients, and then returns to the heart through veins. For the first part of this journey, the movement of the blood is powered by the beating of the heart, but the return journey has no such pump to keep the blood moving along. Instead, the expansion and contraction of the muscles surrounding the veins squeeze the veins and push the blood along. Assisting this process is a series of one-way valves in the veins that prevent the blood from flowing back down. If one or more valves fail to function properly, however, the blood can pool or flow backward. This dilates and stretches the vein, and also makes it impossible for other valves to close properly. When a vein becomes overfilled with blood, it ends up swollen, prominent, and kinked. As time goes on, the vein develops a tortuous and bulging appearance caused by the backflow of blood. This is a varicose vein.

It is not known why some people develop varicose veins and others do not, although the disorder seems to run in families. We do know of certain factors that can contribute to varicose veins, including obesity, lack of regular exercise, chronic constipation, heavy lifting, pregnancy, habitual standing or sitting for long periods, hormonal changes, and heavy metal toxicity. Some women with varicosities experience the greatest difficulty just prior to menstruation.

Varicose veins can lead to a number of other problems, including bleeding under the skin, thrombophlebitis (blood clots in the veins), and tissue breakdown caused by a lack of blood flow in the surrounding area that can result in the formation of an ulcerated area on the skin. Another complication, though rare, can occur due to a bump or cut of the skin over a varicose vein, which may cause the distended vein to bleed profusely. Raising the leg to allow the blood to drain and applying pressure to the site may be necessary to stem the bleeding.

Spider Veins

Spider veins are very tiny blood vessels visible as thin blue lines just under the surface of the skin, usually of the thighs and legs. Though many people associate them with varicose veins, they are not a sign of early varicosities, and are not dangerous. In fact, despite their common name, they are not veins at all, but dilated capillaries or arterioles (tiny blood vessels that connect arteries to capillaries). They are common after pregnancy.

For the most part, spider veins cause no symptoms and can merely be ignored. If you find them unsightly, you can cover them with cosmetics designed for this purpose, or you can talk to your doctor. It is possible to inject the spider veins with a solution that makes them less noticeable. However, you should be aware that this procedure can have side effects, and the fading effect may not last.

Varicose veins are usually easily diagnosed. Your doctor may evaluate their extent by means of manual examination and, possibly, the use of a tourniquet to assess the flow of the blood in the veins.

CONVENTIONAL MEDICINE

■ If your varicose veins are not too troublesome, your physician may recommend that you wear support stockings or elastic bandages from the time you get up until you go to bed. The elasticity of the stockings helps to keep the damaged veins from bulging, and helps reduce the strain on the affected vein.

■ Varicose veins are sometimes treated by sclerotherapy. In this technique, the physician injects a sclerosing (corrosive) chemical into the distended veins. The chemical causes the walls of the veins to fuse together, so they can no longer carry blood. Collateral circulation develops—that is, surrounding veins take over for the ones that have been destroyed—to ensure that blood is returned to the heart as it should be. Sclerotherapy is done on an outpatient basis over the course of two or three visits. For deeper, larger varicosities, a doctor may use ultrasound to guide him or her in locating and injecting the veins.

■ Severe varicose veins can be treated by surgery to strip the affected veins from the leg. The surgery requires only two small incisions, one in the upper thigh and another in the ankle (or the calf, if the affected vein is higher up the leg). After the vein is clamped and cut, a wire is affixed to the freed vein, threaded back down through the vein, and pulled out through the lower incision, bringing the freed vein with it. Both stripping surgery and scleropathy are usually successful. However, varicosities may develop in other veins as time passes.

DIETARY GUIDELINES

■ Eat a well-balanced high-fiber diet. Maximize your intake of steamed green vegetables and fruits. These foods contain phytochemicals that strengthen blood-vessel walls and contribute to the health of the veins.

■ Avoid fried foods and hydrogenated and partially hydrogenated fats and oils. Fats contribute to circulatory problems.

■ Apple-cider vinegar can be used topically to help improve circulation and reduce pain. Saturate a cloth with the vinegar, wring it out slightly, and apply the compress to the affected area for fifteen to twenty minutes. Do this twice daily for one month.

NUTRITIONAL SUPPLEMENTS

■ Black currant seed oil, borage oil, evening primrose oil, and flaxseed oil contain essential fatty acids (EFAs), which help decrease pain. Take 500 to 1,000 milligrams of black currant seed, borage, or evening primrose oil, and/or an equal amount of flaxseed oil, twice daily.

■ Vitamin C and bioflavonoids help improve circulation and reduce pain. Bioflavonoids also strengthen weak blood-vessel walls and improve the health of connective tissue. Three times a day, take a combination formula that provides 1,000 milligrams of vitamin C, 100 milligrams of rutin, and 100 milligrams of mixed bioflavonoids. Some people experience loose stools if they take high doses of vitamin C. If that happens, cut back slightly on the amount you are taking. If you take the recommended dosage without a problem, you can gradually increase your intake to the highest level your body can tolerate.

■ Vitamin E is an excellent blood thinner that helps improve circulation. It also helps reduce pain caused by varicose veins. Begin by taking 200 international units in the morning and another 200 international units in the evening. Over a six-week period, gradually increase the dosage until you are taking 400 international units three times daily. Continue at this level for three weeks, then cut back to 200 international units twice a day.

Note: If you have high blood pressure, limit your intake of supplemental vitamin E to a total of 400 international units daily. If you are taking an anticoagulant (blood thinner), consult your physician before taking supplemental vitamin E.

HERBAL TREATMENT

■ Bilberry has the ability to strengthen vein walls in two ways. First, it acts to strengthen and stabilize the membranes of vein cells; second, it enhances the effectiveness of vitamin C in reducing the fragility of blood vessels. Choose a product containing 25 percent anthocyanidins (also called PCOs) and take 20 to 40 milligrams three times daily. Do not take this herb if you are already taking pine-bark or grape-seed extract, however.

■ Butcher's broom increases circulation to the legs. This herb has a constricting effect on the veins, which makes it remarkably effective in improving circulation. Take 300 to 500 milligrams three times daily.

■ Ginkgo biloba improves circulation and enhances tissue oxygenation. Select a standardized extract of the whole leaf containing 24 percent ginkgo heterosides (sometimes called flavoglycosides) and take 40 milligrams three times daily.

■ Gotu kola improves venous blood flow and speeds the healing of wounds, including skin ulcers. In clinical trials, approximately 80 percent of subjects have reported a lessening of symptoms, including feelings of heaviness in the lower limbs, vein distension, and numbness, while taking it. Choose a standardized extract containing 16 percent triterpenes and take 200 milligrams three times a day.

■ Hawthorn is high in vitamin C and the bioflavonoids, both necessary for good circulation. It also contains zinc and sulfur, trace minerals that are important to healing. Choose an extract standardized to contain 1.8 percent vitexin-2 rhamnosides, and take 100 to 200 milligrams three times a day.

■ Horse chestnut improves vascular tone, reducing vascular leakage. It also helps with leg pain and fatigue. Take 300 milligrams of standardized extract every twelve hours.

■ Pine-bark and grape-seed extracts improve circulation. Take 50 milligrams of either two to three times daily.

HOMEOPATHY

■ Try *Carbo vegetabilis* if your skin looks mottled and "veiny" and your legs are white, with blue, distended veins. You likely also have digestive problems and are easily nauseated, and may suffer pains in the stomach. Take one dose of *Carbo vegetabilis* 30x or 15c three to four times daily, as needed.

■ Choose *Ferrum phosphoricum* if your legs are pale but redden easily, and walking creates enormous fatigue in your legs. The veins appear more reddish than blue, and your face may be pale, even chalky looking. Take one dose of *Ferrum phosphoricum* 12x or 6c three to four times daily, as needed.

■ *Hamamelis virginiana* is for veins that feel bruised and painful. You may also have hemorrhoids. Take one dose of *Hamamelis virginiana* 12x or 6c three to four times daily, as needed, for up to five days. If there is no improvement after five days, discontinue the *Hamamelis* and select another remedy.

BACH FLOWER REMEDIES

Select the remedy that most closely fits your emotional tendencies and concerns, and take it as needed, following the directions on the product label.

■ Hornbeam will help with exhaustion so debilitating that you miss out on a lot of enjoyable activities.

■ Rock Water helps ease a tendency to be inflexible and to have difficulty forgiving faults, whether in others or in yourself.

ACUPRESSURE

For the locations of acupressure points on the body, *see* ADMINISTERING AN ACUPRESSURE TREATMENT in Part Three.

■ Bladder 23, 25, and 27 improve circulation.

■ Gallbladder 30 and 34 improve circulation to the lower body.

■ Liver 3 also improves circulation to the lower body.

AROMATHERAPY

For specific instructions on how to use aromatherapy, *see* PREPARING AROMATHERAPY TREATMENTS in Part Three.

■ Essential oil of geranium, ginger, neroli, and peppermint can help to boost circulation and relieve pain. Add up to three of these oils to a warm bath or massage oil, or blend a few drops in warm or cool water (experiment to see which temperature suits you best) to make comforting compresses. Apply the compresses for fifteen minutes at a time while sitting with your legs elevated. Repeat as often as needed.

GENERAL RECOMMENDATIONS

■ Spend as much time as you can resting with your legs elevated, preferably above the level of your heart. This will help the pooled blood drain back where it belongs. It will also relieve symptoms.

■ If your physician has advised you to wear elastic stockings, elevate your legs so that they are perpendicular to the floor (or your bed) for a few minutes before putting the stockings on to encourage blood that has pooled in the veins to flow out of your legs toward your heart.

■ Standing worsens symptoms. So does sitting for too long. If your occupation requires you to stand or sit for long periods, vary your posture often. Take walking breaks whenever possible.

■ If you are overweight, make every effort to slim down. Excess weight puts tremendous stress on the veins in your legs. *See* OBESITY for suggestions that can help.

■ Constipation can be a factor in varicose veins, because straining in an effort to force a bowel movement puts added pressure on the veins. *See* CONSTIPATION for ways to prevent or, if necessary, relieve this problem.

PREVENTION

■ Exercise. It is physical activity such as walking that causes the muscles surrounding your veins to expand and contract and move the blood back to your heart.

■ Stretch your legs frequently. If you have a sedentary occupation, this may be as simple as walking around your workplace for five minutes every hour.

■ Keep your weight under control. Carrying excess weight stresses your entire circulatory system, especially the fragile veins in your legs.

■ Avoid becoming constipated. Constipation, especially chronic constipation, is a major factor in the development of varicose veins. A high-fiber diet, as recommended under Dietary Guidelines in this entry, is the best preventive "medicine" for constipation.

Vasculitis

Vasculitis is a general term for inflammation of the blood vessels. It is not a disease in itself, but it is an element in many different disorders. Exactly why it accompanies some illnesses is unknown, however. In some cases, it can be a response to infection, such as in endocarditis or syphilis. The hepatitis B and C viruses can be involved in two of the more prominent disorders associated with vasculitis—polyarteritis and cryoglobulinemia. Rarely, an attack of shingles can be followed by vasculitis within the central nervous system. Reactions to certain drugs, notably penicillins, sulfa drugs, and allopurinol (a gout medication) can cause a blood reaction that leads to vasculitis in some people.

Diseases associated with vasculitis include the following:

• Behçet's syndrome. A relatively uncommon disorder, Behçet's syndrome is a chronic illness characterized by mouth sores that resemble canker sores; similar sores that develop in the genital region; pimples, blisters, and other skin lesions; phlebitis; and inflammation of various structures within the eye, which can lead to vision loss and even blindness.

• Cryoglobulinemia. This disorder results in the presence of blood and protein in the urine, abnormal liver function, abdominal pain, and purpura (bleeding into the skin tissues) in the lower extremities.

• Henoch-Schönlein purpura. This disorder affects small blood vessels and is seen more often in children and males than in females. The purpura is usually of the lower extremities, and there may be swelling of the hands and joint pains. There can also be kidney damage and gastrointestinal bleeding. This condition is believed to be related to sensitivity reactions to various substances, including aspirin, food additives, and drug additives.

• Polyarteritis nodosa. This is a condition characterized by inflammation of numerous medium-sized arteries. It can affect the vessels in various areas of the body, most commonly the kidneys, muscles, joints, nerves, heart, and gastrointestinal (GI) tract, causing fever and pain.

• Polymyalgia rheumatica and giant cell arteritis. These are two related illnesses that primarily affect people over age fifty, causing pain and stiffness in the shoulder and pelvis, often accompanied by fever, anemia, and weight loss. The main difference between the two syndromes is that giant cell arteritis, also called temporal arteritis, can also cause scalp and jaw pain, headaches, and visual disturbances. Worse, it can lead to blindness if not treated early.

• Wegener's granulomatosis. This is a dangerous but uncommon vasculitis that affects the respiratory tract and kidneys. If treated early and aggressively, potentially life-threatening kidney failure may be averted. However, the early symptoms of congestion, sinusitis, ear infection, overgrowth of gum tissue, and/or high-pitched breathing sounds may not be tied to serious illness until it is too late.

With any type of vasculitis, there is a danger that the inflamed blood vessels may become blocked, either by the inflammation itself or by a blood clot lodging within a narrowed vessel. If this situation is not resolved promptly, areas of tissue served by that blood vessel can suffer damage or die. The affected vessel may also suffer permanent damage, and aneurysms (weak spots in blood-vessel walls that are prone to rupture) may develop.

CONVENTIONAL TREATMENT

■ The treatment of choice for most types of vasculitis is steroid therapy. Steroids such as cortisone, prednisone (Deltasone), and methylprednisolone (Medrol) are drugs that reduce inflammation quickly. If begun early enough, such therapy can be life-saving.

■ If vasculitis is a result of infectious disease, appropriate antibiotic therapy is prescribed.

■ If Wegener's granulomatosis is caught early, the combination of prednisone and cyclophosphamide (Cytoxan) may bring about a remission. Cyclophosphamide is a cancer chemotherapy drug that can cause serious side effects, including nausea, vomiting, hair loss, multiple organ damage, bladder cancer, and lymphoma, but considering the danger of this disorder, it may be worth the risk.

DIETARY GUIDELINES

■ Make sure your diet includes plenty of green, yellow, red, and orange vegetables and fruits, which are rich sources of carotenoids.

■ Eliminate or reduce the amount of refined sugars and carbohydrates, as well as saturated and hydrogenated or partially hydrogenated fats and oils. These substances contribute to inflammation.

■ Investigate the possibility that hidden food allergies or sensitivities may be contributing to the problem. (*See* ELIMINATION DIET in Part Three.)

NUTRITIONAL SUPPLEMENTS

■ Take a high-potency multivitamin and mineral supplement daily.

■ Flaxseed oil and fish oils contain essential fatty acids that reduce the inflammatory response by inhibiting inflammatory prostaglandins. Take 1 tablespoon (or 1,000 milligrams) twice daily.

■ Take a probiotic supplement such as acidophilus or bifidobacteria twice a day, between meals, as directed on the product label. Probiotics may help to reduce inflammation and also improve collagen formation.

■ Vitamin C and bioflavonoids help to improve circulation and reduce pain. Bioflavonoids also strengthen weak blood-vessel walls and improve the health of connective tissue. Three times a day, take a 1,000 milligrams of vitamin C and 500 milligrams of mixed bioflavonoids. If you develop loose stools, cut back to the highest dosage of vitamin C that you can tolerate.

■ Vitamin E is an antioxidant, helps to improve circulation, and helps to maintain the integrity of cell membranes. Choose a product containing mixed tocopherols and start by taking 200 international units daily, then gradually increase the dosage until you are taking 400 international units in the morning and another 400 international units in the evening.

Note: If you have high blood pressure, limit your intake of supplemental vitamin E to a total of 400 international units daily. If you are taking an anticoagulant (blood thinner), consult your physician before taking vitamin E.

HERBAL TREATMENT

■ Bilberry contains phytochemicals that strengthen blood-vessel walls and stabilize cell membranes. Choose a standardized extract containing 25 percent anthocyanidins (also called PCOs) and take 40 milligrams three times daily.

■ Hawthorn extract enhances circulation and reduces inflammation. Select an extract standardized to contain 1.8 percent vitexin-2 rhamnosides and take 200 milligrams two or three times daily.

■ Horse chestnut may improve the tone of blood vessels. Take 300 milligrams of standardized extract twice a day.

■ Pine-bark and grape-seed extracts reduce inflammation. Take 50 to 100 milligrams of either three times daily.

HOMEOPATHY

■ *Apis mellifica* is helpful for the swelling and pain of inflammation. Take one dose of *Apis mellifica* 12x or 6c three times daily for three days.

■ *Lachesis* helps to relieve inflammation of the vascular system. Take one dose of *Lachesis* 30x or 15c three times daily for three days.

Venereal Disease

See CHLAMYDIA; GONORRHEA; HERPES; HIV DISEASE; SYPHILIS; TRICHOMONIASIS. *Also see under* CANDIDA INFECTION; EPIDIDYMITIS; VAGINITIS; WARTS.

Vertigo

Vertigo is the sensation that you (or your surroundings) are spinning, falling, rolling, and/or tumbling when, in fact, that is not occurring. It can also manifest itself as a much exaggerated feeling of movement when you have shifted position only slightly. It is not the same thing as feeling faint, losing your balance, or feeling "lightheaded." These problems are most often linked to blood pressure, whereas vertigo originates in the vestibular system in the inner ear, which is responsible for maintaining the body's sense of balance.

The most common cause of vertigo is head trauma that causes a shifting of the structures of the inner ear, disturbing the complicated apparatus involved in spatial orientation. Labyrinthitis, or inflammation of the inner ear, can also cause vertigo. (*See* LABYRINTHITIS.) In some cases, tumors, artery malformations, and especially blood-vessel disease in the central nervous system may be causes as well, though these problems usually cause other neurological symptoms in addition to vertigo.

Multiple sclerosis can have vertigo as a component, as can a form of migraine. Probably the best known disease linked to vertigo is Meniere's disease, which can cause attacks of vertigo that last from one to eight hours, along with some hearing loss, tinnitus, and a sensation of pressure within the ear. (See MENIERE'S DISEASE.)

There are a number of tests that may be done to evaluate the functioning of the vestibular system and diagnose vertigo. In one, the caloric test, the inner ear is cooled, then heated, using water at controlled temperatures, and eye movements are monitored by means of an instrument called an electronystagmograph. This is useful for assessing vestibular function because the eyes normally move in a characteristic fashion in response to the change in temperature in the inner ear. Another test that may be done is the rotary chair test. This test also uses measurements of eye movement, but it does so while you sit in a slowly turning chair and focus on a stationary object.

CONVENTIONAL TREATMENT

■ Since vertigo is a symptom, not a disease in itself, treatment depends on the underlying cause. This may involve treatment with antibiotics, surgery to correct an anatomical problem, or other measures.

■ If no underlying cause can be found, treatment focuses on trying to keep you as comfortable as possible for as long as symptoms persist. A number of different medications may be tried, including the antihistamines meclizine (Antivert, Bonine) and dimenhydrinate (Dramamine), the sedatives diazepam (Valium) and prochlorperazine (Compazine), and drugs classified as anticholinergics, such as atropine and scopolamine (in Transderm Scop). However, it is usually recommended that they be used for the shortest period of time possible, because the return of vestibular-system functioning to normal seems to be slowed by the use of these drugs.

■ For acute attacks, bed rest may be helpful, but for chronic vertigo, physical exercise is important. Such activity enhances the ability of the central nervous system to compensate for abnormalities in vestibular function. Your doctor may even advise you to intentionally and repetitively perform the very movements that cause vertigo, up to the point of nausea, so that your body can learn to handle them. This approach is known as *overloading,* and it is similar to a technique used by professional figure skaters and others who must learn to handle rapid spinning motion without becoming dizzy.

■ In some cases, physical therapy protocols may be helpful. Head manipulations may help reposition tiny crystals within the inner ear that are involved with maintaining balance.

DIETARY GUIDELINES

■ Eat lightly. Having too much food in your stomach often worsens the sensation of vertigo.

■ Avoiding fluctuations in your blood-sugar level is important. Highs and lows can exacerbate symptoms. Eat smaller, more frequent meals rather than two or three large ones. For dietary suggestions to keep your blood sugar on an even keel, *see* HYPOGLYCEMIA.

■ Investigate the possibility that food allergies or sensitivities may be contributing to the problem. *See* ELIMINATION DIET in Part Three.

■ Avoid alcohol, caffeine, and greasy fried foods, which put unnecessary stress on the body.

NUTRITIONAL SUPPLEMENTS

■ Bromelain, an enzyme derived from fresh pineapple, can be helpful if vertigo is due to inflammation in the inner ear. Take 400 milligrams three times daily, between meals.

■ Magnesium deficiency can cause symptoms of dizziness. Take 300 milligrams of magnesium citrate, aspartate, or malate twice a day.

■ The B-complex vitamins nourish and help to regulate the nervous system. Take a B-complex supplement that supplies 50 milligrams of each of the major B vitamins two to three times daily.

■ Some correlation has been found between vitamin B_{12} deficiency and vertigo. In addition to the B complex, take 1,000 micrograms of vitamin B_{12} daily for two weeks.

HERBAL TREATMENT

■ Ginger can help to relieve the nausea associated with vertigo. Take a cup of ginger tea with meals.

■ Ginkgo biloba improves circulation to the brain. Choose a standardized extract containing 24 percent ginkgo heterosides (sometimes called flavoglycosides) and take 80 milligrams three times daily.

HOMEOPATHY

■ *Aconite* can help if you experience vertigo on rising from a prone position. Take one dose of *Aconite* 12x or 6c three times daily for up to three days.

■ *Cocculus* is good for symptoms of vertigo and nausea—feeling as if things are whirling about you—especially if these symptoms occur when you are riding in a car or standing up. These symptoms may be accompanied by a headache, and are likely to be worse after swimming or an emotional upset of some kind. If you are a woman, symptoms are likely to be worse after your menstrual period as well. Take one dose of *Cocculus* 12x or 6c three times daily, up to a total of ten doses.

■ *Conium maculatum* is the remedy for vertigo that occurs when you watch moving objects. Take one dose of *Conium maculatum* 30x or 30c three times daily for up to three days.

■ Choose *Gelsemium* if your head feels light and large, and you have the sensation that you are falling. Take one dose of *Gelsemium* 6x three times daily for up to three days.

■ *Petroleum* is helpful if you experience vertigo on getting up from a sitting or prone position. You may also have a headache, and symptoms are usually worse with cold or dampness, or before and after thunderstorms. You feel better with your head elevated. Take one dose of *Petroleum* 30x or 15c three times daily, up to a total of ten doses.

BACH FLOWER REMEDIES

■ Mimulus can help ease feelings of fearfulness, shyness, and timidity, especially if you frequently express fear of particular things. Take this remedy as recommended on the product label.

ACUPRESSURE

For the locations of acupressure points on the body, *see* ADMINISTERING AN ACUPRESSURE TREATMENT in Part Three.

■ The combination of Bladder 60, Kidney 1, Spleen 6, Stomach 36, and Triple Warmer 5 helps to improve circulation and diminish symptoms of vertigo.

AROMATHERAPY

For specific instructions on how to use aromatherapy, *see* PREPARING AROMATHERAPY TREATMENTS in Part Three.

■ Essential oil of orange has a stabilizing effect of the nervous system. Use it as an inhalant or diffuse it into the air.

GENERAL RECOMMENDATIONS

■ Make the transition from lying down to sitting up to standing gradually.

■ Vertigo is often a symptom of an underlying inner-ear disorder. *See* LABYRINTHITIS and/or MENIERE'S DISEASE.

Vocal Cord Nodules

The vocal cords are bands of fibrous tissue suspended across the larynx, or voice box—a structure of cartilage and muscle that forms the opening between the pharynx, or throat, and the trachea, the first section of the lower respiratory tract. When you speak, the sound comes from air being forced over the vocal cords. The pitch of your voice depends on both the length and amount of tension on the cords.

Vocal cord nodules are nonmalignant overgrowths of tissue on the vocal cords. They are primarily a result of continued use of the voice, whether in singing, shouting, yelling, public speaking, or simply talking too much (or too loudly) for too long. Persistent hoarseness without pain is the chief symptom.

In diagnosing vocal cord nodules, a doctor may examine the larynx (voice box) with a fiber-optic scope inserted through the mouth. He or she may also perform a biopsy of tissue in the area to rule out the possibility of laryngeal cancer, which can cause similar symptoms.

CONVENTIONAL TREATMENT

■ The first treatment likely to be recommended is rest. Vocal cord nodules sometimes disappear if the voice is rested for several months. While resting, you should avoid smoky environments and exposure to airborne allergens.

■ If rest is ineffective, surgery may be recommended to remove the nodules. After surgery, your doctor will probably prescribe a course of antibiotics for a week to ten days, together with resting of the voice until the larynx is fully healed.

DIETARY GUIDELINES

■ Drink plenty of pure water, at least eight 8-ounce glasses daily. The drier the laryngeal tissue, the more vulnerable it is.

■ Eat a healthy, well-balanced diet that includes plenty of chlorophyll- and antioxidant-rich vegetables and fruits. These act as natural anti-inflammatories.

NUTRITIONAL SUPPLEMENTS

■ Bee propolis is soothing to mucous membranes of the throat and acts as an immune stimulant. Take 500 milligrams three times daily.

■ Vitamin A is healing to mucous membranes. Take 10,000 international units three times daily.

Note: If you are pregnant, or intend to get pregnant, or if you have liver disease, consult your doctor before taking supplemental vitamin A. Pregnant women should not ingest a total of more than 25,000 international units of supplemental vitamin A *per week* from all sources.

■ Vitamin C stimulates immune function and is a natural antioxidant and anti-inflammatory. Take 500 milligrams three to four times daily.

■ Vitamin E is a natural antioxidant that promotes healing. Start by taking 200 milligrams daily, then gradually work up to 400 international units twice a day, in morning and evening.

Note: If you have high blood pressure, limit your intake of supplemental vitamin E to a total of 400 international units daily. If you are taking an anticoagulant (blood thinner), consult your physician before taking vitamin E.

■ Zinc lozenges help to heal mucous membranes and alleviate discomfort. Take 5 to 10 milligrams four to six times daily.

HERBAL TREATMENT

■ Slippery elm and marshmallow root are soothing to the mucous membranes of the larynx. Take 500 milligrams of slippery elm four times daily and 250 milligrams of marshmallow root three times daily.

HOMEOPATHY

■ *Causticum* is good if you are hoarse and have difficulty with your voice, accompanied by pain in the chest and a sore feeling about the larynx. This remedy is especially effective for singers and public speakers. Take one dose of *Causticum* 30x or 15c three times daily for up to three days.

■ *Phosphorus* is good if you completely lose the ability to talk at times, especially in the evenings. Your larynx may be very painful, especially when you cough, and you may have a nervous cough that is provoked by strong odors. Take one dose of *Phosphorus* 30x or 15c three times daily for up to three days.

ACUPRESSURE

■ Massaging the Ting points—the end points of the fingers and toes—improves circulation throughout the body, especially in the head.

PREVENTION

■ If you must speak in public, use a microphone whenever possible to avoid straining your voice.

■ Take voice or speech lessons to learn how to use your voice without abusing it, and how to make your voice carry with less effort.

■ Don't smoke, and avoid secondhand smoke. Exposure to smoke is harmful to the larynx.

■ Avoid shouting or otherwise straining your voice for long periods—for example, loud continuous cheering at sporting events. If you do overuse your voice, take care to rest it for some period of time afterward to allow your vocal cords to recover.

Vomiting

See NAUSEA AND VOMITING.

Warts

Warts are skin growths caused by viruses. They occur most often on the hands and feet, but can also appear on the face, neck, and genital area. There are different kinds of warts, including common warts, plantar warts, plane warts, and genital warts. Common warts (verruca) appear as raised, sharply outlined, hardened and rough skin. They are brown or gray in color, and may appear in clusters. Plantar warts take the form of hard, round areas set into the soles of the feet and/or undersides of the toes. Plane warts are small, flat, and flesh-colored, and tend to grow in clusters. Genital warts also usually grow in clusters, in the genital or perianal area. They are moist, rubbery, usually pinkish or red in color, and resemble tiny heads of cauliflower.

Warts can occur at any age, but are most common during childhood and adolescence. They have the annoying tendency to recur and can spread from one location to another. All types of warts are contagious, but with the exception of genital warts, which are usually transmitted through sexual contact, warts rarely spread from one person to another. They may or may not be itchy, tender, or painful.

Any kind of wart can be annoying, but most are harmless. Some do become malignant (cancerous), however. Genital warts in particular should be taken seriously, as they are associated with an increased risk of cervical cancer.

CONVENTIONAL TREATMENT

■ Acid treatment is commonly prescribed for common, plane, and plantar warts. When applied topically to warts, a solution of salicylic acid (12 percent) or lactic acid (10 to 17 percent) works to soften and loosen the hardened skin. Such solutions are available over the counter as Wart-Off and Occlusal, among others. The usual recommendation is to dab acid on the wart two or three times daily, then cover it with an adhesive bandage. Acid treatment is a slow, painless way to remove warts, but acid is drying and irritating to the skin, so it must be applied with care to protect the surrounding skin. Acid-impregnated plasters may be easier to use. Sold over the counter as Mediplast, or by prescription as TransPlantar or TransVer-Sal, the plaster is applied to the wart for twenty-four hours at a time, then replaced with a new one every night. This treatment is usually effective if used consistently for a period of ten to fourteen days.

■ Cryotherapy, also called cryosurgery or "freezing" treatment, is another method of removing warts. In this technique, the physician uses a probe containing liquid nitrogen to cool the wart tissue to -20°F. This injures and destroys the cells of the wart, which usually falls off one or two weeks later. Occasionally several treatments are required, especially for plantar warts. This procedure causes a burning sensation on application, and the area may throb for hours afterward.

■ Bleomycin (Blenoxane), a chemotherapy agent used against cancer, is sometimes used for extremely persistent warts. It is injected directly into the wart. This treatment can be painful, but it is usually highly effective.

■ Warts can also be removed surgically by a physician, or by a podiatrist if they are on the foot. This is a relatively painful procedure, however, and may leave a residual scar. Laser therapy is also available. It takes several weeks for the burned tissue to fill in with newly formed tissue, and is therefore usually reserved for warts that have resisted other treatments.

■ The latest research in the war on warts shows that the drug cimetidine (Tagamet), widely used to treat ulcers, is also effective against warts. In one study, almost 70 percent of subjects who took cimetidine for twelve weeks found their warts disappeared for at least a year, and the warts were reduced by 50 percent in another 17 percent. Resesarchers say that the drug appears to fight human papillomaviruses, the class of viruses that causes warts. No adverse side effects were reported.

■ Genital warts may be treated with applications of podophyllin (Podocon-25). This topical agent is a powerful irritant. It is applied to a very small area at a time, and it should be applied only by a physician. This drug can cause serious adverse effects, including nerve problems, blood abnormalities, and even coma and death.

■ A newer agent, podofilox (Condylox), is similar to podophyllin. It is not as powerful, however, so it can be applied at home. Side effects are common, including burning pain, inflammation, skin erosion, and itching.

DIETARY GUIDELINES

■ Avoid foods containing refined sugars and flours. They can foster bacterial and viral growth.

■ Eat lots of green and yellow vegetables. They are high in beta-carotene, which is healing to the skin.

NUTRITIONAL SUPPLEMENTS

■ Beta-carotene, which the body uses to manufacture vitamin A, has antiviral properties. Take 10,000 international units of beta-carotene twice a day for ten days.

■ Vitamin A can be purchased in liquid form or squeezed out of a capsule. Apply the oil topically twice daily for two to three weeks.

■ Vitamin E is a natural antioxidant that is an important maintenance vitamin for anyone with chronic warts. Start by taking 200 international units daily, and gradually increase until you are taking 400 international units once or twice daily.

Note: If you have high blood pressure, limit your intake of supplemental vitamin E to a total of 400 international units daily. If you are taking an anticoagulant (blood thinner), consult your physician before taking supplemental vitamin E.

HERBAL TREATMENT

■ Banana peel contains a substance that is highly effective at destroying warts. Many dermatologists recommend it. Place a small amount of peel against the wart and hold it in place with adhesive tape. Change the peel once or twice daily, as needed. Repeat for two weeks or until the wart is gone.

■ Shiitake mushrooms have immune-stimulating and antiviral effects. Take 300 to 500 milligrams twice daily for one month.

HOMEOPATHY

■ The following homeopathic regimen may help resolve warts:

Days 1–4: Take one dose of *Thuja* 30x or 9c twice daily.
Days 5–9: Take one dose of *Nitricum acidum* 12x or 6c twice daily.

If the wart has not cleared after nine days, consider one of the symptom-specific remedies that follow.

■ If the wart is dry and itchy, take one dose of *Antimonium crudum* 12x or 6c three times daily for up to three days.

■ Use *Causticum* for warts that bleed easily, are flat, and are mostly found on the fingers. Take one dose of *Causticum* 12x or 5c three times a day for up to three days.

■ *Mercurius cyanatus* is especially helpful for plantar warts. Take one dose of *Mercurius cyanatus* 12x or 5c twice daily for up to five days.

■ Apply homeopathic *Thuja* ointment to the warts once daily for three weeks.

GENERAL RECOMMENDATIONS

■ Warts, especially the dry, itchy ones, are tempting to pick at. Don't. It is impossible to "pick off" a wart. Picking and scratching can only cause infection and may cause the warts to spread.

■ Sometimes warts go away on their own. Try using visualization techniques and imagine that the warts are melting away. Some studies suggest that this may have a beneficial effect.

PREVENTION

■ If you have a tendency to develop warts, take 10,000 international units of beta-carotene, 400 international units of vitamin E, 500 milligrams of bioflavonoids, and 25 to 50 milligrams of zinc each day for two to three months. These nutrients can help to keep warts from recurring.

■ Echinacea and goldenseal stimulate the immune system and help to arm the body's defenses against the viral attacks that lead to warts. Take one dose of an echinacea and goldenseal combination formula supplying 250 to 500 milligrams of echinacea and 150 to 300 milligrams of goldenseal three days a week for two weeks. Discontinue it for two weeks; then take it for another two; and so on.

■ The only way to avoid contracting genital warts is to have a monogamous relationship with a partner you know to be free of the condition. Using a condom will not necessarily protect you against genital warts, as these may occur anywhere in the pubic region and they spread readily by means of skin-to-skin contact.

Weight Problems

See ANOREXIA NERVOSA; BULIMIA; OBESITY; UNDERWEIGHT.

Xerophthalmia

See under DRY EYE.

Yeast Infection

See under CANDIDA INFECTION; THRUSH; VAGINITIS.

Part Three

Therapies and Procedures

Techniques for Using
Conventional and Natural Treatment

Introduction

Part One provided an introduction to conventional and natural approaches to health care, plus important issues in diet and nutrition, exercise, and home safety. Part Two provided discussions of specific health problems and available treatments for them. In Part Three, you will find instructions that will help you to implement the various treatments and diagnostic procedures mentioned in Part Two.

Many people, even if they are interested in trying a natural approach to healing, can be put off because it seems so different from the kind of medicine they know—things like poultices, tinctures, and pressure points sound exotic and mysterious. The entries in this section will explain and show how to prepare the various types of herbal treatments, design an elimination diet, apply acupressure, and more. There are also entries that will show such conventional diagnostic procedures as taking your pulse or temperature.

When you become familiar with the techniques and procedures described here, you will be better able to choose and implement health care that combines the best of conventional and natural approaches.

Administering an Acupressure Treatment

The gentle art of acupressure is something you can do at home. Massaging an acupressure point will help relieve symptoms as well as strengthen your body.

Acupressure points are located along lines called meridians that run along the sides of the body. There are twelve of these meridians on each side of the body, each corresponding to and named for a specific organ. Pressure points are identified by numbers that indicate where they fall along a particular meridian. Spleen 6, for example, is the sixth point along the Spleen meridian.

In the entries in Part Two, specific pressure points are recommended for treatment of different disorders. Use the diagrams in Figure 3.1 (pages 588–590) to help you locate specific pressure points on the body. Keep in mind that, except for Conception Vessel points, each point shown actually represents a pair of points—the other is situated in the corresponding location on the opposite side. That is, if a point is illustrated on the left side of the body, the other point of the pair is found in the same place on the right side.

To give or receive an acupressure treatment, choose a time when you are relatively calm and relaxed. Make sure you are warm enough. You can apply pressure directly to the body or through a shirt or light sheet. Breathe deeply for a few moments beforehand to aid relaxation.

Expect the acupressure points relevant to your condition to be somewhat tender to the touch. Use your judgment. Pay attention to what feels good.

When administering acupressure, work the right- and left-side points at the same time whenever possible (if that is not possible, work one side first and then the other). Using your fingers or thumbs, apply *threshold pressure* to the points. This is firm pressure that is just on the verge of being painful; the point is stimulated but the body doesn't tighten up or retract from the pain. It is a "good hurt" feeling.

Apply from one to three minutes of continuous threshold pressure until the pain is relieved. Or apply pressure for ten seconds, release for ten seconds, apply pressure again for ten seconds, and release again; repeat this sequence ten times.

There are two special acupressure techniques suggested for several of the health problems discussed in Part Two:

❏ Four Gates. Four Gates is a traditional Chinese point combination that has been used by acupuncturists for centuries. Working these points with acupressure will enhance relaxation and help relieve pain, nervousness, anxiety, and sleeplessness. Traditional Chinese doctors believe that working these points "opens the gates" of energy flow in the body. For this technique only, work first on one side of the body and then on the other. Apply pressure simultaneously to Liver 3 and Large Intestine 4.

❏ Neck and Shoulder Release. This is another traditional point combination, used to release the trapezius and other neck and shoulder muscles. Apply threshold pressure to Gallbladder 20 on the right and left sides, until you feel the muscle relax. Then do the same with Gallbladder 21.

Preparing Aromatherapy Treatments

The aromatherapy treatments recommended in this book include inhalants, baths, compresses, and massage oils. All start with pure essential oils, which are highly concentrated distilled essences of various parts of plants. Using aromatherapy treatments is very simple. Following are some of the ways you can use essential oils.

• **Bath.** You can also make a luxuriously fragrant aromatherapy bath by filling the tub with water, then adding 3 to 8 drops of the essential oil or oils (up to three different types) of your choice. Swish the water around to blend before getting into the tub. While you soak in the bath, inhale the fragrance rising from the water.

  Note: Do not use more than 1 drop of basil, peppermint, or thyme oil in a bath, and do not use these oils together.

• **Compress.** To prepare a compress, disperse up to 5 drops of oil in 6 cups of water. The water can be either warm or cool, depending on the condition you are treating. Dip a clean cotton cloth or washcloth in the mixture, then wring it out slightly so that it is no longer dripping and apply it to the affected area. Leave it in place for ten to fifteen minutes, or as required.

• **Diffusion.** Diffusing essential oil into the air is another possibility. There are special aromatherapy lamps and diffusers available for this purpose; simply follow the manufacturer's directions. You can also use an ordinary vaporizer; simply fill the vaporizer with warm water, add 1 to 10 drops of essential oil (depending on the size of the room) to the top of the water, and turn the vaporizer on.

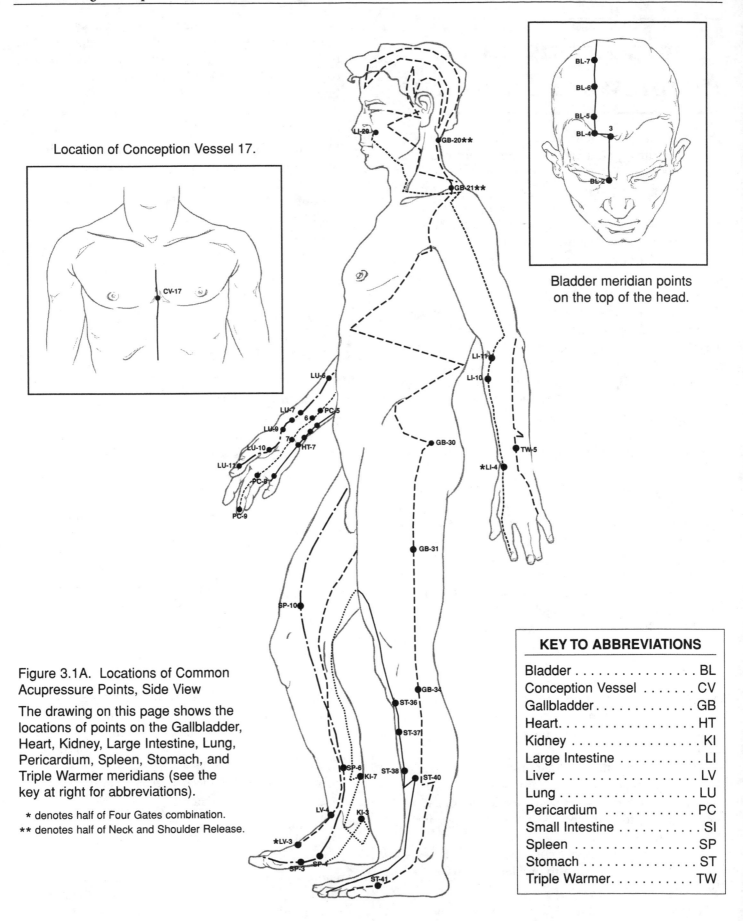

Location of Conception Vessel 17.

Bladder meridian points
on the top of the head.

Figure 3.1A. Locations of Common
Acupressure Points, Side View

The drawing on this page shows the
locations of points on the Gallbladder,
Heart, Kidney, Large Intestine, Lung,
Pericardium, Spleen, Stomach, and
Triple Warmer meridians (see the
key at right for abbreviations).

 * denotes half of Four Gates combination.
** denotes half of Neck and Shoulder Release.

KEY TO ABBREVIATIONS

Bladder	BL
Conception Vessel	CV
Gallbladder	GB
Heart	HT
Kidney	KI
Large Intestine	LI
Liver	LV
Lung	LU
Pericardium	PC
Small Intestine	SI
Spleen	SP
Stomach	ST
Triple Warmer	TW

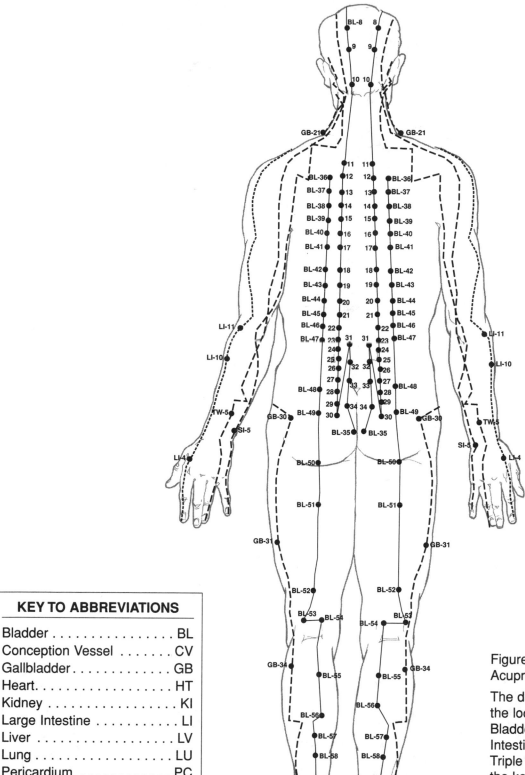

Figure 3.1B. Locations of Common Acupressure Points, Back View

The drawing on this page shows the locations of points on the Bladder, Gallbladder, Large Intestine, Small Intestine, and Triple Warmer meridians (see the key at left for abbreviations).

KEY TO ABBREVIATIONS

Bladder . . . . BL
Conception Vessel CV
Gallbladder . . . . GB
Heart . . . . HT
Kidney . . . . KI
Large Intestine LI
Liver LV
Lung . . . . LU
Pericardium . . . . PC
Small Intestine . . . . SI
Spleen . . . . SP
Stomach . . . . ST
Triple Warmer . . . . TW

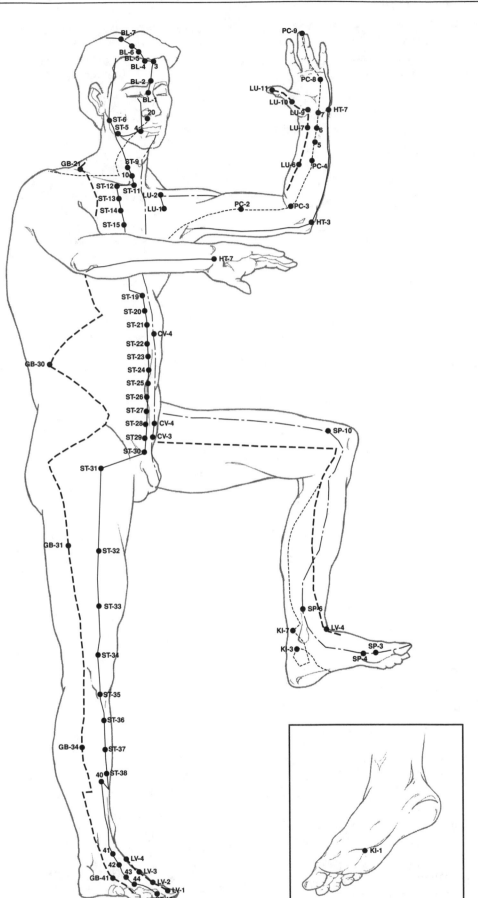

Figure 3.1C. Locations of Common Acupressure Points, Front View

The drawing on this page shows the locations of points on the Bladder, Conception Vessel, Gallbladder, Heart, Kidney, Liver, Lung, Pericardium, Spleen, and Stomach meridians (see the key, below, for abbreviations).

KEY TO ABBREVIATIONS

Bladder	BL
Conception Vessel	CV
Gallbladder	GB
Heart	HT
Kidney	KI
Large Intestine	LI
Liver	LV
Lung	LU
Pericardium	PC
Small Intestine	SI
Spleen	SP
Stomach	ST
Triple Warmer	TW

Location of Kidney 1, on the bottom of the foot.

- **Inhalant.** To use essential oils as inhalants, you have several options. The simplest is just to open the bottle and smell it. You can also place a few drops on a tissue or handkerchief and inhale the aroma that way.

- **Massage oil.** For hands-on aromatherapy, you can add essential oils to massage oil. To make an aromatherapy massage oil, blend the oil or oils (up to three different types) of your choice into a light base oil, such as unprocessed, cold-pressed sesame, soybean, or almond oil. Use up to 5 drops of essential oil per tablespoon of carrier oil (a tablespoon should be more than enough for the average massage).

- **Room spray.** Fill a dark-colored bottle with distilled water. Add 1 to 2 drops of essential oil per ounce of water, seal the lid, and shake to blend. Then spray the air, avoiding objects that might be damaged by water. Shake the bottle again before each use. In hot weather, store the bottle in the refrigerator. You can also use an atomizer to spray essential oils into the air. Use the same type of atomizer you would use for perfume. These are available in many drug and department stores.

- **Shower.** Place 1 or 2 drops of essential oil on a terry washcloth, and rub the cloth over your entire body while in the shower. You can also inhale the scent directly from the washcloth.

- **Steam inhalation treatment.** This is very helpful for opening up congested sinuses and lung passages, helping you to discharge mucus, breathe more easily, and heal faster. Fill your bathroom sink with very hot water and add 2 to 5 drops of essential oil. To keep the water hot and steaming, allow a small, continuous trickle of hot water to flow into the basin (the overflow outlet in your sink should prevent the water from spilling over). Inhale the steam for at least five minutes. As the treated water becomes diluted, add a few more drops of essential oil as needed.

    If it is not feasible to use the bathroom sink for this purpose, use a pot of water heated on the stove to prepare an inhalation treatment. Fill a pot (preferably one that is wide but not too tall) with water. If using whole or dried herbs, add a small handful, heat the water to just short of boiling, remove it from the heat, place it on a tabletop, and add 4 to 5 drops of the oil. Drape a large towel over your head, forming a tent, and lean over the pot. Inhale the steam for at least five minutes. (Be careful that the mixture is not too hot; if it is, it can burn the nasal passages.)

    To help clear lung congestion, take several deep, full breaths of air after an inhalation treatment.

Whatever type of treatment you choose, always remember that a little bit of essential oil goes a long way.

Smell essential oils before you use them; some are more pungent than others, so you may not need as much. In any case, do not exceed the maximum recommended concentration, and do not apply undiluted essential oils directly to your skin, as they can be quite irritating if not properly diluted. And never take essential oils internally. To preserve the potency of essential oils, store them in glass bottles, away from heat, light, and moisture—and, of course, out of the reach of children.

Behavior Modification for Weight Control

Willpower alone is rarely an effective tool for losing weight. Trying to "just say no" when it comes to controlling your appetite, especially if you have an established pattern of overeating, is simply not enough. Instead, you should take advantage of the mind's tendency to follow habits by replacing old habits with new, healthy patterns that support a lifestyle more conducive to change. In psychology, this process is called behavior modification.

Following are a number of behavior-modification tricks to try to help you lose weight. Of course, this technique will probably work best if other members of your household adopt some or all of these measures as well:

- Allow yourself to eat in one room of the house only.

- Do not eat alone.

- Do not do anything else (reading, watching television, etc.) while eating. Concentrate totally on your meal.

- Eat only with utensils—no finger foods.

- Prepare and serve small quantities only.

- Keep only good, nutritious foods on hand.

- Experiment with attractive preparation of the right foods.

- Eat slowly and chew your food thoroughly.

- Swallow all the food in your mouth before taking another bite.

- Introduce planned delays during meals.

- Save one item from each meal to eat later as a snack.

- Except for the saved item, clear your plate directly into the garbage or compost after meals.

- Keep pictures of desired clothing and/or activities on hand.

- Develop a way to get reinforcement for success from other people, including family, friends, other dieters, your physician, and others.

- Plan to reward the achievement of weight-loss goals with a personal gift or a favorite activity (*not* with food!).

Breast Self-Examination

Women who practice regular breast self-examinations are more likely to detect any changes or lumps in their breasts early, when tumors are smaller and more easily cured. Tumors can occur in all areas of breast tissue, but they are more likely in some areas than others. For example, half of all cancers are found in the upper outer quadrant (quarter-section) of the breast, so it is especially important to examine this area thoroughly. Pay special attention to the lymph nodes located in the armpit and the area along the collarbone. The remaining half of breast cancers are found around the nipple (18 percent), in the upper inner quadrant (15 percent), in the lower outer quadrant (11 percent), and in the lower inner quadrant (6 percent).

You should examine your breasts each month, approximately a week after your menstrual period ends (if you no longer have periods, you can do it at any time during the month). Follow the steps below:

1. With your arms at your sides, examine each breast closely in a mirror. Try to memorize its individual contours and appearance so that you can detect any changes that may appear.

2. Squeeze each nipple gently but firmly to determine if there is any discharge.

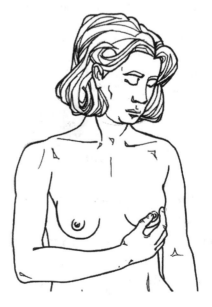

Figure 3.2

3. Closely examine the skin covering your breasts. A localized difference in skin texture can alert you to the presence of a small lump.

4. Raise your left arm, bend your elbow, and rest your hand on the top of your head. Examine your left breast from the front, then turn and examine the breast first from one side and then the other. Notice any changes in contour or appearance. Then raise your right arm and examine your right breast in the same fashion.

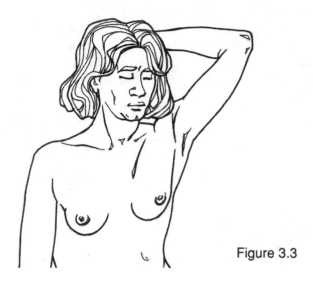

Figure 3.3

5. Lie down on your back with your arms at your sides, with a small pillow supporting your neck and head. Working in a clockwise direction, use the pads of three fingers (index, middle, and ring finger) and move your fingers in either circles or rows to examine your left breast. Check your entire breast, but pay particular attention to the upper outer quadrant, then proceed around the outer area of your entire breast. Then reverse arms and check your right breast.

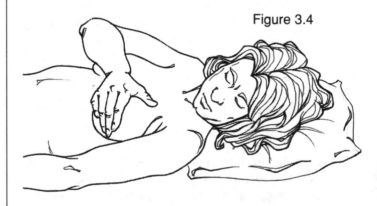

Figure 3.4

6. While still lying down, raise one arm above your head, resting your hand under your neck. This stretches the tissue and makes it easier to find a small lump. Examine the inner portions of your left breast. While in this position, also feel under your armpit, pressing firmly, and check along your collarbone. Then reverse arms and examine your right breast.

If you should find a lump or see any changes in the appearance of one of your breasts, *don't panic*. Remember, many women have fibrous cysts, inflamed sweat glands, and other benign conditions that can cause them to feel lumps in their breasts or armpit area. Detecting a lump does not necessarily mean you have breast cancer. But *do* contact your doctor promptly and schedule an examination. Don't wait. If you do have a cancerous tumor or other problem that requires treatment, early detection and treatment clearly improve the odds of a cure. Besides, waiting will only add to the stress you are experiencing. Call and discuss your concerns with your doctor as soon as possible.

Cardiopulmonary Resuscitation (CPR)

These emergency procedures can sustain life if a person's breathing and/or heart have stopped. When respiration stops, the body begins to be deprived of oxygen, which can cause serious damage. Brain cells begin to die within four to six minutes if they are deprived of oxygen. CPR keeps blood and oxygen circulating in the body. By breathing into the person's lungs and pressing on his or her heart, you can maintain blood flow and oxygen/carbon dioxide exchange to the brain and other organs until the person recovers or until emergency medical personnel arrive to take over.

The outlines of CPR procedures on the following pages are not meant to teach you everything in a time of crisis, but to be used as a refresher for a course on emergency first aid that includes CPR. The authors strongly recommend that anyone who possibly can obtain such training. Courses are usually available through the Red Cross or a local hospital. Reading about the procedures cannot substitute for taking a course and practicing on a mannequin under the guidance of a qualified instructor. Further, these practices are constantly being researched and revised. Stay informed.

In addition to the usual mouth-to-mouth breathing, CPR can involve other procedures in special circumstances, such as giving CPR to a person with a potential spinal-cord injury, mouth-to-nose breathing, mouth-to-nose-and-mouth breathing (as for an infant), and mouth-to-stoma breathing (a stoma is a surgically created opening in the body, such as a tracheostomy or laryngectomy). Only instruction and practice with an instructor in attendance will adequately prepare you to give CPR.

If you see someone lose consciousness, stop breathing, and/or lose his or her pulse, assess the situation quickly, call for emergency help, and initiate CPR in the manner described below.

OPEN THE AIRWAY

1. Place the person on his or her back on the floor, face up.

2. Look to see if there is any foreign material in the individual's mouth. If you can see any foreign material, remove it with your finger, but *do not* sweep your finger blindly through the person's mouth.

3. Tip the person's head back by pushing on the forehead. With your other hand, gently lift the bony part of the jaw. (*See* Figure 3.5.) This positioning opens the airway.

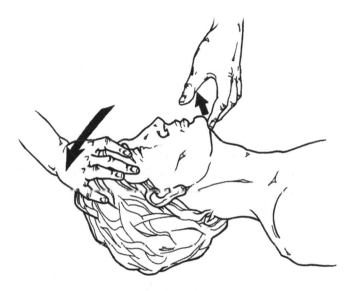

Figure 3.5 Opening the Airway

4. Check for a pulse on the carotid artery, located at the side of the neck. Touch your first two fingers to the Adam's apple. Run your fingers across the neck to the depression between the Adam's apple and the large neck muscle. Press very gently so that you don't interfere with blood flow. Check for breathing by putting your cheek close to the person's mouth to feel for a breath, and watch his or her chest to see if it is rising and falling as in normal breathing. *If the person is not breathing on his or her own, take steps to restore breathing (see step 5). If there is no pulse, initiate full CPR (go to step 9).*

RESTORE BREATHING

5. Once you have the airway open, pinch the person's nostrils closed, cover his or her mouth with yours, and give two slow puffs of air with enough force to cause the chest to rise and fall as in normal breathing. (*See* Figure 3.6.)

6. If your breaths do not cause the person's chest to rise and fall, repeat steps 1 through 3, above, to open the airway again. Give two more puffs of air.

7. If there is still no movement of the chest, the airway is probably blocked. Perform the Heimlich maneuver as follows: Straddle the person, squatting above his or

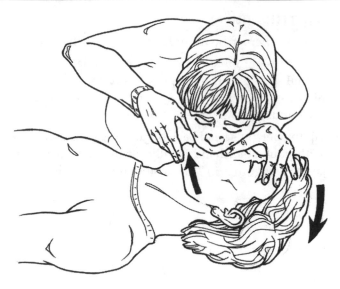

Figure 3.6 Mouth-to-Mouth Breathing

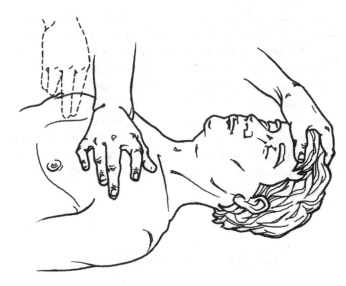

Figure 3.7 Locating the Spot to Give Compressions

her knees. Place the heel of your hand against the abdomen, just above the navel and below the rib cage. Place your other hand on top of the first. Use a quick, forceful *upward* push to force air up through the windpipe. If necessary, continue performing these thrusts until the person coughs up all of the foreign material. Do not stop the procedure until the foreign material is expelled and the person begins coughing, breathing, and talking on his or her own, *or* another person can take over for you, *or* medical help arrives.

8. *If the individual loses his or her pulse during this procedure, initiate full CPR (see step 9).*

FULL CPR

9. Place the person flat on the floor on his or her back. Check for a pulse on the carotid artery again. Only if the person's heart has stopped beating and you cannot feel a pulse can you safely begin CPR. *Never do chest compressions on a person with a heartbeat.*

10. If the person is *not* breathing and *does not* have a pulse, straddle him or her to give compressions. Locate the spot to give compressions by following the rib cage to the place where the ribs and sternum meet. Put your middle finger on this notch and your index finger right next to your middle finger. Notice the placement of your index finger and place the heel of your hand right next to it. (*See* Figure 3.7.) Keep your elbows straight and your shoulders lined up over the person's body. *Keep your fingers off the chest wall.* Maintain this position so that the compressions are done straight up and down on his or her chest. For each compression, push the breastbone straight down $1\frac{1}{2}$ to 2 inches. Do not rock your body. Do not move into the person's chest diagonally. Release the pressure between compressions without taking your hands off his or her chest.

11. Perform cycles of chest compressions and respirations. If you are alone, give 2 breaths after each cycle of 15 compressions, at a rate of 80 to 100 compressions per minute. If there a two rescuers, a complete cycle consists of 5 chest compressions followed by 1 breath. Count aloud to help you maintain a steady rhythm: One one-thousand, two one-thousand, three one-thousand, four one-thousand, and breath, and so on.

12. After giving CPR for one minute, check the person's carotid pulse again. If you feel a pulse, stop doing chest compressions and check for breathing. If there is no pulse, continue performing CPR. Continue to check for a pulse and breathing every few minutes, until emergency medical help arrives. Do not stop CPR until the person starts breathing on his or her own, *or* someone else can take over for you, *or* emergency help arrives.

13. If the person begins breathing on his or her own, discontinue CPR. Once pulse and breathing have been restored and the immediate crisis is over, check and take emergency measures for bleeding, broken bones, or any other injury or problem he or she might have.

Administering a Douche

A douche is one of the most helpful treatments for a vaginal infection, because it works right at the site of the problem. Douches can be made from a variety of ingredients, including medicated products such as Betadine and natural products like herbs, yogurt, and white vinegar. You should use them only if you have an infection or if recommended by your health-care practitioner, however. Excessive douching can cause irritation and infection.

When using a commercial product, prepare the solution according to the directions on the product label. When making an herbal douche, you can use either dried herbs or herbal extracts. If you use the dried form, use 2 ounces of herb for every 4 to 6 ounces of water. Simmer the herb in the water for fifteen minutes, then strain and let the mixture cool to a lukewarm temperature. If you use a tincture, add 5 to 10 drops to a quart of lukewarm water.

Purchase a douche bag or syringe at your local drug store. To administer a standard douche, if you are using a syringe, squat or sit in an empty bathtub and insert the syringe into the vagina. *Gently* squeeze the bag to wash the solution over the tissues. If you are using a bag, sit in an empty bathtub. Hang the bag no more than two feet above your hips. Let the solution fill the tube before inserting the nozzle into your vagina, then allow the solution to flow into and out of the vagina. *Do not* use force or pressure to get the solution into the vagina. The point is to gently cleanse the vaginal tissue.

Some formulas work well as retention douches. These use smaller amounts (no more than about one fluid ounce) of a thicker consistency liquid. As the name implies, a retention douche is retained in the vagina for a period of time. Insert the douche and lie down with your legs elevated for ten minutes (some women do a shoulder stand instead). Afterwards, you can insert a tampon to keep the solution from leaking out, or wear a sanitary pad for the next several hours. Depending on the formula used, a retention douche may be followed with a standard water douche.

Elimination Diet

An elimination diet can help you determine the particular foods to which you are most allergic or sensitive. Once you have identified them, you can eliminate from your diet the things that cause trouble.

Begin by eliminating foods you think may be the source of your symptoms. If you are not sure exactly where to start, start with the foods that most commonly cause a reaction: wheat, citrus fruits and juices, nuts (including peanut butter), dairy products, corn, soy products, and eggs.

Eliminate the suspect foods from your diet for a two-week period. Be aware of the ingredients in manufactured food products. Many of these are likely to contain ingredients that are on your list of suspects. Observe your body carefully during this elimination period. How do you feel?

Do you seem to be breathing more easily? Are your eyes clear instead of itchy and irritated? Are you feeling generally happier and less irritable? Do you have more energy?

After the elimination period, test a food, or class of foods, by putting it back on your menu. For three days, observe how you react (it can take as long as seventy-two hours for a reaction to manifest itself). To make sure you can identify precisely which is the offending food, add back only one food or class of foods every three days, and eat it in as pure a form as possible. For example, to test wheat, have cream of wheat rather than bread, which may contain other allergens.

If eliminating all suspect foods from your diet at one time seems too drastic, try eliminating particular classes of foods one at a time. For example, eliminate all wheat products for a two-week period and see how you react. If your symptoms are not relieved, then eliminate all dairy products as well (and continue to keep wheat off the menu) for the next two-week period, and so on. Continue deleting a food or class of foods until your symptoms improve, and avoid all the deleted foods throughout the entire trial. Once your symptoms improve, you can assume that you are sensitive to the food most recently deleted. You can then add the other foods back into your diet, one at a time, but be alert for any sensitivity or reaction.

Once you have determined which food or foods are causing your reaction, simply keep them off the menu. Read labels carefully to be sure the offending foods are not present as ingredients in the products you buy.

You can also try tracking down food sensitivities by using a diet diary. For three to four weeks, write down everything you eat and when you eat it, along with how you feel and any reactions you have. After the four-week period, you should be able to detect patterns in your responses to different foods.

Starting an Exercise Program

It is difficult to say which is more important for good health, good nutrition or exercise. Eating right and exercising regularly are both requirements for optimum health. For many of the conditions discussed in this book, exercise is recommended both as part of treatment and for prevention.

It has been shown that maintaining a high level of physical fitness can help you stay younger longer. Regular exercise is an important factor in any anti-aging program, and you're never too old—or too young—to start. Regular exercise can help maintain and improve the range of movement of important joints, thus acting both to prevent and alleviate the symptoms of arthritis. It improves coordination and balance, which often deteriorate with age. Exercise also improves flexibility and strengthens muscles, thereby increasing endurance and stamina. Weight-bearing exercise contributes to strong bones, which helps reduce the risk of osteoporosis. Regular exercise leads to a reduction in blood pressure, which reduces the risk of both heart disease and stroke.

Coupled with healthy eating habits, exercise can prevent or help in overcoming obesity, which is a risk factor for many conditions. If you get regular exercise, your body's metabolic rate will increase, with the result that you will burn more calories per minute even when you are sitting still. In addition, regular exercise helps to bring down levels of low-density lipoproteins (LDL, the so-called "bad cholesterol"), while raising levels of high-density lipoproteins (HDL, or "good cholesterol"). Because of its effects on cholesterol levels, and because it strengthens the entire cardiovascular system, regular aerobic exercise protects against heart disease. It also improves breathing and digestion; helps promote regular bowel habits; and strengthens the muscles of the lower back and abdomen, which can help prevent or ease lower back pain. Just as important as the physical effects are the psychological benefits. Exercise is an excellent stress- and anxiety-reducer, and can even relieve the symptoms of more serious psychological conditions, including panic disorder and depression.

The *Journal of the American Medical Association* says that a moderate degree of fitness can be achieved in as little as ten weeks with such easy forms of exercise as walking, bicycling, and gardening Virtually anyone can improve his or her health dramatically simply by making time for some form of exercise he or she enjoys and doing it on a regular basis.

If you love to exercise and do it frequently, you don't need this section. We won't have a whole lot to offer other than to tell you to keep it up (and not to kill yourself doing it). If you're a dyed-in-the-wool jock type, you wouldn't be inclined to make many athletic changes anyway—so exercise, enjoy it, and look at the other sections in this book for ways to take care of your health so you can continue to be active.

If you are just starting out on the road to turning your life around by getting healthy, then exercise may not only be a novelty, it can appear downright intimidating. You look at all the people who are running, cycling, jazzercising, swimming, stair-stepping, or whatever, and many of them don't look like they're having fun. They're sweating, panting—in fact, some look as if they're dying.

It may seem odd to a nonathlete, but these people have chosen to do these things, and they do them because they want to. Maybe they love their new bodies and get

addicted that way; maybe they love the camaraderie, or the challenge, or the "high" exercise can give—or maybe it just feels good when they stop. It doesn't matter. You see these people out there all the time because they are out there all the time . . . because they like being there.

This brings us to a very important point about exercise, which is that you must do something you like, or you will do it for a few days and then quit. If you find you really like sitting on a stationary bike, because you can read or watch the news and get in shape at the same time, do it. If you find yoga rewarding because it gives you an island of calm in a hectic day, do that. Even if working the remote control is the only exercise you get right now, there is some form of exercise out there that you will enjoy. The trick is to find it—and to have it accessible. If you don't have good enough access to do it consistently, you won't do it regularly enough.

So shop around. Find something you like that you can do for at least twenty minutes at a time at least three times a week. Many people find walking an easy way to start. If done consistently, it is a form of exercise that qualifies as both easy and rewarding. The key is consistency. If you walk twenty miles today and no miles at all for the rest of the month, it won't work. A moderate twenty- to thirty-minute walk at least three days a week is what you need. Walking five or six days a week is even better. The body's response to exercise—firmer muscles, a stronger heart, and less body fat—is greatest if you remind your body that you demand those changes every day. If you're short on time, a shorter but faster walk is fine, and is certainly better than skipping the day's exercise altogether. When you walk, wear good walking shoes that provide support and cushioning, and walk briskly, with a rolling stride. Stay tall in your stride and keep your back flat. Keep your elbows bent and swing your arms in rhythym with your steps.

If walking is not for you, there are many more options available. The type of exercise you choose doesn't have to be commonplace, either. Consider tai chi, qi gong, or another martial art form; yoga; a sport such as badminton or tetherball; or even activities like chopping wood or raking leaves—anything that can provide you with physical activity on a regular basis. Or you might consider rebounding exercise. This requires only a single piece of equipment, a mini-trampoline, and is so convenient and easy that even if you steadfastly hate exercise of all kinds, you should be willing at least to tolerate it a few times per week. The value of rebounding exercise goes far beyond its ability to increase heart rate, which all forms of exercise do. Up-and-down motion has a beneficial effect on the cardiovascular system that other forms of exercise cannot match. Running has the same effect, but it is far more traumatic to joints and can even adversely effect soft tissues, depending on the surface you run on. Plus, for most beginners, running is much less enjoyable than bouncing. At the same time, rebounding is a remarkable strength-builder, without seeming to require the extremely hard work weight machines do for most people.

Whatever type of exercise you try, start slowly. Work at an intensity low enough that you cannot even feel it right away, and stay with the activity for twenty to thirty minutes. By the end of that time, you should be feeling some physical exertion—but don't exhaust yourself. As time goes by, you may find yourself wanting to do more, or you may not. If you don't, don't feel you have to increase your workouts, or you will risk getting frustrated and quitting completely. It is far better to know the limits of your tolerance and stick to thirty minutes three days a week.

On the other hand, if the exercise bug bites, you can start thinking about getting more aerobic. This is supposedly the threshold where your cardiovascular system *really* starts getting into shape. There are different theories as to where this point is, but a rule of thumb uses the following equation: Subtract your age from 220. The result is an approximation of your *maximal heart rate,* or the highest number of beats per minute your heart can be expected to take safely. Then calculate 80 percent of your maximal heart rate. This is your *target heart rate.* When you exercise, try to keep your heart beating at the target rate for twenty minutes. It is easiest to measure your heart rate by taking your carotid pulse—the pulse in the carotid artery, in your neck (*see* TAKING YOUR PULSE). Count the beats for one minute, or count the beats for thirty seconds and then double that number to get your heart rate.

In addition to exercise for all-over conditioning and health, you may wish to do other, more specific types of exercise. Strength training and stretching exercises are two examples. Strength exercises are not just for body builders. Studies have shown that working with weights can benefit even senior citizens who have not exercised in years. Of course, if you fall into that category, you should consult with your physician to be sure it is safe for you to begin any type of exercise regimen and, possibly, work with a physical therapist or fitness professional to make sure you are performing the exercises in a way that is both safe and beneficial.

One of the most worried-about parts of the anatomy, among both men and women, is the waistline. (If you have a nice, tight tummy, you can skip this paragraph.) Sit-ups or "crunches" are the usual prescription here. The problem with these exercises is that they simply are not fun. One trick that can help is to do them in bed, first thing in the morning. Try this: Set your alarm to wake you one minute earlier than usual. Then, when it goes off, slide (on your back) down a few inches until your heels catch on the mattress edge at the foot of the bed or your feet reach the footboard. Leave the covers on, put your hands behind your

neck, and do a few sit-ups. You can do them either with your legs straight or bent, as you prefer. You don't even have to open your eyes. Doing that first sit-up will almost certainly be easier than actually climbing out of bed would be, so the sit-up becomes the lesser of two evils at this point. Do as many sit-ups as you can each morning. Even if you can manage only one or two at first, keep in mind that one is better than none, and if you keep with it, soon you will be able to do more. And in a few weeks or months, your stomach should start to feel tighter and you will actually see some results in the mirror.

One word of caution before you begin: If you are over thirty-five and/or have had a sedentary lifestyle for some time, consult with your physician before beginning any new exercise program to be sure that it is safe and appropriate for you.

Glandular Therapy

Some entries in this book recommend glandular extracts to stimulate glands that, for one reason or another, have become "tired" and fail to function as well as they should. Examples include adrenal extract and thyroid extract.

Glands are specialized groups of cells that manufacture and release chemical substances, such as hormones and enzymes, for use in the body. There are two main types of glands: exocrine and endocrine. Exocrine glands are equipped with ducts and release their secretions either onto the skin or into a hollow structure such as the mouth or digestive tract. For example, the salivary glands release their secretions into the mouth; sweat and oil glands release substances through ducts that lead to the surface of the skin. Exocrine glands are also found in the kidneys, the digestive tract, and the breasts.

Endocrine glands release their secretions directly into the bloodstream, even though the organs they target may be quite distant from the area of the body where the manufacturing gland is located. The endocrine glands include the pituitary gland, located at the base of the brain, which supplies hormones that control the functioning of the thyroid gland, the adrenal cortex (part of the adrenal glands), the mammary glands, the ovaries and testes, and other endocrine glands. The thyroid and parathyroid glands, situated at the front of the neck, release hormones that regulate the metabolic processes and heart rate and hormones that stimulate the production of many enzymes that are necessary for muscle tone and vigor. The pancreas, located behind the stomach, releases insulin and glucagon, which regulate the metabolism of carbohydrates. The adrenal glands, situated over the kidneys, produce epinephrine and norepinephrine, which regulate blood pressure and heart rate, as well as hormones that help regulate the body's water balance. This complex gland also manufactures sex hormones, as do the ovaries and testes. The pineal gland, located in the brain, secretes melatonin. The thymus is sometimes referred to as a gland because it was originally believed to be part of the endocrine system, though most scientists now consider it part of the lymphatic system. It plays a key role in the immune system through the production of T-lymphocytes (T-cells).

Hormonal deficiencies can have a wide range of physical effects, depending on the particular hormone or hormones that are lacking. They can also have psychological effects, including a loss of the sense of well-being, increased anxiety, reduce energy, cravings for sweets, poor general health, depression, a decreased sense of vitality, increased social isolation, slower mental processes, and memory loss.

Glandular therapy involves treatment with extracts taken from endocrine glands. Properly prepared glandular can deliver measurable amounts of intact molecules of enzymes, hormones, and other essential substances. They are excellent sources of complete nutrition for the glands.

All systems of the body require nutritional support, and your glands are no exception. The best sources of renewal nutrients for glands that are not functioning at an optimal level are whole, lyophilized glandulars taken from organically-raised clean animals. Research has shown that certain glandular extracts and hormones are effective when taken orally. For example, double-blind clinical studies have shown that taking thymus extract can improve symptoms associated with hay fever, asthma, food allergies, and allergic rhinitis. It is important to choose glandular extracts produced by a reputable manufacturer. Consult with a knowledgeable pharmacist or health-care practitioner for recommendations.

Heimlich Maneuver

If a person gets something stuck in his or her throat but is able to talk or is coughing forcefully, it means that air is getting through the windpipe and no immediate intervention is necessary. As long as the person can breathe, he or she may be able to expel the material without help. But if the person is unable to speak, making high-pitched sounds or gasping for air, turning blue, or clutching at her throat, intervene quickly. Follow the directions below.

Note that slightly different techniques are appropriate for different circumstances. Be aware that the information in this entry is not meant to serve as a substitute for a hands-on course in first aid, but as a review should you ever be called upon to use your first aid training.

STANDARD HEIMLICH MANEUVER

The Heimlich maneuver, named for its developer, Dr. H.J. Heimlich, will expel an object that is lodged in the throat and blocking breathing.

1. Stand (or kneel, in the case of a child or much shorter adult) behind the person who is choking, wrapping your arms around his or her waist.

2. Make a fist with one hand and clasp your other hand over your fist. Position the thumb side of your fist against the person's abdomen, just above the navel and below the rib cage. (*See* Figure 3.8, below.)

3. Use a quick, forceful *upward* push to force air up through the windpipe.

4. Continue performing these thrusts until the person coughs up the foreign material. Do not stop the procedure until all the material is expelled and the person begins coughing, breathing, and talking on his or her own, *or* another person can take over for you, *or* emergency medical help arrives.

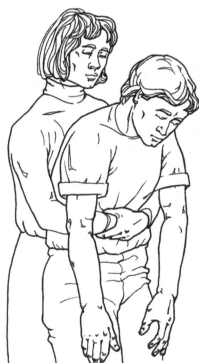

Figure 3.8
Standard Heimlich
Maneuver

ONE-PERSON HEIMLICH MANEUVER

If you are choking and no one is available to assist you, perform the one-person variant of the Hemlich maneuver as follows.

1. Find a stable, blunt object somewhat below chest height—for example, a chair back, countertop edge, or fence post.

2. Place the soft part of your upper abdomen, just below the breastbone, against the object, and relax the area as much as possible.

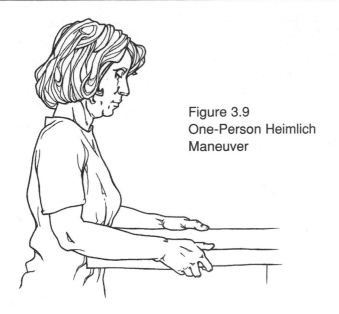

Figure 3.9
One-Person Heimlich
Maneuver

3. Without trying to breathe, thrust your abdomen against the object to rapidly increase pressure under the diaphragm, much as in the standard Heimlich maneuver.

4. Continue doing these thrusts until you expel the foreign material.

Once you have performed the Heimlich maneuver successfully, even if the affected individual seems to be fine, he or she should be examined by a doctor as soon as possible to make sure there has been no damage to the windpipe or abdomen.

Preparing Herbal Treatments

The herbal treatments recommended in this book include teas, baths, compresses, poultices, oils, and ointments. Some require that you start from scratch, while others, especially tablets or capsules, are available ready made. The recipes and directions in this section will teach you how to prepare and use a wide variety of herbal treatments.

HERBAL BATHS

An herbal bath is as much of a treat as it is a treatment. There are several ways to prepare an herbal bath.

If you are using a soluble ingredient, such as baking soda or aloe vera gel, simply dissolve it in hot bath water.

If you are using oatmeal, you can either whirl it into a powder in your blender or bag it (see below). Oatmeal seems soft, but it doesn't dissolve completely unless it has first been very finely milled.

If you are using fresh herbs, you can bag them in a square of cheesecloth or a washcloth. A two- or three-thickness square of cheesecloth is ideal. The loose weave permits maximum release of the herbal essence, yet keeps the parts from floating free in the bath water. One method of bagging herbs is to stitch three sides of a cheesecloth square closed and run a drawstring through the top, or tie the bag closed with a sturdy string. An easier and quicker method is to place a suitable quantity of herbs in the middle of a cheesecloth square. Then simply pull the four corners of the square together and secure them with string. (You can do this with a washcloth or small towel, too, but cheesecloth is easier to manage.) For a full bath, use approximately 6 ounces of dried or fresh herbs.

Fill the tub, placing the bagged herbs under a forceful stream of comfortably hot water. As the tub fills, swish the herbs through the bath water. During the bath, gently squeeze an essence-rich stream of water from the herb bag directly on the part of the body you wish to treat. If you are treating an itchy skin condition, you can *gently* rub the bag across the affected areas, but if you are using dried herbs, you will have to guard against rough parts, which may be irritating.

If you find a particular type of herbal bath especially soothing and comforting, you may want to be ready with a pre-prepared herbal infusion. Soak 6 tablespoons of dried or fresh herbs overnight in 3 cups of water. Start with very hot water and allow it to cool naturally. The following morning, heat the infusion and strain out the residue. No bag is needed; just pour the strained infusion directly into the bath water.

HERBAL INFUSIONS (TEAS)

Medicinal herbs are often administered in tea form. The Chinese, who have a 5,000-year history of herbal medicine, teach that the heat of the water and the taste of the herb enhance its effectiveness. Steeping an herb in hot water draws out the therapeutic essence of the plant.

To prepare hot tea from herbs, measure out 2 heaping tablespoons of fresh herb (or 1 heaping teaspoon of dried) for every cup of tea (unless the label directs otherwise), and place them in a ceramic or glass teapot or cup (plastic and metal containers are not suitable for steeping herbs). For each cup of tea, pour 8 ounces of freshly boiled water over the herbs. Cover the container. As a general rule, teas made with the leaf or flower of the herb should be allowed to steep for five to ten minutes; teas using roots or bark should be simmered for ten minutes and allowed to steep for an additional five minutes. After steeping, strain the tea, cool it to a comfortable temperature, and drink. If you prepare more than one cup of tea at one time, you can keep it at a comfortable sipping temperature in a thermos bottle.

To make an herbal tea from a liquid extract, put about 20 to 40 drops ($\frac{1}{3}$ to $\frac{2}{3}$ teaspoon) of the extract into a cup of HOT water. Let the mixture sit for five minutes to allow some of the alcohol to evaporate.

HERBAL JUICES (JUICED FRESH HERBS)

If you are lucky enough to have a reliable source of fresh herbs and a juicer, you may want to prepare a fresh essence.

Wash the fresh herbs well under cold running water. If necessary, scissor them into pieces of a suitable size. Place the wet herb parts in a juice extractor and whiz them into liquid. The fresh juice may be taken internally in the form of a few drops diluted in tea or spring water. For some conditions, the juice may prove valuable when dabbed externally on the affected parts of the body.

Fresh juices are generally used immediately after extraction. However, if you place the liquid in a small glass bottle, cork it tightly, and refrigerate it, it will keep for several days without an appreciable loss of vital properties.

HERBAL OILS

To prepare a fragrant herbal oil, wash the fresh herbs of your choice and permit them to dry overnight. Place scissored fresh or crumbled dried herbs in a glass bottle or jar. Slowly add light virgin olive oil or almond oil until the oil level is an inch above the herb parts. Cover the container tightly and allow it to stand in a very warm place for two weeks. You may place it near the stove, to gather warmth from cooking, or outside in the sun (but remember to bring it in before night cools the air). Strain the oil before using it.

HERBAL OINTMENTS

There are many very fine herbal ointments and salves available. Purchased ointments and salves are often much more attractive and pleasant to use than the homemade variety. But if you wish to emulate yesterday's herbalists, here's how to make your own herbal ointment.

In a double boiler (preferably ceramic or glass), heat 2 ounces of vegetable lanolin or beeswax until it becomes liquid. Once this base is melted, add 80 to 120 drops of each herbal tincture you want in your salve. Mix them together and pour into a glass container. Refrigerate the mixture and allow it to harden. If you prefer, you can use a very strong herbal tea made with your own fresh or dried herbs instead of a store-bought tincture. Keep a record of your recipes for later use.

HERBAL POULTICES OR COMPRESSES (PULPED)

Only fresh herbs are suitable for making a pulped poultice. Dried herbs do not pulp well. By pulping the herbs directly onto the poultice cloth, you retain all the juices and improve the effectiveness of the poultice.

Place a quantity of fresh herb parts on a clean white cloth (cotton, gauze, linen, and muslin are ideal) several folds thick. Wrap several thicknesses of the cloth over the herbs. Using a rolling pin, thoroughly crush the herbs to a pulp.

Unwrap a layer or two of the cloth, until you uncover a thoroughly wetted area. Apply this to the affected area of the body. To trap the juices and hold the poultice in place, overwrap it well with a woolen cloth or a towel. A pulped compress can remain in place overnight.

HERBAL POULTICES OR COMPRESSES (STEAMED)

A hot herbal poultice can be very comforting. The active ingredients in the herbs will be absorbed through the skin.

Place a steamer, colander, strainer, or sieve over a pot of rapidly boiling water. Layer either chopped fresh or dried herbs in the steamer, reduce the heat to a simmering temperature, and cover the pot. Allow the steam to thoroughly penetrate and wilt the herbs.

After about five minutes, spread the softened and warmed herbs on a clean white, loosely woven cloth, such as cheesecloth, and apply it to the affected area. To hold in the heat, overwrap the poultice in a woolen cloth or a towel. The poultice should remain in place for at least twenty minutes. If you wish, you can leave it on overnight.

HERBAL TINCTURES

Tinctures employ alcohol to draw out and preserve the active properties of an herb. Because tinctures concentrate the essence of herbs, they are commonly taken as drops in tea, or diluted in spring water. Tinctures can also be used in a compress or body massage.

To prepare an herbal tincture at home, loosely fill a glass bottle or jar with herbal parts. If you are using fresh herbs, scissor them into manageable pieces. If you are using dried herbs, crumble them into the container. Add pure spirits, such as vodka, to cover the herbs. Seal the container and allow the tincture to stand in a warm place (between 70° and 80°F) for two weeks. While you are waiting for the tincture to mature, shake the container daily. After two weeks, strain out the herbs and squeeze out the residue.

To remove some of the alcohol from a tincture before taking it, add the suitable number of drops of tincture to $\frac{1}{4}$ cup of very hot water or tea. Most of the alcohol will evaporate away in about five minutes.

Therapeutic Humor

The Bible says, "A cheerful heart is good medicine, but a crushed spirit dries up the bones." That 2,000-year-old "prescription" has since been validated scientifically. New research shows that laughter really is good medicine. You may be surprised to learn that a group of 600 doctors and health-care professionals belong to an organization called the American Association for Therapeutic Humor (AATH). Many of these professionals call laughter a "miracle drug."

Investigation of the effects laughter has on the workings of the brain and body show that humor that provokes laughter has both psychological and physiological effects. It not only reduces levels of stress hormones, but lessens depression and improves mood. Even more important, research shows that laughter stimulates an increase in the activity of defensive immune cells, including T-cells, that attack and kill tumor cells and viruses. It also boosts the activity of the antibodies that defend the body against harmful organisms, and it steps up the production of interferon, a hormone that fights viruses and regulates cell growth.

These solidly documented findings are being taken so seriously that there is a software program in the works designed to help doctors create "laughter prescriptions" tailored to specific individuals. Although humor obviously is not a substitute for appropriate medical treatment of serious health problems, advocates say it can be a useful adjunct in all cases—and it has no unpleasant side effects. The American Association for Therapeutic Humor calls laughter a valuable complementary approach to the practice of traditional medicine.

For advice on ways to use humor in healing, you can contact the American Association for Therapeutic Humor (see the Resources section at the end of the book). Another good resource is *The Courage to Laugh: Humor, Hope and Healing in the Face of Death and Dying,* by Allen Klein (J.P. Tarcher, 1998). A bimonthly journal called *Humor and Health Journal,* published by the Humor and Health Institute, is also available. This publication conducts interviews with well-known proponents of healing humor.

Nasal Saline Flush

Nasal saline flushes, or irrigation, are very useful in the treatment of respiratory allergies and sinus infections. They cleanse the sinuses and the tissues that line the nasal passages, as well as soothing the mucous membranes and thinning mucus.

Dissolve $\frac{1}{4}$ teaspoon of salt and $\frac{1}{8}$ teaspoon of baking soda in 4 ounces of water. Spray the mixture inside your nose with a bulb syringe or instill several drops into your nose with an eyedropper. If you are using this technique to clear nasal congestion, you can then suck out the mucus with a bulb syringe. If you are using it to soothe and moisten the mucous membranes, do not suction out mucus afterward.

Applying a Pressure Bandage

If you are bleeding from a severe external wound, cover it with a clean cloth or gauze and quickly apply firm, steady pressure directly to the site. If there is no clean cloth or gauze immediately available, use your bare hand to apply pressure. Even if the pressure is uncomfortable, applying firm, steady pressure is necessary to stop the bleeding.

If there is no suspicion of a spinal injury or internal bleeding, raise the affected part of the body to above the level of your heart. This will help minimize the amount of blood flowing from the wound. Suspect a spinal cord injury if a you feel weakness, numbness, or paralysis in the extremities; have fallen from a high place; or have been in a car accident. Suspect internal bleeding if you are pale, sweaty, and bleeding from the mouth, nose, or ears; have a very fast or very slow heartbeat; or have a hard, rigid abdomen.

If blood soaks through the cloth pad or gauze, put more cloth or gauze over the old pad and continue applying pressure. It's best not to remove the original blood-soaked pad, as clotting may be disrupted when you try to change the bandage.

Have someone take you to the emergency room of the nearest hospital or call for emergency medical assistance. If neither of these is possible and you must transport yourself, tie cloth or gauze firmly in place over the wound to maintain the pressure. If you must tie on a bandage, check for a pulse beat below the wound to make sure that the tissues below the wound are receiving an adequate supply of blood.

Taking Your Pulse

Taking your pulse is a basic diagnostic procedure that is easily performed. It can be done in several different ways.

TAKING THE BRACHIAL PULSE

This technique is particularly useful if you must take a baby's pulse. Place the tips of your first two fingers on the inner arm above the elbow. Using a precise timer such as the second hand of your watch, count the number of pulses you feel for one minute.

TAKING THE CAROTID PULSE

Feel for a pulse on the carotid artery, located at the side of the neck. Touch your first two fingers to your Adam's apple, and run your fingers across your neck to the depression between the Adam's apple and the large neck muscle.

Using a precise timer such as the second hand of your watch, count the number of beats you feel for one minute, or count for ten seconds and multiply the result by six.

TAKING THE RADIAL PULSE

Another useful place to feel for a pulse is the radial artery, on the thumb side of the wrist. Place either wrist in the palm of the opposite hand, face up. Curl the fingers of the lower hand around the wrist. With your fingertips, feel for a depression toward the "thumb" side of the wrist, and feel for a pulse. Using a precise timer such as the second hand of your watch, count the number of beats you feel for one minute, or count for ten seconds and multiply the result by six.

Relaxation Techniques

There are a number of different techniques that can be helpful when you are restless, ill, under stress (whether physical or mental), or just having trouble falling or staying asleep.

RELAXATION AND VISUALIZATION EXERCISES

The goal of these exercises is to cultivate a sense of physical and emotional relaxation. Situations such as an asthma attack or acute pain can create stress, anxiety, and muscle tension. These reactions in turn make the situation worse. If you have a chronic illness such as asthma, try practicing the exercises consistently so that when needed, you can readily access the exercise.

Sit or lie down in a comfortable position. It is helpful if the environment is quiet. Close your eyes and breathe slowly and deeply. When you breathe out, consciously let go of all of your thoughts of the day. Do this several times. Then begin to release all the tension in your body, moving slowly from your toes to your head. Let your toes feel very heavy and very soft; then let your feet rest and let the floor support them. Continuing to move upward, let go of all the tension in your calves. As you consciously release the tension in each successive body part, allow it to feel very heavy and very soft. Continue working your way up through your entire body, finishing with your head.

For particular health concerns, you can add visualization to this by forming a specific mental picture of such things as your medication traveling to the affected part of your body and imagining that all the sensations of pain and/or illness are disappearing and floating away, or that your body's defenses are taking care of you by fighting to get rid of an affliction such as eczema or psoriasis—whatever type of visualization is appropriate for your situation.

THE RELAXATION RESPONSE

The relaxation response is a natural way to counteract stress. It is also a safe, nontoxic, free, and readily available "tranquilizer" that can be useful if you are having trouble sleeping. Practice the following steps.

1. Sit or lie quietly in a comfortable position.

2. To minimize distraction, close your eyes.

3. Consciously relax all of your muscles, beginning at your feet and progressing upward to your face. To practice "letting go," give a good shake and then relax.

4. Breathe through your nose easily and naturally. On each outgoing breath, say the word *one* silently to yourself. Concentrating on the word *one* helps to keep intrusive thoughts away.

5. Once your muscles are relaxed, continue breathing easily and regularly for ten to fifteen minutes. Sit or lie quietly for several more minutes after you are finished, at first with your eyes closed, then with your eyes open.

If you don't achieve a deep level of relaxation, don't worry. Try to maintain a passive attitude. Relaxation will happen at its own pace. Distracting thoughts will vanish as long as you don't dwell on them. Silently repeating the word *one* helps. With practice, the relaxation response will come with little effort.

This technique can be practiced during the day, but is the most helpful just before bedtime. Because digestion can interfere with the relaxation response, the exercise should not be practiced for two hours after eating.

Rotation Diet

A rotation diet is a diet that can sometimes alleviate problems associated with food allergies or sensitivities in less time than an elimination diet can. Rather than identifying a particular food allergy or sensitivity, the rotation diet provides a way to plan your diet so that you are less at the mercy of food sensitivities. It works on the principle that a person who is allergic to a particular food or class of foods may not show a reaction if those foods are spaced out over a three-day period.

To implement a rotation diet, plan menus so that you do not eat suspect foods or classes of foods more than once during any three-day period. For example, if you suspect that you may be sensitive to wheat, you might vary your breakfast menu as follows:

Day 1: Stone-ground whole wheat toast and a poached egg.

Day 2: Hot oatmeal.

Day 3: A wheat-free muffin.

After three days, the cycle starts again, and you might have a breakfast of wheat toast or a wheat-based cereal.

By following a three-day rotation diet, you may be able to eat all classes of foods without triggering the symptoms of food sensitivity. Of course, if you tend to have a severe reaction, such as hives or wheezing (called *anaphylaxis*), to a particular food, you must eliminate that food from your diet altogether.

Taking Your Temperature

Normal body temperature probably has a much wider range than previously thought. No longer is 98.6°F considered standard. Temperature also varies throughout the day. In general, any temperature above 101°F is considered elevated. However, it is not usually necessary to treat a temperature under 102°F unless it is making you uncomfortable.

There are a number of different ways to take a person's temperature. Two of the simplest ways are by mouth and under the arm. In addition to standard thermometers, there are now digital thermometers available that can take a person's temperature in much less time than the standard models. Another option (highly effective but much more expensive) is a device that measures temperature in the ear.

ORAL METHOD

To take your temperature with a standard oral thermometer, do the following:

1. Shake down the thermometer so that it registers less than 96°F.

2. Place the silver or red end of the thermometer under your tongue or in your cheek. Hold it in place with your fingers. Don't use your teeth to hold it there. Leave the thermometer in place for three minutes.

3. Remove the thermometer from your mouth and read the temperature.

4. After reading your temperature, wash the thermometer with cool water and then rub it with isopropyl rubbing alcohol.

If you notice a crack in the thermometer, throw it out. The mercury it contains is poisonous. If you have just eaten or drunk something warm, are dressed very warmly, or have just been exercising, wait thirty minutes before taking your temperature to be sure you get an accurate reading.

UNDERARM METHOD

If you prefer, you can take your temperature under the arm. This method usually yields a temperature reading approximately 1°F lower than your oral temperature would be. It also does not always give as reliable a reading as the oral method does, so it is best used only as a general indicator.

To take your temperature with the underarm method, do the following:

1. Shake down the thermometer so that it registers less than 96°F.

2. Place the silver or red end of the thermometer against your armpit. Make sure your armpit is dry before placing the thermometer. Leave the thermometer in place for two minutes.

3. Remove the thermometer and read the temperature.

4. After reading the temperature, wash the thermometer with cool water and then rub it with isopropyl rubbing alcohol.

Therapeutic Recipes

Some of the entries in Part Two recommend certain therapeutic foods that can help in different situations. Some of the most useful of these are a soup made with the Chinese herb astragalus and a variety of vegetables; barley or rice water; fresh carrot soup; and a digestive remedy made from kuzu powder and umeboshi plum. All are easy to make.

Astragalus and vegetable soup is excellent for a wide variety of illnesses and conditions. Both astragalus and burdock root help to boost the immune system. Use vegetables that are high in vitamins A and C, such as those suggested in the recipe.

Barley (or rice) water makes a nourishing and strengthening broth that is particularly good during recovery from illness or surgery, when you are not yet up to eating solid foods. Fresh carrot soup is another excellent "starter" food if you have been ill.

Kuzu cream with salt plum is a digestive preparation that is both effective and versatile. It has a delicious flavor and a soothing, thick consistency. It works particularly well for nausea associated with overeating or overindulgence in sweets. It is also excellent for acid indigestion, colds, stomach pains, diarrhea, dysentery, and fever. For an upset stomach or diarrhea, you can take anywhere from 1 tablespoon to ½ cup at a time, in small sips. Repeat every one to three hours throughout the day, as needed.

Astragalus and Vegetable Immune-Boosting Soup

1 astragalus root strip
1 burdock root
$\frac{1}{4}$-inch to 1-inch piece fresh ginger root
10 cups water
$\frac{1}{2}$ teaspoon thyme
$\frac{1}{2}$ teaspoon sage
6 cups vegetables, cut into bite-sized pieces
(good choices include broccoli, cauliflower,
carrots, celery, green peppers, parsley, potatoes,
squash, string beans, and zucchini)
1 cup cooked barley

1. In a glass or stainless-steel pot, simmer the astragalus and burdock root in the water with the thyme and sage for 20 to 30 minutes. Strain out the herbs and use the resulting tea as a broth for the soup.

2. Add the vegetables and barley to the broth and cook. Allow to simmer slowly for 1 hour.

3. Serve warm. You can strain the soup and eat it as a broth, or eat it with all the vegetables. Makes approximately six servings.

Note: If you wish, you can combine steps 1 and 2, adding all the ingredients at one time, and pull the astragalus and burdock root out after the soup has simmered and before serving. This results in a more strongly flavored soup.

Barley or Rice Water

1 cup barley or brown rice
4 cups water

1. In a large glass, enameled, or stainless-steel saucepan, add the grain to the water and bring to a boil over medium heat.

2. Reduce the heat to a simmer and cook, covered or uncovered, for one hour.

3. Remove from heat. Strain out the grain and reserve it for another use. Drink the resulting broth in small sips throughout the day. You can drink it either warm or cool, as you prefer.

Fresh Carrot Soup

$\frac{1}{2}$ to 1 pound fresh organically grown carrots
Water to cover

1. Peel and dice the carrots, and place them in a large glass, enameled, or stainless-steel saucepan. Add water to cover.

2. Bring to a boil over medium heat. Reduce the heat to a simmer and cook until the carrots are very soft, about one hour.

3. Remove from heat. Purée the carrots with the water and enjoy.

Kuzu Cream With Salt Plum

1 cup water
1 salt plum (umeboshi), pitted and minced, *or*
$\frac{1}{2}$ teaspoon umeboshi paste
$1\frac{1}{2}$ tablespoons kuzu powder
$\frac{1}{4}$ cup water
1 teaspoon shoyu (natural soy sauce) *or*
$\frac{1}{4}$ teaspoon grated ginger (optional)

1. In a medium glass, enameled, or stainless-steel saucepan, combine 1 cup water and the salt plum or umeboshi paste. Bring to a boil over medium heat.

2. In a small bowl or measuring cup, dissolve $1\frac{1}{2}$ tablespoons kuzu powder in $\frac{1}{4}$ cup water. (Kuzu powder thickens the mixture. If you find that you prefer a thinner consistency, you may use as little as $1\frac{1}{2}$ teaspoons kuzu powder.)

3. Add the dissolved kuzu powder to the contents of the saucepan, stirring constantly with a fork or wire whisk. Return to a boil.

4. Reduce the heat to low and simmer for 1 minute.

5. Take the mixture off the heat, and allow it to cool to room temperature before serving. Makes about $1\frac{1}{2}$ cups.

6. If desired, add the shoyu or ginger to the mixture along with the dissolved kuzu powder for flavor. Ginger root also soothes the stomach. If you do not have grated ginger, you can substitute $\frac{1}{2}$ teaspoon powdered ginger root, or 12 drops juice from grated ginger root.

Water Purification

With what seems a remarkable increase in natural disasters in recent years—plus the rise in population and pollution—there have been many instances in which municipal water supplies have become unfit to drink. We believe that even the "best" municipal water is suspect (see the discussion of water in DIET AND NUTRITION in Part One), and that you should drink only pure spring water from a reputable source. A time may come, however, when the only source of water available to you is contaminated. To purify water, follow these steps:

1. Remove any sediment or floating material by straining the water through a clean cloth, paper towel, or, preferably, a coffee filter. If you have one, you can use an emergency water-filtering device such as those designed for wilderness camping (available in many sporting-goods stores). These remove far more impurities than simple straining does.

2. Place the filtered water in a large pot and bring it to a rolling boil. Boil for at least five minutes. Boiling not only destroys disease-causing bacteria, viruses, and cysts, but also removes light gases and solvents that vaporize.

3. Add grapefruit-seed extract to the water, following the directions on the product label. Let the water cool, swish it around, then wait at least twenty minutes before using it.

Grapefruit-seed extract, or GSE, is a remarkable purifier. Research has shown it to kill bacteria, fungi, parasites, and even viruses. Very few substances can do all this. What's more, microorganisms seem to have a hard time developing resistance to it. There are many different products available. Choose a concentrated solution of the extract that can be dropped into water being purified. It is extremely bitter, but, fortunately, very little is required for it to be effective. Grapefruit-seed extract has a distinct advantage over chlorine, commonly recommended for purifying water, in that it is not toxic and only tiny amounts are required, making it easily portable. It is a good idea to keep some on hand for emergencies, rather than having to look for it once a crisis occurs.

Appendix

Appendix

References

GENERAL REFERENCE

Brunn, Ruth Dowling, and Bertel Brunn, *The Human Body*, 2nd Ed. (New York, NY: Random House, 1982).

Clayman, Charles B., *American Medical Association Family Medical Guide* (New York, NY: Random House, 1994).

Clayman, Charles B., *American Medical Association Home Medical Encyclopedia* (New York, NY: Random House, 1989).

Davis, Adelle, *Let's Get Well* (New York, NY: New American Library, 1984).

Glanze, W.D., Ed., *The Signet-Mosby Medical Encyclopedia* (New York, NY: Signet Books, 1987).

Guyton, Arthur C., *Textbook of Medical Physiology*, 9th Ed. (Philadelphia, PA: W.B. Saunders Company, 1995).

The Medical Advisor. The Complete Guide to Alternative and Conventional Treatments (Alexandria, VA: Time-Life Books, 1997).

Zand, Janet, Rachel Walton, and Bob Rountree, *A Parent's Guide to Medical Emergencies: First Aid for Your Child* (Garden City Park, NY: Avery Publishing Group, 1997).

Zand, Janet, Rachel Walton, and Bob Rountree, *Smart Medicine for a Healthier Child* (Garden City Park, NY: Avery Publishing Group, 1994).

CONVENTIONAL MEDICINE

Garrett, Laurie, *The Coming Plague* (New York, NY: Penguin Books, 1994).

Merck Manual of Diagnosis and Therapy, The, 16th Ed. (Rahway, NJ: Merck Research Laboratories division of Merck & Co., Inc., 1992).

Physician's Desk Reference, 53rd Ed. (Montvale, NJ: Medical Economics Co., 1999).

Tierney, Lawrence M., Stephen J. McPhee, and Maxine A. Papadakis, eds., *Current Medical Diagnosis and Treatment*, 38th Ed. (Stamford, CT: Appleton & Lange, 1999).

ALTERNATIVE MEDICINE (GENERAL)

Giller, Robert M., and K. Matthews, *Natural Prescriptions* (New York, NY: Carol Southern Books, 1994).

Rosenfeld, Isadore, *Dr. Rosenfeld's Guide to Alternative Medicine* (New York, NY: Random House, 1996).

HERBAL MEDICINE

Blumenthal, Mark, Sr. Ed., *The Complete German Commission E Monographs: Therapeutic Guide to Herbal Medicines* (Austin, TX: American Botanical Council, 1998).

Brinker, Francis J., *Herb Contraindications and Drug Interactions* (Sandy, OR: The Eclectic Institute, 1997).

Gardner, Joy, *Healing Yourself During Pregnancy* (Freedom, CA: The Crossing Press, 1990).

Gladstar, Rosemary, *Herbal Healing for Women* (New York, NY: Fireside, 1993).

Green, James, *The Male Herbal* (Watsonville, CA: The Crossing Press, 1991).

Grieve, M., *A Modern Herbal* (New York, NY: Dover Publications, Inc., 1982).

Griggs, Barbara, *Green Pharmacy: The History and Evolution of Western Medicine* (Rochester, VT: Healing Arts Press, 1991).

Hobbs, Christopher, *Echinacea! The Immune Herb* (Capitola, CA: Botanica Press, 1992).

Hobbs, Christopher, *Ginkgo: The Elixir of Youth* (Capitola, CA: Botanica Press, 1991).

Hobbs, Christopher, *Milk Thistle—The Liver Herb* (Capitola, CA: Botanica Press, 1992).

Hobbs, Christopher, *Natural Liver Therapy* (Capitola, CA: Botanica Press, 1993).

Hobbs, Christopher, *Usnea: The Herbal Antibiotic* (Capitola, CA: Botanica Press, 1990).

Hobbs, Christopher, *Vitex: The Woman's Herb* (Capitola, CA: Botanica Press, 1993).

Hoffmann, David, *The Holistic Herbal* (Longmead, England: Element Books Ltd., 1988).

Hsu, Hong-Yen, *How to Treat Yourself With Chinese Herbs* (Los Angeles, CA: Oriental Healing Arts Institute, 1980).

Hutchens, Alma R., *Indian Herbology of North America* (Boston, MA: Shambhala Publications, 1973).

Johnson, Stewart, *Feverfew* (London, England: Sheldon Press, 1984).

Kaptchuk, Ted, *The Web That Has No Weaver* (New York, NY: Congdon and Weded, 1983).

Lad, Vasant, and David Frawley, *The Yoga of Herbs* (Santa Fe, NM: Lotus Press, 1986).

Lust, John, *The Herb Book* (New York, NY: Bantam Books, 1982).

Marston, M. Maillard, and M. Hamburger, Eds., *Phytochemistry of Plants Used in Traditional Medicine* (New York: Oxford Science Publications, 1995).

McGuffin, Michael, Christopher Hobbs, Roy Upton, and Alicia Goldberg, *American Herbal Products Association's Botanical Safety Handbook* (New York, NY: CRC Press, 1997).

Moore, Michael, *Medicinal Plants of the Desert and Canyon West* (Santa Fe, NM: Museum of New Mexico Press, 1979).

Moore, Michael, *Medicinal Plants of the Mountain West* (Santa Fe, NM: Museum of New Mexico Press, 1979).

Moore, Michael, *Medicinal Plants of the Pacific West* (Santa Fe, NM: Red Crane Books, 1993).

Murray, Michael T., *The Healing Power of Herbs* (Rocklin, CA: Prima Publishing, 1992).

Newall, Carol, Linda Anderson, and J. David Phillipson, *Herbal Medicines: A Guide for Health Care Professionals* (London, England: The Pharmaceutical Press, 1996).

Northrup, Christiane, *Women's Bodies, Women's Wisdom* (New York, NY: Bantam Books, 1994).

Pavarti, Jeannine, *Hygieia, A Woman's Herbal* (Sevier, UT: Freestone Press, 1978).

Pedersen, Mark, *Nutritional Herbology* (Bountiful, UT: Pedersen Publishing, 1987).

Reid, Daniel, *Chinese Herbal Medicine* (Boston, MA: Shambhala Publications, 1993).

Rose, Jeanne, *Herbs and Things* (New York, NY: Grosset and Dunlap, 1975).

Schulick, Paul, *Ginger: Common Spice and Wonder Drug* (Brattleboro, VT: Herbal Free Press, 1994).

Teeguarden, Ron, *Chinese Tonic Herbs* (New York, NY: Japan Publications, 1984).

Tierra, Lesley, *The Herbs of Life* (Freedom, CA: The Crossing Press, 1992).

Tierra, Michael, *Planetary Herbology* (Santa Fe, NM: Lotus Press, 1988).

Tierra, Michael, *The Way of Herbs* (Santa Cruz, CA: Unity Press, 1980).

Weed, Susun, *Wise Women's Herbal for the Childbearing Year* (Woodstock, NY: Ash Tree Publishing, 1985).

Weed, Susun, *Wise Women's Herbal for the Menopausal Years* (Woodstock, NY: Ash Tree Publishing, 1992).

Willard, Terry, *Edible and Medicinal Plants of the Rocky Mountains and Neighboring Territories* (Calgary, Alberta, Canada: Wild Rose Books, 1992).

Wren, R.W., Ed., *Potter's New Cyclopaedia of Botanical Drugs and Preparations* (Sussex, England: Health Sciences Press, 1907).

HOMEOPATHY

Boericke, William, *Materia Medica With Repertory* (Philadelphia, PA: Boericke & Tafel, 1988).

Clark, J.H., *The Prescriber*, 8th Ed. (London, England: Homeopathic Publishing Company, 1952).

Lessell, Colin B., *Homeopathy for Physicians* (Northamptonshire, England: Thorsons Publishers Limited, 1983).

Weiner, Michael, *The Complete Book of Homeopathy* (Garden City Park, NY: Avery Publishing Group, 1989).

CHINESE MEDICINE

A Barefoot Doctor's Manual: The American Translation of the Official Chinese Paramedical Manual (Philadelphia, PA: Running Press, 1977).

Connelly, D.M., *Traditional Acupuncture: The Law of the Five Elements* (Columbia, MD: The Centre for Traditional Acupuncture, 1979).

Jizong, Shi, and Chu Feng Zhu, *The ABC of Traditional Chinese Medicine* (Hong Kong: Hai Feng Publishing Company, 1992).

Lu, Henry C., *Chinese System of Food Cures* (New York, NY: Sterling Publishing Co., Inc., 1986).

BACH FLOWER REMEDIES

Bach, Edward, *Heal Thyself* (Essex, England: C.W. Daniel Company Ltd., 1978).

Bach, Edward, *The Twelve Healers* (Essex, England: C.W. Daniel Company Ltd., 1989).

Jones, T.H., *Dictionary of Bach Flower Remedies* (Essex, England: C.W. Daniel Company Ltd., 1976).

Scheffer, M., *Bach Flower Therapy: Theory and Practice* (Rochester, VT: Healing Arts Press, 1988).

Wheeler, F.J., *The Bach Remedies Repertory* (Essex, England: C.W. Daniel Company Ltd., 1989).

AROMATHERAPY

Damian, Peter, and Kate Damian, *Aromatherapy, Scent and Psyche* (Rochester, VT: Healing Arts Press, 1995).

Wilson, Roberta, *Aromatherapy for Vibrant Health and Beauty* (Garden City Park, NY: Avery Publishing Group, 1994).

Worwood, Valerie Ann, *The Complete Book of Essential Oils and Aromatherapy* (San Rafael, CA: New World Library, 1991).

DIET AND NUTRITION

Abravanel, Elliot D., and E.A. King, *Dr. Abravanel's Body Type Program* (New York, NY: Bantam Books, 1986).

Carper, Jean, *The Food Pharmacy* (New York, NY: Bantam Books, 1988).

Davidson, S., J.E. Passmore, and A.S. Trusswell, *Human Nutrition and Dietetics*, 7th Ed. (New York, NY: Churchill Livingstone, 1979).

Davis, Adelle, *Let's Eat Right to Keep Fit* (New York, NY: New American Library, 1988).

Kirschmann, John D., and L. J. Dunne, *Nutrition Almanac*, 4th Ed. (New York, NY: McGraw-Hill, 1993).

Trenev, Natasha, *Probiotics* (Garden City Park, NY: Avery Publishing Group, 1998).

ACNE

Kligman, A.M., et al., "Oral Vitamin A in Acne Vulgaris," *International Journal of Dermatology* 20 (1981): 278–285.

AGING

Barrett-Connor, E., K.T. Khaw, and S.S. Yen, "A Prospective Study of Dehydroepiandrosterone Sulfate, Mortality and Cardiovascular Disease," *The New England Journal of Medicine* 315 (24) (11 April 1986): 1519–1524.

Conrad, R.A., "An Attempt to Quantify Some Clinical Criteria of Aging," *Journal of Gerontology* 15 (1960): 358–365.

Emanuel, N., "The Principles of Biological Age Determination and Human Viability," *Biological Age, Heredity and Aging—Gerontology and Geriatrics Yearbook 1984* (Kiev, USSR: USSR Gerontological and Geriatrics Society, 1984).

Harman, D., and L.H. Piette, "Free Radical Theory of Aging: Free Radical Reactions in Serum," *Journal of Gerontology* 21 (4) (October 1966): 560–565.

Kleijnen, J., and P. Knipschild, "Ginkgo Biloba," *Lancet* 340 (8828) (7 November 1992): 1, 136–139.

Rai, G.S., M.D., "A Double Blind Placebo Controlled Study of Ginkgo Biloba Extract in Elderly Outpatients With Mild to Moderate Memory Impairment," *Current Medical Research and Opinion* 12 (6) (1991): 350–355.

Shock, N.W., "Physiological and Chronological Age," in *Aging—Its Chemistry*, by A.A. Dietz and V.S. Marcum (Washington: The American Association for Clinical Chemistry, 1980), 3–24.

ALLERGIES

Johnston, Carol S., Ph.D., R.D., et al., "Antihistamine Effects and Complications of Supplemental Vitamin C," *Journal of the American Dietetic Association* 92 (8) (August 1992): 988–989.

ALZHEIMER'S DISEASE

Gibson, G., et al., "Reduced Activities of Thiamine Dependent Frozen Enzymes in the Brains and Peripheral Tissues of Patients with Alzheimer's Disease," *Archives of Neurology* 45 (1988): 836–840.

Heston, L.L., "Alzheimer's Dementia and Down's Syndrome: Genetic Evidence Suggesting an Association in Alzheimer's Disease, Down's Syndrome, and Aging," *Annals of the New York Academy of Sciences* 396 (1982): 29–37.

Imagawa, Masaki, et al., "Coenzyme Q_{10}, Iron and Vitamin B_6 in Genetically Confirmed Alzheimer's Disease," *Lancet* 340 (12 September 1992): 671.

Pettegrew, J., et al., "Clinical and Neurochemical Effects of Acetyl-L-Carnitine in Alzheimer's Disease," *Neurobiology of Aging* 16 (1) (1995): 1–4.

"Zinc Deficiency Tied to Neurofibrillary Tangles in Alzheimer's," *Family Practice News* 20 (20) (15–31 October 1990): 7.

ANEMIA

Beard, John L., et al., "Impaired Thermoregulation and Thyroid Function in Iron Deficiency Anemia," *American Journal of Clinical Nutrition* 52 (1990): 813–819.

Lederle, Frank A., M.D., "Oral Cobalamin for Pernicious Anemia: Medicine's Best Kept Secret," *Journal of the American Medical Association* 265 (1) (2 January 1991): 94–95.

ANOREXIA NERVOSA

Ward, Neil, Ph.D., "Assessment of Zinc Status in Oral Supplementation in Anorexia Nervosa," *Journal of Nutritional Medicine* 1 (1990): 171–177.

ANXIETY DISORDERS

Jussofie, A., et al., "Kavapyrone Enriched Extract from *Piper methysticum* as Modulator of GABA Binding Site in Different Regions of Rat Brain," *Psychopharmacology* 116 (1994): 469–474.

Kinzler, E., et al., "Effect of Kava Extract in Patients with Anxiety, Tension and Excitation States of Non-Psychotic Genesis. Double Blind Study with Placebos over 4 Weeks," *Fortschritte der Arzneimmittelforschung (Progress in Drug Research)* 41 (6) (June 1991): 584–588.

Volz, H.P, and M. Kieser. "Kava Kava Extract WS 1490 Versus Placebo in Anxiety Disorders. A Randomized Placebo Controlled 25 Week Outpatient Trial," *Pharmacopsychiatry* 30 (1997): 1–5.

ARTHRITIS

Drovant, A., et al., "Therapeutic Activity of Oral Glucosamine Sulfate in Osteoarthritis: A Placebo Controlled Double Blind Investigation," *Clinical Therapy* 3 (1980): 260–272.

Morreale, P., et al., "Comparison of the Antiinflammatory Efficacy of Chondroitin Sulfate and Diclofenac Sodium in Patients With Knee Osteoarthritis," *Journal of Rheumatology* 23 (8) (August 1996): 1385–1391.

Patrick, M., S. Hepinstall, and M. Doherty, "Feverfew in Rheumatoid Arthritis: A Double Blind, Placebo Controlled Study," *Annual Rheumatoid Disease Journal* 48 (1989): 547–549.

Zurier, B., "Essential Fatty Acids and Inflammation," *Annals of Rheumatic Diseases* 50 (1991): 745–746.

ASTHMA

Campbell, et al., "Low Levels of Manganese in Bronchial Biopsies from Asthmatic Subjects," *Journal of Allergy and Clinical Immunology* (January 1991): 89.

Flatt, Amber, et al., "Reduced Selenium in Asthmatic Subjects in New Zealand," *Thorax* 45 (1990): 95–99.

Hahn, D.L., R.W. Dodge, and R. Golubjathikov, "Association of Chlamydia Pneumonial (Strain TWAR) Infection with Wheezing, Asthmatic Bronchitis, and Adult Onset Asthma," *Journal of the American Medical Association* 266 (1991): 230–235.

ATHLETE'S FOOT

Buck, D.S., et al., "Comparison of Two Topical Preparations for the Treatment of Onychomycosis: *Melaleuca alternifolia* (Tea Tree) Oil and Clotrimazole," *Journal of Family Practice* 38 (6) (June 1994): 601–605.

BACK PAIN AND STRAIN

Griner, Thomas, *What's Really Wrong With You?* (Garden City Park, NY: Avery Publishing Group, 1996).

CANCER

Barnes, S., et al., "Soybeans Inhibit Mammary Tumors in Models of Breast Cancer," *Progress in Clinical Biological Research* 347 (1990): 239–524.

Block, Gladys, "Vitamin C and Cancer Prevention: The Epidemiologic Evidence," *American Journal of Clinical Nutrition* 53:2 (1991): 270S–282S.

Bunker, V.W., Ph.D., "Selenium Status in Disease: The Role of Selenium as a Therapeutic Agent," *British Journal of Clinical Practice* 44 (8) (1990): 401–404.

Carroll, K.K., "Dietary Factors in Hormone-Dependent Cancers," *Current Concepts in Nutrition*, Vol. 6, *Nutrition and Cancer* (New York, NY: John Wiley and Sons, 1977, pp. 25–40).

Clark, L.C., et al., "Effects of Selenium Supplementation for Cancer Prevention in Patients with Carcinoma of the Skin," *Journal of the American Medical Association* 276:24 (25 December 1997): 1957–1963.

Dorant, E., et al., "Garlic and Its Significance for the Prevention of Cancer: A Critical Review," *British Journal of Cancer* 71 (1993): 383–386.

Ewertz, M., and C. Gill, "Dietary Factors and Breast Cancer Risk in Denmark," *International Journal of Cancer* 46: 779–784.

Giovannucci, E., et al., "Multivitamin Use, Folate and Colon Cancer in Women in the Nurses' Health Study," *Annals of Internal Medicine* 129 (7) (1 October 1998): 517–524.

Kesteloot, H., E. Lesaffre, and J.V. Joossens, "Dietary Fat, Saturated Animal Fat and Cancer Risk," *Preventative Medicine* 20 (1991): 226–236.

Knekt, Paul, et al., "Serum Selenium and Subsequent Risk of Cancer Among Finnish Men and Women," *Journal of the National Cancer Institute* 82 (1990): 864–868.

Kupin, V.I., E.B. Polevaya, and A.M. Sorokin, "Increased Immunologic Reactivity of Lymphocytes in Oncologic Patients Treated with Eleutherococcus Extract," in *New Data on Eleutherococcus: Proceedings of the Second International Symposium on Eleutherococcus*, USSR Academy of Sciences, Moscow, USSR, 1984, 294–300.

Manetta, Alberto, and M.D. Fuchtner, "The Role of Beta Carotene in Cancer Chemoprevention," *Drug Therapy* (July 1992): 55–60.

Moerman, Clara J., et al., "Dietary Sugar Intake in the Etiology of Biliary Tract Cancer," *International Journal of Epidemiology* 22 (1993): 207–214.

Murray, M., "Botanical Monograph—Green Tea," *The American Journal of Natural Medicine* 45 (5) (1997): 18–19.

Palan, Prabhudas, Ph.D., et al., "Decreased Beta Carotene Tissue Levels in Uterine Leiomyomas and Cancers of the Reproductive and Nonreproductive Organs," *American Journal of Obstetrics and Gynecology* 161 (6) (December 1989): Part I 649–652.

Pawlowicz, Z., et al., "Blood Selenium Concentrations and Glutathione Peroxidase Activities in Patients with Breast Cancer and with Advanced Gastrointestinal Cancer," *Journal of Trace Elements, Electrolytes and Health and Disease* 5 (4) (1991): 275–277.

Raloff, J., "Breast Cancer Rise: Due to Dietary Fat?" *Science News*, 21 (April 1990): 245.

Seely, S., and D.F. Horrobin, "Diet and Breast Cancer: The Possible Connection with Sugar Consumption," *Medical Hypotheses* 11 (3) (1983): 319–327.

Yarameko, K.V., "The Main Aspects of the Use of Eleutherococcus Extract in Oncology," in *New Data on Eleutherococcus and Other Adaptogens*, Far Eastern Scientific Center, USSR Academy of Sciences, Vladivostok, USSR, 1981, 75–78.

Ziegler, R.G., "A Review of the Epidemiologic Evidence that Carotenoids Reduce the Risk of Cancer," *Journal of Nutrition* 119 (1989): 116–122.

CANDIDIASIS

Coeugniet, E.K, and R. Kuhnast, "Recurrent Candidiasis: Adjuvant Immunotherapy with Different Formulations of Echinacin," *Therapiewoche* 36 (1986): 3352–3358.

Tadi, Padma R., M.S., et al, "Anticandidal and Anticarcinogenic Potentials for Garlic," *International Clinical Nutritional Review* 10 (4) (October 1990): 423–429.

CARDIOVASCULAR DISEASE

Alfthan, G., and J.T. Salonen, "Association Between Cardiovascular Death and Myocardial Infarction and Serum Selenium," *Lancet* 2 (8291) (25 July 1982): 175–179.

Altschul R., *Niacin in Vascular Disorders and Hyperlipidemia* (Springfield, IL: Charles C. Thomas, 1964).

Altschul, R., A. Hoffer, and J.D. Stephen, "Influence of Nicotinic Acid on Serum Cholesterol in Man," *Archives of Biochemistry and Biophysics* 54 (1955): 558, 559.

Brevetti, G., et al., "Increases in Walking Distance in Patients With Peripheral Vascular Disease Treated With L-Carnitine: A Double-Blind, Crossover Study," *Circulation* 77 (4) (April 1988): 767–773.

Chakrabarty, S., et al., "Protective Role of Ascorbic Acid Against Lipid Peroxidation and Myocardial Injury," *Molecular and Cell Biochemistry* 111 (1992): 41–47.

Cherchi, A., et al., "Effects of L-Carnitine on Exercise Tolerance in Chronic Stable Angina: A Multicenter, Double Blind, Randomized, Placebo Controlled Crossover Study," *International Journal of Clinical Pharmacology, Therapy, and Toxicology* 23 (10) (October 1985): 569–572.

Dyckner, T., et al., "Effect of Magnesium on Blood Pressure," *British Medical Journal* 286 (1983): 1847–1848.

Gerstein, H.C., and S. Yusuf, "Dysglycemia and Risk of Cardiovascular Disease," *Lancet* 347 (9006) (1996): 949–950.

Gleitz, J., et al., "Antithrombotic Action of the Kava Pyrone With and Without Kavain Prepared from *Piper methysticum* on Human Platelets." *Planta Medica* 63 (1997): 27–30.

Gottlieb, Steven S., M.D., et al., "Prognostic Importance of Serum Magnesium Concentration in Patients With Congestive Heart failure," *Journal of the American College of Cardiology* 16 (4) (October 1990): 827–831.

Grundy, S.M., et al., "Influence of Nicotinic Acid on Metabolism of Cholesterol and Triglycerides in Man," *Journal of Lipid Research* 22 (1981): 24–36.

Hampel, Gerhardt, et al., "Selenium Deficiency Inhibits Prostacyclin Release and Enhances Production of Platelet Activating Factor by Human Endothelial Cells," *Biochemica et Biophysica Acta* 1006 (1989): 151–158.

Hennekens, C.H., and J.M. Gaziano, "Antioxidants and heart Disease: Epidemiology and Clinical Evidence," *Clinical Cardiology* 16 (Supplement 1) (1993): 10–15.

Jialal, Isdhwarial, "Inhibition of LDL Oxidation by Beta Carotene," *Circulation* 84 (4) (Supplement II, October 1991/ Abstract 1789): II–449.

Josling, P., A. Walerpa, and J. Grunwals, Eds., "The Action of Garlic in the Pathogenesis of Atherosclerosis: Selected Abstracts from the 4th International Congress on Phytotherapy," *European Journal of Clinical Research* 3A (1992): 1–12.

Juhan-Vague, I., M.C. Alessi, and P. Vague, "Increased Plasma Plasminogen Activator Inhibitor 1 (PAI-I) Levels; A Possible Link Between Insulin Resistance and Atherosclerosis," *Diabetologia* 34 (1991): 457–462.

Kleijnen, J., P. Knipschild, and G. Ter Riet, "Garlic, Onion and Cardiovascular Risk Factors. A Review of Evidence from Human Experiments With Emphasis on Commercially Available Preparations," *British Journal of Clinical Pharmacology* 28 (1989): 535–544.

Knekt, P., et al., "Flavonoid Intake and Coronary Mortality in Finland: A Cohort Study," *British Medical Journal* 312 (1996): 478–481.

Kohashi, N., et al., "Decrease of Taurine in Essential Hypertension," *Japan Heart Journal* 24 (1) (January 1983): 91–102.

Krishna, Gopal, M.D., and Shiv C. Kapoor, Ph.D., "Potassium Depletion Exacerbates Essential Hypertension, *Annals of Internal Medicine* 115 (2) (15 July 1991): 77–83.

Laws, A., et al., "Relation of Fasting Plasma Insulin Concentration to High Density Lipoprotein Cholesterol and Triglyceride Concentration in Men," *Arteriosclerosis, Thrombosis, and Vascular Biology* 11 (6) (1991): 1636–1642.

Lefavi, Robert G., Ph.D., "Has Chromium Been Overlooked as a Hypolipidemic Agent?" *The Nutrition Report* 9 (9) (1991): 65, 72.

Legnani, C., et al., "Effects of a Dried Garlic Preparation on Fibrinolysis and Platelet Aggregation in Health Subjects," *Fortschritte der Arzneimmittelforschung (Progress in Drug Research)* 43 (2) (February 1993): 119–122.

McCarron, D., and D. Morris, "Blood Pressure Response to Oral Calcium in Persons With Mild to Moderate Hypertension," *Annals of Internal Medicine* 103 (1985): 825–831.

Nelson, R.L., et al., "The Effect of Iron on Experimental Colorectal Carcinogenesis," *Anticancer Research* 9:1 (1989): 477–482.

Prescott, Lawrence, Ph.D., "Hypomagnesemia and Sudden Death in CHF Patients," *Practical Cardiology* 16 (6) (June 1990): 8.

Reaven, G.M., "Are Triglycerides Important as a Risk for Coronary Disease?" *Heart Disease and Stroke* 2 (1993): 44–48.

Reaven, P.D., et al., "Effect of Dietary Antioxidant Combinations in Humans. Protection of LDL by Vitamin E But Not by Beta-Carotene," *Arteriosclerosis, Thrombosis, and Vascular Biology* 13 (4) (1993): 590–600.

Roeback, John R., Ph.D., "Effect of Chromium Supplementation on Serum High Density Lipoprotein Cholesterol Levels in Men Taking Beta-Blockers: A Randomized Controlled Trial," *Annals of Internal Medicine* 115 (12) (15 December 1991): 17–24.

Stampfer, M.J., et al., "Vitamin E Consumption and the Risk of Coronary Disease in Men," *The New England Journal of Medicine* 328 (1993): 1450–1456.

Strong, J.P., et al., "Effects of Serum Lipoproteins and Smoking on Atherosclerosis in Young Men and Women: Rationale, Methodology, and Selected Risk Factors," *Cardiovascular Risk Factors* 2 (1993): 22–30.

Strong, J.P., et al., "Pathobiological Determinants of Atherosclerosis in Youth," *Arteriosclerosis, Thrombosis, and Vascular Biology* 17 (1) (January 1997): 95–106.

Tobey, T.A., et al., "Relationship Between Insulin Resistance, Insulin Secretion, Very Low Density Lipoprotein Kinetics and Plasma Triglyceride Levels in Normal Triglyceridemic Men," *Metabolism* 30 (1981): 165–171.

Valdes, Gloria, et al., "Potassium Supplementation Lowers Blood Pressure and Increase Urinary Kallikrein in Essential Hypertensives," *Journal of Human Hypertension* 5 (1991): 91–96.

Yudkin, J., "Dietary Fat and Dietary Sugar in Relation to ischemic Heart Disease and Diabetes," *Lancet* 2 (1964): 4.

Zavaroni, I., et al., "Prevalence of Hyperinsulinaemia in Patients With High Blood Pressure," *Journal of Internal Medicine* 231 (1992): 235–240.

CARPAL TUNNEL SYNDROME

Bernstein, A.L., and J.S. Dienesen, "Effects of Pharmacologic Doses of B$_6$ on Carpal Tunnel Syndrome, Electroencephalographic Results, and Pain," *Journal of the American College of Nutrition* 12 (1) (1988): 73–76.

COMMON COLD

Braunig, B., et al., "*Echinacea purpurea* Root for Strengthening the Immune Response in Flu-like Infections," *Zeitschrift für Phytotherapie (Journal of Phytotherapy)* 13 (1993): 7–13.

Brekhman, I.I., and I.V. Dardymov, "New Substances of Plant Origin Which Increase Non-Specific Resistance," *Annual Review of Pharmacology* 4 (1969): 419–430.

Bucca, C., et al., "Effect of Vitamin C on Transient Increase of Bronchoresponsiveness in Conditions Affecting the Upper Respiratory Airways," in *Beyond Deficiency: New Views on the Function and Health Effects of Vitamins*, New York Academy of Sciences Abstract 16, 9–12 February 1992.

Chu, D.T., et al., "Immunotherapy With Chinese Medicinal Herbs. I. Immune Restoration of Local Xenogenic Graft-Versus-Host Reaction in Cancer Patients by Fractionated *Astragalus membranaceous* in vitro," *Journal of Clinical and Laboratory Immunology* 25 (3) (March 1998): 119–123.

Chu, D.T., et al., "Immunotherapy With Chinese Medicinal Herbs. II. Reversal of Cyclophosphamide-Induced Immune Suppression by Administratoin of Fractionated *Astragalus membranaceous* in vivo," *Journal of Clinical and Laboratory Immunology* 25 (3) (March 1998): 125–129.

Fawzi, W.W., et al., "Vitamin A Supplementation and Child Mortality," *Journal of the American Medical Association* 269 (1993): 898–903.

Fujisara, S., et al., "A Potent Antibacterial Protein in Royal Jelly," *The Journal of Biological Chemistry* 265:19 (5 July 1990): 11,333–11,337.

Gaisbauer, M., et al., "Phagocytic Activity of Granulocytes Using Chemiluminescence Measurement," *Fortschritte der Arzneimmittelforschung (Progress in Drug Research)* 40 (1990) 594–598.

Leutig, B., et al., "Macrophage Activation by the Polysaccharide Arabinogalactan Isolated from Plant Cell Cultures of *Echinacea purpurea*," *Journal of the National Cancer Institute* 81 (9) (3 May 1989): 669–675.

Mossad, S.B., et al., "Zinc Gluconate Lozenges for Treating the Common Cold. A Randomized, Double-Blind, Placebo Controlled Study," *Annals of Internal Medicine* 125 (2) (15 July 1996): 81–88.

Nakayama, T., et al., "Suppression of Oxygen Induced Cytotoxicity by Flavonoids," *Biochemical Pharmacology* 45 (1993): 256–267.

Sawawal, St., et al., "Zinc Supplementation Reduces the Incidence of Acute Lower Respiratory Infection in Infants and Preschool Children," *Pediatrics* 102 (1996): 1–5.

Semba, R.D., "Vitamin A, Immunity and Infection," *Clinical Infectious Disease* 19 (1994): 489–499.

Stimpel, M., et al., "Macrophage Activation and Induction of Macrophage Cytotoxicity by Purified Polysaccharide Fractions from the Plant Echinacea purpurea," *Infection and Immunity* 46 (1984): 845–849.

Thompson, E.H., et al., "Ginger Rhizome: A New Source of Proteolytic Enzyme," *Journal of Food Science* 28 (4) (1973): 652–655.

Zakay-Rones, Z., et al., "Inhibition of Several Strains of Influenza Virus in Vitro and Reduction of Symptoms by an Elderberry Extract (*Sambucus nigra L.*) During an Outbreak of Influenza B Panama," *Journal of Alternative and Complementary Medicine* 1 (4) (1995): 361–369.

Zykov, M.P., and S.F. Protasova, "Prospects of Immunostimulating Vaccination Against Influenza Including the Use of Eleutherococcus and Other Preparations of Plants," in *New Data on Eleutherococcus; Proceedings of the Second International Symposium on Eleutherococcus*, USSR Academy of Sciences, Moscow, USSR, 1984, 164–169.

COUGH

Cygan, F.C., and R. Hansel, "Thyme Species as Cough Medicines," *Zeitschrift für Phytotherapie (Journal of Phytotherapy)* 14 (2) (1993): 104–110.

CONSTIPATION

Passmore, A.P., et al., "Chronic Constipation in Long Stay Elderly Patients. A Comparison of Lactulose and a Senna Fiber Combination," *British Medical Journal* 307 (1993): 769–771.

CONTACT-LENS PROBLEMS

Westerhout, D., "Treatment of Dry Eyes With Aqueous Antioxidant Eye Drops," *Contact Lens Journal* 19 (1989): 165–173.

DEPRESSION

Alpert, J., "Nutrition and Depression: The Role of Folate," *Nutrition Reviews* 55 (5) (1997): 145–149.

Benton, David, and Richard Cook, "Selenium Supplementation Improves Mood in a Double Blind Trial," *Psychopharmacology* 102 (1990): 549–550.

Bergmann, R., J. Duessner, and J. Demling, "Treatment of Mild to Moderate Depressions: A Comparison Between *Hypericum perforatum* and Amitryptiline," *Neurologie/Psychiatrie* 9 (4) (April 1993): 235–240.

Carney, M.W.P., "Vitamin Deficiency and Mental Symptoms," *British Journal of Psychiatry* 156 (1990): 878–882.

Collisson, R.J., "Siberian Ginseng (*Eleutherococcus senticosus*)," *British Journal of Phytotherapy* 2 (1991): 61–71.

Downing, Damien, M.B., B.S., "Cerebral Manifestations of Vitamin B_{12} Deficiency," *Journal of Nutritional Medicine* 2 (1991): 89–90.

Linde, K., et al., "St. John's Wort for Depression—An Overview and Meta-Analysis," *British Medical Journal* 313 (7052) (3 August 1996): 253–258.

Vorbach, E.U., W.D. Hubner, and K.H. Arnold, "Effectiveness and Tolerance of the Hypericum Extract LI 160 in Comparison With Imipramine: Randomized Double-Blind Study With 130 Patients," *Journal of Geriatric Psychiatry and Neurology* Supplement 1 (October 1994): S19–S23.

DIABETES

Abraham, A.S., et al, "The Effects of Chromium Supplementation on Serum Glucose and Lipid in Patients With and Without Non-Insulin-Dependent Diabetes," *Metabolism* 41 (7) (July 1992): 768–771.

Anderson, J.W., et al., "Dietary Fiber and Diabetes: A Comprehensive Review and Practical Application," *Journal of the American Dietetic Association* 87 (9) (1987): 1189–1197.

Honnorat, Jerome, et al., "Effect of Diabetes Type and Treatment on Zinc Status in Diabetes Mellitus," *Biological Trace Element Research* 32 (1992): 311–316.

Paolisso, Guiseppe, et al., "Pharmacologic Doses of Vitamin E Improve Insulin Action in Healthy Subjects and Non-Insulin-Dependent Diabetic Patients," *American Journal of Clinical Nutrition* 57 (1993): 650–656.

Pastors, J.G., et al., "Psyllium Fiber Reduces Rise in Postprandial Glucose and Insulin Concentrations in Patients With Non Insulin Dependent Diabetes," *American Journal of Clinical Nutrition* 53: 1431–1435.

Reichert, R.G., "Evening Primrose Oil and Diabetic Neuropathy," *Quarterly Review of Natural Medicine* (Summer 1995): 141–145.

Shamberger, R.J., "The Insulin-Like Effects of Vanadium," *Journal of Advanced Medicine* 9 (2) (1996): 121–131.

DRY EYES

Westerhout, D., "Treatment of Dry Eyes With Aqueous Antioxidant Eye Drops," *Contact Lens Journal* 19 (1989): 165–173.

ECZEMA

Bordoni, A., et al., "Evening Primrose Oil in the Treatment of Children With Atopic Eczema," *Clinical Research* 14 (1987): 291–297.

Busisnco, L., et al., "Breast Milk From Mothers of Children With Newly Developed Eczema Has Low Levels of Long Chain Polyunsaturated Fatty Acids," *Journal of Clinical Immunology* 91 (1993): 1134–1139.

Horrobin, D.F., and P.F. Morse, "Evening Primrose Oil and Atopic Eczema," letter to the editor, *Lancet* 345 (1995): 260–261.

Manku, M.S., et al., "Essential Fatty Acids in the Plasma Phospholipids of Patients With Atopic Eczema," *British Journal of Dermatology* 110 (1984): 643–648.

EYE INFECTION

Rengstorff, R.H., "Topical Treatment of External Eye Disorders With Preparations Containing Vitamin A," *Practical Optometry* 4 (1993): 163–165.

FATIGUE

Ahlbor, B., et al., "Effect of Potassium-Magnesium Aspartate on the Capacity for Prolonged Exercise in Man," *Acta Physiologica Scandinavica* 74 (1968): 238–245.

Asano, K., et al., "Effect of *Eleutherococcus senticosus* Extract on Human Working Capacity," *Planta Medica* 37 (1986): 175–177.

Fulder, S., "The Drug That Builds Russians," *New Science* 21 (1980): 576–579.

Tintera, J.W., "The Hypoadrenocortical State and Its Management," *New York State Journal of Medicine* 55 (1955): 1869–1876.

FIBROCYSTIC BREAST DISEASE

"Cyclical Breast Pain—What Works and What Doesn't," *Drug Therapeutic Bulletin* 30 (1992): 1–3.

Horrobin, D.F., et al., "Abnormalities in Plasma Essential Fatty Acid Levels in Women With Premenstrual Syndrome and With Nonmalignant Breast Disease," *Journal of Nutritional Medicine* 2 (1991): 259–254.

McFayden, I.J., et al., "Cyclical Breast Pain—Some Observations and the Difficulties in Treatment," *British Journal of Clinical Practice* 46 (1992): 161–164.

Pye, J.K., R.E. Mansel, and L.E. Hughes, "Clinical Experience of Drug Treatment for Mastalgia," *Lancet* 2 (August 1985): 373–377.

HAIR LOSS

Davis, Adelle, *Let's Eat Right to Keep Fit* (New York, NY: New American Library, 1988).

Vachher, P., "Alopecia Areata," *Emergency Medicine* 29 (10) (October 1997): 20–29.

HEADACHE

Grand, E., "Food Allergies and Migraine," *Lancet* 1 (1979): 955–959.

Johnson, E.S., et al., "Efficacy of Feverfew as Prophylactic Treatment of Migraine," *British Medical Journal* 291 (1985): 569–573.

Makheja, A.N., and J.M. Bailery, "A Platelet Phospholipase Inhibitor From the Medicinal Herb Feverfew (*Tanacetum parthenium*)," *Prostaglandins, Leukotrienes, and Medicine* 8 (6) (June 1983): 653–660.

Murphy, J.J., S. Hepinstall, and J.R. Mitchell, "Randomized Double Blind Placebo Controlled Trial of Feverfew in Migraine Prevention," *Lancet* 2 (1988): 189–192.

HIGH BLOOD PRESSURE

Furberg, C.D., et al., "Should Dihydrophyridines Be Used as First Line Drugs in the Treatment of Hypertension? The Con Side," *Archives of Internal Medicine* 155 (13 November 1995): 2157–2161.

Jendryczko, A., and M. Drozdz, "Plasma Retinol, Beta Carotene and Vitamin E Levels in Relation to Future Risk of Preeclampsia," *Zentralblatt für Gynakologie* 111 (16) (1989): 1121–1123.

HIV DISEASE

Abdullah, T.H., et al., "Enhancement of Natural Cell Killer Activity in AIDS With Garlic," *Deutsche Zeitschrift für Onkologie (German Journal of Cancer)* 21: 52–54.

Cathcart, Robert, M.D., "Vitamin C in the Treatment of Acquired Immune Deficiency Syndrome," *Medical Hypotheses* 14 (4) (1984): 423–432.

IRRITABLE BOWEL SYNDROME

Guthrie, et al., "A Controlled Trial of Psychological Treatment for the Irritable Bowel Syndrome," *Gastroenterology* 100 (February 1991): 450–457.

Klauser, A.G., et al., "Functional Diagnostic Workup in Patients With Irritable Bowel Syndrome," *Zeitschrift für Gastroenterologie* 34 (5) (May 1996): 273–278.

Lembo, Tony, et al., "Symptom Duration in Patients With Irritable Bowel Syndrome," *American Journal of Gastroenterology* 91 (5) (May 1996): 898–905.

Shabert, Judy, and Nancy Ehrlich, *The Ultimate Nutrient: Glutamine* (Garden City Park, NY: Avery Publishing Group, 1994).

KIDNEY STONES

Johansson, G., et al., "Effect of Magnesium Hydroxide in Renal Stone Disease," *Journal of the American College of Nutrition* 1 (2) (1982): 179–185.

Murthy, M.S.R., et al., "Effect of Pyridoxine Supplementation on Recurrent Stone Formers," *International Journal of Clinical Pharmacology, Therapy and Toxicology* 20 (9) (September 1982): 434–437.

MACULAR DEGENERATION

Silverstone, B.Z., et al., "Zinc and Copper Metabolism in Patients With Senile Macular Degeneration," *Annals of Ophthalmology* 14 (7) (1985): 419–422.

MANIC-DEPRESSIVE DISORDER

Bowden, C.L., "Maintenance Treatments for Bipolar Disorder," presentation to the 37th annual meeting of the New Clinical Drug Evaluation Unit, Boca Raton, Florida, 27–30 May 1997.

McInnis, M.G., et al., "Anticipation in Bipolar Affective Disorder," *American Journal of Human Genetics* 53 (1993): 385–390.

Milkowitz, D.J., "Psychotherapy in Combination With Drug Treatment for Bipolar Disorder," *Journal of Clinical Psychopharmacology* 16 (Supplement 1) (1996): 56S–66S.

MENOPAUSE

Aldecreutz, Herman, et al., "Dietary Phyto-estrogens and the Menopause in Japan," letter, *Lancet* 339 (1992): 1233.

Chen, J., "Pharmacologic Actions and Therapeutic Uses of Ginseng and Tang Kwei," *International Journal of Chinese Medicine* 1 (3) (1984): 23–27.

Colditz, Graham, et al., "The Use of Estrogens and Progestins and the Risk of Breast Cancer on Postmenopausal Women," *The New England Journal of Medicine* 332 (24) (15 June 1995): 1589–1593.

Kavinsky, N.R., "Vitamin E and the Control of Climacteric Symptoms," *American Western Medicine and Surgery* 4 (1) (1950): 27–32.

Lee, John, *What Your Doctor May Not Tell You About Menopause* (New York: Warner Books, 1996).

Martin, W., "The Miracle of Evening Primrose Oil," *Townsend Letter for Doctors* (November 1992): 990–992.

Prior, Jerilynn, "Progesterone as a Bonetrophic Hormone," *Endocrine Reviews* 11 (2) (May 1990): 387–397.

Setchell, K.D.R., et al., "Nonsteroidal Estrogens of Dietary Origin: Possible Roles in Hormone Dependent Disease," *American Journal of Clinical Nutrition* 40 (September 1984): 569–578.

Tilyard, M.W., et al., "Treatment of Postmenopausal Osteoporosis With Calcitriol or Calcium," *The New England Journal of Medicine* 326 (1992) 357–362.

Warnecke, G., "Psychosomatic Dysfunctions in the Female Climacteric. Clinical Effectiveness and Tolerance of Kava Extract," *Fortschritte der Medizin (Journal of Medicine)* 109 (4) (10 February 1991): 119–122.

NAIL PROBLEMS AND INJURIES

Davis, Adelle, *Let's Eat Right to Keep Fit* (New York, NY: New American Library, 1988).

Davis, Adelle, *Let's Get Well* (New York, NY: New American Library, 1984).

NICOTINE ADDICTION

Braly, James, *Dr. Braly's Optimum Health Program* (New York, NY: Times Books, 1985).

MacKenzie, T.D., C.E. Bartecchi, and R.W. Schrier, "The Human Cost of Tobacco Use." *The New England Journal of Medicine* 330 (14) (7 April 1994): 975–980.

Pekkanen, John, and Anita Bartholomew, "What You Don't Know About Secondhand Smoke." *Reader's Digest* (July 1997): 140–144.

Todd, G.P., *Nutrition, Health, and Disease* (Norfolk, VA: The Donning Co., 1988).

Williams, Roger John. *Nutrition Against Disease* (New York, NY: Bantam, 1973).

Wright, J.V., *Dr. Wright's Guide To Healing With Nutrition* (Emmaus, PA: Rodale Press, 1984).

OSTEOPOROSIS

Abraham, Guy E., M.D., et al., "The Importance of Magnesium in the Management of Primary Postmenopausal Osteoporosis," *Journal of Nutritional Medicine* 2 (1991): 165–178.

Dawson-Hughes, Bess, M.D., "Effect of Vitamin D Supplementation on Wintertime and Overall Bone Loss in Healthy Postmenopausal Women," *Annals of Internal Medicine* 115 (7) (1 October 1991): 505–512.

Hodkinson, H.M., et al., "Sunlight, Vitamin D and Osteomalacia in the Elderly," *Lancet* 1 (1973): 910.

Leach, R.M., et al., "Studies on the Role of Manganese in Bone Formation," *Archives of Biochemistry and Biophysics* 133 (1969): 22–28.

PARASITES, INTESTINAL

Hartung, Robert M. "Parasites: The Hidden Health Menace," *Health Freedom News* (May/June 1997).

Ritchason, Jack, *The Little Herb Encyclopedia* (Springville, UT: Thornwood Books, 1980).

Royal, Penny, *Herbally Yours,* 3rd Ed. (Payson, UT: Sound Nutrition, 1982).

PREMENSTRUAL SYNDROME

Brush, M.G., Ph.D., et al., "Abnormal Essential Fatty Acid Levels in Plasma of Women With Premenstrual Syndrome," *American Journal of Obstetrics and Gynecology* 150 (4) (1984): 363–366.

Cassidy, A., et al., "Biological Effects of a Diet of Soy Protein Rich in Isoflavones on the Menstrual Cycle of Premenopausal Women," *American Journal of Clinical Nutrition* 60 (1994): 333–340.

Facchinetti, Fabio, M.D., et al., "Oral Magnesium Successfully Relieves Premenstrual Mood Changes," *Science News* 138 (27 October 1990): 263.

Horrobin, D.F., "Nutritional and Medical Importance of Gamma Linolenic Acid," *Progress in Lipid Research* 31 (2) (1992): 163–194.

O'Brien, P.M., and H. Massil, "Premenstrual Syndrome: Clinical Studies on Essential Fatty Acids," in *Omega-6 Essential Fatty Acids: Pathophysiology and Roles in Clinical Medicine* (New York: Alan R. Liss, 1990), 523–545.

PROSTATE DISORDERS

Champlault, G., et al., "A Double Blind Trial of an Extract of the Plant *Serenoa repens* in Benign Prostatic Hyperplasia," *British Journal of Clinical Pharmacology* 18 (1984): 461–462.

PSORIASIS

Berth-Jones, J., and R.A.C. Graham-Brown, "Placebo Controlled Study of Essential Fatty Acid Supplementation in Atopic Dermatitis," *Lancet* 341 (1993): 1557–1560.

RAYNAUD'S DISEASE

Fine, Edward J., M.D., "Neurologic Signs of B_{12} Deficiency," *Emergency Medicine*, 15 (July 1992): 198–221.

SKIN CANCER

Liu, Q., et al., "Effect of Green Tea on p52 Mutation in Ultraviolet B Radiation Induced Mouse Skin Tumors," *Carcinogenesis* 19 (7) (1998): 1257–1262.

STRESS

Halliwell, B., "Oxidative Stress, Nutrition and Health: Experimental Strategies for Optimization of Nutritional Antioxidant Intake in Humans," *Free Radical Research* 25 (July 1996): 57–74.

Krehl, J.A., "Protective Effects of Pantothenic Acid for Adrenal Glands," *American Journal of Clinical Nutrition* 11 (1962): 77.

Passwater, Richard A., Ph.D., "The Superantioxidant Plus," in *The Nutrition Superbook: The Antioxidants*, ed. Jean Barilla (New Canaan, CT: Keats Publishing, 1995).

URINARY TRACT INFECTION

Avorn, J., et al., "Reduction of Bacteriuria and Pyuria After Ingestion of Cranberry Juice," *Journal of the American Medical Association* 271 (1994): 751–754.

Bettman, L.R., "Pathogenesis of Urinary Tract Infections: Host Susceptibility and Bacterial Virulence Factors," *Urology* 32 (Supplement) (1988): 9–11.

Blatherwick, N.R., and M.L. Long, "Studies on Urinary Acidity. II. The Increased Acidity Produced by Eating Prunes and Cranberries," *Journal of Biological Chemistry* 57 (1923): 815.

Bodel, P.T., R. Cotran, and E.H. Kass, "Cranberry Juice and the Antibacterial Action of Hippuric Acid," *Journal of Laboratory and Clinical Medicine* 54 (1959): 881–888.

Ofek, I., et al., "Anti-*Escherichia coli* Adhesion Activity of Cranberry and Blueberry Juices," *The New England Journal of Medicine* 324 (1991): 1599.

Papas, P.N., C.A. Brusch, and G.C. Ceresia, "Cranberry Juice in the Treatment of Urinary Tract Infections," *Southwestern Medicine* 47 (1) (January 1966): 17–20.

Sobota, A.E., "Inhibition of Bacterial Adherence by Cranberry Juice: Potential Use for the Treatment of Urinary Tract Infections," *Journal of Urology* 131 (1984): 1013–1016.

Zafiri, D., et al., "Inhibitory Activity of Cranberry Juice on Adherence of Type I and Type P Fimbriated *Escherichia coli* to Eucaryotic Cells," *Antimicrobial Agents of Chemotherapy* 33 (1989): 92–980.

EXERCISE

Carter, Albert, *The New Miracles of Rebound Exercise* (Scottsdale, AZ: ALM Publishers, 1988).

Fenton, Mark, "How to Be a Fitness Walker," *Walking Magazine*, April 1977, 47–55.

WATER PURIFICATION

Mindell, Earl, and W.H. Lee, *The Vitamin Robbers* (New Canaan, CT: Keats Publishing, Inc., 1983).

Sachs, Allan, *Grapefruit Seed Extract* (Mendocino, CA: Life Rhythm Publishing, 1997).

Shaper, A.G., "Soft Water, Heart Attacks, and Stroke," *Journal of the American Medical Association* 230 (1) (7 October 1974): 130–131.

Glossary

absorption. In nutrition, the process by which nutrients are absorbed through the intestinal tract into the bloodstream for use by the body. If nutrients are not properly absorbed, nutritional deficiencies can result.

acidophilus. *Lactobacillus acidophilus.* A species of bacteria that is normally found in a healthy intestine.

acute illness. An illness that comes on quickly and causes relatively severe symptoms, but is of limited duration.

adeno-. Pertaining to a gland (prefix).

adrenal gland. One of two glands located above the kidneys that secrete a number of key hormones, including epinephrine and cortisol.

-algia. Pain (suffix).

allergen. An ordinarily harmless substance that provokes an allergic response in a sensitive individual.

allergy. An immunological response to a certain substance or substances that causes an individual to develop sneezing, hives, or some other reaction when he or she comes into contact with it or ingests it.

amino acid. One of twenty-two known organic acids that contain nitrogen and serve as building blocks for the production of protein in the body; most are synthesized in the liver, but eight of them cannot be. Because they must be taken in through the diet, these are called *essential amino acids.*

analgesic. A substance that alleviates pain.

anemia. A condition in which the blood is incapable of transporting sufficient oxygen to the body tissues, caused by an unusually low number of red blood cells, too little hemoglobin in the red blood cells, or low blood volume.

anesthetic. A substance that causes the loss of sensation, especially the ability to feel pain.

angina. A condition characterized by chest pain that is usually brought on and made worse by exertion, and relieved by rest. It results from inadequate blood supply to the heart, usually due to coronary artery disease.

antacid. A substance that neutralizes acid in the digestive tract, especially the stomach.

anterior. In or toward the front.

antibiotic. A substance capable of killing or inhibiting the growth of microorganisms, especially bacteria.

antibody. A protein created by the immune system, in response to the presence of a foreign organism or toxin, that is capable of destroying or neutralizing the invader.

anticonvulsant. A substance that prevents or relieves seizures.

antiemetic. A drug designed to ease nausea and stop vomiting.

antigen. A substance that stimulates the production of an antibody.

antihistamine. A substance that blocks the action of histamines.

antioxidant. A substance that blocks oxidation reactions in the body, some of which can lead to cellular dysfunction and destruction. Antioxidant nutrients include beta-carotene, vitamin C, vitamin E, and selenium. Other antioxidants include the amino acid glutathione and the enzymes superoxide dismutase (SOD), peroxidase, and catalase.

antipyretic. A substance that lowers fever.

antispasmodic. A substance that relieves or prevents spasms and cramping.

appestat. The area of the brain that controls appetite, probably located in the hypothalamus.

arrhythmia. An irregular heartbeat. Some arrhythmias are benign; others are quite dangerous.

arteri/arterio-. Pertaining to an artery or arteries (prefix).

arteriosclerosis. Medical term for hardening of the arteries; a condition in which the walls of the arteries thicken and stiffen, impairing circulation.

arthr-/arthro-. Pertaining to or one or more joints (prefix).

articular. Pertaining to one or more joints.

ascorbate. A mineral salt of ascorbic acid (a chemical combination of vitamin C with a mineral). In this form, vitamin C is buffered, making it less acidic and therefore less irritating to the intestinal tract.

astringent. A substance that tends to draw together or tighten tissues.

atherosclerosis. A type of arteriosclerosis caused by the deposition of fatty plaques on the interior walls of the arteries.

atopic. Used to refer to conditions, especially allergies, that develop as a result of an inherited predisposition.

auricular. Pertaining to the ear.

autoimmune disorder. A condition in which the immune system attacks the body's own tissues and interferes with normal functioning.

bacteremia. A bacterial infection in the blood.

bacteria. Single-celled microorganisms. Some bacteria cause disease; others live in the body and are necessary for normal functioning and help to defend against invasions from harmful microorganisms.

behavior modification. The use of techniques such as conditioning, basic learning, and habit-creation to alter behavior.

benign. In medicine, used to refer to conditions that do not pose any threat to health or well-being. Also used to refer to cells, especially those growing in inappropriate locations, that are not cancerous. The word comes from the Latin *benignus*, meaning "good."

beta-carotene. A nutrient related to vitamin A that is used by the body to manufacture vitamin A as needed.

bile. A bitter yellowish substance manufactured by the liver that is necessary for the digestion and absorption of fats.

biofeedback. A technique that involves monitoring the body's processes, especially involuntary ones such as heartbeat, to help an individual become more aware of his or her physical responses and gain mastery over them. It is especially helpful for the management of such conditions as migraine and chronic pain.

bioflavonoid. Any of a diverse group of compounds found in most plants—in fruits and vegetables, usually next to the peel; in trees, in the bark. Bioflavonoids can act as antioxidants, immune-system regulators, and anti-inflammatory agents.

biopsy. Removal and examination of a sample of living tissue.

blood count. A basic diagnostic test that involves examining a sample of blood to determine the number of red blood cells, white blood cells, and platelets.

blood-brain barrier. A protective mechanism involving the capillaries and certain other cells of the brain that keeps many substances, especially water-based substances, from passing out of the blood vessels and into brain tissue.

botulism. A type of food poisoning caused by the ingestion of botulin, a toxin manufactured by the bacteria *Clostridium botulinum.*

bradycardia. Abnormally slow heartbeat.

brewer's yeast. A type of yeast that is a source of B-complex vitamins.

bronchi. The two main branches of the trachea (windpipe) that lead to the lungs.

bronchiole. The small, thin-walled air passages that branch off from the bronchi in the lungs.

bronchodilator. A substance that causes the air passages to relax and widen.

candida. Yeastlike fungus that can cause infections, most commonly in the mouth, the digestive tract, and the vagina.

capillaries. Tiny blood vessels that deliver nutrients to the cells and remove wastes from the cells.

carbohydrate. Any of the many organic substances, almost all of plant origin, that are composed of carbon, hydrogen, and oxygen, and that serve as the body's major source of energy.

carcinogen. An agent that causes the body to develop cancer.

cardiac. Pertaining to the heart.

carditis. Inflammation of the heart tissue.

carotenoid. Any of a group of yellow to red plant pigments. Many have valuable antioxidant properties; some can be converted into vitamin A in the body. Examples include alpha-, beta-, and gamma-carotene; lutein; and lycopene.

CAT scan. *See* Computerized axial tomography scan.

cauterization. A procedure in which an electrical current, laser beam, or silver nitrate stick is applied directly to a broken blood vessel to solidify blood and stop bleeding.

cell. A very small but complex organic unit consisting of a nucleus, cytoplasm, and surrounding cell membrane. All living tissues are composed of cells.

cellulose. An indigestible carbohydrate found mostly in the outer layers of fruits and vegetables.

cephalgia. Medical term for headache.

cephalo-. Pertaining to the head (prefix).

cerebral. Pertaining to the brain.

cervical. (1) Pertaining to the neck. (2) Pertaining to the narrow lower part of the uterus that joins with the vagina.

chalazion. A tiny cyst that appears as a small bump on the rim of the eyelid.

chemotherapy. The use of chemicals to treat disease, especially the treatment of cancer by means of toxic chemicals that destroy cancerous cells.

chiropractic. A system of healing based on the belief that many disorders can be traced to misalignments (called subluxations) of the spinal vertebrae and other joints. Chiropractors use physical manipulation techniques to restore proper alignment and, therefore, normal health and functioning.

chlorophyll. The green pigment in many plant tissues; taken as a dietary supplement, it is a source of magnesium and trace elements.

cholesterol. A substance that is an important constituent in cell walls and precursor of certain hormones. It also facilitates the transport of fatty acids in the body.

chondro-. Pertaining to cartilage (prefix).

chronic illness. An illness, whether mild or severe, that lasts or recurs consistently for a long period of time, or throughout the life of an individual.

CMV. *See* Cytomegalovirus.

coenzyme. A substance, usually containing a vitamin or mineral, that an enzyme must combine with in order to perform its appointed function in the body.

colic. Spasm in certain organs or structures, such as the intestines, uterus, or bile ducts, that is accompanied by pain.

complete protein. A source of dietary protein that contains a full complement of amino acids, especially the eight that the body cannot produce on its own.

complex carbohydrate. A carbohydrate that includes fiber, which slows the release of sugar from the carbohydrate into the bloodstream and provides dietary fiber as well. Sources of complex carbohydrate include whole grains, fruits, and vegetables.

complication. A secondary infection, reaction, or other development that occurs during an illness, usually making recovery more difficult and/or longer.

computerized axial tomography scan (CAT scan or CT scan). A diagnostic test that uses computers and x-rays to construct a three-dimensional picture of the body's structures and organs.

congenital. Present from birth, but not necessarily inherited.

conjunctiva. The transparent mucous membrane that lines the eyeball and inner surface of the eyelid.

contraindication. A reason why a drug or other treatment should *not* be used in a particular circumstance.

contusion. A bruise or injury in which the skin is not broken.

costal. Pertaining to the ribs.

corticosteroid. A steroid hormone produced by the adrenal gland, or a synthetic version of such a hormone.

coryza. Medical term for the nasal symptoms of the common cold.

cranial. Pertaining to the skull.

cruciferous vegetables. A group of vegetables including broccoli, Brussels sprouts, cabbage, cauliflower, turnips, and rutabagas, vegetables that have been found to contain cancer-fighting substances.

CT scan. *See* Computerized axial tomography scan.

cutaneous. Pertaining to the skin.

cystoscope. An instrument used to examine the ureters and bladder.

cyt-/cyto-. Pertaining to a cell or cells (prefix).

cytomegalovirus (CMV). A common virus of the herpes family that can cause disease in infants and in people with compromised immune systems.

-dactyl-. Pertaining to a finger or toe (prefix or suffix).

decongestant. A substance that reduces nasal congestion and swelling by constricting the blood vessels in the nasal membranes.

dementia. An acquired impairment in mental functioning that may be manifested in significant problems with learning and memory, language ability, orientation, visuospatial skills, reasoning, abstract thinking, and the ability to make calculations, as well as mood swings and personality changes. It can be either static or progressive, depending on the cause.

demulcent. Soothing, especially to mucous membranes.

deoxyribonucleic acid (DNA). Substance in the nuclei of all the cells of the body that contains the cells' genetic blueprints and determine the types of life form into which the cells will develop.

dermal. Pertaining to the skin.

dermatitis. Inflammation of the skin.

dermis. The layer of the skin that lies underneath the epidermis and contains blood and lymphatic vessels as well as sweat- and oil-producing glands.

desensitization. A treatment sometimes recommended for allergies in which gradually increasing amounts of diluted allergen are injected into the skin with the intent of stimulating the body to develop resistance to it.

disinfectant. A substance or agent that kills or neutralizes disease-causing microorganisms.

diuretic. A substance that increases the excretion of urine.

DNA. *See* Deoxyribonucleic acid.

dys-. Improper or abnormal (prefix).

dysmenorrhea. Medical term for menstrual cramps or pain.

dyspepsia. Medical term for indigestion.

dyspnea. Medical term for shortness of breath.

eardrum. The thin membrane that separates the middle ear from the outer ear. Also called the *tympanic membrane*.

eating disorder. A disorder characterized by a distorted body image, fear of gaining weight, obsession with food, and/or abnormal habits relating to the handling of food.

EBV. *See* Epstein-Barr virus.

ECG. *See* Electrocardiography.

echocardiogram. A diagnostic test that uses ultrasound to detect structural and functional abnormalities of the heart.

-ectomy. Surgical removal of (suffix).

edema. Swelling that results from an accumulation of fluid in tissue.

EEG. *See* Electroencephalography.

EKG. *See* Electrocardiography.

electrocardiography (EKG or ECG). A type of testing that monitors heart function by tracing the conduction of electrical impulses associated with heart activity.

electroencephalograpy (EEG). A type of testing used to measure brain-wave activity.

electrolyte. A form of sodium, magnesium, calcium, potassium, or other mineral that is used by the body to regulate the maintenance of fluid balance in the cells.

electromyelography (EMG). A type of testing used to measure the electrical activity in the muscles to determine whether both the muscles and the nerves that serve those muscles are functioning properly.

ELISA. *See* Enzyme-linked immunoadsorbent assay.

embolus. A tiny mass, such as a clot or air bubble, that travels through the bloodstream. Emboli have the potential to lodge at narrowed places, blocking blood flow.

emetic. A substance that induces vomiting.

EMG. *See* Electromyelography.

-emia. Pertaining to the blood (suffix).

emulsion. A substance that consists of two liquids that do not mix, such as oil and water; the two do not combine, but one is present as small globules in suspension in the other.

encephalitis. An inflammation of the brain.

endemic. Native to or prevalent in a particular geographic area. Often used to describe diseases.

endo-. Inside (prefix).

endocrine system. The system of glands that secrete hormones into the bloodstream to regulate or initiate various bodily processes; these include the pituitary, thyroid, and adrenal glands, as well as the pancreas, ovaries, and testes.

endorphin. Any of a number of hormonelike substances found primarily in the brain. One function of endorphins is to suppress the sensation of pain by binding to the same receptors in the brain that narcotic drugs do.

endoscope. An instrument used to examine the interior of hollow organs.

enteric. Pertaining to the small intestine.

enzyme. A protein that serves as a catalyst, causing or accelerating chemical reactions in the body without being consumed.

enzyme-linked immunoadsorbent assay (ELISA). A test that determines the presence of a particular protein, such as an antibody, in the blood or other fluid. It is the type of test most often used to look for antibodies to HIV, the virus that causes AIDS.

epidemic. Used to describe an outbreak of disease that spreads rapidly and extensively, or with unusually high incidence.

epidermis. The outer layer of the skin.

Epstein-Barr virus (EBV). A member of the herpes family of viruses and the agent that causes mononucleosis.

erythema. Medical term for reddening, especially of the skin.

erythro-. Red (prefix).

essential. In nutrition, used to refer to substances, such as amino acids, that the body requires but cannot manufacture on its own, and that therefore must be supplied through the diet.

eustachian tube. A structure that connects the middle ear to the nasal cavity and the throat, and through which secretions drain away from the ear and into the nose and throat.

excision. Surgical cutting away and/or removal of tissue.

expectorant. A substance that thins secretions and makes it easier to expel them from the respiratory tract.

extra-. Outside (prefix).

extract. A concentrated essence, as of an herb, made by leaching the active properties out with either alcohol or water.

fat cell. A cell in which fat is stored in the body.

fat-soluble. Capable of dissolving in the same organic solvents as fats and oils.

fatty acid. Any of the many organic acids of which fats and oils are composed.

fever of unknown origin (FUO). A body temperature elevated to above 101°F for three weeks or more for which no cause can be found.

fiber. The indigestible portion of plant foods.

fibrosis. A condition characterized by excessive formation of fibrous tissue. Depending on where in the body this happens, it can cause normally elastic tissue to stiffen, which in turn can lead to problems with the functioning of that tissue.

fistula. An opening or passageway between two organs or body parts that should not exist; it may be the result of injury, disease, or a congenital defect.

flavonoid. *See* bioflavonoid.

free radical. An atom, molecule, or fragment of a molecule that has at least one unpaired electron, making it highly unstable and ready to react with other atoms or molecules in its vicinity. Because they join so readily with other substances, free radicals can attack cells and cause damage to the body at the cellular level. Free radicals come from many sources, including normal metabolism as well as exposure to radiation, pollutants, and high levels of dietary fat, especially fats that have been subjected to heat.

free-radical scavenger. A substance that removes, destroys, or neutralizes free radicals.

fungus. A low form of plant life, most often a microscopically small organism. Some types of fungus are capable of causing infection. Candidiasis and athlete's foot are two examples of diseases caused by fungal infection.

FUO. *See* Fever of unknown origin.

gastric. Pertaining to the stomach.

gastric lavage. Also called stomach pumping, this is a procedure used to remove toxic substances from the stomach by means of a tube that is inserted through the nose and into the stomach.

gastrointestinal tract. A general term for the stomach and intestines, which together make up the digestive system.

genetic. Inherited.

gland. An organ that manufactures and secretes substances, such as hormones, that are not needed for its own functioning, but are used in other parts of the body.

globulin. A type of protein found in the blood. Certain globulins contain disease-fighting antibodies.

glucose. A simple sugar that is the principal source of energy for the body's cells.

gluten. A protein found in wheat, rye, barley, and oats.

glycogen. A complex carbohydrate that is the primary form in which glucose is stored in the body (mainly in the liver and muscles). It is converted back into glucose as needed to supply energy.

heavy metal. A metallic element whose specific gravity (a measurement of mass) is greater than 5.0. Some heavy metals, including lead and mercury, are extremely toxic.

hematocrit. The percentage of blood volume that is composed of red blood cells.

hematology. Medical specialty dealing with the study and treatment of disorders of the blood.

hematoma. A bulge or swelling that is filled with blood; usually forms as a result of a break in a blood vessel under the skin.

hemoglobin. The iron-containing red pigment in the blood required for the transport of oxygen.

hemorrhage. Profuse or abnormal bleeding.

hepatic. Pertaining to the liver.

hernia. A condition in which part of an internal organ protrudes through an abnormal opening in the wall of tissue that is supposed to contain it.

herpes. A group of viruses characterized by their tendency to cause skin eruptions or blisters. They include herpes simplex viruses 1 and 2 (HSV1 and HSV2) as well as the varicella-zoster and Epstein-Barr viruses.

hist-/histo-. Pertaining to tissue (prefix).

histamine. A chemical produced by the immune system in response to contact with an allergen. Histamines cause bronchial tube muscles to constrict, small blood vessels to dilate, and secretions from mucous membranes to increase, all of which result in the sneezing, itching, and discomfort of an allergic reaction.

HIV. *See* Human immunodeficiency virus.

Hodgkin's disease. A type of lymphoma (cancer of the lymphatic system).

hormone. A substance produced by one of the endocrine glands to regulate a specific bodily function.

host. An organism in or on which another organism or microorganism lives, and from which the parasite takes its nourishment.

human immunodeficiency virus (HIV). The virus that causes AIDS. HIV is actually a category of viruses, not a single one. The most common forms are designated HIV-1 and HIV-2.

hydro-. Water (prefix).

hydrogenation. A chemical process used to turn liquid oils into more solid form by bombarding the oil molecules with hydrogen. This destroys the nutritional properties of the oil and also results in the formation of cis- and trans-fatty acids, a type of strangely altered fatty acid that does not occur in nature, and that has effects in the body like those of saturated fats.

hydrolyzed protein. A common food additive that is a source of hidden gluten in food products, a hazard for people with celiac disease.

hyper-. Too much or too high (prefix).

hypertension. High blood pressure.

hypo-. Too little or too low (prefix).

hypotension. Low blood pressure.

hypothalamus. The portion of the brain that regulates body temperature and other metabolic processes, including the hunger response.

hyster-. Pertaining to the uterus (prefix).

idiopathic. Used to refer to a disease whose cause is unknown.

immune deficiency. Failure of the immune system to function normally in response to disease or infection.

immune globulin. A protein manufactured by certain white blood cells and found in body fluids and on mucous membranes. Immune globulins function as antibodies in the body's immune response.

immune system. The complex or organs, cells, tissues, and proteins that work in a coordinated manner to fight off invaders such as viruses and harmful bacteria.

immunity. The condition of being able to resist or overcome infection or disease.

incubation period. The period of time between exposure to an infectious disease and the appearance of symptoms, during which infection is developing.

infection. An invasion of the body by organisms such as viruses, harmful bacteria, or fungi that results in disease.

infestation. An invasion of the body by parasites such as insects, worms, or protozoa.

inflammation. A reaction to illness or injury characterized by swelling and redness.

infusion. A preparation made by steeping herbs in hot water; tea.

inguinal. Concerning or located in the groin.

insulin. A hormone produced by the pancreas that is necessary for the metabolism of carbohydrates, especially sugar.

interaction. A term describing the effects of two different substances in the presence of each other; interactions can occur between one drug and another drug, between drugs and foods, and so on.

interferon. A protein produced by the immune system in response to the presence of a virus that can prevent the virus from reproducing or infecting other cells.

international unit (IU). A unit of potency based on an accepted international standard. The potency of vitamin A and E supplements, among others, is usually measured in international units.

intestinal flora. The "friendly" bacteria normally present in the intestines that are necessary for the digestion and absorption of certain nutrients.

intolerance. In nutrition, the inability to digest a particular food, usually due to a lack or deficiency of certain enzymes.

intradermal testing. Testing for allergies that is performed by injecting the skin with suspected allergens at timed intervals.

intravenous. A term describing the administration of drugs or fluids by means of a small needle inserted directly in a vein.

intravenous pyelography (IVP). A testing procedure used to diagnose problems of the kidneys and urinary tract. It involves the intravenous injection of a dye followed by x-ray photographs to track its progress through the system.

ischemia. The condition of being starved for blood. Ischemia affecting the heart or brain can cause a heart attack or stroke.

-itis. Inflammation of (suffix).

IU. *See* International unit.

IVP. *See* Intravenous pyelography.

jaundice. Visible yellowing of the skin and eyes that occurs when bile is not processed properly and so accumulates in those tissues.

ketoacidosis. A complication of diabetes, caused by a high blood sugar episode, that can lead to loss of consciousness, coma, or even death if not properly and promptly treated.

laceration. An injury in which tissue is torn.

lactobacilli. "Friendly" bacteria that are capable of fermenting milk sugar; taken as a supplement, they help to establish healthy flora in the intestines, aiding digestion and increasing the body's resistance to certain types of infection.

laser. An instrument that focuses highly amplified light waves. Lasers are used in surgery, particularly eye surgery, and also in dentistry. (*Laser* stands for *l*ight *a*mplification *s*timulated by *e*mission of *r*adiation.)

laxative. A substance that tends to stimulate the bowels to move.

leukemia. A cancer of the blood-producing tissues, especially the bone marrow and lymph nodes, resulting in abundance of white blood cells. It can be either acute (most common in children) or chronic (most common in adults).

ligament. A cord of fibrous tissue that connects one bone with another.

limbic system. A group of deep brain structures that, among other things, transmit the perception of pain to the brain and generate an emotional reaction to it.

lipid. Any of a group of fat-soluble organic substances. Often used interchangeably with *fat*.

lipoprotein. A type of protein molecule that incorporates a lipid. Lipoproteins function as a means of transporting lipids in water-based substances such as blood and lymph.

lipotropic. One of a group of substances, including choline, inositol, and methionine, that prevent the accumulation of abnormal or excessive levels of fat in the liver. They also help to control blood-sugar levels and enhance fat and carbohydrate metabolism.

lower respiratory tract. Usually refers to the trachea (the windpipe), the bronchi, the bronchioles, and the lungs.

lumbar. Pertaining to the lower back, between the bottom of the rib cage and the pelvis.

lymph. The clear fluid in which all of the body's cells are bathed. It provides nourishment to the cells and collects waste products given off by the cells.

lymph node. One of many small structures located in the lymph vessels that produce lymphocytes (white blood cells) and remove foreign materials from the lymph stream.

lymphadenopathy. Medical term for swollen lymph nodes ("swollen glands").

lymphocyte. A type of white blood cell that is a crucial component of the immune system.

lymphoma. A cancer of the lymphatic system.

magnetic resonance imaging (MRI). A diagnostic technique involving the use of radio waves and magnetic forces to produce detailed images of the body's internal organs and structures.

malignant. In medicine, used to refer to conditions that are threatening to life; also used to refer to cells or groups of cells that are cancerous and likely to spread. The word comes from the Latin *malignus,* meaning "evil."

mcg. *See* Microgram.

-megaly. Enlargement of (suffix).

menarche. The onset of menstruation.

meninges. The three thin membranes that cover the brain and spinal cord.

menopause. The cessation of menstruation, caused by a decrease in the production of the sex hormones estrogen and progesterone.

metabolic rate. The rate at which the body carries out metabolic functions.

metabolism. The term for the entire complex of physical and chemical processes that are necessary to sustain life; these include the breaking down of certain substances (such as foods, to release energy) and the synthesis of others (such as proteins for growth and repair of tissues).

metabolite. A substance produced as a result of a metabolic process.

mg. *See* Milligram.

microgram (mcg). A measurement of weight equivalent to 1/1,000 milligram (or 1/1,000,000 gram).

micronutrient. A nutrient required in small amounts, such as a vitamin or mineral.

microorganism. A microscopically small organism, such as a bacterium, fungus, or protozoan.

milligram (mg). A measurement of weight equivalent to 1/1,000 gram.

mineral. An inorganic substance, such as calcium, magnesium, or sodium. Many minerals are required by the body for proper functioning.

monilia. An infectious fungus also known as candida.

MRI. *See* Magnetic resonance imaging.

mucous membrane. A membrane that lines one of the hollow organs of the body, such as the nose, mouth, stomach, intestines, bronchial tubes, anus, and vagina.

myelo-. Pertaining to bone marrow (prefix).

myo-. Pertaining to muscle (prefix).

narcotic. A powerful drug that blocks the perception of pain by binding with receptors in the central nervous system. It is this interaction with body chemistry that makes narcotics addictive.

naturopathy. A system of medicine that uses herbs and other natural methods to stimulate the body to heal itself without the use of drugs.

neoplasm. Medical term for a tumor.

nephro-. Pertaining to the kidneys (prefix).

neural. Pertaining to nerves.

neuropathy. A complex of symptoms caused by abnormalities in nerve function. Symptoms may include tingling or numbness, especially in the hands or feet, followed by gradual, progressive muscle weakness.

neurotransmitter. A chemical that transmits impulses between neurons (nerve cells) in the brain and nervous system.

nonsteroidal anti-inflammatory drug (NSAID). Any of a class of drugs often used as painkillers for mild to moderate pain; some are available by prescription only.

NSAID. *See* nonsteroidal anti-inflammatory drug.

nucleic acid. And of a class of compounds found in all viruses and plant and animal cells. RNA and DNA are two principal types.

nutraceutical. A food- or nutrient-based product or supplement designed and/or used for a specific therapeutic purpose.

occult blood test. A test that detects the presence of blood in bodily excretions such as stool, sputum, or urine. It is most often used in screening for cancer.

-oma. Tumor (suffix).

oncology. Medical specialty dealing with the study and treatment of different types of cancer.

-opia. Vision (suffix).

organic. A term used to describe foods that are grown without the use of synthetic chemicals, such as pesticides, herbicides, and hormones.

orientation. A normal awareness of and relationship to one's surroundings, including the ability to comprehend time, people, and place.

-osis. Condition (suffix).

osseo-. Pertaining to bone (prefix).

osteo-. Pertaining to bone (prefix).

-otomy. Surgical incision into (suffix).

oxidation. Technically, a chemical reaction in which oxygen reacts with another substance, causing a chemical transformation of the substance. Also sometimes used to refer to chemical reactions not involving oxygen, but that involve a similar process and lead to similar results. Many oxidation reactions result in some type of spoilage or deterioration.

oximeter. A device that is placed on a toe or finger to measure the amount of oxygen being transported by the blood.

Pap test. Microscopic examination of cells collected from the vagina and cervix to test for signs of cancer (*Pap* is short for *Papanicolaou,* the name of the man who developed the test).

parasite. An organism or microorganism that lives in or on, and takes nourishment from, another organism.

parotid gland. One of the two saliva-producing glands

located in the back of the mouth, below and in front of the ears.

peak flow meter. An instrument used to measure changes in breathing capacity by determining how much air is exerted with a full exhalation.

-penia. Deficiency of (suffix).

peptic. Pertaining to digestion.

peri-. Around (prefix).

peritoneum. The membrane that lines the entire abdominal cavity and folds to surround the abdominal organs.

pH. A scale used to measure relative acidity or alkalinity. The pH scale runs from 0 to 14; a pH of 7 is considered neutral, while numbers below 7 denote increasing acidity and numbers above 7 denote increasing alkalinity. (*pH* stands for *potential of hydrogen.*)

pharyngitis. A medical term for sore throat.

phenylketonuria. A condition in which the body fails to produce the enzyme required to convert the amino acid phenylalanine into another amino acid, tyrosine, which is part of the process of normal protein metabolism.

phleb-/phlebo-. Pertaining to veins (prefix).

pituitary. A gland located at the base of the brain that secretes hormones that regulate growth and metabolism, as well as coordinating the actions of other endocrine glands.

-plasty. Surgical repair (suffix).

-plegia. Paralysis (suffix).

pneumo-. Pertaining to the lungs (prefix).

poly-. More than one (prefix).

posterior. In or toward the back.

postnasal drip. A condition in which nasal mucus flows down through the throat, rather than being discharged through the nostrils, often as a result of allergy or chronic infection.

presby-. Related to aging (prefix).

proctology. Medical specialty dealing with the study and treatment of disorders of the colon, rectum, and anus.

prognosis. A prediction as to the course and/or outcome of an illness.

projectile vomiting. Vomiting so violent that vomit is ejected in a forceful stream and lands at a distance from the mouth.

propolis. A resinous substance collected by bees; used as a dietary supplement or salve, it has antibacterial properties that aid in fighting infection.

prostaglandins. Hormonelike body chemicals that act in extremely low concentrations on local target organs. For example, prostaglandins secreted by the uterine lining cause the smooth muscle of the uterus to contract.

prostate-specific antigen test (PSA test). A blood test that is used to detect problems with the prostate gland, including cancer.

protein. A nitrogen-containing compound that is an essential constituent of all animal and vegetable tissues, necessary for growth and repair.

protocol. A course of medical treatment.

protozoan. Any of a group of single-celled microorganisms, such as amoebas.

pruritus. Medical term for itching.

PSA test. *See* Prostate-specific antigen test.

pulmonary. Pertaining to the lungs.

purulent. Containing or causing the production of pus.

pyro-. Pertaining to fever (prefix).

radiation therapy. A type of treatment for cancer in which radiation is used to kill cancerous tissues; also called radiotherapy.

radioallergosorbent test (RAST). A blood test that measures levels of specific antibodies produced by the body's immune system, used to test for allergic reactions.

rapid eye movement (REM). A term used to describe a phase of the sleep cycle in which the eyes move rapidly and in a jerky motion, and during which dreaming takes place.

RAST. *See* Radioallergosorbent test.

rebound effect. A situation in which a person who has been treated for a particular symptom or illness, particularly with drug therapy, experiences worse symptoms after the treatment is stopped than he or she had initially.

red blood cells. Blood cells that contain hemoglobin and transport oxygen and carbon dioxide.

reflux. A condition in which a substance flows backward, instead of in the intended direction. For example, urine can flow backwards up through the urethra to the bladder, and sometimes through the ureters to the kidneys, instead of moving out of the body.

REM. *See* Rapid eye movement.

remission. Lessening or reversal of the signs and symptoms of disease. This term is used primarily in connection with serious and/or chronic illnesses such as cancer and multiple sclerosis.

renal. Pertaining to the kidneys.

rhino-. Pertaining to the nose (prefix).

ribonucleic acid (RNA). A complex protein found in plant and animal cells, as well as viruses, that carries coded genetic information.

RNA. *See* Ribonucleic acid.

saturated fat. A type of fat characterized by its inability to incorporate additional hydrogen atoms. Saturated fats are solid at room temperature, like butter or lard. They are found primarily in foods of animal origin, such as meat and dairy products. A diet high in saturated fats has been implicated in the development of heart disease and certain types of cancer; experts recommend keeping consumption of saturated fats to a minimum.

scratch test. An allergy test that involves placing a small amount of a suspected allergen on a lightly scratched area of skin.

sebaceous glands. Glands in the skin that secrete sebum.

sebum. The oily lubricating secretion produced by glands in the skin.

secondary infection. An infection that develops after and is made possible by the presence or effect of a previous infection or inflammation, but is not necessarily directly caused by it.

seizure. A sudden and temporary change in brain function resulting in changes in consciousness, uncontrollable contractions of groups of muscles, and/or other symptoms.

sensitivity. A tendency to react to the presence of a particular agent or substance.

septic sore throat. A sore throat resulting from bacterial infection; strep throat.

serotonin. A neurotransmitter that, among other things, is responsible for regulating the mechanisms of normal sleep.

serum. The fluid portion of the blood.

simple carbohydrate. A type of carbohydrate that, owing to its chemical structure, is rapidly digested and absorbed into the bloodstream. Sugars are simple carbohydrates.

sinus. Any of four pairs of open spaces within the bones of the skull, located behind the bridge of the nose, back in the upper nose, in the forehead, and under the eyes.

spinal tap. A procedure in which a small amount of spinal fluid is withdrawn for examination by means of a needle inserted into a space between two vertebrae.

spirochete. Any of a number of different harmful bacteria species characterized by their slender spiral shape.

stenosis. Narrowing or constriction, especially of a tube-like structure.

steroid. Any of a group of fat-soluble organic compounds with a characteristic chemical composition; a number of different hormones, drugs, and other substances—including cholesterol—are classified as steroids.

streptococcus. A genus of bacteria, many members of which cause disease (including strep throat and scarlet fever) by destroying red blood cells.

subcutaneous. Under the skin.

symptom-specific. Designed to treat a particular symptom or set of symptoms.

syncope. Temporary loss of consciousness; fainting.

syndrome. Not a recognized disease as such, but a group of signs and symptoms that together form a condition that has a predictable outcome or requires special treatment.

systemic. Pertaining to the entire body.

tachycardia. Abnormally fast heartbeat.

tendon. A cord of fibrous tissue that connects a bone with a muscle.

teratogen. An agent that causes malformation of an embryo or fetus.

thoracic. Pertaining to the chest.

thrombo-. Pertaining to a blood clot (prefix).

thrombus. A clot that forms in a blood vessel.

tincture. A concentrated essence made by using alcohol to extract and concentrate the active properties of a substance, such as an herb.

tonsils. Two small masses of lymphatic tissue located at the back of the throat that are believed to help the body defend against respiratory infection.

topical. Applied to the surface of the body.

toxin. A substance that is poisonous to the body.

toxoid. An ordinarily poisonous substance that has been treated to remove its dangerous properties, but that remains capable of stimulating the body to develop protective antitoxins.

trace element. A substance, most commonly a mineral, required by the body in minute amounts.

tremor. Involuntary trembling.

triglyceride. A type of fat consisting of three fatty acids plus glycerol. Triglycerides are the form in which fat is stored in the body, and are the primary type of lipid in the diet as well.

tuberculin test. A test used to determine if a person has been exposed to or is infected with tuberculosis.

tumor. An abnormal mass of tissue that serves no function.

tympanic membrane. *See* Eardrum.

type-A personality. A personality that tends to be impatient and aggressive. Persons with type-A personalities have stronger stress reactions than most people, and may be more susceptible to cardiovascular disease and other health problems.

type-B personality. A personality that tends to be relaxed and patient, and less reactive to stress. People with type-B personalities may be less prone to develop stress-related illnesses such as high blood pressure and heart disease.

ultrasound. The use of ultra-high-frequency sound waves as a diagnostic tool or for medical treatment.

unsaturated fat. A type of fat characterized chemically by an ability to incorporate additional hydrogen atoms. Unsaturated fats are liquid at room temperature. They come from vegetable sources and are good sources of essential fatty acids. Oils high in unsaturated fats include canola oil, corn oil, olive oil, sunflower oil, and safflower oil.

upper respiratory tract. Usually refers to the nose and nasal passages, the throat, and the larynx (the voice box).

urticaria. Medical term for hives.

vaccine. A substance administered to induce the body to develop immunity against a disease without developing the disease itself.

vascular. Pertaining to blood vessels.

vaso-. Pertaining to blood vessels (prefix).

venom. A poisonous substance produced by animals, such as certain snakes and insects.

vestibular apparatus. The structure of the inner ear responsible for maintaining the body's sense of balance and equilibrium.

villi. Microscopic hairlike "fingers" lining the walls of the intestinal tract that absorb and transport fluids and nutrients.

virus. Any of a large class of minute parasitic organic structures that consist of a protein coat and a core of genetic material and that are capable of infecting plants and animals by reproducing within their cells. Because they cannot reproduce outside of a host organisms cells, viruses are not technically considered living organisms.

visualization. A technique that involves consciously using the mind to influence the health and functioning of the body.

vital signs. Basic indicators of an individual's health status, including pulse, breathing, blood pressure, and body temperature.

vitamin. Any of approximately fifteen organic micronutrients required by the body that must be obtained through diet.

water-soluble. Capable of dissolving in water or water-based fluids.

white blood cells. Blood cells that function in fighting infection and in wound repair. An elevated white blood cell count is often a sign of infection or disease.

withdrawal. The process of adjustment that occurs when the use of a habit-forming substance to which the body has been accustomed is discontinued.

yeast. A single-celled organism that can cause infection in various parts of the body, most commonly the mouth (thrush), the vagina (vaginitis), or the gastrointestinal tract.

Common Medical Abbreviations

bid. Twice a day.
BP. Blood pressure.
CBC. Complete blood count.
CNS. Central nervous system.
CPR. Cardiopulmonary resuscitation.
CSF. Cerebrospinal fluid.
ENT. Ear, nose, and throat.
FUO. Fever of unknown origin.
GI. Gastrointestinal.
GU. Genitourinary.
Hb or Hgb. Hemoglobin.
Hct. Hematocrit.
hs. Hour of sleep (i.e., bedtime).
IU. International unit.
IV. Intravenous.
mcg. Microgram.

mg. Milligram.
MI. Myocardial infarction (heart attack).
mL. Milliliter.
mm. Millimeter.
NSAID. Nonsteroidal anti-inflammatory drug.
OTC. Over-the-counter.
po. Orally.
ppm. Parts per million.
prn. As needed.
q. Every.
qid. Four times a day.
RBC. Red blood cell.
tid. Three times a day.
URI. Upper respiratory infection.
UTI. Urinary tract infection.
WBC. White blood cell.

Resources

RECOMMENDED SUPPLIERS

The following list of suppliers is included so that you can find and use the remedies recommended in this book. It is not intended to be an exhaustive list of all possible sources of these products. Rather, we recommend them because we have found their products to be of good quality. Please be aware that addresses and phone numbers are subject to change.

Herbal Products

Advantage Nutrition
37 Forrester Street
Pittsburgh, PA 15207
888–422–1710
Website: http://www.advantage-rx.com

Enzymatic Therapy
825 Challenger Drive
Green Bay, WI 54311
800–783–2286
E-mail: etmail@enzy.com
Website: http://www.enzy.com

Herb Pharmacy
20260 Williams Highway
Williams, OR 97544
541–846–6262

Nature's Herbs
600 East Quality Drive
American Fork, UT 84003
800–437–2257 or 801–763–0700; fax 801–763–0789
Website: http://www.naturesherb.com

Nature's Way Products
P.O. Box 4000
Springville, UT 84663
800–962–8873 or 801–489–1500; fax 801–489–1700
Website: http://www.naturesway.com

Pharmanex
75 West Center
Provo, UT 84601
800–800–0260 or 801–345–9800; fax 800–800–0259
Website: http://www.pharmanex.com

Wild River Herbs
P.O. Box 3876
Jackson, WY 83001
307–733–6731

Zand Herbal Formulas
1772 14th Street, Suite 230
Boulder, CO 80302
303–786–8558; fax 303–786–9435
Website: http://www.zand.com

Homeopathic Remedies

Boericke and Tafel, Inc.
2381 Circadian Way
Santa Rosa, CA 95407
707–571–8202; fax 707–571–8237

Boiron
6 Campus Boulevard
Newtown Square, PA 19073
800–BLU–TUBE or 610–325–7464; fax 610–325–7480

Dolisos America, Inc.
3014 Rigel Avenue
Las Vegas, NV 89102
702–871–7153; fax 702–871–9670
Website: http://dolisos.com

Hahnemann Pharmacy
1940 Fourth Street
San Rafael, CA 94901
510–527–3003

Heel Inc./BHI
11600 Cochiti Road Southeast
Albuquerque, NM 87123
505–293–3843
Website: http://www.heelbhi.com

Homeopathic Educational Services
2124 Kittredge Street
Berkeley, CA 94704
510–649–8930; fax 510–649–1955
Website: http://www.homeopathic.com

Luyties Pharmacal Company
4200 Laclede Avenue
St. Louis, MO 63108
800–325–8080; fax 314–535–9600
Website: http://www.1800homeopathy.com

Standard Homeopathic Company
P.O. Box 61067
154 West 131st Street
Los Angeles, CA 90061
310–768–0700; fax 310–516–8579
Website: http://www.hylands.com

Nutritional Supplements

Advanced Medical Nutrition
2247 National Avenue
Hayward, CA 94545
510–783–6969; fax 510–783–8196
E-mail: custserv@amni.com
Website: http://www.amni.com
Products sold only through physicians.

Alacer Corporation
19631 Pauling
Foot Hill Ranch, CA 92610
800–854–0249 or 949–454–3900; fax 949–951–7235
Website: http://www.alacercorp.com

Amrion Labs
6565 O'Dell Place
Boulder, CO 80301
303–530–2525; fax 303–530–2592
Website: http://www.amrion.com

Enzymatic Therapy
825 Challenger Drive
Green Bay, WI 54311
800–783–2286
E-mail: etmail@enzy.com
Website: http://www.enzy.com

Ethical Nutrients
971 Calle Negocio
San Clemente, CA 92673
800–668–8743 or 800–621–6070

Miracle Exclusives Inc.
64 Seaview Boulevard
Port Washington, NY 11050
516–621–3333; fax 516–621–1997
E-mail: miracle-exc@juno.com
Website: http://www.miracleexclusives.com

Natren, Inc.
P.O. Box 7448
Thousand Oaks, CA 91359
800–992–3323; fax 805–371–4742
Website: http://www.natren.com

Nutrabiotic
P.O. Box 238
Lakeport, CA 95453
800–225–4345; fax 707–263–7844

Professional Health Products Ltd.
Industrial Park
Sewickley, PA 15143
800–929–4133 or 412–741–6351; fax 412–741–6372
Website: http://www.phpltd.com

Rainbow Light Nutritional Systems
207 McPherson Street
P.O. Box 600
Santa Cruz, CA 95061
800–635–1233 or 831–429–9089; fax 831–429–0189

Solgar Vitamin and Herb Company
500 Willow Tree Road
Leonia, NJ 07605
201–944–2311; fax 201–944–7351
Website: http://www.solgar.com

Twinlab
2120 Smithtown Avenue
Ronkonkoma, NY 11779
800–645–5626 or 516–467–3140
Website: http://www.twinlab.com

UAS Labs
5610 Rowland Road, Suite 110
Minnetonka, MN 55345
800–422–3371
E-mail: dash@uaslabs.com

Wakunaga of America Company, Ltd.
23501 Madero
Mission Viejo, CA 92691–2744
800–421–2998 or 949–855–2776; fax 949–458–2764
Website: http://www.kyolic.com

Essential Oils

Aroma Vera
5901 Rodeo Road
Los Angeles, CA 90016–4312
800–669–9514 or 310–280–0407; fax 310–280–0395
Website: http://www.aromavera.com

Leydet Aromatics
P.O. Box 2354
Fair Oaks, CA 95628
916–965–7546
Website: http://www.leydet.com

Original Swiss Aromatics
P.O. Box 6842
San Rafael, CA 94903
415–459–3998

Prima Fleur Botanicals
1525 East Francisco Boulevard
San Rafael, CA 94901
415–455–0957; fax 415–455–0956

Santa Fe Botanical Fragrances, Inc.
P.O. Box 282
Santa Fe, NM 87504
505–473–1717
E-mail: sfragrance@aol.com

Source Vital
3637 West Alabama, Suite 240
Houston, TX 77027
800–880–6457 or 713–622–2190; fax 713–622–2010
Website: http://www.sourcevital.com

Organic Foods by Mail Order

French Meadow Bakery
2610 Lyndale Avenue South
Minneapolis, MN 55408
612–870–4740; fax 612–870–0907
E-mail: info@frenchmeadow.com
Website: http://www.frenchmeadow.com

Gold Mine Natural Food Company
3419 Hancock Street
San Diego, CA 92110
800–475–3663 or 619–296–8536; fax 619–296–9756

Lundberg Family Farms
P.O. Box 369
Richvale, CA 95974
530–882–4551; fax 530–882–4500
Website: http://www.lundberg.com

Mountain Ark Trading Company
799 Old Leicester Highway
Asheville, NC 28806
800–643–8909; fax 828–252–9479

Organic Foods Express
11711B Parklawn Drive
Rockville, MD 20852
301–816–4944; fax 301–816–3247

Walnut Acres
Penns Creek, PA 17862
717–837–0601; fax 570–837–1146
Website: http://www.walnutacres.com

Other

Great Smokies Diagnostic Laboratory
63 Zillicoa Street
Asheville, NC 28801
800–522–4762
Website: http://www.greatsmokies-lab.com

Performs laboratory tests for intestinal parasites, including comprehensive digestive stool analysis (CDSA); vaginosis profile; microbiology analysis; and parasitology studies.

Medic Alert
2323 Colorado Avenue
Turlock, CA 95382
800–432–5378
Hotline: 800–344–3226; 800–468–1020 (from California);
   209–668–3333 (from Alaska or Hawaii);
   fax 209–669–2495
Website: http://www.medicalert.org
Provides bracelets that warn about serious chronic medical conditions such as severe allergies, diabetes, and epilepsy.

Sawyer Products
605 7th Avenue North
Safety Harbor, FL 34695
800–356–7811; fax 727–725–1954
Website: http://www.sawyerproducts.com
Manufacturer of The Extractor venom extraction kit.

Sun Precautions
2815 Wetmore Avenue
Everett, WA 98201
800–882–7860
E-mail: SPF30plus@aol.com
Website: http://www.sunprecautions.com
Manufacturer of Solumbra sun-protective clothing.

ORGANIZATIONS

The following organizations can answer questions, provide referrals, and tell you how to find more information. Some organizations sell literature or offer classes and workshops to help you broaden your understanding of natural medicine. Be aware that addresses and telephone numbers are subject to change.

Acupuncture, Acupressure, and Massage

Acupressure Institute
1533 Shattuck Avenue
Berkeley, CA 94709
510–845–1059 (in California) 800–442–2232 (elsewhere);
   fax 510–845–1496
E-mail: info@acupressure.com
Website: http://www.acupressure.com

American Association of Oriental Medicine
433 Front Street
Catasauqua, PA 18032
610–266–1433; fax 610–264–2768
E-mail: aaom1@aol.com (note first "1" is the numeral one)
Website: http://www.aaom.org

American Massage Therapy Association
820 Davis Street, Suite 100
Evanston, IL 60201-4444
847–864–0123
E-mail: info@inet.amtamassage.org
Website: http://www.amtamassage.org

American Physical Therapy Association
1111 North Fairfax Street
Alexandria, VA 22314
800–999–2782
Website: http://www.apta.org

National Acupuncture and Oriental Medicine Alliance
14637 Starr Road SE
Olalla, WA 98359
253–851–6896
Website: http://www.acuall.org

National Certification Commission for Acupuncture and Oriental Medicine
P.O. Box 97075
Washington, DC 20090–7075
703–548–9004
E-mail: ncaa@compuserve.com
Website: http://www.nccaom.org

Alternative Medicine (General)

American Association of Naturopathic Physicians
601 Valley Street, Suite 105
Seattle, WA 98109
206–298–0125
E-mail: 74602.3715@compuserve.com
website: http://www.naturopathic.org

American Chiropractic Association
1701 Clarendon Boulevard
Arlington, VA 22209
703–276–8800
E-mail: memberinfo@amerchiro.org
Website: http://www.amerchiro.org

American Holistic Health Association
P.O. Box 17400
Anaheim, CA 92817–7400
714–779–6152
E-mail: ahha@healthy.net
Website: http://www.ahha.org

American Osteopathic Association
142 East Ontario Street
Chicago, IL 60611–2864
800–621–1773 or 312–202–8061
E-mail: info@aoa-net.org
Website: http://www.am-osteo-assn.org

Bastyr University of Naturopathic Medicine
144 NE 54th Street
Seattle, WA 98103
425–823–1300
Website: http://www.bastyr.edu

Foundation for the Advancement of Innovative Medicine (FAIM)
100 Airport Executive Park, No. 105
Nanuet, NY 10954
914–371–3246; fax 914–371–4790
E-mail:faim@fcc.net
Website: http://www.faim.org

National Center for Complementary and Alternative Medicine
P.O. Box 8218
Silver Spring, MD 20907-8218
888–644–6226; fax 301–495–4957
E-mail: nccam-info@altmedinfo.org
Website: http://www.altmed.od.nih.gov

Bach Flower Remedies

Nelson Bach USA Ltd.
Wilmington Technology Park
100 Research Drive
Wilmington, MA 01887
800–319–9151 or 978–988–3833; fax 978–988–0233
Website: http://www.nelsonbach.com

Biofeedback/Hypnosis

American Board of Hypnotherapy
16842 Von Karman Avenue, Suite 475
Irvine, CA 92606
800–634–9766; fax 714–251–4632
E-mail: aih@ix.netcom.com
Website: http://www.hypnosis.com

American Society of Clinical Hypnosis
33 West Grand Avenue, No. 402
Chicago, IL 60610
847–297–3317
Website: http://www.asch.net

Association for Applied Psychophysiology and Biofeedback
10200 West 44th Avenue, Suite 304
Wheat Ridge, CO 80033–2840
800–477–8892 or 303–422–8436; fax 303–422–8894
E-mail: aapb@resourcenter.com
Website: http://www.aapb.org

Biofeedback Certification Institute of America
10200 West 44th Avenue, Suite 310
Wheat Ridge, CO 80033
303–420–2902
E-mail: bcia@resourcenter.com

Society for Clinical and Experimental Hypnosis
2201 Haeder Road
Pullman, WA 99163
509–332–7555; fax 509–332–5907
E-mail: sceh@pullman.com
Website: http://sunsite.utk.edu/JCEH/scehframe.htm

Diet, Nutrition, and Food Safety

California Certified Organic Farmers (CCOF)
1115 Mission Street
Santa Cruz, CA 95060
831–423–2263
Website: http://www.ccof.org

Campaign for Food Safety
860 Highway 61
Little Marais, MN 55614
218–226–4164; fax 218–226–4157
E-mail: alliance@mr.net
Website: http://www.purefood.org

Center for Science in the Public Interest
1875 Connecticut Avenue, NW
Washington, DC 20009
202–332–9110
Website: http://www.cspinet.org

Colorado Department of Agriculture (CDA)
700 Kipling Street, No. 4000
Lakewood, CO 80215–5894
303–239–4100; fax 303–239–4125
Website: http://www.ag.state.co.us/DPI

Florida Certified Organic Growers and Consumers, Inc.
   (FOG)
P.O. Box 12311
Gainesville, FL 32604
352–377–6343; fax 352–377–8363
E-mail: FOGoffice@aol.com
Website: http://www.floridaplants.com/FOG

Food and Water, Inc.
389 Vermont Route 215
Walden, VT 05873
800–EAT–SAFE or 802–563–3300

Mothers and Others for Pesticide Limits
40 West 20th Street
New York, NY 10011
212–242–0010
E-mail: mothers@mothers.org

Water Quality Association
4151 Naperville Road
Lisle, IL 60532
630–505–0160; fax 630–505–9637
E-mail: wqa@mail.wqa.org
Website: http://www.wqa.org

Herbal Medicine

American Botanical Council
P.O. Box 144345
Austin, TX 78714–4345
512–331–8868; fax 512–926–2345
E-mail: custserv@herbalgram.org
Website: http://www.herbalgram.org

American Herbalists Guild
P.O. Box 70
Roosevelt, UT 84066
435–722–8434; fax 435–722–8452
E-mail: ahgoffice@earthlink.net
Website: http://www.healthy.net.herbalists

Herb Research Foundation
1007 Pearl Street, Suite 200
Boulder, CO 80302
303–449–2265
E-mail: info@herbs.org
Website: http://www.herbs.org

Homeopathy

Foundation for Homeopathic Education and Research
   and Homeopathic Educational Services
2124 Kittredge Street
Berkeley, CA 94704
510–649–8930 or 510–649–0294
E-mail: mail@homeopathic.com
Website: http://www.homeopathic.com

Homeopathic Academy of Naturopathic Physicians
   (HANP)
12132 SE Foster Place
Portland, OR 97266
503–761–3298
E-mail: e-hanp@igc.apc.org
Website: ttp://www.healthworld.com/associations/pa/
   Homeopathic/hanp/index.html

National Center for Homeopathy
801 North Fairfax Street, Suite 306
Alexandria, VA 22314
703–548-7790; fax 703–548–7792
Website: http://www.homeopathic.org

Relaxation/Meditation

Academy for Guided Imagery
P.O. Box 2070
Mill Valley, CA 94942
800–726–2070
E-mail: agil1996@aol.com
Website: http://www.healthy.net/agi

Institute of Noetic Sciences
475 Gate Five Road, Suite 300
Sausalito, CA 94965
415–331–5650; fax 415–331–5673
E-mail: Webmaster@noetic.org
Website: http://www.noetic.org

Therapeutic Humor

American Association for Therapeutic Humor (AATH)
222 South Meramec, Suite 303
St. Louis, MO 63105
314–863–6232; fax 314–863–6457
website: http://www.aath.org

Humor and Health Institute
P.O. Box 16814
Jackson, MS 39236-6814
601–957–0075; fax 601–977–0423
website: http://www.intop.net~jrdunn

Specific Health Issues

Adult Children of Alcoholics (ACoA)
P.O. Box 3216
Torrance, CA 90510
310–534–1815
E-mail: info@AdultChildren.org
Website: http://www.AdultChildren.org

AIDS Hot Line
800–342–AIDS

Alateen
200 Park Avenue South, Room 814
New York, NY 10003
212–254–7230 or 212–254–7236

Alcohol and Drug Helpline
800–252–6465

Alcoholics Anonymous
475 Riverside Drive
New York, NY 10115
212–870–3400
Website: http://www.aa.org

Alexander Graham Bell Association for the Deaf
3417 Volta Place NW
Washington, DC 20007–2778
202–337–5220
E-mail: agbell2@aol.com
Website: http://www.agbell.org

Alzheimer's Association
919 North Michigan Avenue, Suite 1000
Chicago, IL 60611
800–272–3900 or 312–335–8700
Website: http://www.alz.org

American Academy of Allergy, Asthma, and Immunology
611 East Wells Street
Milwaukee, WI 53202
800–822–ASMA or 414–272–6071
Website: http://www.aaaai.org

American Academy of Dermatology
930 North Meacham Road
P.O. Box 4014
Schaumburg, IL 60173–4965
847–330–9830; fax 847–330–0050
Website: http://www.aad.org

American Academy of Ophthalmology
655 Beach Street
San Francisco, CA 94109-1336
415–561–8500; fax 415–561–8533
Website: http://www.eyenet.org

American Academy of Otolaryngology—
    Head and Neck Surgery
1 Prince Street
Alexandria, VA 22314
703–836–4444; fax 703–683–5100
Website: http://www.entnet.org

American Academy of Pain Management
13947 Mono Way #A
Sonora, CA 95370
209–533–9744; fax 209–533–9750
E-mail: aapm@aapainmanage.org
Website: http://www.aapainmanage.org

American Anorexia/Bulimia Association (AABA)
165 West 46th Street, No. 1108
New York, NY 10036
212–575–6200; fax 212–719–0193
Website: http://www.aabainc.org

The American Cancer Society
1599 Clifton Road, NE
Atlanta, GA 30329
800–ACS–2345; fax 212–719–0193
Website: http://www.cancer.org

American Chronic Pain Association
P.O. Box 850
Rocklin, CA 95677
916–632–0922; fax 916–632–3208
E-mail: acpa@pacbell.net
Website: http://www.theacpa.org

American College of Advancement in Medicine (ACAM)
23121 Verdugo Drive, No. 204
Laguna Hills, CA 92653
800–532–3688; fax 949–455–9679
E-mail: acam@acam.org
Website: http://www.acam.org

American Council for Headache Education (ACHE)
19 Mantua Road
Mount Royal, NJ 08061
609–423–0258 (in New Jersey) 800–255–ACHE (elsewhere);
    fax 609–423–0082
E-mail: achehq@talley.com
Website: http://www.achenet.org

American Dental Association
211 East Chicago Avenue
Chicago, IL 60611
312–440–2500; fax 312–440–7494
Website: http://www.ada.org

American Diabetes Association
1600 Duke Street
Alexandria, VA 22314
800–232–3472 or 703–549–1500; fax 703–549–6995
E-mail: customerservice@diabetes.org
Website: http://www.diabetes.org

American Foundation for AIDS Research (AMFAR)
120 Wall Street, 13th Floor
New York, NY 10005
212–806–1600; fax 212–806–1601
E-mail: amfar@amfar.org

American Foundation for Urologic Disease, Inc.
1128 North Charles Street
Baltimore, MD 21201
410–468–1800; fax 410–468–1808
E-mail: admin@afud.org
Website: www.afud.org

American Health Foundation
320 East 43rd Street
New York, NY 10017
212–953–1900; fax 212–687–2339
Website: http://www.ahf.org

American Hearing Research Foundation
55 East Washington Street, Suite 2022
Chicago, IL 60602
312–726–9670; fax 312–726–9695

American Heart Association
7272 Greenville Avenue
Dallas, TX 75231
214–373–6300
E-mail: inquire@heart.org
Website: http://www.americanheart.org

American Liver Foundation
1425 Pompton Avenue
Cedar Grove, NJ 07009
800–223–0179 or 973–256–2550; fax 973–256–3214
E-mail: info@liverfoundation.org
Website: http://www.liverfoundation.org

American Lung Association
1740 Broadway
New York, NY 10019
800–LUNG–USA or 212–315–8700; fax 212–265–5642
E-mail: info@lungusa.org
Website: http://www.lungusa.org

American Pain Society
4700 West Lake Avenue
Glenview, IL 60025
847–375–4715; fax 847–375–4777
E-mail: info@ampainsoc.org
Website: http://www.ampainsoc.org

American Parkinson Association
1250 Hylan Boulevard
Staten Island, NY 10305
800–223–2732; fax 718–981–4399
E-mail: apda@admin.con2.com
Website: http://www.apdaparkinson.com

The American Psychiatric Association
1400 K Street NW
Washington, DC 20005
202–682–6000; fax 202–682–6850
E-mail: apa@psych.org
Website: http://www.psych.org

American Psychological Association
750 First Street NE
Washington, DC 20002-4242
800–964–2000 or 202–336–5500
E-mail: helping@qpq.org
Website: http://www.apa.org

American Social Health Association
P.O. Box 13827
Research Triangle Park, NC 27709
919–361–8400; fax 919–361–8425
Information about sexually transmitted diseases.

American Society for Reproductive Medicine
1209 Montgomery Highway
Birmingham, AL 35216
205–978–5000; fax 205–978–5005
Website: http://www.asrm.org

American Speech-Language-Hearing Association
10801 Rockville Pike
Rockville, MD 20852
800–498–2071 or 301–897–5700
    or 301–897–8682;
    fax 301–571–0457
Website: http://www.asha.org

American Tinnitus Association
P.O. Box 5
Portland, OR 97207
501–248–9985; fax 503–248–0024
E-mail: tinnitus@ata.org
Website: http://www.ata.org

Arthritis Foundation
1330 West Peachtree Street
Atlanta, GA 30309
800–283–7800 or 404–872–7100; fax 404–872–0457
E-mail: help@arthritis.org
Website: http://www.arthritis.org

Asthma and Allergy Foundations of America
1125 15th Street NW, Suite 502
Washington, DC 20005
800–7–ASTHMA or 202–466–7643; fax 202–466–8940
E-mail: info@aafa.org
Website: http://www.aafa.org

Better Hearing Institute
5021-B Backlick Road
Annandale, VA 22003
703–642–0580; fax 703–750–9302
E-mail: mail@betterhearing.org
Website: http://www.betterhearing.org

Brain Injury Association
105 North Alfred Street
Alexandria, VA 22314
703–236–6000
Hotline: 800–444–6443; fax 703–236–6001
Website: http://www.biausa.org

Bulimia Anorexia Treatment and Education Center
615 North New Ballas Road
St. Louis, MO 63141
314–569–6565

Cancer Information Service
National Cancer Institute
Building 31, Room 10A24
9000 Rockville Pike
Bethesda, MD 20892
Hotline: 800–4–CANCER
Website: http://www.nci.nih.gov

Celiac Disease Foundation
13251 Ventura Boulevard, Suite 1
Studio City, CA 91604–1838
818–990–2354; fax 818–990–2379
E-mail: cdf@celiac.org
Website: http://www.celiac.org

Center for Medical Consumers and Health Care
   Information
237 Thompson Street
New York, NY 10012
212–674–7105
Website: http://www.medicalconsumers.org

Centers for Disease Control and Prevention (CDC)
1600 Clifton Road NE
Atlanta, GA 30333
404–639–3311
Website: http://www.cdc.gov

Children of Aging Parents (CAPS)
1609 Woodburne Road, Suite 302A
Levittown, PA 19057
215-945–6900; fax 215–945–8720
Website: http://www.careguide.net

Chronic Fatigue and Immune Dysfunction Syndrome
   (CFIDS) Association of America
P.O. Box 220398
Charlotte, NC 28222–0398
800–442–3437; fax 704–365–9755
E-mail: info@cfids.org
Website: http://www.cfids.org

Crohn's and Colitis Foundation of America
386 Park Avenue South, 17th Floor
New York, NY 10016–8804
800–932–2423 or 800–343–3637 or 212–685–3440;
   fax 212–779–4098
Website: http://www.ccfa.org

Depression After Delivery (DAD)
P.O. Box 1282
Morrisville, PA 19067
800–944–4PPD

Endometriosis Association
8585 North 76th Place
Milwaukee, WI 53223
800–992–ENDO (in the U.S.) 800–426–2ENDO (in Canada)
E-mail: endo@endometriosisassn.org
Website: endometriosisassn.org

Epilepsy Foundation of America
4351 Garden City Drive
Landover, MD 20785–2267
800–213–5821 or 800–332–1000 or 301–459–3700
E-mail: postmaster@efa.org
Website: http://www.efa.org
Website: http://www.epilepsyfoundation.org

Fertility Research Foundation
875 Park Avenue
New York, NY 10021
212–744–5500; fax 212–744–6536
E-mail: frfbaby@msn.com

Food Allergy Network
10400 Eaton Place, Suite 107
Fairfax, VA 20030
703–691–3179; fax 703–691–2713
E-mail: fan@worldweb.net
Website: http://www.foodallergy.org

Foundation for Alternative Cancer Therapies (FACT)
P.O. Box 1242, Old Chelsea Station
New York, NY 10113
212–741–2790

Foundation for Fighting Blindness/
   Retinitis Pigmentosa Foundation
Executive Plaza One, Suite 800
11350 McCormich Road
Hunt Valley, MD 21031–1014
800–683–5555; fax 410–771–9470
Website: http://www.blindness.org

Gay Men's Health Crisis
119 West 24th Street
New York, NY 10011-1913
212–807–6655; TTY 212–645–7470
Website: http://www.gmhc.org
HIV and AIDS issues.

Herpes Resource Center
P.O. Box 13827
Research Triangle Park, NC 27709
919–361–8488
Website: http://www.ashastd.org

House Ear Institute
2100 West 3rd Street, 5th Floor
Los Angeles, CA 90057
213–483-4431; fax 213–483–8789
Website: http://www.hei.org

Immune Deficiency Foundation
25 West Chesapeake Avenue, Suite 206
Towson, MD 21204
800–296–4433 or 410–321–6647; fax 410–321–9165
Website: http://www.primaryimmune.org

Impotence Foundation
P.O. Box 60260
Santa Barbara, CA 93160
800–221–5517

Institute of Parasitic Diseases
3530 East Indian School Road, Suite 3
Phoenix, Arizona 85018
602–955–4211; fax 602–955–4102
E-mail: omaramin@aol.com

International College of Applied Kinesiology
6405 Metcalf Avenue, Suite 503
Shawnee Mission, KS 66202–3929
913–384–5336; fax 913–384–5112
E-mail: icak@usa.net
Website: http://www.icak.com

Joslin Diabetes Center in Massachusetts
One Joslin Place
Boston, MA 02215
617–732–2400; fax 617–732–2500
Website: http://www.joslin.org

Leukemia Society of America
600 Third Avenue
New York, NY 10016
212–573–8484; fax 212–856–9686
Website: http://www.leukemia.org

Life Extension Foundation
P.O. Box 229120
Hollywood, FL 33022
800–544–4440 or 800–841–5433; fax 954–761–9199
E-mail: lef@lef.org
Website: http://www.lef.org

Lupus Foundation of America
1300 Piccard Drive, Suite 200
Rockville, MD 20850–4303
800–558–0121 or 301–670–9292; fax 301–670–7486
Website: http://www.lupus.org/lupus

Lyme Disease Foundation
1 Financial Plaza
Hartford, CT 06103
800–886–LYME; fax 800–525–8425
E-mail: lymefnd@aol.com
Website: http://www.lyme.org

Medicare Hot Line
800–638–6833

Medicine OnLine
Foot of Broad Street
Stratford, CT 06615
203–375–7300; fax 203–375–6699
E-mail: ultitech@meds.com
Website: http://www.meds.com

Meniere's Network
Ear Foundation
1817 Patterson Street
Nashville, TN 37203
615–329-7807; fax 615–329–7935
Website: http://www.earfoundation.org

Multiple Sclerosis Foundation
6350 North Andrews Avenue
Fort Lauderdale, FL 33309
800–441–7055; fax 954–351–0630
E-mail: mssupport@msfacts.org
Website: http://www.msfacts.org

Myasthenia Gravis Foundation of America, Inc.
222 South Riverside Plaza, Suite 1540
Chicago, IL 60606
800–541–5454; fax 312–258–0461
E-mail: mgfa@aol.com
Website: http://www.myasthenia.org

Narcolepsy and Sleep Disorders: An International
  Newsletter
P.O. Box 51113
Palo Alto, CA 94303-9559
831–646–2055; fax 831–646–2055
Website: http://www.narcolepsy.com

Narcolepsy Network
277 Fairfield Road, Suite 310B
Fairfield, NJ 07004
973–276–0115; fax 973–227–8224
E-mail: narnet@aol.com
Website: http://www.websciences.org/narnet

National Adrenal Disease Foundation
505 Northern Boulevard, Suite 200
Great Neck, NY 11021
516–487–4992; fax 516–887–6997
E-mail: nadf@aol.com

National Aging Information Center
500 E Street SW, Suite 910
Washington, DC 20024–2710
202–554–9800

National Alliance of Breast Cancer Organizations (NABCO)
9 East 37th Street, 10th Floor
New York, NY 10016
800–719–9154
E-mail: NABCOinfo@aol.com
Website: http://www.nabco.org/

National Alopecia Areata Foundation
P.O. Box 150760
San Rafael, CA 94915
415–456-4644; fax 415–456-4274
Website: http://www.alopeciareata.com

National Association for Anorexia Nervosa
  and Associated Disorders
P.O. Box 7
Highland Park, IL 60035
847–831–3438; fax 847–433–4632
E-mail: ANAD20@aol.com
Website: http://www.members.aol.com/anad20/index.html

National Association for Continence
P.O. Box 8310
Spartanburg, SC 29307
800–BLADDER or 803–579–7900; fax 864–579–7902
Website: http://www.nafc.org

National Breast Cancer Coalition
1707 L Street, NW, Suite 1060
Washington, D.C. 20036
202–296–7477; fax 202–265–6854
E-mail: clhain@natlbcc.org
Website: http://www.natlbcc.org/

National Chronic Pain Outreach Association
7979 Old Georgetown Road, Suite 100
Bethesda, MD 20814–2429
301–652–4948; fax 301–907–0745
Website: http://www.brain.mgh.harvard.edu:100/
  ncpainoa.htm

National Clearinghouse for Alcohol and
  Drug Information
11426–28 Rockville Pike
Rockville, MD 20852
800–729–6686 or 301–468–2600; fax 301–468–6433
Website: http://www.health.org

National Cocaine Hot Line
800–COCAINE

National Council on Aging
409 Third Street SW, 2nd Floor
Washington, DC 20024
202–479–1200; fax 202–479–0735
Website: http://www.NCOA.org

National Council on Alcoholism and Drug
  Dependence
352 Park Avenue South, 8th Floor
New York, NY 10013
800–622–2255

National Diabetes Information Clearinghouse
  (NDIC)
1 Information Way
Bethesda, MD 20892–3560
301–654–3327; fax 301–907–8906
E-mail: ndic@info.niddk.nih.gov
Website: http://www.niddk.nih.gov

National Digestive Diseases Information Clearinghouse
(NDIC)
2 Information Way
Bethesda, MD 20892–3560
301–654–3810; fax 301–907–8906
E-mail: nddic@info.niddk.nih.gov
Website: http://www. niddk.nih.gov

National Eating Disorders Organization
6655 South Yale
Tulsa, OK 74136
918–481–4044; fax 918–481–4076
Website: http://www.laureate.com

National Eye Institute (NEI)
National Institutes of Health
Building 31, Room 6A32
31 Center Drive, MSC 2510
Bethesda, MD 20892–2510
301–496–5248; fax 301–402–1065
E-mail: 2020@nei.nih.gov
Website: http://www.nei.nih.gov

National Foundation for Depressive Illness
P.O. Box 2257
New York, NY 10116
800–248–4344

National Headache Foundation
428 West St. James Place, 2nd Floor
Chicago, IL 60614
888–643–5552
Website: http://www.headaches.org

National Health Information Clearinghouse
P.O. Box 1133
Washington, DC 20013–1133
Hotline: 800–336–4797; fax 301–984–4256
E-mail: nhicinfo@health.org
Website: http://nhic-nt.health.org

National Hemophilia Foundation (NHF)
116 West 32nd Street, 11th Floor
New York, NY 10001
212–328–3700; fax 212–328–3777
Website: http://www.hemophilia.org

National Hospice Organization
1901 North Moore Street
Suite 901
Arlington, VA 22209
703–243-5900; fax 703–525–5762
E-mail: drsnho@cais.com
Website: http://www.nho.org

National Institute on Deafness and Other Communication
Disorders (NIDCD) Information Clearinghouse
1 Communication Avenue
Bethesda, MD 20892-3456
800–241–1044; TTY 800–241–1055; fax 301–907–8830
E-mail: nidcdinfo@nidcd.nih.gov
Website: http://www.nih.gov/nidcd

National Institute of Neurological Disorders and Stroke
Building #31, Room 8A06
31 Center Drive
Bethesda, MD 20892-2540
301–496–5751; fax 301–402–2186
Website: http://www.ninds.nih.gov

National Jewish Center's Lung Line
800–222–5864 or 303–355–5864

National Kidney Foundation
30 East 33rd Street, Suite 1100
New York, NY 10016
800–622–9010; fax 212–779–0068
Website: http://www.kidney.org

National Lymphedema Network
2211 Post Street, Suite 404
San Francisco, CA 94115-3427
415–921–1306
Hotline: 800–541–3259; fax 415–921–4284
E-mail: nln@lymphnet.org
Website: http://www.lymphnet.org

National Multiple Sclerosis Society
733 Third Avenue
New York, NY 10017
800–344–4867 or 212–986–3240; fax 212–986–7981
E-mail: nat@nmss.org
Website: http://www.nmss.org

National Organization for Rare Disorders
100 Route 37, P.O. Box 8923
New Fairfield, CT 06812–8923
800–999–6673 or 203–746–6518; fax 203–746–6481
E-mail: orphan@raredisease.org
Website: http: //www.rarediseases.org

National Osteoporosis Foundation (NOF)
1150 17th Street NW, Suite 500
Washington, DC 20036–4603
800–223–9994 or 202–223–2225; fax 202–223–2237
E-mail: nofmail@nof.org
Website: http://www.nof.org

National Parkinson Foundation (NFP)
1501 NW 9th Avenue
Miami, FL 33136–1494
800–327–4545 or 305–547–6666; fax 305–243–4403
E-mail: mailbox@npf.med.miami.edu
Website: http://www.parkinson.org

National Pesticide Telecommunications Network
800–858–7378

National Psoriasis Foundation
6600 SW 92nd Avenue, Suite 300
Portland, OR 97223
800–723–9166 or 503–244–7404; fax 503–245–0626
E-mail: getinfo@npfusa.org
Website: http://www.psoriasis.org

National Rosacea Society
800 South NW Highway 200
Barrington, IL 60010
847–382–8971; fax 847–382–5567
E-mail: rosaceas@aol.com
Website: http://www.rosacea.org

National Sjögren's Syndrome Association
5815 North Black Canyon Highway, Suite 103
Phoenix, AZ 85015–2200
602–433–9844
Website: http://www.sjogrens.org

National Stroke Association
96 Inverness Drive East, Suite I
Englewood, CO 80112
800–STROKES; fax 303–649–1328
E-mail: info@stroke.org
Website: http://www.stroke.org

Parkinson Support Group of America
11376 Cherry Hill Road, Suite 204
Beltsville, MD 20705
301–937–1545

People Against Cancer
P.O. Box 10
Otho, IA 50569
800–662–2623; fax 515–972–4415
E-mail: nocancer@ix.netcom.com
Website: http://www.dodgenet.com/nocancer

Planned Parenthood Federation of America
810 Seventh Avenue
New York, NY 10019
212–541–7800; fax 212–245–1845
Website: http://www.plannedparenthood.org

Women's Health America, Inc., PMS Access
P.O. Box 259690
Madison, WI 53725
800–222–4767; fax 888–898–7412
E-mail: wha@womenshealth.com
Website: http://www.womenshealth.com

Postpartum Support International
927 North Kellogg Avenue
Santa Barbara, CA 93111
Voice mail: 805–967–7636; fax 805–967–0608
Website: http://www.iup.edu/an/postpartum

Project Inform
205 13th Street, Suite 2001
San Francisco, CA 94103
Hotline: 800–822–7422
Administration: 415–558–8669; fax 415–558–0684
Website: http://www.projinf.org
HIV and AIDS issues.

Prostate Cancer Survivor Support Group
US TOO International, Inc.
930 North York Road, Suite 50
Hinsdale, IL 60521-2993
800–808–7866 or 630–323–1002; fax 630–323–1003
E-mail: ustoo@ustoo.com
Website: http://www.ustoo.com

Scleroderma Foundation
89 Newbury Street
Danvers, MA 01923
800–422–1113; fax 978–750–9902
E-mail: sfinfo@scleroderma.org
Website: http://www.scleroderma.org

Self-Help for Hard of Hearing People
7910 Woodmont Avenue, Suite 1200
Bethesda, MD 20814
301–657–2248; fax 301–913–9413
E-mail: national@shhh.org
Website: http://www.shhh.org

SHARE (Self Help for Women with Breast or
    Ovarian Cancer)
1501 Broadway, Suite 1720
New York, NY 10036
212–719–0364
Hotline: 212–382–2111 (English);
    212–719–4454 (Spanish);
    fax 212–869–3431
Website: http://www.sharecancersupport.org

The Simon Foundation for Continence
P.O. Box 835
Wilmette, IL 60091
800–237–4666

Sjögren's Syndrome Foundation
333 North Broadway, Suite 200
Jericho, NY 11753
516–933–6365; fax 516–933–6368
E-mail: ssf@idt.net
Website: http://www.sjogrens.com

Skin Cancer Foundation
245 Fifth Avenue, Suite 1403
New York, NY 10016
212–725–5176; fax 212–725–5751
E-mail: info@skincancer.org

Thyroid Foundation of America
Ruth Sleeper Hall—RSL 350
40 Parkman Street
Boston, MA 02114–2698
800–832–8321

United Ostomy Association
19772 MacArthur Boulevard, Suite 200
Irvine, CA 92612
800–826–0826 or 714–660–8624; fax 949–660–9262
E-mail: uoa@deltanet.com
Website: http://www.uoa.org

Vestibular Disorders Association
P.O. Box 4467
Portland, OR 97208-4467
Voice mail: 503–229–7705; fax 503–229–8064
E-mail: veda@vestibular.org
Website: http://www.teleport.com/~veda

Y-ME National Breast Cancer Organization
212 West Van Buren Street, 5th Floor
Chicago, IL 60607-3908
800–221–2141; fax 312–294–8597
Website: http://www.y-me.org

Other

American Self-Help Clearinghouse
Saint Clare's Health Services
25 Pocono Road
Denville, NJ 07834
973–625–9565; fax 973–625–8848
E-mail: ASHC@cybernex.net
Website: http://www.cmhc.com/selfhelp/
Tracks 700 different support groups throughout the country and publishes "The Self-Help Sourcebook," which offers advice on setting up your own support group.

National Library of Medicine
8600 Rockville Pike
Bethesda, MD 20894
888–346–3656 or 301–496–6308
Website: http://www.nlm.nih.gov
Provides free access to Medline's database of over 9 million references, abstracts, and journal articles.

Bibliography for Further Reading

GENERAL REFERENCE

Brunn, Ruth Dowling, and Bertel Brunn. *The Human Body*, 2nd Ed. New York, NY: Random House, 1982.

Dox, Ida G., B. John Melloni, and Gilbert M. Eisner. *The HarperCollins Illustrated Medical Dictionary*. New York, NY: Harper Collins, 1993.

The Medical Advisor. The Complete Guide to Alternative and Conventional Treatments. Alexandria, VA: Time-Life Books, 1997.

Stewart, Felicia H. *Understanding Your Body*. New York, NY: Bantam, 1987.

CONVENTIONAL MEDICINE

Berkow, Robert, Ed. in Chief. *The Merck Manual of Medical Information, Home Edition*. Whitehouse Station, NJ: Merck Research Laboratories, 1997.

Clayman, Charles B. *American Medical Association Family Medical Guide*. New York, NY: Random House, 1994.

Clayman, Charles B. *American Medical Association Home Medical Encyclopedia*. New York, NY: Random House, 1989.

Graedon, Joe. *The People's Pharmacy*. New York, NY: St. Martin's Press, 1996.

Graedon, Joe. *Deadly Drug Interactions*. New York, NY: St. Martin's Press, 1995.

The PDR Family Guide to Prescription Drugs, 6th Ed. Montvale, NJ: Medical Economics Data, 1998.

Pinkney, Cathey, and Edward R. Pinckney. *The Patient's Guide to Medical Tests*. New York, NY: Facts on File, 1987.

Silverman, Harold M., Ed. in Chief. *The Pill Book*, 7th Ed. New York, NY: Bantam Books, 1996.

ALTERNATIVE MEDICINE (GENERAL)

Balch, James F., and Phyllis A. Balch. *Prescription for Nutritional Healing*, 2nd Ed. Garden City Park, NY: Avery Publishing Group, 1997.

Braly, James. *Dr. Braly's Optimum Health Program*. New York, NY: Times Books, 1985.

Davis, Adelle. *Let's Get Well*. New York, NY: New American Library, 1984.

Giller, Robert M., and K. Matthews. *Natural Prescriptions*. New York, NY: Carol Southern Books, 1994.

Rosenfeld, Isadore. *Dr. Rosenfeld's Guide to Alternative Medicine*. New York, NY: Random House, 1996.

Trattler, R. *Better Health Through Natural Healing*. New York, NY: McGraw-Hill, 1985.

HERBAL MEDICINE

Castleman, M. *The Healing Herbs*. Emmaus, PA: Rodale Press, 1991.

Gardner, Joy. *Healing Yourself During Pregnancy*. Freedom, CA: The Crossing Press, 1990.

Gladstar, Rosemary. *Herbal Healing for Women*. New York: Fireside, 1993.

Green, James. *The Male Herbal*. Watsonville, CA: The Crossing Press, 1991.

Grieve, M. *A Modern Herbal*. New York, NY: Dover Publications, Inc., 1982.

Griggs, Barbara. *Green Pharmacy: The History and Evolution of Western Medicine*. Rochester, VT: Healing Arts Press, 1991.

Hobbs, Christopher. *Echinacea! The Immune Herb*. Capitola, CA: Botanica Press, 1992.

Hobbs, Christopher. *Ginkgo: The Elixir of Youth*. Capitola, CA: Botanica Press, 1991.

Hobbs, Christopher. *Milk Thistle—The Liver Herb*. Capitola, CA: Botanica Press, 1992.

Hobbs, Christopher. *Natural Liver Therapy*. Capitola, CA: Botanica Press, 1993.

Hobbs, Christopher. *Usnea: The Herbal Antibiotic*. Capitola, CA: Botanica Press, 1990.

Hobbs, Christopher. *Vitex: The Woman's Herb*. Capitola, CA: Botanica Press, 1993.

Hoffmann, David. *The Holistic Herbal*. Longmead, England: Element Books Ltd., 1988.

Hsu, Hong-Yen. *How to Treat Yourself With Chinese Herbs*. Los Angeles, CA: Oriental Healing Arts Institute, 1980.

Johnson, Stewart. *Feverfew*. London, England: Sheldon Press, 1984.

Kaptchuk, Ted. *The Web That Has No Weaver.* New York, NY: Congdon and Weded, 1983.

Lad, Vasant, and David Frawley. *The Yoga of Herbs.* Santa Fe, NM: Lotus Press, 1986.

McGuffin, Michael, Christopher Hobbs, Roy Upton, and Alicia Goldberg. *American Herbal Products Association's Botanical Safety Handbook.* New York, NY: CRC Press, 1997.

Moore, Michael. *Medicinal Plants of the Desert and Canyon West.* Santa Fe, NM: Museum of New Mexico Press, 1979.

Moore, Michael. *Medicinal Plants of the Mountain West.* Santa Fe, NM: Museum of New Mexico Press, 1993.

Moore, Michael. *Medicinal Plants of the Moutain West.* Santa Fe, NM: Museum of New Mexico Press, 1979.

Murray, Michael T. *The Healing Power of Herbs.* Rocklin, CA: Prima Publishing, 1992.

Northrup, Christiane. *Women's Bodies, Women's Wisdom.* New York, NY: Bantam Books, 1994.

Pavarti, Jeannine. *Hygieia, A Woman's Herbal.* Sevier, UT: Freestone Press, 1978.

Pedersen, Mark. *Nutritional Herbology.* Bountiful, UT: Pedersen Publishing, 1987.

Reid, Daniel. *Chinese Herbal Medicine.* Boston, MA: Shambhala Publications, 1993.

Ritchason, Jack. *The Little Herb Encyclopedia.* Springville, UT: Thornwood Books, 1980.

Rose, Jeanne. *Herbs and Things.* New York, NY: Grosset and Dunlap, 1975.

Schulick, Paul. *Ginger: Common Spice and Wonder Drug.* Brattleboro, VT: Herbal Free Press, 1994.

Teeguarden, Ron. *Chinese Tonic Herbs.* New York, NY: Japan Publications, 1984.

Tierra, Lesley. *The Herbs of Life.* Freedom, CA: The Crossing Press, 1992.

Tierra, Michael. *Planetary Herbology.* Santa Fe, NM: Lotus Press, 1988.

Tierra, Michael. *The Way of Herbs.* Santa Cruz, CA: Unity Press, 1980.

Weed, Susan. *Wise Women's Herbal for the Childbearing Year.* Woodstock, NY: Ash Tree Publishing, 1985.

Weed, Susan. *Wise Women's Herbal for the Menopausal Years.* Woodstock, NY: Ash Tree Publishing, 1992.

HOMEOPATHY

Cummings, S., and D. Ullman. *Everybody's Guide to Homeopathic Medicines.* Los Angeles, CA: J.P. Tarcher, 1984.

Panos, Maisemond B., and J. Heimlich. *Homeopathic Medicine at Home.* Los Angeles, CA: J.P. Tarcher, 1982.

Stevenson, J.H. *Helping Yourself With Homeopathic Remedies.* San Francisco, CA: Thorsons, 1976.

Weiner, Michael. *The Complete Book of Homeopathy.* Garden City Park, NY: Avery Publishing Group, 1989.

CHINESE MEDICINE

A Barefoot Doctor's Manual: The American Translation of the Official Chinese Paramedical Manual. Philadelphia, PA: Running Press, 1977.

Jizong, Shi, and Chu Feng Zhu. *The ABC of Traditional Chinese Medicine.* Hong Kong: Hai Feng Publishing Company, 1992.

Lu, Henry C. *Chinese System of Food Cures.* New York, NY: Sterling Publishing Co., Inc., 1986.

RELAXATION AND MASSAGE

Achterberg, Jeanne. *Imagery in Healing.* Boston, MA: Shambhala Publications, 1995.

Benson, H. *The Relaxation Response.* New York, NY: Outlet Books, 1993.

Fine, Donald I. *Transcendental Meditation.* New York, NY: Roth Robert, 1998.

Goleman, Daniel, and Joel Gurin, Eds. *Mind-Body Medicine: How to Use Your Mind for Better Health.* Yonkers, NY: Consumer Reports Books, 1993.

Iyengar, Geeta S. *A Gem for Women.* Spokane, WA: Timeless Books, 1990.

BACH FLOWER REMEDIES

Bach, Edward. *Heal Thyself.* Essex, England: C.W. Daniel Company Ltd., 1978.

Bach, Edward. *The Twelve Healers.* Essex, England: C.W. Daniel Company Ltd., 1978.

Scheffer, M. *Bach Flower Therapy: Theory and Practice.* Rochester, VT: Healing Arts Press, 1988.

AROMATHERAPY

Damian, Peter, and Kate Damian. *Aromatherapy: Scent and Psyche.* Rochester, VT: Healing Arts Press, 1995.

Wilson, Roberta. *Aromatherapy for Vibrant Health and Beauty.* Garden City Park, NY: Avery Publishing Group, 1994.

DIET AND NUTRITION

Abrahamson, E.M., and A.W. Pezet. *Body, Mind and Sugar.* New York, NY: Jove, 1971.

Abravanel, Elliot D., and E.A. King. *Dr. Abravanel's Body Type Program.* New York, NY: Bantam Books, 1986.

Adams, Ruth, and Frank Murray. *Body, Mind and the B Vitamins.* New York, NY: Larchmont Books, 1975.

Appleton, Nancy. *Lick the Sugar Habit,* 2nd Ed. Garden City Park, NY: Avery Publishing Group, 1996.

Carper, Jean. *The Food Pharmacy*. New York, NY: Bantam Books, 1988.

Cheraskin, E., W.M. Ringsdorf, and J.W. Clark. *Diet and Disease*. New Canaan, CT: Keats Publishing, Inc., 1977.

Crook, W.G. *Tracking Down Hidden Food Allergies*. Jackson, TN: Professional Books, 1978.

Davis, Adelle. *Let's Eat Right to Keep Fit*. New York, NY: New American Library, 1988.

Deskins, Barbara, and Jean E. Anderson. *The Nutrition Bible: The Comprehensive, No-Nonsense Guide to Foods, Nutrients, Additives, Preservatives, Pollutants and Everything Else We Eat and Drink*. New York, NY: William Morrow & Co., 1997.

Kirschmann, John D., and L. J. Dunne. *Nutrition Almanac*, 4th Ed. New York, NY: McGraw-Hill, 1996.

Lieberman, Shari, and Nancy Bruning. *The Real Vitamin and Mineral Book*, 2nd Ed. Garden City Park, NY: Avery Publishing Group, 1997.

Messinger, Lisa. *Why Should I Eat Better?* Garden City Park, NY: Avery Publishing Group, 1993.

Mindell, Earl, and W.H. Lee. *The Vitamin Robbers*. New Canaan, CT: Keats Publishing, Inc., 1983.

Null, Gary, and Steve Null. *The Complete Handbook of Nutrition*. New York, NY: Dell, 1973.

Passwater, Richard A. *The New Supernutrition*. New York: Pocket Books, 1995.

Pauling, Linus. *Vitamin C and the Common Cold*. New York, NY: Bantam, 1971.

Simone, Charles. *Cancer and Nutrition*. Garden City Park, NY: Avery Publishing Group, 1992.

Todd, G.P. *Nutrition, Health, and Disease*. Norfolk, VA: The Donning Co., 1988.

Trenev, Natasha, *Probiotics*. Garden City Park, NY: Avery Publishing Group, 1998.

Williams, Roger John. *Nutrition Against Disease*. New York, NY: Bantam, 1973.

Wright, J.V. *Dr. Wright's Guide to Healing With Nutrition*. Emmaus, PA: Rodale Press, 1984.

EXERCISE

Carter, Albert. *The New Miracles of Rebound Exercise*. Scottsdale, AZ: ALM Publishers, 1988.

Fenton, Mark. "How to Be a Fitness Walker." *Walking Magazine*, April 1977: 47–55.

SPECIFIC HEALTH ISSUES

Ahlgrimm, Marla, and John M. Kells. *The HRT Solution*. Garden City Park, NY: Avery Publishing Group, 1999.

American Council on Headache Education, with Lynne M.

Constantine and Suzanne Scott. *Migraine: The Complete Guide*. New York, NY: Dell, 1994.

Balch, James F., and Morton Walker. *Heartburn and What to Do About It*. Garden City Park, NY: Avery Publishing Group, 1998.

Bell, David S., and Stev Donev. *Curing Fatigue: A Step-by-Step Plan to Uncover and Eliminate the Causes of Chronic Fatigue*. Emmaus, PA: Rodale Press, 1993.

Cauldill, Margaret A. *Managing Pain Before It Manages You*. New York, NY: Guilford Press, 1995.

Combs, Alec. *Hearing Loss Help*. San Luis Obispo, CA: Impact Publishers, 1991.

Corey, David, and Stan Solomon. *Pain: Free Yourself for Life*. New York, NY: NAL-Dutton, 1989.

Crook, William. *The Yeast Connection and the Woman*. Jackson, TN: Professional Books, 1995.

D'Alonzo, T.L. *Your Eyes: A Comprehensive Look at the Understanding and Treatment of Vision Problems*. Clifton Heights, PA: Avanti Publishing, 1991.

Diamond, W. John, and W. Lee Cowden, with Burton Goldberg. *An Alternative Medicine Definitive Guide to Cancer*. Tiburon, CA: Future Medicine Publishing, Inc., 1997.

Donoghue, Paul J., and Mary E. Siegel. *Sick and Tired of Feeling Sick and Tired: Living With Invisible Chronic Illness*. New York, NY: W.W. Norton & Co., 1992.

Eisenstein, Phyllis, and Samuel M. Scheiner. *Overcoming the Pain of Inflammatory Arthritis*. Garden City Park, NY: Avery Publishing Group, 1997.

Evans, Richard A. *Making the Right Choice: Treatment Options in Cancer Surgery*. Garden City Park, NY: Avery Publishing Group, 1995.

Fogler, Janet. *Improving Your Memory: How to Remember What You're Starting to Forget*. Baltimore, MD: Johns Hopkins University Press, 1994.

Hales, Diane R. *Caring for the Mind: The Comprehensive Guide to Mental Health*. New York, NY: Bantam Boos, 1994.

Hartung, Robert M. "Parasites: The Hidden Health Menace." *Health Freedom News*, May/June 1997.

Heber, David. *Natural Remedies for a Healthy Heart*. Garden City Park, NY: Avery Publishing Group, 1998.

Heston, Leonard L. *Mending Minds: A Guide to the New Psychiatry of Depression, Anxiety, and Other Mental Disorders*. New York, NY: W.H. Freeman, 1992.

Jeffries, William. *Safe Uses of Cortisol*, 2nd Ed. Springfield, IL: Charles C. Thomas Publisher Ltd., 1996.

Krumholz, Harlan M., and Robert H. Phillips. *No If's, And's, or Butts: The Smoker's Guide to Quitting*. Garden City Park, NY: Avery Publishing Group, 1993.

Lahita, Robert G., and Robert H. Phillips. *Lupus: Everything You Need to Know*. Garden City Park, NY: Avery Publishing Group, 1998.

Lane, I. William, and Linda Comac. *The Skin Cancer Answer.* Garden City Park, NY: Avery Publishing Group, 1999.

Lee, John R. *What Your Doctor May Not Tell You About Menopause.* New York: Warner Books, 1996.

Mark, Vernon H. *Reversing Memory Loss: Proven Methods for Regaining, Strengthening, and Preserving Your Memory.* Boston, MA: Houghton-Mifflin, 1992.

Marks, Edith, with Rita Montauredes. *Coping With Glaucoma.* Garden City Park, NY: Avery Publishing Group, 1997.

McIlwain, Harris H., Fruce Fulgham, Debra Fulgham, and Joel C. Silverfield. *Winning With Back Pain.* New York, NY: John Wiley & Sons, 1994.

Rapoport, Alan, and Fred D. Sheftell. *Headache Relief.* New York, NY: Fireside Books, 1991.

Sahelian, Ray, and Victoria Dolby Toews. *The Common Cold Cure.* Garden City Park, NY: Avery Publishing Group, 1999.

Saper, Joel R. *Help for Headaches: A Guide to Understanding Their Causes and Finding the Best Methods of Treatment.* New York, NY: Warner Books, 1987.

Sarno, John. *Healing Back Pain: The Mind-Body Connection.* New York, NY: Warner Books, 1991.

Simone, Charles B. *Breast Health.* Garden City Park, NY: Avery Publishing Group, 1995.

Swank, Roy, and Barbara Brewer Dugan. *The Multiple Sclerosis Diet Book.* New York, NY: Doubleday, 1987.

Stoler, Diane Roberts, and Barbara Albers Hill. *Coping With Mild Traumatic Brain Injury.* Garden City Park, NY: Avery Publishing Group, 1998.

Swirsky, Joan, and Diane Sackett Nannery. *Coping With Lymphedema.* Garden City Park, NY: Avery Publishing Group, 1998.

Wright, J.V., and John Morgenthaler. *Natural Hormone Replacement.* Petaluma, CA: Smart Publications, 1997.

OTHER TOPICS

Buist, Robert. *Food Chemical Sensitivity.* Garden City Park, NY: Avery Publishing Group, 1988.

Crose, Royda. *Why Women Liver Longer Than Men. . . and What Men Can Learn From Them.* San Francisco, CA: Jossey-Bass Publishers, 1997.

Dadd, Debra Lynn. *Nontoxic, Natural, and Earthwise.* Los Angeles, CA: J.P. Tarcher Inc., 1990.

Garrett, Laurie. *The Coming Plague.* New York, NY: Penguin Books, 1994.

Klein, Allen. *The Courage to Laugh: Humor, Hope and Healing in the Face of Death and Dying.* Los Angeles, CA: J.P. Tarcher, 1998.

Levenstein, Mary Kerney. *Everyday Cancer Risks and How to Avoid Them.* Garden City Park, NY: Avery Publishing Group, 1992.

Stutz, David, and Bernard Feder. *The Savvy Patient: How to Be an Active Participant in Your Medical Care.* Yonkers, NY: Consumer Reports Books, 1990.

White, Barbara J., and Edward J. Madara, Eds. *The Self-Help Sourcebook: Finding and Forming Mutual Aid Self-Help Groups.* Denville, NJ: Self-Help Clearing House, 1995.

Index

OTHER AVERY BOOKS OF INTEREST

A Parents Guide to Safe and Effective Relief
of Common Childhood Disorders Using
Nutritional Supplements, Herbs, Homeopathy,
Acupressure, Diet, and Conventional Medicine

SMART MEDICINE FOR A HEALTHIER CHILD

A PRACTICAL A-TO-Z
REFERENCE TO **CHILD**
NATURAL AND
CONVENTIONAL **JANET ZAND**, LAc, OM
TREATMENTS FOR **RACHEL WALTON**, RN
INFANTS & CHILDREN **BOB ROUNTREE**, MD

480 pages
ISBN 0-89529-545-8
$19.95

A QUICK AND EASY-TO-USE HANDBOOK TO
THE MOST COMMON CHILDHOOD ACCIDENTS

A Parent's Guide to Medical Emergencies

FIRST AID FOR YOUR CHILD

What You Need to Know

Janet Zand, OMD Robert Rountree, MD Rachel Walton, RN
BESTSELLING AUTHORS OF SMART MEDICINE FOR A HEALTHIER CHILD

196 pages
ISBN 0-89529-736-1
$11.95

OTHER AVERY BOOKS OF INTEREST

A RESOURCE OF REMEDIES USING CONVENTIONAL, NUTRITIONAL, AND HOMEOPATHIC EYE CARE

SMART MEDICINE FOR YOUR EYES

280 pages
ISBN 0-89529-870-8
$17.95

A GUIDE TO SAFE AND EFFECTIVE RELIEF OF COMMON EYE DISORDERS

Dr. Jeffrey Anshel

A NO NONSENSE GUIDE TO USING H.R.T., HERBS, VITAMINS, FOODS, AND NATURAL SUPPLEMENTS TO EASE THE DISCOMFORT OF MENOPAUSE

SMART MEDICINE for MENOPAUSE

Hormone Replacement Therapy and its Natural Alternatives

SANDRA CABOT, MD

From the Bestselling Author of Women's Health

208 pages
ISBN 0-89529-628-4
$9.95